Basic & Clinical
Endocrinology

a LANGE medical book

Basic & Clinical
Endocrinology

fifth edition

Edited by

Francis S. Greenspan, MD
Clinical Professor of Medicine and Radiology
Chief, Thyroid Clinic, Division of Endocrinology,
Department of Medicine
University of California, San Francisco

Gordon J. Strewler, MD
Professor of Medicine, Harvard Medical School
Chief, Department of Medicine
Brockton/West Roxbury Veterans Administration Medical Center
West Roxbury, Massachusetts

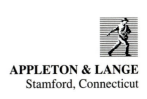

APPLETON & LANGE
Stamford, Connecticut

Notice: The authors and the publisher of this volume have taken care to make certain that the doses of drugs and schedules of treatment are correct and compatible with the standards generally accepted at the time of publication. Nevertheless, as new information becomes available, changes in treatment and in the use of drugs become necessary. The reader is advised to carefully consult the instruction and information material included in the package insert of each drug or therapeutic agent before administration. This advice is especially important when using, administering, or recommending new or infrequently used drugs. The authors and publisher disclaim all responsibility for any liability, loss, injury, or damage incurred as a consequence, directly or indirectly, of the use and application of any of the contents of the volume.

97 98 99 00 01 / 10 9 8 7 6 5 4 3 2 1

Prentice Hall International (UK) Limited, *London*
Prentice Hall of Australia Pty. Limited, *Sydney*
Prentice Hall Canada, Inc., *Toronto*
Prentice Hall Hispanoamericana, S.A., *Mexico*
Prentice Hall of India Private Limited, *New Delhi*
Prentice Hall of Japan, Inc., *Tokyo*
Simon & Schuster Asia Pte. Ltd., *Singapore*
Editora Prentice Hall do Brasil Ltda., *Rio de Janeiro*
Prentice Hall *Upper Saddle River, New Jersey*

ISSN 0891-2068

Acquisitions Editor: Shelley Reinhardt
Production Editor: Chris Langan
Designer: Mary Skudlarek
Associate Art Manager: Maggie Belis Darrow
Art Coordinator: Becky Hainz-Baxter

Printed in the USA

ISBN 0-8385-0588-0

90000

9 780838 505885

Table of Contents

Authors .... **xiii**

Preface .... **xv**

1. Introduction to Endocrinology **1**

John D. Baxter, MD

The Endocrine System 1
Paracrine & Autocrine Actions 3
Chemical Composition of Hormones 3
Vitamins & Hormones 4
Hormones & Oncogenes 5
Hormones & the Immune System 5
Eicosanoids: Prostaglandins, Thromboxanes,
   Leukotrienes, & Related Compounds 5
Mechanisms of Hormone Action 6
   Hormone Receptors 6
   Regulation of Responsiveness to Hormones 7
   Interactions Between Hormone Response
      Systems 7
Classes of Hormone Action 8
   Use of Receptors for Classifying the Types of
      Hormone Actions 8
   Classification of Hormones by the Types of
      Ligands 9
Endocrine & Nervous System Relationships:
   Neuroendocrinology 10
   Neurotransmitters & Hormones 10
   Hypothalamic-Pituitary Relationships 11
Gene Expression & Recombinant DNA in
   Endocrinology & Metabolism 13
Evolution of the Endocrine System 14
   Cellular Control Networks & the Origins of
      Regulatory Chemicals 15
   The Origins of Hormones 15
   Intracellular Communication 15
   Evolution of Genes Involved in the Endocrine
      System 15
   Integrative Networks 16
   Evolution of the Endocrine Glands 16
Hormone Synthesis & Release 17
Hormone Transport 17
   Steroid Hormones & Vitamin D 17
   Thyroid Hormones 17

Polypeptide Hormones 18
Regulation of Plasma-Binding Proteins 18
Metabolism & Elimination of Hormones 19
   Peptide Hormones 19
   Steroid Hormones & Vitamin D 19
   Thyroid Hormones 20
   Catecholamines 20
   Eicosanoid Metabolism 20
Regulation of the Endocrine System 20
Actions of Hormones 21
   Developmental Effects 21
   Cell Growth & Cancer 21
   Central Nervous System Effects 22
   Effects on Metabolism 22
   Effects on Cardiovascular & Renal Function 22
   Effects of Mineral & Water Metabolism 23
   Effects on Skeletal Functions 23
   Effects on Reproductive Function 23
   Release of Other Hormones 23
   Effects on Immunologic Functions 23
Disorders of the Endocrine System 24
   Hypofunction 24
   Hyperfunction 25
   Defects in Sensitivity to Hormones 25
   Syndromes of Hormone Excess Due to
      Administration of Exogenous Hormone
      or Medication 27
   Disorders of the Endocrine Glands Not
      Associated With Disease 27
Approach to the Patient With Endocrine Disease 27
   History & Physical Examination 28
   Laboratory Studies 28
   Screening for Endocrine Diseases 33
   Treatment of Endocrine Diseases 34
Uses of Hormones in Therapy of Nonendocrine
   Disease 35
References 36

2. Hormone Synthesis & Release **39**

Vishwanath R. Lingappa, MD, PhD, & Synthia H. Mellon, PhD

Overview of Hormone Biosynthesis 39
Membrane Vesicle-Mediated Hormone Export 40
Hormone Export Not Mediated by Membrane
   Vesicles 49

Metabolism, Transport, Elimination, & Regulation of
   Hormones 54
References 57

3. Mechanisms of Hormone Action 58
David G. Gardner, MD

Receptors 58
  Neurotransmitter & Peptide Hormone
    Receptors 60
  Seven-Transmembrane Receptors 61
  G Protein Transducers 61
  Effectors 62
  G Protein-Linked Receptors & Human
    Disease 65
  Growth Factor Receptors 66
  Cytokine Receptors 67

Guanylyl Cyclase-Linked Receptors 68
Nuclear Action of Peptide Hormones 70
Nuclear Receptors 70
  Steroid Receptor Family 70
  Thyroid Receptor Family 72
Nongenomic Effects of the Steroid Hormones 73
Steroid & Thyroid Hormone Receptor Resistance
  Syndromes 74
References 74

4. Autoimmunity & Endocrine Disease 76
Judith A. Shizuru, MD, PhD

Components of the Immune System 76
The Autoimmune Response 88

References 93

5. Hypothalamus & Pituitary 95
David C. Aron, MS, MD, James W. Findling, MD, & J. Blake Tyrrell, MD

Hypothalamic Hormones 100
Anterior Pituitary Hormones 104
  ACTH & Related Peptides 104
  Growth Hormone 106
  Prolactin 108
  Thyrotropin 110
  Gonadotropins: LH & FSH 112
Endocrinologic Evaluation of the Hypothalamic-
  Pituitary Axis 114
  Evaluation of ACTH 114
  Evaluation of Growth Hormone 115
  Evaluation of Prolactin 116
  Evaluation of TSH 116
  Evaluation of LH & FSH 117
  Problems in Evaluation of the Hypothalamic-
    Pituitary Axis 117
  Effects of Pharmacologic Agents on
    Hypothalamic-Pituitary Functions 118

Endocrine Tests of Hypothalamic-Pituitary
  Function 118
  Neuroradiologic Evaluation 118
Pituitary & Hypothalamic Disorders 122
  Empty Sella Syndrome 123
  Hypothalamic Dysfunction 124
  Hypopituitarism 125
  Pituitary Adenomas 130
Posterior Pituitary Hormones 146
  Antidiuretic Hormone 146
  Oxytocin 147
  Control of Water Balance 147
  Diabetes Insipidus 149
  Syndrome of Inappropriate Secretion of
    Antidiuretic Hormone 152
References 154

6. Growth 157
Dennis M. Styne, MD

Normal Growth 157
  Intrauterine Growth 157
  Postnatal Growth 158
  Measurement of Growth 168
  Skeletal (Bone) Age 170
Disorders of Growth 170

Short Stature Due to Nonendocrine Causes 170
Short Stature Due to Endocrine Disorders 176
The Diagnosis of Short Stature 187
Tall Stature Due to Nonendocrine Causes 188
Tall Stature Due to Endocrine Causes 189
References 189

7. The Thyroid Gland 192
Francis S. Greenspan, MD

Anatomy & Histology 192
Physiology 194
  Iodine Metabolism 194
  Thyroid Hormone Synthesis & Secretion 196
  Abnormalities in Thyroid Hormone Synthesis
    & Release 200
  Thyroid Hormone Transport 201
  Metabolism of Thyroid Hormones 204
  Control of Thyroid Function 207

Action of Thyroid Hormones 213
Physiologic Changes in Thyroid Function 215
Thyroid Autoimmunity 217
Tests of Thyroid Function 218
  Tests of Thyroid Hormones in Blood 218
  Evaluation of the Hypothalamic-Pituitary-
    Thyroid Axis 219
  Iodine Metabolism & Biosynthetic Activity 220
  Thyroid Imaging 220

Thyroid Biopsy 223
Effects of Thyroid Hormones on Peripheral
    Tissues 223
Measurement of Thyroid Autoantibodies 223
Summary: Clinical Use of Thyroid Function
    Tests 224
Disorders of the Thyroid 214
    Hypothyroidism 225

Hyperthyroidism & Thyrotoxicosis 233
Thyroid Hormone Resistance Syndromes 243
Nontoxic Goiter 244
Thyroiditis 246
Effects of Ionizing Radiation on the Thyroid
    Gland 249
Thyroid Nodules & Thyroid Cancer 250
References 259

8. Mineral Metabolism & Metabolic Bone Disease **263**

Gordon J. Strewler, MD

Cellular & Extracellular Calcium Metabolism 263
Parathyroid Hormone 264
Calcitonin 269
Vitamin D 271
Integrated Control of Mineral Homeostasis 274
Medullary Thyroid Carcinoma 274
Hypercalcemia 276

Hypocalcemia 286
Bone Anatomy & Remodeling 290
Osteoporosis 295
Osteomalacia 304
Paget's Disease of Bone 308
Renal Osteodystrophy 311
References 313

9. Glucocorticoids & Adrenal Androgens **317**

James W. Findling, MD, David C. Aron, MS, MD, & J. Blake Tyrrell, MD

Embryology & Anatomy 317
Biosynthesis of Cortisol & Adrenal Androgens 320
Circulation of Cortisol & Adrenal Androgens 324
Metabolism of Cortisol & Adrenal Androgens 325
Biologic Effects 326
    Glucocorticoids 326
    Adrenal Androgens 329
    Laboratory Evaluation 330

Disorders of Adrenocortical Insufficiency 334
    Primary Adrenocortical Insufficiency (Addison's
        Disease) 334
    Secondary Adrenocortical Insufficiency 338
    Cushing's Syndrome 343
    Hirsutism & Virilism 354
    Incidental Adrenal Mass 354
References 356

10. Endocrine Hypertension **359**

Burl R. Don, MD, Edward G. Biglieri, MD, & Morris Schambelan, MD

Hypertension of Adrenal Origin 359
Hypertension of Renal Origin 371

Other Hormone Systems & Hypertension 377
References 379

11. Adrenal Medulla **381**

Alan Goldfien, MD

Anatomy 381
Hormones of the Adrenal Medulla 382
    Catecholamines 382
    Other Hormones 391
Disorders of Adrenal Medullary Function 392

Hypofunction 392
Hyperfunction 393
Pheochromocytoma 393
References 401

12. Testes **403**

Glenn D. Braunstein, MD

Anatomy & Structure-Function Relationships 403
    Testes 403
    Accessory Structures 405
Physiology of the Male Reproductive System 405
    Gonadal Steroids 405
    Control of Testicular Function 408
Evaluation of Male Gonadal Function 409
Pharmacology of Drugs Used to Treat Male
        Gonadal Disorders 414
    Androgens 414
    Gonadotropins 414
    Gonadotropin-Releasing Hormone 415
Clinical Male Gonadal Disorders 415

Klinefelter's Syndrome 415
Bilateral Anorchia 417
Leydig Cell Aplasia 418
Cryptorchidism 419
Noonan's Syndrome 420
Myotonic Dystrophy 421
Adult Seminiferous Tubule Failure 421
Adult Leydig Cell Failure 423
Impotence 423
Male Infertility 425
Gynecomastia 427
Testicular Tumors 429
References 432

13. Ovaries 434

Alan Goldfien, MD

Anatomy of the Ovaries 434
Hormones of the Ovary 435
  Steroid Hormones 435
  Relaxin 441
  Other Ovarian Hormones & Regulatory
    Substances 441
The Menstrual Cycle 441
  Hormonal Profiles During the Menstrual
    Cycle 441
  The Ovarian Cycle 444
  Hormone Interaction & Regulation During the
    Menstrual Cycle 446
Cyclic Changes in the Female Reproductive
    Tract 448
  Histology of the Endometrium Throughout
    the Menstrual Cycle 448
  Cervical Mucus 450
  Vaginal Epithelium 450
Extragenital Symptoms Associated With Menstrual
    Function 452
  Premenstrual Syndrome 452
  Dysmenorrhea 453
Disorders of Ovarian & Menstrual Function 453
  Amenorrhea in the Absence of Sexual
    Maturation 454
  Amenorrhea in Patients With Normal Secondary
    Sex Characteristics 455
  Disorders of Androgen Metabolism 460

Hirsutism 463
  Anovulatory Bleeding 468
Ovulation Induction 469
  Clomiphene Citrate 469
  Human Menopausal Gonadotropins 469
  Gonadotropin-Releasing Hormone 470
  Bromocriptine 470
Therapeutic Use of Ovarian Hormones & Their
    Synthetic Analogs 470
  Treatment of Primary Hypogonadism 470
  Ovarian Suppression 470
  Threatened Abortion 471
  Inadequate Luteal Phase 471
  Diagnostic Uses 471
Inhibitors of Ovarian Function 471
  Gonadotropin-Releasing Hormone Analogs
    & Antagonists 471
  Antiestrogens 471
  Danazol 472
  Antiprogestins 472
  Antiandrogens 472
Menopause 473
  Hormonal Changes 473
  Clinical Manifestations of Menopause 474
  Management of Menopause 476
Hormonal Contraception 477
Infertility 482
References 484

14. Abnormalities of Sexual Determination & Differentiation 487

Felix A. Conte, MD, & Melvin M. Grumbach, MD

Normal Sex Differentiation 487
Testicular & Ovarian Differentiation 491
Psychosexual Differentiation 493
Abnormal Sex Differentiation 497
Seminiferous Tubule Dysgenesis:
    Chromatin-positive Klinefelter's Syndrome
    & Its Variants 497
Syndrome Of Gonadal Dysgenesis: Turner's
    Syndrome & Its Variants 499
46,XX & 46,XY Gonadal Dysgenesis 501

True Hermaphroditism 503
Female Pseudohermaphroditism 503
P450 Aromatase Deficiency 508
Maternal Androgens & Progestogens 508
Male Pseudohermaphroditism 508
Unclassified Forms of Abnormal Sexual
    Development in Males 516
Management of Patients With Intersex
    Problems 517
References 519

15. Puberty 521

Dennis M. Styne, MD

Physiology of Puberty 521
Delayed Puberty or Absent Puberty 530

Precocious Puberty 539
References 545

16. The Endocrinology of Pregnancy 548

Robert N. Taylor, MD, PhD, & Mary C. Martin, MD

Conception & Implantation 548
Fetal-Placental-Decidual Unit 549
Polypeptide Hormones 552
Steroid Hormones 553
Maternal Adaptation to Pregnancy 554
Fetal Endocrinology 558
Endocrine Control of Parturition 559
Endocrinology of the Puerperium 560
Endocrine Disorders of Pregnancy 562

Pregnancy & Pituitary Adenomas 562
Pregnancy & Breast Cancer 563
Hypertensive Disorders of Pregnancy 564
Hyperthyroidism in Pregnancy 565
Hypothyroidism in Pregnancy 566
Diabetes Mellitus & Pregnancy
    (by John L. Kitzmiller, MD) 566
References 572

17. Regulatory Peptides of the Gut 575

Sean J. Mulvihill, MD, & Haile T. Debas, MD

Gastrin 575
Cholecystokinin 580
Secretin 581
Somatostatin 582
Bombesin & Gastrin-Releasing Peptide 582
Calcitonin Gene-Related Peptide 583
Gastric Inhibitory Peptide 583
Vasoactive Intestinal Polypeptide 583
Galanin 584
Substance P 584
Enkephalins 585
Neurotensin 585
Motilin 585
Pancreatic Polypeptide Family 586
Enteroglucagon 586

Abnormalities of Regulatory Peptides in Diseases
of the Gastrointestinal Tract 586
Duodenal Ulcer 586
Motility Disorders of the Gastrointestinal
Tract 587
Inflammatory Bowel Disease 587
Neuroendocrine Tumors of the Gut 588
Multiple Endocrine Neoplasia Syndromes 588
Zollinger-Ellison Syndrome 588
Vipoma 589
Glucagonoma 589
Carcinoid Tumors & Carcinoid Syndrome 589
Miscellaneous Tumors 590
Clinical Uses of Gut Peptides 591
References 591

18. Pancreatic Hormones & Diabetes Mellitus 595

John H. Karam, MD

The Endocrine Pancreas 595
Anatomy & Histology 595
Hormones of the Endocrine Pancreas 596
Insulin 596
Glucagon 602
Somatostatin 604
Pancreatic Polypeptide 605
Diabetes Mellitus 605
Classification 605
Type I: Insulin-Dependent (Immune-
Dependent) Diabetes Mellitus
(IDDM) 605
Type II: Non-Insulin-Dependent (Non-
Immune-Dependent) Diabetes Mellitus
(NIDDM) 608
Secondary Diabetes 611
Clinical Features of Diabetes Mellitus 612
Type I Diabetes (IDDM) 612
Type II Diabetes (NIDDM) 613
Laboratory Findings in Diabetes Mellitus 614
Urinalysis 614
Blood Glucose Testing 615
Serum Ketone Determinations 616
Glycosylated Hemoglobin Assays 616
Capillary Morphometry 617
Lipoproteins in Diabetes 617
Diagnosis of Diabetes Mellitus 617
Simple Diagnostic Test by Fasting Plasma
Glucose 617
Oral Glucose Tolerance Test 618
Insulin Levels 618

Intravenous Glucose Tolerance Test 618
Treatment of Diabetes Mellitus 619
Available Treatment Regimens 620
Diet 620
Oral Hypoglycemic Drugs 622
Insulin 627
Steps in the Management of the Diabetic
Patient 632
Acute Complications of Diabetes Mellitus 641
Hypoglycemia 641
Coma 644
Diabetic Ketoacidosis 645
Hyperglycemic, Hyperosmolar, Nonketotic
State 650
Hypoglycemic Coma 651
Lactic Acidosis 652
Chronic Complications of Diabetes Mellitus 653
Ophthalmologic Complications 654
Renal Complications 655
Neurologic Complications 656
Cardiovascular Complications 658
Skin Changes 659
Bone & Joint Complications 659
Infection 659
Surgery in the Diabetic Patient 659
Diabetics Regulated by Diet Alone 659
Diabetics Taking Oral Hypoglycemia
Agents 659
Diabetics Taking Insulin 660
Prognosis for Patients With Diabetes Mellitus 660
References 661

19. Hypoglycemic Disorders 664

John H. Karam, MD

Pathophysiology of the Counterregulatory Response
to Neuroglycopenia 664
Classification of Hypoglycemic Disorders 668
Clinical Presentation of Hypoglycemia 669
Specific Hypoglycemic Disorders 670
Symptomatic Fasting Hypoglycemia With
Hyperinsulinism 670

Insulin Reaction 670
Sulfonylurea Overdose 671
Surreptitious Insulin or Sulfonylurea
Administration 672
Autoimmune Hypoglycemia 672
Pentamidine-Induced Hypoglycemia 672
Pancreatic B Cell Tumors 672

Symptomatic Fasting Hypoglycemia Without
Hyperinsulinism 676
Disorders Associated With Low Hepatic
Glucose Output 676
Ethanol Hypoglycemia 676
Nonpancreatic Tumors 677

Nonfasting Hypoglycemia 677
Postgastrectomy Alimentary
Hypoglycemia 677
Functional Alimentary Hypoglycemia 677
Late Hypoglycemia 678
References 678

20. Disorders of Lipoprotein Metabolism **680**

John P. Kane, MD, PhD, & Mary J. Malloy, MD

Arteriosclerosis 680
Overview of Lipid Transport 681
Differentiation of Disorders of Lipoprotein
Metabolism 687
Clinical Descriptions of Primary & Secondary
Disorders of Lipoprotein Metabolism 689
The Hypertriglyceridemias 689
Primary Hypertriglyceridemia 690
Secondary Hypertriglyceridemia 692
The Primary Hypercholesterolemias 696
Familial Hypercholesterolemia 696
Familial Combined Hypercholes-
terolemia 696
Lp(a) Hyperlipoproteinemia 697
Familial Ligand-Defective Apo B 697
Secondary Hypercholesterolemia 698
Hypothyroidism 698
Nephrosis 698
Immunoglobulin Disorders 698
Anorexia Nervosa 698
Cholestasis 698

The Primary Hypolipidemias 699
Primary Hypolipidemia Due to Deficiency of
High-density Lipoproteins 699
Primary Hypolipidemia Due to Deficiency of
Apo-B-Containing Lipoproteins 699
Secondary Hypolipidemia 701
Other Disorders of Lipoprotein Metabolism 701
The Lipodystrophies 701
Rare Disorders 702
Treatment Of Hyperlipidemia 703
Dietary Factors in the Management of
Lipoprotein Disorders 703
Drugs Used in Treatment of
Hyperlipoproteinemia 705
Niacin 706
Gemfibrozil 707
HMG-CoA Reductase Inhibitors 707
Combined Drug Therapy 707
Possible Untoward Consequences of Lipid-
lowering Therapy 708
References 709

21. Obesity **710**

George A. Bray, MD

Genetic Factors Predisposing to Obesity 710
Nutrient Balance Model 711
Treatment of Obesity 721

Summary 723
References 723

22. Hormones & Cancer **724**

Debasish Tripathy, MD, & Christopher C. Benz, MD

Effects of Hormones on Tumors 724
Growth Promotion & Malignant
Transformation 724
Tumor Growth Mediated by Autocrine
& Paracrine Factors 726
Steroid-Dependent Tumors 727
Tumors Affecting Endocrine Status 727
Nonsecretory Tumors 727
Secretory Tumors 727
Treatment-Induced Endocrinopathy 728
Endocrine Therapy for Cancer 729

Steroid Receptors & Treatment 729
Primary Modalities of Endocrine Intervention 730
Combination Endocrine Therapy 731
Chemo-Endocrine Therapy 732
Clinical Problems 732
Breast Cancer in Women 732
Breast Cancer in Men 736
Endometrial Cancer 736
Prostatic Cancer 738
Miscellaneous Tumors 739
References 739

23. Humoral Manifestations of Malignancy **741**

Gordon J. Strewler, MD

General Concept of Ectopic Hormone
Secretion 741
Malignancy-Associated Hypercalcemia 743
The Syndrome of Inappropriate ADH Secretion 747

Cushing's Syndrome 747
Non-Islet-Cell Tumors & Hypoglycemia 748
Other Hormones Secreted by Tumors 749
References 750

24. Syndromes Involving Multiple Endocrine Glands **753**

Leonard J. Deftos, MD, JD, & John J. Nolan, MB, Bch, MRCPI

Multiple Endocrine Neoplasia 753
  Multiple Endocrine Neoplasia Type I 754
  Multiple Endocrine Neoplasia Types IIa
    & IIb 755
  Other Multiple Endocrine Neoplasias 759
  Management of Patients With Multiple Endocrine
    Neoplasia (MEN) Syndromes 759
  Genetic Diagnosis 759
Failure of Multiple Endocrine Glands 759

Prototypical Autoimmune Endocrinopathy:
  Addison's Disease 761
Clinical & Immunologic Heterogeneity 762
Management of Patients With Failure of Multiple
  Endocrine Glands 765
Genetic Aspects of Autoimmune Disorders 766
Nonautoimmune Endocrine Failure 767
References 767

25. Geriatric Endocrinology **770**

Susan L. Greenspan, MD, & Neil M. Resnick, MD

Thyroid Function & Disease 770
  Disorders of the Thyroid Gland 771
    Hyperthyroidism 771
    Hypothyroidism 773
    Multinodular Goiter 774
    Thyroid Nodules & Cancer 774
Carbohydrate Intolerance & Diabetes Mellitus 774
  Aging & the Physiology of Carbohydrate
    Intolerance 774
  Diabetes Mellitus 775
  Nonketotic Hyperosmolar Coma 776
Osteoporosis & Calcium Homeostasis 776
  Osteoporosis 776

Hyperparathyroidism 781
Changes in Water Balance 782
  Hypernatremia 782
  Hyponatremia 782
  Hyporeninemic Hypoaldosteronism 782
Glucocorticoids & Stress 782
  Disorders Of The Hypothalamic-Pituitary-
    Adrenal Axis 783
    Abnormal Response to Stress 783
    Adrenal Insufficiency 783
Changes in Reproductive Function in Men 784
Benign Prostatic Hyperplasia 784
References 785

Appendix: Table of Normal Hormone Reference Ranges **788**

Index **799**

Authors

David C. Aron, MS, MD
Professor of Medicine, Division of Clinical and Molecular Endocrinology, Case Western Reserve University School of Medicine, Cleveland; Acting Chief, Medical Service, Veterans Affairs Medical Center, Cleveland, Ohio.

John D. Baxter, MD
Professor of Medicine, Director of the Metabolic Research Unit; Chief, Division of Endocrinology, Parnassus and Mt Zion Campuses, University of California, San Francisco.

Christopher C. Benz, MD
Professor of Medicine, Cancer Research Institute, Division of Hematology/Oncology, University of California, San Francisco.

Edward G. Biglieri, MD
Professor of Medicine Emeritus, University of California, San Francisco.

Glenn D. Braunstein, MD
Professor of Medicine, School of Medicine, University of California, Los Angeles; Chairman, Department of Medicine, Cedars-Sinai Medical Center, Los Angeles.

George A. Bray, MD
Professor of Medicine, Pennington Biomedical Research Center, Louisiana State University, Baton Rouge.

Felix A. Conte, MD
Professor of Pediatrics, University of California, San Francisco.

Haile T. Debas, MD, FRCS(C)
Dean, School of Medicine; Maurice Galante Distinguished Professor of Surgery, University of California, San Francisco.

Leonard J. Deftos, MD, JD
Professor of Medicine, University of California, San Diego; San Diego Veterans Affairs Medical Center, La Jolla.

Burl R. Don, MD
Associate Professor of Medicine, University of California, San Francisco; Associate Director, University of California Renal Center, San Francisco.

James W. Findling, MD
Clinical Professor of Medicine, Medical College of Wisconsin; Director, Endocrine-Diabetes Center, St. Luke's Medical Center, Milwaukee, Wisconsin.

David G. Gardner, MD
Professor of Medicine, Department of Medicine and Metabolic Research Unit, University of California, San Francisco.

Alan Goldfien, MD
Professor Emeritus, Departments of Medicine, and Obstetrics and Gynecology and Reproductive Sciences, Cardiovascular Research Institute, University of California, San Francisco.

Francis S. Greenspan, MD, FACP
Clinical Professor of Medicine and Radiology; Chief, Thyroid Clinic, Division of Endocrinology, Department of Medicine, University of California, San Francisco.

Susan L. Greenspan, MD
Assistant Professor of Medicine, Harvard Medical School, Boston; Director, Osteoporosis Prevention and Treatment Center, Beth Israel Deaconess Medical Center, Boston, Massachusetts.

Melvin M. Grumbach, MD
Edward B. Shaw Professor of Pediatrics and Chairman Emeritus, Department of Pediatrics, University of California, San Francisco.

John P. Kane, MD, PhD
Professor of Medicine, Biochemistry, and Biophysics, Cardiovascular Research Institute; Director, Lipid Clinic, University of California, San Francisco.

John H. Karam, MD
Professor of Medicine Emeritus, University of California, San Francisco.

Vishwanath R. Lingappa, MD, PhD
Professor of Physiology and Medicine, University of California, San Francisco.

Mary J. Malloy, MD
Clinical Professor of Medicine and Pediatrics; Director, Pediatric Lipid Clinic, University of California, San Francisco.

Mary C. Martin, MD
Associate Professor, Department of Obstetrics and Gynecology and Reproductive Sciences, University of California, San Francisco.

Synthia H. Mellon, PhD
Associate Professor, Department of Obstetrics and Gynecology and Reproductive Sciences, The Reproductive Endocrinology Center and The Metabolic Research Unit, University of California, San Francisco.

Sean J. Mulvihill, MD
Associate Professor of Surgery; Chief, Division of General Surgery, University of California, San Francisco.

John J. Nolan, MB, BCh, MRCPI
Lecturer in Endocrinology, Trinity College, Dublin, Ireland; Consultant Endocrinologist, St. James Hospital, Dublin, Ireland.

Neil M. Resnick, MD
Associate Professor of Medicine, Harvard Medical School, Boston, Massachusetts.

Morris Schambelan, MD
Professor of Medicine, University of California, San Francisco; Chief, Division of Endocrinology, San Francisco General Hospital.

Judith A. Shizuru, MD, PhD
Assistant Professor of Medicine (Acting), Division of Bone Marrow Transplantation, Stanford University School of Medicine, Stanford, California.

Gordon J. Strewler, MD
Professor of Medicine, Harvard Medical School, Chief, Department of Medicine, Brockton/West Roxbury Veterans Administration Medical Center, West Roxbury, Massachusetts.

Dennis M. Styne, MD
Professor and Chair, Department of Pediatrics, University of California, Davis, Medical Center, Sacramento.

Robert N. Taylor, MD, PhD
Associate Professor of Obstetrics & Gynecology, Department of Obstetrics and Gynecology and Reproductive Sciences, University of California, San Francisco.

Debasish Tripathy, MD
Assistant Professor of Medicine, University of California, San Francisco.

J. Blake Tyrrell, MD
Clinical Professor of Medicine; Chief, Clinical Endocrinology and Metabolism, Metabolic Research Unit, University of California, San Francisco.

Preface

The fifth edition of *Basic & Clinical Endocrinology* is a major contribution to the study of the science of endocrinology and the practice of medicine in this area of specialization. Endocrinology is moving rapidly both in elucidation of molecular mechanisms and in improved techniques of diagnosis and therapy. Keeping up with this activity requires updating of texts at fairly short intervals. All of the chapters in this new edition have been reviewed and revised, and new chapters have been added on hormone synthesis and release, mechanisms of hormone action, and endocrine autoimmunity. The reader will find this book an excellent source for current concepts of endocrine pathophysiology. The student and clinician will find clearly outlined the modern techniques for diagnosis and treatment of endocrine disorders.

All of the artwork has been redone and now makes use of color, allowing better visualization of important material. Abundant use of cartoons, flow diagrams, and tables facilitates understanding of complicated systems and therapeutic options.

It has been a joy and an honor to have had the opportunity to participate with our outstanding authors in the development of this new edition.

Francis S. Greenspan, MD
Gordon J. Strewler, MD

San Francisco and West Roxbury
March 1997

Introduction to Endocrinology

1

John D. Baxter, MD

THE ENDOCRINE SYSTEM

The endocrine and nervous systems are the major means by which the body transmits information between different cells and tissues (Figure 1–1). This information results in regulation of most bodily functions. The term "endocrine" denotes internal secretion of biologically active substances—in contrast to "exocrine," which is secretion outside the body, eg, through sweat glands or ducts that lead into the gastrointestinal tract. The endocrine system uses hormones to convey its information. A hormone is typi-

---

ACRONYMS USED IN THIS CHAPTER

ACTH	Adrenocorticotropic hormone; corticotropin	**HRE**	Hormone response element	
ADH	Antidiuretic hormone; vasopressin	**IDDM**	Insulin dependent diabetes mellitus	
ADP	Adenosine diphosphate	**IGF-1**	Insulin-like growth factor-1	
ANP	Atrial natriuretic peptide	**IGF-2**	Insulin-like growth factor-2	
AP1	Transcription factor AP1	**LDL**	Low-density lipoprotein	
ATP	Adenosine triphosphate	**LH**	Luteinizing hormone	
cAMP	Cyclic AMP, cyclic adenosine monophosphate	**MAO**	Monamine oxidase	
		MEN	Multiple endocrine neoplasia	
CBG	Corticosteroid-binding globulin; transcortin	**MRI**	Magnetic resonance imaging	
		mRNA	Messenger RNA	
CCK	Cholecystokinin	**NIDDM**	Non-insulin-dependent diabetes mellitus	
CG	Chorionic gonadotropin			
cGMP	Guanosine 3',5'-cyclic monophosphate, cyclic GMP	**PCR**	Polymerase chain reaction	
		PGDF	Platelet-derived growth factor	
CGRH	Calcitonin gene-related hormone	**PRL**	Prolactin	
COMT	Catechol-O-methyltransferase	**PTH**	Parathyroid hormone	
CRH	Corticotropin-releasing hormone	**RFLP**	Restriction fragment length polymorphism	
CS	Chorionic somatomammotropin, placental lactogen			
		RNA	Ribonucleic acid	
DNA	Deoxyribonucleic acid	**SHBG**	Sex hormone-binding globulin	
EGF	Epidermal growth factor	**TBG**	Thyroid hormone-binding globulin	
ELISA	Enzyme-linked immunosorbent assay	**TBPA**	Thyroid hormone-binding prealbumin; transthyretin	
ERE	Estrogen response element	**TGFα, TGFβ**	Transforming growth factors α and β	
FGF	Fibroblast growth factor			
FSH	Follicle-stimulating hormone	**TRH**	Thyrotropin-releasing hormone	
GABA	γ-Aminobutyric acid	**TSH**	Thyroid-stimulating hormone, thyrotropin	
GH	Growth hormone			
GnRH	Gonadotropin-releasing hormone	**VIP**	Vasoactive intestinal peptide	
GRH	Growth hormone-releasing hormone	**VMA**	Vanillylmandelic acid	

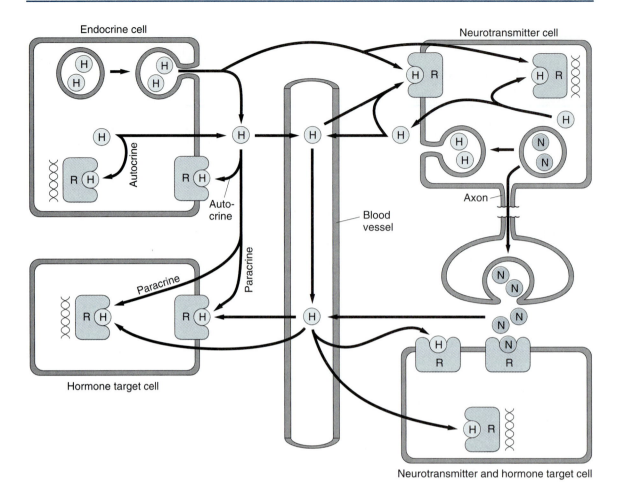

Figure 1–1. Actions of hormones and neurotransmitters and their interrelationships. Both endocrine and neurotransmitter cells release hormones that they synthesize either from secretory vesicles or by diffusion. These hormones may act on the same cell in which they are produced (autocrine) without leaving the cell or after their release and subsequent binding to receptors in or on the cell. They may act on other target cells in their vicinity, including neurotransmitter cells, without entering the circulation (paracrine). They may go to the target cell through the circulation (hormonal). Neurotransmitter cells produce neurotransmitters that are released at nerve terminals. These same neurotransmitters can be released to act as hormones through the synaptic junctions or directly by the cell. (H, hormone; R, receptor; N, neurotransmitter.)

cally defined as a substance released by an endocrine gland and transported through the bloodstream to another tissue where it acts to regulate functions of the target tissue. These actions are mediated by binding of the hormone to receptor molecules (Chapter 3). The receptors must (1) distinguish the hormone from all of the millions of other molecules to which they are exposed and (2) transmit the binding information into postreceptor events. Hormones are allosteric effectors that alter the conformations of the receptor proteins to which they bind.

The endocrine system is diverse and complex, with varied and sophisticated mechanisms that control hormone synthesis, release, and activation, transport in the circulation, and metabolism and delivery to the surface or interior of cells upon which they act. Other mechanisms regulate the sensitivity of cells to hormones in target tissues and the specific responses elicited by hormones.

In addition to these traditional functions of the system, a more expanded view of hormone action must be taken. Many actions of hormones occur in autocrine, paracrine, or juxtacrine fashions in which the hormones do not enter the circulation (Figure 1–1, and see below). Molecules that are usually not considered hormones, such as lymphokines, act as hormones. Tissues such as the kidney, liver, and heart, ordinarily not considered to be endocrine glands, produce and release hormones. Complex interrelationships exist between the nervous, immune, and other systems. Interrelationships between the endocrine and nervous systems are briefly described below and to some extent in Chapter 5 (hypothalamus and pituitary gland) and Chapter 11 (the adrenal medulla). Relationships between the endocrine and immunologic systems are discussed briefly below and in more detail in Chapter 4. Also described are the class of molecules termed "eicosanoids," including the prostaglandins and prostacyclins, which have numerous relationships with the endocrine system.

This chapter provides an overview of the field of endocrinology in general terms, including basic science and principles that are important for diagnosis and management of patients with endocrine disease.

PARACRINE & AUTOCRINE ACTIONS

As mentioned above, hormones not only reach target tissues through the circulation but also act locally in the vicinity in which they are released (Figure 1–1). When they act locally on cells other than those that produce them, the action is called "paracrine," as illustrated by the actions of sex steroids in the ovary, angiotensin II in the kidney, and platelet-derived growth factor released by platelets. As a variant of

this action, the hormone in the membrane of one cell can interact directly with a receptor on a juxtaposed cell. This is seen, for example, with some hematopoietic growth factors and is termed "juxtacrine" regulation. The hormone can also act on the cell in which it is produced, a phenomenon referred to as "autocrine"; in this case, the hormone may be released by the cell and then act on it, or it may act inside the cell without ever being released. For example, insulin released by the pancreatic islet B cells can inhibit insulin release by the same cells, and somatostatin can inhibit its release from pancreatic D cells (Chapter 18). Autocrine actions appear to be especially important with cancer cells that synthesize various oncogene products which act in the same cell to stimulate cell division and promote the overall growth of the cancer.

CHEMICAL COMPOSITION OF HORMONES

Hormones are derived from the major classes of compounds used by the body for general functional purposes (Figures 1–2 and 1–3; see also Chapter 2). In fact, derivatives of all types of small molecules act as regulatory ligands for autocrine, paracrine, juxtacrine, or endocrine actions, or in the mediation of

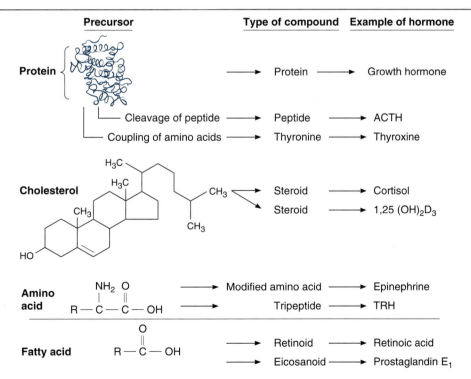

Figure 1–2. Precursors of hormones. Shown are representations of the sources of the major hormones, with examples of the molecular types of derivatives and hormones that reflect each chemical type.

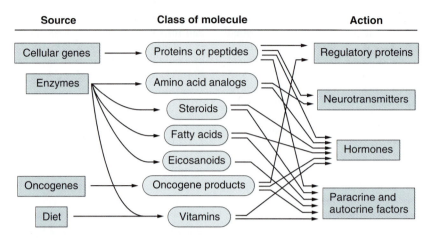

Source	Class of molecule	Action

Figure 1–3. Relations between the source, class of molecules, and actions of various species of molecules involved in the endocrine system. These molecules are or become hormones, eicosanoids, oncogene products, and vitamins. Normal genes encode proteins that are regulatory proteins, neurotransmitters, hormones, and paracrine or autocrine factors (or polypeptides from which these are derived). Normal genes also encode enzymes that participate in generating amino acid analogs that can be neurotransmitters, hormones, and autocrine or paracrine factors, steroids that can be hormones or autocrine or paracrine factors, or eicosanoids that can be autocrine or paracrine factors. Oncogenes encode proteins that can be regulatory proteins, hormones, or autocrine or paracrine factors. Vitamins can be obtained from the diet or in some cases synthesized by the body, and the latter can act as hormones or as autocrine or paracrine factors.

actions of hormones. Although the major hormones that are necessary for life and for which deficiency states can occur through destruction of the endocrine gland have been identified, new hormones are still being discovered, and it is certain that a number of hormones have not yet been identified.

Nuclear receptors provide an example of the explosion of information in the field. These receptors bind the steroid hormones, thyroid hormones, retinoids, and vitamin D (Chapter 3). However, over 100 different genes encode molecules in this "superfamily," far more than is accounted for by the major classes of hormones listed above. Many new ligands that bind to various nuclear receptor family members are being identified, such as certain fatty acids and retinoids, but ligands for most of the proteins in the family have not yet been identified. It appears likely that many more hormones or other ligands that act in autocrine and paracrine fashions will be identified in the future, although it is not currently known whether most of the molecules in this superfamily of proteins will turn out to bind hormones. Similarly, many new cell surface receptors have been identified in recent years, and it appears that a number of additional cell surface receptors will also be identified in the future.

Thus, hormones can be proteins (including glycoproteins), smaller peptides or peptide derivatives, amino acid analogs, or lipids. Polypeptide hormones are direct translation products of specific mRNAs, cleavage products of larger precursor proteins, or modified peptides. Catecholamines and thyroid hormones are derivatives of amino acids. Steroid hormones and vitamin D are derived from cholesterol. Retinoids are derived from carotenoids in the diet that are modified by the body. Eicosanoids such as prostaglandins, prostacyclins, and leukotrienes are related to hormones (see below) and are derived from fatty acids. Whereas hormones are referred to as such when their structures are known, they are sometimes called "factors" when their activities have been isolated but their structures are not known.

VITAMINS & HORMONES

Classically, vitamins (Figure 1–3) are defined as essential substances that are required in small quantities from the diet that are not utilized by the body as fuels, like foods, but mostly serve as mediators of various processes in the body. Although this definition is generally acceptable, it should also be recognized that in some cases "vitamins" can also be produced by the body. For example, vitamin D is produced endogenously in individuals who have sufficient exposure to sunlight and is a required vitamin only when there is inadequate exposure to sunlight (Chapter 8). Furthermore, the final active product of the vitamin may be a derivative of the ingested vitamin. This is the case for vitamin D and for the retinoids. Vitamins can act by mechanisms similar to those of hormones. For example, $1,25(OH)_2$-cholecalciferol ($1,25\text{-}(OH)_2D_3$) and the retinoids (retinoic acid, 9-*cis*-retinoic acid, and others) act through receptors of the same family as the steroid and thyroid hormones. (See above and Chapter 3.)

HORMONES & ONCOGENES

Oncogenes are cancer-promoting genes (see Chapter 22 and Figure 1–3). These genes are commonly either altered (eg, by mutation), or overexpressed versions of normal cellular genes. They were originally described in cancer-promoting viruses that appear to have derived their oncogenes from their host's cellular genes. In many cases, oncogenes are analogs either of hormones, hormone receptors, or molecules involved in transmitting hormone actions. Viral oncogenes are designated by "*v-*" and the normal cellular counterparts by "*c-.*" The *v-erb*A oncogene from the chicken erythroleukemia virus is similar to the thyroid hormone receptor (sometimes thus designated as *c-erb*A), and the *v-erb*B oncogene is similar to the epidermal growth factor (EGF) receptor (*c-erb*B). It is usual for the oncogene to have a function different from its normal cellular counterpart. Thus, for example, unlike the thyroid hormone receptor, the *v-erb* A oncogene product (*v-erb* A) does not bind thyroid hormone and in general is a transcriptional repressor. Other examples of oncogenes and the types of products they encode are H-*ras* and K-*ras*, guanylyl nucleotide binding proteins involved in intracellular signaling; *abl*, tyrosine kinase; *jun*, a subunit of the AP1 transcription factor; and *sis*, the platelet-derived growth factor (PDGF) B chain. The mechanisms of action of these products are described in Chapters 3 and 22.

HORMONES & THE IMMUNE SYSTEM

Many of the complex interrelationships between the endocrine and immune systems are described in Chapter 4 and are simplistically illustrated in Figure 1–4. The response of the immune system to foreign substances and the lack of response to substances produced by the body involve ligand-receptor actions that are similar to the mechanisms of hormone action described in Chapter 3. Whereas cell-cell interactions participate in more steps with the immune system than with the endocrine system, major regulation also occurs through release of chemical signals by either cells of the immune system or by tissues that ordinarily are not considered to be part of the immune system that act either systemically or locally.

Thus, immunologically competent cells release cytokines that can stimulate growth, regulate specific processes, destroy target cells through cytotoxic lymphokines, and mediate suppressor cell effects to block B cells from producing antibodies. For exam-

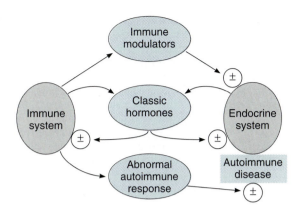

Figure 1–4. Interrelations between the endocrine and immune systems. The "plus or minus" signs indicate that the influences can be stimulatory or inhibitory.

ple, activated T lymphocytes release lymphokines that attract macrophages and neutrophils to an area of infection. Various complement proteins act in a paracrine fashion by attracting and activating macrophages. Interleukins, interferons, tumor necrosis factor, plasminogen activator, and other peptides are representative of these factors. In some cases, peptides traditionally considered as hormones (eg, corticotropin [ACTH], prolactin [PRL]) are produced by cells of the immune system. Their roles are currently being deciphered. Finally, substances released by cells of the immune system can affect the function of the endocrine system and the release of hormones. For example, tumor necrosis factor can affect the release and metabolism of thyroid hormones.

There is also extensive regulation of the immune system by hormones. This topic is addressed in a subsequent section of this chapter on the actions of hormones (see Effects on Immunologic Functions).

As discussed in Chapter 4 and below in the section on disorders of the endocrine system, autoimmune-induced disorders of the endocrine glands comprise a major component of endocrine practice. These include both autoimmune destruction of glands as is seen with insulin-dependent diabetes mellitus (IDDM) (Chapter 18) and the most common form of Addison's disease (Chapter 9)—and, less commonly, autoimmune stimulation, as is seen with the most common form of hyperthyroidism (Chapter 7).

EICOSANOIDS: PROSTAGLANDINS, THROMBOXANES, LEUKOTRIENES, & RELATED COMPOUNDS

Eicosanoids (including prostaglandins; Figures 1–2 and 1–3) are derived from polyunsaturated fatty acids with 18-, 20-, or 22-carbon skeletons. Among these, arachidonic acid (*cis*-5,8,11,14-eicosatetraenoic acid) is the most important and abundant precursor for the various eicosanoids in humans. Derivatives of these substances include prostaglandins, prostacyclins, leukotrienes, and thromboxanes. These fatty acid derivatives are produced by most cells, released with little storage, cleared rapidly from the circulation, and thought to act predominantly in a paracrine or autocrine fashion. They have mechanisms of action similar to those of hormones; they were previously thought to act exclusively through cell surface receptors (discussed below), but more recently some of these compounds have been found to interact with nuclear receptors. Eicosanoid synthesis is frequently stimulated in response to hormones, and in these instances, these molecules mediate hormone action. For example, changes in prostaglandin synthesis are a common feature of hormones acting on the kidney. Eicosanoids can also regulate hormone release and actions. For example, prostaglandin E (PGE) compounds inhibit the release of growth hormone (GH) and PRL from the pituitary. Eicosanoids affect essentially every type of cell in some way, including effects on hemostasis, smooth muscle contraction, calcium ion mobilization, renal and reproductive function, and traumatic, inflammatory, immunologic, vascular, airway, and gut responses.

MECHANISMS OF HORMONE ACTION

Detailed mechanisms of hormone action are discussed in Chapter 3. Once a hormone reaches a target tissue, the tissue needs to recognize it and distinguish it from the myriad of other chemicals to which the cell is exposed. This recognition event must be transmitted into an appropriate response. These processes are mediated by hormone receptors that bind hormones specifically and with high affinity.

HORMONE RECEPTORS

Hormone receptors are present either on the cell surface or inside the cell. As discussed earlier in this chapter, the continued application of newer techniques of molecular biology to this field is resulting in identification of many new hormone receptors and the ligands that bind to them.

Cell Surface Receptors

In general, cell surface receptors mediate actions of polypeptide hormones, catecholamines, and prostaglandins. These receptors may be single

polypeptide chains or may have up to four subunits. A large class of receptors have seven transmembrane domains; these mediate actions of catecholamines, prostaglandins, ACTH, glucagon, parathyroid hormone (PTH) and other hormones. Other receptors have one or two transmembrane domains, as is seen with the family of tetrameric receptors as represented by the insulin receptor and the huge family of receptors represented by the growth hormone and many cytokine receptors. Some "receptors" with single polypeptide chains also serve to transport hormones into the cell for degradation or intercellular actions. These are represented by the low-density lipoprotein (LDL) and some of the atrial natriuretic peptide (ANP) receptors. These molecules are often called "transporters" rather than receptors.

Binding of hormones by cell surface receptors results in triggering of so-called "second messenger" signaling. Thus, with the seven transmembrane receptors, binding is coupled to interactions with guanylyl nucleotide binding "G proteins" and other proteins that in turn regulate processes such as generation of or inhibition of production of cyclic AMP (cAMP), cyclic GMP (cGMP), regulation of the intracellular levels of calcium ion, or regulation of C kinase activity. Other receptors either have or are coupled to tyrosine kinase activity, as occurs with the receptors that include those for EGF, guanylyl cyclase activating activity as is seen with one class of ANP receptors, or other types of kinase activities.

Molecules such as cAMP, cGMP, and Ca^{2+} themselves bind to other proteins with the result that other kinases are activated. For example, cAMP binds to a protein complex that results in dissociation and thereby activation of a serine and threonine kinase catalytic unit. The kinases then can phosphorylate substrates on diverse proteins with a spectrum of effects. In some cases, the substrates are themselves enzymes involved in metabolism, such as those involved in glycogen deposition, whereas in other cases a cascade of additional regulatory events is set in motion such that the final hormone response involves a different protein. The modified protein can be a regulatory protein. As examples, second messenger-induced phosphorylations can modify transcription factors with resultant influences on gene expression (Chapter 3).

Nuclear Receptors

Hormones that act inside the cell bind to one of the receptors that is a member of a huge superfamily of receptors comprising over 100 different members. These receptors mediate actions of steroid hormones, vitamin D, thyroid hormones, retinoids, and a number of other ligands, including various fatty acids and eicosanoids. As discussed above in the section on chemical composition of hormones, new ligands for nuclear receptors are being identified at a rapid pace, and these ligands will probably turn out to act variously as hormones and in autocrine and paracrine fashions.

Nuclear receptors are ligand-regulated transcription factors. They have generally similar structures and functions, though various receptors show some differences in the details of their actions, especially in their states and functions in the unliganded state. For example, unliganded steroid receptors are associated with heat shock proteins and are present in either the cytosol or the nucleus. Ligand binding promotes dissociation of the heat shock proteins, following which the receptor units dimerize and then bind to the nucleus, usually to DNA elements termed hormone response elements (HREs), but sometimes they are tethered to other proteins that are bound to DNA. Bound in these ways, the hormone-receptor complexes usually stimulate but sometimes repress transcription of specific genes. With other receptors such as the thyroid hormone and retinoid receptors, the unliganded receptors are bound to DNA or tethered to other proteins where they can suppress (particularly common with thyroid hormone receptors), stimulate, or have no influence on transcription. With the thyroid hormone receptor, ligand binding promotes dissociation of a repressor protein, thereby relieving repression, and also promotes binding of so-called coactivator proteins that are involved in stimulating transcription.

It is surprising that all hormones known to act inside the cell bind to a member of the class of nuclear receptors, given that these receptors represent only one of a large number of classes of transcription factors. Thus, it is possible that hormones and other paracrine or autocrine factors will be found that act by binding to other types of transcription factors, even if there are no clear examples of this to date. However, the dioxin receptor is a nuclear transcription factor composed of two subunits; this receptor mediates actions of dioxin, and it is likely that there is a naturally occurring endogenous ligand that binds to it.

REGULATION OF RESPONSIVENESS TO HORMONES

Responsiveness to hormones is extensively regulated, though it varies extensively with individual responses (Figure 1–5). Down-regulation by the homologous ligand of responsiveness is a general feature of hormones that bind to cell surface receptors, though occasionally the effect is up-regulation. Such down-regulation occurs through ligand-induced decreases in receptor levels and activity. However, postreceptor events also can blunt hormone responsiveness. Most typically, this occurs through phosphorylations, induced by the hormone of proteins involved in transmitting hormone responses. In addition, the effects of hormone action, as reflected by insulin's effect on blood glucose, can also influence the overall hormone response.

Down-regulation by nuclear receptor family members is more varied, sometimes occurs only to a very modest extent, and usually occurs through inhibition by the homologous ligand bound to its cognate receptor of transcription of the receptor gene. There are also cases of heterologous regulation, and in some cases there is positive control. For example, there is strong regulation of progesterone receptor levels by estrogens in breast tissue (Chapter 22). As occurs with cell surface receptors, responsiveness to hormones that act through nuclear receptors can also be regulated at a number of postreceptor loci.

INTERACTIONS BETWEEN HORMONE RESPONSE SYSTEMS

Interactions between various hormone response systems are extensive. The regulation of hormone responsiveness by homologous and heterologous hormones is discussed in the preceding section. Hormones can also show crossover in terms of the receptors or effector systems they use (Figure 1–6).

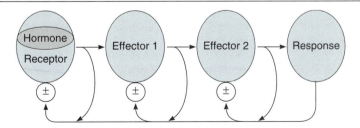

Figure 1–5. Hormone responsiveness by homologous hormone-receptor complexes can occur at multiple loci. Shown are feedback loops that are usually negative but can be positive and that regulate responsiveness through effects on the receptor, effector, or response limbs on any of the elements of the response network. The "plus or minus" signs indicate that the influences can be stimulatory or inhibitory.

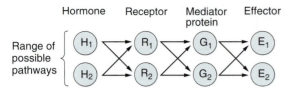

Figure 1–6. Possible pathways of transmission of hormonal signals. Each hormone can work through one or more receptors; each hormone-receptor complex can work through one or more mediator proteins (either G proteins or other signaling mechanism), and each mediating protein or enzyme activated by hormone-receptor complexes can affect one or more effector functions.

Crossover in terms of receptors is discussed in the following section on classes of hormone action. Crossover in terms of effector systems occurs with most classes of hormones. Thus, several classes of hormones utilize cAMP, Ca^{2+}, and C kinase as second messengers; and several nuclear receptors can utilize the same HRE or be tethered to the DNA through the same proteins, as is seen with the AP1 transcription factor complex (Chapter 3).

Synergistic and antagonistic interactions between various hormone response networks forms a critical component of endocrine control and of regulation in general. Figure 1–7 illustrates a synergistic hormone response. Commonly, the effect on either of two hormones on a given response is minor, but when two hormones are given there is a major response. Many variations can also be observed. Furthermore, the effect of one hormone can be inhibitory but overcome by the second hormone that may or may not have a significant effect alone. These synergistic or antagonistic interactions can occur between any of the types of responses, ie, with nuclear receptor-nuclear receptor, membrane receptor-membrane receptor, and nu-

clear receptor-membrane receptor networks. Such interactions provide for a wide array of combinatorial possibilities that greatly enhance the ability of hormones to exert influences that range from subtle fine tuning of metabolism to major changes in gene expression.

CLASSES OF HORMONE ACTION

The author classifies hormones and hormone analogs in two ways (Figure 1–8). The first is with respect to the function of the ligand according to whether it binds to a given receptor and whether it drives the receptor into postbinding events that result in receptor action. This classification separates hormones into agonist, antagonist or partial agonist-partial antagonist, mixed agonist-antagonist, or inactive compounds. The second way classifies the function of the hormone according to the types of responses it mediates and according to the type of receptor through which the ligand acts. With the use of these two means, a compound that is an agonist and produces effects on breast tissue through binding to the estrogen receptor is said to be an estrogen receptor agonist. Conversely, when a compound binds to the estrogen receptor, allows the receptor to remain in a functionally inactive state, and blocks the binding and the actions of estrogens, it is said to be an estrogen receptor antagonist.

USE OF RECEPTORS FOR CLASSIFYING THE TYPES OF HORMONE ACTIONS

Traditionally, hormones were classified according to their effects. For example, glucocorticoids were named for their carbohydrate-regulating activities, mineralocorticoids for their salt-regulating activities, and pituitary tropic hormones for the types of tropism they exerted. Other hormones were named for the gland from which they were released (eg, parathyroid hormone). Whereas naming hormones for effects they were first found to elicit is reasonable, classification according to types of action can pose several problems. First, effects initially described for the hormone may later be found not to be its major effects. Actions of glucocorticoids, for instance, are diverse, and those on carbohydrate metabolism comprise only a subset. Second, several different hormones can have the same effects through the same receptor that generally is associated with only one of the hormones (Figures 1–6 and 1–8); thus, both the "glucocorticoid" cortisol and the "mineralocorticoid" aldosterone can regulate min-

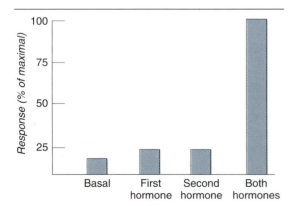

Figure 1–7. Schematic representation of a synergistic hormone response. Note that in this case neither hormone has a major effect alone.

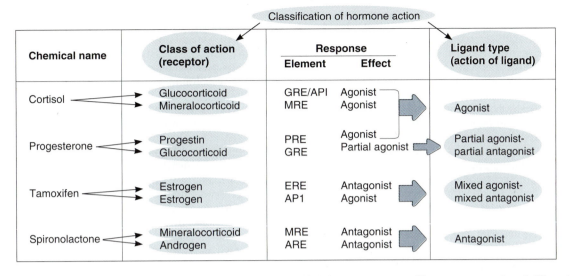

Figure 1–8. Classification of actions of ligands that interact with hormone receptors. Shown are examples of different types of ligands with classification of the type of ligand and the receptors through which they interact. (GRE, glucocorticoid response element; AP1, transcription factor 1; MRE, mineralocorticoid response element; PRE, progesterone response element; ERE, estrogen response element; ARE, androgen response element.)

eral metabolism by interactions with mineralocorticoid receptors; insulin can act similarly to insulin-like growth factors-1 and 2 (IGF-1 and IGF-2) by binding to IGF-1 receptors; and chorionic gonadotropin (CG) can act like thyroid-stimulating hormone (TSH) by binding to TSH receptors. In addition to interactions of different hormones with the same receptor, two hormones can have the same effect through interactions with different receptors. For example, both glucocorticoids and insulin can promote glycogen deposition through different mechanisms. Classification according to the gland can also be confusing given that in general most glands (eg, adrenal, pancreas) produce more than one hormone.

This confusion is avoided by utilizing the receptor for classification of hormone action, a system that is unambiguous, more rigorous, and simpler to use (Figure 1–8). Furthermore, use of the receptor poses no problem with initial naming of a class of hormones for a given type of action, since definition of actions mediated by the receptor acknowledges the spectrum of receptor-mediated actions while preserving the historical name. This system was established and has been used by pharmacologists from the time the concept of receptor was established and before receptors were even proved experimentally. Use of this classification for catecholamine actions through α- and β-adrenergic receptors, and other subclasses of these are most familiar to clinicians and scientists. Thus, whereas most actions of cortisol are mediated through glucocorticoid receptors, when this steroid acts through mineralocorticoid receptors, that action should be termed a mineralocorticoid action of cortisol.

CLASSIFICATION OF HORMONES BY THE TYPES OF LIGANDS: AGONISTS, ANTAGONISTS, PARTIAL AGONISTS/PARTIAL ANTAGONISTS, & INACTIVE COMPOUNDS

Classification of ligands as agonists, partial agonists-partial antagonists, antagonists, or inactive compounds has been utilized for both hormones and drugs. The author has also introduced an additional classification of mixed agonist-antagonist compounds to account for newer information about mechanisms of action of various ligands whose properties do not fit these categories.

Inactive Compounds

Compounds that do not bind to receptors have neither agonist nor antagonist activity and are said to be inactive compounds.

Agonist

An agonist is a compound that binds to a receptor and transmits binding into a hormone response. Most naturally produced ligands that bind to receptors function as agonists. All known major hormones are full agonists. However, a number of hormone analogs that are chemically synthesized by chemical or recombinant means have been produced. In some cases these compounds have more activity than the natural hormone. Examples include the synthetic glucocorticoids such as prednisone, dexamethasone, and triamcinolone that are used extensively to suppress inflammatory and immunologic responses (Chapter 9).

Antagonist

An antagonist is a compound that binds to a given receptor and does not transmit the binding into a receptor response. The binding of an antagonist also blocks binding of agonists and thereby prevents their actions, thus defining the term antagonist.

Although compounds with antagonist activity are produced by the body, in general these circulate at levels too low to be effective. As an example, progesterone, which acts as an agonist through binding to progesterone receptors, can have antagonist actions through either mineralocorticoid or glucocorticoid receptors. However, progesterone binds to the glucocorticoid and mineralocorticoid receptors with an affinity that is much weaker than that for the progesterone receptor such that the concentrations of progesterone which accumulate under ordinary circumstances are too low for the steroid to substantially occupy the mineralocorticoid or glucocorticoid receptors.

Partial Agonist-Partial Antagonist

Partial agonists-partial antagonists are compounds that bind to receptors and yield a response that is less than that of a full agonist even at ligand concentrations that fully saturate the receptors. As a result, when the concentration of partial agonist is sufficient both to occupy many or all of the receptors and to block the binding of an agonist, the partial agonist will suppress the agonist response but only to the level induced by the partial agonist alone. In this case, the partial agonist is also acting as an antagonist, thereby justifying its designation as a partial antagonist. These compounds are also naturally produced, although—as in the case of antagonists—the author is unaware of examples where their occupancy of receptors is important in endogenous circumstances. For example, the mineralocorticoid steroid deoxycorticosterone is a glucocorticoid partial agonist-partial agonist, but at the low levels of this compound that circulate in the circulation it probably does not substantially occupy glucocorticoid receptors. Understanding the existence of partial agonists has been important for pharmaceutical design, and many promising antagonist compounds have been rejected because they have too much partial agonist activity.

Mixed or Heterologous Agonists-Antagonists

This classification has been introduced to accommodate compounds that act in different ways through the same receptor type in different contexts. Thus, these compounds can act with more agonist activities in some contexts and with more antagonist activities in other contexts, and the extent to which the compound is has agonist, partial agonist-partial antagonist, or antagonist activities may vary in the different contexts. As an example, the estrogen "antagonist" tamoxifen acts mostly as an estrogen antagonist in breast tissue but has mostly estrogen agonist actions in bone and uterus. This property is exploited clinically in the utilization of this drug, since the effects on both bone and breast are useful. In this case, tamoxifen acts as an antagonist when it is bound to an estrogen response element (ERE), whereas it acts as an agonist when it acts through the AP1 transcription factor. The exploitation of these properties is opening new vistas in pharmaceutical development.

Mechanisms of Agonist & Antagonist Actions

The mechanisms of agonist and antagonist hormone action are addressed in Chapter 3. In general, unliganded, inactive receptors are in a conformational state that does not enable them to transmit postbinding information into receptor responses. Agonists bind to receptors and bring about conformational changes that induce them to transmit postbinding information into hormone responses. In general, these changes result in dissociation of proteins from the receptor, binding of other proteins by the receptors, or the capability of the receptors to be modified such as through phosphorylation. By this formulation, a partial agonist would induce only a subpopulation of the receptors to undergo the agonist-like conformational changes. For the mixed agonist-mixed antagonist compounds, the relevant changes would be induced in some contexts but not others. This may occur in a variety of ways. For nuclear receptors, for example, the ligand actually induces several different changes simultaneously, and some ligands may induce only a subset of these changes. Thus, certain changes may be required for agonist activity in a given context, but other changes required for agonist activity in another context would not be induced by the mixed compound. In other cases, the extent of agonist-induced changes may be influenced by other factors in the cell that may vary according to their presence, activities, or levels.

ENDOCRINE & NERVOUS SYSTEM RELATIONSHIPS: NEUROENDOCRINOLOGY

NEUROTRANSMITTERS & HORMONES

Traditionally, the endocrine system has been distinguished from the nervous system by the fact that the nervous system is connected to its target tissues through neurons that carry and transmit chemical signals (Figure 1–1). Thus, the neurotransmitter, which mediates the synaptic transmission between two neurons, is synthesized in the cell body of the neuron and travels down the axon, where it is stored in synaptic vesicles and released upon depolarization. Neuron-to-neuron interaction occurs at the synapse, where the neurotransmitter is released and binds to specific receptors on the postsynaptic neuron. Examples of neurotransmitter receptors are the α_1-, α_2-, β_1-, and β_2-adrenergic, muscarinic cholinergic, and nicotinic cholinergic receptors and the serotonergic, dopaminergic, and γ-aminobutyric acid (GABA) receptors. These vary in their relative levels in different parts of the brain. Thus, the neurotransmitter acts in the vicinity of the target, does not travel through the circulation, and in this sense acts in a paracrine fashion. By this means, the nervous system can release high concentrations of the transmitter to the target and avoid releasing the transmitter at other loci. The concentration of the neurotransmitter at the synapse is also rapidly decreased through degradation or reuptake by the surrounding tissues. A given neuron may have multiple inputs through both multiple synapses and several different neurotransmitters. These inputs can be synergistic or antagonistic. A neuromodulator is a substance that is released in the vicinity of the synapse and augments or blocks the release of the neurotransmitter. A given neuron may also release more than one neurotransmitter. A common pattern in this respect is the concomitant release of a bioamine and a neuropeptide. Thus, parasympathetic nerves contain both acetylcholine and vasoactive intestinal polypeptide (VIP), and sympathetic nerves can contain both norepinephrine and neuropeptide Y.

By contrast, when a hormone circulates, it is in general distributed to all tissues, and reliance is placed on the receptor to generate responses in specific cells and to distinguish the hormone from all the other myriad molecules to which it is exposed (Figure 1–1).

However, similarities between the two systems blur the distinctions. Neuroendocrinology is the discipline that takes as its subject matter the interactions between the nervous and endocrine systems. The same molecule can be a neurotransmitter and a hormone (Figure 1–1). Catecholamines released by the adrenal medulla are hormones (Chapter 11), and when released by the nerve terminals they are neurotransmitters. A number of hormones and hormone receptors are produced in the central nervous system. For example, there is more thyrotropin-releasing hormone (TRH) outside the hypothalamus, which is ordinarily considered to be the major site of its production, than inside. The neurotransmitter actions of TRH include increased motor activity, arousal, tremor, and enhanced peripheral sympathetic activity. Dopamine, corticotropin-releasing hormone (CRH), calcitonin gene-related hormone (CGRH), somatostatin, gonadotropin-releasing hormone (GnRH), VIP, gastrin, secretin, cholecystokinin, and other hormones and their receptors are found in various parts of the brain, and all are both hormones and neurotransmitters. Neurosteroids are produced by the brain to act locally. Interestingly, some hypothalamic hormones—growth hormone-releasing hormone (GRH), for example—are not found in the brain outside the hypothalamus even though GRH is found in many tissues outside the central nervous system and pituitary (pancreas, thyroid gland, lung, gastrointestinal tract, and kidney). Both hormones and neurotransmitters are also present in various tissues generally considered to be neither endocrine nor neural.

Mechanisms of actions of hormones and neurotransmitters are similar. For example, receptors for adrenergic receptors are similar in the central nervous system and the peripheral tissues, and neurotransmitters utilize the same signaling pathways through cAMP, Ca^{2+}, protein kinase C, and phosphoinositide turnover. Neurons may have hormone receptors in regions distinct from the region of the synapse.

HYPOTHALAMIC-PITUITARY RELATIONSHIPS

The primary neuroendocrine interface is at the hypothalamus and pituitary. Chapter 5 describes anatomic relations between the hypothalamus and pituitary and regulation of the relevant hormones. The hypothalamus contains several nuclei of neuronal cells; within these nuclei are groups of specialized cells that release a particular hormone or hormones. The hypothalamus also regulates other brain functions, including temperature, appetite, thirst, sexual behavior, defensive reactions such as rage and fear, and body rhythms; it has extensive communications with other brain regions.

The hypothalamus contains two types of neurosecretory cells that propagate action potentials, release hormones, and are regulated by both hormonal and central nervous system input. Neurohypophysial neurons traverse the hypothalamic-pituitary stalk and release vasopressin (ADH) and oxytocin from nerve endings in the posterior pituitary; hypophysiotropic neurons release hormones into the median eminence and thence into the hypothalamic-pituitary vessels.

Hypothalamic Neurotransmitters

Hypothalamic neurotransmitters, like those elsewhere in the central nervous system, are simple amino acids, bioamines, or peptides, though other entities may also exist. Amino acids include glutamate and glycine; little is known about their influences on the endocrine system. Bioamines include dopamine, norepinephrine, epinephrine, serotonin, acetylcholine, GABA, and histamine. Dopamine regulates prolactin release and has complex influences on somatostatin release (see Chapter 5 and below). Noradrenergic neurons release norepinephrine and couple neuroendocrine with autonomic systems; they do not directly affect pituitary function. Serotonin may be made in the pituitary and may be involved in generating circadian rhythms. GABA is present in more cells of the hypothalamus than any other transmitter—and in the median eminence and posterior pituitary—and is probably an inhibitory neurotransmitter. The roles of epinephrine, acetylcholine, and histamine are less well defined, though epinephrine may stimulate pituitary hormone release. Neuropeptides include VIP, substance P, neurotensin, components of the renin-angiotensin system, cholecystokinin (CCK), opioid peptides, ANP and related peptides, galanin, endothelin, and neuropeptide Y. VIP, also found in the pituitary, stimulates the release of several pituitary hormones, including prolactin, growth hormone, and ACTH, and has vasodilator and excitatory actions in the central nervous system. Substance P stimulates prolactin and inhibits CRH-stimulated ACTH release and is a pain neurotransmitter in peripheral nerves. Neurotensin is a systemic vasodilator, can cause hypothermia when injected centrally, and can affect glucagon, somatostatin, growth hormone, and prolactin release. Roles of components of the renin-angiotensin system in the central nervous system are not well defined. Cholecystokinin may affect satiety and prolactin release. The opioid peptides such as β-endorphin, metenkephalin and leu-enkephalin, and dynorphin are produced in the pituitary and in the periphery, have receptors distributed throughout the central nervous system, mediate analgesic and behavioral responses, and can affect ACTH, growth hormone, and prolactin release, but overall they do not appear to have a major role in neuroendocrine regulation. The roles of other neuropeptides are less well understood.

Hypothalamic-Anterior Pituitary Relations

Vessels of a hypophysial-pituitary portal system deliver blood from the median eminence of the hypothalamus to the anterior pituitary (there may be some flow in the opposite direction) (Figure 5–2). This system delivers hormones released from hypothalamic neuronal axons in the median eminence to the anterior pituitary (adenohypophysis); this gland has little nervous innervation and is dominantly dependent on vascular delivery of hormones for regulation of its functions. Hypophysiotropic hormones regulate hormone release from the anterior pituitary. Stimulating hormones (releasing hormones) include TRH, GnRH, CRH, GRH, prolactin-releasing factor, and ADH. Inhibitory hormones include somatostatin and dopamine. Some releasing hormones can regulate levels of more than one hormone, and more than one releasing hormone can affect a pituitary hormone. Thus, TRH stimulates both TSH and prolactin re-

lease, and ACTH release is stimulated by both CRH and vasopressin. The anterior pituitary also produces several other endocrine proteins such as renin, chorionic gonadotropin, chromogranin A, and neuromedin and in some cases hypothalamic peptides such as VIP and TRH.

Release of anterior pituitary hormones is regulated by three different means (Figure 1–9). First, spontaneous rhythms originating in the brain promote basal hormone release. This release is dominantly pulsatile, as illustrated by the patterns of luteinizing hormone (LH) and follicle-stimulating hormone (FSH) release, though the pattern can vary. The amplitude and frequency of the pulses are governed by several factors, including intrinsic properties of the cells and rhythms established by the central nervous system. These rhythms can be ultradian (shorter than a day), circadian (approximately 24 hour periodicity), or infradian (periodicity > 24 hours). The suprachiasmatic nucleus appears to play a major role in the rhythms

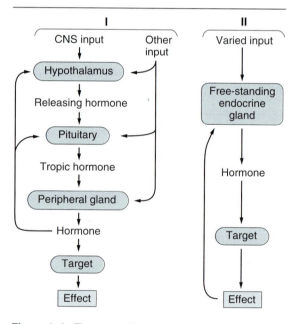

Figure 1–9. The two major types of control of endocrine gland function. *I:* The hypothalamic-pituitary-target gland systems involve the release of a series of hormones beginning with central nervous system regulation of releasing hormones from the hypothalamus that stimulate the pituitary to release tropic hormones which act on peripheral glands to release hormones. These hormones can be regulated by other factors. The hormones from the peripheral glands exert feedback control on the hypothalamus and pituitary. *II:* Free-standing endocrine glands (eg, parathyroid and islet cells) release hormones that stimulate a target tissue to produce an effect (eg, a rise in calcium or fall in blood sugar) which in turn modifies the function of the gland.

and has extensive interconnections with the hypothalamus. The pituitary hormones have mainly circadian rhythms, which are influenced by a number of factors and especially the sleep-wake cycle. Second, hormones from the peripheral glands and perhaps the pituitary regulate pituitary hormone release through feedback loops. Thus, cortisol, thyroid hormone, and estrogens inhibit the release of their tropic hormones: ACTH, TSH, and LH, respectively. Third, intervening influences such as stress, nutritional influences, illnesses, and other hormones can influence hormone release. Thus, stress increases the release of ACTH, growth hormone, and prolactin, and systemic illness can suppress the hypothalamic-pituitary-thyroid axis and the release of gonadotropins. Immunomodulatory substances such as interleukin-1 and interleukin-2 and epinephrine can increase CRH and ACTH release; and angiotensin II, interleukin-2, cholecystokinin, and oxytocin can stimulate ACTH release. The thymic hormone thymosin b4, whose secretion may be decreased with estrogens, can increase GnRH release.

PRL and GH are both regulated by releasing hormones (prolactin-releasing factor and GRH, respectively) and by inhibitory hormones (dopamine and somatostatin, respectively). The inhibitory hormone is more dominant with PRL, whereas the stimulatory hormone is more dominant for GH; hypothalamic lesions that disrupt delivery of hormones to the anterior pituitary result in elevated prolactin and depressed growth hormone levels (Chapter 5). GH and PRL do not act like other endocrine glands that feedback-regulate their release, but IGF-1, produced in response to GH, feeds back to inhibit GH release. Feedback influences can be directed at the pituitary, hypothalamus, or, typically, at both.

Tropic anterior pituitary hormones (ACTH, FSH, LH, TSH) stimulate in their cognate target glands (adrenals, gonads, and thyroid gland) both release of target hormones and other functions. In these cases, hormones from the target glands regulate the releasing hormones mostly through negative feedback but sometimes through positive feedback, as with estradiol-release of both the hypothalamic and the pituitary hormone. The gonads also produce other hormones—inhibin, follistatin, and activin—that also regulate tropic hormone release. These regulatory networks tend to control hormone levels within a narrow range (see the chapters on the various glands or systems). The level of hormone maintained by the regulatory influence is referred to as the set point.

Hypothalamic-Posterior Pituitary Relations

The posterior pituitary (Chapter 5), or neurohypophysis, is an extension of the hypothalamus and is composed mostly of neural tissue. Nerve terminals from axons that originate in the hypothalamus are located in the gland. These release hormones, vasopressin and oxytocin, into the circulation.

The Pineal Gland

The pineal gland provides an interface free of the blood-brain barrier between the brain, the cerebral circulation, and the cerebrospinal fluid. The gland indirectly receives photosensory information that influences its production of melatonin, derived from serotonin. In animals, melatonin can have antireproductive functions, block GnRH-induced LH release, and have other effects on hormone release. It has received considerable recent attention for its role in regulating circadian rhythms, but its role in humans is not well defined.

GENE EXPRESSION & RECOMBINANT DNA IN ENDOCRINOLOGY & METABOLISM: MOLECULAR BASIS FOR FUNCTION OF THE SYSTEM AND GENETIC ENDOCRINE DISEASE

Advances resulting from the cloning, expression and study of genes that encode proteins involved in the endocrine system has had an enormous impact on endocrinology. These genes encode proteins that are hormones, hormone receptors, and mediators of hormone action as well as those involved in hormone synthesis, release, and metabolism and many other functions. Some contributions of recombinant DNA technology are listed in Table 1–1. Recombinant DNA technology has provided therapeutic products such as GH and insulin and diagnostic materials such as polypeptide hormones. Most importantly, it has provided information about the function of the endocrine system in health and disease. Elucidation of mechanisms that regulate gene expression in general has provided insights into mechanisms of hormone action (see Chapter 3) and regulation of the entire system as detailed for individual systems in subsequent chapters of this book. Conversely, insights gained from studies of the mechanisms of hormone synthesis and release and of hormone action have contributed substantially to overall understanding of gene expression.

Many endocrine diseases have a strong genetic component. This apples not only to rare syndromes, such as the defects in steroid biosynthesis (Chapters 9, 10, 12, 13, and 14) and mutations in hormone genes, such as in the GH gene (Chapter 6); it also applies to more common problems such as hypertension (Chapter 10) and non-insulin-dependent diabetes mellitus (NIDDM; Chapter 18). Thus, understanding

Table 1–1. Impact of molecular biology and recombinant DNA technology on endocrinology.

Information about all aspects of endocrinology, including:
Production and regulation of hormones
Mechanisms of hormone action
Actions of hormones
Mechanisms of disease

Diagnosis of endocrine diseases:
Information gained from studies using the technology
Reagents from recombinant products (eg, polypeptide hormones)
DNA analysis, including restriction fragment length polymorphism (RFLP) and polymerase chain reaction (PCR) techniques

Treatment of endocrine disease:
Information gained from studies using the technology
Production of hormones and hormone analogs used for therapy (growth hormone, insulin, growth factors, etc)
Materials for determination of three-dimensional structures of drug targets (eg, renin, growth hormone receptor, nuclear receptors, polypeptides, signaling molecules such as *ras*)
Technology for gene therapy

gained from general studies of the mechanisms of genetic diseases extends to understand of endocrinologic concepts as well. Many of the mechanisms of genetic disease are discussed in the chapters that follow. The defects can be severe, resulting in complete hormone deficiency, such as of GH (Chapter 5) or steroid hormones (Chapters 9, 10, 12, 13, and 14), and life-threatening maladies such as severe hypertension (Chapter 10) or endocrine neoplasia (Chapter 24). There can also be more subtle abnormalities, including many as yet undefined, which increase susceptibility to developing disease with age, as is the case with NIDDM (Chapter 18).

The specific genetic defects that occur are similar to those that generate other genetic diseases. Thus, there can be nucleotide substitutions in the DNA that alter the amino acid encoded by a gene or create a translational stop codon. These can be seen with mutated polypeptide hormones such as insulin or growth hormone, with transcription factors such as the Pit-1 factor that regulates the GH gene, or with hormone receptors as in the testicular feminization syndrome (Chapter 14). Such simple mutations can also affect the ability of a gene to be regulated. There can be deletions of all or of parts of genes that result in a complete loss of the gene's function, as with deletions of polypeptide genes such as growth hormone (Chapter 5), hormone receptors, or enzymes involved in hormone synthesis. The latter, for example, can be observed in congenital adrenal hyperplasia (Chapters 9, 12, 13, and 14). There can be insertions of other genes or rearrangements between genes, and generation of new genes with different functions. The latter are seen with profound alterations in the function of

cells when growth factor or related genes are rearranged under control of a new gene with generation of malignancy (Chapters 22 and 24), or with a form of hypertension where the enzyme that promotes production of aldosterone is inserted into the regulatory region of another gene that is controlled by ACTH (Chapter 10).

In addition to the more obvious genetic diseases, there is growing recognition of more subtle variations between individuals that contribute heavily to endocrine disease. For example, the defect that causes NIDDM occurs commonly in the population, and the progression to overt diabetes may be heavily influenced by other genetic components.

EVOLUTION OF THE ENDOCRINE SYSTEM

Consideration of the evolution of the endocrine system may provide a broader framework for understanding why hormones, systems for regulation of hormone levels, and signaling systems have emerged; how these may become deranged in disease; and what may be the prospects for discovery of new hormones and mechanisms. A schematic representation of some of the events in evolution of the endocrine system is provided in Figure 1–10.

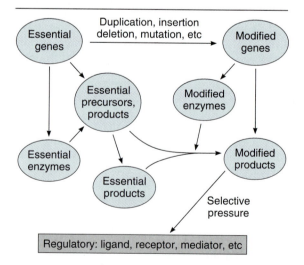

Figure 1–10. Steps in the evolution of the endocrine system, with duplications and mutations of genes that encode essential enzymes and other products that result in new genes which encode products involved in endocrine control.

CELLULAR CONTROL NETWORKS & THE ORIGINS OF REGULATORY CHEMICALS

The endocrine system probably had its origins with intracellular communication in lower forms. For example, cAMP and protein phosphorylation reactions that mediate hormone actions in humans exert regulatory roles in bacteria. These mechanisms have been preserved in evolution and also extended in higher species to establish response systems for hormones. Simple control systems in bacteria are used for regulation of metabolism within the bacterium, which are analogous to hormone response networks; and for responses to the external environment, such as chemotactic stimuli, which are analogous to endocrine control.

Regulatory chemicals produced by bacteria are typically modified analogs of essential molecules, as noted by Tomkins over 20 years ago in his article entitled "The Metabolic Code." For example, cAMP is derived from ATP. Tomkins noted that it would be difficult for ATP to be a regulatory molecule, since marked variations in ATP levels that might be required for regulation might impair cellular function. He speculated that substances such as cAMP were originally generated as by-products of ATP and that once that a mechanism for regulation of cAMP generation evolved, the molecule could then perform some regulatory function. cAMP generation might have increased, for example, during "idling" of ATP hydrolysis to ADP, but it might also have occurred when a mutation or change in regulation of a preexisting protein occurred, such that a new enzyme that specifically produced cAMP was formed. This type of process could be considered as a primitive and simple form of "complex" regulation, as distinct from "simple" regulation, eg, inhibition of an enzyme by its product. In the example described, cAMP formation might then be signaled by idling of ATP hydrolysis. Therefore, a regulatory system might be established if the cell learned to regulate processes that overcame the reason for the idling. In this example of complex regulation, cAMP production could be regulated independently of ATP production or hydrolysis, thereby giving the organism much greater flexibility for control. Indeed, Tomkins called cAMP a "symbol" that is produced in response to the "signal," glucose deprivation, by bacteria. In bacteria, the symbol, cAMP, in turn induces enzymes that metabolize alternative substrates such as lactose to overcome the deficiency of glucose.

The response limb for cAMP in bacteria is a transcription factor whose activity is affected by cAMP binding. This could have arisen, for example, by combining a derivative of a primitive nucleotide binding site with that for a DNA binding protein or in other analogous ways.

THE ORIGINS OF HORMONES

Hormones are also derived from more essential compounds and macromolecules. Thus, peptides are derived from proteins, steroids from cholesterol, and catecholamines and thyroid hormones from amino acids (Chapter 2). In fact, all major classes of molecules that exist in mammalian cells are precursors of molecules that are either hormones or are involved in transmission of hormone action. Control of production of these compounds may originally have been by processes analogous to that described above for cAMP. For example, steroid production might originally have been controlled by processes that affected cholesterol synthesis or utilization, eg, by signals that affect cell growth. Thyroid or catecholamine production might be regulated by processes that affected amino acid or protein metabolism. Once the original hormones, the precursors to today's hormones, were generated, modifications of them gave the additional needed properties in terms of ability to be secreted, specificity for receptor binding, bioavailability (including binding to transport proteins), and ability to be degraded or cleared.

INTRACELLULAR COMMUNICATION

Once hormones interact with receptors in or on the target cells, intracellular communication events are initiated. These can involve modification reactions such as phosphorylation, or they may affect gene expression or ion transport. In bacteria, these could have been simple mechanisms; however, in higher organisms, more sophisticated means have been developed not only to release hormones, sometimes in a specific direction, but to regulate their release. The common thread is that the same intracellular control networks could be used in the target cells.

EVOLUTION OF GENES INVOLVED IN THE ENDOCRINE SYSTEM

Genes evolved to encode all aspects of the endocrine system: enzymes involved in hormone synthesis, processing, release, transport, and metabolism; hormone receptors; proteins involved in signaling hormone-receptor actions; and other proteins. Genes evolve through duplications of ancestral genes, rearrangements of genes, movements of parts of genes to the same or other genes, and specific mutations. For example, it appears that polypeptide hormone genes are composed of parts of several different primitive precursor genes and that duplications of these genes or portions of them, insertions from other genes, and subsequent mutations were used to generate the gene that encodes the final product. In addition, families of genes evolved by duplications and additional modifications. Examples of families of genes include the GH, PRL, and placental lactogen (chorionic somatomammotropin) family and the glycoprotein hormones that share the same α subunit and have homologous β subunits. Genes involved in the synthesis of other classes of hormones and encoding hormone receptors probably evolved in a similar way. For example, there are similarities in some genes involved in steroid hormone biosynthesis. As alluded to in the earlier section on types of hormones, over 100 different genes encode the nuclear receptor superfamily that include those for receptors for the steroid hormones, thyroid hormones, retinoids, and vitamin D; these genes appear to have evolved from a common evolutionary precursor gene through duplications, mutations, and insertions from other genes. Genes encode receptors for GH and PRL and belong to a large family that includes the receptors for many cytokines and hematopoietic factors.

The organization of genes with introns and exons has probably facilitated movement of DNA segments during evolution. The inserted segment could contain nucleotides that are either coding sequences, ie, for the amino acids in a protein, or alternatively could contain regulatory sequences that influence gene expression. Introns facilitate such rearrangements by allowing genetic events to be somewhat imprecise. For example, insertion of a segment with an exon flanked by two introns into an intron of an existing gene would result in an altered mRNA product that would be translated into a protein containing the new amino acids encoded by the added exon. For this event, breaks in the DNA need to occur somewhere in the middle of the intron in segments that do not contain critical control structures such as those that affect RNA processing. Without introns, such insertions would be much more difficult to achieve without compromising the original gene. By modifying existing genes and either deleting or adding other segments that have special functions, such evolutionary events have resulted in tremendous diversity and specialization of all of the functions of the human endocrine system.

INTEGRATIVE NETWORKS

Integrative networks have also evolved. For example, coordinated responses regulate cardiovascular functions, metabolism, and other processes. These processes involve integrated actions of a given hormone within the same cell and in different tissues and complementary or counterbalancing multihormonal influences, sometimes overlapping and not always in the same direction. Integrative networks probably developed in several ways. For example, once a hormone learned to regulate a given response,

eg, glucose metabolism, it might have been easy for it to evolve to regulate other processes for which the influence on glucose was either advantageous or not detrimental. For example, glucocorticoids "learned" to regulate glucose metabolism. These hormones may have been an "anxiety" stimulus for preparation for starvation, and one response would be to increase glucose production and glycogen storage. It might then have been easy for the hormones to incorporate other actions, such as those on lipid and amino acid metabolism, that were complementary in this setting. Such networks, once established, would probably be relatively stable evolutionarily. However, they could be modified and expanded, and gene duplications could allow complementary and even antagonistic hormones and response networks to diverge from these networks that would better serve the host. Hormones with counterbalancing actions could then develop in an analogous fashion. Thus, the hormones gradually established the complex patterns that are seen today.

EVOLUTION OF THE ENDOCRINE GLANDS

In primitive systems, cell-cell communication occurred through the release of substances into the media to act on adjacent cells, ie, paracrine control. Many also developed primitive nervous systems that ultimately evolved into today's more complicated ones. Although the nervous system remains an excellent means for intercellular communication, this system alone was not optimal for all of the types of regulation that were possible. At least two additional control mechanisms evolved. First, signals released by cells that were acting in paracrine or autocrine fashions were allowed to travel through the circulation to act as hormones. Second, nerve cells became endocrine cells by secreting hormones themselves, as now occurs with the nervous system (as discussed in the earlier sections on endocrine, nervous, and hypothalamic-pituitary relations), or by allowing neurotransmitters to move farther than the synapse and act as hormones or in a paracrine fashion. Examples of the latter are the posterior pituitary and the adrenal medulla, where nerve terminals release vasopressin and oxytocin and epinephrine, respectively. Whereas in most cases endocrine glands release hormones for systemic availability, in limited circumstances anatomic structures have formed that allow more local delivery. This is observed in the portal system of the hypothalamus and pituitary and with insulin and glucagon delivery first to the liver. An additional specialization in this regard was the development of a large component of the endocrine system, the pituitary, in proximity to the central nervous system, where it could be centrally controlled.

HORMONE SYNTHESIS & RELEASE

Details of the synthesis of individual classes of hormones are provided in Chapter 2 and in the chapters on those hormones. Since hormones are analogs of molecules used generally for cellular function—proteins and smaller peptides, cholesterol derivatives, amino acid analogs, and other fat derivatives (Figure 1–2)—overall hormone synthesis involves either utilization of the same machinery that is used to produce the general class of compounds or it uses enzymes that modify the compounds.

Thus, protein hormones such as growth hormone, prolactin, and PTH are produced in a manner analogous to the production of any protein that is secreted. The glycoprotein hormones, TSH, LH, FSH, and CG, contain two protein chains bound tightly together. One chain is common among the four hormones, whereas the second chain is unique. Insulin is derived from proinsulin following cleavage of a prosegment that leaves two peptide chains connected by disulfide bonds. Smaller peptides such as ACTH, CRH, and glucagon are produced by cleavage of a larger protein by specific proteases. Other molecules with unique structures, such as the cyclic tripeptide TRH, involve specialized enzymes.

Various processes are used for producing amino acid analogs such as thyroid hormones or catecholamines. Thyroid hormones contain two phenolic rings connected by an oxygen and an alanine side chain. Iodine moieties are connected to the phenolic rings. These hormones are produced in the thyroid gland through iodination of tyrosine residues contained in a large protein, thyroglobulin, followed by condensation of two iodotyrosine residues. Catecholamine production involves modifications of phenylalanine.

Steroid hormones are produced in a series of reactions that start with cholesterol. These reactions involve cleavage of residues of the side chain of cholesterol to yield pregnenolone, followed by a variety of modifications that include hydroxylations, other cleavage reactions, and modification of the ring structures.

In many cases, the form of the hormone released by the endocrine gland is not the hormone form that is active in the target tissue. Thus, for thyroid hormones, there is deiodination of the major form of thyroid hormone released from the gland, $3,5,3',5'$-tetraiodo-L-thyronine (thyroxine; T_4) to the more active $3,5,3'$-triiodo-L-thyronine (triiodothyronine; T_3) both in peripheral tissues and in the thyroid gland. Testosterone is reduced to dihydrotestosterone in target tissues. The major active form of vitamin D re-sults from hydroxylation reactions that occur dominantly in the liver and kidney. These types of conversions are also illustrated in Figure 1–11.

HORMONE TRANSPORT

Hormones circulate both free and bound to plasma proteins (Figure 1–12). There are major differences between the various hormones in the extent of their association with the plasma proteins. In general, the binding of hormones to plasma is through noncovalent interactions, though cholesterol is considered to be bound through ester bonds to phosphatidylcholine. However, even in this case, the esterified cholesterol is bound through noncovalent interactions with the lipoprotein particles (Chapter 20).

STEROID HORMONES & VITAMIN D

All steroid hormones are bound to plasma proteins to some extent through either high-affinity binding to specific globulins or relatively low-affinity and non-specific binding to proteins such as albumin. The major binding proteins are corticosteroid-binding globulin (CBG; transcortin), which binds both cortisol and progesterone (Chapter 9), and sex hormone-binding globulin (SHBG), which binds testosterone and estradiol (testosterone more tightly than estradiol; Chapters 12 and 13). These proteins are present in sufficient concentrations that over 90% of the total cortisol and about 98% of the testosterone and estradiol are bound. Levels of their binding capacities in some cases exceed only slightly the normal concentrations of the steroid, so that with higher levels a much higher proportion of the hormone can be free. With cortisol, for example, the CBG capacity for cortisol is about 25 mg/dL (690 ng/dL). Aldosterone does not bind to a specific protein, with the result that only about 50% of the plasma aldosterone is bound. Vitamin D circulates mostly bound to vitamin D-binding protein (Chapter 8). This protein binds 25-$(OH)D_3$ more tightly than $1,25$-$(OH)_2D_3$ or previtamin D_3.

THYROID HORMONES

Thyroid hormones circulate bound to plasma proteins such that 0.04% of the T_4 and 0.4% of the T_3 are free (Chapter 7). About 68% of the T_4 and 80% of the T_3 are bound by the glycoprotein thyroid hormone-binding globulin (TBG). About 11% of the T_4

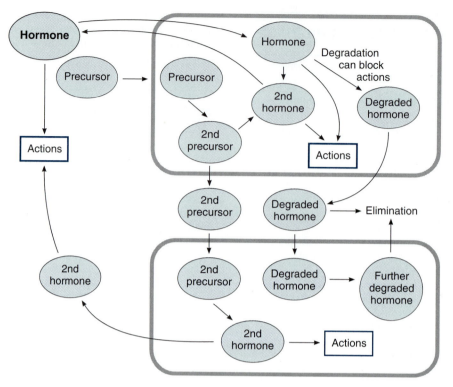

Figure 1–11. Hormone metabolism. Shown are various pathways along which hormones are metabolized and the effects of those pathways with production of additional precursors; production of more active hormones for local or systemic actions; selective degradation of hormones to prevent local actions; and degradation to inactive forms that are eliminated.

and 9% of the T_3 are bound to transthyretin (thyroid hormone-binding prealbumin; TBPA). The remainder is bound to albumin.

POLYPEPTIDE HORMONES

Many polypeptide hormones circulate at low concentrations unbound to other proteins, though there are exceptions. Exceptions include several different IGF-1-binding proteins that bind IGF-1 (Chapter 6). Vasopressin and oxytocin are bound to neurophysins (Chapter 5). Growth hormone binds to a protein that is identical to the hormone-binding portion of the growth hormone receptor (Chapter 6).

REGULATION OF PLASMA-BINDING PROTEINS

The levels of plasma-binding proteins can vary with both disease states and drug therapy (Chapters 5, 7, 12, and 13). For example, CBG, SHBG, and TBG levels are increased by estrogens. SHBG levels

are increased by thyroid hormones, and SHBG and TBG levels are decreased by androgens.

Role of Plasma Binding

An understanding the roles of plasma binding of hormones is just emerging. In general, hormones are sufficiently soluble to circulate unassociated at levels at which they are highly active, such that the transport protein is not required for transport per se. Cholesterol may be an exception if it is considered to be a hormone. With steroid and thyroid hormones, deficiency states characterized by genetic defects with very low levels of transport proteins are not associated with clinical abnormalities. For example, deletion of the mouse transthyretin gene, which encodes the protein responsible for most of the thyroid hormone binding in the plasma of this species did not result in detectable phenotypic abnormalities. Thus, there is no evidence that these proteins are essential.

In most cases, (1) it is the free hormone that is available for binding to receptors and therefore represents the active hormone; (2) the levels of free hormone dictate the magnitude of feedback inhibition and related regulatory influences that control hor-

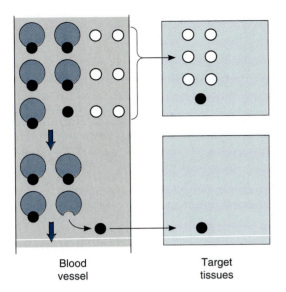

Figure 1–12. Role of plasma binding in delivery of hormones to peripheral tissues. Shown are examples with a hormone that is bound (solid circles) to a plasma protein (large circles) and a hormone that is not plasma-bound (open circles). With the hormone that binds to plasma proteins, only the free hormone (a fraction of the total) is available for tissue uptake, whereas with the hormone that is not bound all of the hormone present is available for uptake. With the plasma-bound hormone, as the blood moves to more distal portions of the tissue, additional hormone dissociates from the plasma-binding protein and is available for tissue uptake.

Blood
vessel

Target
tissues

mone release (see below); (3) the free levels of hormones determine the rates of their clearance; and (4) clinical states of hormone excess and deficiency correlate best with free levels of hormones. The latter is a critical consideration in many cases, eg, with states of adrenal (Chapter 9) or thyroid hormone (Chapter 7) excess and deficiency and with hypercalcemic and hypocalcemic states (Chapter 8). With these hormones and Ca^{2+}, factors that affect the levels of plasma-binding proteins can elevate or depress the total hormone or Ca^{2+} levels without affecting the free hormone levels, or the changes could mask pathologic hormone excess or deficiency states. These considerations are discussed later.

One of the most important roles for transport proteins may be to facilitate an even delivery of hormones to the target tissues (Figure 1–12). In a tissue such as liver, for example, a hormone that is totally free might be completely sequestered as the blood flows through the proximal portions of the tissue, whereas if it were mostly bound, then only the free, unbound hormone would be sequestered in proximal portions of the tissue, and as this occurred and the blood moves more distally, release of additional hor-

mone from the bound fraction would make hormone available for these regions.

Plasma binding also in general increases the half-life of the hormone in the circulation.

METABOLISM & ELIMINATION OF HORMONES

Metabolism of hormones and their precursors is utilized to generate more active forms from precursor or less active hormones and to degrade hormones to inactive forms (Figure 1–11). Most of the elimination of hormones is through degradation, though elimination of some of the intact hormone also occurs in a few cases.

PEPTIDE HORMONES

In general, peptide hormones have short half-lives (a few minutes) in the circulation, as occurs with ACTH, insulin, glucagon, PTH, and the releasing hormones. As has been said, the glycosylated glycoprotein hormones are more stable, and CG has a half-life of several hours. Although there may be some degradation of the hormone by proteases in the circulation, the major mechanism for hormone degradation is binding by cell surface receptors for the hormone or through nonreceptor cell surface hormone-binding sites, with subsequent uptake into the cell (internalization; see below) and degradation by enzymes in the cell membrane or inside the cell. A number of specific enzymes mediate these processes, which differ for the various hormones. In addition, several steps may be involved. The first of these may inactivate the hormone, and this can be due—eg, in the case of insulin—to reduction of disulfide bonds in the protein. An important source for these enzymes is the lysosome, which may fuse with endocytosed vesicles to expose its enzyme's contents and its acid environment to the internalized hormone-receptor complex. An advantage of the short circulating half-lives of some classes of hormones is that the duration of the response can be relatively brief. In addition, the persistent presence of significant levels of many classes of hormones that act on the cell surface results in down-regulation of the responsiveness to the hormone that may not be desirable.

STEROID HORMONES & VITAMIN D

The hydrophobic steroid hormones and the D vitamins are filtered by the kidney and generally reabsorbed. For example, about 1% of the cortisol produced daily ends up in the urine (Chapter 9). These compounds are ordinarily handled by metabolizing them to inactive species and to more water-soluble forms that are more effectively eliminated. The free steroid fraction is accessible to metabolic inactivation. The inactivations are accomplished by converting hydroxyl groups to keto groups, reducing double bonds, and conjugating the steroids with glucuronide and sulfate groups. Over 50 different steroid metabolites have been described. Production of active hormones by metabolism in peripheral tissues, as is seen with androgens, estrogens, and vitamin D, is discussed above in the section on hormone synthesis.

Metabolism in peripheral tissues can dictate the type of steroid that binds to the receptor (Figure 1–11). Aldosterone is ordinarily the major mineralocorticoid hormone responsible for the salt-retaining actions of the steroid hormones. This steroid binds to the mineralocorticoid receptor only about ten times more tightly than cortisol, whose total and free concentrations in the circulation are about 1000 times and 100 times (respectively) those of aldosterone, such that cortisol should ordinarily be the main occupant of the mineralocorticoid receptors. This occurs in tissues such as the brain and pituitary, but in the kidney, cortisol is avidly converted to the essentially inactive cortisone and perhaps other steroids (Chapter 9); some types of licorice or congenital defects can block the conversion and result in mineralocorticoid excess states that are due to cortisol (Chapter 10). Dihydrotestosterone production from testosterone in androgen-responsive tissues governs access of this steroid to its cognate receptor (Chapter 12).

THYROID HORMONES

Metabolism of thyroid hormones is discussed in Chapter 7. The circulating half-lives of T_4 (7 days) and T_3 (about 1 day) are longer than for most hormones. These differences are due to the higher affinity of T_4 than T_3 for TBG. The hormones are degraded to inactive forms by microsomal deiodinases. The type I deiodinase is prevalent in most peripheral tissues, including liver and kidney, and is responsible for most of the production of T_3. A type II deiodinase present in the pituitary and central nervous system is involved in generating T_3 for feedback inhibition of TSH release. The deiodinases also convert reverse T_3 (3,3′,5′-triiodo-L-thyronine) to 3,3′-T_2 (3,3′-diiodo-L-thyronine). 5-Deiodinases act on T_4 to generate reverse T_3 and on T_3 to generate 3,3′-T_2. Deaminations and decarboxylations of the alanine side chains as well as conjugations with glucuronic acid and sulfate groups are also involved in degrading thyroid hormones.

CATECHOLAMINES

Metabolism of catecholamines is discussed in Chapter 11. These compounds are cleared rapidly, with half-lives of 1–2 minutes. Clearance is primarily by cellular uptake and metabolism, and only about 2–3% of the norepinephrine that enters the circulation is excreted in the urine. Furthermore, a significant amount of the catecholamine metabolites in the circulation reflects catecholamines whose degradation occurred within adrenergic neuron terminals, a point of importance for interpreting clinical data. Catecholamines are degraded by two principal routes: catechol-*O*-methyltransferase (COMT) and monoamine oxidase (MAO). Measurement of some of the metabolites—normetanephrine, metanephrine, and vanillylmandelic acid (VMA)—can be useful in evaluating possible catecholamine overproduction.

EICOSANOID METABOLISM

Prostaglandins are rapidly metabolized—within seconds—by enzymes that are widely distributed. Prominent in the metabolism is oxidation of the 15-hydroxyl group of the prostaglandin that renders the molecule inactive. Subsequently, other reactions involve both oxidations and reductions.

REGULATION OF THE ENDOCRINE SYSTEM

The effective concentration of a hormone is determined by rates of its production, delivery to the target tissue, and degradation. All of these processes are finely regulated to achieve the physiologic level of the hormone, although the importance of the steps differs with various hormones. By far the most highly regulated process is hormone production, which is controlled at the level of synthesis in all cases and release in many cases. With many classes of hormones, the short half-lives of the hormones provide means of terminating the responses and thus preventing excessive responses. The latter are also blunted by negative regulation of both hormone responsiveness (discussed below) and release, as well as by other factors. In many cases the other factors are also hormones. For example, in stress, glucocorticoids produced in excess probably blunt actions of a number of hormones that would otherwise be harmful (Chapter 9). Thus, when actions and half-lives of hormones are short, the hormone response can be terminated by simply stopping release of the hormone. An exception is thyroid hormone, which has a long half-life (Chapter 7). Details of controls of the individual systems are provided in subsequent chapters on the various glands and systems.

There are a number of different patterns of regulation of hormone release. Many hormones are linked to the hypothalamic-pituitary axis (discussed in detail in the section on neuroendocrinology; Figure 1–9). These involve both classic feedback loops by hormones that are released by peripheral glands (cortisol, thyroid hormone, etc) and more subtle controls, as is seen with GH and PRL.

However, many other systems are more freestanding. This is illustrated by the parathyroid glands (Chapter 5) (Figure 1–9) and by the pancreatic islets (Chapter 18). With the parathyroid glands, the Ca^{2+} concentration that is increased in plasma by the hormone exerts a dominant feedback inhibition on the release of PTH. With insulin, depression of the glucose levels in response to insulin action results in cessation of the stimulus to release more insulin. In addition, in both cases, release of the hormone and the overall state of the gland is influenced by numerous other factors.

Stimuli to regulate hormone production include essentially all of the types of regulatory molecules, including hormones such as the tropic hormones and counterregulatory hormones (discussed above), traditional growth factors, eicosanoids, and ions. For example, potassium ion is an important regulator of the adrenal zona glomerulosa. Production of various eicosanoids is regulated by local factors acting on cells in which these products are released. For example, tropic stimulation of most endocrine glands results in enhancement of eicosanoid production.

Production of hormones is regulated at multiple levels. First, synthesis of the hormone can be regulated at the level of transcription, as is commonly seen with the polypeptide hormones or enzymes involved in synthesis of other hormones such as the steroids. It can also be affected by posttranscriptional mechanisms. Second, release of the hormone stored in secretory granules from tissues that contain the regulated secretory pathway is regulated by secretagogues, as was discussed in the section on hormone synthesis. Secretory cells can store peptide hormones in sufficient quantity so that the amount released over a short period can exceed the rate of synthesis of the hormone. Third, stimulation of endocrine glands by tropic hormones and other factors such as growth factors can increase the number and size of cells that are actively producing the hormone.

ACTIONS OF HORMONES

Hormones affect all tissues and organ systems of the body and are important from very early in embryonic development throughout life. Details of the actions of various hormones are described in subsequent chapters of this book, but some general patterns are summarized in this section.

DEVELOPMENTAL EFFECTS

Hormones influence development of the fetus and the child. These actions are extensive, with effects on essentially all organs and systems of the body. Cretinism resulting from severe hypothyroidism (Chapter 7), dwarfism resulting from growth hormone deficiency (Chapter 6), and inability to develop and survive with an enzyme defect that results in inability to make steroid hormones (Chapter 9) illustrate the profound effects of different classes of hormones on development. Hormones exert major influences on sexual development, as is illustrated by the failure of male sexual development in the androgen-deficient state (Chapter 14).

CELL GROWTH & CANCER

Hormones are important for the growth of a number of cell types. Prominent examples are actions of tropic factors that regulate growth of various endocrine glands, eg, actions of ACTH and angiotensin II on the adrenal gland (Chapter 9), TSH on the thyroid gland (Chapter 7), and LH and FSH on the ovary (Chapter 13) and testis (Chapter 12). Peptide hormones such as growth hormone, IGF-1, and IGF-2 directly stimulate both linear growth and cellular proliferation in other tissues (Chapter 6). Other peptides such as fibroblast growth factor (FGF), platelet-derived growth factor (PGDF), and transforming growth factors α and β (TGFα and TGFβ) are growth factors both in multiple tissues and in endocrine glands. Thyroid hormones can stimulate the growth of several tissues (Chapter 7). Steroid hormones can both inhibit and stimulate cell growth. For example, glucocorticoids inhibit the growth of several cell types and even kill some lymphocyte cell types, whereas estradiol and testosterone and dihydrotestosterone can stimulate growth of breast and prostatic tissues, respectively (Chapter 22). Compounds that inhibit estrogen and androgen action are used to treat breast and prostate cancers (Chapter 22; Table 1–2). Hormones have extensive interrelation-

Table 1–2. Examples of hormone antagonists used in therapy.

Antagonist to	Use
Progesterone	Contraceptive, abortion
Glucocorticoid	Spontaneous Cushing's syndrome
Mineralocorticoid	Primary and secondary mineralocorticoid excess
Androgen	Prostate cancer
Estrogen	Breast cancer
GnRH	Prostate cancer
β-Adrenergic	Hypertension, hyperthyroidism
Prostaglandin	Acute and chronic inflammatory disease

ships with cancer, as described in Chapter 22. Prostatic, breast, endometrial, and other cancers can be dependent on steroid hormones. Thyroid cancers can be dependent on and influenced by TSH. Many oncogenes are analogs of growth factors or growth factor receptors, as described above in the earlier section on hormones and oncogenes and in Chapter 22.

CENTRAL NERVOUS SYSTEM EFFECTS

Many interrelationships between the endocrine and nervous systems are described in the earlier section on endocrine and central nervous system relationships and in Chapter 5 on the hypothalamus and pituitary. Hormones act as neurotransmitters, and neurotransmitters are extensively involved in regulating endocrine functions. Hormones also regulate a number of other functions in the central nervous system such as mood, appetite, memory, and cognitive function. Hormones can also have secondary influences on the central nervous system through their effects on general metabolism. Examples of profound mental abnormalities with hormone excess or deficient states that serve to underscore how hormones influence the nervous system include slowed mentation that can progress to frank coma with severe hypothyroidism (Chapter 7); psychosis that can occur with glucocorticoid excess; and coma that can occur with hypoglycemia due to insulin excess (Chapter 19).

EFFECTS ON METABOLISM

Hormones regulate metabolism of all major classes of chemicals. Carbohydrate, fat, protein, amino acid, and nucleic acid metabolism are tightly regulated by insulin, glucagon, somatostatin, growth hormone, catecholamines (epinephrine, norepinephrine), thyroid hormones, glucocorticoids, and other hormones (Chapters 6, 7, 9, 18, and 21). These interactions are coordinated in a complex way to provide for finely tuned regulation and responsiveness to circumstances such as stress or starvation. Insulin is dominant in lowering blood glucose and in stimulating metabolism of glucose and synthesis of fat, proteins, and nucleic acids. By contrast, cortisol, glucagon, catecholamines, and growth hormone tend to elevate the blood sugar by diverse mechanisms. However, these hormones differ in the patterns of their effects on protein, fat, and nucleic acid metabolism. A number of different enzymes and specific processes are affected by hormones. These include regulation of the uptake of glucose, amino acids, nucleosides, and other small molecules. For example, insulin increases glucose uptake by promoting redistribution of glucose transporters to the plasma membrane. Enzymes regulated include, among others, those involved in gluconeogenesis, lipolysis, glycogen synthesis, amino acid metabolism and synthesis, and lipid synthesis.

EFFECTS ON CARDIOVASCULAR & RENAL FUNCTION

Hormones are extensively involved in regulation of cardiovascular and renal function. The renin-angiotensin system, atrial natriuretic peptide, endothelins, catecholamines, steroid hormones, thyroid hormone, prostaglandins, kinins, modulators of immunologic and inflammatory reactions, substance P, calcitonin gene-related hormone, and other substances all can profoundly affect this system. These can affect heart rate and contractility. Effects of hormones on blood pressure are complex, with varied influences on arteries and veins having both constrictor and dilator functions (see also Chapter 10). The growth factor properties of hormones can influence cardiovascular development, muscular hypertrophy, and muscular hyperplasia and are involved in pathologic processes leading to hypertensive vascular changes, atherosclerosis, heart failure, and cardiac hypertrophy (see also Chapters 10 and 20). Hormones influence renal function by regulating renal blood flow, glomerular filtration rate, and the transport of ions, water, and other chemicals. Hormones regulate both active and passive transport processes through activation of channels, stimulating the synthesis of new channels, providing greater energy for active transport, or promoting redistribution of channels. Drugs that block many of these systems, such as converting enzyme inhibitors, β-adrenergic blockers, and mineralocorticoid hormone antagonists, are used extensively in therapy (Table 1–2).

EFFECTS ON MINERAL & WATER METABOLISM

Hormones are intimately involved in both mineral and water metabolism. Regulation of calcium and phosphate ion concentrations is discussed in the following section. A major regulator of serum osmolality and water excretion is vasopressin (Chapter 5). The mineralocorticoid aldosterone has emerged as a dominant regulator of serum sodium and potassium and to some extent chloride and bicarbonate ion concentrations and balance Chapters 5 and 10). Ionic balance is also regulated by other hormones, including ANP, insulin, glucagon, catecholamines, angiotensin II, and PTH.

EFFECTS ON SKELETAL FUNCTIONS

Bone is in a continuing state of remodeling under complex control by hormones and other factors (Chapter 8). These actions control both growth of bone, through actions of IGF-1, and bone mineralization, through influences on both the matrix and mineral phase. Examples of influences include effects of parathyroid hormone on bone remodeling, actions of vitamin D overall on calcium metabolism, effects of estrogens to prevent osteoporosis, and osteoporosis due to glucocorticoid excess.

EFFECTS ON REPRODUCTIVE FUNCTION

The role of gonadotropins in regulating ovarian and testicular function and the secretion of hormones from these organs is mentioned above. The male sex steroids, testosterone and dihydrotestosterone, regulate development of male sexual characteristics such as penile and prostate growth, voice, and muscular development and affect libido and sexual behavior (Chapters 12 and 14). The female sex steroids regulate functions of female reproductive organs, including the menstrual cycle and ovulation (Chapter 13). Pregnancy is regulated extensively by hormones (Chapter 16). Hormones are critical for egg and sperm development, preparation of the uterus for conception and implantation, and development of the fetus. The placenta itself produces a number of hormones, some of which are mostly unique (chorionic somatomammotropin, placental lactogen; CS) and others that are also produced abundantly by other glands (progesterone and other steroid hormones; Chapters 13 and 16).

RELEASE OF OTHER HORMONES

Hormones are extensively involved in regulating the production and release of the homologous hormone and of other hormones. These aspects are described in the earlier sections on neuroendocrinology, synthesis of hormones, regulation of the endocrine system, and mechanisms of hormone action.

EFFECTS ON IMMUNOLOGIC FUNCTIONS

There is extensive regulation of the immune system by hormones. The glucocorticoids and sex steroids are the hormones whose immunologic effects are best understood. Thyroid hormone, GH, catecholamines, PRL, and other hormones have all been reported to influence immunologic or inflammatory functions, but the roles of these and of other hormones are still being defined (see also Chapter 4). The major hormone class known to affect lymphokines is the glucocorticoids, which can blunt immunologic and inflammatory responses at high doses. This action forms the basis for the extensive use of glucocorticoids to suppress inflammatory and immunologic responses. The role of a normal level of glucocorticoid is still being elucidated. The sex steroids affect the immune response generally in a suppressive way. Castration in animals can result in enlargement of lymph nodes and spleen, more severe graft-versus-host disease, increased skin graft rejection, and stimulation of in vitro T lymphocyte mitogen responsiveness. These effects are mainly on cellular immune responses; influences on humoral responses are less clear. Estrogens may stimulate antibody production, and females tend to have higher levels of the major immunoglobulin classes under both basal and stimulated conditions than males. Females tend to have a higher incidence of autoimmune diseases and more active cellular and humoral immune responses than males. These differences (sometimes referred to as sexual dimorphisms) are not observed before puberty.

Pregnancy, with its associated changes in a number of hormones, commonly results in amelioration of autoimmune diseases. The mechanisms for these changes are not known. It is noteworthy that the peptide hormone whose concentrations are the highest reported to date for any hormone is chorionic somatomammotropin (CS), which has weak GH and PRL activities. Could this hormone have some immunoregulatory roles? Pregnancy tends to suppress the cellular but not the humoral immune responses, and this may contribute to prevention of maternal rejection of fetal tissues. Susceptibility to a number of viral and fungal diseases is increased in pregnancy. This immunosuppression is most pronounced in the second and third trimesters of pregnancy. By about 3–6 months postpartum, there is a rebound, with a reduction in sex steroid levels and an increase in the incidence of autoimmune diseases.

DISORDERS OF THE ENDOCRINE SYSTEM

The classic disorders of the endocrine system result principally in states of excess or deficiency of hormones due to hyperfunction or hypofunction of the glands. However, there is a growing awareness that variations in sensitivity to hormones also play a major role in disease states. The endocrinologist is also confronted with specific tumors and other problems such as iatrogenic syndromes. The types of abnormalities that in principle can occur are illustrated in Figure 1–13.

HYPOFUNCTION (Figure 1–13)

Destruction of the Gland

A common mechanism for glandular hypofunction is destruction of the gland. The most common cause of destruction of endocrine glands is autoimmune disease (Chapter 4). This is seen in most cases of IDDM (Chapter 18), hypothyroidism (Chapter 7), adrenal insufficiency (Chapter 9), and gonadal failure (Chapters 12 and 13). A polyglandular failure syndrome (Schmidt's syndrome) results from autoimmune destruction of several different endocrine glands in the same patient (Chapter 24). The immunologic damage also results in other abnormalities, including pernicious anemia and vitiligo. Destruction of the pituitary gland is usually due to a tumor, ischemia, or autoimmune hypophysitis (Chapter 5). Hypofunction of any of the endocrine glands may result from damage by neoplasms, infection, or hemorrhage.

Extraglandular Disorders

Endocrine hypofunction can be due to defects outside traditional glands. In some cases, these are simply due to damage to tissues which are not ordinarily considered to be endocrine glands that either produce the hormones involved or convert hormone precursors to active forms. These disorders can be considered simply as derangements of "endocrine glands" that happen to be organs with other major functions. Thus, renal disease can result in defective conversion of $25(OH)D_3$ to $1,25(OH)_2D_3$ with consequent abnormalities in calcium and phosphate balance (Chapter 8), damage to the renin-producing juxtaglomerular cells can result in hyporeninemic hypoaldosteronism (Chapter 9), and damage to erythropoietin-producing cells can result in anemia. In

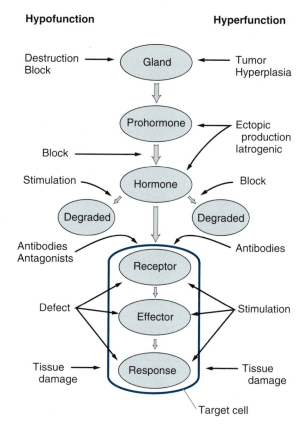

Figure 1–13. Causes of hypofunction and hyperfunction of the endocrine system. (Reprinted from Baxter JD in: *Cecil's Textbook of Medicine.* Wyngaarden JB, Smith LH Jr [editors]. Saunders, 1985.)

congenital 5α-reductase deficiency, there is impaired dihydrotestosterone production from testosterone in androgen target tissues, resulting in partial androgen deficiency (Chapter 14). Alternatively, this disorder could be classified as a defect of hormone biosynthesis (see below).

In some cases, factors that influence hormone degradation or sensitivity can precipitate or aggravate hormone deficiency when there is preexisting insufficient reserve in the endocrine gland. For example, glucocorticoid therapy increases the need for insulin and can precipitate latent diabetes mellitus or aggravate existing diabetes (Chapter 18). Thyroid hormones increase the metabolism of cortisol, and treatment of hypothyroidism with thyroid hormone can unmask latent adrenal deficiency (Chapter 9). Treatment with the anticonvulsant phenytoin can accelerate the degradation of glucocorticoids and increase the need for these hormones (Chapter 9).

Specific Defects In Hormone Biosynthesis

Endocrine hypofunction can be due to congenital defects in hormone synthesis. The types of mutations that can produce these defects were briefly summarized in the earlier section on gene expression and recombinant DNA in endocrinology and metabolism. These can be due to defects in genes that encode hormones, regulate hormone production, and encode hormone-producing enzymes or are involved in hormone metabolism. The 21-hydroxylase syndrome that results in defective cortisol production is one of the most common defined genetic diseases (Chapter 9). Other congenital adrenal gland defects include the 11β- and 18-hydroxylase syndromes (Chapters 9 and 10). Congenital defects also occur with the thyroid gland (Chapter 7). Dietary iodine deficiency results in deficient thyroid hormone biosynthesis and afflicts millions of people worldwide (Chapter 7). Mutations in genes encoding polypeptide hormones can lead to hormone deficiency due to decreased production of the hormone or production of a defective hormone. Forms of growth deficiency can result from mutations or deletions in the GH gene, defective production of GRH, or mutations in the gene for the transcription factor Pit-1, which regulates GH synthesis (Chapter 6). A rare form of diabetes mellitus results from a mutation in the insulin gene with consequent defective insulin (Chapter 18).

HYPERFUNCTION
(Figure 1–13)

Hyperfunction of endocrine glands results usually from tumors, hyperplasia, or autoimmune stimulation.

Tumors that produce excess hormone can occur in any of the endocrine glands. Tumors of the pituitary can lead to overproduction of the major classes of hormones of this gland (ACTH, GH, PRL, TSH, LH, FSH, etc; Chapter 5). In general, these tumors produce predominantly one of the hormones. Overproduction of the tropic hormones leads to stimulation of other glands, as is reflected by the cortisol excess due to pituitary ACTH-producing tumors or the rare syndrome of hyperthyroidism due to pituitary TSH-producing tumors. Tumors of the parathyroid glands can overproduce PTH (Chapter 8); thyroid parafollicular cells, calcitonin (Chapter 7); thyroid follicular cells, thyroglobulin, or thyroid hormone (Chapter 7); pancreatic islets, insulin (Chapter 19), or glucagon; adrenals, cortisol, aldosterone, deoxycorticosterone, androgens, and other steroids (Chapters 9 and 10); of the stomach, gastrin; of the kidney, renin or erythropoietin; etc. There are also syndromes of multiple endocrine neoplasia, in which there is a predisposition to develop tumors of several glands (Chapter 24). However, most tumors of the thyroid gland do not overproduce thyroid hormone (Chapter 7). Similarly, it is rare for ovarian or testicular tumors to overproduce steroids or for posterior pituitary tumors to overproduce oxytocin or vasopressin.

There can also be ectopic production of hormones by tumors of many types of tissues that ordinarily do not produce the hormone (Chapter 23). With rare exceptions, ectopically produced hormones are polypeptide hormones and include ACTH, PTH, ADH, FSH, LH, calcitonin, various releasing hormones, GH, and PRL. However, some polypeptide hormones such as insulin are rarely if ever expressed ectopically.

Hyperplasia, with increased cellularity and hormone overproduction, is seen with most endocrine glands. Hyperplasia of the parathyroid glands is commonly seen in renal failure, where depression of serum calcium ion levels stimulates the gland (Chapter 8). Less commonly, hyperplasia of the parathyroid glands occurs as a result of a specific genetic defect. Hyperplasia is commonly seen with the adrenal glomerulosa, where it results in aldosterone excess and the syndrome of primary aldosteronism (Chapter 10). Hyperplasia of the adrenal fasciculata and reticularis results in cortisol excess and Cushing's syndrome (Chapter 9). Hyperplasia of the fasciculata and reticularis is almost always due to a pituitary ACTH-producing tumor, as mentioned above. The cause of hyperplasia of the adrenal glomerulosa is not known, and the disorder is therefore referred to as idiopathic hyperplasia, or idiopathic aldosteronism. Hyperplasia of the thyroid gland is common and may be due to autoimmune stimulation of the gland (see below), iodine deficiency with impaired T_4 synthesis and subsequent TSH hypersecretion, and nodular goiter due to genetic biosynthetic abnormalities (Chapter 7). Hyperplasia of the ovaries is very common and results in the polycystic ovary syndrome, with abnormalities in ovarian steroid production; the causes of this syndrome are poorly understood (Chapter 13).

Autoimmune stimulation resulting in hyperfunction is seen most commonly with hyperthyroidism (Chapters 4 and 7). In this case, antibodies are produced that bind to and activate the TSH receptor on the gland. Hyperinsulinism due to autoimmune attack on the pancreatic B cells can be seen transiently early in the course of development of IDDM (Chapter 18). The mechanism for the stimulation in this case is unclear. Otherwise, autoimmune stimulation leading to hyperfunction of endocrine glands is rare.

DEFECTS IN SENSITIVITY TO HORMONES

Genetic and acquired defects in sensitivity to hormones were traditionally considered to be problems encountered only uncommonly by the endocrinologist. However, as more insights were gained into the pathogenesis of disorders such as NIDDM and hypertension, it has become clear that defects in sensitivity to hormones play a crucial role in these common disorders. Such defects are also responsible for a number of uncommon diseases and probably play a major role in many endocrine diseases. Most of these disorders result in resistance to the hormone. Resistance may be due to a number of different types of defects, such as in the hormone receptor, functions distal to the receptor, or influences extrinsic to the receptor-response pathway.

There are a number of disorders of primary resistance to hormones due to receptor defects. Characterized genetic defects in receptors that cause syndromes of resistance include those for glucocorticoids, thyroid hormones, androgens, estrogens, vitamin D, PTH, ADH, GH, insulin, and TSH.

Defects in responsiveness to hormones that are due to gene mutations whose products are involved in postreceptor events are in general less well understood. An exception is the syndrome of pseudohypoparathyroidism, in which mutations occur in the gene encoding the guanylyl nucleotide binding protein that links PTH-receptor binding to activation of adenylyl cyclase (Chapter 8). Hormone resistance due to poorly understood mechanisms but distal to the receptor in the hormone response element occurs in NIDDM, the most common form of diabetes mellitus (Chapter 18). In NIDDM there is both resistance to insulin and impaired release of insulin in response to glucose. With NIDDM, weight reduction and diet can commonly normalize these manifestations, suggesting that the problem is one of impaired adaptation, perhaps due to excessive down-regulation of responsiveness to stimuli. The so-called syndrome X is manifested by excessive insulin resistance with overlap into NIDDM, hyperlipidemia with increased triglycerides and cholesterol, and hypertension. This syndrome is also commonly observed in obese individuals and appears to account for much of the hypertension in Western societies. In hypertension, there are also variations in sensitivity to salt, angiotensin II, the release of renin in response to various stimuli, and to other effectors. Although the mechanisms for the differences are poorly understood, substantial insights into disorders such as these should come from a better understanding of the mechanisms of variations in sensitivity to hormones. A schematic representation of how resistance to hormones at postreceptor loci with either excessive or impaired down-regulation might occur is illustrated in Figure 1–14.

Acquired resistance to hormones can occur in several different ways. It can exist when there is frank disease that damages the target tissue and interferes with its ability to respond to the hormone, as is seen with renal disease and insensitivity to vasopressin,

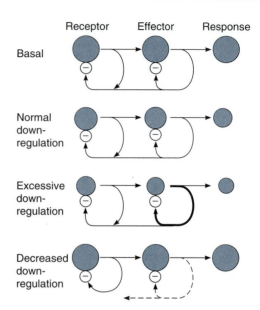

Figure 1–14. Hypothetical scheme for generation of diseases of hyperresponsiveness or hyporesponsiveness to hormones through excessive or impaired down-regulation. The top row indicates the response network before down-regulation occurs. The second row indicates the magnitude of the response network with normal down-regulation. The third row indicates a situation with excessive down-regulation due to a defect in the effector arm of the response with normal receptor function; the sizes of the circles reflect the influence, and the increased size of the arrow reflects the enhanced down-regulation. The fourth row depicts a situation with decreased down-regulation at the effector arm of the response. The dotted arrow reflects the decreased down-regulation, and the larger response circles, compared with the second panel, reflect the increased response resulting from the decreased down-regulation.

and liver disease and insensitivity to glucagon. It can occur as a result of excess production of other hormones or substances that promote hormone resistance. Thus, stress responses, hyperglycemia, and states that increase the levels of GH, cortisol, or glucagon all lead to insulin resistance that can aggravate or precipitate NIDDM (Chapter 18). Acquired resistance to the homologous or other hormones may also occur in the course of therapy with these hormones. This is particularly true with GnRH analogs (Chapter 22) and calcitonin and sometimes occurs with glucocorticoids. In fact, the acquired resistance with GnRH analogs forms the basis for their use in prostate cancer. In this setting, the GnRH-induced down-regulation of GnRH responsiveness shuts down FSH and LH release with the desired consequent reduction in testosterone production. Immunologic mechanisms can lead to acquired resistance, as can occur with antibodies produced to hormones (eg, with insulin or GH therapy), or receptors (eg, to insulin receptors; Chapter 18).

The clinical presentations of these syndromes show considerable variations. In the classic hormone resistance syndromes, there are elevated or normal hormone levels with clinical manifestations of hormone deficiency and failure of hormonal replacement to correct the disorder. However, resistance can be partial, with some response to higher hormone doses and a more subtle clinical presentation. Thus, in some cases, the syndromes simply resemble hormone deficiency states, as is the case with testicular feminization syndrome (androgen insensitivity; Chapter 14), rickets (vitamin D insensitivity; Chapter 8), and nephrogenic diabetes insipidus (ADH insensitivity). However, there can be wide variations in the clinical presentations. As an example, manifestations due to mutations of the androgen receptor gene can vary from a phenotypic female with a male genotype to mild androgen deficiency with impotence in an otherwise normal appearing male (Chapter 14).

In many cases, secondary hormone hypersecretion compensates largely for the defect, and the clinical presentation is more complex. Elevated hormone levels occur in hormone resistance syndromes because of absence of the usual feedback inhibition of hormone release resulting from the resistance or manifestations of it. For example, in the syndrome of generalized resistance to thyroid hormone (Chapter 7), the clinical presentation may have features of euthyroidism, hyperthyroidism (tachycardia, poor attention), and hypothyroidism (poor growth). In this syndrome, there is a mutation in one of the genes for the β form of the thyroid hormone receptor, but the remaining β receptors encoded by the second gene and the α-receptors encoded by separate genes are normal. The abnormal β-gene results in a decrease in the usual pituitary feedback by thyroid hormone and compensatory hypersecretion of thyroid hormone. The elevated thyroid hormone levels compensate for the defect through actions through the normal α and β receptors and in some cases by binding to the mutated receptors. Thus, thyroid hormone-regulated functions normally mediated through the α receptors are hyperstimulated, and functions mediated through the β receptors can be stimulated normally or may be understimulated in cases where a normal complement of β receptors is required and the elevated hormone cannot overcome the defect in the mutated receptors.

Such hyperstimulation of the endocrine glands in some cases results in overproduction of other hormones that in turn account for the major sequelae of the state. Mutations that lead to a reduced affinity for binding of cortisol to the glucocorticoid receptor result in a compensatory ACTH hypersecretion. Whereas the resulting hypercortisolemia compensates for the defect, increases in other steroids such as deoxycorticosterone and testosterone can promote mineralocorticoid hypertension and hirsutism.

Primary hyperresponsiveness to hormones has rarely been encountered. This may occur in low-renin hypertension in humans and in primary aldosteronism with hyperplasia that may be a variant of primary aldosteronism. Acquired hypersensitivity can be observed, as with catecholamine hypersensitivity in hyperthyroidism and increased sensitivity to insulin with cortisol deficiency.

SYNDROMES OF HORMONE EXCESS DUE TO ADMINISTRATION OF EXOGENOUS HORMONE OR MEDICATION

Syndromes of hormone excess can result from deliberate or inadvertent administration of exogenous hormones. Examples of deliberate administration are administration of glucocorticoids to patients producing Cushing's syndrome, or administration of high doses of thyroid hormone to suppress a malignancy of the gland producing hyperthyroidism. Deliberate androgen excess occurs in athletes who take steroids with androgen activity to improve performance. As an example of inadvertent administration, the author has observed Cushing's syndrome in a patient who received glucocorticoids but was not told she had been given a glucocorticoid. Outbreaks of hyperthyroidism have occurred when hamburger meat has been consumed that was contaminated by thyroid gland tissue in the beef (Chapter 7). Some nasal sprays have contained substances with mineralocorticoid activity that produce a mineralocorticoid excess state (Chapter 10).

DISORDERS OF THE ENDOCRINE GLANDS NOT ASSOCIATED WITH DISEASE

Endocrine glands can be affected by diseases just like other tissues of the body, and these can cause problems unrelated to the endocrine excess or deficiency state. For example, pituitary tumors can cause increased intracranial pressure or neurologic or ocular problems or may lead to infections when they extend outside the sella turcica (Chapter 5). Thyroid tumors or large goiters can cause local problems in the neck (Chapter 7).

APPROACH TO THE PATIENT WITH ENDOCRINE DISEASE

As is the case with all medical specialists, the endocrinologist hopes primarily to prevent diseases and their sequelae and, when this is impossible, to detect and treat disease at an early stage. Treatment of diseases at late stages is neither as easy nor as successful as with earlier stages. Thus, whereas endocrine diseases are generally most easily recognizable in their more extreme forms, it is hoped that few patients will progress to that level. Instead, the physician should be aware of the subtle early manifestations of endocrine disease and strive for early diagnosis with the aid of sophisticated laboratory tests. Early diagnosis can also be facilitated by screening for endocrine diseases in certain cases (discussed below).

Several general principles should be considered in evaluating endocrine diseases. Symptoms and signs are commonly vague and attributable to anxiety or depression or to common nonendocrine causes. The subtle early presentation of these disorders can be masked even further by counterregulatory actions by the body to compensate for the hormonal deficiency. The clinical presentation of a given condition can differ depending on its chronicity, and a severe deficiency state can present as an acute and severe problem in a patient in whom chronic manifestations of the disorder have not had time to develop. The clinician must make decisions about whether treatment should be instituted immediately, before time-consuming tests leading to definitive diagnosis have been completed. In spite of emphasis on early diagnosis, it is sometimes difficult to arrive at a clear diagnosis, and the procedures needed to make a definitive diagnosis may have more risk than the disease over a short period of time. In such cases, a decision to follow the patient must be made. For example, this sometimes occurs with ACTH-dependent Cushing's syndrome, where the differentiation between an occult carcinoid tumor and a small pituitary adenoma as the source of ACTH hypersecretion would require risky invasive procedures (Chapter 9).

In today's environment of cost containment, the efficiency of diagnosis must be a priority. Although today's tests may involve spending at an unprecedented level, they also allow for efficiency of diagnosis at an unprecedented level. Thus, by combining the most efficient use of tests based on the history and physical examination with sound clinical judgment, diagnosis and management of endocrine disease should be better, quicker, and cheaper than ever before.

HISTORY & PHYSICAL EXAMINATION

A carefully performed history and physical examination can provide information that cannot be obtained from laboratory testing. Some diagnoses, such as hypertension, are based on the physical examination alone. Even in cases where the history and physical are unrevealing, they enable the physician to select appropriate laboratory tests and avoid unneces-

sary testing. Most specialists have a fund of stories about consultations on extensively studied patients where simply elicited symptoms or signs that were overlooked would have led to a clear diagnosis. Thus, a carefully performed history and physical examination should address issues that will lead to the diagnosis and to the plan of approach. These activities should also reveal information about how much tissue damage or physical deformity has occurred, how long the disease has been present, the effect the various manifestations have had on the patient, and relevant data from the social, family, and personal histories that will facilitate evaluation and management.

Manifestations of endocrine disease that are frequently due to nonendocrine or unknown causes (Table 1–3) include tiredness, malaise, weakness, headache, anorexia, depression, weight gain or loss, bruising, constipation, and many others. Thus, weight loss is a common manifestation of hyperthyroidism, though most people with weight loss suffer from a condition other than hyperthyroidism (Chapter 7). Adrenal insufficiency is a rare disease and an even rarer cause of nausea (Chapter 9).

LABORATORY STUDIES

Laboratory evaluations are critical both for making and confirming endocrine diagnoses and to rule out specific diagnoses. The growing sophistication of these tests has led physicians to place increasing reliance on them. However, these tests cannot replace good clinical judgment that utilizes all available information in making clinical decisions. Laboratory tests in general measure either the level of the hormone in some body fluid, the sequelae of the hormone, or the sequelae of the process that contributed to the hormonal abnormality. The tests can be performed under random or basal conditions, precisely defined conditions, or in response to some provocative stimulus. In measuring hormone levels, the sensitivity of the assay refers to the lowest concentration of the hormone that can be accurately detected, and the specificity refers to the extent to which cross-reacting species that are not intended for the measurement are scored inappropriately as the hormone in the assay.

Measurements of Hormone Levels: Basal Levels

Immunologic assays have become the dominant technology utilized to measure levels of hormones in body fluids, even though there are other ways to measure them. Most measurements are made on blood or urine samples. The hormone is measured either directly from the samples or following extraction and purification. Most measurements are of the active hormone, though measurement of either a metabolite or precursor of the hormone or a con-

Table 1–3. Examples of manifestations of endocrine disease. (The manifestations do not occur in all cases, and the severity can vary markedly.)

Abdominal pain	Addisonian crisis; diabetic ketoacidosis; hyperparathyroidism
Amenorrhea or oligomenorrhea	Adrenal insufficiency, adrenogenital syndrome, anorexia nervosa, Cushing's syndrome, hyperprolactinemic states, hypopituitarism, hypothyroidism, menopause, ovarian failure, polycystic ovaries, pseudohermaphroditic syndromes
Anemia	Adrenal insufficiency, gonadal insufficiency, hypothyroidism, hyperparathyroidism, panhypopituitarism
Anorexia	Addison's disease, diabetic ketoacidosis, hypercalcemia (eg, hyperparathyroidism), hypothyroidism
Constipation	Diabetic neuropathy, hypercalcemia, hypothyroidism, pheochromocytoma
Depression	Adrenal insufficiency, Cushing's syndrome, hypercalcemic states, hypoglycemia, hypothyroidism
Diarrhea	Hyperthyroidism, metastatic carcinoid tumors, metastatic medullary thyroid carcinoma
Fever	Adrenal insufficiency, hyperthyroidism (severe: thyroid storm), hypothalamic disease
Hair changes	Decreased body hair (hypothyroidism, hypopituitarism, Cushing's syndrome, thyrotoxicosis); hirsutism (androgen excess states, Cushing's syndrome, acromegaly)
Headache	Hypertensive episodes with pheochromocytoma, hypoglycemia, pituitary tumors
Hypothermia	Hypoglycemia, hypothyroidism
Libido changes	Adrenal insufficiency, Cushing's syndrome, hypercalcemia, hyperprolactinemia, hyperthyroidism, hypokalemia, hypopituitarism, hypothyroidism, poorly controlled diabetes mellitus
Nervousness	Cushing's syndrome, hyperthyroidism
Polyuria	Diabetes insipidus, diabetes mellitus, hypercalcemia, hypokalemia
Skin changes	Acanthosis nigricans (obesity, polycystic ovaries, severe insulin resistance, Cushing's syndrome, acromegaly), acne (androgen excess), hyperpigmentation (adrenal insufficiency, Nelson's syndrome), dry (hypothyroidism), hypopigmentation (panhypopituitarism), striae, plethora, bruising, ecchymoses (Cushing's syndrome), vitiligo (autoimmune thyroid disease, Addison's disease)
Weakness and fatigue	Addison's disease, Cushing's syndrome, diabetes mellitus, hypokalemia (eg, primary aldosteronism, Bartter's syndrome), hypothyroidism, hyperthyroidism, hypercalcemia (eg, hyperparathyroidism, panchypopituitarism, pheochromocytoma)

(continued)

Table 1–3. (continued)

Weight gain	Central nervous system disease, Cushing's syndrome, hypothyroidism, insulinoma, pituitary tumors
Weight loss	Adrenal insufficiency, anorexia nervosa, endocrine cancer, hyperthyroidism, insulin-dependent diabetes mellitus, panhypopituitarism, pheochromocytoma

comitantly released substance sometimes provides the best information. Thus, in assessing vitamin D status, it is usually more informative to measure the precursor hormone, 25(OH)D, even though the final active hormone is 1,25(OH)$_2$D (Chapter 8). In 21-hydroxylase syndrome, the clinical problem is a deficiency of cortisol or aldosterone, whereas the most sensitive measurement is of the plasma 17α-hydroxyprogesterone level, a precursor of cortisol (Chapter 9). In looking for a pheochromocytoma, levels of metabolites of epinephrine are sometimes as informative as those of epinephrine, the active hormone (Chapter 11).

Plasma & Urine Assays

Assays of hormones in blood samples—plasma or serum—will indicate the level of hormone at that time. For hormones with long half-lives whose levels do not change rapidly (eg, thyroxine), measurements from samples taken randomly provide an integrated assessment of hormonal status. For hormones with shorter half-lives, such as epinephrine or cortisol, the assay will provide information only for the time of sample collection. Thus, with a pheochromocytoma that episodically releases epinephrine, elevated plasma epinephrine levels would be found only during periods of release and not between them (Chapter 11). Spontaneous Cushing's disease can be associated with an increased number of pulses of cortisol release with normal plasma cortisol levels between pulses (Chapter 9). In early Addison's disease, the number of pulses of cortisol release can be decreased, but occasional releases can occur that result in plasma cortisol levels which can be transiently in the normal range (Chapter 9).

Urine assays are generally restricted to measurement of levels of steroid and catecholamine hormones or metabolites and are not generally useful for polypeptide hormones that are either not cleared or are unstable. The collection period can be a random sample or, more often, a timed collection (usually 24 hours). Interpretations of urinary measurements must account for the fact that urinary levels reflect renal handling of the hormone. Urine measurements were utilized even more frequently in the past because larger quantities of the hormone could be obtained in many cases. However, with the high sensitivities of today's immunoassays, this advantage of urine is disappearing, and blood measurements are usually preferred. An advantage of urinary assays is that they can provide an integrated assessment of hormonal status. With cortisol, for example, only about 1–3% of the hormone released by the adrenal gland appears in the urine, but measurement of the urine cortisol in a 24-hour "urine free cortisol" sample provides an excellent assessment of the integrated production of cortisol (Chapter 9). This is important, since cortisol is released episodically, and a random plasma cortisol can be in the normal range in the face of mild to moderate Cushing's disease. Urinary assays are frequently used to document aldosterone excess in primary aldosteronism (Chapter 10) and epinephrine excess in pheochromocytoma (Chapter 11).

Free Hormone Levels

As discussed in an earlier section on plasma binding, many hormones circulate bound to plasma proteins, and in general it is the free hormone fraction that is biologically relevant. Thus, assessment of free hormone levels is more critical than that of total hormone levels. Tests that measure free hormone levels can utilize equilibrium dialysis, ultrafiltration, competitive binding, and other means. Although such tests are not commonly employed, their use may increase. A reflection of this is an increasing use of measurements of plasma free thyroxine (Chapter 7) and serum ionized Ca^{2+} levels (see Chapter 8).

Immunoassays

Hormone immunoassays utilize antibodies with high affinity to the hormone, raised in animals. The antibodies can be polyclonal or monoclonal. If the human hormone to which the antibody is to be raised is different enough from that in the animal, the unmodified hormone can be used to raise the antibodies. However, for hormones that have conserved structures and high homology with the animal hormone—and especially with very small hormones such as steroids or releasing factors that are not very immunogenic—the hormone is used as a hapten and linked to a highly immunogenic molecule or in other ways incorporated into a larger molecule for raising antibodies. In general, a given animal will produce a number of different antibodies to a given antigen, each from a clone of antibody producing B lymphocytes—thus the term "polyclonal antibodies." Within this mixture of antibodies, there can be many antibodies with extremely high affinities for the hormone, and these will provide a high level of sensitivity in a subsequent radioimmunoassay.

Monoclonal antibodies are obtained by several means; they are commonly obtained by injecting the antigen into a mouse or rat or by incubating it with cells in vitro. The animal spleen or cells incubated in vitro are then immortalized by fusing them to myeloma cells or transforming them with tumor viruses. This produces a number of clones of antibody-producing cells. The clones are then screened with the hormone antigen until a suitable antibody-producing clone is found. A major disadvantage of monoclonal antibodies is that many of the antibodies have a low affinity for the hormone, and considerable screening is necessary to obtain a high-affinity antibody. In addition, each antibody reacts with only one epitope on the antigen, and these antibodies are not as useful for traditional reagent-limiting assays. However, these antibodies are critical for the "sandwich assays" described below.

In traditional assays, the antigen is labeled in order to detect its binding to the antibody. The antigen must be labeled in such a way that this does not block its binding to the antibody. Immunoassays traditionally utilized radiolabeled hormones as the antigen. Most commonly, this was radiolabeled iodine, which can be obtained with a very high specific activity of radioactivity. However, the disadvantages with radioactivity in terms of shelf life and escalating expense for disposal have led to increasing use of nonisotopic means to perform immunoassays. For these, the antigen is linked to an enzyme, fluorescent label, chemiluminescent label, or latex particle that can be agglutinated with the antigen, or in some other way so that it can be detected. The enzyme-linked immunosorbent assays (ELISAs) that utilize antibody-coated microtiter plates and an enzyme-labeled reporter antibody are sometimes as sensitive as radioimmunoassays.

In practice, measurement of hormone levels by immunoassay involves incubating the plasma or urine sample or an extract with the antisera and then measuring the levels of antigen-antibody complexes by one of several means. The classic immunoassays utilize very high-affinity antibodies immobilized (at low concentrations to permit maximal sensitivity) on the surface of a test tube, polystyrene bead, or paramagnetic particle. The unknown sample and the antibody are incubated, and the labeled antigen is added either at zero time or later. A standard curve is prepared using the antibody and a known concentration of hormone. From this curve, the extent of inhibition by the added hormone of the binding of the labeled hormone is plotted, usually as the ratio of bound to free hormone as a function of the log of the total hormone concentration, which ordinarily gives a sigmoid curve (Figure 1–15). Alternatively, a log-logit plot can be used to linearize the data (Figure 1–15). The level of hormone in the sample is obtained by relating the value to the standard curve.

A recent modification of immunoassays is the sandwich technique, which utilizes two different monoclonal antibodies each of which recognizes a separate but different portion of the hormone. This aspect limits the technique, as it is difficult to utilize it for small molecules for which separable reactive

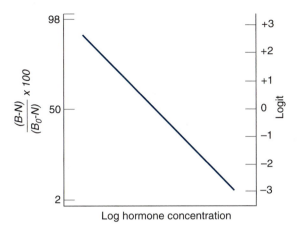

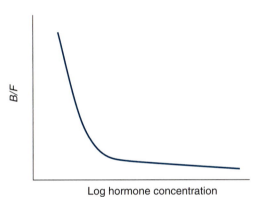

Figure 1–15. Standard curve of hormone radioimmunoassay. (B, counts bound; F, free counts; N, nonspecific count; B_0, maximum number of counts bound when only antibody and labeled hormone are incubated. (Reproduced, with permission, from Vaitukaitis J in: *Hormone Assays in Endocrinology and Metabolism,* 2nd ed. Felig P et al [editors]. McGraw-Hill, 1987.)

domains cannot be obtained. The assay is performed by using the first antibody, attached—preferably in excess relative to the amount of hormone in the sample—to a solid support matrix to adsorb the hormone to be assayed. After removal of the plasma and washing, the second (labeled) antibody is then incubated with the bound hormone-first antibody complex. The amount of binding of the second antibody is proportionate to the concentration of hormone in the sample. Use of the two antibodies results in a markedly enhanced specificity with a great reduction in background levels, thus improving both sensitivity and specificity of the assay.

Nonimmunologic Assays

Nonimmunologic assays include chemical assays, which take advantage of chemically reactive groups in the molecule; bioassays, which assess the activity of the hormone incubated with cells or tissues in vitro or injected into an animal; and receptor-binding and other assays, which exploit the high affinity of the hormone for receptors or other molecules such as plasma-binding proteins. These assays are rarely used. The fact that assays which substitute for or complement immunoassays have not come into general use indicates the power of immunoassays. For example, immunoassays are in general superior to receptor assays because antibodies can be obtained that have much higher affinities for hormones than receptors. An example of a receptor assay is one using cultured cells of a thyroid tumor (FRTL-5 cells) that contain TSH receptors, to detect antibodies to these receptors that occur in Graves' disease.

Diagnosis of Genetic Disease Using DNA

Methods for diagnosis of genetic diseases using DNA analyses are improving rapidly, although these are still used uncommonly. Thus, DNA can be obtained from cells from peripheral blood, fractionated, and then hybridized with a specific probe or sequenced. In the rare case where the mutation to be detected is known, such a procedure can lead to rapid and accurate diagnosis in the general population. This is the case with sickle cell anemia, in which a single mutation in one codon is present in all individuals with the disease. However, even in this case other diagnostic measures are currently easier to perform. By contrast, with almost all other genetic diseases, multiple different mutations lead to the same disease, and screening for any one mutation would miss most individuals in the population. Thus, for assessing genetic diseases in a general population, it is usually easier to measure the phenotype that results from the mutation. For example, the 21-hydroxylase deficiency syndrome is due to a number of different mutations, and it is simpler to measure 21-hydroxyprogesterone levels (Chapter 9) than to examine DNA samples for a large number of mutations.

A circumstance where DNA analysis will be used increasingly is with specific families, in whom the same mutation is present in all family members and it is desired to know whether a given family member has inherited that particular mutation. Endocrine diseases where this may come into increasing use are the multiple endocrine neoplasia (MEN) syndromes, where the specific defects are being defined (Chapter 24). Thus, it is now becoming possible to ascertain which family members have inherited the defect. Thus, people who have inherited the defect can be advised in regard to appropriate follow-up or preventive surgery, and those without the defect can be spared unnecessary anxiety and testing.

Two types of DNA analyses are generally performed. The first is direct examination of the defect by sequence analysis. Thus, the region of interest in a given DNA sample can be amplified using polymerase chain reaction (PCR) methodology. PCR utilizes primer DNAs that initiate DNA replication at specific sequences that ordinarily flank the region of interest. Inclusion of a heat-stable DNA polymerase allows for replication of the DNA sequences between the primer sites and for multiple rounds of replication, yielding a large number of copies of the region of interest. The amplified DNA can then be sequenced or examined by hybridization with a specific probe.

The second method is termed restriction fragment length polymorphisms (RFLPs) and is illustrated in Figure 1–16. This method utilizes restriction enzymes that cut the DNA at regions near the gene of

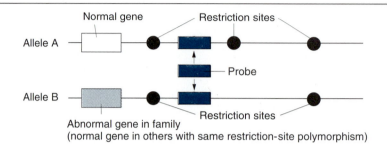

Figure 1–16. Diagnosis of genetic diseases. Shown in the top portion are two representative alleles with differences in a restriction site (nothing to do with the disease). In this example, the loss of the site in allele B is linked to a mutation that results in disease. Note that the allele B associated with the defective gene may be present with the missing restriction site in other unaffected individuals. Shown in the middle portion are representations of gel analysis results that distinguish the two alleles (in this case RFLPs). Shown at the bottom is an analysis of a family with the disease. Boxes represent males, circles females. Dark boxes or circles depict people who are or were afflicted. A diagonal line through the box or square indicates that the individual is deceased. Note that the disease always segregates with the B allele but that in the family depicted at far right, a B allele contributed by the unafflicted persons does not contain the defective gene.

interest. Because many sites are naturally polymorphic, ie, the DNA sequence of the site shows natural variation, inheritance of the site in a given family can be linked to the presence of any normal or mutated gene in the vicinity of the site. By following the inheritance of such polymorphisms that are linked in families, the presence of a mutated gene can be predicted with great accuracy.

Indirect Measurements of Hormonal Status

Measurement of hormonal status can in some circumstances be even more important than measuring the levels of the hormone and in many situations provides critical complementary information. Even when hormone levels are measured, it is common to obtain at least one index of the effects of the hormone in evaluating an endocrine disease. The blood glucose level is generally more useful than the plasma insulin level in diagnosing and treating diabetes mellitus (Chapter 18). Plasma insulin levels can be high in the face of frank hyperglycemia in non-insulin-dependent diabetes mellitus, and in insulin-dependent diabetes mellitus insulin levels are a much less reliable index of diabetic status than the blood glucose (Chapter 18). Measurement of the serum calcium level is critical for evaluating hyperparathyroidism (Chapter 8). Measurement of plasma renin levels is critical for evaluating primary aldosteronism, in which plasma renin levels are suppressed (Chapter 10). The most common cause of elevated aldosterone levels is dehydration, exercise, diuretic therapy, and other conditions that produce secondary aldosteronism; in these settings, the plasma renin levels tend to be high rather than low (Chapter 9).

Provocative Tests

In many cases, the level of a hormone or parameter affected by a hormone is best interpreted following some provocative challenge, although increasingly, more sophisticated ways to bypass the need for such tests are being developed. For example, with thyroid disease, provocative tests are rarely needed (Chapter 7), whereas with adrenal insufficiency or glucocorticoid excess (Chapter 9), heavy reliance is placed on such tests. With thyroid disease, slow clearance of the hormone results in basal levels of hormone that are highly informative, whereas the pulsatile nature of cortisol release results in fluctuating plasma cortisol levels that need to be measured under more defined conditions. This problem is bypassed in evaluation of adrenal insufficiency by administering an analog of ACTH that maximally stimulates the adrenal (Chapter 9). Diagnosis of Cushing's disease reflects a different type of problem (Chapter 9). Once cortisol hypersecretion has been documented, the cause must be identified. The clinician takes advantage of the fact that release of ACTH (and consequently of cortisol that is measured) by pituitary mi-

croadenomas is suppressed by the glucocorticoid dexamethasone to a greater extent than is the release of cortisol by adrenal tumors or of ACTH by ectopic ACTH-producing tumors. Similarly, GnRH analogs (which stimulate FSH and LH release), TRH (which stimulates both prolactin and TSH release), and insulin hypoglycemia (which stimulates the release of ACTH and GH) can be used to evaluate pituitary reserve (Chapter 5). In evaluating primary aldosteronism, provocative stimuli (diuresis, change in posture, inhibition of converting enzyme) are sometimes used to increase renin release (Chapter 10).

Imaging Studies

Imaging studies are gaining increasing usage in diagnosis and follow-up of endocrine diseases. MRI and CT have been especially important in this regard. These procedures allow visualization of endocrine glands and tumors of them at a much greater resolution than in the past. These procedures have been especially useful for evaluation of tumors of the pituitary and adrenals (Chapters 5 and 9). Scanning of the thyroid gland using radioactive iodine has been useful for evaluation of functioning nodules of this gland (Chapter 7). The endocrinologist can also resort to other sophisticated procedures that involve selective sampling from particular sites. For example, selective venous catheterization of the petrosal sinuses can be particularly useful in detecting ACTH hypersecretion in Cushing's disease (Chapter 9), and selective sampling of the renal veins can be helpful in the diagnosis of renovascular hypertension.

Biopsy Procedures

Although biopsy procedures are uncommonly used for evaluation of most endocrine diseases, they are occasionally useful to diagnose neoplasia. However, an exception is the use of fine-needle biopsy of the thyroid gland (Chapter 7) that has had a major impact on evaluation of thyroid nodules.

SCREENING FOR ENDOCRINE DISEASES

Some endocrine diseases are sufficiently common that screening for them should be part of usual clinical practice. This is particularly true for hypertension, thyroid disease (Chapter 7), and diabetes (Chapter 18). Thus, the blood pressure should be measured as part of any physical examination, and when hypertension is inappropriate, evaluation for a secondary form of the disorder should be instituted (Chapter 10). Thyroid disease has a prevalence of around 3% in women under the age of 60 and an even greater prevalence in both men and women of older ages. The clinical presentations, especially in milder forms, are frequently subtle and missed by the physician. Whereas there is no clear consensus for recommending for screening with serum TSH levels, such recommendations may ultimately emerge, given the increasing awareness of the incidence of thyroid disease and of the detrimental sequelae of subclinical disease (Chapter 7). Blood glucose levels should be determined in everyone at some interval. Even though hyperparathyroidism and hypercalcemia of malignancy are of much lower incidence than thyroid disease or diabetes mellitus, for example, determinations of serum calcium ion levels can be easily obtained as part of an automated panel of tests (Chapter 8). Finally, clues to endocrine diseases can be obtained from other abnormalities detected in screening, eg, blood counts and serum electrolyte measurements.

Clinical Interpretation of Laboratory Tests

Many salient points in interpreting laboratory tests are mentioned in the preceding sections; these and other points can be summarized as follows:

(1) Any result must be interpreted in light of clinical knowledge of the patient using data from the history and physical examination.

(2) Basal levels of hormones or peripheral effects of hormones must be interpreted in light of the way the hormone is released and controlled.

(3) Hormone levels must in many cases be interpreted in conjunction with information from other tests that reflect the patient's status: serum PTH levels in conjunction with serum calcium levels (Chapter 8); serum aldosterone levels in conjunction with plasma renin levels (Chapters 9 and 10); serum gonadotropin levels in conjunction with serum estradiol (Chapters 13 and 14) or testosterone (Chapters 12 and 14) levels; etc.

(4) Occasionally, urinary measurements are superior to plasma tests for assaying the integrated release of hormone.

(5) Ranges of normal values can vary from one laboratory to the next. The range for the laboratory utilized should be employed.

(6) Laboratory tests must be interpreted with knowledge of the value of the test. Reported normal ranges for tests cannot be used as absolute reflections of excess or deficiency states and must be interpreted in light of the clinical situation.

(7) Occasionally, laboratory test results are interfered with by extraneous or contaminating substances. For example, in illness, lipids in the plasma sometimes interfere with measurement of thyroid hormone-binding capacity (Chapter 7). In pregnancy, CG can cross-react in the TSH assay (Chapter 7). Antibodies generated when hormones are used in therapy (insulin, GH, etc) can lead to great increases in the total hormone owing to their sequestration of the hormone.

(8) Provocative tests are sometimes necessary.

(9) Imaging studies may help with the diagnosis, especially with respect to the source of hormone hypersecretion.

TREATMENT OF ENDOCRINE DISEASES

Treatment of hormone deficiency states requires, ideally, replacement with the hormone in a manner that mimics the physiologic setting. In many cases, a reasonable approximation of the physiologic status can be achieved by administering the hormone itself or an analog of it. Thus, treatment of hypothyroidism with thyroxine, adrenal insufficiency with cortisol, and the menopause with estrogen-containing preparations have proved to be highly effective. In other cases, there are problems with replacement therapy. Whereas recombinant GH is available to treat GH deficiency, it still must be injected and is expensive. A useful form of PTH is not available to treat hypoparathyroidism; effective PTH therapy will probably require a long-acting PTH preparation. For this disorder, patients are treated in less than ideal fashion with high doses of vitamin D and calcium (Chapter 8). Although insulin therapy will effectively control the hyperglycemia and prevent acidosis in most patients with diabetes mellitus, the long-term complications of the disease still occur with most regimes utilized today (Chapter 18). These result, at least in part, from the fact that we do not replace insulin in an ideal manner. When the hormone is injected subcutaneously, it is not delivered first to the liver; the kinetics of the injected hormone do not mimic accurately enough the physiologic release of insulin; and in many cases the delicate balance desired of normalization of blood glucose and avoidance of hypoglycemia cannot be achieved. For diseases such as IDDM, there is a major need for alternative approaches such as might ultimately be achieved through gene transfer, islet transplantation, mechanical pumps linked to glucose sensors, improved versions of insulin, or other means.

Since NIDDM, Addison's disease, hypothyroidism, and many other endocrine deficiency states result from autoimmune destruction of the gland (Chapter 4), there is a clear need for means to predict the emergence of the condition and to prevent the damage in the first place. It is already clear that measurement of the levels of certain antibodies with IDDM, thyroid disease, and other endocrine deficiency states can be used to predict the development of the disorder before there is major destruction of the gland. In the future, when means are available to prevent progression of the autoimmune disorder, these antibody or other measurements of immunologic processes will be used increasingly in screening procedures to detect the disease process and to prevent destruction of the gland.

For hormone excess states, treatment is ordinarily directed at the cause of the excess, usually a tumor or autoimmune condition. Tumors are removed when possible. Improvements in overall surgical techniques have markedly decreased the mortality and morbidity rates resulting from surgical removal of tumors of the endocrine system. In addition, alternative and less invasive approaches are supplanting the need for traditional surgery. For example, laparoscopic surgical techniques are being used increasingly for removal of tumors inside the abdomen. We cannot yet treat the autoimmune condition that results in hyperthyroidism, so therapy is directed at reducing the secretions of the thyroid gland by pharmacologic blockade, radioiodine therapy, or surgical removal (Chapter 7). Hormone production may also be blocked by pharmacologic means in many other instances. For example, with prolactin hypersecretion, use of the dopamine receptor agonist bromocriptine is commonly preferred to surgical removal of a small prolactinoma (Chapter 5). Octreotide acetate, a somatostatin analog, is sometimes used to block GH hypersecretion (Chapter 5). Inhibitors of steroid production such as ketoconazole are used to treat states in which the source of excess steroid production cannot be removed or found (Chapter 9).

In many cases, it is necessary to control the sequelae of hormone excess by alternative means. Thus, β-adrenergic blockers are useful to control sequelae of hyperthyroidism (Chapter 7), α-adrenergic blockers to control sequelae of pheochromocytoma (Chapter 11), mineralocorticoid antagonists to control blood pressure and hypokalemia in primary aldosteronism (Chapter 10), and inhibitors of cholesterol

biosynthesis to treat hypercholesterolemia, as with familial hypercholesterolemia (Chapter 20). With hypertension, a number of modalities are available to block hormone systems. Examples are angiotensin-converting enzyme inhibitors to block the renin-angiotensin system, calcium channel or β-adrenergic blockers to inhibit second messenger signaling, or diuretics to lower blood volume.

USES OF HORMONES IN THERAPY OF NONENDOCRINE DISEASE

The diverse actions of hormones have allowed them to be used extensively in therapy. Hormone antagonists are also used extensively. Hormone action is blocked in some cases with the use of enzyme inhibitors. Tables 1–2 and 1–4 present examples of hormone and hormone analog agonists (including eicosanoids) and antagonists, respectively, that are used in therapy. The most extensively used agonists are probably the glucocorticoids that are given to millions of Americans annually, largely to suppress inflammatory and immunologic responses. That the glucocorticoids would have this application came as a great surprise to the medical world, and Hench, Kendall, and Reichstein received the Nobel Prize for this discovery about 1 year after cortisone was first given to a patient with rheumatoid arthritis. Given this unexpected application, it is likely that uses of hormones for therapy will be greatly expanded over the next 20 years. For example, it is likely that the use of GH will be considerably expanded as informa-

Table 1–4. Hormones used in endocrinologic management for other than replacement.

Hormone or Analogue	Use	Evaluation
Glucocorticoid	Suppression of inflammatory or immune responses	
Growth hormone	Small stature	Wasting syndromes Osteoporosis
PTH		Osteoporosis
IGF-1		Osteoporosis Wasting syndromes
Octreotide acetate	Inhibition of GH release Diarrhea	Neuroendocrine tumors
Progesterone Estrogens Testosterone	Contraception Prostate cancer Breast cancer	
Prostaglandins	Induce labor, terminate pregnancy, maintain patent ductus artenosus at surgery	

tion from more clinical trials becomes available. This hormone may blunt some of the nitrogen wasting that occurs with glucocorticoid therapy and other states.

Extensively used hormone antagonists include the β-adrenergic blocking agents and the mixed estrogen antagonist tamoxifen (Table 1–2).

REFERENCES*

General
Alberts B et al: *Molecular Biology of the Cell,* 3rd ed. Garland, 1994.

Baxter JD et al: Introduction to the endocrine system. In: *Endocrinology and Metabolism,* 3rd ed. Felig P, Baxter JD, Frohman LA (editors). McGraw-Hill, 1995.

Frohman L et al: The clinical manifestations of endocrine disease. In: *Endocrinology and Metabolism,* 3rd ed. Felig P, Baxter JD, Frohman LA (editors). McGraw-Hill, 1995.

Sporn MB, Roberts AB: Autocrine secretion—10 years later. Ann Intern Med 1992;117:408.

Stryer L: *Biochemistry,* 4th ed. Freeman, 1995.

Assays as Diagnostic Procedures
Diamandis EP, Christopolos TK: *Immunoassay.* Academic Press, 1996.

Ekins R: Measurement of free hormones in blood. Endocr Rev 1990;11:5.

Feldman H, Rodbard D: Mathematical theory of radioimmunoassay. In: *Principles of Competitive Protein Binding Assay.* Odell WD, Daughaday WH (editors). Lippincott, 1971.

Pekary AE, Hershman JM: Hormone assays. In: *Endocrinology and Metabolism,* 3rd ed. Felig P, Baxter JD, Frohman LA (editors). McGraw-Hill, 1995.

Evolution of the Endocrine System
Alberts B et al: *Molecular Biology of the Cell,* 3rd ed. Garland, 1994.

Baxter JD et al: Introduction to the endocrine system. In: *Endocrinology and Metabolism,* 3rd ed. Felig P, Baxter JD, Frohman LA (editors). McGraw-Hill, 1995.

Baxter JD, Rousseau GG: Glucocorticoids and the metabolic code. In: *Glucocorticoid Hormone Action.* Baxter JD, Rousseau GG (editors). Springer, 1979.

Howard JC: Molecular evolution: How old is a polymorphism? Nature 1988;332;588.

Stryer L: *Biochemistry,* 4th ed. Freeman, 1995.

Tomkins GM: The metabolic code. Science 1975;189: 760.

Hormone Actions and Mechanisms
Bagatell CJ, Bremner WJ: Androgens in men—uses and abuses. N Engl J Med 1996;334:707.

Baird PN et al: Cytokine receptor genes: Structure, chromosomal location, and involvement in human disease. Leuk Lymphoma 1995;18:373.

Benz CC: Hormone-responsive tumors. In: *Endocrinology and Metabolism,* 3rd ed. Felig P, Baxter JD, Frohman LA (editors). McGraw-Hill, 1995.

Sun H, Tonks NK: The coordinated action of protein tyrosine phosphatases and kinases in cell signaling. Trends Biochem Sci 1994;19:480.

Soderling TR: Protein kinases and phosphatases: Regulation by autoinhibitory domains. Biotechnol Appl Biochem 1993;18:185.

Sucov HM, Evans RM: Retinoic acid and retinoic acid receptors in development. Mol Neurobiol 1995; 10:169.

Tallarida RJ: Receptor discrimination and control of agonist-antagonist binding. Am J Physiol 1995;269:379.

Hormone Metabolism and Regulation of the Endocrine System
Baxter JD et al: The endocrinology of hypertension. In: *Endocrinology and Metabolism,* 3rd ed. Felig P, Baxter JD, Frohman LA (editors). McGraw-Hill, 1995.

Glaser KB: Regulation of phospholipase A_2 enzymes: Selective inhibitors and their pharmacological potential. Adv Pharmacol 1995;32:31.

Levine JE et al: Amplitude and frequency modulation of pulsatile luteinizing hormone-releasing hormone release. Cell Mol Neurobiol 1995;15:117.

Monder C, White PC: 11β-Hydroxysteroid dehydrogenase. Vitam Horm 1993;47:187.

Ross AC: Overview of retinoid metabolism. J Nutr 1993 Feb, 123(2 Suppl):346.

Hormone Resistance and Mechanisms of Diseases
Auchus RJ, Fuqua SA: Clinical syndromes of hormone receptor mutations: Hormone resistance and independence. Semin Cell Biol 1994;5:127.

Baxter JD et al: The endocrinology of hypertension. In: *Endocrinology and Metabolism,* 3rd ed. Felig P, Baxter JD, Frohman LA (editors). McGraw-Hill, 1995.

Hewison M, O'Riordan JL: Hormone-nuclear receptor interactions in health and disease: Vitamin D resistance. Baillieres Clin Endocrinol Metab 1994;8:305.

Jameson JL: Mechanisms by which thyroid hormone receptor mutations cause clinical syndromes of resistance to thyroid hormone. Thyroid 1994;4:485.

Komesaroff PA, Funder JW; Fuller PJ. Hormone-nuclear receptor interactions in health and disease: Mineralocorticoid resistance. Baillieres Clin Endocrinol Metab 1994;8:333.

---

*Additional details pertaining to subjects taken up in this chapter are provided in subsequent chapters, to which extensive references are made in the text. The following references are included to direct the reader to further information about issues that may not be discussed in as great detail in this book.

Lifton RP: Genetic determinants of human hypertension. Proc Natl Acad Sci U S A 1995;92:8545.

Muller-Wieland D et al: Molecular biology of insulin resistance. Exper Clin Endocrinol 1993;101:17.

Raymond JR: Hereditary and acquired defects in signaling through the hormone-receptor-G protein complex. (Editorial.) Am J Psychiatry 1994;266:F163.

Ross RJ, Chew SL: Acquired growth hormone resistance. Eur J Endocrinol 1995;132:655.

Schmidt TJ, Meyer AS: Autoregulation of corticosteroid receptors: How, when, where, and why? Receptor 1994;4:229.

Sluyser M: Hormone resistance in cancer: The role of abnormal steroid receptors. Crit Rev Oncog 1994; 5:539.

Taylor SI et al: Polycystic ovary syndrome: Relationship to growth hormone, insulin-like growth factor-I, and insulin. Curr Opin Obstet Gynecol 1994;6:279.

Immunoendocrinology

Daynes RA et al: Steroids as regulators of the mammalian immune response. J Invest Dermatol 1995; 105:14S.

Foxwell BM, Barrett K, Feldman M: Cytokine receptors: Structure and signal transduction. Clin Exp Immunol 1992;90:161.

Logan A: Endocrinology and the immune system. Lancet 1992;340:420.

Murphy WJ et al: Effects of growth hormone and prolactin immune development and function. Life Sci 1995;57:1.

Shurtz-Swirski R et al: Parathyroid hormone and the cellular immune system. Nephron 1995;70:21.

Wilder RL: Neuroendocrine-immune system interactions and autoimmunity. Annu Rev Immunol 1995; 13:307.

Neuroendocrinology

Acher R, Chauvet J: The neurohypophysial endocrine regulatory cascade: Precursors, mediators, receptors and effectors. Front Neuroendocrinol 1995;16:237.

Martin JB, Reichlin S: *Clinical Neuroendocrinology,* 2nd ed. Davis, 1987.

Molitch ME: Neuroendocrinology. In: *Endocrinology and Metabolism,* 3rd ed. Felig P, Baxter JD, Frohman LA (editors). McGraw-Hill, 1995.

Reppert SM, Weaver DR: Melatonin madness. Cell 1995;83:1059.

Rupprecht R et al: Neurosteroids: Molecular mechanisms of action and psychopharmacological significance. J Steroid Biochem Mol Biol 1996;56:1.

Veldhuis JD (editor): Neuroendocrinology I. Med Clin North Am 1992;21:767; Neuroendocrinology II. Med Clin North Am 1993;22:1.

Pharmacology; Agonist and Antagonist Therapy

Cumming DC: Hormones and athletic performance. In: *Endocrinology and Metabolism,* 3rd ed. Felig P, Baxter JD, Frohman LA (editors). McGraw-Hill, 1995.

Gilman AG et al (editors): *Goodman and Gilman's The Pharmacological Basis of Therapeutics,* 9th ed. McGraw-Hill, 1996.

Jensen EV: Steroid hormone antagonists: Summary and future challenges. Ann N Y Acad Sci 1995;761:1.

Katzung BG: *Basic and Clinical Pharmacology,* 6th ed. Appleton & Lange, 1995.

McLeod DG. Antiandrogenic drugs. Cancer 1993;71(3 Suppl):1046.

Sudduth SL, Koronkowski MJ. Finasteride: the first 5 alpha-reductase inhibitor. Pharmacotherapy 1993; 13:309; discussion 325.

Tyrrell JB: Glucocorticoid therapy. In: *Endocrinology and Metabolism,* 3rd ed. Felig P, Baxter JD, Frohman LA (editors). McGraw-Hill, 1995.

Plasma Binding

Baumann G: Growth hormone binding to a circulating receptor fragment: The concept of receptor shedding and receptor splicing. Exper Clin Endocrinol Diabetes 1995;103:2.

Behan DP et al: Corticotropin releasing factor (CRF) binding protein: A novel regulator of CRF and related peptides. Front Neuroendocrinol 1995;16:362.

Brann DW et al: Emerging diversities in the mechanism of action of steroid hormones. J Steroid Biochem Mol Biol 1995;52:113.

Dunger DB et al: Insulin-like growth factors (IGFs) and IGF-I treatment in the adolescent with insulin-dependent diabetes mellitus. Metabolism 1995;44:119.

Episkopou V et al: Disruption of the transthyretin gene results in mice with depressed levels of plasma retinol and thyroid hormone. Proc Natl Acad Sci U S A 1993;90:2375.

Farnsworth WE: Roles of estrogen and SHBG in prostate physiology. Prostate 1996;28:17.

Hammond GL: Molecular properties of corticosteroid binding globulin and the sex-steroid binding proteins. Endocr Rev 1990;11:65.

Herve F: Drug binding in plasma: A summary of recent trends in the study of drug and hormone binding. Clin Pharmacokinet 1994;26:44.

Joseph DR: Structure, function, and regulation of androgen-binding protein/sex hormone-binding globulin. Vitam Horm 1994;49:197.

Mendel CM et al: Uptake of thyroxine by the perfused rat liver: Implications for the free hormone hypothesis. Am J Physiol 1988;255:E110.

Schreiber G: Hormone delivery systems to the brain: Transthyretin. Exper Clin Endocrinol Diab 1995; 103:75.

Sumida C: Fatty acids: Ancestral ligands and modern co-regulators of the steroid hormone receptor cell signalling pathway. Prostaglandins Leukot Essent Fatty Acids 1995;52:137.

Recombinant DNA and Molecular Biology

Alcamo IE: *DNA Technology: The Awesome Skill.* Brown, 1966.

Aldhous P: Fast tracks to disease genes. Science 1994;265:2008.

Gardner DG, Gertz BJ: Gene expression and recombinant DNA in endocrinology and metabolism. In: *Endocrinology and Metabolism,* 3rd ed. Felig P, Baxter JD, Frohman LA (editors). McGraw-Hill, 1995.

Glick BR, Pasternak JJ: *Molecular Biotechnology: Principles and Applications of Recombinant DNA.* ASM Press, 1994.

Lander ES, Schork NJ: Genetic dissection of complex traits. Science 1994;265:2037.

Todd JA: Genetic analysis of type 1 diabetes using whole genome approaches. Proc Natl Acad Sci U S A 1995;92:8560.

Leiden JM: Gene therapy: Promise, pitfalls and prognosis. N Engl J Med 1995;333:871.

Shuldiner AR: Transgenic animals. N Engl J Med 1996; 334:653.

Watson JD et al: *Recombinant DNA*. Freeman, 1992.

Hormone Synthesis & Release

2

Vishwanath R. Lingappa, MD, PhD, & Synthia H. Mellon, PhD

OVERVIEW OF HORMONE BIOSYNTHESIS

Any molecule delivered via the bloodstream that can be recognized by a receptor in or on a target cell in a manner that conveys information can, in principle, be used by the body as a hormone. In the course of evolution, an incredible variety of molecules have been utilized as hormones by various organisms. With this diversity of hormone structure comes a corresponding variety in modes of hormone biosynthesis. In this chapter, we shall summarize current concepts of hormone synthesis and release.

Hormones can be divided into two broad classes (Figure 2–1). Some are stored in membrane vesicles. These hormones are released from an endocrine cell by fusion of membrane vesicles with the plasma membrane, typically in response to a stimulus for secretion that may or may not be coupled with the stimulus for hormone synthesis. Hormones of this class may be synthesized and then stored for later release. The second broad class of hormones are those that are secreted immediately upon synthesis in a manner not mediated by membrane vesicle fusion. For these hormones, there is typically no distinction between the stimulus for synthesis and the stimulus for release—hence, control over synthesis is the major means known for regulating their secretion.

The **polypeptide hormones** are the most prominent example of hormones whose release is vesicle-mediated, and their secretion involves transit through multiple membrane-delimited compartments of the classic secretory pathway (see below). However, the vesicle-mediated pathway is also used for the secretion of a number of nonpolypeptide hormones and neurotransmitters such as catecholamines (eg, dopamine) and γ-aminobutyric acid (GABA). These small molecules do not undergo the full range of intracellular trafficking events involving multiple compartments that is seen in protein secretion. Rather, vesicles recycle after a round of vesicle fusion by a process known as **endocytosis.** These nonpolypeptide hormones, either newly synthesized or taken up by specific transporters from outside the cell, are pumped back into the vesicle from

ACRONYMS USED IN THIS CHAPTER	
ACAT	Acyl-coenzyme A cholesterol acyltransferase
ACTH	Adrenocorticotropic hormone
ATP	Adenosine triphosphate
CBG	Corticosteroid-binding globulin
COP	Coat-associated protein
EGF	Epidermal growth factor
ER	Endoplasmic reticulum
GABA	Gamma-aminobutyric acid
GDP	Guanosine diphosphate
GTP	Guanosine triphosphate
HDL	High-density lipoprotein
HETE	Hydroxyeicosatetraenoic acid
HPETE	Hydroxyperoxyeicosatetraenoic acid
LDL	Low-density lipoprotein
M-6-P	Mannose-6-phosphate
NAC	Nascent chain-associated complex
NSF	*N*-Ethyl maleimide-sensitive factor
POMC	Proopiomelanocortin
SCP-2	Sterol carrier protein-2
SHBG	Sex hormone-binding globulin
SNAP	Soluble NSF-attachment protein
SRP	Signal recognition particle
StAR	Steroidogenic acute regulator
TBG	Thyroid hormone-binding globulin
TGN	*Trans* Golgi network
t-SNARE	Target membrane SNAP receptor
TRAM	Translocating chain-associated membrane protein
TSH	Thyroid-stimulating hormone
v-SNARE	Vesicle membrane SNAP protein

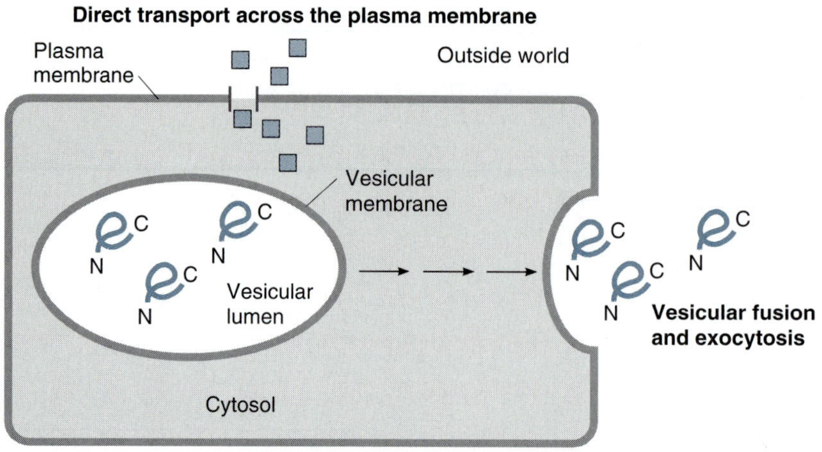

Direct transport across the plasma membrane

Figure 2–1. Vesicular and nonvesicular modes of hormone secretion. Schematic diagram of a cell, indicating that some hormones are transported in vesicles to the cell surface and released in quanta upon fusion of the vesicle with the plasma membrane, while other hormones are transported directly across the plasma membrane either by specific transporters or by diffusion. Vesicular secretion can be regulated separately at the level of synthesis and of release, while control over synthesis is the only known way to regulate hormones released in a nonvesicular manner. Examples of hormones secreted in a vesicle-mediated fashion are most polypeptide hormones and catecholamines. Examples of hormones released in a nonvesicular manner are the eicosanoids, steroids, and thyroid hormones.

the cytosol in preparation for another round of vesicle fusion and secretion. As will be summarized below, tremendous progress has been made in recent years in our understanding of the molecular mechanisms of vesicular traffic involved in biosynthesis and release of both peptide and nonpeptide hormones.

Classes of hormones released by other than vesicle-mediated mechanisms include the **steroids (glucocorticoids, androgens, estrogens** and **mineralocorticoids,** all derived from cholesterol) and the **eicosanoids** (a family of fatty acid-derived signaling molecules that include the **prostaglandins**). Exactly how non-vesicle-mediated release occurs is not as well understood as vesicular secretion. Historically, simple diffusion was assumed to be the mechanism both for release from the hormone-producing cells and for entry into target cells. In recent years, however, specific transporters have been implicated in directing some of these classes of molecules out of the cell. Whether all non-vesicle fusion-mediated secretion will prove to be driven by transporters and directed through specific channels or whether some hormones leave the cell solely by diffusion remains a subject for future investigation.

MEMBRANE VESICLE-MEDIATED HORMONE EXPORT

With the exception of a very small number of proteins synthesized within the mitochondrial matrix and in plants, within chloroplasts, most proteins made in eukaryotic cells are synthesized on ribosomes in the cytoplasm. Proteins that reside in the cytoplasm are not secreted out of cells. The presence of cytosolic proteins outside of cells is usually due to cell damage or death. Thus, specialized mechanisms must exist to discriminate between newly synthesized proteins that are destined to be secreted and those which are to remain in the cytoplasm.

The polypeptide hormones are an important subset of secretory proteins, and the classic secretory pathway by which they leave the cell is the best-understood mechanism of hormone export. It appears to be the mechanism used for most but not all polypeptide hormones and can be separated into early and late events. The early events involve getting a newly synthesized secretory protein into the luminal space of the **endoplasmic reticulum (ER),** a membrane-delimited compartment. The late events involve the transport of that protein from the ER lumen to the lumen of other membrane-delimited compartments, including the **Golgi apparatus** and subsequently to **secretory granules** and ultimately, upon fusion of a secretory granule with the plasma membrane, out of the cell. Whereas the early events involve direct transfer of individual secretory polypeptides across a lipid bilayer (the ER membrane), the later events move secretory proteins exclusively by budding of membrane vesicles from one compartment and their fusion with another, such that the protein cargo moves from vesicle to vesicle without ever again actually crossing a lipid bilayer directly (Figure 2–1).

Targeting to the Membrane of the Endoplasmic Reticulum

The early events of polypeptide hormone targeting to and translocation across the ER membrane generally occur while the protein is still being synthesized. The mechanism that appears to have evolved as the major pathway of ER translocation in eukaryotes involves a **signal sequence** found in nascent secretory proteins (Figure 2–2). The signal sequence is a sequence of amino acid residues encoded in the mRNA, usually, but not always, at the 5' end and thus usually occurring at the amino terminal. The signal sequence typically emerges from the ribosome as part of the nascent protein chain and is quickly bound by a cytoplasmic ribonucleoprotein complex composed of six polypeptides and a small RNA termed **signal recognition particle (SRP)**. "Professional" secretory tissues such as endocrine glands often contain a substantial amount of "rough" ER visible under the electron microscope, so-called because of the presence of ribosomes bound to the ER membrane that are targeted by SRP.

SRP serves in two ways to facilitate translocation of nascent secretory proteins across the ER membrane. First, binding of SRP to both the signal sequence and the ribosome slows the rate of chain elongation, thereby increasing the "window" of time during which the chain can find the cytoplasmic face of the ER while still nascent and thus still able to be translocated into the lumen. Most proteins cannot be translocated after their synthesis has been completed and they have been released from the ribosome. In part this is because most chains are translocation competent only when they are unfolded. In part, the cotranslational requirement also reflects a role for the ribosome in opening the channels through which translocation occurs (see below). Second, when bound to a signal sequence, SRP undergoes conformational changes resulting in high affinity for a receptor on the ER membrane (termed the **SRP recep-**

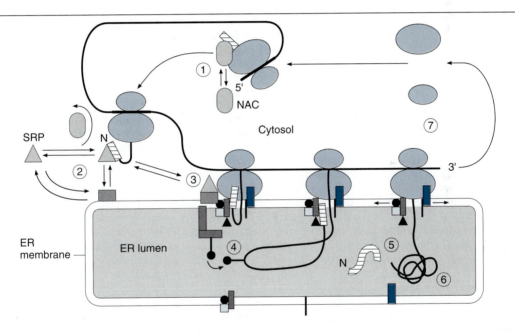

Figure 2–2. Translocation of nascent polypeptide hormones across the ER membrane. Key steps in polypeptide hormone biosynthesis and secretion are indicated by the circled numbers. (1) Ribosomes from the free cytoplasmic pool initiate translation of mRNA encoding secretory proteins. A protein complex termed nascent chain associated complex (NAC) appears to prevent inappropriate or premature targeting of the nascent chain. (2) The initial codons encode a signal sequence that emerges from the ribosome and will serve to target the nascent secretory chain to the ER membrane by virtue of the affinity of a cytosolic particle termed signal recognition particle (SRP) for both the signal sequence and a receptor in the ER membrane. SRP binding displaces NAC from the nascent chain; SRP docking to the ER membrane displaces the nascent chain from SRP. (3) Assembly of a channel across the ER membrane provides a pathway for the nascent growing chain to enter the ER lumen. Translocation involves a ribosome-membrane junction sufficiently "tight" to shield the nascent growing chain from the cytoplasm, thereby preventing the cytoplasm from being secreted into the ER lumen. (4) During translocation, the chain is subject to a host of co-translational modifications including the addition of carbohydrates which are transferred as a preformed structure composed of 11 carbohydrate residues from lipid carriers to the protein. (5) Translocation-associated events in polypeptide hormone biogenesis usually include cleavage of the signal sequence. (6) As the chain emerges into the ER lumen, folding occurs, governed by molecular chaperones in the ER lumen. (7) After completion of protein synthesis, the ribosome subunits are released back into the free cytosolic pool, the channel disassembles or closes, and the folded chain is localized to the ER lumen.

tor), thereby targeting the nascent chain to the correct subcellular location. Upon binding the SRP receptor, SRP undergoes another conformational change that releases the signal sequence and the ribosome, allowing the rate of chain elongation to increase and freeing the signal sequence and nascent chain to interact with other proteins in the ER membrane. During the same time, a firm ribosome membrane junction forms by interacting with receptor proteins. This helps to keep the channel open for translocation and forms a tight seal to prevent the cytosol from leaking across the ER membrane.

Some of the proteins that compose both SRP and the SRP receptor are GTP binding proteins, and it appears that cycles of GDP-GTP exchange and GTP hydrolysis serve to ensure the fidelity of targeting and the unidirectionality of several of the early events in translocation, including (1) signal recognition by SRP, (2) targeting of the nascent ribosome-signal sequence-SRP complex to the SRP receptor, (3) assembly of the translocation channel, and (4) release of SRP to participate in another round of targeting.

Recently, a protein complex termed the **nascent chain-associated complex (NAC)** has been described that binds both secretory and nonsecretory nascent chains as they are being synthesized. SRP subsequently displaces NAC from nascent secretory proteins by recognition of the signal sequence and the ribosome. This may be a mechanism to improve the fidelity of targeting.

Finally, a non-SRP-mediated pathway of targeting has been described in yeast. The full significance of this finding remains to be established. However, it is consistent with the concept that crucial biologic recognition systems have evolved a degree of redundancy in case (for whatever reason) the primary recognition system should fail. Thus, SRP-deficient yeast mutants are viable but grow slowly. Some proteins in these mutants are severely affected by lack of SRP while others appear largely unaffected, presumably because they can target to the ER membrane as efficiently by non-SRP mediated mechanisms.

Translocation Across the ER Membrane

Once targeted to the ER membrane, the nascent chain must somehow traverse the ER membrane, which is otherwise a nearly impenetrable barrier to movement of most proteins from the cytosol to the ER lumen. Upon release from SRP, the correctly targeted signal sequence appears to interact with other proteins in the ER membrane to open a channel to the ER lumen. The growing polypeptide chain—but not the proteins or even the ions in the cytosol—has access to the channel. The nascent chain is translocated through this channel into the lumen of the ER, tightly shielded from the cytosol by the ribosome-membrane junction. Recent studies suggest that a

form of regulation involves transiently breaking the ribosome membrane junction directed by particular sequences present in some nascent proteins. As a consequence, translocation across the ER membrane is interrupted and specific domains of nascent secretory proteins are exposed to the cytoplasm prior to reestablishment of a tight ribosome-membrane junction and resumption of translocation.

In addition to the GTP hydrolysis-dependent steps of targeting, subsequent steps of translocation also appear to involve ATP hydrolysis. The precise role of the energy requirement of chain translocation—apart from that involving GTP hydrolysis for targeting—remains unclear. Perhaps the energy of ATP hydrolysis is needed to form or maintain the channel in an open conformation or to actually pull the chain across the membrane, as has been suggested for protein secretion in bacteria. Alternatively, ATP may be hydrolyzed as part of the action of molecular chaperones acting on the chain in the ER lumen, and the actual translocation may even occur by brownian motion without any requirement for ATP hydrolysis. Major progress has been made in recent years in identifying ER membrane proteins involved in nascent chain translocation across the ER membrane. It appears that at least two membrane protein complexes, the heterodimeric SRP receptor and the heterotrimeric Sec 61p complex, are involved in translocation of every protein. A third membrane protein, termed translocating chain-associated membrane protein (TRAM), is involved in translocation of most but not all proteins. Roles for other accessory proteins in translocation of specific subsets of polypeptides or in more complex modification events associated with translocation have been suggested but not yet proved. Recent studies have strongly suggested that the translocation channel in eukaryotes is an aqueous protein-lined, protein-conducting pore. Yet lipids appear to have at least transient access to the nascent chain during its translocation, perhaps reflecting the dynamic and transient nature of a channel rapidly assembled and disassembled from component subunits.

Upon completion of secretory protein synthesis, the ribosomal subunits release from the cytoplasmic side of the ER membrane and the transmembrane channel disassembles or in some other way closes, leaving the newly synthesized secretory protein localized to the luminal space of the ER with no way to return to the cytosol (Figure 2–2).

Co- & Posttranslational Modification of Proteins

During translocation across the ER, subsequently within the ER lumen, and in a variety of later membrane-delimited compartments, newly synthesized proteins may be subject to literally dozens of possible processing events that often vary from protein to protein, tissue to tissue, and species to species. Only a small number of the many possible modifications actually occur on any given protein, and some proteins appear to receive no modifications at all. In the few modifications that have been well studied, it appears that either primary amino acid sequence motifs or secondary or tertiary structural features of a particular newly synthesized protein are recognized by the enzymes that carry out these modifications. Some of these modifications are covalent, eg, proteolytic removal of the signal sequence disulfide bond formation and addition of various moieties to amino acid side chains (eg, carbohydrates). Other modifications are noncovalent, such as proper folding of newly synthesized polypeptides under the supervision of families of proteins termed **molecular chaperones** that are present in the cytosol, ER membrane, and ER lumen.

Perhaps the best-understood posttranslational modification is a subset of carbohydrate addition termed N-linked glycosylation (Figure 2–2). This form of glycosylation occurs on selected asparagine residues during translocation of the nascent chain into the ER lumen. The carbohydrate units consist of up to 14 sugars that are assembled in a tree-like structure on lipid transporters called **dolichols.** The entire sugar tree is then transferred en bloc to selected asparagine residues of the nascent protein as it enters the ER lumen (hence the term "N-linked" glycosylation). Subsequently, the individual sugars that compose the sugar tree are modified, with some removed and others added, in the ER and in more distal compartments of the secretory pathway.

In most cases, the precise functions of the various covalent co- and posttranslational modifications, including N-linked glycosylation, are unknown. However, as will be discussed below, two important roles for N-linked carbohydrates in facilitating proper sorting and traffic of some proteins through the secretory pathway have been discovered. In other cases, changes in carbohydrates have been shown to alter the activity of particular hormones once secreted, either by affecting the affinity of binding to hormone receptors or by altering the clearance from the bloodstream and hence the half-life and effective concentration of the particular hormone in blood.

Quality Control by the ER

Within the ER lumen, molecular chaperones not only facilitate proper folding of the newly arrived polypeptide, they also assess the outcome of folding. Often, as a result of interaction with molecular chaperones, proteins deemed improperly folded are not allowed to leave the ER, even though, in at least some cases, those proteins appear sufficiently well folded to be capable of physiologic function in vitro. This "quality control" function appears to be a major role of the ER in the scheme of protein biogenesis. Whether the molecular chaperones that carry out these recognition events for protein folding and quality control also play a role in the actual translo-

cation of proteins into the ER lumen remains controversial.

In the case of one particular ER molecular chaperone, termed **calnexin,** trimming of the glucose units at the end of the N-linked carbohydrate tree appears to serve as a monitor of the need for further chaperone action for at least some newly synthesized proteins. Calnexin binds these unfolded chains upon trimming of the outer two of the three glucose residues found on the N-linked carbohydrate tree. Like other molecular chaperones, calnexin uses the energy from cycles of ATP hydrolysis to prevent misfolding of the newly synthesized protein. Upon completion of proper folding, the final glucose is trimmed, calnexin is released, and the protein is transported in vesicles out of the ER. If proper folding, as defined by the quality control machinery, is not achieved, glucose may be added back and multiple cycles of calnexin binding, folding, sugar trimming, and release allowed to occur. Calnexin is unusual among the molecular chaperones in that it recognizes the polar carbohydrate. In the case of most other molecular chaperones, hydrophobic interactions are the important determinants of interaction with substrates.

In a number of cases, proteins deemed to be improperly folded by the quality control machinery are not only prevented from leaving the ER, they are rapidly degraded there as well. Some data suggest that in the case of some particularly complex secretory and integral membrane polypeptides, rapid degradation in the ER can be a point of regulation of protein biogenesis, multisubunit assembly, and secretion.

Post-ER Vesicular Traffic in the Secretory Pathway

Translocation across the ER membrane is the only time that a secretory protein directly crosses a lipid bilayer. All subsequent trafficking steps involve the pinching off of a membrane vesicle containing a cargo of newly synthesized protein from one membrane-delimited compartment and its transfer to another membrane compartment by fusion of the vesicle. Ultimately, vesicles fuse to the plasma membrane (exocytosis) or to the lysosome (lysosomal targeting; Figure 2–3). Concomitantly with traffic of vesicles through the secretory pathway, a recycling of membrane must occur. Both vesicular and tubular pathways of membrane recycling have been proposed (Figure 2–3).

The exact number of membrane compartments in the secretory pathway has yet to be determined. Indeed, in some cases the distinction between one compartment and the next may be largely semantic. At the least, all secretory proteins are transported in vesicles from their site of synthesis in the ER to a post-ER "intermediate" compartment from which vesicles deliver them to the Golgi apparatus. Within

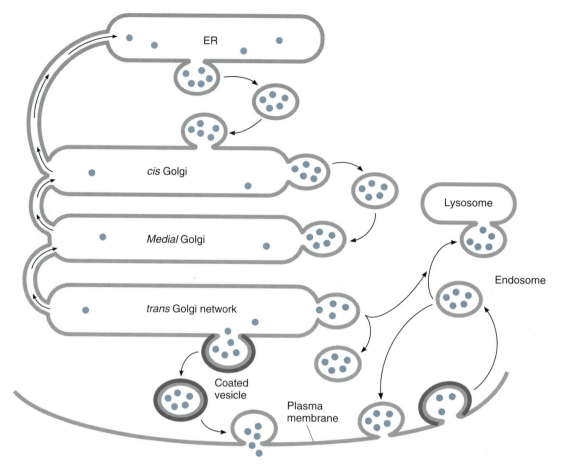

Figure 2–3. Membrane traffic in hormone-secreting cells. Polypeptide hormones travel through a variety of membrane compartments of the secretory pathway, with transport mediated by the fission and fusion of vesicles. Newly synthesized polypeptide hormones exit the ER and travel in vesicles to the Golgi apparatus. Vesicles transport the proteins through the Golgi apparatus to the *trans*-Golgi network whence other vesicles transport the proteins to either the regulated or constitutive secretory pathways or to lysosomes for degradation. In addition to forward transport, a pathway of retrograde transport, perhaps largely mediated by tubules rather than vesicles, returns membrane and some proteins to earlier compartments, including the ER and Golgi stacks. Endocytosis is the set of membrane-delimited trafficking pathways whereby hormones bound to receptors at the cell surface are internalized and transported either to the lysosome for degradation or back to the cell surface for rerelease. The pathways of endocytosis and biogenesis can overlap in key compartments and share common features of mechanism—eg, the role of "coat" proteins in forming and targeting vesicles from *trans*-Golgi network to plasma membrane during protein biogenesis and from plasma membrane to lysosome in endocytosis.

the Golgi, they are transferred serially from the so-called *cis* Golgi network to the medial Golgi stack, to the *trans* Golgi stack, and finally to the *trans* Golgi network (TGN) membrane cisternae. Each serial compartment is operationally defined by localization of specific enzymes (such as those involved in modifying carbohydrates) to a particular subset of membranes. As more compartment-specific genes are cloned and monospecific antibodies generated to modifying enzymes, it is likely that additional subcompartments will be operationally distinguished within the currently understood secretory pathway. However, not every protein that traverses the secre-

tory pathway receives a modification in any particular compartment as far as is known.

Trafficking of proteins through the vesicular stages of the secretory pathway involves recognition events both in the lumen, such as that described above for calnexin, and recognition events in the cytosol. The cytosolic recognition events involve cytoplasmically disposed domains of proteins within the vesicular membrane. Various families of small and large GTP binding proteins have been implicated in control of these cytosolic recognition processes.

In a manner analogous to the mechanism targeting the nascent secretory protein to the ER membrane described above, cycles of GTP for GDP exchange followed by GTP hydrolysis ensure correct vesicle formation, docking, and fusion to the correct target compartment. Other GTP-binding proteins confer unidirectionality on the membrane fusion event which is itself mediated by a "fusion machine" assembled from various proteins including some in the cytosol and some that were also involved in vesicle formation and targeting.

Differences in adapter proteins (including some that bind and hydrolyze GTP) and surface receptor proteins termed **v-SNARES** with cognate binding sites (termed **t-SNARES**) on the correct membrane of destination are believed to mediate the correct targeting of vesicles throughout the secretory pathway (Figure 2–4).

In some cases, various "coats" composed of specific proteins form on the outside of membranes, allowing them to be pinched off to form vesicles. Vesicles of different sizes, containing different classes of proteins as their cargo and destined for different subcellular fates, are often observed to have different coats or different adapter proteins that mediate assembly of a particular coat, permitting the resulting vesicle to be selectively targeted to the correct membrane destination. Recent work demonstrates that phosphatidylinositol transfer proteins greatly stimulate the formation of vesicles from the TGN. These findings suggest a role for these negatively charged phospholipids in vesicle formation, perhaps by inducing membrane curvature or by recruiting coat proteins and other cytosolic components.

Membrane Trafficking Steps Prior to Sorting of Cargo

Through the TGN, the cargo contained within the vesicles that move from compartment to compartment is nonspecific, meaning that no sorting of content proteins has occurred. Thus, for example, a vesicle leaving the *cis* Golgi and targeted to the medial Golgi will contain a mixture of newly synthesized proteins including enzymes to be localized within the **lysosome** (an acidic membrane-bound organelle containing various hydrolytic enzymes that are active at low pH), proteins to be secreted continuously and proteins to be secreted only in response to specific stimuli (ie, hormones). Likewise, the membrane of this vesicle contains various classes of membrane proteins with different destinations (eg, those targeted selectively to the apical plasma membrane and others targeted exclusively to the basolateral plasma membrane). While the cargo delivered to the TGN is nonspecific, the pathway followed by the vesicles is not. A vesicle derived from the *cis* Golgi must be selectively targeted to the medial Golgi and not the *trans* stack or back to the ER or to the plasma membrane. A separate pathway of vesicular transport is involved in "recycling" of membrane containers by return from *cis* Golgi to ER, etc. This recycling pathway is also used to return so-called resident proteins (such as calnexin) that need to be retained in a particular compartment. It appears that at least one of the mechanisms involved is not retention per se but rather efficient *retrieval* of wayward polypeptides from the subsequent compartment. The coats of the

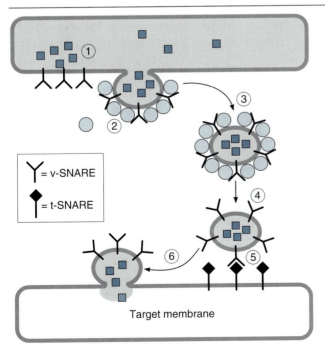

Figure 2–4. SNARE hypothesis for intracellular vesicular traffic. Vesicular traffic requires a means of discrimination on both sides of a membrane so that (1) products destined for one fate can be sorted from those with another, and (2) so that the sorted molecules can be correctly targeted to the correct subsequent membrane compartment. This includes a role for coat proteins that associate with the surface of a compartment to form or pinch off vesicles. (3) Once vesicles have formed, their trafficking is governed by recognition events between molecules termed v-SNARES on their surface with molecules termed t-SNARES on the surface of the target membrane. Before localization of cargo to the target compartment can be consummated, several events must occur in concert with v-SNARE-t-SNARE interaction, including uncoating (4), docking (5), and fusion (6). These events can be constitutive or regulated simply by placing one or more of them under control of a signal-transduction pathway.

intra-Golgi vesicles with nonspecific cargo and involved in recycling contain a protein termed **COP I.** The coats of vesicles involved in ER to *cis* Golgi traffic contain a protein termed **COP II.**

Despite the nonspecific nature of their cargo, vesicle recognition events are probably occurring within the lumen of the ER and Golgi stack. For example, it was recently noted that some membrane proteins are concentrated in the intermediate compartment between ER and Golgi, strongly suggesting the occurrence of selective luminal recognition events. Whether this is true for all proteins or only for a subset within the nonspecific cargo remains to be determined.

A large body of evidence, summarized above, supports the notion that transfer from *cis* to medial to *trans* Golgi and TGN cisternae involves budding of vesicles from one compartment and their fusion to the next compartment within the Golgi apparatus. However, controversy has emerged as to the relative role of vesicles versus tubules of membranes that may connect one compartment with the next and whether one versus the other mechanism is involved in "forward" transport versus the return of "empty" membrane containers back to their compartment of origin. If tubular connections rather than membrane vesicles emerge as the major means of forward intra-Golgi traffic, the concept of relatively fixed compartments between which newly synthesized proteins are moved may have to be at least partially revised in favor of a more dynamic "maturational" model for membrane flow within the Golgi apparatus.

Sorting of Vesicle Cargo at the TGN

Unlike most vesicular transport from ER to TGN, true sorting occurs upon exit from the TGN. Vesicles leaving the TGN are heterogeneous with respect to both their cargo and their destination. Some vesicles are loaded with exclusively lysosomal enzymes and are targeted selectively to an acidic endosomal compartment in a pathway that will lead eventually to the lysosome or to a compartment which becomes a lysosome.

Other vesicles lead to the **regulated secretory pathway,** where the final vesicular fusion event of a secretory granule fusing to the plasma membrane to release the secretory proteins happens only upon specific stimulation. Thus, the stimulus to insulin release via the regulated secretory pathway is hypoglycemia; that of parathyroid hormone release is hypocalcemia; that of renin release includes adrenergic neural stimulation; etc. Some of the vesicles that are released by the regulated secretory pathway first condense their contents into a concentrated precipitate of secretory product and proteoglycans. These vesicles are termed secretory granules (see below). Other regulated secretory vesicles are morphologically distinguishable in that their contents do not undergo concentration.

However, they do display stimulus-secretion coupling, the sine qua non of the regulated secretory pathway.

Still other vesicles, including those containing many membrane proteins, enter the **constitutive secretory pathway.** The constitutive pathway differs from the regulated pathway in that nothing prevents the final vesicle from fusing with the plasma membrane as soon as the vesicle has formed and been targeted—ie, no stimulus is required to overcome a pre-existing block that prevents vesicle fusion to the plasma membrane in the absence of stimulus.

In addition to segregating content proteins with different subsequent vesicular destinations, the TGN sorting step sets in motion another set of posttranslational modifications. For example, the proteolytic processing of proinsulin to insulin and of proopiomelanocortin (POMC) into adrenocorticotropic hormone (ACTH) and other active peptides is initiated in the TGN and continues in the vesicles targeted to the regulated secretory pathway (see below).

The sorting event that occurs at the TGN is probably mediated by similar interactions on the cytosolic side of the vesicles as were just described for the vesicular transport of nonselective cargo—as well as by additional interactions that specifically connect the sorting event occurring on the luminal side with a particular targeting event on the cytosolic side. The best-defined of these TGN sorting events is that involved in diverting lysosomal enzymes from the common secretory pathway to the lysosome.

Lysosomal Enzyme Sorting

The lysosome is a membrane-delimited organelle in which various hydrolytic enzymes with an acid pH optimum are found. These enzymes—proteases, DNases, RNases, lipases, and the like—are used to break down macromolecules into recyclable building blocks that can be transported to the cytosol or elsewhere for reuse.

The lysosomal hydrolases that ultimately reside within the lysosome start out in the ER lumen, where they are glycosylated along with many other secretory proteins. Once in the *cis* Golgi, however, lysosomal enzymes are specifically recognized by an *N*-acetylglucosamine (GlcNAc) phosphotransferase, resulting in the addition of a GlcNAc phosphate moiety to the terminal mannose residue of their N-linked carbohydrate tree (exposed upon trimming of the glucose residues discussed above). Unlike the signal sequence, the recognition of lysosomal enzymes by GlcNAc phosphotransferase is not based on binding of a linear sequence of amino acid residues but is rather a function of affinity for a so-called **signal patch** composed of amino acid residues from different parts of the molecule that come together upon three-dimensional folding of the protein. This is an important experimental point since a single linear peptide is easy to define and manipulate, while a targeting-sorting signal composed of disparate parts of a protein is more difficult to analyze.

A subsequent enzyme removes the GlcNAc, exposing mannose 6-phosphate (M6P), which specifically binds a luminally disposed domain of the transmembrane M6P receptor found in the TGN. The cytosolically disposed domain of the transmembrane M6P receptor binds a specific adapter protein that catalyses coat formation, vesicle budding, and targeting toward a prelysosomal, early endosomal compartment. Upon fusion with this membrane, the M6P receptor and the lysosomal enzymes it has bound are exposed to a slightly acidic environment in which M6P—and therefore the lysosomal enzymes—has much lower affinity for the M6P receptor, resulting in dissociation of lysosomal enzymes from the M6P receptor. Once dissociation has occurred, the receptor is free to recycle back to the TGN, leaving the lysosomal enzymes in the endosomal compartment, which can either fuse to late endosomes and ultimately to lysosomes or "mature" into first a late endosome and then into a lysosome. Recent data support the maturational model for the relationship of endosomes to lysosomes.

Note that the presence of an intermediate acidic compartment between TGN and lysosomes allowed recycling of M6P receptors without subjecting them to the potentially damaging lysosomal environment. While the M6P receptor pathway provides a framework for understanding one possible way in which sorting occurs, it is likely that other ways to sort lysosomal enzymes will also be found since patients with I cell disease, in which a mutant GlcNAc phosphotransferase fails to tag lysosomal enzymes, are observed to secrete their lysosomal enzymes from only some tissues (eg, fibroblasts but not liver). In liver and other tissues, lysosomal enzymes are correctly localized to the lysosome despite lack of the M6P tag, suggesting the existence of an alternative pathway for lysosomal enzyme recognition and sorting.

Regulated Secretion

Much of the recent progress in understanding the pathway of regulated secretion by which most hormones are released on specific stimulation comes from work on the molecular events of synaptic transmission, which can be viewed as a specific example of regulated secretion. Synaptic transmission occurs extremely quickly, placing limits on the number and nature of interactions, including simple diffusion, that can occur between stimulus and secretion. A number of proteins in the synaptic vesicular membrane have been identified and cloned, and functions have been ascribed to most. Many of these proteins are also found in neuroendocrine cells and are not exclusively neuronal proteins.

In both neurons and neuroendocrine cells, regulated secretion is dependent on an elevation of intracellular calcium. However, calcium probably acts at a number of different steps in each, involving both high- and low-affinity calcium receptor proteins. These steps probably include priming or docking of vesicles as well as vesicle fusion itself. They may also include events such as local disassembly of cytoskeletal proteins to allow secretory granules to dock at the plasma membrane. To date, the precise differences between neuronal and neuroendocrine-regulated secretion have not been fully resolved. More importantly, however, it is now recognized that a number of proteins are involved in both of these two modes of regulated protein secretion.

Some of the proteins involved probably play a regulatory role but appear not to be required for exocytosis per se, based on studies of transgenic knockout mice and *Drosophila* and *Caenorhabditis elegans* mutations. This group includes the proteins Rab3a, unc18, synapsin, and synaptotagmin. This conclusion, however, is clouded by the possibility that multiple genes encoding functionally related products exist and that another gene product is at least partially able to offset the lack of a deleted or mutated gene.

Other proteins are clearly essential components of the universal machinery for vesicular exocytosis. These include gene products specifically cleaved by the clostridial neurotoxins that inhibit regulated secretion from both neurons and neuroendocrine cells. Synaptobrevin, syntaxin, and synaptosome-associated protein 25 are examples of this second group.

Finally, a number of proteins such as *N*-ethyl maleimide-sensitive factor (NSF) and SNAPs (discussed earlier) clearly associate with the neurotoxin substrates. Based on this association, synaptobrevin, syntaxin, and synaptosome-associated protein 25 can be viewed as SNAP receptors (SNAREs). Thus, regulated secretion in both neurons (synaptic transmission) and in neuroendocrine cells can be unified under the SNARE hypothesis described earlier for other steps of vesicular transport (Figure 2–4). The novel twist in this hypothesis to accommodate regulated secretion is that the ability of the secretory vesicle v-SNARE to dock with the plasma membrane t-SNARE is dependent on the calcium-signaling step that triggers secretion. In the next few years, this hypothesis is likely to be tested, and if it is fully validated in either neuronal or neuroendocrine systems, a number of unanswered questions can be resolved.

Regulation of Hormone Release After Exocytosis

Upon condensation into secretory granules, the vesicle content exists as a crystalline precipitate and is no longer osmotically active, a property that facilitates their storage in the regulated secretory pathway. Upon fusion of such a secretory granule to the plasma membrane, the insoluble content must dissolve into the extracellular medium. It appears that the ionic composition of the extracellular fluid can significantly influence the rate of phase transition of the insoluble proteoglycan matrix and hence dissolution and effective release of secretory products. This phenomenon is likely to be an important point of regulation in systems where pulse frequency and amplitude of secretion are important properties (eg, release of neurotransmitters).

POMC Processing & Secretion

Recently there has been progress in understanding the nature of the sorting signal on an individual hormone that accounts for how those molecules are segregated in the TGN from lysosomal, constitutive secretory, and other pathways. In the case of POMC, a specific conformational motif responsible for sorting to the regulated secretory pathway has been identified. It is composed of a 13-amino-acid amphipathic loop close to the amino terminal of the polypeptide and appears to be stabilized by a disulfide bridge. Presumably this feature is recognized in the lumen by transmembrane receptors whose cytoplasmic tails recognize adaptin-type proteins responsible for coat assembly, vesicle formation, and proper targeting to the appropriate domain of the plasma membrane.

During this transport process, the vesicles "mature" into secretory granules. Key features of this maturation step include proteolysis (eg, in the case of POMC, where a small peptide, ACTH, will be released from the much larger precursor) and concentration. The concentration step is such that often the regulated secretory cargo forms crystalline arrays of precipitated protein within the granule lumen. Upon stimulation, when the granule fuses to the plasma membrane, the exocytosed product is diluted and dissolves into the bloodstream.

Endocytosis & Recycling

In addition to transport and correct localization of newly synthesized hormones and receptors, vesicular membrane trafficking events are involved in important responses to hormones. In parallel with the pathway of membrane vesicles from ER to plasma membrane is a pathway that leads from the plasma membrane back to various compartments, including the TGN and perhaps even the ER. In part this represents the need to recycle membrane. Note that the volume of regulated secretion in endocrine cells is such that the entire intracellular membrane system would be consumed and localized to the plasma membrane literally in minutes if there were no way to recycle the "empty" membrane containers after use. Not only is there such a pathway, but it probably operates in reverse between each forward compartment (ie, from plasma membrane to TGN, from TGN to *trans* Golgi, from *trans* to medial Golgi, from medial to *cis* Golgi, from *cis* Golgi to intermediate compartment, and from intermediate compartment to ER).

However, endocytosis is not simply a means of re-

covering "empty" containers. It provides a means for the cell to take up valuable nutrients and to "sample" the environment. Such is the case for endocytosis of low-density lipoproteins via LDL receptors that are internalized as coated vesicles from coated pits on the plasma membrane of hepatocytes.

Finally, of particular interest for endocrinology, endocytosis provides a means of responding to hormones and other signals. Endocytosis of a vesicle from the plasma membrane places hormone receptors in a protected space where they can no longer be activated by external hormone. This is one (of several) molecular bases of receptor down-regulation and tachyphylaxis to drugs.

Whereas some receptors enter the coated pits only when bound to ligand (eg, EGF receptor), others enter constantly whether ligand-bound or not. In some cases, both ligand and receptor are targeted from the endosome to the lysosomes and degraded (eg, EGF and its receptor). In other cases, dissociation of ligand from receptor in an intermediate acidic compartment allows the receptor to be recycled and only the cargo to be sent to the lysosome (eg, LDL receptor).

One difference from the biosynthetic flow of membranes is that different machinery is involved in vesicle formation from the plasma membrane, which is much more rigid than intracellular membrane compartments by virtue of having cytoskeletal elements bound on the inside and extracellular matrix bound on the outside. Thus, the microtubule-associated protein dynamin has recently been implicated in driving vesicular invagination, constriction, and pinching off from the plasma membrane.

Recently, noncoated invaginations termed **caveolae** have been noted to occur at the plasma membrane and have been implicated in such hormone-related events as translocation of the insulin-sensitive isoform of the glucose transporter to the cell surface upon insulin stimulation.

As mentioned earlier, a complicating issue in vesicular dynamics is whether different gene products can, at least partially, perform each other's function, hence obscuring the consequences of knockout experiments to assess the role of a particular protein in trafficking events. A better understanding of these features of membrane vesicular dynamics is likely to emerge in the coming years. Some of the differences in pathways defined by the presence or absence of a particular protein may prove to be largely semantic owing to complementary functional activity of another protein despite morphologic, structural, or antigenic differences. In other cases, differences in protein composition may reflect important mechanistic differences in the pathways of vesicular traffic. The importance of recent progress is that such differences in trafficking pathways are no longer the subject of speculation but rather are being detected and studied and the genes associated with them cloned and their expression manipulated.

Secretion of Catecholamines, GABA, & Other Nonpolypeptide Neurotransmitters

Nonpolypeptide products that are released by fusion of vesicles such as catecholamines, acetylcholine, and GABA represent a variation on the theme of recycling through the endocytotic pathway. The vesicles containing these neurotransmitters are loaded with their product by transporters that engage in direct uptake from the cytosol. Loaded vesicles fuse with the plasma membrane in a regulated fashion coupled with a stimulus and usually mediated by a rise in intracellular free calcium. Subsequently, the membrane container is reendocytosed, reloaded, and subjected to another cycle of triggered fusion and content release, as with other forms of stimulus-coupled secretion. Several members of a related family of transporters involved in uptake of these small molecules from the cytosol have been identified.

Secretion of Thyroid Hormone

Thyroid hormone is an example of a hormone whose biogenesis involves a hybrid of vesicular and nonvesicular trafficking. It is synthesized initially as a large polypeptide precursor, termed **thyroglobulin,** which is assembled into a dimer, iodinated, and modified in the classic secretory pathway before constitutive exocytosis across the apical plasma membrane. Iodinated thyroglobulin is stored outside of the cell in the thyroid follicle lumen and is termed **colloid.** Upon appropriate stimulation by thyroid-stimulating hormone (TSH), colloid is taken up by endocytosis and transported across the cell in vesicles that fuse to the basolateral plasma membrane. This variant of endocytosis, in which a product is taken up and delivered from one side of a cell to the other in a polarized fashion, is termed **transcytosis.** During transcytosis, the thyroglobulin is degraded by proteases to release active thyroid hormone. Remarkably, out of approximately 6600 amino acid residues comprising the thyroglobulin dimer, six pairs of iodinated, modified tyrosines are released as thyroid hormone, containing either three or four iodines (T_3 or T_4). Thyroid hormone released from the large polypeptide precursor during transcytosis is able to cross the vesicular membrane and the plasma membrane directly and hence is released immediately upon synthesis in a non-vesicle-mediated manner.

Relevance of Membrane Traffic to Disease

Given the complexities of hormone biogenesis and the many gene products involved in synthesis, maturation, and trafficking of hormones, it should not be surprising that defects in membrane trafficking are prominent among those genetic diseases whose molecular basis is well understood. Thus, a common genetic disease, cystic fibrosis, is due to mutations in a membrane protein. As a result of this mutation, this protein is unable to leave the ER despite the fact that it remains functional. Presumably, this is a case in which the ER quality control machinery acts as a "double-edged sword": Preventing export from the ER of a slightly misfolded protein causes a much more severe disease due to a complete lack of the protein at its proper location, the plasma membrane. Similarly, α_1-antiprotease deficiency, which results in emphysema, is due to a trafficking defect in which the misfolded protein fails to leave the ER.

In most cases, our understanding of acquired disorders, including degenerative diseases, does not extend to the relative importance of disorders of trafficking. However, proteins that undergo complex trafficking pathways, including growth factors and hormone receptors, are central to many of these disorders, suggesting that important connections are yet to be discovered.

An emerging principle of cellular pathophysiology seems to be that for the most important pathways, cells have evolved backup systems that can to some extent maintain crucial functions. Thus, yeasts lacking SRP are sick and have substantial defects in translocation across the ER but survive thanks to non-SRP-mediated backup systems. Thus, patients with I cell disease have correct lysosomal localization of lysosomal enzymes in some tissues even though all tissues lack the GlcNAc phosphotransferase necessary to generate the ligand for the M6P receptor. Two consequences of this principle are that important trafficking defects are apt to be acquired rather than inherited and that identification of these lesions will prove extremely difficult and will require a more intimate understanding of the complex regulation of normal trafficking in the absence of disease.

HORMONE EXPORT NOT MEDIATED BY MEMBRANE VESICLES

1. STEROID HORMONES

Steroid hormones are mainly synthesized in the adrenals, gonads, and placenta. Recent experiments indicate that steroids are synthesized in the nervous system as well, and other tissues may also synthesize steroid hormones in much smaller quantities. The overall pathway for the synthesis of all steroid hormones is similar (Figure 2–5). Tissue-specific, cell-specific, and even subcellular compartment-specific differences in the expression of particular steroidogenic enzymes regulate the particular pattern of steroid hormone synthesized.

Chemistry

All steroids are derived from pregnenolone (Figure 2–5). Pregnenolone, naturally occurring progestins, glucocorticoids, and mineralocorticoids contain 21 carbons and are referred to as C-21 steroids.

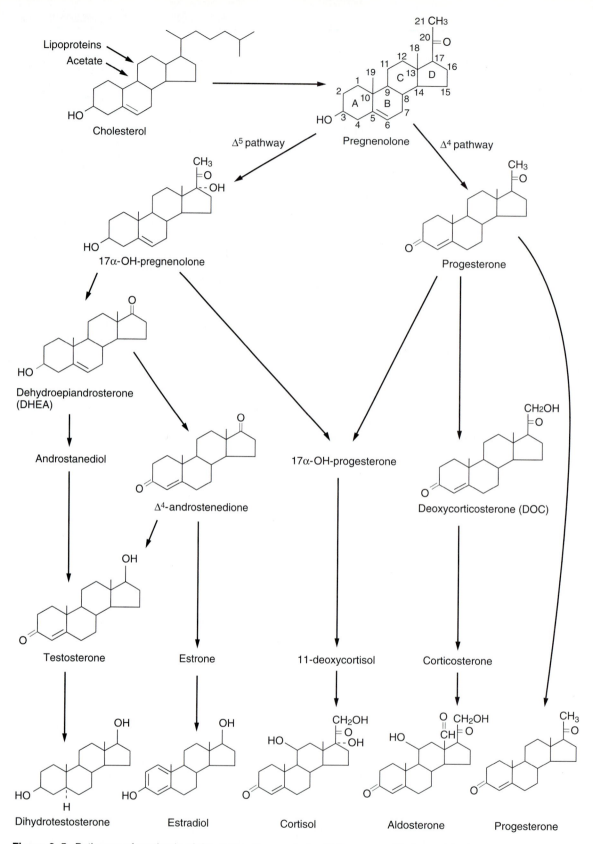

Figure 2–5. Pathways of synthesis of the major classes of steroid hormones. Cholesterol is derived from acetate by synthesis or from lipoprotein particles. The numbering of the steroid molecule is shown for pregnenolone. The major pathways thought to be used are shown. (See also Figures 9–4, 12–2, 13–4, and 14–13.)

Androgens and estrogens have two less carbons, and are therefore C-19 steroids. The different rings of the steroid structure are designated A–D, and the numbering of each carbon atom is useful in understanding how the different steroid-synthesizing enzymes modify the steroids at particular locations. All steroids have the basic cyclopentanoperhydrophenanthrene ring (four-ring) structure, and all have a single unsaturated carbon-carbon double bond except for the estrogens, in which the A ring is aromatized. Pregnenolone and other steroids called A-5 steroids have this double bond between carbons 5 and 6, while progesterone, glucocorticoids, mineralocorticoids, and androgens are called A-4 steroids and have this double bond between carbons 4 and 5.

Steroids are given both chemical and trivial names. As the chemical names are often cumbersome, trivial names are commonly used. For example, the chemical name for progesterone is pregn-4-ene-3,20-dione, cortisol is 11β,17α,21-trihydroxypregn-4-ene-3,20-dione, etc. Chemical names are given in a particular order: hydroxyl groups, aldehyde groups, core ring structure, and aldehydes or ketones. The core ring structure is given a name based on the number of carbons it contains. Thus, C-27 steroids are cholestanes, C-21 steroids are pregnanes, C-19 steroids are androstanes, and C-18 steroids are estranes. Like all chemical names, a saturated structure is given the suffix *-ane* while an unsaturated structure is given the suffix *-ene*.

In addition to the trivial names for the steroid hormones, steroids may be given a letter abbreviation. These are the names of the steroids as they were originally identified by chromatography by the chemists who first isolated and characterized them about 50 years ago. Therefore, cortisol may be called compound F; cortisone, compound E; corticosterone, compound B, etc. The trivial names and systematic names of some natural and synthetic steroids are listed in Table 2–1. (See also Chapters 9, 10, 12, and 13.)

Cholesterol Synthesis & Uptake

All steroid hormones are synthesized from the precursor cholesterol. There are three sources of cholesterol for use in steroid hormone synthesis: de novo

Table 2–1. Trivial and chemical names of some natural and synthetic steroids.

Trivial Name	(Other Names)	Chemical Name
Aldosterone	Electrocortin	11β,21-Dihydroxy-3,20-dioxo-4-pregnen-18-al
Corticosterone	Compound B	11β,21-Dihydroxy-4-pregnene-3,20-dione
Cortisol	Hydrocortisone, compound F	11β,17α,21-Trihydroxy-4-pregnene-3,20-dione
Cortisone	Compound E	17α,21-Dihydroxy-4-pregnene-3,11,20-trione
Dehydroepiandrosterone	Prasterone, DHEA	3β-Hydroxy-5-androsten-17-one
11-Deoxycorticosterone	DOC	21-Hydrox-4-pregnene-3,20-dione
11-Deoxy-17-hydroxycorticosterone	11-Deoxycortisol, cortexolone, compound S	17α,21-Dihydroxy-4-pregnene-3,20-dione
Estradiol		1,3,5(10)-Estratriene-3,17β-diol
Pregnenolone		3β-Hydroxy-5-pregnen-20-one
Progesterone		4-Pregnene-3,20-dione
Testosterone		17β-Hydroxy-4-androsten-3-one
Allopregnanolone	3α,5α-Tetrahydroprogesterone, THP	5α-Pregnan-3α-ol-20-one
Dexamethasone		9α-Fluoro-11β,17α,21-trihydroxy-16α-methylpregna-1,4-diene-3,20-dione
Betamethasone		9α-Fluoro-11β,17α,21-trihydroxy-16β-methylpregna-1,4-diene-3,20-dione
Prednisone		17α,21-Dihydroxypregna-1,4-diene-3,11,20-trione
Prednisolone		11β,17α,21-Trihydroxypregna-1,4-diene-3,20-dione
Spironolactone	Aldactone, Verospiron	4,17α-Pregnen-21-carboxylicic acid-17β-ol-3-one-7α-thiol-21,17 γ-lactone, 7-acetate
Triamcinolone		9α-Fluoro-11β,16α,17α,21-tetrahydroxypregna-1,4-diene-3,20-dione

synthesis from acetate, pools of cholesterol esters in steroidogenic tissues, and dietary sources. About 80% of the cholesterol used for steroid hormone synthesis comes from dietary cholesterol, transported in human plasma as low-density lipoprotein (LDL) particles. In rats and other species, cholesterol is transported as high-density lipoprotein (HDL) particles. Uptake of LDL cholesterol is enhanced by ACTH treatment, which increases the activity of LDL receptors and uptake of LDL cholesterol. The majority of LDL cholesterol uptake is by receptor-mediated endocytosis via coated pits, and less than 10% enters the cell independently of this mechanism. HDL cholesterol uptake, however, occurs by receptor-independent mechanisms.

Intracellular Cholesterol Storage & Transport

Several factors have been identified as being important in cholesterol mobilization within steroidogenic tissues. Cholesterol is esterified to polyunsaturated fatty acids in the endoplasmic reticulum by acyl-CoA:cholesterol acyltransferase (ACAT), and accumulated cholesteryl esters form lipid droplets. These fatty acid esters are hydrolyzed to free cholesterol by cholesteryl esterase (sterol ester hydrolase). Tissue-specific tropic hormones (eg, ACTH, LH, and FSH) stimulate the esterase and inhibit the acyltransferase, resulting in increased accumulation of free cholesterol. Some steroids, such as pregnenolone, testosterone, and estradiol, can be reesterified to form fatty acid esters. Pregnenolone fatty acid esters form biosynthetic intermediates in the synthesis of adrenal steroids, and testosterone and estradiol fatty acid esters can accumulate in target tissues and behave as endogenous long-acting androgens and estrogens.

Steroid Hormone Synthesis

The first step in steroid hormone synthesis, the conversion of cholesterol to pregnenolone, occurs in the mitochondria. However, cholesterol does not enter the mitochondria freely but rather must be carried through the cytoplasm to the inner mitochondrial membrane. Free cholesterol, which would be insoluble free in the aqueous cytoplasm, binds to sterol carrier protein 2 (SCP-2), which plays a major role in its transport to the mitochondria. Once there, cholesterol must traverse the outer mitochondrial membrane and the intermembrane space to reach the inner mitochondrial membrane, where the first steroid hydroxylating enzyme, P450scc, resides. A newly characterized protein, given the name StAR (steroidogenic acute regulator), functions to assist cholesterol in this transport.

Cytochromes P450

Most steroidogenic enzymes are members of the cytochrome P450 group of oxidases. All of these enzymes have molecular masses of about 50 kDa and contain a single heme group. They are called "P450" ("pigment" 450) because they all exhibit a characteristic absorbance at 450 nm upon reduction with carbon monoxide. The mechanism by which all the steroidogenic P450s function is identical. They all reduce atmospheric oxygen with electrons from NADPH. These electrons reach the P450 by one or more protein intermediates. For the mitochondrial P450s, two protein intermediates, adrenodoxin reductase and adrenodoxin, are involved. For the microsomal P450s, one protein intermediate, P450 reductase, is involved (Figure 2–6).

The synthesis of all steroid hormones from cholesterol involves one or more of six distinct cytochromes P450 (Figure 2–6), which are expressed in compartment- and tissue-specific patterns, thereby accounting for the differences in compartment- and tissue-specific steroids (eg, made in mitochondria versus ER, and in adrenal versus gonads versus placenta). Many of the steroid hydroxylases have multiple enzymatic activities. Purification of the proteins and cloning of the cDNAs encoding these proteins has rigorously demonstrated that these activities indeed reside within single proteins.

Neurosteroidogenesis

In the brain, the expression of the steroidogenic enzymes is developmentally and regionally regulated, ensuring the regulated synthesis of specific neurosteroids. The sites of synthesis suggest that their steroidal products may have many diverse functions. These include coordinating environmental cues and behavior, sensorimotor functions, neuronal targeting and survival, and development and organization of the nervous system.

2. VITAMIN D

The active form of vitamin D—1,25-$(OH)_2$-cholecalciferol (1,25-$[OH]_2D_3$)—is derived from vitamin D_3 (cholecalciferol; Chapter 8). Cholecalciferol is obtained either from the diet or from the conversion of 7-dehydrocholesterol (present in the skin) in response to ultraviolet irradiation via a 6,7-*cis* isomer intermediate (provitamin D). Vitamin D_2 (ergocalciferol), which is present in plants and differs from vitamin D_3 in having a double bond at C_{22} and C_{23}, a methyl group at C_{24}, and several features of the A ring of the molecule, also serves as a precursor of active vitamin D products. The ultimate vitamin D products are a mixture of compounds derived from these two compounds and can vary depending on the dietary intake (Chapter 8). Vitamins D_2 and D_3 are transported, bound to a vitamin D transport protein, to the liver, where the actions of a microsomal cytochrome P450c25 convert them to 25-hydroxy derivatives—25-OH-cholecalciferol (25-$[OH]D_3$) for vitamin D_3. 25-$(OH)D_3$ then circulates bound to an

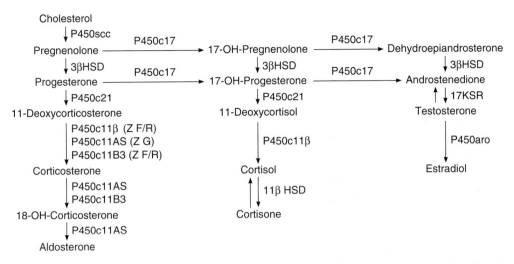

Figure 2–6. Principal steroidogenic pathways in classic endocrine tissues. Other steroids, such as steroid sulfates and lipoidal derivatives, are also produced. The names for each enzyme are shown by each reaction. P450scc, mitochondrial cholesterol side-chain cleavage enzyme, mediates 20α hydroxylation, 22 hydroxylation, and scission of the C20–22 bond; 3β HSD, a non-P450 enzyme bound to the endoplasmic reticulum, mediates both 3β-hydroxysteroid dehydrogenase and A5–A4 isomerase activities; P450c21 in the endoplasmic reticulum mediates 21-hydroxylation; P450c11β, mitochondrial 11-hydroxylase in the adrenal fasciculata-reticularis, mediates 11-hydroxylation; P450c11AS, mitochondrial aldosterone synthase in the adrenal glomerulosa, mediates 11-hydroxylation, 18-hydroxylation, and 18-oxidation; P450c11B3, mitochondrial 11,18-hydroxylase in the adrenal fasciculata-reticularis that is expressed only from day 6 to day 36 after birth; P450c17 in the endoplasmic reticulum mediates both 17α-hydroxylation and scission of the C17,20 bond; 17KSR, a non-P450 enzyme of the endoplasmic reticulum, produces testosterone, which may be converted to estradiol by P450arom in the endoplasmic reticulum, which mediates aromatization of the A ring of the steroid nucleus. 11βHSD is a non-P450 enzyme that inactivates cortisol in target organs by conversion to cortisone. (Z F/R, zonae fasciculata and reticularis; ZG, zona glomerulosa.)

α-globulin transport protein; in the proximal tubular cells of the kidney, 25-(OH)D$_3$ is converted to 1,25-(OH)$_2$D$_3$ by the actions of a mitochondrial cytochrome P450c1α (see Chapter 8). This latter step is rate-limiting for overall 1,25-(OH)$_2$D$_3$ production and is regulated chiefly by PTH and phosphate ions. States of vitamin D deficiency are best assessed by measuring 25-(OH)D$_3$ levels in serum.

3. EICOSANOIDS

Arachidonic acid is the most important and abundant precursor of the various eicosanoids in humans and is rate-limiting for eicosanoid synthesis (Figure 2–7). Arachidonic acid is formed from linoleic acid (18:2n-6; an essential fatty acid) in most cases through desaturation and elongation to homo-γ linoleic acid (20:5n-3) and subsequent desaturation. Whereas eicosanoids are not stored by cells, arachidonic acid precursor stores are present in membrane lipids, from which it is released in response to various stimuli through actions of phospholipases. Phospholipase A$_2$ or both phospholipase C and diglyceride lipase catalyze the cleavage of esterified arachidonic acid from the 2 position of glycerophospholipids in the lipid bilayer of the cell (Figure 2–7).

The lipid content of the various cells differs, and this results in different patterns of eicosanoid production from different cell types. Phospholipase A$_2$ activity in vitro can be strongly inhibited by glucocorticoids through the induction of proteins called lipocortins; this may contribute to glucocorticoid suppression of certain inflammatory reactions, but the importance of this block in humans is not established.

Arachidonic acid can be converted to the endoperoxide prostaglandin H$_2$, which is the precursor to the prostaglandins, prostacyclins, and thromboxanes, or it can be acted on by other lipoxygenases to form the leukotrienes and other eicosanoids such as HETE. For prostaglandin synthesis, cyclooxygenase (also called endoperoxide synthetase) converts arachidonic acid to the unstable endoperoxide PGG$_2$, which is rapidly reduced to PGH$_2$. Cyclooxygenase is widely distributed throughout the body (except for erythrocytes and lymphocytes) and is inhibited by aspirin, indomethacin, and other nonsteroidal anti-inflammatory agents. In some tissues, PGH$_2$ can be converted to other prostaglandins (eg, PGD$_2$, PGE$_2$, PGF$_2$ [via PGE$_2$]) in reactions involving prostaglandin synthetases. Similarly, prostacyclin synthetase, which is prevalent in endothelial and smooth muscle cells, fibroblasts, and macrophages, can convert PGH$_2$ to prostacyclins, and thromboxane synthetase, prevalent

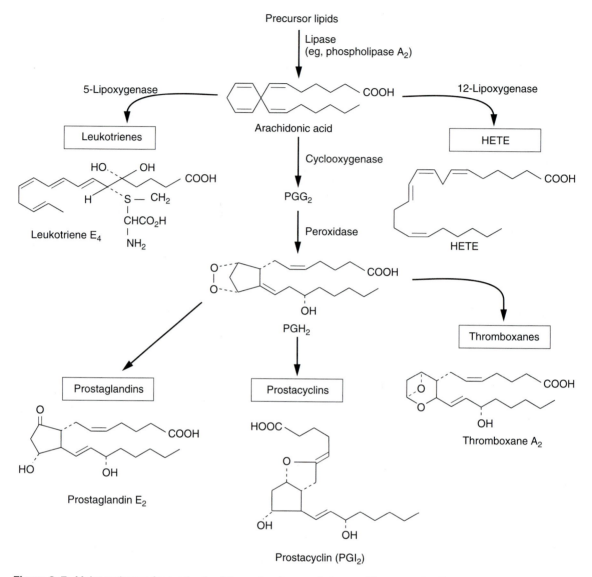

Figure 2–7. Major pathways for synthesis of the major classes of eicosanoids: prostaglandins, prostacyclins, thromboxanes, and leukotrienes. All steps in the pathways are not shown. Below each pathway, enclosed by boxes, is a representative compound of the class. (HETE, hydroxyeicosatetraenoic acid; PGG_2, prostaglandin G_2; PGH_2, prostaglandin H_2.)

in platelets and macrophages, can convert PGH_2 to thromboxanes (eg, thromboxane A_2. Arachidonic acid metabolism by 5-lipoxygenase results in leukotriene production, and metabolism by 12-lipoxygenase results in 12HPETE (hydroxyperoxy-eicosatetraenoic acid) that is converted to HETE. Arachidonic acid can also be oxygenated by cytochrome P450 monoxygenases to various omega oxidation products and epoxides and derivatives that may have biologic activities.

Historically, it has been believed that prostaglandins, like steroids, simply diffused across membranes. Recently, however, a prostaglandin transporter has been identified, suggesting specific uptake of these products by target tissues.

METABOLISM, TRANSPORT, ELIMINATION, & REGULATION OF HORMONES

Hormones circulate both free and bound to plasma proteins. There are major differences between the various hormones in the extent of their association with the plasma proteins. In general, the binding of hormones to plasma is through noncovalent interactions, although cholesterol is considered to be bound through ester bonds to phosphatidylcholine. However, even in this case, the esterified cholesterol is bound through hydrophobic interactions to the lipoprotein particles.

Metabolism of
Polypeptide Hormones

Most polypeptide hormones circulate at low concentrations unbound to other proteins, although there are exceptions. For example, there are several different IGF-1-binding proteins that bind IGF-1. Vasopressin and oxytocin are bound to neurophysins. Growth hormone binds to a protein that is identical to the hormone-binding portion of the growth hormone receptor.

In general, peptide hormones have short half-lives (a few minutes) in the circulation, as occurs with ACTH, insulin, glucagon, PTH, and the releasing hormones. As has been said, the glycosylated glycoprotein hormones are more stable, and chorionic gonadotropin has a half-life of several hours. Although there may be some degradation of the hormone by proteases in the circulation, the major mechanism for hormone degradation is binding by cell surface receptors for the hormone or through non-receptor cell surface hormone-binding sites, with subsequent uptake into the cell (internalization; see below) and degradation by enzymes in the cell membrane or inside the cell. A number of specific enzymes mediate these processes, which differ for the various hormones. In addition, several steps may be involved. The first of these may inactivate the hormone, and this can be due—eg, in the case of insulin—to reduction of disulfide bonds in the protein. An important overall source for these enzymes is the lysosome, which may fuse with endocytosed vesicles to expose its enzyme contents and its acid environment to the internalized hormone-receptor complex. An advantage of the short circulating half-lives of some classes of hormones is that the duration of the response can be relatively short. In addition, the persistent presence of significant levels of many classes of hormones that act on the cell surface results in down-regulation of the responsiveness to the hormone that may not be desirable.

Metabolism of Steroid Hormones
& Vitamin D

All of the steroid hormones are bound to plasma proteins to some extent, with high-affinity binding to specific globulins and relatively low-affinity and nonspecific binding to proteins such as albumin. The major specific binding proteins are corticosteroid-binding globulin (CBG; transcortin), which binds both cortisol and progesterone, and sex hormone-binding globulin (SHBG), which binds testosterone and estradiol (testosterone more tightly than estradiol). These proteins are present in sufficient concen-

trations so that over 90% of the total cortisol and about 98% of the testosterone and estradiol are bound. The levels of their binding capacities in some cases exceed only slightly the normal concentrations of the steroid, so that with higher levels a much higher proportion of the hormone can be free. For example, the CBG capacity for cortisol is about 25 mg/dL (690 nmol/L). Aldosterone does not bind to a specific protein, with the result that only about 50% of the plasma aldosterone is bound. Vitamin D circulates mostly bound to vitamin D-binding protein. This protein binds $25\text{-}(OH)D_3$ more tightly than $1,25\text{-}(OH)_2D_3$ or vitamin D_3.

The hydrophobic steroid hormones and the D vitamins are filtered by the kidney and generally reabsorbed. For example, about 1% of the cortisol produced daily ends up in the urine. These compounds are ordinarily handled by metabolizing them to inactive species and to more water-soluble forms that are more effectively eliminated. The free steroid fraction is accessible to metabolic inactivation. The inactivations are accomplished by converting hydroxyl groups to keto groups, reducing double bonds, and conjugating the steroids with glucuronide and sulfate groups. Over 50 different steroid metabolites have been described.

The production of active hormones by metabolism in peripheral tissues, as is seen with androgens, estrogens, and vitamin D, is discussed above in the section on hormone synthesis. In addition, metabolism in peripheral tissues can direct the type of steroid that binds to the receptor. Aldosterone is ordinarily the major mineralocorticoid hormone responsible for the salt-retaining actions of the steroid hormones. This steroid binds to the mineralocorticoid receptor only about ten times more tightly than cortisol, whose total and free concentrations in the circulation are about 1000 times and 100 times (respectively) those of aldosterone; thus, cortisol should ordinarily be the main occupant of the mineralocorticoid receptors. This in fact occurs in tissues such as the brain and pituitary, but in the kidney, cortisol is avidly converted to the essentially inactive cortisone and perhaps other species; some types of licorice or congenital defects can block the conversion and result in a mineralocorticoid excess state that is due to cortisol (Chapter 10).

Metabolism of Thyroid Hormones

Thyroid hormones circulate bound to plasma proteins such that 0.04% of the T_4 and 0.4% of the T_3 are free. About 68% of the T_4 and 80% of the T_3 are bound by the glycoprotein thyroid hormone-binding globulin (TBG). About 11% of the T_4 and 9% of the T_3 are bound to transthyretin (thyroid hormone-binding prealbumin; TBPA). The remainder is bound to albumin.

The metabolism of thyroid hormones is discussed in Chapter 7. The circulating halflives of T_4 (7 days) and T_3 (about 1 day) are longer than for most hormones. These differences are due to the higher affinity of T_4 than T_3 for TBG. The hormones are degraded to inactive forms by microsomal deiodinases. The type I 5'deiodinase is prevalent in most peripheral tissues, including liver and kidney, and is responsible for most of the production of T_3. A type II 5'-deiodinase present in the pituitary and central nervous system is involved in generating T_3 for feedback inhibition of TSH release. The 5'-deiodinases also convert reverse T_3 (3,3',5'-L-triiodothyronine) to 3,3'-T_2 (3,3'-diiodothyronine). 5-Deiodinases act on T_4 to generate reverse T_3 and on T_3 to generate 3,3'-T_2. Deaminations and decarboxylations of the alanine side chains as well as conjugations with glucuronic acid and sulfate groups are also involved in degrading thyroid hormones. (See Chapter 7.)

Metabolism of Catecholamines

The metabolism of the catecholamines is discussed in Chapter 11. These compounds are cleared rapidly, with half-lives of 1–2 minutes. Clearance is primarily by cellular uptake and metabolism, and only about 2–3% of the norepinephrine that enters the circulation is excreted in the urine. Furthermore, a significant amount of the catecholamine metabolites in the circulation reflect catecholamines whose degradation occurred within adrenergic neuron terminals, a point of importance for interpreting clinical data. The catecholamines are degraded by two principal routes, catechol-O-methyltransferase (COMT) and monoamine oxidase (MAO). The measurement of some of the metabolites—normetanephrine, metanephrine, and vanillylmandelic acid (VMA)—can be useful in evaluating cases of possible catecholamine overproduction.

Metabolism of Eicosanoids

Prostaglandins are rapidly metabolized within seconds by enzymes that are widely distributed. Prominent in the metabolism is oxidation of the 15-hydroxyl group of the prostaglandin that renders the molecule inactive. Subsequent other reactions involve both oxidations and reductions.

Regulation of Hormone Binding Proteins in Plasma

The levels of the plasma binding proteins can vary with both disease states and drug therapy. For example, CBG, SHBG, and TBG levels are increased by estrogens. SHBG levels are increased by thyroid hormones, and SHBG and TBG levels are decreased by androgens.

An understanding of the roles of plasma binding of hormones is just emerging. In general, the hormones are sufficiently soluble to circulate unassociated at levels at which they are highly active. Cholesterol may be an exception if it is considered a hormone. With the steroid and thyroid hormones, deficiency states characterized by genetic defects with very low levels of transport proteins are not associated with clinical abnormalities. Recently, the transthyretin gene, which encodes the protein responsible for most of the thyroid hormone binding in the plasma of mice, was deleted in the species and the animals were phenotypically normal. Thus, there is no evidence that these binding proteins are essential.

In most cases, it is the free hormone that is active; the free levels of the hormone are responsible for the feedback and related regulatory influences that control hormone release (see below); the free levels of hormones are related to the rates of their clearance; and clinical states correlate best with the free levels of hormones. The latter is a critical consideration in many cases, as with states of adrenal or thyroid hormone excess and deficiency. With these hormones, factors that affect the levels of plasma binding proteins can spuriously elevate or depress the total hormone levels in otherwise normal individuals, or the changes could mask pathologic hormone excess or deficiency states. These considerations are discussed in Chapters 7 and 9. However, transport proteins may greatly facilitate an even delivery of hormones to the target tissues. In a tissue such as the liver, for example, a hormone that is totally free would be completely sequestered as the blood flows through the proximal portions of the tissue, whereas if it were mostly bound, the free hormone would be sequestered in proximal portions and additional hormone would be available for more distal portions through the dissociation of plasma-bound hormone to facilitate more even delivery. With polypeptide hormones, plasma binding can increase the half-life of the hormone in the circulation; it may also facilitate its delivery into the target tissues.

Overall Regulation of the Endocrine System

The effective concentration of a hormone is determined by the rates of its production, delivery to the target tissue, and degradation. All of these processes are finely regulated to achieve the physiologic level of the hormone. However, the importance of the steps may differ in some cases. By far the most highly regulated process is hormone production. With many classes of hormones, the short half-lives of the hormones provide means of terminating the responses and thus preventing excessive responses. The latter are also blunted by negative regulation of both hormone responsiveness (discussed below) and release, as well as by other factors. For example, in stress, glucocorticoids produced in excess probably blunt the actions of a number of hormones that would otherwise be harmful (Chapter 9). Thus, when the actions and half-lives of the hormones are short, the hormone response can be terminated by simply stopping release of the hormone. An exception is thyroid hormone, with its long half-life. Details of the controls of the individual systems are provided in later chapters.

There are a number of different patterns of regulation of hormone release. Many hormones are linked to the hypothalamic-pituitary axis (discussed in detail in the section on neuroendocrinology; Figure 5–10). These involve both classic feedback loops by hormones that are released by peripheral glands (cortisol, thyroid hormone, etc) and more subtle control, as is seen with GH and PRL. However, many other systems are more free-standing. This is illustrated by the parathyroid glands (Chapter 8) and by the pancreatic islets (Chapter 18). With the parathyroid glands, the Ca^{2+} concentration that is increased in the plasma by the hormone exerts a dominant feedback inhibition on the release of PTH. With insulin, depression of glucose levels in response to insulin action results in cessation of the stimulus to release more insulin. In addition, in both cases, the release of the hormone and the overall state of the gland are influenced by numerous other factors.

The stimuli to regulate hormone production include essentially all of the types of regulatory molecules, including hormones such as the tropic hormones and counterregulatory hormones (discussed above), traditional growth factors, eicosanoids, and ions. For example, potassium ion is an important regulator of the adrenal zona glomerulosa. The production of the various eicosanoids is regulated by local factors acting on the cells in which these products are released. For example, tropic stimulation of most endocrine glands results in enhancement of eicosanoid production.

The production of hormones is regulated at multiple levels. First, synthesis of the hormone can be regulated at the level of transcription, as is commonly seen with the polypeptide hormones or the enzymes involved in the synthesis of other hormones such as the steroids. It can also be affected by posttranscriptional mechanisms. Second, release of the hormone stored in secretory granules from tissues that contain the regulated secretory pathway is regulated by secretagogues, as was discussed in the section on hormone synthesis. The secretory cells can store the peptide hormones in sufficient quantity so that the amount released over a short period can exceed the rate of synthesis of the hormone. And third, stimulation of endocrine glands by tropic hormones and other substances such as growth factors can increase the number and size of cells that are actively producing the hormone.

REFERENCES

Alberts B et al: *Molecular Biology of the Cell,* 3rd ed. Garland, 1994.

Baranski TJ et al: Generation of a lysosomal enzyme targeting signal in the secretory protein pepsinogen. Cell 1990;63:281.

Burgoyne RD, Morgan A: Ca^{2+} and secretory-vesicle dynamics. Trends Neurosci 1995;18:191.

Cool DR et al: Identification of the sorting signal motif within proopiomelanocortin for the regulated secretory pathway. J Biol Chem 1995;270:8723.

Crowley KS et al: Secretory proteins move through the endoplasmic reticulum membrane via an aqueous, gated pore. Cell 1994;78:461.

Dunphy W, Rothman JE: Compartmental organization of the Golgi stack. Cell 1995;42:13.

Gorlich D, Rapoport TA: Protein translocation into proteoliposomes reconstituted from purified components of the endoplasmic reticulum membrane. Cell 1993;75:615.

Hann BC, Walter P: The signal recognition particle in *S cerevisiae.* Cell 1991;67:131.

Hebert DN et al: Glucose trimming and reglucosylation determine glycoprotein association with calnexin in the ER. Cell 1995;81:425.

Hinshaw JE, Schmid SL: Dynamin self-assembles into rings suggesting a mechanism for coated vesicle budding. Nature 1995;374:190. (N)

Ikonen E et al: Different requirements for NSF, SNAP and Rab proteins in apical and basolateral transport in MDCK cells. Cell 1995;81:571.

Kanai N et al: Identification and characterization of a prostaglandin transporter. Science 1995;268:866.

Lingappa VR: More than just a channel: Provocative new features of protein traffic across the ER membrane. Cell 1991;65:527.

Mellman I, Simons K: The Golgi complex: in vitro veritas? Cell 1992;68:829.

Mellon SH: Neurosteroids: Biochemistry, modes of action, and clinical relevance. J Clin Endocrinol Metab 1994;78:1003.

Miller WL: Molecular biology of steroid hormone synthesis. Endocr Rev 1988;9:295.

Ohashi M et al: A role for phosphatidylinositol transfer protein in secretory vesicle formation. Nature 1995; 377:544.

Omura T, Morohashi K: Gene regulation of steroidogenesis. J Steroid Biochem Mol Biol 1995;53:19.

Rothman JE: Mechanism of intracellular protein transport. Nature 1994;372:55.

Simon S, Blobel G: A protein conducting channel in the ER. Cell 1991;65:371.

Sudhof TC: The synaptic vesicle cycle: A cascade of protein-protein interactions. Nature 1995;375:645.

Walter P, Johnson AE: Signal sequence recognition and protein targeting to the endoplasmic reticulum membrane. Annu Rev Cell Biol 1994;10:87.

White PC: Genetic diseases of steroid metabolism. Vitam Horm 1994;49:131.

3

Mechanisms of Hormone Action

David G. Gardner, MD

Hormones produce their biologic effects through interaction with high-affinity receptors which are, in turn, linked to one or more effector systems within the cell. These effectors involve many different components of the cell's metabolic machinery, ranging from ion transport at the cell surface to stimulation of the nuclear transcriptional apparatus. Steroids and thyroid hormones exert their effects in the cell nucleus, although regulatory activity in the extranuclear compartment has also been documented. Peptide hormones and neurotransmitters, on the other hand, trigger a plethora of signaling activity in the cytoplasmic and membrane compartments while at the same time exerting parallel effects on the transcriptional apparatus. The discussion that follows will focus on the primary signaling systems employed by selected hormonal agonists and attempt to identify examples where aberrant signaling results in human disease.

RECEPTORS

The biologic activity of individual hormones is dependent upon their interactions with specific high-affinity receptors on the surfaces of target cells. The receptors, in turn, are linked to signaling effector systems responsible for generating the observed biologic response. Receptors therefore convey not only specificity of the response (ie, cells lacking receptors lack responsivenss to the hormone) but also the means for activating the effector mechanism. In general, receptors for the peptide hormones and neurotransmitters are aligned on the cell surface while those for the steroid hormones, thyroid hormone, and vitamin D are found in the cytoplasmic or nuclear compartments.

Interactions between the hormone ligand and its receptor are governed by the laws of mass action:

$$[H] + [R] \underset{k_{-1}}{\overset{k_{+1}}{\rightleftarrows}} [HR]$$

where [H] is the hormone concentration, [R] is the receptor concentration, [HR] is the concentration of the hormone-receptor complex and k_{+1} and k_{-1} are the rate constants for [HR] formation and dissociation respectively. Thus, at equilibrium,

$$k_{+1}[H][R] = k_{-1}[HR]$$

or

$$\frac{[H][R]}{[HR]} = \frac{k_{-1}}{k_{+1}} = K_D$$

where K_D is the equilibrium dissociation constant which defines the affinity of the hormone-receptor interaction (ie, the lower the dissociation constant, the higher the affinity). Assuming that total receptor concentration $R_o = [HR] + [R]$, this equation can be rearranged to give

$$\frac{[HR]}{[H]} = -\left(\frac{[HR]}{K_D}\right) + \frac{R_o}{K_D}$$

This is the Scatchard equation and states that when bound over free ligand (ie, [HR]/[H]) is plotted against bound ligand (ie, [HR]), the slope of the line is defined by $-1/K_D$, the y-intercept by R_o/K_D and the x-intercept by R_o (Figure 3–1). When [HR] = $R_o/2$, [H] = K_D; therefore, the K_D is also the concentration of hormone [H] at which one-half of the available receptors are occupied. Thus, knowledge of bound and free ligand concentrations, which can be determined experimentally, provides information regarding the affinity of the receptor for its ligand and the total concentration of receptor in the preparation.

Agents that bind to receptors with high affinity are classified as either agonists or antagonists based on the functional outcome of this receptor-ligand interaction. Agonists are ligands that trigger the effector mechanisms and produce biologic effects. Antagonists bind to the receptor but do not activate the effector mechanisms. Since they occupy receptor and block association with the agonist, they antagonize the functional activity of the latter. Partial agonists bind to the recep-

ACRONYMS USED IN THIS CHAPTER

ACTH	Adrenocorticotropin
βARK	β-Adrenergic receptor kinase
cAMP	Cyclic adenosine-3′,5′-monophosphate
cGMP	Cyclic guanosine-3′,5′-monophosphate
CNP	C-type natriuretic peptide
CREB	cAMP response element-binding protein
DAG	Diacylglycerol
EGF	Epidermal growth factor
ER	Estrogen receptor
ERK	Extracellular signal-regulated kinase
FAD	Flavin adenine dinucleotide
FGF	Fibroblast growth factor
FMN	Flavin mononucleotide
GAP	GTPase-activating protein
GDP	Guanosine diphosphate
GH	Growth hormone
GR	Glucocorticoid receptor
GRB2	Growth factor receptor-bound protein-2
GRH	Growth hormone-releasing hormone
GTP	Guanosine triphosphate
HRE	Hormone response element
HSP	Heat shock protein
IGF	Insulin-like growth factor
IP_3	Inositol 1,4,5-trisphosphate
IP_4	Inositol 1,3,4,5-tetrakis-phosphate
JAK	Janus kinase
LH	Luteinizing hormone
MAPK	Mitogen-activated protein kinase
MR	Mineralocorticoid receptor
MSH	Melanocyte-stimulating hormone
NPR	Natriuretic peptide receptor
PDGF	Platelet-derived growth factor
PIP_2	Phosphoinositol bisphosphate
PKA	cAMP-dependent protein kinase
PKC	Protein kinase C
PKG	cGMP-dependent protein kinase
PLC_β	Phospholipase C beta
PLC_γ	Phospholipase C gamma
PLC_{PC}	Phosphatidylcholine-selective phospholipase
PR	Progesterone receptor
PTH	Parathyroid hormone
RAR	Retinoic acid receptor
RE	Response element
RSK	Ribosomal S6 kinase
RXR	Retinoid X receptor
SIE	sis-inducible element
SOS	Son-of-sevenless
SR	Steroid receptor
SRE	Serum response element
SRF	Serum response factor
TAF	TBP associated factor
TBP	TATA binding protein
TFIIB	Transcription factor IIB
TPA	12-0-Tetradecanoyl-phorbol 13-acetate
TR	Thyroid hormone receptor
TRE	TPA response element
TSH	Thyroid-stimulating hormone
V2	Type 2 vasopressin receptor
VDR	Vitamin D receptor

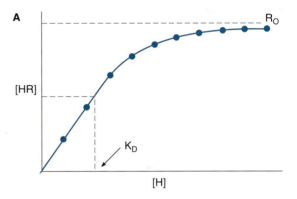

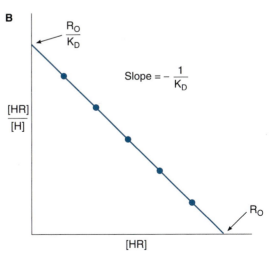

Figure 3–1. Ligand saturation **(A)** and Scatchard analysis **(B)** of a hypothetical hormone receptor interaction. K_D represents the dissociation constant; R_o the total receptor concentration; [HR] and [H] the bound and free ligand, respectively. Note in **A** that the K_D is the concentration [H] at which half of available receptors are occupied.

tor but possess limited ability to activate the effector mechanisms. In different circumstances, partial agonists demonstrate variable biologic activity. For example, when employed alone, they may display weak activating activity, whereas their use together with a full agonist may lead to inhibition of function since the latter is displaced from the receptor molecule by a ligand with lower intrinsic activity.

In some systems, receptors are available in a surplus which is severalfold higher than that required to elicit a maximal biologic response. Such spare receptor systems, though they superficially appear redundant, are designed to rectify a mismatch between low circulating ligand levels and a relatively low affinity ligand-receptor interaction. Thus, by increasing the number of available receptors, the system is guaranteed a sufficient number of liganded receptor units to activate downstream effector systems fully, despite operating at subsaturating levels of ligand.

NEUROTRANSMITTER & PEPTIDE HORMONE RECEPTORS

As mentioned above, neurotransmitter and peptide hormones interact predominantly with receptors scattered on the plasma membrane at the cell surface. These receptors fall into four major groups (Table 3–1). The first includes the so-called serpentine or "seven-transmembrane-domain" receptors. These receptors each contain an amino terminal extracellular domain followed by seven hydrophobic amino acid segments, each of which is believed to span the membrane bilayer (Figure 3–2). The seventh of

Table 3–1. Major subdivisions of the neurotransmitter-peptide hormone receptor families. Receptors have been subdivided based on shared structural and functional similarities. (–) denotes a negative effect on cyclase activity. Abbreviations follow conventional nomenclature.

Receptor Type	Examples	
Seven-transmembrane domain	β-Adrenergic	TRH
	PTH	ACTH
	LH	MSH
	TSH	Glucagon
	GRH	Dopamine
	α_2-Adrenergic (–)	
	Somatostatin (–)	
Single-transmembrane domain Growth factor receptors	Insulin	
	IGF	
	EGF	
	PDGF	
Cytokine receptors	Growth hormone	
	Prolactin	
	Erythropoietin	
	CSF	
Guanylyl cyclase-linked receptors	Natriuretic peptides	

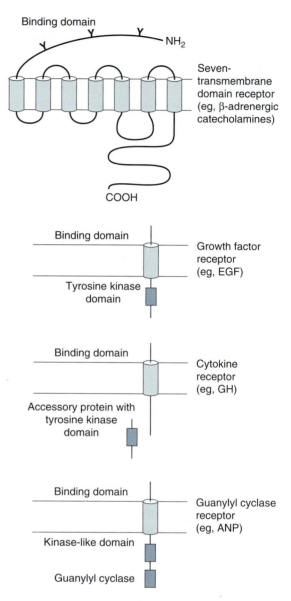

Figure 3–2. Structural schematics of different classes of membrane-associated hormone receptors. Representative ligands are presented in parentheses. (EGF, epidermal growth factor; GH, growth hormone; ANP, atrial natriuretic peptide.)

these, in turn, is followed by a hydrophilic carboxyl terminal domain that resides within the cytoplasmic compartment. As a group, they share a dependence on the G protein transducers (see below) to realize many of their biologic effects. A second group includes the single-transmembrane domain receptors that harbor intrinsic tyrosine kinase activity. This includes the insulin, IGF, and EGF receptors. A third group, which is functionally similar to the second group, is characterized by a large extracellular binding domain followed by a single membrane-spanning segment and a cytoplasmic tail. These receptors do not possess intrinsic tyrosine kinase activity but appear to function through interaction with soluble transducer molecules which do possess such activity. Prolactin and growth hormone are included in this group. A fourth group, which includes the natriuretic peptide receptors, operates through activation of a particulate guanylyl cyclase and synthesis of cGMP. The cyclase is covalently attached at the carboxyl terminal of the ligand-binding domain and thus represents an intrinsic part of the receptor molecule.

SEVEN-TRANSMEMBRANE RECEPTORS

The prototypical receptor in this group is the β-adrenergic receptor. Structurally, this receptor conforms to the schema presented in Figure 3–2. Selected amino acids within the membrane-spanning domains appear to be important for ligand recognition. The intracytoplasmic loops, particularly the third loop extending from transmembrane (TM) domain 5 to 6, as well as the carboxyl terminal tail are also important for receptor function, providing the molecular interfaces required for interaction with the G protein transducers described below. The carboxyl terminal region also harbors the substrate site for the β-adrenergic receptor kinase (βARK) which is responsible for desensitization of this receptor. Receptors for LH, ACTH, PTH, α-adrenergic agonists, dopamine, MSH, and glucagon have a structural topology similar to that described for the β-adrenergic receptor.

G PROTEIN TRANSDUCERS

The heterotrimeric G proteins link the seven-transmembrane domain receptors with the effector proteins responsible for producing changes in cellular function. These G proteins are heterogeneous (Table 3–2) with different subtypes (G_s, G_i, G_q, G_o, etc) capable of interacting not only with different types of receptors but with different effector molecules as well. The β-adrenergic receptor, for example, preferentially interacts with the heterotrimeric G protein G_s, which in turn selectively interacts with and stimulates the enzymatic effector adenylyl cyclase. Consequently, one of the most predictable effects of β-adrenergic receptor occupancy with a catecholamine ligand is stimulation of adenylyl cyclase activity and increased cellular cAMP levels. However, many receptors can interact with several different G proteins, and a given G protein may interact with a number of different receptors. The α-adrenergic receptor, for example, can interact with either G_i or G_q, which in turn couples with different effector molecules (adenylyl cyclase and phospholipase C, re-

Table 3–2. G protein subunits selectively interact with specific receptor and effector mechanisms.

G Protein Subunit	Associated Receptors	Effector
α_s	β-Adrenergic TSH Clucagon	Adenylyl cyclase Ca^{2+} channels
α_i	α_2-Adrenergic Muscarinic (type II)	Adenylyl cyclase Ca^{2+} channels K^+ channels
α_q	α_1-Adrenergic	PLCβ
β/α		Adenylyl cyclase (+ or –) PLC Supports βARK-mediated receptor phosphorylation and desensitization

spectively) to produce distinct biologic effects. Conversely, G_s interacts with LH, PTH and a number of other receptors in addition to the β-adrenergic receptor, while G_i couples to a number of different effectors (eg, adenylyl cyclase as well as G protein-coupled potassium channels in the plasma membrane). This type of flexibility in the signaling process engenders a tremendous diversity of responses which are dependent upon the types of receptors, G proteins, and effector molecules available in a particular target cell. This, together with the extensive regulatory interactions that take place between the individual signaling systems may serve to tailor an individual response to the specific needs of the target cell.

The mechanistic underpinnings of the G proteins are detailed in Figure 3–3. Each G protein consists of a GTP-GDP binding subunit, termed the α subunit, as well as two less diversified subunits, the β and γ subunits. The identity of the individual G protein is determined by the nature of the α subunit. In the quiescent state, the α subunit is bound to GDP in a trimeric complex that includes the β and γ subunits. Addition of the ligand to the relevant receptor results in association of the liganded receptor with the α subunit and dissociation of GDP and the β/γ subunits from the complex. Subsequently, GTP binds to the guanine nucleotide binding site on the α subunit, promoting dissociation of the hormone-receptor complex (as well as a reduction in the affinity of the receptor for its ligand) and "activation" of the α subunit. Activated α subunit associates with the relevant effector molecule (adenylyl cyclase, phospholipase C, etc), triggering an increase in the activity of the latter (eg, generation of cAMP from ATP or hydrolysis of phosphoinositide lipids in the membrane). The GTP is subsequently hydrolyzed to GDP, permitting the reassociation of the α and β/γ subunits and completion of the cycle. Though the β/γ subunits commonly function in an inhibitory role (ie, controlling

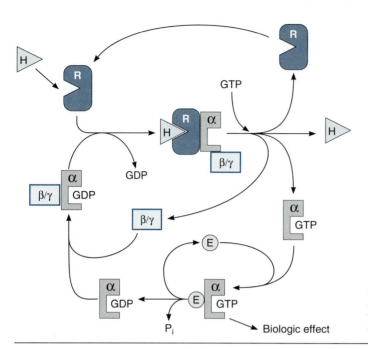

Figure 3–3. G protein-mediated signal transduction. α and β/γ subunits of a representative G protein are depicted. (R, hormone receptor; H, hormonal ligand; E, effector.)

the activity of the functional α subunit), they also appear to possess independent regulatory activity of their own, including stimulation of ion channel activity, activation of phospholipase C ($\beta2$ isoform), regulation of adenylyl cyclase, and stimulation of phosphodiesterase activity.

Specific toxins can perturb the G protein transduction system. Cholera toxin, for example, ADP-ribosylates Arg^{201} on the α subunit of G_s, resulting in a dramatic decrease in GTP hydrolysis. This results in an extremely long-lived α subunit-GTP complex that leads to persistent activation of the downstream effector, in this case adenylyl cyclase. Pertussis toxin, on the other hand, fosters ADP-ribosylation of a cysteine residue near the carboxyl terminal of the α subunit of G_i. This leads to uncoupling of the G protein mechanism and diminished activity of downstream G_i-linked effectors.

EFFECTORS

Numerous effectors have been linked to the G protein-coupled receptors. A number of these are presented in Table 3–2. There are a great many other G proteins, not dealt with here, which are coupled to physical or biochemical stimuli but have very limited involvement in hormone action. As discussed above, adenylyl cyclase, perhaps the best-studied of the group, is activated by G_s (Figure 3–4). This activation results in a transient increase in intracellular cAMP levels. cAMP binds to the inhibitory regulatory subunit of inactive protein kinase A (PKA) and promotes its dissociation from the complex, thereby permitting enhanced activity of the catalytic subunit. The latter phosphorylates a variety of cellular substrates, among them the hepatic phosphorylase kinase that initiates the enzymatic cascade which results in enhanced glycogenolysis and the nuclear transcription factor CREB (cAMP response element binding protein), which mediates many of the known transcriptional responses to cAMP (and to some extent calcium) in the nuclear compartment. Other transcription factors are also known to be phosphorylated by PKA.

Phospholipase C beta (PLC_β) is a second effector system that has been studied extensively. The enzyme is activated through G_q-mediated transduction of signals generated by a wide array of hormone-receptor complexes, including those for angiotensin II, α-adrenergic agonists, and endothelin. Activation of the enzyme leads to cleavage of phosphoinositol 4,5-bisphosphate in the plasma membrane to generate inositol 1,4,5-trisphosphate (IP_3) and diacylglycerol (Figure 3–5). The former interacts with a specific receptor present on the endoplasmic reticulum membrane to promote release of Ca^{2+} into the cytoplasmic compartment. The increased calcium, in turn, may activate protein kinases, promote secretion, or foster contractile function. Depletion of intracellular calcium pools by IP_3 results in enhanced uptake of calcium across the plasma membrane (perhaps through generation of IP_4 [1,3,4,5-tetrakisphosphate]), thereby activating a second, albeit indirect,

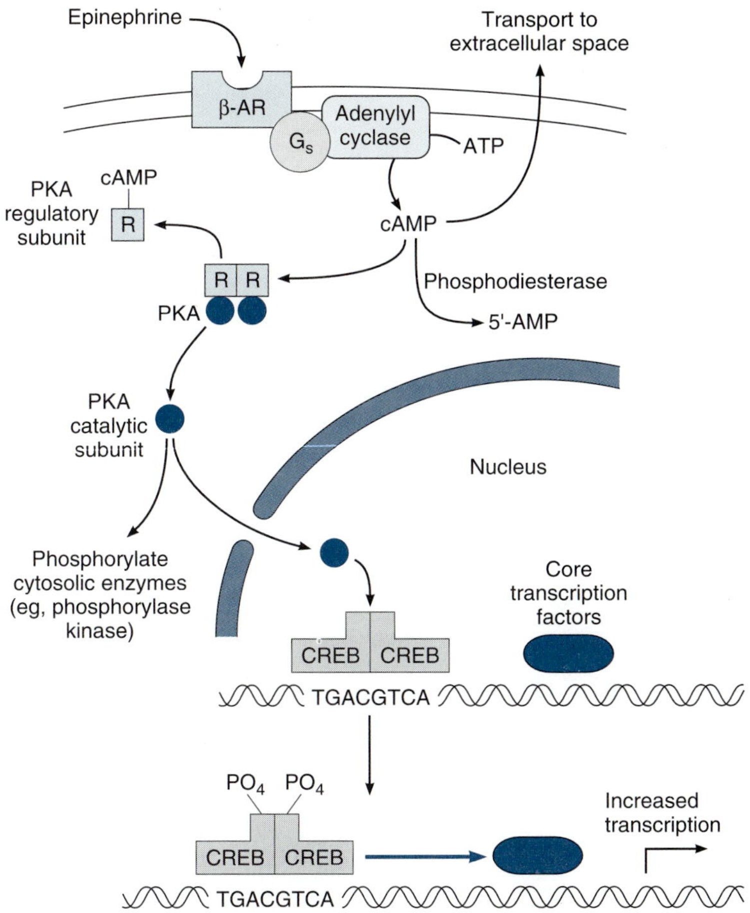

Figure 3–4. β-Adrenergic receptor signaling in the cytoplasmic and nuclear compartments. The cyclic AMP response element binding protein (CREB) is depicted bound to a consensus CRE in the basal state. Phosphorylation of this protein leads to activation of the juxtaposed core transcriptional machinery.

signaling mechanism that serves to increase intracellular calcium levels even further. Diacylglycerol (DAG) functions as an activator of protein kinase C (PKC) within the cell. Several different isoenzymatic forms of PKC (eg, α, β, γ) exist in a given cell type. A number of these are calcium-dependent, a property which, given the IP_3 activity mentioned above, provides the opportunity for a synergistic interaction of the two signaling pathways driven by PLC_β activity. However, not all protein kinase C activity derives from the breakdown of PIP_2 substrate. Metabolism of phosphatidylcholine by PLC_{PC} leads to the generation of phosphocholine and DAG. This latter pathway is believed to be responsible for the more protracted elevations in PKC activity seen following exposure to agonist. Other phospholipases may also be important in hormone-dependent signaling. Phospholipase D employs phosphatidylcholine as a substrate to generate choline and phosphatidic acid. The latter may serve as a precursor for subsequent DAG formation. As with PLC_{PC} above, no IP_3 is generated as a consequence of this reaction. Phospholipase A_2 triggers release of arachidonic acid, a precursor of prostaglandins, leukotrienes, endoperoxides, and thromboxanes, all signaling molecules in their own right. The relative contribution of these other phospholipases to hormone-mediated signal transduction and the role of the idiosyncratic products (phosphocholine, phosphatidic acid, etc) in conveying regulatory information remains an area of active research.

Following activation of the effector mechanism, additional events can be triggered that truncate the signal and protect the target cell from overstimulation by the agonist. In most cases, these events are more prominent with hormones which bind to receptors on the cell surface. They are accomplished by receptor desensitization and down-regulation as well as through modulation of postreceptor mechanisms. These processes have been best studied for the β-adrenergic receptor. In this case, desensitization, which takes place in a matter of seconds to minutes following application of agonist, is effected by cAMP-dependent phosphorylation of amino acid residues located in the cytoplasmic domain of the re-

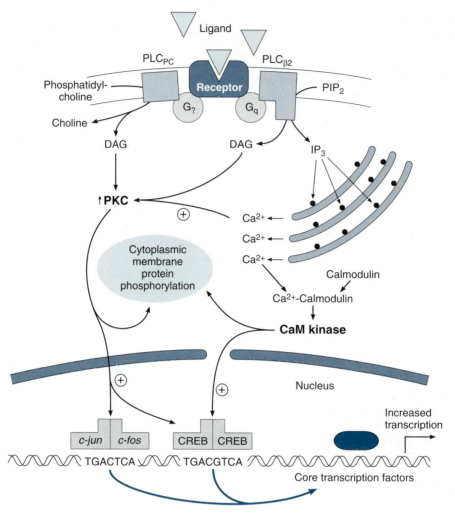

Figure 3–5. PLC$_\beta$-coupled receptor signaling in the cytoplasmic and nuclear compartments. (PLC, phospholipase; PC, phosphatidylcholine; DAG, diacylglycerol; PKC, protein kinase C.)

ceptor. These phosphorylations are carried out by the β-adrenergic receptor kinase (βARK) and, in part, by protein kinase A (PKA). They foster a rapid uncoupling of the receptor from the G$_s$ transducer protein, effectively terminating the signaling event (Figure 3–6). This abrogation of the signaling process is further amplified by a second protein, arrestin, which associates with the βARK-phosphorylated receptor and precludes further association with the G protein. The process is rapidly reversible following removal of agonist. A presumptive receptor phosphatase removes the phosphate and restores receptor sensitivity. Down-regulation of receptor levels follows continued exposure to high levels of agonist. It involves the internalization and subsequent proteolysis of receptor protein and, by definition, is not readily reversible. New protein synthesis is required to regenerate receptor on the cell surface. While at least one

component of down-regulation may be cAMP-dependent, the process appears more clearly tied to successful engagement of the G protein coupling mechanism since forskolin, which directly activates the catalytic activity of adenylyl cyclase, and exogenous cAMP only partially reproduce the effect. It is believed that this coupling may unmask an otherwise protected amino acid sequence in the receptor which targets it for internalization and subsequent destruction. Over the longer term, exposure to high levels of agonist leads to a decrease in steady-state receptor transcript levels, implying reduced synthesis of the receptor protein. Thus, the acute internalization event is followed by a reduction in new receptor synthesis to ensure that steady-state receptor levels—and therefore sensitivity to the agonist—are reduced and the target cell protected from the detrimental effects of overstimulation.

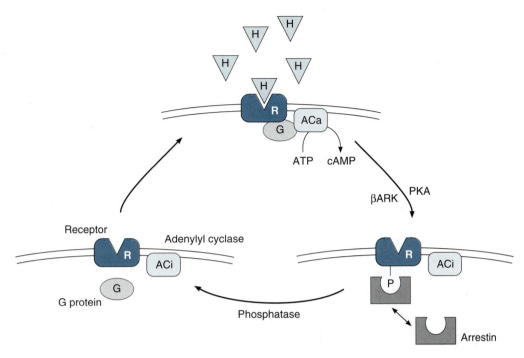

Figure 3–6. Kinase-dependent desensitization of the ligand-receptor complex. Schema shown is that for the β-adrenergic receptor, but similar systems probably exist for other types of G protein-linked receptors. (βARK identifies the β-adrenergic receptor kinase; PKA, protein kinase A; ACa, active adenylyl cyclase; ACi, inactive cyclase.)

G PROTEIN-LINKED RECEPTORS & HUMAN DISEASE

There are a number of well-documented examples where heritable or acquired defects in the peptide hormone receptors or their associated G proteins result in clinical disease. As mentioned above, the bacterial disease cholera is characterized by the production of a toxin which selectively ADP-ribosylates a key arginine residue in the α subunit of the G_s protein (Arg[201] in the 394-amino-acid protein), resulting in inhibition of intrinsic GTPase activity and constitutive activation of the associated adenylyl cyclase effector. This results in persistent transepithelial transport of chloride ion and water into the intestinal lumen, producing the watery diarrhea and severe intravascular volume contraction associated with this disease. Interestingly, a subset of growth hormone-producing pituitary tumors (ie, somatotropinomas with attendant clinical acromegaly) possess a mutation of the same arginine residue (Arg[201]) or an alternative mutation at Gln[227]. Both mutations lead to impaired GTP hydrolysis and persistent activation of the linked adenylyl cyclase. A similar activating mutation (ie, at Arg[201]) has been found in selected thyroid adenomas and in McCune-Albright syndrome, a disorder characterized by variations in skin pigmentation (ie, café au lait spots), polyostotic bone lesions, precocious puberty, thyroid adenomas, adrenal

hyperplasia, and growth hormone-producing adenomas of the pituitary gland. In this case, the defect arises early in embryogenesis, giving rise to a mosaic phenotype in the adult (ie, not all cells harbor the defective gene). Amplification of the melanocyte-stimulating hormone-, luteinizing hormone-, and GRH-dependent signaling mechanisms has been postulated to explain the pigmentation abnormalities, precocious puberty and somatotropinomas, respectively. Activating mutations of $G_{i2\alpha}$ have also been described in ovarian and adrenal tumors.

Albright's hereditary osteodystrophy, or pseudohypoparathyroidism (type I), is characterized by a number of inactivating mutations in the $G_s\alpha$ protein, including an Arg[385] to His[385] mutation that effectively uncouples the liganded receptor from the adenylyl cyclase effector. In addition to the disturbance in calcium and phosphate homeostasis seen in these patients resulting from impaired parathyroid hormone activity, there is also a reduction in TSH and LH activity, much as one might predict given the linkage of these receptors to the same G_s-dependent adenylyl cyclase mechanism. Loss of function mutations in the V2 (vasopressin), TSH, and ACTH receptors has been associated with heritable forms of nephrogenic diabetes insipidus, thyroid deficiency, and adrenal insufficiency, respectively. Activating mutations in the TSH receptor have been associated with neonatal thyrotoxicosis, while analogous activating mutations in the LH receptor have been linked to pseudo-precocious puberty and testotoxicosis, reflecting ligand-independent activation of the LH receptor on the testicular Leydig cell and consequent overproduction of the virilizing hormone testosterone. More recently, a novel mutation has been described in two unrelated male patients that resulted in a seemingly paradoxic phenotype of pseudohypoparathyroidism and testotoxicosis. These individuals appear to have a temperature-sensitive mutation in the alpha subunit of the G_s protein. At the cooler temperatures found in the scrotal testes, the mutation results in an increase in adenylyl cyclase activity and LH-independent Leydig cell stimulation (ie, testotoxicosis). However, at normal core temperature, the protein is inactivated, resulting in a phenotype suggestive of hormonal resistance similar to that seen in pseudohypoparathyroidism.

GROWTH FACTOR RECEPTORS

The growth factor receptors differ from those described above both structurally and functionally. Unlike the G protein-associated receptors, these proteins span the membrane only once and acquire their signaling ability, at least in part, through activation of tyrosine kinase activity, which is intrinsic to the individual receptor molecules. The insulin and IGF receptors fall within this group as do those for the autocrine or paracrine regulators platelet-derived growth factor (PDGF), fibroblast growth factor (FGF), and epidermal growth factor (EGF). Signaling is initiated by the association of ligand (eg, insulin) with the receptor's extracellular domain (Figure 3–7) and subsequent receptor dimerization. This results in phosphorylation of tyrosines both on the receptor itself as well as on nonreceptor substrates. It is

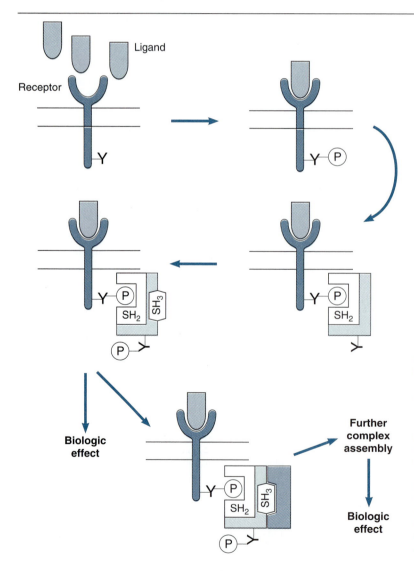

Figure 3–7. Signaling by tyrosine kinase-containing growth factor receptor. Receptors depicted here as monomers for simplicity; typically dimerization of receptors follows association with ligand. Autophosphorylation of one or more critically positioned tyrosine residues in the receptor leads to association with accessory proteins or effectors through SH2 domains present on the latter. In some cases an SH3 domain present on the same protein leads to recruitment of yet other proteins leading to further complex assembly.

assumed that phosphorylation of these substrates result in a cascade of activation events, similar to those described for the G protein-coupled systems, which contribute to perturbations in the intracellular phenotype. The autophosphorylation of the receptor molecules themselves has been studied extensively and provided some intriguing insights into the mechanisms that underlie signal transduction by this group of proteins.

Tyrosine phosphorylation takes place at specific locations in the receptor molecule. Once phosphorylated, these sites associate, in highly specific fashion, with a variety of accessory proteins that possess independent signaling capability. These include phospholipase Cγ (PLCγ), phosphoinositol (PI) 3′ kinase, GTPase-activating protein (GAP), and growth factor receptor-bound protein-2 (GRB2). These interactions are fostered by the presence of highly conserved type 2 *src* homology (based on sequence homology to the *src* proto-oncogene) domains (SH2) in each of the accessory molecules. Each individual SH2 domain displays specificity for the contextual amino acids surrounding the phosphotyrosine residues in the receptor molecule. Thus, in the PDGF receptor, for example, the SH2 domain of PLCγ associates selectively with Tyr^{977} and Tyr^{989} while that of PI 3′ kinase associates with Tyr^{708} and Tyr^{719}. Such associations may provide a means of directly activating the signaling molecule in question, perhaps through a change in steric conformation. Alternatively, they may facilitate the sequestration of these accessory proteins in or near the plasma membrane compartment, in close proximity to key substrates (eg, membrane lipids in the case of PLC_γ) or other important regulatory proteins. While some of these associations trigger immediate signaling events, others (eg, GRB2) may act largely to provide the scaffolding needed to construct a more complex signaling apparatus (Figure 3–8). In the case of GRB2, another accessory protein (son-of-sevenless; SOS) associates with the receptor-GRB2 complex through a type 3 *src* homology (SH3) domain present in the latter. This domain recognizes a sequence of proline-rich amino acids present in the SOS protein. SOS, in turn, facilitates assembly of the *ras-raf*-MEKK complex which permits activation of downstream effectors like mitogen-activated protein kinase (MAPK) kinase. This latter kinase, which possesses both serine-threonine and tyrosine kinase activity, activates the p42 and p44 MAPKs (also called extracellular signal-regulated kinases; ERKs). MAPK acts upon a variety of substrates within the cell, including the RSK kinases which, in turn, lead to phosphorylation of the ribosomal S6 protein. These phosphorylation reactions (and their amplification in those instances where the MAPK substrate is a kinase itself) often lead to protean changes in the phenotype of the target cells. Once again, diversity of response is controlled by contextual sequences around individual phosphotyrosine residues that determine the types of accessory proteins which will be brought into the signaling complex.

CYTOKINE RECEPTORS

These include the receptors for a variety of cytokines, erythropoietin, colony-stimulating factor, growth hormone, and prolactin. These receptors have a single internal hydrophobic stretch of amino acids, suggesting that they span the membrane but once (Figure 3–9). Interestingly, alternative splicing of the GH receptor gene primary transcript results in a foreshortened "receptor" that lacks the membrane anchor

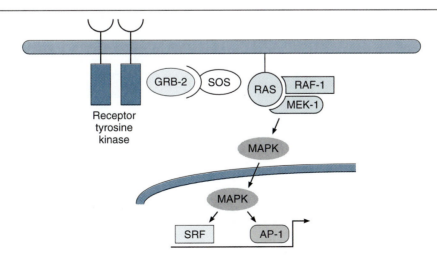

Figure 3–8. Growth factor-dependent pathway. Assembly of the components involved in the *ras/raf*/MEK/MAPK signaling mechanism.

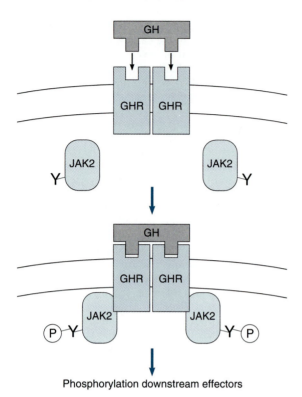

Figure 3–9. Signaling by the growth hormone receptor. Different portions of a single growth hormone molecule associate with homologous regions of two independent growth hormone receptor (GHR) molecules. This is believed to lead to the recruitment of the accessory protein JAK2 and activation of downstream effectors.

and carboxyl terminal domain of the protein. This "receptor" is secreted and serves to bind GH in the extracellular space. Unlike the growth factor receptors described above, GH receptors lack a tyrosine kinase domain. Their mechanism of action is not per-

fectly understood but may involve the participation of signaling intermediates, like JAK2, a protein that possesses intrinsic tyrosine kinase activity. The association of JAK2 with the liganded GH receptor presumably provokes a conformational change in JAK2 and activation of its tyrosine kinase catalytic activity. This, in turn, triggers downstream signaling events, including activation of MAPK and the S6 kinase (RSK) family.

GUANYLYL CYCLASE-LINKED RECEPTORS

Activation of guanylyl cyclase-dependent signaling cascades can occur through two independent mechanisms. The first involves activation of the soluble guanylyl cyclase, a heme-containing enzyme that is activated by the gas nitric oxide (NO) generated in the same or neighboring cells. NO is produced by the enzyme nitric oxide synthase. NO synthase exists as three different isozymes in selected body tissues (Figure 3–10). Constitutive forms of NO synthase are produced in endothelial and neuronal cells. The endothelial enzyme possesses binding sites for FAD and FMN as well as calcium and appears to require calcium for optimal activity. Agents like bradykinin and acetylcholine, which interact with receptors on the surface of endothelial cells and increase intracellular calcium levels, trigger an increase in constitutive NO synthase activity with consequent generation of NO and activation of soluble guanylyl cyclase activity in neighboring vascular smooth muscle cells (Figure 3–11). Thus, in this instance, the cGMP-dependent vasodilatory activity of acetylcholine requires sequential waves of signaling activity in two different cell types to realize the ultimate physiologic effect.

The inducible (i) form of NO synthase is found predominantly in inflammatory cells of the immune system although it has also been reported to be pres-

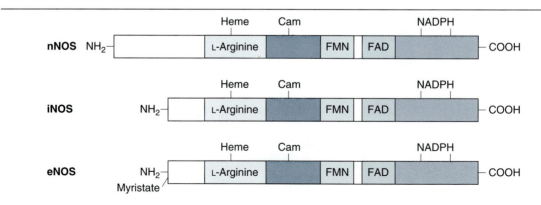

Figure 3–10. Structural schematics of the neural (n), inducible (i) and endothelial (e) forms of nitric oxide synthase (NOS). Bindings sites for calmodulin (Cam), heme, FMN, FAD, NAPDH, and the arginine substrate are indicated.

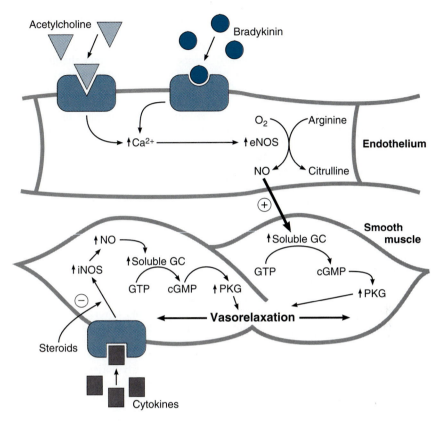

Figure 3–11. Signaling through the endothelial (e) and inducible (i) nitric oxide synthases (NOS) in the vascular wall. Activation of eNOS in the endothelial cell or iNOS in the vascular smooth muscle cell leads to an increase in NO and stimulation of soluble guanylyl cyclase (GC) activity. Subsequent elevations in cGMP activate cGMP-dependent protein kinase (PKG) and promote vasorelaxation.

ent in vascular smooth muscle cells of the vascular wall. Unlike the endothelial form of NO synthase, expression of iNO synthase is low in the basal state. Treatment of cells with a variety of cytokines triggers an increase in new iNO synthase synthesis (hence, the inducible component of iNO synthase activity), probably through activation of specific *cis* elements in the iNO synthase promoter. Thus, hormones, cytokines, or growth factors with the capacity for induction of iNO synthase activity may direct at least a portion of their signaling activity through a cGMP-dependent pathway.

A third mechanism for increasing cGMP levels within target cells involves the activation of particulate guanylyl cyclases. From an endocrine standpoint, this involves predominantly the natriuretic peptide receptors (NPR). NPR-A is a single-transmembrane-domain receptor (about 130 kDa) with a large extracellular domain that provides ligand recognition and binding. This is followed by a hydrophobic transmembrane domain and a large intracellular domain which harbors the signaling func-

tion. The amino terminal portion of this intracellular region contains a kinase-like ATP-binding domain that is involved in regulating cyclase activity while the carboxyl terminal domain contains the catalytic core of the particulate guanylyl cyclase. It is believed that association of ligand with the extracellular domain leads to a conformational change in the receptor that arrests the tonic inhibitory control of the kinase-like domain and permits activation of guanylyl cyclase activity. NPR-B, the product of a separate gene, has a similar topology and a relatively high level of sequence homology to the NPR-A gene product; however, while NPR-A responds predominantly to the cardiac atrial natriuretic peptide (ANP), NPR-B is activated by the C-type NP (CNP), a peptide found in the central nervous system, endothelium, and reproductive tissues but not in the heart. Thus, segregated expression of the ligand and its cognate receptor convey a high level of response specificity to these two systems despite the fact that they share a common final effector mechanism.

NUCLEAR ACTION OF PEPTIDE HORMONES

Although the initial targets of peptide hormone receptor signaling appear to be confined to the cytoplasm, it is clear that these receptors can also have profound effects on nuclear transcriptional activity. They accomplish this through the same mechanisms they employ to regulate enzymatic activity in the cytoplasmic compartment (eg, through activation of kinases and phosphatases). In this case, however, the ultimate targets are transcription factors that govern the expression of target genes. Examples include hormonal activation of c-*jun* and c-*fos,* nuclear transcription factors which make up the heterodimeric AP-1 complex. This complex has been shown to alter the expression of a wide variety of eukaryotic genes through association with a specific recognition element, termed the phorbol ester (TPA)-response element (TRE), present within the DNA sequence of their respective promoters. Other growth factor receptors that employ the MAPK-dependent signaling mechanism appear to target the serum response factor (SRF) and its associated ternary complex proteins. Posttranslational modification of these transcription factors is believed to amplify the signal that traffics from this complex, when associated with the cognate serum response element (SRE), to the core transcriptional apparatus. cAMP-dependent activation of protein kinase A results in the phosphorylation of a nuclear protein CREB (cAMP-response element binding protein) at Ser[119], an event which results in enhanced transcriptional activity of closely positioned promoters. Growth hormone is known to induce the phosphorylation of an 84 kDa and a 97 kDa protein in target cells. These proteins have been shown to associate with the sis-inducible element (SIE) in the c-*fos* promoter and to play a role in signaling cytokine activity which traffics through this element. It remains to be demonstrated that these proteins play a similar functional role in mediating GH-dependent effects.

NUCLEAR RECEPTORS

The nuclear receptors, which include those for the glucocorticoids, mineralocorticoids, androgens, progesterone, estrogens, thyroid hormone, and vitamin D, differ from the receptors of the surface membrane described above in that they are soluble receptors with a proclivity for employing transcriptional regulation as a means of promoting their biologic effects. Thus, though some receptors are compartmentalized in the cytoplasm (eg, glucocorticoid receptor) while others are confined to the nucleus (eg, thyroid hormone receptor), they all operate within the nuclear chromatin to initiate the signaling cascade. These receptors can be grouped into two major subtypes based on shared structural and functional properties. The first, the steroid receptor family, includes the prototypical glucocorticoid receptor (GR) and the receptors for mineralocorticoids (MR), androgens (AR), and progesterone (PR). The second, the thyroid receptor family, includes the thyroid hormone receptor (TR), estrogen (ER), retinoic acid (RAR and RXR), and vitamin D (VDR) receptors. In addition, there are more than 100 so-called orphan receptors that bear structural homology to members of the extended nuclear receptor family. For most of these the "ligand" is unknown, and their functional roles in the regulation of gene expression have yet to be determined.

STEROID RECEPTOR FAMILY

Steroid receptors (ie, GR, MR, AR, and PR), under basal conditions, exist as cytoplasmic, multimeric complexes that include the heat shock proteins hsp 90, hsp 70, and hsp 56. The estrogen receptor (ER), though demonstrating similar association with heat shock proteins, is largely confined to the nuclear compartment. Association of the steroid ligand with the receptor results in dissociation of the heat shock proteins. This in turn exposes a nuclear translocation signal previously buried in the receptor structure and initiates transport of the receptor to the nucleus, where it associates with the hormone response element (Figure 3–12).

Each of the family members has been cloned and sequenced, and consequently we know a great deal about their structure and function (Figure 3–13). Each has an extended amino terminus of varying length and limited sequence homology to other family members. This region is believed to participate in the transactivation function through which the individual receptors promote increased gene transcription. Significant variability in the length of the amino terminal regions of the different receptors suggests potential differences in their respective mechanisms for transcriptional regulation. The amino terminal is followed by a basic region that has a high degree of homology to similarly positioned regions in both the steroid and thyroid receptor gene families. This basic region encodes two zinc finger motifs (Figure 3–14) which have been shown to establish contacts in the major groove of the cognate DNA recognition element (see below). Based on crystallographic data collected for the DNA binding region of the GR, we know that the amino acid sequence lying between the first and second fingers (ie, recognition helix) is responsible for establishing specific contacts with the DNA. The second finger provides the stabilizing contacts that increase the affinity of the receptor for DNA. Following the basic region is the carboxyl terminal domain of the protein. This domain is responsible for binding of the relevant ligand, receptor dimerization or heterodimerization, and association with the heat shock proteins. It also contributes to the

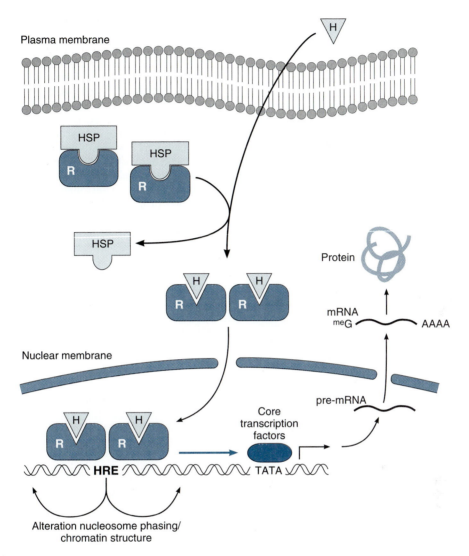

Figure 3–12. Signaling through the steroid receptor complex. Similar mechanisms are employed by members of the TR gene family, though most of the latter are concentrated in the nuclear compartment and are not associated with the heat shock protein complex prior to binding ligand. (^{me}G, methyl guanosine.)

ligand-dependent transactivation function that drives transcriptional activity. Interestingly, in selected cases, nonligands have been shown to be capable of activating steroid receptors. Dopamine activates the progesterone receptor and increases PR-dependent transcriptional activity, probably through a phosphorylation event which elicits a conformational change similar to that produced by the association of the receptor with progesterone.

The DNA-binding regions of these receptors contact DNA through a canonical hormone recognition element (HRE) which is described in Table 3–3. Interestingly, each receptor in the individual subfamily binds to the same recognition element with high affinity. Thus, specificity of hormone action must be established either by contextual DNA sequence lying outside the recognition element or by other, nonreceptor DNA-protein interactions positioned in close proximity to the element. Interestingly, the GR—and probably other steroid hormone receptors—is capable of binding to DNA sequence lacking the classic HRE. Originally described in the mouse proliferin gene promoter, these composite elements associate with heterologous complexes containing GR, as well as components of the AP-1 transcription factor complex (ie, c-*jun* and c-*fos*), and display unique regulatory activity at the level of contiguously positioned promoters. One such composite element, for example, directs very specific transcriptional effects depending on whether the GR or the MR is included in the complex.

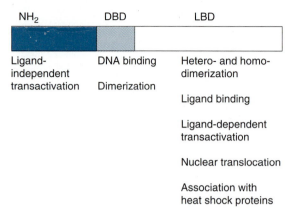

NH₂   DBD   LBD

Ligand-independent transactivation	DNA binding	Hetero- and homo-dimerization
	Dimerization	Ligand binding
		Ligand-dependent transactivation
		Nuclear translocation
		Association with heat shock proteins

Figure 3–13. Structural schematic of a representative steroid receptor molecule. Separate designations are given to the amino terminal (NH$_2$), DNA-binding (DBD) and ligand-binding (LBD) domains. Functional activity associated with each of these individual domains, as determined by mutagenesis studies, are indicated below.

Several steroids, particularly the glucocorticoids and estrogens, have been reported to have independent effects on the stability of target gene transcripts. At this point it is unclear what role the hormone receptors play in this process and whether transcript stabilization is tied mechanistically to the enhancement of transcriptional activity.

THYROID RECEPTOR FAMILY

Included in this group are the thyroid hormone receptor, the retinoic acid receptors, the estrogen receptor, and the vitamin D receptor. They share a high degree of homology to the proto-oncogene c-*erb*A and high affinity for a common DNA recognition site (Table 3–3). With the exception of the ER, they do not associate with the heat shock proteins, and they are constitutively bound to chromatin in the cell nucleus. Specificity of binding for each of the individual receptors is, once again, probably conferred by a contextual sequence surrounding this element, the orientation of the elements (eg, direct repeats or inverted repeats or palindromes), the polarity (ie, 5′ in contrast to 3′ position on two successive repeats), and the number and nature of the spacing nucleotides separating the repeats.

The estrogen receptor binds to its RE as a homodimer, while the VDR, RAR, RXR, and TR prefer binding as heterodimers. The nature of the heterodimeric partners has provided some intriguing insights into the biology of these receptors. The most prevalent TR-associated partners appear to be the retinoid X receptors. These receptors, which form high-affinity associations with 9-*cis* retinoic acid, also form heterodimeric complexes with VDR and RAR. In individual cases where it has been examined, heterodimerization with RXR amplifies both the DNA binding and the functional activity of these

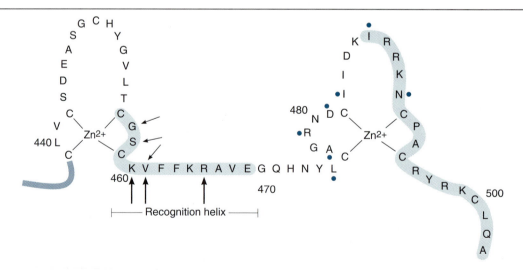

Figure 3–14. Schema of the two zinc fingers, together with coordinated zinc ion, which make up the DNA-binding domain of the glucocorticoid receptor (amino acids are numbered relative to the full length receptor). Shaded regions denote two alpha helical structures which are oriented perpendicularly to one another in the receptor molecule. The first of these, the recognition helix, makes contact with bases in the major groove of the DNA. Large arrows identify amino acids which contact specific bases in the glucocorticoid response element (GRE). Lighter arrows identify amino acids that confer specificity for the GRE; selective substitutions at these positions can shift receptor specificity to other response elements. Dots identify amino acids making specific contacts with the phosphate backbone of DNA. (Modified from Luisi BF et al. Reprinted, with permission, from Nature 1991;352:498. Copyright © Macmillan Magazines Ltd.)

Table 3–3. DNA recognition elements for major classes of nuclear hormone receptors. Elements represent consensus sequences selected to emphasize the modular nature of the half-sites and their capacity for palindrome generation. Sequences read in the 5′ to 3′ direction. N denotes a spacer nucleoside (either A, G, C, or T). Half-sites are identified by the overlying arrows. The TRE is arrayed as a direct repeat but may also exist as a palindrome or an inverted palindrome. A variable number of spacer nucleotides are positioned between the two direct repeats, depending on the type of hormone receptor. Three, four, and five nucleosides (ie, n = 3, 4, or 5) are preferred for binding of the VDR, TR, or RAR, respectively.

Element	Recognition Sequence	Receptor
HRE	$\xrightarrow{\hspace{1cm}}$ $\xleftarrow{\hspace{1cm}}$ AGAACANNNTGTTCT	Glucocorticoid Mineralocorticoid Progesterone Androgen
ERE	$\xrightarrow{\hspace{1cm}}$ $\xleftarrow{\hspace{1cm}}$ AGGTCANNNTGACCT	Estrogen
TRE	$\xleftarrow{\hspace{1cm}}$ $\xleftarrow{\hspace{1cm}}$ AGGTCA(N)$_n$AGGTCA	Vitamin D Thyroid hormone Retinoic acids

liver, kidney, and central nervous system. They are believed to signal most of the developmental and thermogenic effects of thyroid hormone in the whole animal. TR β2, a splice variant of the TR β gene, is found in the rodent pituitary gland, where it may subserve a specific regulatory function (eg, control of TSH secretion). TR α2, an alternatively spliced product of the TR α gene, lacks the hormone binding domain at the carboxyl terminal of the molecule and thus is not a true thyroid hormone receptor. While under certain experimental conditions TR α2 can block the activity of other members of the TR family, its physiologic role, if one exists, remains undefined. Similar heterogeneity exists in the retinoid receptor family. There are three isoforms for both the RXR and RAR. Collectively, these receptors are thought to play an important role in morphogenesis, but the function of the individual isoforms remains only poorly defined.

NONGENOMIC EFFECTS OF THE STEROID HORMONES

While steroids exert most of their biologic activity through direct genomic effects, there are several lines of evidence suggesting that this does not provide a complete picture of steroid hormone action. There are several examples which, for kinetic or experimental reasons, do not fit the classic paradigm associated with a transcriptional regulatory mechanism. Included within this group are the early water imbibition of the uterus associated with estrogen administration, the rapid suppression of ACTH secretion following steroid administration, the modulation of oocyte maturation by progesterone, and regulation of calcium channel function by 1,25-(OH)$_2$ vitamin D. While we still do not completely understand the mechanisms underlying these nongenomic effects, their potential importance in mediating steroid or thyroid hormone action may, in selected instances, approach that of their more conventional genomic counterparts.

Neurosteroids represent another class of nontraditional hormonal agonists with unique biologic activity. Some of these are native steroids (eg, progesterone), while others are conjugated derivatives or metabolites of the native steroids (eg, dihydroprogesterone). These agonists have been identified in the central nervous system and in some instances shown to have potent biologic activity. It is believed that they operate through interaction with the receptor for γ-aminobutyric acid, a molecule that increases neuronal membrane conductance to chloride ion. This has the net effect of hyperpolarizing the cellular

other receptors. Thus, the ability to form such heterodimeric complexes may add significantly to the flexibility and potency of these hormone receptor systems in regulating gene expression. Interestingly, the positioning (5′ versus 3′) of the participant proteins on the RE is important in determining the functional outcome of the association. In most of those situations linked to transcriptional activation, RXR seems to prefer the upstream (5′) position in the dimeric complex. Thus, diversity of response is engendered by the selection of recognition elements (eg, monomeric versus dimeric versus oligomeric sites) and by the choice and positioning of the dimeric partner (eg, homodimer versus heterodimer) where applicable.

The mechanism underlying SR- (or TR family member)-dependent transcriptional activation remains undefined, though in some cases physical contacts have been identified between the hormone receptors and proteins of the basal transcription complex (eg, TFIIB or TBP) in vitro. Interactions of the liganded receptors with these proteins or, perhaps, the more selective TAFs (TATA-binding protein–associated factors) may provide the requisite trigger to permit initiation and subsequent elongation of the RNA chain.

While the glucocorticoid receptor is encoded by a single gene, there are two genes for the TR (α and β). TR α1 and TR β1 appear to be the dominant forms of TR in the body. Although considerable overlap exists in their tissue distribution, TR α1 is enriched in skeletal muscle, brown fat, and the central nervous system, while TR β1 is found in the

membrane and suppressing neuronal excitability. Interactions that promote receptor activity would be predicted to produce sedative-hypnotic effects in the whole animal, while inhibitory interactions would be expected to lead to a state of central nervous system excitation.

STEROID & THYROID HORMONE RECEPTOR RESISTANCE SYNDROMES

Heritable defects in these receptors have been linked to the pathophysiology of a number of hormone resistance syndromes. These syndromes are characterized by a clinical phenotype suggesting hormone deficiency, by elevated levels of the circulating hormone ligand, and increased (or inappropriately detectable) levels of the relevant trophic regulatory hormone (eg, ACTH, TSH, FSH, or LH). Point mutations in the zinc fingers of the DNA-binding domain as well the ligand-binding domain of the vitamin D receptor leads to a form of vitamin D-dependent rickets (type II) characterized by typical rachitic bone lesions, secondary hyperparathyroidism, and alopecia. It is inherited as an autosomal recessive disorder. Molecular defects scattered along the full length of the androgen receptor, though concentrated in the ligand-binding domain, have been linked to syndromes characterized by varying degrees of androgen resistance ranging from infertility to the full-blown testicular feminization syndrome. Clinical severity, in this case, is thought to be related to the severity of the functional impairment which the mutation imposes on the receptor. Since the androgen receptor is located on the X chromosome, these disorders are inherited in an X-linked fashion. Defects in the glucocorticoid receptor are less common, perhaps reflecting the life-threatening nature of derangements in this system. However, mutations have been identified that impact negatively on receptor function. Clinical presentations in these cases have been domi-

nated by signs and symptoms referable to adrenal androgen (eg, hirsutism and sexual precocity) and mineralocorticoid (low renin hypertension) overproduction. This presumably results from defective steroid-mediated suppression of ACTH secretion and adrenal hyperplasia as ACTH rises in a futile attempt to restore glucocorticoid activity at the periphery. Resistance to thyroid hormone has been linked to a large number of mutations scattered along the full length of the β form of the receptor, although, once again, there is a concentration of mutations in the ligand-binding domain. No mutations in the α form of the receptor have been linked to a hormone-resistant phenotype. The clinical presentation of thyroid hormone resistance extends from the more typical mild attention deficit syndromes to full-blown hypothyroidism with impaired growth. Different target tissues harboring the mutant receptors display variable sensitivity to thyroid hormone, with some tissues (eg, pituitary) displaying profound resistance and others (eg, heart) responding in a fashion suggesting hyperstimulation with thyroid hormone (ie, thyrotoxicosis). These syndromes are rather unique in that they are inherited as autosomal dominant disorders, presumably reflecting the ability of the mutated receptors to interfere with receptors produced from the normal allele, either by binding to the RE with higher affinity than the wild-type receptors and precluding access of the latter to target genes or by forming inactive heterodimers with the wild-type receptor proteins. Defects in the estrogen receptor are rare, perhaps reflecting the critical role estrogens play in regulating lipoprotein metabolism. However, one male patient has been described who harbors a mutation within the ligand-binding domain of the estrogen receptor. His clinical presentation was characterized by infertility as well as osteopenia, suggesting important roles for estrogens in the maintenance of spermatogenesis as well as bone growth even in male subjects. A syndrome of mineralocorticoid resistance, or pseudohypoaldosteronism, has been described in a number of independent kindreds. The mineralocorticoid receptor appears to be structurally intact in these individuals, implying that the problem lies either with regulation of receptor levels or with events that occur downstream of the ligand-receptor interaction.

REFERENCES

G Protein-Coupled Receptors

Caron MG, Lefkowitz RJ: Catecholamine receptors: Structure, function and regulation. Rec Prog Horm Res 1993;48:277.

Clark AJL, Weber A: Molecular insights into inherited ACTH resistance syndromes. Trends Endocrinol Metab 1994;5:209.

Collins S, Caron MG, Lefkowitz RJ: From ligand bind-

ing to gene expression: New insights into the regulation of G-protein-coupled receptors. Trends Biochem Sci 1992;17:37.

Hepler JR, Gilman AG: G proteins. Trends Biochem Sci 1992;17:383.

Iiri T et al:Rapid GDP release from G$_s\alpha$ in patients with gain and loss of endocrine function. Nature 1994; 371:164.

Palczewski K, Benovic JL: G-protein-coupled receptor kinases. Trends Biochem Sci 1991;16:387.

Spiegel AM, Weinstein LS, Shenker A: Abnormalities in G protein-coupled signal transduction pathways in human disease. J Clin Invest 1993;92:1119.

Effectors

Asaoka Y et al: Protein kinase C, calcium and phospholipid degradation. Trends Biochem Sci 1992;17:414.

Balla T, Catt KJ: Phosphoinositides and calcium signaling. Trends Endocrinol Metab 1994;5:250.

Liscovitch M: Crosstalk among multiple signal-activated phospholipases. Trends Biochem Sci 1992;17:393.

Meyer TE, Habener JF: Cyclic adenosine 3',5'-monophosphate response element binding protein (CREB) and related transcription-activation deoxyribonucleic acid-binding proteins. Endocr Rev 1993; 14:269.

Sterweis PC, Smrcka AV: Regulation of phospholipase C by G proteins. Trends Biochem Sci 1992;17:502.

Tyrosine Kinase-Coupled Receptors

Mathews LS: Molecular biology of growth hormone receptors. Trends Endocrinol Metab 1991;2:176.

Mussachchio A, Wilmanns M, Saraste M: Structure and function of the SH3 domain. Prog Biophys Molec Biol 1994;61:283.

Nishida E, Gotoh Y: The MAP kinase cascade is essential for diverse signal transduction pathways. Trends Biochem Sci 1993;18:128.

Pazin MJ, Williams LT: Triggering signaling cascades by receptor tyrosine kinases. Trends Biochem Sci 1992;17:374.

Pelech SL, Sanghera JS: Mitogen-activated protein kinases: versatile transducers for cell signaling. Trends Biochem Sci 1992;17:233.

Roupas P, Herington AC: Postreceptor signaling mechanisms for growth hormone. Trends Endocrinol Metab 1994;5:154.

Guanylyl Cyclase-Linked Receptors

Drewett JG, Garbers DL: The family of guanylyl cyclase receptors and their ligands. Endocr Rev 1994;15:135.

Knowles RG, Moncada S: Nitric oxide as a signal in blood vessels. Trends Biochem Sci 1992;17:399.

Sessa WC: The nitric oxide synthase family of proteins. J Vasc Res 1994;31:131.

Steroid Receptors

Carson-Jurica MA, Schrader WT, O'Malley BW: Steroid receptor family: Structure and functions. Endocr Rev 1990;11:201.

Freedman LP, Luisi BF: On the mechanism of DNA binding by nuclear hormone receptors: A structural and functional perspective. J Cell Biochem 1993; 51:140.

Glass CK: Differential recognition of target genes by nuclear receptor monomers, dimers and heterodimers. Endocr Rev 1994;15:391.

Miner JN, Yamamoto KR: Regulatory crosstalk at composite response elements. Trends Biochem Sci 1991;16:423.

Robel P, Baulieu E-E: Neurosteroids. Trends Endocrinol Metab 1994;5:1.

Wehling M: Nongenomic actions of steroid hormones. Trends Endocrinol Metab 1994;5:347.

Autoimmunity & Endocrine Disease

Judith A. Shizuru, MD, PhD

The primary role of the immune system is defensive. Thus, it is critical that the system be exquisitely specific. It must be able to distinguish normal self components from nonself and, after making that distinction, destroy foreign invaders or other pathologic processes (eg, neoplasms) that might harm the body. Autoimmune disease occurs when there is breakdown in the signals that mediate host recognition. The result of such breakdown in **self-tolerance** is activation of the effectors of host defense and subsequent tissue destruction. Theoretically, all tissue types, including all endocrine organs, are at risk; however, it is not known why certain organs are targets of autoimmune destruction more commonly than others. Autoimmune responses are generally sustained and persistent, with manifestations of chronic tissue damage, presumably because self-antigens are continually produced on the targeted tissue and diminution of the response does not occur until after the cells involved in antigen production are destroyed.

COMPONENTS OF THE IMMUNE SYSTEM

Immune Cells

Similar to the endocrine system, the immune system is an interactive network of cells and soluble molecules communicating through receptors and second messengers. The principal cellular components are T and B lymphocytes; antigen-presenting cells (APCs), including macrophages and dendritic cells and other cells of the reticuloendothelial system; and an array of nonspecific inflammatory cells such as natural killer (NK) cells and granulocytes. While these numerous cells types participate in host defenses, T and B lymphocytes may be viewed as the gatekeepers of the immune response since they have both the most highly developed capacity to distinguish self antigens from nonself antigens and the ability to activate downstream effector mechanisms. T cells predominate in **cell-mediated immunity,** while B cells that secrete **immunoglobulins** (also called **antibodies**) predominate in **humoral re-**

ACRONYMS USED IN THIS CHAPTER	
APC	Antigen-presenting cell
BSA	Bovine serum albumin
CD	Cluster designation
EAT	Experimental autoimmune thyroiditis
GAD	Glutamic acid decarboxylase
γ-IFN	Gamma interferon
HLA	Human leukocyte antigen
IDDM	Insulin-dependent diabetes mellitus
IL	Interleukin
mAbs	Monoclonal antibodies
NK	Natural killer
MHC	Major histocompatibility complex
NOD	Nonobese diabetic
TCR	T cell receptor
TNF	Tumor necrosis factor
TSH	Thyroid-stimulating hormone

sponses. T cells may be subdivided into two major functional subsets that correspond with expression of the CD4 or CD8 co-receptor molecules. CD4 expression generally correlates with helper-inducer activity, whereas CD8 expression correlates with suppressor-cytotoxic activity.

Molecules of Immune Recognition

Also analogous to the endocrine system, receptor-ligand interactions mediate the activity of immune cells. However, what distinguishes the receptor-ligand components of the immune system from all other physiologic systems is the high degree of structural diversity that the major types of immune receptors possess in order to be able to recognize an unlimited number of foreign antigens. These major receptor types include the gene products of the **major histocompatibility complex (MHC), immunoglobulins,** and the antigen-specific **T cell receptor (TCR).**

A. MHC Molecules: The major histocompatibility complex consists of a linked set of genes encoding the major glycoproteins involved in antigen presentation (Figure 4–1). MHC is the generic name for this gene cluster, and homologous regions have been found in all vertebrate species studied to date. In humans, the MHC is referred to as **human leukocyte antigen (HLA).** The HLA region extends over 4×10^6 base pairs and contains at least 50 genes located on the short arm of chromosome 6. There are three major types of MHC molecules: **class I, class II,** and **class III.** Class I- and class II-encoded molecules are structurally similar cell surface glycoproteins that bind peptide fragments and whose function is to deliver peptide derived from foreign antigens to the cell surface for recognition by T lymphocytes. The class III region encodes an assortment of proteins that are structurally and functionally distinct from the class I and class II molecules. The class III MHC-encoded proteins include some of the components of the complement system and certain cytokines, and although they participate in immune responses, they play a lesser role in autoimmunity and will not be discussed further as a group.

Class I and class II MHC molecules were first identified as important in transplantation rejection, an observation that relates both to their central role in inducing immune responses and to another important feature, which is their high degree of **genetic variability,** or **polymorphism.** This polymorphism is reflected as differences in MHC genes between individuals in a species (Table 4–1). In addition, there are several genes that encode MHC molecules, and these gene products are co-dominantly expressed, so that an individual cell can express several different MHC molecules. In humans there are three class I MHC genes—**HLA-A, HLA-B,** and **HLA-C**—that each encode a single α chain. The class I-encoded α chains span the plasma membrane, and each is noncovalently associated on the cell surface with a non-MHC-encoded molecule called β_2 microglobulin (Figure 4–2A). For class II, there are three pairs of MHC genes that encode an α and β chain, both of which span the membrane and are noncovalently associated on the cell surface (Figure 4–2B). The pairs are designated **HLA-DR, HLA-DP,** and **HLA-DQ** and are tightly linked. Although class I and class II MHC molecules are readily distinguished by their subunit structure, they are closely related in overall three-dimensional structure. Both classes of molecules have α helices at their distal surface which serve as binding sites for a number of different peptides (Figure 4–3), and both classes function to bind peptides for presentation to T cells. The two classes differ importantly with regard to the cellular compartments from which the antigenic peptides are derived and the types of T cells to which they present the antigen (Figure 4–4). Antigenic fragments from pathogens that reside in the cytosolic compartment such as viruses or intracellular bacteria are brought to the cell surface by class I MHC molecules, where the peptide:MHC complex is recognized by CD8 T cells. Pathogens that enter cells through the vesicular compartment, ie, via endocytosis, are processed in acidified vesicles, and their antigenic fragments are bound and brought to the surface by class II MHC molecules, where the peptide:MHC complex is recognized by CD4 T cells. The two MHC classes also differ in their tissue distribution. Class I MHC molecules are expressed by all nucleated cells, whereas class II MHC molecules are expressed only on certain hematopoietic cells, the so-called professional antigen-presenting cells (APCs).

B. Lymphocyte Antigen Receptors: The membrane-bound form of **immunoglobulins** and **T cell receptor** complexes comprise the antigen-specific receptors on B and T lymphocytes, respectively (Figure 4–5). Ligation of these receptors sends a critical signal to the naive lymphocyte to proliferate and differentiate. Since virtually any foreign substance

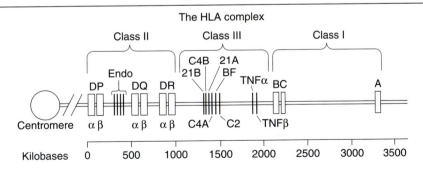

Figure 4–1. Gene organization of the human MHC complex. Regions encoding the three classes of MHC proteins are indicated by braces. "Endo" denotes a cluster of genes within the class II region that encode molecules involved in processing and transport of endogenous antigens. Class III proteins are unrelated to classes I and II and are not involved in antigen presentation. Among proteins encoded in the class III region are tumor necrosis factors α and β and complement factors C2, C4, B, and F. (Reproduced, with permission, from Stites DP, Terr AI, Parslow TG: *Basic & Clinical Immunology,* 8th ed. Appleton & Lange, 1994.)

Table 4–1. HLA antigen specificities.[1,2]

A	B	C	DR	DQ	DP
A1	B5	Cw1	DR1	DQ1	DPw1
A2	B7	Cw2	DR103	DQ2	DPw2
A203	B703	Cw3	DR2	DQ3	DPw3
A210	B8	Cw4	DR3	DQ4	DPw4
A3	B12	Cw5	DR4	DQ5(1)	DPw5
A9	B13	Cw6	DR5	DQ6(1)	DPw6
A10	B14	Cw7	DR6	DQ7(3)	
A11	B15	Cw8	DR7	DQ8(3)	
A19	B16	Cw9(w3)	DR8	DQ9(3)	
A23(9)	B17	Cw10(w3)	DR9		
A24(9)	B18		DR10		
A2403	B21		DR11(5)		
A25(10)	B22		DR12(5)		
A26(10)	B27		DR13(6)		
A28	B35		DR14(6)		
A29(19)	B37		DR1403		
A30(19)	B38(16)		DR1404		
A31(19)	B39(16)		DR15(2)		
A32(19)	B3901		DR16(2)		
A33(19)	B3902		DR17(3)		
A34(10)	B40		DR18(3)		
A36	B4005				
A43	B41		DR51		
A66(10)	B42				
A68(28)	B44(12)		DR52		
A69(28)	B45(12)				
A74(19)	B46		DR53		
	B47				
	B48				
	B49(21)				
	B50(21)				
	B51(5)				
	B5102				
	B5103				
	B52(5)				
	B53				
	B54(22)				
	B55(22)				
	B56(22)				
	B57(17)				
	B58(17)				
	B59				
	B60(40)				
	B61(40)				
	B62(15)				
	B63(15)				
	B64(14)				
	B65(14)				
	B67				
	B70				
	B71(70)				
	B72(70)				
	B73				
	B75(15)				
	B76(15)				
	B77(15)				
	B7801				
	Bw4				
	Bw6				

[1]Reproduced, with permission, from Stites DP, Terr AI, Parslow TG: *Basic & Clinical Immunology,* 8th ed. Appleton & Lange, 1994.
[2]Antigens as recognized by the World Health Organization. Antigens listed in parentheses are the broad antigens; antigens followed by broad antigens in parentheses are the antigen splits. Antigens of the Dw series are omitted.

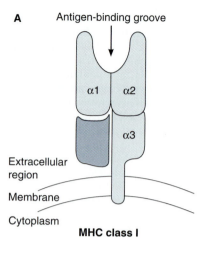

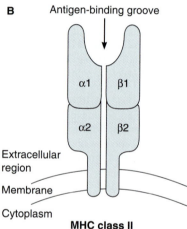

Figure 4–2. Schematic representation of class I and class II MHC molecules. *A:* MHC class I molecules are encoded by a single α chain with three extracellular domains designated α1, α2, and α3. The α chain is noncovalently associated with β_2-microglobulin (β_2m). The binding site for immunogenic peptides is formed by the cleft between the α1 and α2 domains. *B:* MHC class II molecules are encoded by an α and a β chain that are noncovalently associated on the cell surface. The binding site for immunogenic peptides is formed by the cleft between the α1 and β1 domains.

can elicit an immune response, an enormous number of receptors that recognize different antigens must be generated. As a collective population, lymphocytes can produce an almost infinite range of receptors with recognition sites for different antigens; however, each individual lymphocyte carries a receptor of one and only one specificity. Lymphocytes that share the same receptor specificity are thought to arise from a common progenitor cell and thus are said to belong to the same **clone.** To achieve the immense receptor diversity, immunoglobulins and TCR genes utilize a strategy of **somatic recombination.**

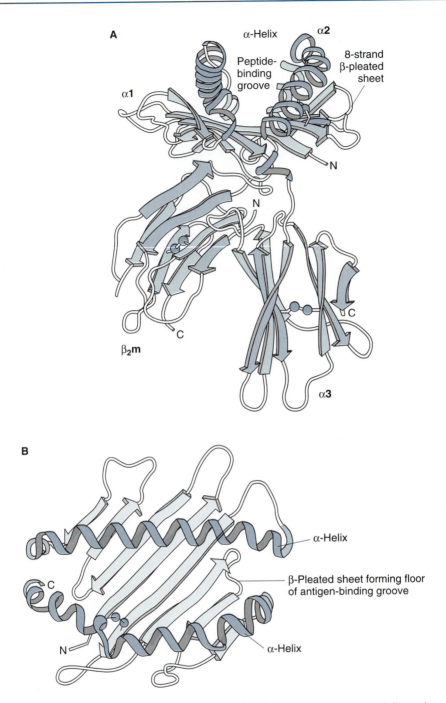

Figure 4–3. Diagrammatic structure of a class I HLA molecule based upon x-ray crystallography. **A:** Side view of the whole molecule, which is mostly comprised of a β-pleated sheet structure, but the peptide binding groove is formed by a pair of α-helices from the α1 and α2 domains. The β-sheet structure forms the floor and the two α-helices form the walls of the groove. **B:** The peptide-binding groove from a view looking down on the molecule from above. (Modified and reproduced, with permission, from Bjorkman PJ et al: Structure of the human class I histocompatibility antigen HLA-A2. Nature 1987:329:506.)

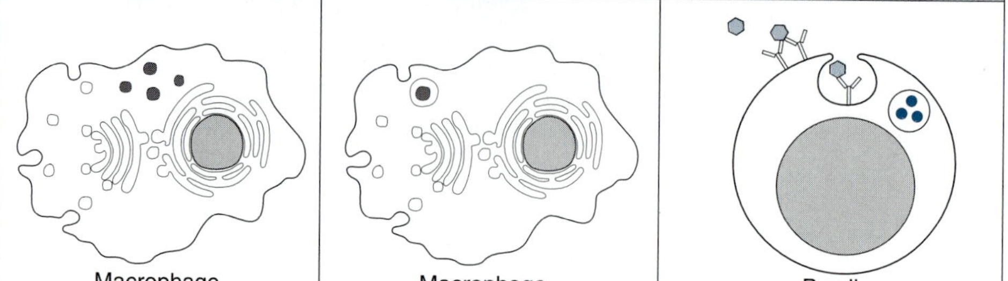

A. Cytosolic pathogens	B. Intravesicular pathogens	C. Extracellular pathogens and toxins
Macrophage	Macrophage	B cell

	A. Cytosolic pathogens	B. Intravesicular pathogens	C. Extracellular pathogens and toxins
Degraded in:	Cytoplasm	Acidified vesicles	Acidified vesicles
Peptides bind to:	MHC class I	MHC class II	MHC class II
Presented to:	CD8 T cells	CD4 T cells	CD4 T cells
Effect on presenting cell:	Cell death	Activation of macrophages to kill intravesicular bacteria and parasites	Activation of B cells to secrete Ig to eliminate extracellular bacteria and toxins

Figure 4–4. Processing and presentation of pathogens is dependent upon whether they enter the cytoplasmic or vesicular compartment of a cell. Peptide antigens derived from self-components can also be bound to and presented by MHC molecules. *A:* Cytosolic antigens are bound to MHC class I molecules for presentation to CD8 cells. *B:* Antigens taken up into endosomes are bound to MHC class II molecules for presentation to CD4 cells. *C:* Extracellular antigens can be taken up into B lymphocytes by the membrane-bound form of immunoglobulins and processed in the vesicular compartment for presentation by MHC class II molecules. (Reproduced, with permission, from Janeway CA Jr, Travers P: *Immunobiology: The Immune System in Health and Disease.* Current Biology Ltd. Garland, 1994.)

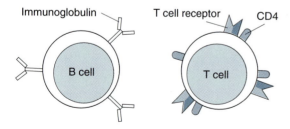

Figure 4–5. The antigen-specific receptors on lymphocytes. For B cells, the receptor is the membrane-bound form of immunoglobulin, which is found in a complex with two other transmembrane glycoproteins designated Igα and Igβ. For T cells, the receptor is designated the α/β T cell receptor, which is stably associated with a complex of molecules designated as CD3 (not shown). The co-receptors designated CD4 or CD8 (not shown) subdivide T cells into two major functional classes, and their expression is mutually exclusive in circulating T cells. CD4 and CD8 associate with TCR only during antigen recognition.

This means that the polypeptide chains that make up the these receptors are encoded by gene segments that rearrange during lymphocyte development. In this regard, immunoglobulins and T cell receptor genes differ from nearly all other human genes. For other genes the germline arrangement of coding sequences (**exons**) and noncoding sequences (**introns**) is the same in primitive and mature cells, and only after the gene is transcribed are the exons joined by RNA splicing. In contrast, for immunoglobulins and T cell receptors, a number of small exon cassettes encoding specific portions of the receptor molecules are sequentially arranged on the germline gene, and during lymphocyte development the cassettes are joined together with permanent excision of the intervening DNA (Figure 4–6). The gene segments that correspond to the so-called **variable region** of these receptors are present in multiple copy but differ slightly in nucleotide sequence. Therefore, diversity in the immunoglobulin and TCR repertoire is created by the selection of different combinations of gene

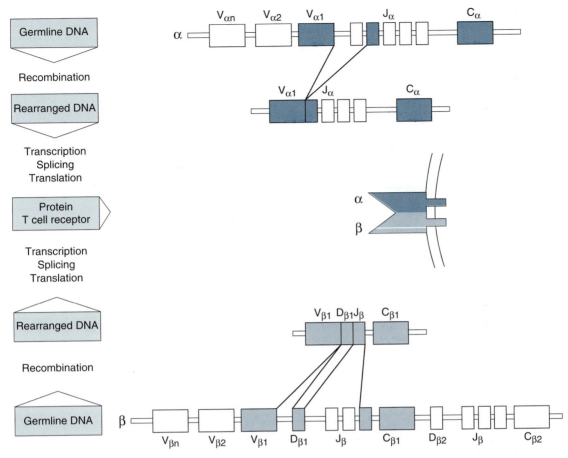

Figure 4–6: Rearrangement of the TCR α and β genes to form a functional receptor. The α and β gene locus contains multiple discrete segments, only some of which are shown here. During T cell development, the TCR α and β gene segments rearrange by somatic recombination so that one of the V_α segments pairs with a single J_α segment, and a V_β segment pairs with a single D_β and J_β segment. The C (constant) segments are brought together with the rearranged segments by transcription and splicing to generate the functional mRNA that will be translated into the α and β protein chains.

segments which are joined together by random recombination to construct the functional receptor. In addition, joining of the gene segments is imprecise, thus introducing further diversity in the sequences at these junctions. As a consequence of somatic recombination, each individual lymphocyte expresses a receptor of unique specificity, and all progeny arising from that cell inherit the genes encoding for the same specificity.

There are important differences in the way immunoglobulins and T cell receptors recognize antigens. Only certain portions of a given molecule, called **epitopes,** are recognized and bound by immunoglobulins or T cells. Epitope recognition by immunoglobulins is relatively straightforward and involves a bimolecular interaction that occurs in solution. The antigenic epitope for a single immunoglobulin generally encompasses about 3–20 amino acids or sugar residues and can either be a

portion of a molecule in its three-dimensional native state (composed of amino acids brought together by protein folding) or a linear sequence. In contrast, T cell epitopes are more complex, since the T cell receptor recognizes small peptide fragments only if they are bound to self-encoded MHC molecules on the cell surface (Figure 4–7A). Thus, T cells show no preference for epitopes that lie on the surface (as opposed to the interior) of globular proteins and rarely recognize specific conformation features of the native antigen.

Co-receptors & Accessory Molecules

In addition to the three types of major receptors described above, there are a large number of co-receptors and accessory surface molecules that subserve immune cell functions (Table 4–2). These other molecules function in three general ways: (1) to act

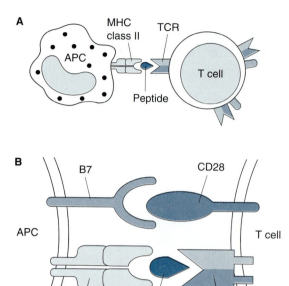

Figure 4–7. Model for antigen recognition by T cells. *A:* Here a CD4 T cell is engaged in recognition of its cognate antigen, composed of a small peptide bound to a class II MHC molecule presented on the surface of an antigen-presenting cell (APC). *B:* As described in the text, recognition of the cognate antigen alone is insufficient for activation of T cells. Rather, a second co-stimulatory signal is required to be delivered simultaneously with antigen recognition in order to achieve activation. At least under certain conditions, the CD28 receptor receives the second signal delivered by the APC via the B7 ligand.

Table 4–2. Some important co-receptors on T lymphocytes.[1]

Marker	Major Function or Significance
T cell receptor	Antigen binding
CD3 complex	Signal transduction from T cell receptor; lineage-specific marker
CD2, CD5, CD7	Lineage-specific markers
CD4	Subset-specific marker (mainly on helper cells); interaction with class II MHC proteins
CD8	Subset specific marker (mainly on cytotoxic cells); interaction with Class I MHC proteins
IL-2 receptor Class II MHC proteins Transferrin receptor CD25, CD29, CD54, CD69 CD40 ligand (CD40L)	Activation-specific markers
IL-1 receptor IL-6 receptor TNFα receptor	Other cytokine receptors
Fc receptors	Immunoglobulin binding
LFA-1, ICAM-1	Cell-cell adhesion molecules
CD28	Receptor for co-stimulating signal delivered by B7.1 and B7.2 activation of naive T cells

[1]Modified and reproduced, with permission, from Stites DP, Terr AI, Parslow TG: *Basic & Clinical Immunology,* 8th ed. Appleton & Lange, 1994.

as co-stimulatory molecules that transduce signals across the plasma membrane, (2) to enhance adhesion between cells, and (3) to guide the migration of immune cells through lymph nodes and to their target tissues. The TCR itself is stably associated on the T cell surface with a complex of proteins collectively known as **CD3.** The CD3 complex is composed of five distinct, invariant proteins that have cytoplasmic extensions important in signal transduction.

Perhaps the best-known co-receptor molecules are **CD4** and **CD8,** which are expressed on the surfaces of T cells and subdivide T cells into two mutually exclusive subsets that differ with regard to the MHC molecules they recognize and differ in effector functions. During antigen recognition, CD4 and CD8 associate with components of the TCR-CD3 complex and participate in both adhesion and signal transduction. CD4, found on the surface of helper-inducer T cells, binds to an invariant part of the MHC class II molecule at a proximal membrane site and distal to the peptide binding cleft. The CD4 cytoplasmic domain interacts strongly with a tyrosine kinase called lck, or p56^{lck}, through which the CD4 molecule participates in signal transduction. CD8, found on the

surface of cytotoxic T cells, similarly binds to a membrane proximal region of the class I MHC molecule, and its cytoplasmic tail also binds lck. The CD8 co-receptor has been shown to increase the sensitivity to antigen presented by class I MHC molecules by about 100-fold.

An important ligand that acts together with the peptide:MHC complex to co-stimulate T cells is **B7** (Figure 4–7B). B7 is a homodimeric member of the immunoglobulin superfamily of proteins that is found on the antigen-presenting cells capable of stimulating T cell activation and growth. The receptor for B7 on T lymphocytes is **CD28.** Ligation of CD28 by B7 or by antibodies directed against CD28 will act as a T cell co-stimulus, while antibodies to B7 that block binding to CD28 inhibit T cell responses. In naive T cells, CD28 is the only receptor for B7; but following activation, T cells express an additional receptor called **CTLA-4** that binds B7 with higher affinity.

Adhesion molecules participate in all aspects of immune cell-cell interactions, including the initial interactions of a lymphocyte with an antigen-presenting cell, the trafficking of lymphocyte through tissues, and the homing of cells to their target tissues. The main classes of adhesion molecules that are known to play a part in lymphocyte interactions are the **selectins,** the **integrins,** members of the **immunoglobulin superfamily,** and certain **mucin-like molecules.**

Soluble Mediators

The soluble components in an immune response include the secreted form of **immunoglobulins** and **cytokines.** Immunoglobulins, or **antibodies,** are the antigen-specific protein products made by mature B lymphocytes. The secreted and transmembrane

forms of an antibody coexist in the same B cell, and the two forms arise because of alternative RNA processing during antibody production (Figure 4–8). Both forms share the same receptor specificity. As described above, the transmembrane form is the antigen-specific B cell receptor involved in antigen processing and signal transduction, while the secreted antibody molecule carries out effector functions. The secreted antibody molecule has two structurally and functionally separable regions. The **variable region** binds to antigen, while the other segment, called the **heavy chain constant region,** binds to a variety of molecules that aid in the disposal of a bound

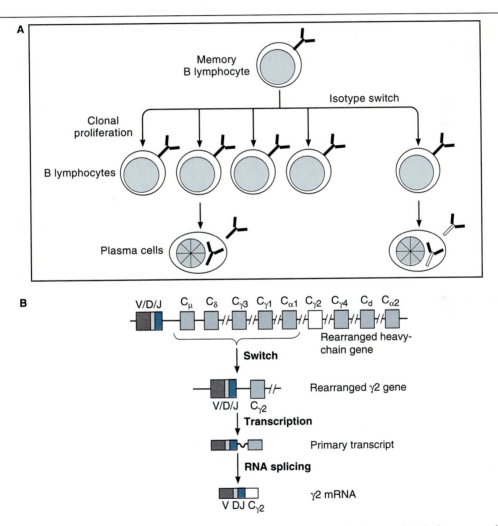

Figure 4–8. The transformation of surface bound immunoglobulin to secreted the immunoglobulin form occurs following B lymphocyte activation via process of heavy chain isotype switching. Circulating resting B cells express IgM and IgD on their surface. The activation of B cells by cytokines made by CD4 helper T cells results in the DNA rearrangement so that the V/D/J exons are brought into close association with the selected heavy locus. **A:** During clonal proliferation of activated B cells, some of the progeny develop into memory cells, whereas others undergo heavy chain class switching and become immunoglobulin secreting plasma cells. **B:** Example of heavy chain class switching to produce a functional immunoglobulin of the Igγ2 isotype. (Reproduced, with permission, from Stites DP, Terr AI, Parslow TG [editors]: *Basic & Clinical Immunology,* 8th ed. Appleton & Lange, 1994.)

pathogen. There are five major classes of heavy chain constant regions that are referred to as **isotypes** and are designated **IgM, IgD, IgG, IgE,** and **IgA.** Each isotype binds different receptors (ie, complement) and in that way determines the effector function of the antibody molecule. Although an individual B cell can produce antibodies of only a single isotype, daughter cells can express antibodies of different heavy chain classes. This change in heavy chain type occurs via a specialized process of DNA rearrangement termed **isotype switching.**

Cytokines are extraordinarily potent molecules that act on target cells to influence activation, growth, and differentiation. Although somewhat analogous to endocrine hormones, they are produced by many types of immune cells and therefore exhibit less restricted tissue specificity than endocrine hormones. At least 100 cytokines have been identified to date. Table 4–3 lists some of the better-characterized cytokines and their currently known effects.

Controls Against Lymphocyte Self-Reactivity

The specificity of an immune response is determined by the appropriate activation of circulating naive lymphocytes. In order to ensure that lymphocyte responses and the downstream effector mechanisms they control are directed against foreign antigens and not normal self tissues, a number of obstacles must be overcome before lymphocytes can differentiate and proliferate. Thus, there are three general mechanisms by which the immune system controls against self-reactivity. These steps in lymphocyte regulation are termed **clonal deletion, anergy,** and **active suppression** (Figure 4–9).

A. Clonal Deletion: During development, all lymphocytes undergo a rigorous selection process to delete potentially self-reactive cells. The progenitor cells for both T and B cell lineages arise in the bone marrow. For T cells, the precursor cells leave the bone marrow and migrate to the thymus, a **central lymphoid organ** that provides the specialized microenvironment where T cell maturation and selection can occur. Developing T cells that are potentially self-reactive—ie, those cells with TCRs that bind too strongly to self-peptides—plus self-MHC molecules are eliminated, a process termed **negative selection** or **clonal deletion.** Only those T cells that have receptors with the potential of recognizing self-MHC molecules plus foreign peptide can leave the thymus and enter the bloodstream **(positive selection).** Immature B cells that express immunoglobulin receptors which bind too strongly to components of self either die within the bone marrow or become impaired in their ability to respond to antigen. The latter state of antigen nonreactivity (discussed below) is called **anergy.**

B. Anergy: The second level of control against nonspecific or self-reactive immune responses is the

requirement necessary to achieve lymphocyte activation. The immature lymphocytes that are allowed to continue their development leave the central lymphoid organs and enter the peripheral circulation as naive cells. These naive cells survey the body for pathogens by trafficking through the blood, lymphatics, and lymphoid organs. Each circulating lymphocyte expresses a receptor specific for a particular antigen, called its **cognate antigen.** A critical event in lymphocyte activation is the interaction of its antigen-specific receptor with its cognate antigen; however, this interaction is not by itself sufficient to induce naive lymphocytes to divide and differentiate into effector cells. Other **co-stimulatory signals** are required to be delivered simultaneously to engagement of the antigen receptor. Antigen recognition in the absence of these co-stimulatory signals leads to a state of lymphocyte unresponsiveness (anergy), wherein a lymphocyte that has been rendered anergic cannot respond to its cognate antigen if encountered at a later time. Anergy has been observed in both B cells and T cells.

B. Suppression: A third way that unwanted immune responses can be controlled is through cell populations that function to actively suppress lymphocyte activity. It has been demonstrated in a number of experimental models that certain CD8 T cells can suppress the reactivity of other T cells in an antigen-specific fashion. Such active suppression appears to be dominant and is mediated by so-called **suppressor cells.** As an example, transfer of CD8 T cells from mice that have been made tolerant to a specific antigen can suppress the immune response in naive mice that are challenged with the specific antigen but not other antigens. Although the existence of suppressor populations is no longer as controversial as in recent years, the mechanism by which these cells function remains uncertain.

The Immune Response

A. Requirements for Activation: Induction of antigen-specific immune responses follows a complex and orchestrated cascade of events (Figure 4–10). The first critical step in the activation of the response requires the processing of antigen for presentation to CD4 helper-inducer T lymphocytes. CD4 T cells are central in the induction of immune responses because they form the critical link between recognition of foreign antigen and the activation of effector mechanisms that destroy the antigen source. Most effector cells rely upon the co-stimulatory signals provided by activated helper CD4 T cells in order to proliferate and differentiate. The co-stimulatory signals provided by the helper CD4 cells are in the form of direct receptor:ligand interactions or via cytokines which they secrete.

Because the consequences of nonspecific or inappropriate stimulation of naive CD4 T cells are potentially disastrous, a number of criteria must be met to

Table 4–3. Major properties of human interleukins and other immunoregulatory cytokines.[1]

	Earlier Terms	Principal Cell Source	Principal Effects[2]
Interleukins IL-1 α and β	Lymphocyte-activating factor, B cell activating factor, hematopoietin	Macrophages, other APCs, other somatic cells	Costimulation of APCs and T cells B cell proliferation and Ig production Acute-phase response of liver (see Table 9–3) Phagocyte activation Inflammation and fever Hematopoiesis
IL-2	T cell growth factor	Activated TH1 cells, Tc cells, NK cells	Proliferation of activated T cells NK and Tc cell functions B cell proliferation and IgG2 expression
IL-3	Multi-colony-stimulating factor	T lymphocytes	Growth of early hematopoietic progenitors
IL-4	B cells growth factor I, B cell stimulatory factor I	TH2 cells, mast cells	B cell proliferation, IgE expression, and class II MHC expression TH2- and Tc-cell proliferation and functions Eosinophil and mast cell growth and function Inhibition of monokine production
IL-5		TH2 cells, mast cells	Eosinophil growth and function
IL-6	IFN-β2, hepatocyte-stimulating factor, hybridoma growth factor	Activated TH2 cells, APCs, other somatic cells	Synergistic effects with IL-1 or TNF to costimulate T cells Acute-phase response of liver (see Table 9–3) B-cell proliferation and Ig production Thrombopoiesis (see Table 9–4)
IL-7		Thymic and marrow stromal cells	T and B lymphopoiesis Tc cell functions
IL-8		Macrophages, other somatic cells	Chemoattractant for neutrophils and T cells (see Table 9–5)
IL-9		Cultured T cells	Some hematopoietic and thymopoietic effects
IL-10	Cytokine synthesis inhibitory factor	Activated TH2, CD8 T, and B lymphocytes, macrophages	Inhibition of cytokine production by TH1 cells, NK cells, and APCs Promotion of B cell proliferation and antibody responses Suppression of cellular immunity Mast cell growth
IL-11		Stromal cells	Synergistic effects on hematopoiesis and thrombopoiesis
IL-12	Cytotoxic lymphocyte maturation factor, NK cell stimulatory factor	B cells, macrophages	Proliferation and function of activated Tc and NK cells IFN γ production TH1 cell induction; suppresses TH2 cell functions Promotion of cell-mediated immune responses
IL-13		TH2 cells	IL-4-like effects
Other cytokines TNFα	Cachectin	Activated macrophages, other somatic cells	IL-1-like effects (see Table 9–2) Vascular thrombosis and tumor necrosis
TNFβ	Lymphotoxin	Activated TH1 cells	IL-1-like effects (see Table 9–2) Vascular thrombosis and tumor necrosis
INF α and β	Leukocyte interferons, type I interferons	Macrophages; neutrophils, other somatic cells	Antiviral effects Induction of class I MHC on all somatic cells Activation of macrophages and NK cells

(continued)

Table 4–3. Major properties of human interleukins and other immunoregulatory cytokines.[1] (continued)

	Earlier Terms	Principal Cell Source	Principal Effects[2]
Other cytokines (cont'd.)			
INFγ	Immune interferon, type II interferon	Activated TH1 and NK cells	Induction of class I MHC on all somatic cells Induction of class II MHC on APCs and somatic cells Activation of macrophages, neutrophils, and NK cells Promotion of cell-mediated immunity (inhibits TH2 cells) Induction of high endothelial venules Antiviral effects
TGFβ		Activated T lymphocytes, platelets, macrophages, other somatic cells	Anti-inflammatory (suppression of cytokine production and class II MHC expression) Anti-proliferative for macrophages and lymphocytes Promotion of B-cell expression of IgA Promotion of fibroblast proliferation and wound healing

[1]Reproduced, with permission, from Stites DP, Terr AI, Parslow TG: Basic & Clinical Immunology, 8th ed. Appleton & Lange, 1994.
[2]All of the listed processes are enhanced unless otherwise indicated.

activate these cells. Thus, only certain specialized cells, called professional antigen-presenting cells (APCs) can fulfill all of the requirements needed for CD4 T cell activation. The professional APCs include B lymphocytes, macrophages, and dendritic cells. As part of their function, the APCs take up exogenous foreign antigen by endocytosis. The antigen is processed intracellularly via trafficking through acidified vesicles, and within the vesicles the resultant peptide fragments are bound to class II MHC molecules. Macrophages and dendritic cells take up antigen with very little specificity, whereas B lymphocytes bind native antigen through their antigen-specific surface immunoglobulins. The most important event in activation of a CD4 T cell is encounter with its cognate antigen, which consists of the appropriate peptide bound to a self-MHC class II molecule, and only professional APCs normally express high levels of class II MHC molecules on their surfaces.

In addition to the binding of a TCR with its cognate antigen, activation cannot be achieved unless this interaction is accompanied by the simultaneous delivery of a co-stimulatory signal. In the absence of

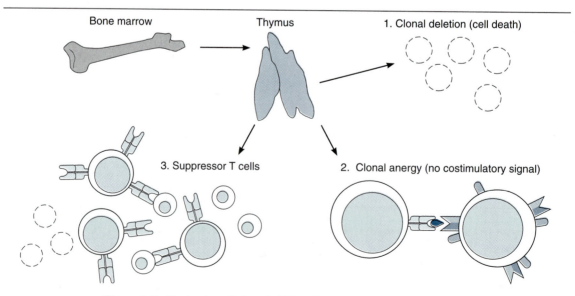

Figure 4–9. Mechanisms that control T lymphocyte self-reactivity (see text).

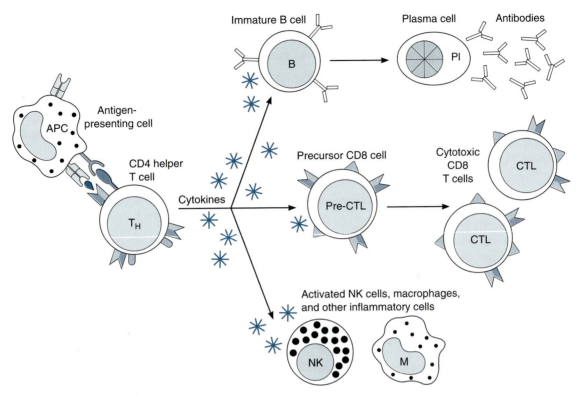

Figure 4–10. Schematic representation of the immune response cascade. Professional APCs present peptide antigens bound to class II MHC molecules to CD4 T helper cells. T cells require co-stimulation with a second signal provided by the B7/CD28 interaction. Once activation of CD4 T cells occurs, these cells produce and secrete a number of cytokines, and the downstream effector mechanisms are turned on via these cytokines and by direct interaction with the effectors cells (eg, B lymphocytes).

the co-stimulatory signal, engagement of the antigen receptor will lead to anergy. Again, only professional APCs can deliver the appropriate co-stimulatory signals to CD4 T cells. B7 (described above) is the best-characterized of the co-stimulatory molecules expressed on APCs, and its expression is either constitutive or inducible. B7 is the ligand for the CD28 receptor expressed on T cells. As a result of the combined effects of TCR and CD28 ligation, naive CD4 T cells are stimulated to rapidly proliferate and differentiate. As part of this process, they begin to express new receptor molecules and synthesize and secrete a number of cytokines. One of the most important cytokines is **interleukin-2 (IL-2).** The production of IL-2 determines whether a CD4 T cell will proliferate and continue along its differentiation pathway. IL-2 functions both as a growth factor that influences the activation state of other T cells and as an **autocrine hormone** that induces the synthesis and expression of a high-affinity IL-2 receptor on the CD4 T cell itself. Signaling through the high-affinity IL-2 receptor triggers the cells to progress through the remainder of the cell cycle. The importance of IL-2 in inducing and sustaining immune responses is

underscored by the fact that certain powerful immunosuppressant drugs such as **cyclosporine** and **tacrolimus** exert their influence by blocking IL-2 production. These agents act by inhibiting the signaling pathway through the TCR.

Following CD4 T cell stimulation and production of IL-2, these cells differentiate into two distinct populations that are distinguishable by the cytokines they produce. One population produces γ-IFN, TNFβ, and IL-2 and the other produces IL-4 and its congeners. These subpopulations have been designated T helper 1 (T_H1) and T helper 2 (T_H2) cells, respectively. T_H1 cells produce cytokines that drive inflammation or cell-mediated immunity, while T_H2 cells, which elaborate cytokines critical to B lymphocyte differentiation, provide help for antibody production. It is clear that these CD4 T cell subsets can regulate the growth and effector functions of the opposite T cell subset.

B. Activation of Effector Mechanisms: Cellular and humoral mechanisms carry out the effector phase of an immune response by destroying the pathogenic organisms that bear the target antigens. Effector cell populations include mature B cells, activated cytotoxic T cells, and other inflammatory cells such as natural killer (NK) and phagocytic cells. The humoral components of the effector phase include antibodies, complement proteins, and cytokines.

1. B cell responses–The differentiation pathway for a naive B cell following an encounter with antigen is to become a mature antibody-secreting plasma cell. Almost all naive B cells are dependent upon CD4 helper T cells to deliver the activating signals that drive this process. The way this interaction is thought to occur is that the B cell initiates the process by its antigen-presenting cell functions. Complex antigen is bound and internalized via its antibody receptors and undergoes intracellular processing so that antigen fragments associate with class II MHC molecules for appropriate presentation to CD4 T cells. When the B cell encounters a CD4 T cell with specificity for one of its peptide:MHC class II complexes, direct cell-cell interaction will occur. Such T and B cell interactions are synergistic, since B cells can express the co-stimulatory molecules B7.1 and B7.2, while CD4 T cells not only secrete cytokines necessary for B cell clonal expansion and differentiation but also express a ligand called **CD40 ligand** that binds to the B cell surface receptor **CD40.** Ligation of CD40 helps to drive naive B cells into cell cycle. Among the cytokines produced by CD4 T cells that directly affect B cell development are **IL-4, IL-5,** and **IL-6.** IL-4 works synergistically with CD40 ligation to drive the expansion of a B cell clone prior to antibody production. IL-5 and IL-6 contribute to the later stages of B cell activation.

2. Cytotoxic T call responses–Because MHC class I molecules are ubiquitously expressed on all nucleated cells, theoretically most cells can be recognized and destroyed by CD8 cytotoxic cells. However, activation of CD8 cells is dependent upon simultaneous ligation of the TCR with its peptide antigen bound to a self-MHC class I molecule and upon help provided by CD4 cells. CD4 T cells are thought to provide help either in the form of cytokines, especially by IL-2, or by inducing the expression of the co-stimulatory molecule B7 on an APC that has engaged a CD8 cell via its TCR.

3. Nonspecific inflammatory responses–Activated CD4 T cells also induce an array of antigen-nonspecific effector mechanisms. T_H1 cells interact with resting macrophages directly and deliver the co-stimulatory cytokine γ-IFN to convert them to activated macrophages that are much more efficient at killing their ingested targets. The cumulative effects of cytokines made by T and B cells and by macrophages induce the activation state of other cells such as natural killer (NK) cells. Furthermore, certain cytokines can change the expression of adhesion molecules on the endothelial cells, thus attracting more cells of the immune system to an inflamed site.

THE AUTOIMMUNE RESPONSE

The definition of an autoimmune disease is one in which self antigens become targets for immune destruction and the response is directed either against a single tissue type or a very limited number of tissues. Antibodies, activated T or B lymphocytes, and nonspecific inflammatory cells have been found to predominate in certain autoimmune lesions, and on that basis either humoral or cellular mechanisms have been judged to be the cause of the underlying clinical disease. Thus, traditionally, immunologic diseases are categorized as types I–IV **hypersensitivity responses.** Types II–IV are involved in autoimmune tissue damage, where type II responses are mediated by antigen-specific antibodies, type III responses by immune complex deposition, and type IV responses are cell-mediated. Type I responses are mediated by antibodies of the IgE isotype and are considered allergic responses, not involved in autoimmunity. In the context of endocrine autoimmune syndromes, only types II and IV appear to be relevant, and (conveniently), the two best-studied endocrine autoimmune disorders—Graves' disease, in which autoantibodies directed against the TSH receptor have been shown to be pathologic; and insulin-dependent diabetes mellitus (IDDM), in which the insulin-producing cells of the pancreas have been destroyed by cellular infiltrates—are prototypical for type II and type IV responses, respectively. However, all that having been said, it should be emphasized that these classifications do not in fact illuminate the more fundamental and important issue of what it is that triggers autoimmune responses, since by the time an autoimmune process becomes clinically evident and classifiable by this scheme, the initiating events are obscured by the downstream effector mechanisms causing the actual tissue damage. At least for reactions of types II, III, and IV, there appears to be a common pathway by which autoreactive lymphocyte clones develop and escape the controls that enforce self-tolerance. From our current understanding of how the immune system functions and from the cumulative experience with a number of autoimmune syndromes, it is apparent that loss of T cell tolerance is the central pathogenic event.

Genetic Factors in Autoimmune Disease

How and why loss of immune self-tolerance occurs is not known, but both genetic and environmental factors appear to be necessary. Epidemiologic studies demonstrate that susceptibility to most autoimmune diseases has a significant genetic component. Using IDDM as an example, there is a clear association with race and susceptibility to disease. The incidence of IDDM is approximately 40 times higher in Finland than in Japan. Familial studies also demonstrate a strong underlying genetic component, since the lifetime risk of developing IDDM in the United States is 0.4%, whereas in relatives of diabetic patients the risk is substantially higher (Table 4–4). Furthermore, certain inbred rodent strains reliably develop spontaneous autoimmune diabetes.

The inheritance pattern of autoimmune disorders is complex, however. These diseases are polygenic, arising from several independently segregating genes, and to date the only clear-cut consistent genetic marker for susceptibility to any autoimmune disease has been the MHC genotype. A further level of complexity in autoimmune disease pathogenesis is that environmental factors also play a critical role. The evidence for this comes from studies of monozygotic twins which show that the concordance rates for autoimmune disorders are imperfect, ranging from 25% to 75% depending on the specific disease. Again using IDDM as an example, monozygotic twins show less than a 50% concordance.

The Role of the MHC in Autoimmunity

A. MHC Association With Disease Susceptibility: The most clearly established genetic association for predisposition to autoimmune disease is the genotype of the MHC. This correlation has been noted since the mid 1970s. Initially, associations were made with the class I MHC type and the spondyloarthropathies. For example, ankylosing spondylitis was found to be strongly associated with the class I HLA-B27 allele. Later, however, many other diseases (Table 4–5), including Graves' disease and IDDM, were found to be associated with HLA class II DR specificities. In the last 20 years, the technology of HLA typing has advanced from serologic assays to the more sensitive molecular-based assays that can detect variations at the nucleotide level. As this technology for HLA genotyping has become more precise, such that specific regions of the MHC can be examined, the associations have become stronger. For example, in IDDM, up to 95% of Caucasians developing IDDM express the HLA alleles DR3 or DR4 versus about 40% of normal individuals, and individuals heterozygous for both DR3 and DR4 have the highest risk of IDDM development.

Table 4–4. Familial inheritance of diabetes mellitus.[1]

Diabetes Mellitus in–	IDDM
Parents	4%
Father	6%
Mother	2%
Sibling	5–7%
HLA-identical	20%
Dizygotic twins	Same as sibs
Monozygotic twins	25–40%
General population	0.3–0.5%

[1]Modified and reproduced, with permission, from Atkinson MA, Maclaren NK: The pathogenesis of insulin-dependent diabetes mellitus. N Engl J Med 1994;334:1428.

Table 4–5. Associations of HLA genotype with autoimmune disease.

Disease	HLA Allele	Relative Risk[1]
Ankylosing spondylitis	B27	87
Reiter's syndrome	B27	40
Goodpasture's syndrome	DR2	16
Multiple sclerosis	DR2	5
Graves' disease	DR3	4
Hashimoto's thyroiditis	DR5	3
Insulin-dependent diabetes mellitus	DR3 and DR4	3

[1]Chance that a person who is heterozygous for the indicated allele will develop the disease compared with the number that would be expected, given the prevalence of that allele in the general population.

Subsequent to these observations, it has been shown that, in fact, the DQ rather than the DR genotype is a more specific marker of IDDM susceptibility and that the previous correlation with HLA-DR is due to the fact that DR and DQ are the product of closely linked genes. Thus, for IDDM, the highest-risk DQ alleles, DQα1*0501/DQβ1*0201 and DQα1*0301/DQβ1*0302, are invariably found with the DR3 and DR4 genotype, respectively. Individuals heterozygous for these two DQ alleles have the highest risk of IDDM development. Such individuals comprise 2% of the general United States population but 40% of patients with IDDM.

A similar evolution in the association of HLA type and disease susceptibility has occurred for Graves' disease. Graves' disease was among the first autoimmune disorders noted to have an association with HLA haplotypes, and the initial association was with the MHC class I genotype HLA-B8. Later, however, it became evident that the stronger association was with HLA-DR3, which is tightly linked to HLA-B8.

B. Function of MHC in Disease Pathogenesis: Although genetic associations have been clearly established between autoimmune disease and certain MHC haplotypes, the way in which the MHC molecules contribute to development of autoimmunity remains hypothetical. In light of the essential role played by MHC molecules in antigen presentation to T cells and in the selection of T cells during development—and given that all autoimmune responses involve T lymphocytes—the theory with the strongest support involves aberrations in the presentation of antigenic peptides to T cells. It is known that polymorphic differences in the amino acids that form the walls of the peptide-binding groove can result in profound differences in the binding affinity of self peptides and in the conformation of the peptide-MHC complex. In addition, other polymorphic residues of the MHC molecule that vary between MHC haplotypes also make direct contact with T cell receptors and affect antigen recognition. Thus, MHC:peptide-restricted recognition reflects the combined effects of differences in peptide binding and of direct contact between allotypic portions of the MHC molecule. It is possible that certain haplotypes make certain self antigens appear foreign when the two are combined or that these haplotypes generate a strong enough immune response to self antigens to overcome T cell suppression.

Support for this hypothesis comes from sequence analysis of HLA-DR and DQ genes from individuals with IDDM. The sequence studies have suggested that there is a critical single amino acid at position 57 on the DQβ chain that confers either susceptibility or resistance to IDDM. An aspartic acid, as is present in most persons at that position, has been shown to decrease the risk of IDDM, whereas the presence of other amino acids at position 57 is associated with increased risk. Further evidence for the importance of this single amino acid change is found in spontaneous autoimmune nonobese diabetic (NOD) mice. These mice show a similar replacement of serine for aspartic acid at position 57 of the homologous mouse I-Aβ chain. In humans, amino acid 57 is located at the distal end of the DQβ chain and is part of the peptide-binding cleft of the DQ molecule. Aspartic acid, the protective amino acid at this position, forms a salt bridge with a residue on the opposite side of the binding cleft, and replacement of an uncharged residue at this position disrupts salt bridge formation.

The hypothesis just presented presumes that the association with autoimmune disease and MHC haplotype derives directly from the function of the MHC gene products. While this hypothesis has been amply supported by data from both humans and rodents, it is not conclusively proved. Disease association clearly maps to the MHC region; however, contained within this region are a number of other genes. An alternative hypothesis is that the MHC haplotype serves as a marker only and that the true (and as yet undetermined) disease-associated genes are linked to the MHC alleles.

The Role of the Environment

Although there are clear associations with the development of autoimmune disease and an individual's genetic makeup, the fact that only 25–75% of identical twins develop the same disease suggests that environmental factors contribute significantly to the autoimmune pathogenesis. Even more convincing evidence for the importance of the environment on disease pathogenesis comes from rodent models that reliably develop autoimmune syndromes. For example, NOD mice develop a spontaneous autoimmune diabetes with many features in common with human IDDM. These mice demonstrate a lymphocyte-mediated destruction of their pancreatic islets beginning in young adulthood that can progress over a period of several weeks to overt hyperglycemia. These mice are highly inbred and thus genetically identical but even so, not all NOD mice develop frank diabetes. Disease prevalence varies from nil to 100% between established colonies.

The environmental factors thought to have greatest influence on disease development include infectious agents and diet. Of the infectious pathogens, viruses have been the strongest candidates. In humans there are known associations between certain viral infections and IDDM. Up to 20% of children that are prenatally infected with rubella develop IDDM, and the risk of IDDM development is increased in individuals with the high-risk MHC loci. Children with congenital rubella also have an increased incidence of other autoimmune immune disorders, including thyroiditis and agammaglobulinemia. Coxsackievirus B4 has also been implicated epidemiologically with development of IDDM.

The importance of diet in the development of autoimmunity remains controversial. In IDDM the best-studied example showing a positive correlation with diet and disease susceptibility is from reports that children who were breast-fed as infants have a significantly lower incidence of IDDM than those that were fed cow's milk. One of the major components of cow's milk protein is bovine serum albumin (BSA), and there is a known homology between BSA and an islet B cell protein. Children and young adults with new-onset IDDM have been shown to have high-titer antibodies to BSA. Thus, it has been proposed that the presence of BSA in the diet can lead to IDDM via a mechanism of molecular mimicry to an islet cell protein. An alternative explanation is that contained within human breast milk is a substance that acts to make infants tolerant to self components. A body of evidence demonstrates that orally administered antigens can induce peripheral immune tolerance. Selected antigens have been administered orally to a broad spectrum of mice with autoimmune disorders, including NOD mice that were fed porcine insulin. The data in the animal models were so compelling that this approach was tried in small studies in humans with multiple sclerosis and rheumatoid arthritis. The positive results achieved in these human trials have led to large multicenter trials.

How environmental factors function to induce an autoimmune response remains speculative. It is important to note that exposure to environmental pathogens and other antigens does not always result in disease. In fact, it has been shown in the NOD mouse model of diabetes that exposure to pathogens can act in a protective manner. In colonies where the mice are bred under germ-free conditions, the incidence of diabetes is significantly higher than in colonies where the mice are exposed to greater numbers of pathogens. Immunologic tolerance is not preprogrammed into the germline but is acquired during maturation of the cells of the immune system, especially lymphocytes. Thus, for each individual the repertoire of immunoglobulin and T cell receptors is assembled during lymphocyte ontogeny by exposure to self antigens and antigens in the environment. Furthermore, receptor assembly is a stochastic process. Therefore, the immune response to a particular antigen will be different between individuals even if they are genetically identical.

The Role of T & B Lymphocytes in Autoimmunity

Autoimmune disorders become clinically evident only after significant tissue damage already exists. Therefore, it has not been possible to study the early events in autoimmune pathogenesis in patients. Much of our understanding of the early stages of autoimmunity is extrapolated from what is known about the way the immune system normally functions in fighting environmental pathogens and in resisting transplanted organs. Animal models of spontaneous or experimentally induced autoimmune syndromes have also offered invaluable insights into the pathogenic mechanisms. The cumulative evidence suggests that all autoimmune diseases involve, at the outset, loss of T cell tolerance to a tissue-specific antigen and that—with inappropriate activation of T cell clones—a self-reactive immune response is amplified and perpetuated. Lymphocyte transfer studies in autoimmune mouse models in which unfractionated T cells or T cell subsets have been shown to transfer disease into nonautoimmune strains or accelerate disease in young, unaffected mice have provided the most direct evidence for the primary role of T lymphocytes.

Consistent with their important role in the induction of normal immune responses, CD4 T cells have been shown to be the primary mediators of autoimmune pathogenesis in a number of different autoimmune mouse models, since treatment of such mice with monoclonal antibodies directed against the CD4 molecule can prevent the development of disease. Recent evidence suggests that interactions between the T_H1 and T_H2 CD4 T cell subpopulations determines whether or not a potentially autoreactive stimulus results in a benign immune response or in the progression and perpetuation of autoimmune tissue destruction. In experimental models, responses that are dominated by the T_H1 subset have a higher correlation with autoimmunity than those dominated by the T_H2 cells. CD8 T cells participate directly in tissue destruction along with other more nonspecific effector mechanisms of cell-mediated responses following activation by T_H1 CD4 cells.

There is evidence in most autoimmune immune syndromes that B lymphocyte-mediated humoral responses are also activated. Autoantibodies directed against a number of tissue-specific antigens may be found in the sera of affected patients, and the appearance of such autoantibodies may precede the development of overt disease by years. However, the anti-bodies often do not appear to contribute to the clinical syndrome but are regarded as markers of an underlying disease process. Whether or not an autoantibody contributes significantly to the autoimmune disease depends upon the target antigen and the epitope against which the antibody is directed. This is best demonstrated by the spectrum of tissue-specific antibody abnormalities seen in autoimmune thyroid diseases. For example, the hallmark for the diagnosis of Hashimoto's disease is the presence of circulating autoantibodies to thyroglobulin and thyroid peroxidase. However, the disease is not caused by these antibodies—rather, the disease is due to a cell-mediated lymphocytic infiltration that almost completely replaces the normal architecture of the thyroid gland. In contrast, in Graves' disease, there is a predominance of antibodies directed against the TSH receptor that directly stimulate the production of excessive thyroid hormone and are the cause for the clinical manifestations of hyperthyroidism. For patients with IDDM, a number of pancreatic islet antigens may be found in patients' sera none of which contribute significantly to the destruction of islet cells or the development of hyperglycemia. Interestingly, it has been shown in both autoimmune thyroiditis and IDDM that similar disease-associated autoantibodies may be found in the sera of healthy first-degree relatives. Regardless of their role in disease pathogenesis, the induction and perpetuation of autoantibody production is dependent upon stimulation by T_H2 CD4 T cells.

Models for the Induction of Autoimmunity

Several hypotheses have been put forward to explain the pathogenesis of autoimmune disease. Based upon the cumulative data that link autoimmune responses with the MHC and the important role that T cells play in the induction and perpetuation of all immune responses, these hypotheses have focused mainly on loss of T cell tolerance, either through inappropriate presentation of self-antigens to T cells or the failure to eliminate or silence self-reactive T cell clones. Although T cells undergo a rigorous selection process during development in the thymus, it is thought that such clonal deletion is imperfect and that circulating self-reactive naive T cells exist which are controlled by the mechanisms of peripheral tolerance. Most self peptides cannot serve either as autoantigens or induce tolerance (central or peripheral) simply because they are presented at levels that are too low to be detectable by naive T cells. However, a few self peptides that fail to induce tolerance may be present at high enough levels to be recognized by T cells. It is likely that only certain peptides can act as autoantigens, since there are relatively few distinct autoimmune syndromes, and individuals with a particular autoimmune disease seem to recognize the same antigen. Autoimmunity may result if an APC picks up one of these peptides and presents it as an antigen. Once a tissue-specific peptide is presented by a cell with co-stimulatory potential, T cells specific for the autoantigen can be activated and home to the tissues where they produce tissue damage.

Such a hypothesis has been born out by a number of animal models of experimentally induced autoimmune disease. Experimental autoimmune thyroiditis results after immunization of animals with thyroglobulin. In good-responder mice, immunization with thyroglobulin alone produces the syndrome, and in other strains an adjuvant is required with the immunization to achieve disease expression. The significance of adjuvant administration is that these agents are known to induce co-stimulatory molecules on macrophages and B lymphocytes, thus increasing the likelihood that the antigen with which it is administered is presented in an immunogenic rather than a tolerogenic fashion, as might occur in the absence of co-stimulatory signals. The following two hypotheses suggest the events that might induce autoimmune responses to develop spontaneously.

A. Molecular Mimicry: The hypothesis of molecular mimicry suggests that immune responses directed against infectious agents can cross-react with self antigens, causing autoimmune destruction. Thus, the inciting antigen could be a bacterium- or virus-derived protein that shares an amino acid sequence with a prevalent tissue-specific protein (Figure 4–11). Antibodies or cytotoxic T cells directed against the pathogen will also selectively destroy the normal tissue that expresses the cross-reactive protein. Support for this hypothesis comes from well-known clinical syndromes where infection with a specific agent leads to a particular disease, such as is the case with rheumatic fever, which can follow group A streptococcal infections. For endocrine disorders, the best examples are from studies in IDDM, where correlations exist between congenital rubella and coxsackievirus B4. For rubella, it has been shown that an immunogenic epitope on the virus capsid protein has structural similarities to an islet B cell protein. In the case of coxsackievirus B4, there is a striking amino acid sequence homology with an enzyme found within B cells called glutamic acid decarboxylase (GAD). Autoantibodies against GAD may be found in the serum of prediabetic and diabetic patients.

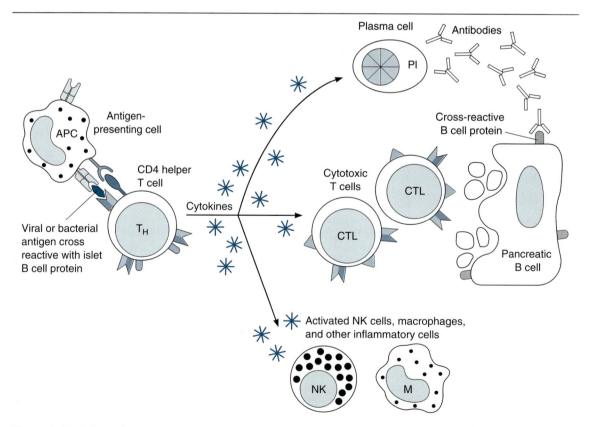

Figure 4–11. Schematic representation of the way in which an autoimmune response might develop against a pancreatic B cell-specific antigen by the mechanism of molecular mimicry. Here a peptide antigen derived from a viral or bacterial pathogen that cross-reacts with a similar peptide on the surface of B cells is presented in an immunogenic way to a CD4 T cell. The resultant immune response is directed against both the pathogen and the B cells.

B. Tissue Injury: An alternative hypothesis to explain the induction of an autoimmune response is that the target tissue itself is injured, either by organisms trophic for the tissue or by agents such as chemicals or drugs. In the setting of tissue injury, a localized inflammatory response will be generated. During tissue inflammation, the release of chemoattractants and cytokines can attract a variety of effector cells to the area, including macrophages, lymphocytes, and nonspecific inflammatory cells. Cytokines are also known to increase the expression of adhesion molecules on the vascular endothelium so that lymphocytes and other effector cells will home to and extravasate into the target tissue. The injured cells might release tissue-specific antigens or be engulfed by APCs already present in the area, resulting in the presentation of self antigen at a high enough level to act as an immunogen.

Inappropriate Expression of MHC Molecules

The local actions of cytokines, and in particular γ-IFN, can induce the expression of class II MHC molecules on the surface of tissue parenchymal cells that do not normally express these molecules. In an earlier hypothesis, it was suggested that such an aberrant expression of class II MHC molecules might allow the parenchymal cells to act as antigen-presenting cells and present their own cellular proteins as antigens that would otherwise be undetectable. This hypothesis originated in observations made in autoimmune thyroiditis, where it was noted that thyroid parenchymal cells, which do not normally express MHC class II molecules, were found to express these molecules at high levels. Subsequently, it has been determined that antigen presentation by cells which lack the ability to deliver a co-stimulatory signal (nonprofessional APCs) will result in T cell unresponsiveness, or anergy, rather than activation. Thus, it is currently believed that the induced expression of class II MHC molecules by parenchymal cells serves to protect normal tissues rather than to provoke an autoimmune attack.

Animal Models

A number of animal models of autoimmune disorders have contributed significantly to our understanding of disease pathogenesis. For autoimmune endocrine diseases, the focus has been primarily on IDDM and autoimmune thyroid disease, though autoimmune adrenal and gonadal disorders exist in mice. The NOD mouse and experimental autoimmune thyroiditis (EAT) have been described above.

There are three major types of animal autoimmune disorders: (1) those that appear to arise spontaneously, such as the NOD mouse;(2) those that are induced by immunization with the tissue-specific proteins, such as in EAT; and (3) those that are created by genetic engineering technology. Of the latter, many transgenic mice have been designed to test broader theories for the loss of self-tolerance, and the majority of these studies have focused on IDDM as the disease model. Specifically, the cause of autoimmune diabetes has been studied by creating transgenic mice that express regulatory molecules of the immune system in islet B cells. B cell-specific expression is achieved by constructing chimeric transgenes in which the insulin promoter is fused to the selected gene, so that gene expression is controlled by the insulin promoter. The molecules that have been constitutively expressed in B cells include MHC class I and class II molecules, cytokines, oncogenes, and even viruses. Transgenic mice have also been created that can express only one type of T cell receptor which was derived from an islet specific T cell clone.

Many of the concepts described in this chapter regarding the causes of autoimmunity have either originated from or been confirmed by observations made in these animal models. Here, only a few examples will be cited. The essential role of the MHC and T lymphocytes in autoimmune pathogenesis was confirmed in animals that develop spontaneous autoimmune syndromes. The notion that aberrant expression of MHC molecules in non-APCs can induce tolerance rather than immunity was derived directly from studies in transgenic mice that expressed class II MHC molecules in parenchymal cells. Finally, the more recent hypothesis that T_H1 cells may play the dominant role over T_H2 cells in autoimmune disease was based upon studies in T cell receptor transgenic mice. Given the power of this approach it can be expected that in the next several years a greatly expanded understanding of all aspects of the autoimmunity will be achieved.

REFERENCES

Abbas AK, Licktman AH, Pober JS: *Cellular and Molecular Immunology.* Saunders, 1991.

Atkinson MA, Maclaren NK: The pathogenesis of insulin-dependent diabetes mellitus. N Engl J Med 1994;331: 1428.

Bowman MA, Leiter EH, Atkinson MA: Prevention of diabetes in the NOD mouse: Implications for the therapeutic intervention in human disease. Immunol Today 1994; 15:115.

Fathman CG, Myers BD: Cyclosporine therapy for autoimmune disease. N Engl J Med 1992;326;1693.

Gepts W: Pathologic anatomy of the pancreas in juvenile diabetes mellitus. Diabetes 1965:14;619.

Janeway CA Jr, Travers P: *Immunobiology: The Immune System in Health and Disease*. Current Biology Ltd. Garland, 1994.

Katz J, Wang B, Haskins K, Benoist C, Mathis D: Following a diabetogenic T cell from genesis through pathogenesis. Cell 1993;74:1089–1100.

Kendall-Taylor P (editor): Autoimmune endocrine disease. Bailliere's Clin Endocrin and Metab 1995;9(1):1–199.

Moller G (editor): Models of autoimmunity. Immunol Rev 1993;118:1–310.

Shizuru JA et al: Immunotherapy of the nonobese diabetic mouse: treatment with an antibody to T-helper lymphocytes. Science 1988;240:659.

Shizuru JA, Sarvetnick N: Transgenic mice for the study of diabetes mellitus. Trends Endocrin Metab 1991;2:97.

Wicker LS, Todd JA, Peterson LB: Genetic control of autoimmune diabetes in the NOD mouse. Ann Rev Immunol 1993;13:179–200.

Hypothalamus & Pituitary

5

David C. Aron, MS, MD, James W. Findling, MD, & J. Blake Tyrrell, MD

The hypothalamus and pituitary gland form a unit which exerts control over the function of several endocrine glands—thyroid, adrenals, and gonads—as well as a wide range of physiologic activities. This unit constitutes a paradigm of neuroendocrinology—brain-endocrine interactions. The actions and interactions of the endocrine and nervous systems whereby the nervous system regulates the endocrine system and endocrine activity modulates the activity of the central nervous system constitute the major regulatory mechanisms for virtually all physiologic activities. The immune system also interacts with both endocrine and nervous systems (see Chapter 4). These neuroendocrine interactions are also important in disease pathophysiology. This chapter will review the normal functions of the pituitary gland, the neuroendocrine control mechanisms of the hypothalamus and their disorders.

Nerve cells and endocrine gland cells which are both involved in cell-to-cell communication share certain characteristic features—secretion of chemical messengers (neurotransmitters or hormones) and electrical activity. A single chemical messenger—peptide or amine—can be secreted by neurons as a neurotransmitter or neural hormone and by endocrine gland cells as a classic hormone. Examples of such multifunctional chemical messengers are shown in Table 5–1. The cell-to-cell communication may occur by four mechanisms: (1) neural communication via synaptic junctions; (2) endocrine communication via circulating hormones; (3) paracrine communication via messengers that diffuse in the interstitial fluid to adjacent target cells (without entering the bloodstream); and (4) autocrine communication via messengers that diffuse in the interstitial fluid to where the messengers act on the cells that secreted them (Figure 5–1). The two major mechanisms of neural regulation of endocrine function are direct innervation and neurosecretion (neural secretion of hormones). The adrenal medulla, kidney, parathyroid gland, and pancreatic islets are endocrine tissues which receive direct autonomic innervation (see Chapters 8, 10, 11, and 18). An example of neurosecretory regulation is the hormonal secretion of cer-

ACRONYMS USED IN THIS CHAPTER	
ACTH	Adrenocorticotropic hormone
ADH	Antidiuretic hormone (vasopressin)
cAMP	Cyclic adenosine monophosphate
CLIP	Corticotropin-like intermediate lobe peptide
CRH	Corticotropin-releasing hormone
DI	Diabetes insipidus
FSH	Follicle-stimulating hormone
GABA	Gamma-aminobutyric acid
GAP	GnRH-associated peptide
GH	Growth hormone (somatrotropin)
GHBP	Growth hormone-inding protein
GnRH	Gonadotropin-releasing hormone
GRH	Growth hormone-releasing hormone
hGH	Human growth hormone
hMG	Human menopausal gonadotropin
LH	Luteinizing hormone
β-LPH	β-Lipotropin
LPH	Lipotropin
MEN	Multiple endocrine neoplasia
MRI	Magnetic resonance imaging
MSH	Melanocyte-stimulating hormone
PIH	Prolactin-inhibiting hormone
PRH	Prolactin-releasing hormone
PRL	Prolactin
SHBG	Sex hormone-binding globulin
SIADH	Syndrome of inappropriate secretion of antidiuretic hormone
TRH	Thyrotropin-releasing hormone
TSH	Thyroid-stimulating hormone (thyrotropin)
VIP	Vasoactive intestinal polypeptide

Table 5–1. Neuroendocrine messengers: Substances that function as neurotransmitters, neural hormones, and classic hormones.

	Neuro-transmitter (Present in Nerve Endings)	Hormone Secreted by Neurons	Hormone Secreted by Endocrine Cells
Dopamine	+	+	+
Norepinephrine	+	+	+
Epinephrine	+		+
Somatostatin	+	+	+
Gonadotropin-releasing hormone (GnRH)	+	+	+
Thyrotropin-releasing hormone (TRH)	+	+	
Oxytocin	+	+	+
Vasopressin	+	+	+
Vasoactive intestinal polypeptide (VIP)	+	+	
Cholecystokinin (CCK)	+		+
Glucagon	+		+
Enkephalins	+		+
Pro-opiomelanocortin derivatives	+		+
Other anterior pituitary hormones	+		+

tain hypothalamic nuclei into the portal hypophysial vessels, which regulate the hormone-secreting cells of the anterior lobe of the pituitary. Another example of neurosecretory regulation is the posterior lobe of the pituitary gland, which is made up of the endings of neurons whose cell bodies reside in hypothalamic nuclei. These neurons secrete vasopressin and oxytocin into the general circulation.

Anatomy & Embryology

The anatomic relationships between the pituitary and the main nuclei of the hypothalamus are shown in Figure 5–2. The posterior lobe of the pituitary (neurohypophysis) is of neural origin, arising embryologically as an evagination of the ventral hypothalamus and the third ventricle. The neurohypophysis consists of the axons and nerve endings of neurons whose cell bodies reside in the supraoptic and paraventricular nuclei of the hypothalamus and supporting tissues. This hypothalamo-neurohypophysial nerve tract contains approximately 100,000 nerve fibers. Repeated swellings along the nerve fibers ranging in thickness from 1 to 50 μm constitute the nerve terminals.

The human fetal anterior pituitary anlage is initially recognizable at 4–5 weeks of gestation, and rapid cytologic differentiation leads to a mature hypothalamic-pituitary unit at 20 weeks. The anterior pituitary (adenohypophysis) originates from Rathke's pouch, an ectodermal evagination of the oropharynx, and migrates to join the neurohypophysis. The portion of Rathke's pouch in contact with the neurohypophysis develops less extensively and forms the intermediate lobe. This lobe remains intact in some species, but in humans its cells become interspersed with those of the anterior lobe and develop the capacity to synthesize and secrete pro-opiomelanocortin and adrenocorticotropic hormone (ACTH). Remnants of Rathke's pouch may persist at the boundary of the neurohypophysis, resulting in small colloid cysts. In addition, cells may persist in the lower portion of Rathke's pouch beneath the sphenoid bone, the pharyngeal pituitary. These cells have the potential to secrete hormones and have been reported to undergo adenomatous change.

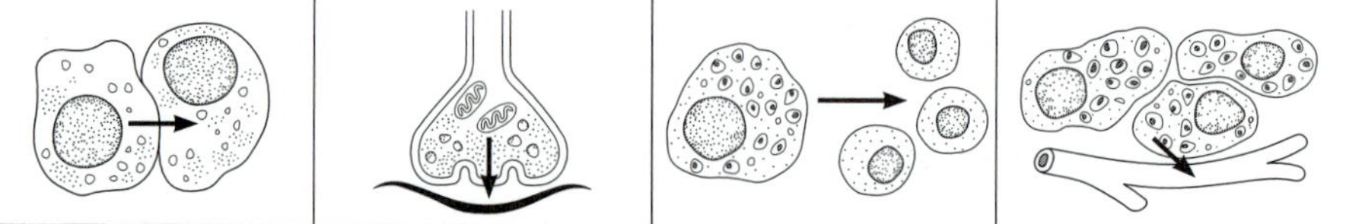

	GAP JUNCTIONS	SYNAPTIC	PARACRINE	ENDOCRINE
Message transmission	Directly from cell to cell	Across synaptic cleft	By diffusion in interstitial fluid	By circulating body fluids
Local or general	Local	Local	Locally diffuse	General
Specificity depends on	Anatomic location	Anatomic location and receptors	Receptors	Receptors

Figure 5–1. Intercellular communication by chemical mediators.

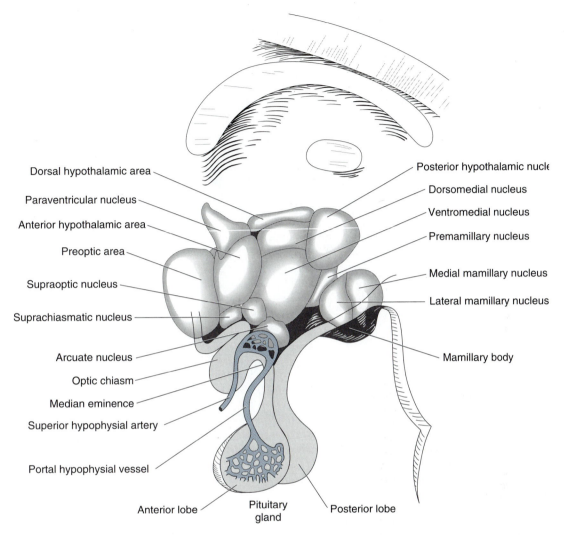

Dorsal hypothalamic area

Paraventricular nucleus

Anterior hypothalamic area

Preoptic area

Supraoptic nucleus

Suprachiasmatic nucleus

Arcuate nucleus

Optic chiasm

Median eminence

Superior hypophysial artery

Portal hypophysial vessel

Anterior lobe

Pituitary gland

Posterior lobe

Posterior hypothalamic nucle

Dorsomedial nucleus

Ventromedial nucleus

Premamillary nucleus

Medial mamillary nucleus

Lateral mamillary nucleus

Mamillary body

Figure 5–2. The human hypothalamus, with a superimposed diagrammatic representation of the portal hypophysial vessels. (Reproduced, with permission, from Ganong WF: *Review of Medical Physiology,* 15th ed. Appleton & Lange, 1993.)

The pituitary gland itself lies at the base of the skull in a portion of the sphenoid bone called the sella turcica ("Turkish saddle"). The anterior portion, the tuberculum sellae, is flanked by posterior projections of the sphenoid wings, the anterior clinoid processes; the dorsum sellae forms the posterior wall, and its upper corners project into the posterior clinoid processes. The gland is surrounded by dura, and the roof is formed by a reflection of the dura attached to the clinoid processes, the diaphragma sellae. The arachnoid membrane and, therefore, cerebrospinal fluid are prevented from entering the sella turcica by the diaphragma sellae. The pituitary stalk and its blood vessels pass through an opening in this diaphragm. The lateral walls of the gland are in direct apposition to the cavernous sinuses and separated from them by dural membranes. The optic chiasm lies 5–10 mm above the diaphragma sellae and anterior to the stalk (Figure 5–3).

The size of the pituitary gland, of which the anterior lobe constitutes two-thirds, varies considerably. It measures approximately 15 × 10 × 6 mm and weighs 500–900 mg; it may double in size during pregnancy. The sella turcica tends to conform to the shape and size of the gland, and for that reason there is considerable variability in its contour.

Blood Supply

The anterior pituitary is the most richly vascularized of all mammalian tissues, receiving 0.8 mL/g/min from a portal circulation connecting the median eminence of the hypothalamus and the anterior pituitary. Arterial blood is supplied from the internal carotid arteries via the superior, middle, and

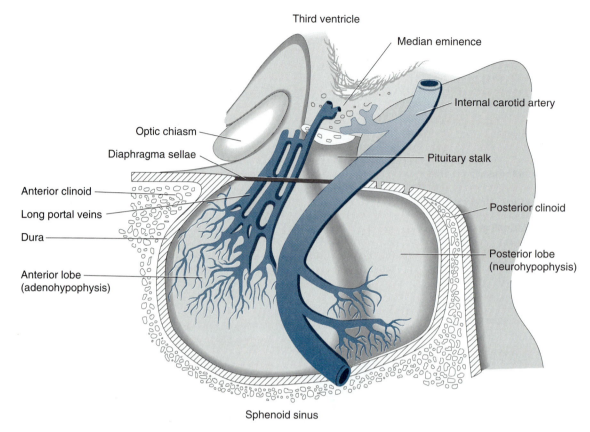

Figure 5–3. Anatomic relationships and blood supply of the pituitary gland. (Reproduced, with permission, from Frohman LA: Diseases of the anterior pituitary. In: *Endocrinology and Metabolism,* 3rd ed. Felig P, Baxter JD, Frohman LA [editors]. McGraw-Hill, 1995.)

inferior hypophysial arteries. The superior hypophysial arteries form a capillary network in the median eminence of the hypothalamus that recombines in long portal veins draining down the pituitary stalk to the anterior lobe, where they break up into another capillary network and re-form into venous channels. The pituitary stalk and the posterior pituitary are supplied directly from branches of the middle and inferior hypophysial arteries (Figures 5–2 and 5–3).

Venous drainage of the pituitary, the route through which anterior pituitary hormones reach the systemic circulation, is variable, but venous channels eventually drain via the cavernous sinus posteriorly into the superior and inferior petrosal sinuses to the jugular bulb and vein (Figure 5–4). The axons of the neurohypophysis terminate on capillaries that drain via the posterior lobe veins and the cavernous sinuses to the general circulation. The hypophysial-portal system of capillaries allows control of anterior pituitary function by the hypothalamic hypophyseotropic hormones secreted into the portal hypophysial vessels. This provides a short, direct connection to the anterior pituitary from the ventral hypothalamus and the

median eminence. (Figure 5–5). There may also be retrograde blood flow between the pituitary and hypothalamus, providing a possible means of direct feedback between pituitary hormones and their neuroendocrine control.

Histology

Anterior pituitary cells were originally classified as acidophils, basophils, and chromophobe cells. Immunocytochemical and electron microscopic techniques now permit classification of cells by their specific secretory products: somatotrophs (growth hormone [GH]-secreting cells), lactotrophs (prolactin [PRL]-secreting cells), thyrotrophs (cells secreting thyroid-stimulating hormone [thyrotropin; TSH]), corticotrophs (cells secreting adrenocorticotropic hormone [corticotropin; ACTH] and related peptides), and gonadotrophs (luteinizing hormone [LH]- and follicle-stimulating hormone [FSH]-secreting cells). Development of the capacity for expression of hormone secretion depends upon a variety of factors including the transcription factor Pit-1. Abnormalities of this factor have been associated with the development of hypopituitarism. Although traditionally

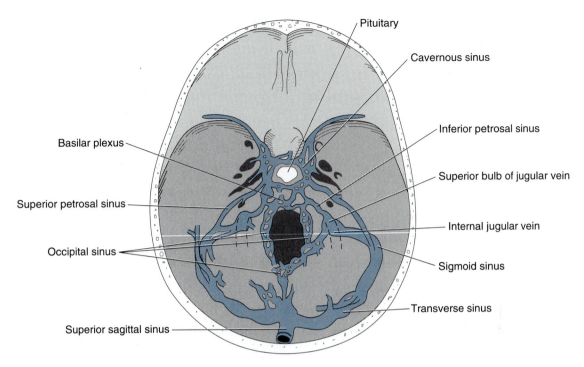

Figure 5–4. Venous drainage of the pituitary gland—the route by which adenohypophysial hormones reach the systemic circulation. (Reproduced, with permission, from Findling JW et al: Selective venous sampling for ACTH in Cushing's syndrome: Differentiation between Cushing's disease and the ectopic ACTH syndrome. Ann Intern Med 1981; 94:647.)

the pituitary has been conceptualized as a gland with distinct and highly specialized cells that respond to specific hypothalamic and peripheral hormones, it has become clear that local (ie, paracrine) factors also play a role in normal pituitary physiology.

A. Somatotrophs: The GH-secreting cells are acidophilic in standard hematoxylin and eosin preparations and are usually located in the lateral portions of the anterior lobe. Granule size by electron microscopy is 150–600 nm in diameter. These cells account for about 50% of the adenohypophysial cells.

B. Lactotrophs: The PRL-secreting cell is a second but distinct acidophil-staining cell randomly distributed in the anterior pituitary is. These cells account for 10–25% of anterior pituitary cells. Granule size averages approximately 550 nm on electron microscopy. There are two types of lactotrophs: sparsely granulated and densely granulated. These cells proliferate during pregnancy as a result of elevated estrogen levels and account for the twofold increase in gland size.

C. Thyrotrophs: These TSH-secreting cells, because of their glycoprotein product, are basophilic and also show a positive reaction with periodic acid-Schiff (PAS) stain. Thyrotrophs are the least common pituitary cell type, making up less than 10% of adenohypophysial cells. The thyrotroph granules are small (50–100 nm); these cells are usually located in the anteromedial and anterolateral portions of the gland. During states of primary thyroid failure, the cells demonstrate marked hypertrophy, increasing overall gland size.

D. Corticotrophs: ACTH and its related peptides (see below) are secreted by basophilic cells that are embryologically of intermediate lobe origin and usually located in the anteromedial portion of the gland. Corticotrophs represent 15–20% of adenohypophysial cells. Electron microscopy shows that these secretory granules are about 360 nm in diameter. In states of glucocorticoid excess, corticotrophs undergo degranulation and a microtubular hyalinization known as Crooke's hyaline degeneration.

E. Gonadotrophs: LH and FSH originate from basophil-staining cells, whose secretory granules are about 200 nm in diameter. These cells constitute 10–15% of anterior pituitary cells, and they are located throughout the entire anterior lobe. They become hypertrophied and cause the gland to enlarge during states of primary gonadal failure such as menopause, Klinefelter's syndrome, and Turner's syndrome.

F. Other Cell Types: Despite immunocytochemical staining with antibodies directed against all of the known anterior pituitary hormones, some cells remain unstained. These are chromophobes by conventional staining methods, but electron microscopy

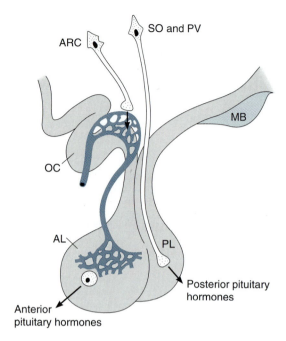

Figure 5–5. Secretion of hypothalamic hormones. The hormones of the posterior lobe (PL) are released into the general circulation from the endings of supraoptic and paraventricular neurons, whereas hypophyseotropic hormones are secreted into the portal hypophysial circulation from the endings of arcuate and other hypothalamic neurons. (AL, anterior lobe; MB, mamillary bodies; OC, optic chiasm.)

has identified secretory granules in many of them. These cells have been called null cells; they may give rise to nonfunctioning adenomas. It is not certain whether they represent undifferentiated primitive secretory cells or whether they produce as yet unidentified hormones, such as adrenal androgen-stimulating hormone, ovarian growth factor, or aldosterone-stimulating factor. Mammosomatotrophs contain both GH and PRL; these bihormonal cells are most often seen in pituitary tumors. Human chorionic gonadotropin is also secreted by the anterior pituitary gland, but its cell of origin and physiologic significance are uncertain.

HYPOTHALAMIC HORMONES

The hypothalamic hormones can be divided into those secreted into hypophysial portal blood vessels and those secreted by the neurohypophysis directly into the general circulation. The eight known hypo-thalamic hormones are listed with their structures in Table 5–2.

Hypophyseotropic Hormones

The hypophyseotropic hormones which regulate the secretion of anterior pituitary hormones include growth hormone releasing hormone (GRH), somatostatin, dopamine, thyrotropin releasing hormone (TRH), corticotropin-releasing hormone (CRH), and gonadotropin-releasing hormone (GnRH). Most of the anterior pituitary hormones are controlled by stimulatory hormones, but growth hormone and especially prolactin are also regulated by inhibitory hormones. Some hypophyseotropic hormones are multifunctional. The hormones of the hypothalamus are secreted episodically and not continuously, and in some cases—eg, CRH and TRH—there is an underlying circadian rhythm.

A. GRH: GRH stimulates growth hormone (GH) secretion by somatotrophs. GRH-secreting neurons are located in the arcuate nuclei (Figure 5–2), and axons terminate in the external layer of the median eminence. Two peptides (of 40 and 44 amino acids) with potent GH-releasing activity were isolated from separate pancreatic tumors in patients with clinical manifestations of growth hormone excess (acromegaly) associated with somatotroph hyperplasia (see below). GRH is synthesized from a larger precursor of 107 or 108 amino acids. These precursors differ by the presence or absence of a serine at position 103. The function of other secretory products derived from this precursor is unknown. Full biologic activity of these releasing factors appears to reside in the 1–29 amino acid sequence of the amino terminal portion of the molecule. Human GRH is strikingly similar to many gastrointestinal peptides, including secretin, gastrin, vasoactive intestinal polypeptide (VIP), and gastric inhibitory peptide. Like CRH, GRH has a rather long half-life (50 minutes).

B. Somatostatin: Somatostatin inhibits the secretion of GH and TSH. Somatostatin-secreting cells are located in the periventricular region immediately above the optic chiasm (Figure 5–2) with nerve endings found diffusely in the external layer of the median eminence.

Somatostatin, a tetradecapeptide, has been found not only in the hypothalamus but also in the D cells of the pancreatic islets, the gastrointestinal mucosa, and the C-cells (parafollicular cells) of the thyroid. The somatostatin precursor has 116 amino acids. Processing of the carboxyl terminal region of preprosomatostatin results in the generation of the tetradecapeptide somatostatin 14 and an amino terminal extended form containing 28 amino acid residues (somatostatin 28). Somatostatin 14 is the major species in the hypothalamus, while somatostatin 28 is found in the gut. Processing of somatostatin 28 produces somatostatin 14 and a duodecapeptide from the

Table 5–2. Hypothalamic hormones.

Hormone	Structure
Posterior pituitary hormones	
Arginine vasopressin	$\lceil$—S———————S—$\rceil$ Cys-Tyr-Phe-Gln-Asn-Cys-Pro-Arg-Gly-NH$_2$
Oxytocin	$\lceil$—S———————S—$\rceil$ Cys-Tyr-Ile-Gln-Asn-Cys-Pro-Leu-Gly-NH$_2$
Hypophyseotropic hormones Thyrotropin-releasing hormone (TRH)	(pyro)Glu-His-Pro-NH$_2$
Gonadotropin-releasing hormone (GnRH)	(pyro)Glu-His-Trp-Ser-Tyr-Gly-Leu-Arg-Pro-Gly-NH$_2$
Somatostatin[1]	———————S———————————S——————— Ala-Gly-Cys-Lys-Asn-Phe-Phe-Trp-Lys-Thr-Phe-Thr-Ser-Cys
Growth hormone-releasing hormone (GRH)	Tyr-Ala-Asp-Ala-Ile-Phe-Thr-Asn-Ser-Tyr-Arg-Lys-Val-Leu-Gly-Gln-Leu-Ser- Ala-Arg-Lys-Leu-Gln-Asp-Ile-Met-Ser-Arg-Gln-Gln-Gly-Glu-Ser-Asn-Gln-Glu- Arg-Gly-Ala-Arg-Ala-Arg-Leu-NH$_2$
Prolactin-inhibiting hormone-(PIH, dopamine)	
Corticotropin-releasing hormone (CRH)	Ser-Gln-Glu-Pro-Pro-Ile-Ser-Leu-Asp-Leu-Thr-Phe-His-Leu-Leu-Arg-Glu-Val- Leu-Glu-Met-Thr-Lys-Ala-Asp-Gln-Leu-Ala-Gln-Gln-Ala-His-Ser-Asn-Arg-Lys- Leu-Leu-Asp-Ile-Ala-NH$_2$

[1]In addition to the tetradecapeptide shown here (somatostatin 14), an amino terminal extended molecule (somatostatin 28) and a 12-amino-acid form (somatostatin 28 [1–12]) are found in most tissues.

amino terminal extension (somatostatin 28 [1–12]). The function of this latter peptide is unknown. In addition to its profound inhibitory effect on GH secretion, somatostatin also has important inhibitory influences on many other hormones, including insulin, glucagon, gastrin, secretin, and VIP. This inhibitory hypothalamic peptide plays a role in the physiologic secretion of TSH by augmenting the direct inhibitory effect of thyroid hormone on the thyrotrophs; administration of anti-somatostatin antibodies results in a rise in circulating TSH level.

C. Dopamine: Dopamine, the primary prolactin-inhibitory hormone (PIH), is found in the portal circulation and binds to dopamine receptors in lactotrophs. The hypothalamic control of PRL secretion, unlike that of the other pituitary hormones, is predominantly inhibitory. Thus, disruption of the hypothalamic-pituitary connection by stalk section, hypothalamic lesions, or pituitary autotransplantation increases PRL secretion. Dopamine-secreting neurons (tuberoinfundibular dopaminergic system) are located in the arcuate nuclei and their axons terminate in the external layer of the median eminence, primarily in the same area as the GnRH endings (laterally) and to a lesser extent medially (Figure 5–2). The neurotransmitter gamma-aminobutyric acid (GABA) and cholinergic pathways also appear to inhibit PRL release.

D. Prolactin-Releasing Factors: The best-studied PRL-releasing factor is thyrotropin-releasing hormone (see below) However, there are several dis-

cordant responses, suggesting that TRH is not the only PRL-releasing factor. The PRL increase associated with sleep, during stress, and after nipple stimulation or suckling is not accompanied by an increase in TRH or TSH. Another hypothalamic peptide, VIP, stimulates PRL release in humans. Serotonergic pathways may also stimulate PRL secretion, as demonstrated by the increased PRL secretion after the administration of serotonin precursors and by the reduction of secretion following treatment with serotonin antagonists.

E. Thyrotropin-Releasing Hormone (TRH): TRH, a tripeptide, is the major hypothalamic factor in TSH secretion. Human TRH is synthesized from a large precursor of 242 amino acids that contains six copies of TRH. TRH-secreting neurons are located in the medial portions of the paraventricular nuclei (Figure 5–2), and their axons terminate in the medial portion of the external layer of the median eminence. TRH has been found in the hypothalamus as well as the portal blood; perfusion of pituitary stalk vessels with TRH evokes TSH release, and interruption of the hypothalamic-pituitary portal vessels decreases TSH secretion.

F. Corticotropin-Releasing hormone (CRH): CRH, a 41-amino-acid peptide, stimulates the secretion of adrenocorticotropic hormone (ACTH) and other products of its precursor molecule, pro-opiomelanocortin. The structure of human CRH is identical to that of rat CRH. CRH is synthesized from a precursor of 196 amino acids. CRH has a long plasma half-life (approximately 60 minutes), and both ADH and angiotensin II potentiate CRH-mediated secretion of ACTH. In contrast, oxytocin inhibits CRH-mediated ACTH secretion. CRH-secreting neurons are found in the anterior portion of the paraventricular nuclei just lateral to the TRH-secreting neurons; their nerve endings are found in all parts of the external layer of the median eminence. CRH is also secreted from human placenta. The level of this hormone increases significantly during late pregnancy and delivery. In addition, a specific CRH-binding protein (CRHBP) has been described in both serum and in intracellular locations within a variety of cells. It is likely that CRHBPs modulate the actions of CRH.

G. Gonadotropin-Releasing Hormone (GnRH): The secretion of Luteinizing Hormone (LH) and follicle-stimulating hormone (FSH) is controlled by a single stimulatory hypothalamic hormone, gonadotropin-releasing hormone (GnRH). GnRH is a linear decapeptide that stimulates only LH and FSH; it has no effect on other pituitary hormones except in some patients with acromegaly and Cushing's disease (see below). The precursor of GnRH—proGnRH—contains 92 amino acids. ProGnRH also contains the sequence of a 56-amino-acid polypeptide called GnRH-associated peptide (GAP). This secretory product exhibits prolactin-inhibiting activity, but its physiologic role is unknown. GnRH-secreting neurons are located primarily in the in preoptic area of the anterior hypothalamus and their nerve terminal are found in the lateral portions of the external layer of the median eminence adjacent to the pituitary stalk (Figure 5–2).

Posterior Pituitary Hormones

The hypothalamo-neurohypophysial system secretes two nonapeptides: antidiuretic hormone (ADH) (also known as arginine vasopressin) and oxytocin. They are synthesized in large cell bodies of neurons (magnocellular neurons) in the supraoptic nuclei and the lateral and superior parts of the paraventricular nuclei (Figure 5–2). ADH is an important regulator of water balance; it also is a potent vasoconstrictor and plays a role in regulation of cardiovascular function. Oxytocin causes contraction of smooth muscle, especially of the myoepithelial cells that line the ducts of the mammary gland, thus causing milk ejection.

ADH and oxytocin are basic nonapeptides (MW 1084 and 1007, respectively) characterized by a ring structure with a disulfide linkage (see Table 5–2). They are synthesized by separate cells (ie, there is no co-secretion or synthesis) from prohormones which contain both the peptide and an associated binding peptide or neurophysin specific for the hormone: neurophysin II for ADH and neurophysin I for oxytocin. Since the hormone and neurophysin are synthesized from the same prohormone, defects in gene expression result in deficiency of both products. For example, the Brattleboro rat has a deficiency of ADH and neurophysin II (but not of oxytocin and neurophysin I). Following synthesis and initial processing, secretory granules containing the prohormone migrate by axoplasmic flow (2–3 mm/h) to the nerve endings of the posterior lobe. In the secretory granules, further processing produces the mature nonapeptide and its neurophysin, which are co-secreted in equimolar amounts by exocytosis. Action potentials that reach the nerve endings increase the Ca^{2+} influx and initiate hormone secretion.

Neuroendocrinology: The Hypothalamus as Part of a Larger System

The hypothalamus is involved in many nonendocrine functions such as regulation of body temperature and food intake and is connected with many other parts of the nervous system. The brain itself is influenced by both direct and indirect hormonal effects. Steroid and thyroid hormones cross the blood-brain barrier and produce specific receptor-mediated actions (see Chapters 7 and 9). Peptides in the general circulation which do not cross the blood brain barrier elicit their effects indirectly eg insulin-mediated changes in blood glucose concentration. In addition, communication between the general circulation and the brain may take place via the circumventricular organs, which are located outside the blood brain barrier (see below). Moreover, hypothalamic hormones in extrahypothalamic brain function as neurotransmitters or neurohormones. They are also found in other tissues where they function as hormones (endocrine, paracrine, or autocrine). For example, somatostatin-containing neurons are widely distributed in the nervous system. They are also found in the pancreatic islets (D cells), the gastrointestinal mucosa, and the C cells of the thyroid gland (parafollicular cells). Somatostatin is not only secreted into the general circulation and diffuses locally—it is also secreted into the lumen of the gut, where it may affect gut secretion. A hormone with this activity has been called a "lumone." Hormones common to the brain, pituitary, and gastrointestinal tract include not only TRH and somatostatin but also vasoactive intestinal polypeptide (VIP) and peptides derived from pro-opiomelanocortin (see Chapter 17).

Hypothalamic function is regulated both by hormone-mediated signals—eg, negative feedback—and by neural inputs from a wide variety of sources. These nerve signals are mediated by neurotransmitters including acetylcholine, dopamine, norepinephrine, epinephrine, serotonin, gamma-aminobutyric acid, and opioids. The hypothalamus can be considered a final common pathway by which signals from multiple systems reach the anterior pituitary. For example, cytokines that play a role in the response to infection, such as the interleukins, are also involved in regulation of the hypothalamic-pituitary-adrenal axis. This system of immunoneuroendocrine interactions is important in the organism's response to a variety of stresses.

The hypothalamus also sends signals to other parts of the nervous system. For example, while the major nerve tracts of the magnocellular neurons containing vasopressin and oxytocin terminate in the posterior pituitary, nerve fibers from the paraventricular and supraoptic nuclei project to many other parts of the nervous system. In the brain stem, vasopressinergic neurons are involved in the autonomic regulation of blood pressure. Similar neurons project to the gray matter and are implicated in higher cortical functions. Fibers terminating in the median eminence permit release of ADH into the hypophysial-portal system; delivery of ADH in high concentrations to the anterior pituitary may facilitate its involvement in the regulation of ACTH secretion. Magnocellular neurons also project to the choroid plexus where they may release ADH into the cerebrospinal fluid. In addition to magnocellular neurons, the paraventricular nuclei contain cells with smaller cell bodies—parvicellular neurons. Such neurons are also found in other regions of the nervous system and may contain other peptides such as CRH and TRH.

The Pineal Gland & the Circumventricular Organs

The circumventricular organs are secretory midline brain structures that arise from the ependymal cell lining of the ventricular system (Figure 5–6). These organs are located adjacent to the third ventricle—subfornical organ, subcommissural organ, oganum vasculosum of the lamina terminalis, pineal, and part of the median eminence—and at the roof of the fourth ventricle—area postrema (Figure 5–6). The tissues of these organs have relatively large interstitial spaces and have fenestrated capillaries which being highly permeable, permit diffusion of large molecules from the general circulation; elsewhere in the brain tight capillary endothelial junctions prevent such diffusion—the blood-brain barrier. For example, angiotensin II (see Chapter 10) is involved in the regulation of water intake, blood pressure, and secretion of vasopressin. In addition to its peripheral effects, circulating angiotensin II acts on the subfornical organ resulting in an increased in water intake.

The pineal gland, considered by the 17th century French philosopher Descartes to be the seat of the soul, is located at the roof of the posterior portion of the third ventricle. The pineal gland in humans and other mammals has no direct neural connections with the brain except for sympathetic innervation via the superior cervical ganglion. The pineal gland secretes

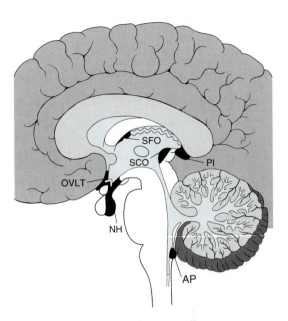

Figure 5–6. Circumventricular organs. The neurohypophysis (NH) and adjacent median eminence, the organum vasculosum of the lamina terminalis (OVLT), the subfornical organ (SFO), and the area postrema (AP) are shown projected on a sagittal section of the human brain. The pineal (PI) and the subcommissural organ (SCO) are also shown but probably do not function as circumventricular organs. (Reproduced, with permission, from Ganong WF: *Review of Medical Physiology,* 15th ed. Appleton & Lange, 1993.)

melatonin, an indole synthesized from serotonin by 5-methoxylation and *N*-acetylation (Figure 5–7). The pineal releases melatonin into the general circulation and into the cerebrospinal fluid. Melatonin secretion is regulated by the sympathetic nervous system and is increased in response to hypoglycemia and darkness. The pineal also contains other bioactive peptides and amines including TRH, somatostatin, GnRH, and norepinephrine. The physiologic roles of the pineal remain to be elucidated, but they involve regulation of gonadal function and development and chronobiologic rhythms.

The pineal gland may be the site of pineal cell tumors (pinealomas) or germ cell tumors (germinomas). Neurologic signs and symptoms are the predominant clinical manifestations, eg, increased intracranial pressure, visual abnormalities, ataxia, and Parinaud's syndrome—upward gaze palsy, absent pupillary light reflex, paralysis of convergence, and wide based gait. Endocrine manifestations result primarily from deficiency of hypothalamic hormones (diabetes insipidus, hypopituitarism, or disorders of gonadal development). Treatment involves surgical removal or decompression, radiation therapy, and hormone replacement (see below).

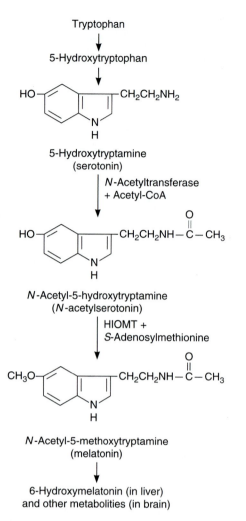

Tryptophan

5-Hydroxytryptophan

5-Hydroxytryptamine
(serotonin)

N-Acetyltransferase
+ Acetyl-CoA

N-Acetyl-5-hydroxytryptamine
(*N*-acetylserotonin)

HIOMT +
S-Adenosylmethionine

N-Acetyl-5-methoxytryptamine
(melatonin)

6-Hydroxymelatonin (in liver)
and other metabolities (in brain)

Figure 5–7. Formation and metabolism of melatonin. (HIOMT, hydroxyindole-O-methyltransferase.) (Reproduced, with permission, from Ganong WF: *Review of Medical Physiology,* 15th ed. Appleton & Lange, 1993.)

ANTERIOR PITUITARY HORMONES

The six major anterior pituitary hormones—ACTH, GH, PRL, TSH, LH, and FSH—may be classified into three groups: corticotropin-related peptides (ACTH, LPH, melanocyte-stimulating hormone [MSH], and endorphins); the somatomammotropins (GH and PRL), which are also peptides; and the glycoproteins (LH, FSH, and TSH). The chemical features of these hormones are illustrated in Table 5–3

ACTH & RELATED PEPTIDES

Biosynthesis

ACTH is a 39-amino-acid peptide hormone (MW 4500) processed from a large precursor molecule, pro-opiomelanocortin (POMC) (MW 28,500). Within the corticotroph, a single mRNA directs the synthesis and processing of POMC into smaller biologically active fragments (Figure 5–8) which include β-LPH, α-MSH, β-MSH, β-endorphin, and the amino terminal fragment of pro-opiomelanocortin. Most of these peptides are glycosylated, which accounts for differences in the reporting of molecular weights. These carbohydrate moieties are responsible for the basophilic staining of corticotrophs.

Two of these fragments are contained within the structure of ACTH: α-MSH is identical to $ACTH_{1-13}$, and corticotropin-like intermediate lobe peptide (CLIP) represents $ACTH_{18-39}$ (Figure 5–8). Although these fragments are found in species with developed intermediate lobes (eg, the rat), they are not secreted as separate hormones in humans. β-Lipotropin, a fragment with 91 amino acids (1–91), is secreted by the corticotroph in equimolar quantities with ACTH. Within the β-LPH molecule exists the amino acid sequence for β-MSH (41–58), γ-LPH (1–58), and β-endorphin (61–91).

The amino terminal fragment (131 amino acids) of pro-opiomelanocortin has been isolated and sequenced. The first 76 amino acids of this Amino terminal sequence appear to be the physiologically relevant form of this fragment. Plasma levels of this peptide increase in response to hypoglycemic stress. It may be an adrenal growth factor and may potentiate ACTH action on steroidogenesis.

Function

ACTH stimulates the secretion of glucocorticoids, mineralocorticoids, and androgenic steroids from the adrenal cortex (see Chapters 9 and 10). The amino terminal end (residues 1–18) is responsible for this biologic activity. ACTH binds to receptors on the adrenal cortex and provokes steroidogenesis through the mediation of cAMP.

The hyperpigmentation observed in states of ACTH hypersecretion (eg, Addison's disease, Nelson's syndrome) appears to be primarily due to ACTH. Because α- and β-MSH do not exist as separate hormones in humans, the exact cause of this increased pigmentation remains unclear.

The physiologic function of β-LPH and its family of peptide hormones, including β-endorphin, is not completely understood. However, both β-LPH and β-endorphin have the same secretory dynamics as ACTH; they increase in response to stress, hypoglycemia, and metyrapone and are suppressible with glucocorticoids. These hormones, including the Amino terminal fragment, also parallel ACTH in dis-

Table 5–3. Characteristics of anterior pituitary hormones.[1]

Pituitary Hormone	Molecular Weight	Amino Acids	Other Features
I. Corticotropin-lipotropin ACTH	4,500	39	All of these hormones are derived from a common precursor.
β-Lipotropin	11,200	91	
β-Endorphin	4,000	31	
II. Glycoprotein LH	29,000	Alpha subunit: 89 Beta subunit: 115	All have 2 subunits, with the alpha subunit being identical in each and the beta subunit conferring biologic specificity.
FSH	29,000	Alpha subunit: 89 Beta subunit: 115	
TSH	28,000	Alpha subunit: 89 Beta subunit: 112	
III. Somatomammotropin GH	21,500	191	Evolved from a common hormone.
PRL	22,000	198	

[1]Adapted from Frohman LA: Diseases of the anterior pituitary. In: *Endocrinology and Metabolism.* Felig P et al (editors). McGraw-Hill, 1981.

ease states—eg, they are elevated in Addison's disease, Cushing's disease, and Nelson's syndrome and suppressed by glucocorticord excess. Furthermore, there is evidence that β-endorphin acts as an "endogenous opiate," suggesting a role in pain appreciation. It may affect the endocrine regulation of other pituitary hormones and perhaps also the neural control of breathing.

Measurement

The development of an immunoradiometric assay using monoclonal antibodies has provided a sensitive and practical clinical ACTH assay for the evaluation of pituitary-adrenal disorders. The basal morning concentration ranges from 9 to 52 pg/mL (2.2–11 pmol/L). Its short plasma half-life (7–12 minutes) and episodic secretion cause wide and rapid fluctuations both in its plasma concentration and in that of cortisol.

Although β-LPH has a longer half-life than ACTH and is more stable in plasma, its measurement has not been extensively utilized. Current data suggest that the normal concentration of β-LPH is 10–40 pg/mL (1–4 pmol/L).

Secretion

The physiologic secretion of ACTH is mediated through neural influences by means of a complex of hormones, the most important of which is corticotropin-releasing hormone (CRH) (Figure 5–9).

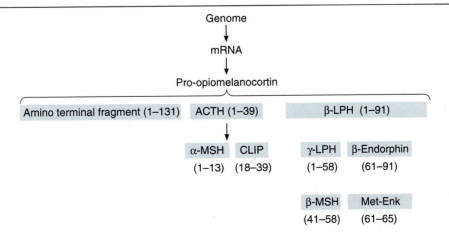

Figure 5–8. The processing of pro-opiomelanocortin (MW 28,500) into its biologically active peptide hormones. Abbreviations are expanded in the text.

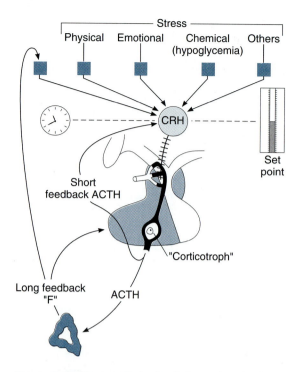

Figure 5–9. The hypothalamic-pituitary-adrenal axis, illustrating negative feedback by cortisol ("F") at the hypothalamic and pituitary levels. A short negative feedback loop of ACTH on the secretion of corticotropin-releasing hormone (CRH) also exists. (Reproduced, with permission, from Gwinup G, Johnson B: Clinical testing of the hypothalamic-pituitary-adrenocortical system in states of hypo- and hypercortisolism. Metabolism 1975;24:777.)

CRH stimulates ACTH in a pulsatile manner: Diurnal rhythmicity causes a peak before awakening and a decline as the day progresses. The diurnal rhythm is a reflection of neural control and provokes concordant diurnal secretion of cortisol from the adrenal cortex (Figure 5–10). This episodic release of ACTH is independent of circulating cortisol levels—ie, the magnitude of an ACTH impulse is not related to preceding plasma cortisol levels. An example is the persistence of diurnal rhythm in patients with primary adrenal failure (Addison's disease). ACTH secretion also increases in response to feeding in both humans and animals.

Many stresses stimulate ACTH, often superseding the normal diurnal rhythmicity. Physical, emotional, and chemical stresses such as pain, trauma, hypoxia, acute hypoglycemia, cold exposure, surgery, depression, and pyrogen and vasopressin administration have all been shown to stimulate ACTH and cortisol secretion. The increase in ACTH levels during stress is mediated by vasopressin as well as CRH. Although physiologic cortisol levels do not blunt the ACTH response to stress, exogenous corticosteroids in high doses suppress it.

Negative feedback of cortisol and synthetic glucocorticoids on ACTH secretion occurs at both the hypothalamic and pituitary levels via two mechanisms: "Fast feedback" is sensitive to the rate of change in cortisol levels, while "slow feedback" is sensitive to the absolute cortisol level. The first mechanism is probably nonnuclear; ie, this phenomenon occurs too rapidly to be explained by the influence of corticosteroids on nuclear transcription of the specific mRNA responsible for ACTH. "Slow feedback," occurring later, may be explained by a nuclear-mediated mechanism and a subsequent decrease in synthesis of ACTH. This latter form of negative feedback is the type probed by the clinical dexamethasone suppression test. In addition to the negative feedback of corticoids, ACTH also inhibits its own secretion (short loop feedback).

GROWTH HORMONE

Biosynthesis

Growth hormone (GH; somatotropin) is a 191-amino-acid polypeptide hormone (MW 21,500) synthesized and secreted by the somatotrophs of the anterior pituitary. Its larger precursor peptide, preGH (MW 28,000), is also secreted but has no physiologic significance.

Function

The primary function of growth hormone (somatotropin) is promotion of linear growth. Its basic metabolic effects serve to achieve this result, but most of the growth-promoting effects are mediated by insulin-like growth factor 1 (IGF-1; also known as somatomedin C) (see Chapter 6).

Growth hormone, via IGF-1, increases protein synthesis by enhancing amino acid uptake and directly accelerating the transcription and translation of mRNA. In addition, GH tends to decrease protein catabolism by mobilizing fat as a more efficient fuel source: It directly causes the release of fatty acids from adipose tissue and enhances their conversion to acetyl-CO, from which energy is derived. This protein-sparing effect is an important mechanism by which GH promotes growth and development.

GH also affects carbohydrate metabolism. In excess, it decreases carbohydrate utilization and impairs glucose uptake into cells. This GH-induced insulin resistance appears to be due to a postreceptor impairment in insulin action. These events result in glucose intolerance and secondary hyperinsulinism.

Measurement

GH circulates unbound in plasma and has a half-life of 20–50 minutes. The healthy adult secretes approximately 400 μg/d (18.6 nmol/d); in contrast, young adolescents secrete about 700 μg/d (32.5 nmol/d).

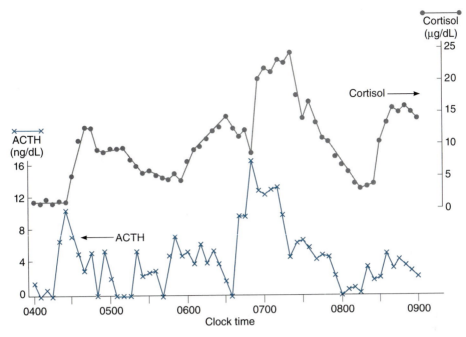

Figure 5–10. The episodic, pulsatile pattern of ACTH secretion and its concordance with cortisol secretion in a healthy human subject during the early morning. (Reproduced, with permission, from Gallagher TF et al: ACTH and cortisol secretory patterns in man. J Clin Endocrinol Metab 1973;36:1058.)

The early morning GH concentration in fasting adults is less than 5 ng/mL (230 pmol/L) and usually less than 2 ng/mL (90 pmol/L). There are no significant sex differences.

Concentrations of IGF-1 are determined by radioreceptor assays or radioimmunoassays. Determining the levels of these mediators of GH action may result in more accurate assessment of the biologic activity of GH (see Chapter 6). Growth hormone-binding proteins (GHBPs) include a high-affinity GHBP that represents the extracellular portion of the GH receptor and a low-affinity species. About half of circulating GH is bound to GHBPs. Measurement of serum concentrations of the high-affinity GHBP provides an index of GH receptor concentrations.

Secretion

The secretion of GH is mediated by two hypothalamic hormones: growth hormone-releasing hormone (GRH) and somatostatin (growth hormone-inhibiting hormone). These hypothalamic influences are tightly regulated by an integrated system of neural, metabolic, and hormonal factors. Because neither GRH nor somatostatin can be measured directly, the net result of any factor on GH secretion must be considered as the sum of its effects on these hypothalamic hormones. Table 5–4 summarizes the many factors that affect GH secretion in physiologic, pharmacologic, and pathologic states.

A. GRH: Both the 40- and the 44-amino-acid forms of GRH are present in the human hypothalamus; however, whether one of these forms is more important physiologically is not clear. GRH stimulates cAMP production by somatotrophs and stimulates both GH synthesis and secretion. The effects of GRH are partially blocked by somatostatin. The administration of GRH to normal humans leads to rapid release of GH (within minutes); levels peak at 30 minutes and are sustained for 60–120 minutes.

Other peptide hormones such as ADH, ACTH, and α-MSH may act as GH-releasing factors when present in pharmacologic amounts. Even thyrotropin- and gonadotropin-releasing hormones (TRH and GnRH) often cause GH secretion in patients with acromegaly; however, it is not certain whether any of these effects are mediated by the hypothalamus or represent direct effects on the somatotroph.

B. Somatostatin: Somatostatin, a tetradecapeptide, is a potent inhibitor of GH secretion. It decreases cAMP production in GH-secreting cells and inhibits both basal and stimulated GH secretion. Somatostatin secretion is increased by elevated levels of GH and IGF-1. A long-acting analog of somatostatin, octreotide acetate, has been used therapeutically in the management of GH excess and in conditions such as pancreatic and carcinoid tumors that cause diarrhea.

C. Neural Control: The neural control of basal GH secretion results in irregular and intermittent re-

Table 5–4. Factors affecting growth hormone secretion.[1]

Increase	Decrease[2]
Physiologic	
Sleep	Postprandial hyperglycemia
Exercise	Elevated free fatty acids
Stress (physical or psychologic)	
Postprandial:	
Hyperaminoacidemia	
Hypoglycemia (relative)	
Pharmacologic	
Hypoglycemia:	Hormones:
Absolute: insulin or 2-deoxyglucose	Somatostatin
	Growth hormone
Relative: postglucagon	Progesterone
Hormones:	Glucocorticoids
GRH	Neurotransmitters, etc:
Peptide (ACTH, α-MSH, vasopressin)	Alpha-adrenergic antagonists (phentolamine)
Estrogen	Beta-adrenergic agonists (isoproterenol)
Neurotransmitters, etc:	Serotonin antagonists (methysergide)
Alpha-adrenergic agonists (clonidine)	Dopamine antagonists (phenothiazines)
Beta-adrenergic antagonists (propranolol)	
Serotonin precursors	
Dopamine agonists (levodopa, apomorphine, bromocriptine)	
GABA agonists (muscimol)	
Potassium infusion	
Pyrogens (*Pseudomonas* endotoxin)	
Pathologic	
Protein depletion and starvation	Obesity
Anorexia nervosa	Acromegaly: dopamine agonists
Ectopic production of GRH	Hypo- and hyperthyroidism
Chronic renal failure	
Acromegaly:	
TRH	
GnRH	

[1]Modified and reproduced, with permission, from Frohman LA: Diseases of the anterior pituitary. In: *Endocrinology and Metabolism*, Felig P et al (editors). McGraw-Hill, 1981.
[2]Suppressive effects of some factors can be demonstrated only in the presence of a stimulus.

lease associated with sleep and varying with age. Peak levels occur 1–4 hours after the onset of sleep (during stages 3 and 4) (Figure 5–11). These nocturnal sleep bursts, which account for nearly 70% of daily GH secretion, are greater in children and tend to decrease with age. Glucose infusion will not suppress this episodic release. Emotional, physical, and chemical stress, including surgery, trauma, exercise, electroshock therapy, and pyrogen administration, provoke GH release; and impairment of secretion, leading to growth failure, has been well documented in children with severe emotional deprivation (see Chapter 6).

D. Metabolic Control: The metabolic factors affecting GH secretion include all fuel substrates: carbohydrate, protein, and fat. Glucose administration, orally or intravenously, lowers GH in healthy subjects and provides a simple physiologic maneuver useful in the diagnosis of acromegaly (see below). In contrast, hypoglycemia stimulates GH release. This effect depends on intracellular glycopenia, since the administration of 2-deoxyglucose (a glucose analog that causes intracellular glucose deficiency) also increases GH. This response to hypoglycemia depends on both the rate of change in blood glucose and the absolute level attained.

A protein meal or intravenous infusion of amino acids (eg, arginine) causes GH release. Paradoxically, states of protein-calorie malnutrition also increase GH, possibly as a result of decreased IGF-1 production and lack of inhibitory feedback.

Fatty acids suppress GH responses to certain stimuli, including arginine and hypoglycemia. Fasting stimulates GH secretion, possibly as a means of mobilizing fat as an energy source and preventing protein loss.

E. Effects of Other Hormones: Responses to stimuli are blunted in states of cortisol excess and during hypo- and hyperthyroidism. Estrogen enhances GH secretion in response to stimulation.

F. Effects of Neuropharmacologic Agents: Many neurotransmitters and neuropharmacologic agents affect GH secretion. Biogenic amine agonists and antagonists act at the hypothalamic level and alter GRH or somatostatin release. Dopaminergic, alpha-adrenergic, and serotonergic agents all stimulate GH release.

Dopamine agonists such as levodopa, apomorphine, and bromocriptine increase GH secretion, whereas dopaminergic antagonists such as phenothiazines inhibit GH. The effect of levodopa, a precursor of both norepinephrine and dopamine, may be mediated by its conversion to norepinephrine, since its effect is blocked by the alpha-adrenergic antagonist phentolamine. Moreover, phentolamine suppresses GH release in response to other stimuli such as hypoglycemia, exercise, and arginine, emphasizing the importance of alpha-adrenergic mechanisms in modulating GH secretion.

Beta-adrenergic agonists inhibit GH, and beta-adrenergic antagonists such as propranolol enhance secretion to provocative stimuli.

PROLACTIN

Biosynthesis

Prolactin (PRL) is a 198-amino-acid polypeptide hormone (MW 22,000) synthesized and secreted from the lactotrophs of the anterior pituitary. Despite evolution from an ancestral hormone common to GH

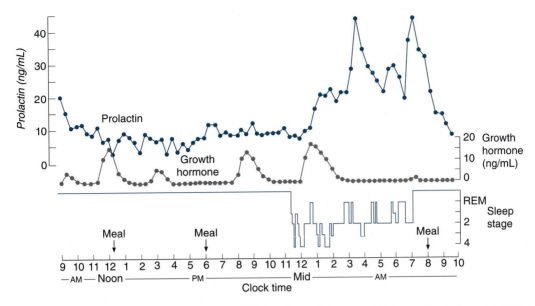

Figure 5–11. Sleep-associated changes in prolactin (PRL) and growth hormone (GH) secretion in humans. Peak levels of GH occur during sleep stages 3 or 4; the increase in PRL is observed 1–2 hours after sleep begins and is not associated with a specific sleep phase. (Reproduced, with permission, from Sassin JF et al: Human prolactin: 24-hour pattern with increased release during sleep. Science 1972;177:1205.)

and human placental lactogen (hPL), PRL shares only 16% of its residues with the former and 13% with hPL. A precursor molecule (MW 40,000–50,000) is also secreted and may constitute 8–20% of the PRL plasma immunoreactivity in healthy persons and in patients with PRL-secreting pituitary tumors.

Function

PRL stimulates lactation in the postpartum period (see Chapter 16). During pregnancy, PRL secretion increases and, in concert with many other hormones (estrogen, progesterone, hPL, insulin, and cortisol), promotes additional breast development in preparation for milk production. Despite its importance during pregnancy, PRL has not been demonstrated to play a role in the development of normal breast tissue in humans. During pregnancy, estrogen enhances breast development but blunts the effect of PRL on lactation; the decrease in both estrogen and progesterone after parturition allows initiation of lactation. Accordingly, galactorrhea may accompany the discontinuance of oral contraceptives or estrogen therapy. Although basal PRL secretion falls in the postpartum period, lactation is maintained by persistent breast suckling.

PRL levels are very high in the fetus and in newborn infants, declining during the first few months of life.

Although PRL does not appear to play a physiologic role in the regulation of gonadal function, hy-

perprolactinemia in humans leads to hypogonadism. In women, initially there is a shortening of the luteal phase; subsequently, anovulation, oligomenorrhea or amenorrhea, and infertility occur. In men, PRL excess leads to decreased testosterone synthesis and decreased spermatogenesis, which clinically present as decreased libido, impotence, and infertility. The exact mechanisms of PRL inhibition of gonadal function are unclear, but the principal one appears to be alteration of hypothalamic-pituitary control of gonadotropin secretion. Basal LH and FSH levels are normal or subnormal; however, their pulsatile secretion is decreased and the midcycle LH surge is suppressed in women. Gonadotropin reserve, as assessed with GnRH, is usually normal or even exaggerated.

Measurement

The PRL secretory rate is approximately 400 μg/d (18.6 nmol/d). The hormone is cleared by the liver (75%) and the kidney (25%), and its half-time of disappearance from plasma is about 50 minutes.

Basal levels of PRL in adults vary considerably, with a mean of 13 ng/mL (0.6 nmol/L) in women and 5 ng/mL (0.23 nmol/L) in men. The upper range of normal in most laboratories is 15–20 ng/mL (0.7–0.9 nmol/L).

Secretion

The hypothalamic control of PRL secretion is predominantly inhibitory, and dopamine is the most important inhibitory factor. The administration of dopamine or its precursor levodopa, either in vitro or in vivo, inhibits PRL release; drugs that block dopamine receptors (eg, phenothiazines, metoclopramide) or cause hypothalamic dopamine depletion (reserpine, methyldopa) stimulate PRL release. The physiologic, pathologic, and pharmacologic factors influencing PRL secretion are listed in Table 5–5.

A. Prolactin-Releasing Factors: TRH is a potent prolactin-releasing factor that evokes release of PRL at a threshold dose similar to that which stimulates release of TSH. An exaggerated response of both TSH and PRL to TRH is observed in primary hypothyroidism, and their responses are blunted in hyperthyroidism. In addition, PRL secretion is also stimulated by VIP and serotonergic pathways.

B. Episodic and Sleep-Related Secretion: PRL secretion is episodic. An increase is observed 60–90 minutes after sleep begins but, in contrast to GH, is not associated with a specific sleep phase. Peak levels are usually attained between 4 and 7 AM (Figure 5–11). This sleep-associated augmentation of

PRL release is not part of a circadian rhythm, like that of ACTH; it is related strictly to the sleeping period regardless of when it occurs during the day.

C. Other Stimuli: Stresses, including surgery, exercise, hypoglycemia, and acute myocardial infarction, cause significant elevation of PRL levels. Nipple stimulation in nonpregnant women also increases PRL. This neurogenic reflex may also occur from chest wall injury such as mechanical trauma, burns, surgery, and herpes zoster of thoracic dermatomes. This reflex discharge of PRL is abolished by denervation of the nipple or by spinal cord or brain stem lesions.

D. Effects of Other Hormones: Many hormones influence PRL release. Estrogens augment basal and stimulated PRL secretion after 2–3 days of use (an effect that is of special clinical importance in patients with PRL-secreting pituitary adenomas); glucocorticoids tend to suppress TRH-induced PRL secretion; and thyroid hormone administration may blunt the PRL response to TRH.

E. Effects of Pharmacologic Agents: (Table 5–5.) Many pharmacologic agents alter PRL secretion. Dopamine agonists (eg, bromocriptine) decrease secretion, forming the basis for their use in states of PRL excess. Dopamine antagonists (eg, phenothiazines) augment PRL release. There is good correlation between the antipsychotic potency of these drugs and their hyperprolactinemic response, perhaps related to the extent of dopamine antagonism. Serotonin agonists will enhance PRL secretion; serotonin receptor blockers suppress stress- and nursing-associated PRL release.

Table 5–5. Factors affecting prolactin secretion.

Increase	Decrease
Physiologic	
Pregnancy	
Nursing	
Nipple stimulation	
Exercise	
Stress (hypoglycemia)	
Sleep	
Seizures	
Neonatal	
Pharmacologic	
TRH	Dopamine agonists (levo-
Estrogen	dopa, apomorphine,
VIP	bromocriptine, pergolide)
Dopamine antagonists (phe-	GABA
nothiazines, haloperidol,	
metoclopramide, reser-	
pine, methyldopa, amox-	
apine, opiates)	
Opioids	
Monoamine oxidase inhibi-	
tors	
Cimetidine (intravenous)	
Verapamil	
Licorice	
Pathologic	
Pituitary tumors	Pseudohypoparathyroidism
Hypothalamic/pituitary stalk	Pituitary destruction or re-
lesions	moval
Neuraxis irradiation	Lymphocytic hypophysitis
Chest wall lesions	
Spinal cord lesions	
Hypothyroidism	
Chronic renal failure	
Severe liver disease	

THYROTROPIN

Biosynthesis

Thyrotropin (thyroid-stimulating hormone, TSH) is a glycoprotein (MW 28,000) composed of two noncovalently linked alpha and beta subunits. The structure of the alpha subunit of TSH resembles that of the other glycoprotein molecules—FSH, LH, and human chorionic gonadotropin (hCG)—but the beta subunit differs in these glycoproteins and is responsible for their biologic and immunologic specificity. The peptides of these subunits appear to be synthesized separately and united before the carbohydrate groups are attached. The intact molecule is then secreted, as are small amounts of nonlinked subunits.

Function

The beta subunit of TSH attaches to high-affinity receptors in the thyroid, stimulating iodide uptake, hormonogenesis, and release of T_4 and T_3. This occurs through activation of adenylyl cyclase and the generation of cAMP. TSH secretion also causes an increase in gland size and vascularity by promoting mRNA and protein synthesis. (For a more detailed description, see Chapter 7.)

Measurement

TSH circulates unbound in the blood with a half-life of 50–60 minutes. With ultrasensitive immunoradiometric assays for measuring TSH concentration, the normal range is usually 0.5–5.0 µU/mL (0.5–5.0 m U/L). These new assays are helpful in the diagnosis of primary hypothyroidism and hyperthyroidism; however, TSH levels alone cannot be used to evaluate pituitary or hypothalamic hypothyroidism.

The alpha subunit can be detected in about 80% of normals, with a range of 0.5–2 ng/mL. Plasma alpha subunit levels increase after administration of TRH in normal subjects, and basal levels are elevated in primary hypothyroidism, primary hypogonadism, and in patients with gonadotropin-secreting or pure alpha subunit-secreting pituitary adenomas.

Secretion

The secretion of TSH is controlled by both stimulatory (TRH) and inhibitory (somatostatin) influences from the hypothalamus and in addition is modulated by the feedback inhibition of thyroid hormone on the hypothalamic-pituitary axis (Figures 5–12 and 7–21).

A. TRH: The response of TSH to TRH is modulated by the circulating concentration of thyroid hormones. Small changes in serum levels (even within the physiologic range) cause substantial alterations in the TSH response to TRH. As shown in Figure 5–13, the administration of T_3 (15 µg) and T_4 (60 µg) to healthy persons for 3–4 weeks suppresses the TSH response to TRH despite only small increases in circulating T_3 and T_4 levels. Thus, the secretion of TSH is inversely proportionate to the concentration of thyroid hormone.

The set point (the level at which TSH secretion is maintained) is determined by TRH. Deviations from this set point result in appropriate changes in TSH release. Administration of TRH increases TSH within 2 minutes, and this response is blocked by previous T_3 administration; however, larger doses of TRH may overcome this blockade—suggesting that both T_3 and TRH act at the pituitary level to influence TSH secretion. In addition, T_3 and T_4 inhibit mRNA for TRH synthesis in the hypothalamus, indicating that a negative feedback mechanism operates at this level also.

B. Somatostatin: This inhibitory hypothalamic peptide augments the direct inhibitory effect of thyroid hormone on the thyrotrophs. Infusion of somatostatin blunts the early morning TSH surge and will suppress high levels of TSH in primary hypothyroidism. Octreotide acetate, a long-acting somatostatin analog, has been used successfully to inhibit TSH secretion in some patients with TSH-secreting pituitary tumors.

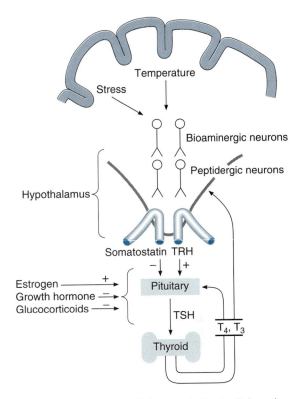

Figure 5–12. Diagram of the hypothalamic-pituitary-thyroid axis, illustrating the negative feedback of thyroid hormones (T_4, T_3) predominantly at the pituitary level. Hypothalamic factors may stimulate (TRH) or suppress (somatostatin) TSH secretion. Estrogen, GH, and glucocorticoids influence the effects of TRH on TSH secretion. (Reproduced, with permission, from Martin JB, Reichlin S, Brown GM: *Clinical Neuroendocrinology.* Davis, 1977.)

C. Neural Control: In addition to these hypothalamic influences on TSH secretion, neurally mediated factors may be important. Dopamine physiologically inhibits TSH secretion. Intravenous dopamine administration will decrease TSH in both healthy and hypothyroid subjects as well as blunt the TSH response to TRH. Thus, as expected, dopaminergic agonists such as bromocriptine inhibit TSH secretion and dopaminergic antagonists such as metaclopramide increase TSH secretion in euthyroid subjects. Bromocriptine has also been effective in the management of some TSH-secreting pituitary tumors.

D. Effects of Cortisol and Estrogens: Glucocorticoid excess has been shown to impair the sensitivity of the pituitary to TRH and to be able to lower serum TSH to undetectable levels. However, estrogens increase the sensitivity of the thyrotroph to TRH; women have a greater TSH response to TRH than men do, and pretreatment of men with estradiol will increase their TRH-induced TSH response. (See also Chapter 7 and Table 7–6.)

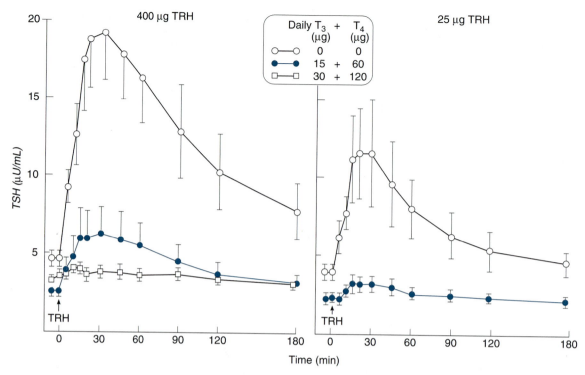

Figure 5–13. Administration of small doses of T_3 (15 μg) and T_4 (60 μg) healthy subjects inhibits the TSH response to 2 doses (400 μg, left; 25 μg, right) of TRH (protirelin). (Reproduced, with permission, from Snyder PJ, Utiger RD: Inhibition of thyrotropin-releasing hormone by small quantities of thyroid hormones. J Clin Invest 1972;51:2077.)

GONADOTROPINS: LUTEINIZING HORMONE, FOLLICLE-STIMULATING HORMONE

Biosynthesis

Luteinizing hormone (LH) and follicle-stimulating hormone (FSH) are glycoprotein gonadotropins composed of alpha and beta subunits and secreted by the same cell. The specific beta subunit confers on these hormones their unique biologic activity, as it does with TSH and hCG. The biologic activity of hCG, a placental glycoprotein, closely resembles that of LH. Human menopausal gonadotropin (hMG, menotropins)—an altered mixture of pituitary gonadotropins recovered from the urine of postmenopausal women—is a preparation with FSH-like activity. Menotropins and chorionic gonadotropin are used clinically for induction of spermatogenesis or ovulation (see Chapters 12 and 13).

Function

LH and FSH bind to receptors in the ovary and testis and regulate gonadal function by promoting sex steroid production and gametogenesis.

In men, LH stimulates testosterone production from the interstitial cells of the testes (Leydig cells). Maturation of spermatozoa, however, requires both LH and FSH. FSH stimulates testicular growth and enhances the production of an androgen-binding protein by the Sertoli cells, which are a component of the testicular tubule necessary for sustaining the maturing sperm cell. This androgen-binding protein causes high local concentrations of testosterone near the sperm, an essential factor in the development of normal spermatogenesis (see Chapter 12).

In women, LH stimulates estrogen and progesterone production from the ovary. A surge of LH in the mid menstrual cycle is responsible for ovulation, and continued LH secretion subsequently stimulates the corpus luteum to produce progesterone by enhancing the conversion of cholesterol to pregnenolone. Development of the ovarian follicle is largely under FSH control, and the secretion of estrogen from this follicle is dependent on both FSH and LH.

Measurement

The normal levels of LH and FSH vary with the age of the subject (see Appendix). They are low before puberty and elevated in postmenopausal women. A nocturnal rise of LH in boys and the cyclic secretion of FSH and LH in girls usually herald the onset of puberty before clinical signs are apparent. In women, LH and FSH vary during the menstrual cycle; during the initial phase of the cycle (follicular), LH steadily increases, with a midcycle surge that initiates ovulation. FSH, on the other hand, initially rises and then decreases during the later follicular phase until the midcycle surge, which is concordant with LH. Both LH and FSH levels fall steadily after ovulation (Figure 5–14). (See Chapter 13.)

LH and FSH levels in men are similar to those in women during the follicular phase. The alpha subunit, shared by all the pituitary glycoprotein hormones, can also be measured (see TSH) and will rise following GnRH administration. The normal responses of LH and FSH to GnRH are shown in Table 5–6.

Secretion

The secretion of LH and FSH is controlled by gonadotropin-releasing hormone (GnRH), which maintains basal gonadotropin secretion, generates the phasic release of gonadotropins for ovulation, and determines the onset of puberty.

A. Episodic Secretion: In both males and females, secretion of LH and FSH is episodic, with secretory bursts that occur each hour and are mediated by a concordant episodic release of GnRH. The amplitude of these secretory surges is greater in patients with primary hypogonadism. The pulsatile nature of GnRH release is critical for sustaining gonadotropin secretion. A continuous, prolonged infusion of GnRH in women evokes an initial increase in LH and FSH followed by prolonged suppression of gonadotropin secretion. This phenomenon may be explained by down-regulation of GnRH receptors on the pituitary gonadotrophs. Consequently, long-acting synthetic analogs of GnRH may be used clinically to suppress LH and FSH secretion in conditions such as precocious puberty.

B. Positive Feedback: Circulating sex steroids affect GnRH secretion and thus LH and FSH secretion by both positive and negative (inhibitory) feedback mechanisms. During the menstrual cycle, estrogens provide a positive influence on GnRH effects on LH and FSH secretion, and the rise in estrogen during the follicular phase is the stimulus for the LH and FSH ovulatory surge. This phenomenon suggests that the secretion of estrogen is to some extent influenced by an intrinsic ovarian cycle. Progesterone amplifies the duration of the LH and FSH surge and augments the effect of estrogen. After this midcycle surge, the developed egg leaves the ovary. Ovulation occurs approximately 10–12 hours after the LH peak and 24–36 hours after the estradiol peak. The remaining follicular cells in the ovary are converted, under the influence of LH, to a progesterone-secreting structure, the corpus luteum. After about 12 days, the corpus luteum involutes, resulting in decreased estro-

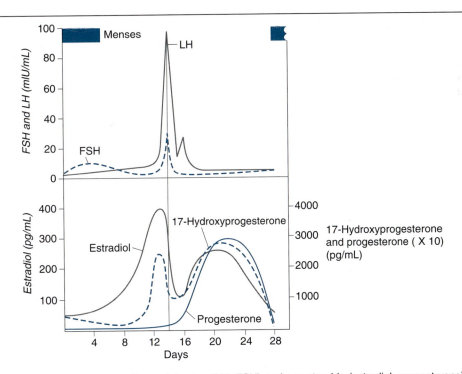

Figure 5–14. The secretory pattern of gonadotropins (LH, FSH) and sex steroids (estradiol, progesterone) during the normal female menstrual cycle. A midcycle surge of LH and FSH, stimulated by the rise in estradiol during the follicular phase, results in ovulation. After ovulation, the luteinized follicle secretes progesterone. (Reproduced, with permission, from Odell WD, Moyer DL: *Physiology of Reproduction.* Mosby, 1971.)

Table 5–6. Normal gonadotropin responses (± SD) to GnRH (100 μg).

	Mean Maximum Exchange LH		Mean Maximum Exchange FSH	
	(μg/L)	(IU/L)	(μg/L)	(IU/L)
Women				
Follicular phase	2.1 ± 0.4	17 ± 3	1.0 ± 0.3	3 ± 1
Around LH peak	20.8 ± 6.2	162 ± 49	2.7 ± 1.0	8 ± 3
Luteal phase	6.3 ± 1.0	49 ± 8	1.0 ± 0.1	3 ± 0.4
Men				
Age 18–40	4.1 ± 0.8	32 ± 6	1.0 ± 0.3	3 ± 1
Age over 65	2.9 ± 0.5	23 ± 4	1.0 ± 0.3	3 ± 1

Conversion factors: For LH (LER 960), 1 ng = 7.8 mIU; for FSH (LER 869), 1 ng = 3 mIU.

gen and progesterone levels and then uterine bleeding. (See Chapter 13.)

C. Negative Feedback: Negative feedback effects of sex steroids on gonadotropin secretion also occur. In women, primary gonadal failure or menopause results in elevations of LH and FSH, which can be suppressed with long-term, high-dose estrogen therapy. However, a shorter duration of low-dose estrogen may enhance the LH response to GnRH. In men, primary gonadal failure with low circulating testosterone levels is also associated with elevated gonadotropins. However, testosterone is not the sole inhibitor of gonadotropin secretion in men, since selective destruction of the tubules (eg, by cyclophosphamide therapy) results in azoospermia and elevation of only FSH.

Inhibin, a polypeptide (MW 32,000) secreted by the Sertoli cells of the seminiferous tubules, is the major factor that inhibits FSH secretion by negative feedback. Inhibin, which has been purified and sequenced by analysis of its complementary DNA, consists of separate alpha and beta subunits connected by a disulfide bridge. Androgens stimulate inhibin production; this peptide may help to locally regulate spermatogenesis.

ENDOCRINOLOGIC EVALUATION OF THE HYPOTHALAMIC-PITUITARY AXIS

The precise assessment of the hypothalamic-pituitary axis has been made possible by radioimmunoassays of the major anterior pituitary hormones and their specific target gland hormones. In addition, four synthetic hypothalamic hormones: TRH (protirelin) and GnRH (gonadorelin), which are available commercially; and the more recently synthesized ovine CRH and human GRH (GRH-40 and GRH-44) can be used to assess hypothalamic-pituitary reserve.

This section describes the principles involved in testing each pituitary hormone as well as special situations (eg, drugs, obesity) that may interfere with pituitary function or pituitary testing. Specific protocols for performing and interpreting diagnostic procedures are outlined at the end of this section. The clinical manifestations of either hypo- or hypersecretion of anterior pituitary hormones are discussed in subsequent sections.

EVALUATION OF ACTH

ACTH deficiency leads to adrenocortical insufficiency, characterized by decreased secretion of cortisol and the adrenal androgens; aldosterone secretion, controlled primarily by the renin-angiotensin axis, is usually maintained.

Plasma ACTH Levels

Basal ACTH measurements are usually unreliable indicators of pituitary secretory reserve, since its short plasma half-life and episodic secretion result in wide fluctuations in plasma levels. Therefore, the interpretation of plasma ACTH levels requires the simultaneous assessment of cortisol secretion by the adrenal cortex. These measurements are of greatest utility in differentiating primary and secondary adrenocortical insufficiency and in establishing the etiology of Cushing's syndrome (see the later section on Cushing's disease and also Chapter 9).

Evaluation of ACTH Deficiency

In evaluating ACTH deficiency, measurement of basal cortisol levels is also unreliable. Although morning cortisol values are usually less than 10 μg/dL (280 nmol/L) in states of diminished pituitary ACTH reserve, such low levels also occur in normal subjects because of the episodic nature of ACTH secretion. In addition, patients with ACTH deficiency following removal of ACTH-secreting pituitary adenomas or withdrawal of synthetic glucocorticoid therapy may have basal cortisol values exceeding 10 μg/dL (276 nmol/L) that fail to increase in response to a stressful stimulus. Consequently, the diagnosis of ACTH hyposecretion (secondary adrenal insufficiency) must be established by provocative testing of the reserve capacity of the hypothalamic-pituitary axis.

Adrenal Stimulation

Since adrenal atrophy develops as a consequence of prolonged ACTH deficiency, the initial and most convenient approach to evaluation of the hypothalamic-pituitary-adrenal axis is assessment of the plasma cortisol response to synthetic ACTH (cosyntropin). In normal individuals, injection of cosyntropin (250 μg) causes a rapid increase (within 30 minutes) of cortisol to at least 20 μg/dL (550 nmol/L), and this response usually correlates with the cortisol response to insulin-induced hypoglycemia. A subnormal cortisol response to ACTH confirms adrenocortical insufficiency. However, a normal response does not directly evaluate the ability of the hypothalamic-pituitary axis to respond to stress (see Chapter 9). Thus, patients withdrawn from long-term glucocorticoid therapy may have an adequate increase in cortisol following exogenous ACTH that precedes complete recovery of the hypothalamic-pituitary-adrenal axis. Therefore, such patients should receive glucocorticoids during periods of stress for at least 1 year after steroids are discontinued, unless the hypothalamic-pituitary axis is shown to be responsive to stress as described below. Use of a 1 μg dose of ACTH is better able to detect secondary adrenal insufficiency than the 250 μg dose. This low-dose test will probably supplant the high-dose version.

Pituitary Stimulation

Direct evaluation of pituitary ACTH reserve can be performed by means of insulin-induced hypoglycemia, metyrapone administration, or CRH stimulation. These studies are unnecessary if the cortisol response to rapid ACTH stimulation is subnormal.

A. Insulin-Induced Hypoglycemia: The stimulus of neuroglycopenia associated with hypoglycemia (blood glucose < 40 mg/dL) evokes a stress-mediated activation of the hypothalamic-pituitary-adrenal axis. Subjects should experience adrenergic symptoms (diaphoresis, tachycardia, weakness, headache) associated with the fall in blood sugar. In normal persons, plasma cortisol increases to more than 20 μg/dL (550 mmol/L, indicating normal ACTH reserve. Although plasma ACTH also rises, its determination has not proved to be as useful, since pulsatile secretion requires frequent sampling, and the normal response is not well standardized. Although insulin-induced hypoglycemia most reliably predicts ACTH secretory capacity in times of stress, it is rarely performed at present since the procedure requires a physician's presence and is contraindicated in elderly patients, patients with cerebrovascular or cardiovascular disease, and those with seizure disorders. It should be used with caution in patients in whom diminished adrenal reserve is suspected, since severe hypoglycemia may occur; in these patients, the test should always be preceded by the ACTH adrenal stimulation test.

B. Metyrapone Stimulation: Metyrapone administration is an alternative method for assessing ACTH secretory reserve. Metyrapone inhibits P450c11 (11β-hydroxylase), the enzyme that catalyzes the final step in cortisol biosynthesis (see Chapter 9). The inhibition of cortisol secretion interrupts negative feedback on the hypothalamic-pituitary axis, resulting in a compensatory increase in ACTH. The increase in ACTH secretion stimulates increased steroid biosynthesis proximal to P450c11, and the increase can be detected as an increase in the precursor steroid (11-deoxycortisol) in plasma. The overnight test is preferred because of its simplicity; it is performed by administering 30 mg/kg of metyrapone orally at midnight. Plasma 11-deoxycortisol is determined the following morning and rises to more than 7 μg/dL (0.19 μmol/L) in healthy individuals. Again the test should be used cautiously in patients with suspected adrenal insufficiency and should be preceded by a rapid ACTH stimulation test (see above). The traditional 3-day metyrapone test is rarely used at present. The limited availability of oral metyrapone has decreased the use of this test.

C. CRH Stimulation: Ovine CRH administered intravenously is used to assess ACTH secretory dynamics. In healthy subjects, CRH (1 μg/kg) provokes a peak ACTH response within 15 minutes and a peak cortisol response within 30–60 minutes. This dose may be associated with mild flushing, occasional shortness of breath, tachycardia, and hypotension. Patients with primary adrenal insufficiency have elevated basal ACTH levels and exaggerated responses to CRH. Secondary adrenal insufficiency results in an absent ACTH response to CRH in patients with pituitary corticotroph destruction; however, in patients with hypothalamic dysfunction, there is a prolonged and augmented ACTH response to CRH with a delayed peak.

ACTH Hypersecretion

ACTH hypersecretion is manifested by adrenocortical hyperfunction (Cushing's syndrome). The diagnosis and differential diagnosis of ACTH hypersecretion are outlined in a later section on Cushing's disease and also in Chapter 9.

EVALUATION OF GROWTH HORMONE

The evaluation of GH secretory reserve is important in the assessment of children with short stature and in adults with suspected hypopituitarism.

Provocative tests are necessary because basal levels of GH are usually low and do not distinguish between normal and GH-deficient conditions.

Insulin-Induced Hypoglycemia

The most reliable stimulus of GH secretion is insulin-induced hypoglycemia. In normal individuals, GH levels will increase to more than 10 ng/mL (460 pmol/L) after adequate hypoglycemia is achieved. Since 10% of normal individuals fail to respond to hypoglycemia, other stimulatory tests may be necessary.

Tests with Levodopa, Arginine, & Other Stimuli

GH rises after oral administration of levodopa, a precursor of dopamine and norepinephrine that readily crosses the blood-brain barrier. About 80% of healthy subjects have a GH response greater than 6 ng/mL (280 pmol/L), and the mean maximal response is 28 ng/mL (1300 pmol/L). This test is safer than insulin-induced hypoglycemia in older patients. An Arginine infusion will raise GH in 70% of healthy individuals. Pretreatment with estrogen will enhance this response in many of the nonresponders, most of whom are men. Other stimuli, such as propranolol and glucagon, have also been utilized in assessing GH secretory capacity.

GRH Test

Both forms of human GRH (GRH-40 and GRH-44) have been used to evaluate GH secretory capacity. A dose of GRH (1 μg/kg) promptly stimulates GH; the mean peak is 10–15 ng/mL (460–700 pmol/L) at 30–60 minutes in healthy subjects. There is usually a small increase in IGF-1 levels 24 hours after the administration of GRH.

GH Hypersecretion

The evaluation of GH hypersecretion is discussed in the section on acromegaly and is most conveniently assessed by suppression testing with oral glucose.

EVALUATION OF PROLACTIN

PRL secretion by the pituitary is the most resistant to local damage, and decreased PRL secretory reserve indicates severe intrinsic pituitary disease.

Prolactin Reserve

The administration of TRH is the simplest and most reliable means of assessing PRL reserve. Although the response of PRL to TRH varies somewhat according to sex and age (Table 5–7), PRL levels usually increase twofold 15–30 minutes after TRH administration. In addition, insulin-induced hypoglycemia will evoke a stress-related increase in PRL.

Table 5–7. Normal responses to TSH and prolactin to TRH (500 μg).

	TSH	
	(μU/mL)	(mU/L)
Maximum Δ TSH		
Women and men aged < 40	≥ 6	≥ 6
Men aged 40–79	≥ 2	≥ 2
Time of maximum Δ TSH (min)	≤ 45	

	Prolactin	
	(ng/mL)	(pmol/L)
Basal, men and women	< 15	< 681
Maximum Δ prolactin		
Men aged 20–39	25–49	681–1818
Men aged 40–59	19–50	454–2272
Men aged 60–79	5–90	227–4090
Women aged 20–39	30–120	1383–5454
Women aged 40–59	20–120	909–5454
Women aged 60–79	10–100	454–4545

[1]Reproduced, with permission, from Snyder PJ et al: Diagnostic value of thyrotrophin-releasing hormone in pituitary and hypothalamic diseases: Assessment of thyrotrophin and pro-

PRL Hypersecretion

PRL hypersecretion is a common endocrine problem. Its evaluation is discussed in the section on prolactinomas.

EVALUATION OF TSH

Basal Measurements

The laboratory evaluation of TSH secretory reserve begins with an assessment of target gland secretion; thyroid function tests (free thyroxine [FT_4]) should be obtained. Normal thyroid function studies in a clinically euthyroid patient indicate adequate TSH secretion, and no further studies are warranted. Laboratory evidence of hypothyroidism requires measurement of a TSH level. With primary thyroid gland failure, the TSH level will be elevated; low or normal TSH in the presence of hypothyroidism suggests hypothalamic-pituitary dysfunction.

TRH Test

In healthy subjects, protirelin produces an increase of TSH of at least 6 μU/mL (6 mU/L) within 15–30 minutes (Table 5–7). In patients with primary hypothyroidism, an elevated TSH level confirms the diagnosis; thus, the TRH test is not indicated. Patients with secondary hypothyroidism have normal to low basal TSH levels, and an impaired or absent TSH response in these patients implicates hypothalamic-pituitary failure. Patients with hypothalamic disease often show a delayed TSH response (60–120 minutes) to TRH (see Figure 7–25) and, less commonly, an exaggerated TSH increase. Unlike gonadotropic function, prolonged TRH deficiency does not impair

TSH responsiveness. Many patients with hypothyroidism due to pituitary disease have normal responses to TRH, or responses that resemble hypothalamic dysfunction. Accordingly, the TRH test is not always a reliable way to differentiate pituitary from hypothalamic disease.

Responsiveness to TRH is often impaired in patients with hypothalamic pituitary disease (eg, acromegaly, Cushing's syndrome) who are euthyroid. Since GH or cortisol excess may decrease the TSH response to TRH, an absent response does not always indicate destruction of thyrotrophs. (See also Chapter 7.)

EVALUATION OF LH & FSH

Testosterone & Estrogen Levels

The evaluation of gonadotropin function also requires assessment of target gland secretory function, and measurement of gonadal steroids (testosterone in men, estradiol in women) is useful in the diagnosis of hypogonadism. In women, the presence of regular menstrual cycles is strong evidence that the hypothalamic-pituitary-gonadal axis is intact. Estradiol levels rarely fall below 50 pg/mL (180 pmol/L), even during the early follicular phase. A level of less than 30 pg/mL (110 pmol/L) in the presence of oligomenorrhea or amenorrhea is indicative of gonadal failure. In men, serum testosterone (normal range, 300–1000 ng/dL (10–35 nmol/L) is a sensitive index of gonadal function.

LH & FSH Levels

In the presence of gonadal insufficiency, high LH and FSH levels are a sign of primary gonadal disease; low or normal LH and FSH suggest hypothalamic-pituitary dysfunction (hypogonadotropic hypogonadism).

GnRH Test

LH and FSH secretory reserves may be assessed with the use of synthetic GnRH (gonadorelin). Administration of GnRH causes a prompt increase in plasma LH and a lesser and slower increase in FSH (for normal responses, see Table 5–6). The LH response to GnRH is lowest during the follicular phase and greatest during the ovulatory surge. Normal subjects may have no FSH response to GnRH. On the other hand, in prepubertal children and in some patients with hyperprolactinemia, the FSH response is greater than that of LH.

A single GnRH test does not distinguish hypothalamic from pituitary disease. Patients with disturbances of the hypothalamus and pituitary may have an absent, normal, or exaggerated gonadotropin response to GnRH. Hypothalamic disease with long-standing GnRH deficiency results in an absent LH response to GnRH, but normal responsiveness may be restored with more prolonged and intermittent stimulation.

Clomiphene Test

Clomiphene citrate, an antiestrogen that blocks estrogen receptors, causes a state of functional estrogen deficiency resulting in GnRH and gonadotropin release. The occurrence of a normal menstrual period approximately 12 days after administration of the drug or evidence of ovulation by basal body temperature constitutes a normal response. Failure of LH levels to increase after 5–10 days of clomiphene in a patient with a normal GnRH test suggests hypothalamic disease. (See Chapter 13.)

PROBLEMS IN EVALUATION OF THE HYPOTHALAMIC-PITUITARY AXIS

This section briefly outlines some of the disorders and conditions that may cause confusion and lead to misinterpretation of pituitary function tests. The effects of drugs are described in the next section.

Obesity

GH dynamics are impaired in many obese patients; all provocative stimuli, including insulin-induced hypoglycemia, arginine, levodopa, and glucagon plus propranolol, often fail to provoke GH secretion. The GH response to GRH is also impaired in obesity and improves with weight loss. Obesity may increase urinary 17-hydroxycorticosteroid levels and the cortisol secretory rate, however, urinary free cortisol excretion is unchanged. Plasma cortisol demonstrates normal diurnal variation and responds to hypoglycemia. The cortisol response to CRH is also blunted in obesity.

Diabetes Mellitus

Although glucose normally suppresses GH secretion, most type I diabetic individuals have normal or elevated GH levels that often do not rise further in response to hypoglycemia or arginine. Levodopa will increase GH in some diabetic patients, and even a dopamine infusion (which produces no GH change in nondiabetic subjects, since it does not cross the blood-brain barrier) will stimulate GH in diabetic patients. Despite the increased GH secretion in patients with inadequately controlled diabetes, the GH response to GRH in insulin-dependent diabetic patients is similar to that of nondiabetic subjects. IGF-1 levels are low in insulin-deficient diabetes despite the elevated GH levels.

Uremia

Basal levels of GH, PRL, LH, FSH, TSH, and free cortisol tend to be elevated, for the most part owing to prolongation of their plasma half-life. GH may paradoxically increase following glucose administration and is often hyperresponsive to a hypoglycemic stimulus. Although the administration of TRH (protirelin) has no effect on GH secretion in healthy subjects, the drug may increase GH in patients with chronic renal failure. The response of PRL to TRH is blunted and prolonged. Gonadotropin response to synthetic GnRH usually remains intact. Dexamethasone suppression of cortisol may be impaired.

Starvation & Anorexia Nervosa

GH secretion increases with fasting and malnutrition, and such conditions may cause a paradoxical increase in GH following glucose administration. Severe starvation, such as occurs in patients with anorexia nervosa, may result in low levels of gonadal steroids. LH and FSH responses to GnRH may be intact despite a state of functional hypogonadotropic hypogonadism. Cortisol levels may be increased and fail to suppress adequately with dexamethasone. PRL and TSH dynamics are usually normal despite a marked decrease in circulating total thyroid hormones (see Chapter 7).

Depression

Depression may alter the ability of dexamethasone to suppress plasma cortisol and may elevate cortisol secretion; the response to insulin-induced hypoglycemia usually remains intact. The ACTH response to CRH is blunted in endogenous depression. Some depressed patients also have abnormal GH dynamics: TRH may increase GH, and hypoglycemia or levodopa may fail to increase GH. These patients may also show blunted TSH responses to TRH.

EFFECTS OF PHARMACOLOGIC AGENTS ON HYPOTHALAMIC-PITUITARY FUNCTION

Glucocorticoid excess impairs the GH response to hypoglycemia, the TSH response to TRH, and the LH response to GnRH. Estrogens tend to augment GH dynamics as well as the PRL and TSH response to TRH. Estrogens increase plasma cortisol secondary to a rise in corticosteroid-binding globulin and may result in inadequate suppression with dexamethasone.

Phenytoin enhances the metabolism of dexamethasone, making studies with this agent difficult to interpret. Phenothiazines may blunt the GH response to hypoglycemia and levodopa and frequently cause hyperprolactinemia. The many other pharmacologic agents that increase PRL secretion are listed in Table 5-5.

Narcotics, including heroin, morphine, and methadone, may all raise PRL levels and suppress GH and cortisol response to hypoglycemia.

In chronic alcoholics, alcohol excess or withdrawal may increase cortisol levels and cause inadequate dexamethasone suppression and an impaired cortisol increase after hypoglycemia.

ENDOCRINE TESTS OF HYPOTHALAMIC-PITUITARY FUNCTION

Methods for performing endocrine tests and their normal responses are summarized in Table 5-8. The indications for and the clinical utility of these procedures are described in the preceding section and will be mentioned again in the section on pituitary and hypothalamic disorders.

NEURORADIOLOGIC EVALUATION

Symptoms of pituitary hormone excess or deficiency, headache, or visual disturbance lead the clinician to consider a hypothalamic-pituitary disorder. In this setting, accurate neuroradiologic assessment of the hypothalamus and pituitary is essential in confirming the existence and defining the extent of hypothalamic-pituitary lesions; however, the diagnosis of such lesions should be based on both endocrine and radiologic criteria. This is because variability of pituitary anatomy in the normal population may lead to false-positive interpretations. Furthermore, patients with pituitary microadenomas may have normal neuroradiologic studies. Imaging studies must be interpreted in light of the fact that 10–20% of the general population harbor nonfunctional and asymptomatic pituitary microadenomas.

MRI is the current procedure of choice for imaging the hypothalamus and pituitary. It has superseded the use of CT since it allows better definition of normal structures and has better resolution in defining tumors. Arteriography is rarely utilized at present except in patients with intrasellar or parasellar aneurysms.

Magnetic Resonance Imaging (MRI)

Imaging is performed in sagittal and coronal planes at 1.5–2 mm intervals. This allows clear definition of hypothalamic and pituitary anatomy and can accurately visualize lesions as small as 3–5 mm. The use of the heavy-metal contrast agent gadolinium allows even more precise differentiation of small pituitary adenomas from normal anterior pituitary tissue and other adjacent structures as shown in Figure 5–15.

A. Normal Anatomy: The normal anterior pituitary is 5–7 mm in height and approximately 10 mm in its lateral dimensions. The superior margin is flat or concave but may be upwardly convex with a height of 10–12 mm in healthy menstruating young women. The floor of the sella turcica is formed by the bony

Table 5–8. Endocrine tests of hypothalamic-pituitary function.

	Method	Sample Collection	Possible Side Effects; Contraindications	Interpretation
Rapid ACTH stimulation test (cosyntropin test)	Administer synthetic $ACTH_{1-24}$ (cosyntropin), 250 μg intravenously or intramuscularly. The test may be performed at any time of the day or night and does not require fasting. The low-dose test is performed in the same manner except that 1 μg of synthetic $ACTH_{1-24}$ is administered.	Obtain samples for plasma cortisol at 0 and 30 minutes or at 0 and 60 minutes.	Rare allergic reactions have been reported.	A normal response is a peak plasma cortisol level > 20 μg/dL (550 nmol/L). In the low-dose test, the normal response is a peak plasma cortisol level > 20 μg/dL (550 nmol/L) at 30 minutes.
Insulin hypoglycemia test	Give nothing by mouth after midnight. Start an intravenous infusion with normal saline solution. Regular insulin is given intravenously in a dose sufficient to cause adequate hypoglycemia (blood glucose < 40 mg/dL). The dose is 0.1–0.15 unit/kg (healthy subjects); 0.2–0.3 unit/kg (obese subjects or those with Cushing's syndrome or acromegaly); 0.05 unit/kg (patients with suspected hypopituitarism).	Collect blood for glucose determinations every 15 minutes during the study. Samples of GH and cortisol are obtained at 0, 30, 45, 60, 75, and 90 minutes.	A physician must be in attendance. Symptomatic hypoglycemia (diaphoresis, headache, tachycardia, weakness) is necessary for adequate stimulation and occurs 20–35 minutes after insulin is administered in most patients. If severe central nervous system signs or symptoms occur, intravenous glucose (25–50 mL of 50% glucose) should be given immediately; otherwise, the test can be terminated with a meal or with oral glucose. This test is contraindicated in the elderly or in patients with cardiovascular or cerebrovascular disease and seizure disorders.	Symptomatic hypoglycemia and a fall in blood glucose to less than 40 mg/dL (2.2 mmol/L) will increase GH to a maximal level greater than 10 ng/mL (460 pmol/L); some investigators regard an increment of 6 ng/mL (280 pmol/L) as normal. Plasma cortisol should increase to a peak level of at least 20 μg/dL (550 nmol/L).
Metyrapone tests	Metyrapone is given orally between 11 and 12 PM with a snack to minimize gastrointestinal discomfort. The dose is 30 mg/kg.	Blood for plasma 11-deoxycortisol and cortisol determinations is obtained at 8 AM the morning after metyrapone is given.	Gastrointestinal upset may occur. Adrenal insufficiency may occur. Metyrapone should not be used in sick patients or those in whom primary adrenal insufficiency is suspected.	Serum 11-deoxycortisol should increase to > 7 μg/dL (0.19 μmol/l). Cortisol should be < 10 μg/dL (0.28 μmol/L) in order to ensure adequate inhibition of 11β-hydroxylation.
Levodopa test	The patient should be fasting and at bed rest after midnight. Levodopa, 500 mg, is given by mouth.	Blood samples for plasma GH determinations are obtained at 0, 30, and 60 minutes.	Nausea and vomiting may occur 45–60 minutes after levodopa is given. This test is safer than the insulin hypoglycemia test in older patients.	A normal response is a maximal level of GH greater than 6 ng/mL (280 pmol/L); however, the peak response is usually more than 20 ng/mL (930 pmol/L).
Arginine infusion test	The patient should be fasting after midnight. Give arginine hydrochloride, 0.5 g/kg intravenously, up to a maximum of 30 g over 30 minutes. Pretreatment with estrogen in postmenopausal women and in men can also be done.	Blood for plasma GH determinations is collected at 0, 30, 60, 90, and 120 minutes. Arginine infusion also stimulates insulin and glucagon.	Nausea and vomiting may occur. This test is contraindicated in patients with severe liver disease, renal disease, or acidosis.	The response is greater in women than in men. The lower limit of normal for the peak GH response is 6 ng/mL (280 pmol/L) is non-estrogen-treated patients and 10 ng/mL (460 pmol/L) in estrogen-treated patients and premenopausal women.

(continued)

Table 5–8. Endocrine tests of hypothalamic-pituitary function. (continued)

	Method	Sample Collection	Possible Side Effects; Contraindications	Interpretation
Glucose-growth hormone suppression test	The patient should be fasting after midnight. Give glucose, 75–100 g orally	GH and glucose should be determined at 0, 30, and 60 minutes after glucose administration.	Patients may complain of nausea after the large glucose load.	GH levels are suppressed to less than 2 ng/mL (90 pmol/L). in healthy subjects. Failure of adequate suppression or a paradoxic rise may be seen in acromegaly, starvation, protein-calorie malnutrition, and anorexia nervosa.
TRH test	Fasting is not required, but since nausea may occur, it is preferred. Give protirelin, 500 μg intravenously over 15–30 seconds. The patient should be kept supine, since slight hypertension or hypotension may occur. Protirelin is supplied in vials of 500 μg, although 400 μg will evoke normal responses.	Blood for determination of plasma, TSH, PRL, or GH (in the case of suspected acromegaly) is obtained at 0, 30, and 60 minutes; a 90-minute sample for TSH may be necessary in cases of suspected tertiary hypothyroidism. An abbreviated test utilizes samples taken at 0 and 30 minutes only.	No serious complications have been reported. Most patients complain of a sensation of urinary urgency and a metallic taste in the mouth; other symptoms include flushing, palpitations, and nausea. These symptoms occur within 1–2 minutes of the injection and last 5 minutes at most.	Normal TSH and PRL responses to TRH are outlined in Table 5–7. GH should not increase in healthy subjects.
GnRH test	The patient should be at rest but need not be fasting. Give GnRH (gonadorelin), 100 μg intravenously, over 15 seconds.	Blood samples for LH and FSH determinations are taken at 0, 30, and 60 minutes. Since the FSH response is somewhat delayed, a 90-minute specimen may be necessary.	Side effects are rare, and no contraindications have been reported.	This response is dependent on sex and the time of the menstrual cycle. Table 5–6 illustrates the mean maximal change in LH and FSH after GnRH administration. An increase of LH of 1.3–2.6 μg/L (12–23 IU/L) is considered to be normal; FSH usually responds more slowly and less markedly. FSH may not increase even in healthy subjects.
Clomiphene test	Clomiphene is administered orally. For women, give 100 mg daily for 5 days (being on day 5 of the cycle if the patient is menstruating); for men, give 100 mg daily for 7–10 days.	Blood for LH and FSH determinations is drawn before and after clomiphene is given.	This drug may, of course, stimulate ovulation, and women should be advised accordingly.	In women, LH and FSH levels peak on the fifth day to a level above the normal range. After the fifth day, LH and FSH levels decline. In men, LH should double after 1 week; FSH will also increase, but to a lesser extent.
CRH test	CRH (1 μg/kg) is given intravenously as a bolus injection.	Blood samples for ACTH and cortisol are taken at 0, 15, 30, and 60 minutes.	Flushing often occurs. Transient tachycardia and hypotension have also been reported.	The ACTH response is dependent on the assay utilized and occurs 15 minutes after CRH is administered. The peak cortisol response occurs at 30–60 minutes and is usually greater than 10 μg/dL (280 nmol/L).
GRH test	GRH (1 μg/kg) is given intravenously as a bolus injection.	Blood samples for GH are drawn at 0, 30, and 60 minutes.	Mild flushing and a metallic taste or smell occur in a few patients.	The range of normal responses is wide. Most patients have a peak GH response of greater than 10 ng/mL (460 pmol/L) at 30–60 minutes.

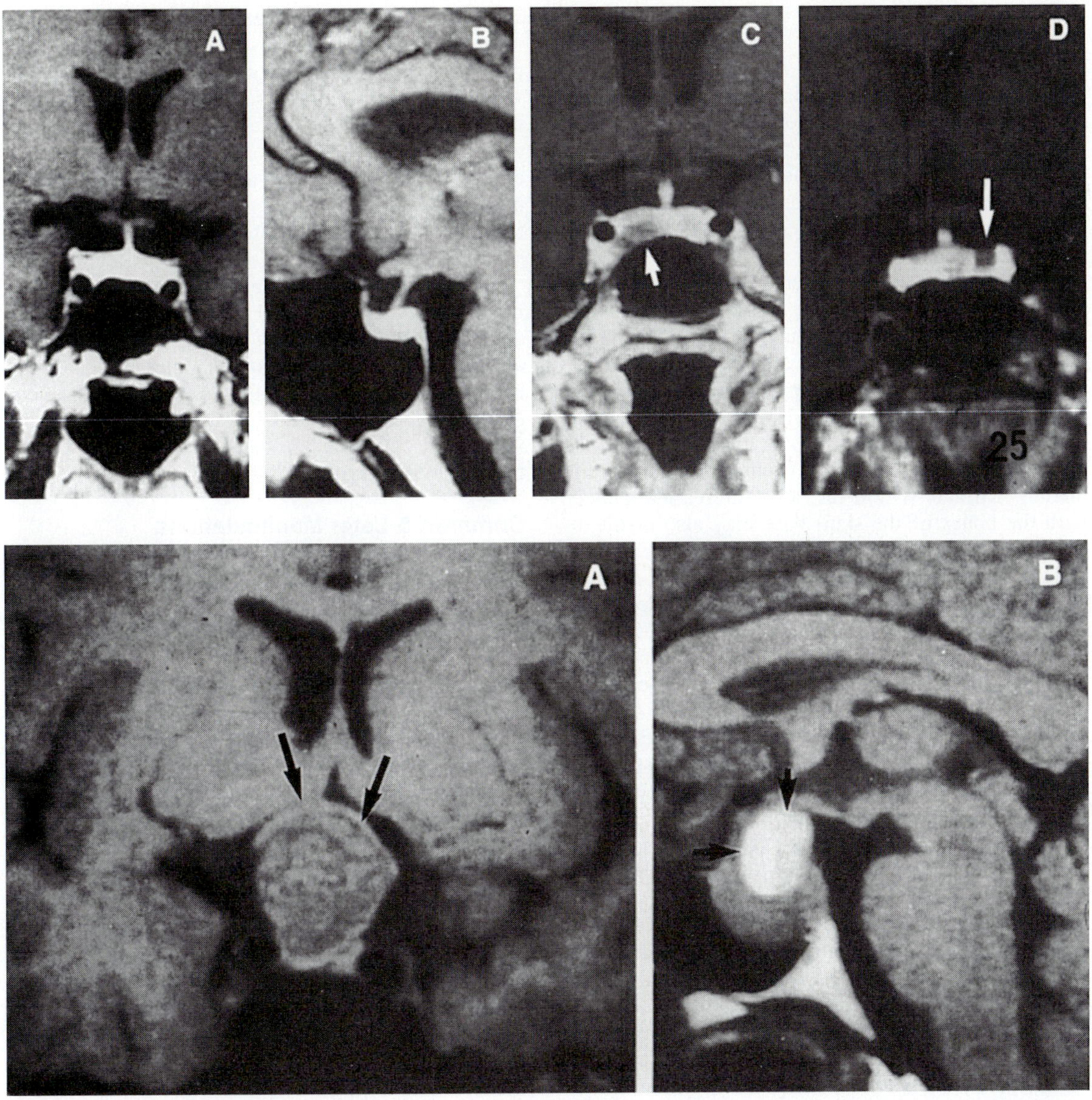

Figure 5–15. **Upper Panel:** Gadolinium-enhanced magnetic resonance images are shown of the pituitary gland. **A and B:** Coronal and sagittal images show the normal, uniformly enhancing pituitary stalk and pituitary gland. **C:** A pituitary microadenoma appears as a low-intensity lesion in the inferior aspect of the right lobe of the gland (arrow). **D:** The pituitary microadenoma appears as a low-intensity lesion between the left lobe of the pituitary and the left cavernous sinus (arrow). (Photographs courtesy of David Norman, MD.) **Lower Panel: A:** The coronal magnetic resonance (MR) image shows a large nonfunctioning pituitary adenoma (arrows) with pronounced suprasellar extension and chiasmal compression. **B:** A sagittal MR image of another large pituitary adenoma shows spontaneous hemorrhage within the suprasellar portion of the adenoma (arrows). (Photographs courtesy of David Norman, MD.) (Reproduced, with permission, from Western Journal of Medicine 1995;162:342, 350.)

roof of the sphenoid sinus, and its lateral margins are formed by the dural membranes of the cavernous sinuses, which contain the carotid arteries and the third, fourth, and sixth cranial nerves. The posterior pituitary appears on MRI as a high-signal-intensity structure, the "posterior pituitary bright spot," which is absent in patients with diabetes insipidus. The pituitary stalk, which is normally in the midline, is 2–3 mm in diameter and 5–7 mm in length. The pituitary stalk joins the inferior hypothalamus below the third ventricle and posterior to the optic chiasm. All of these normal structures are readily visualized with MRI; the normal pituitary and the pituitary stalk show increased signal intensity with gadolinium.

B. Microadenomas: These lesions, which range from 2 mm to 10 mm in diameter, appear as low-signal-intensity lesions with MRI and do not usually enhance with gadolinium. Adenomas less than 5 mm in diameter may not be visualized and do not usually alter the normal pituitary contour. Lesions greater than 5 mm in diameter create a unilateral convex superior gland margin and usually cause deviation of the pituitary stalk toward the side opposite the adenoma.

MRI scans must be interpreted with caution, since minor abnormalities occur in 10% of patients who have had incidental high-resolution scans but no clinical pituitary disease. These abnormalities may of course represent the clinically insignificant pituitary abnormalities which occur in 10–20% of the general population, and they may also be due to small intrapituitary cysts, which usually occur in the pars intermedia. Artifacts within the sella turcica associated with the bones of the skull base may also result in misinterpretation of imaging studies. Finally, many patients with pituitary microadenomas have normal high-resolution MRI scans. Therefore, despite increased accuracy of neuroradiologic diagnosis, the presence or absence of a small pituitary tumor and the decision concerning its treatment must be based on the entire clinical picture.

C Macroadenomas: Pituitary adenomas greater than 10 mm in diameter are readily visualized with MRI scans, and the scan will also define the adjacent structures and degree of extension of the lesion. Thus, larger tumors show compression of the normal pituitary and distortion of the pituitary stalk. Adenomas larger than 1.5 cm frequently have suprasellar extension, and MRI scans show compression and upward displacement of the optic chiasm. Less commonly, there is lateral extension and invasion of the cavernous sinus.

D Other Uses: High-resolution MRI scanning is also a valuable tool in the diagnosis of empty sella syndrome, hypothalamic tumors, and other parasellar lesions.

PITUITARY & HYPOTHALAMIC DISORDERS

Hypothalamic-pituitary lesions present with a variety of manifestations, including pituitary hormone hypersecretion and hyposecretion, sellar enlargement, and visual loss. The approach to evaluation should be designed to ensure early diagnosis at a stage when the lesions are amenable to therapy.

Etiology & Early Manifestations

In adults, the commonest cause of hypothalamic-pituitary dysfunction is a pituitary adenoma, of which the great majority are hypersecreting. Thus, the earliest symptoms of such tumors are due to endocrinologic abnormalities, and these precede sellar enlargement and local manifestations such as headache and visual loss, which are late manifestations seen only in patients with larger tumors or suprasellar extension.

In children, pituitary adenomas are uncommon; the most frequent structural lesions causing hypothalamic-pituitary dysfunction are craniopharyngiomas and other hypothalamic tumors. These also usually manifest as endocrine disturbances (low GH levels, delayed puberty, diabetes insipidus) prior to the development of headache, visual loss, or other central nervous system symptoms.

Common & Later Manifestations

A. Pituitary Hypersecretion: PRL is the hormone most commonly secreted in excess amounts by pituitary adenomas, and it is usually elevated in patients with hypothalamic disorders as well. Thus, PRL measurement is essential in evaluating patients with suspected pituitary disorders and should be performed in patients presenting with galactorrhea, gonadal dysfunction, secondary gonadotropin deficiency, or enlargement of the sella turcica. Hypersecretion of GH or ACTH leads to the more characteristic syndromes of acromegaly and Cushing's disease (see below).

B. Pituitary Insufficiency: Although panhypopituitarism is a classic manifestation of pituitary adenomas, it is present in less than 20% of patients in current large series because of earlier diagnosis of these lesions.

At present, the earliest clinical manifestation of a pituitary adenoma in adults is hypogonadism secondary to elevated levels of PRL, GH, or ACTH and cortisol. The hypogonadism in these patients is due to interference with the secretion of GnRH rather than to destruction of anterior pituitary tissue. Thus, patients with hypogonadism should first be screened with FSH/LH measurements to exclude primary gonadal failure (elevated FSH/LH) and those with hypogonadotropic hypogonadism should have serum PRL levels measured and be examined for clinical evidence of GH or ACTH and cortisol excess.

In children, short stature is the most frequent clinical presentation of hypothalamic-pituitary dysfunction; in these patients, GH deficiency should be considered.

TSH or ACTH deficiency is relatively unusual in current series of patients and usually indicates panhypopituitarism. Thus, patients with secondary hypothyroidism or hypoadrenalism should undergo a complete assessment of pituitary function and neuroradiologic studies, since panhypopituitarism and large pituitary tumors are common in this setting. PRL measurement is again essential, since prolactinomas are the most frequent pituitary tumors in adults.

C. Enlarged Sella Turcica: Patients may present with enlargement of the sella turcica, which may be noted on radiographs performed for head trauma or on sinus series. These patients usually have either a pituitary adenoma or empty sella syndrome. Evaluation should include clinical assessment of pituitary dysfunction and measurements of PRL and thyroid and adrenal function. Pituitary function is usually normal in the empty sella syndrome; this diagnosis can be confirmed by MRI or CT scanning. Patients with clinical or laboratory evidence of pituitary dysfunction usually have a pituitary adenoma.

D. Visual Field Defects: Patients presenting with bitemporal hemianopsia or unexplained visual field defects or visual loss should be considered to have a pituitary or hypothalamic disorder until proved otherwise. The initial steps in diagnosis should be neuro-ophthalmologic evaluation and neuroradiologic studies with MRI or CT scanning, which will reveal the tumor if one is present. These patients should also have PRL measurements and be assessed for anterior pituitary insufficiency, which is especially common with large pituitary adenomas.

In addition to causing visual field defects, large pituitary lesions may occasionally extend laterally into the cavernous sinus, compromising the function of the third, fourth, or sixth cranial nerve, leading to diplopia.

E. Diabetes Insipidus: Diabetes insipidus is a common manifestation of hypothalamic lesions but is rare in primary pituitary lesions. Diagnostic evaluation is described later. In addition, all patients should undergo radiologic evaluation and assessment of anterior pituitary function.

EMPTY SELLA SYNDROME

Etiology & Incidence

The empty sella syndrome occurs when the subarachnoid space extends into the sella turcica, partially filling it with cerebrospinal fluid. This process causes remodeling and enlargement of the sella turcica and flattening of the pituitary gland.

Primary empty sella syndrome resulting from congenital incompetence of the diaphragma sellae (Figure 5–16) is common, with an incidence in autopsy series ranging from 5% to 23%. It is the most frequent cause of enlarged sella turcica. An empty sella is also commonly seen after pituitary surgery or radiation therapy and may also occur following postpartum pituitary infarction (Sheehan's syndrome). In addition, both PRL-secreting and GH-secreting pituitary adenomas may undergo subclinical hemorrhagic infarction and cause contraction of the overlying suprasellar cistern downward into the sella. Therefore, the presence of an empty sella does not exclude the possibility of a coexisting pituitary tumor.

Pathogenesis

The pathogenesis of primary empty sella syndrome is uncertain. It has been postulated that increased cerebrospinal fluid pressure leads to herniation of arachnoid through the diaphragma sellae. A mesenchymal defect may be present in some patients, re-

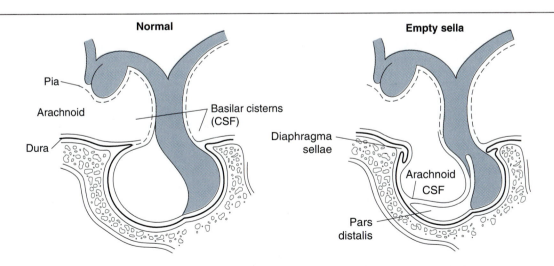

Figure 5–16. Representation of the normal relationship of the meninges to the pituitary gland *(left)* and the findings in the empty sella *(right)* as the arachnoid membrane herniates through the incompetent diaphragma sellae. (Reproduced, with permission, from Jordan RM, Kendall JW, Kerber CW: The primary empty sella syndrome: Analysis of the clinical characteristics, radiographic features, pituitary function, and cerebrospinal fluid adenohypophysial hormone concentrations. Am J Med 1977;62:569.)

sulting in hypoplasia of the sellar diaphragm. A kindred has been described in which both primary empty sella syndrome and Rieger's anomaly of the anterior chamber of the eye (a developmental abnormality of mesenchymal origin involving the iris) occurred in an autosomal dominant fashion.

Clinical Features

A. Symptoms and Signs: Most patients are middle-aged obese women. Many have systemic hypertension; benign intracranial hypertension may also occur. Although 48% of patients complain of headache, this feature may have only initiated the evaluation (ie, skull x-rays), and its relationship with the empty sella is probably coincidental. Serious clinical manifestations are uncommon. Spontaneous cerebrospinal fluid rhinorrhea and visual field impairment may rarely occur.

B. Laboratory Findings: Tests of anterior pituitary function are almost always normal, though some patients have hyperprolactinemia. This observation correlates well with histologic immunocytochemical studies of the pituitary gland in patients with the syndrome. Such studies have demonstrated that the remodeled pituitary gland contains adequate amounts of all six adenohypophysial hormones. TSH, GH, and gonadotropin secretory reserves have rarely been reported to be impaired; however, pituitary hypofunction in such cases may result from subclinical pituitary ischemic damage followed by contraction of glandular tissue and a secondary empty sella.

Endocrine function studies should be performed to exclude pituitary hormone insufficiency or a hypersecretory pituitary adenoma.

Diagnosis

The diagnosis of the empty sella syndrome can be readily confirmed by MRI or CT scanning, either of which demonstrates the presence of cerebrospinal fluid in the sella turcica.

HYPOTHALAMIC DYSFUNCTION

Hypothalamic dysfunction is most often caused by tumors, of which craniopharyngioma is the most common in children, adolescents, and young adults. In older adults, primary central nervous system tumors and those arising from hypothalamic (epidermoid and dermoid tumors) and pineal structures (pinealomas) are more common. Other causes of hypothalamic-pituitary dysfunction are discussed below in the section on hypopituitarism.

Clinical Features

A. Craniopharyngioma: The initial symptoms of craniopharyngioma in children and adolescents are predominantly endocrinologic; however, these manifestations are frequently unrecognized, and at diagnosis over 80% of patients have hypothalamic-pituitary endocrine deficiencies. These endocrine abnormalities may precede presenting symptoms by months or years; GH deficiency is most common, with about 50% of patients having growth retardation and approximately 70% decreased GH responses to stimulation at diagnosis. Gonadotropin deficiency leading to absent or arrested puberty is usual in older children and adolescents; TSH and ACTH deficiency is less common, and diabetes insipidus is present in about 15%.

Symptoms leading to the diagnosis are, unfortunately, frequently neurologic and due to the mass effect of the expanding tumor. Symptoms of increased intracranial pressure such as headache and vomiting are present in about 40%; decreased visual acuity or visual field defects are the presenting symptoms in another 35%. Plain films of the skull reveal intrasellar or suprasellar calcification in 75% of these children. MRI or CT scans confirm the tumor in virtually all patients; in 95%, the tumor is suprasellar.

In adults, craniopharyngiomas have similar presentations; ie, the diagnosis is usually reached as a result of investigation of symptoms of increased intracranial pressure, headache, or visual loss. However, endocrine manifestations—especially hypogonadism, diabetes insipidus, or other deficiencies of anterior pituitary hormones—usually precede these late manifestations. Intrasellar or suprasellar calcification is less common in adults (for unknown reasons), but scans again readily demonstrate the tumors, which in adults are almost always both intrasellar and suprasellar.

B. Other Tumors: Other hypothalamic or pineal tumors and primary central nervous system tumors involving the hypothalamus have variable presentations in both children and adults. Thus, presentation is with headache, visual loss, symptoms of increased intracranial pressure, growth failure, various degrees of hypopituitarism, or diabetes insipidus. Endocrine deficiencies usually precede neurologic manifestations. Hypothalamic tumors in childhood may present with precocious puberty.

C. Other Manifestations of Hypothalamic Dysfunction: Lesions in the hypothalamus can cause many other abnormalities, including disorders of consciousness, behavior, thirst, appetite, and temperature regulation. These abnormalities are usually accompanied by hypopituitarism and diabetes insipidus.

Somnolence can occur with hypothalamic lesions, as can a variety of changes in emotional behavior. Decreased or absent thirst may occur and predispose these patients to dehydration. When diminished thirst accompanies diabetes insipidus, fluid balance is difficult to control. Hypothalamic dysfunction may also cause increased thirst, leading to polydipsia and polyuria that may mimic diabetes insipidus. Obesity is common in patients with hypothalamic tumors because of hyperphagia, decreased satiety, and decreased activity. Anorexia and weight loss are unusual manifestations of these tumors.

Temperature regulation can also be disordered in these patients. Sustained or, less commonly, paroxysmal hyperthermia can occur following acute injury due to trauma, hemorrhage, or craniotomy. This problem usually lasts less than 2 weeks. Poikilothermia, the inability to adjust to changes in ambient temperature, can occur in patients with bilateral hypothalamic lesions. These patients most frequently exhibit hypothermia but can also develop hyperthermia during hot weather. A few patients manifest sustained hypothermia due to anterior hypothalamic lesions.

Diagnosis

Patients with suspected hypothalamic tumors should have MRI or CT scans to determine the extent and nature of the tumor. Complete assessment of anterior pituitary function is necessary in these patients, since deficiencies are present in the great majority (see section on hypopituitarism below) and the evaluation will establish the requirements for replacement therapy. PRL levels should also be determined, since most hypothalamic lesions cause hyperprolactinemia either by hypothalamic injury or by damage to the pituitary stalk.

Treatment

Treatment depends upon the type of tumor. Since complete resection of craniopharyngioma is usually not feasible, this tumor is best managed by limited neurosurgical removal of accessible tumor and decompression of cysts, followed by conventional radiotherapy. Patients treated by this method have a recurrence rate of approximately 20%; with surgery alone, the recurrence rate approximates 80%.

Other hypothalamic tumors are usually not completely resectable; however, biopsy is indicated to arrive at a histologic diagnosis.

HYPOPITUITARISM

Hypopituitarism is manifested by diminished or absent secretion of one or more pituitary hormones. The development of signs and symptoms is often slow and insidious, depending on the rate of onset and the magnitude of hypothalamic-pituitary damage—factors that are influenced by the underlying pathogenesis. Hypopituitarism is either a primary event caused by destruction of the anterior pituitary gland or a secondary phenomenon resulting from deficiency of hypothalamic stimulatory (or inhibitory) factors normally acting on the pituitary. Although provocative endocrine testing is useful in evaluating anterior pituitary gland function, it is not always pos-

sible (even with the use of hypothalamic releasing hormones) to distinguish between a pituitary and a hypothalamic lesion. Treatment and prognosis depend on the extent of hypofunction, the underlying cause, and the location of the lesion in the hypothalamic-pituitary axis.

Etiology

The etiologic considerations in hypopituitarism are diverse. As shown below and in Table 5–9, a helpful mnemonic device is the phrase "nine I's": Invasive, Infarction, Infiltrative, Injury, Immunologic, Iatrogenic, Infectious, Idiopathic, and Isolated. Most of these lesions may cause pituitary or hypothalamic failure (or both). Establishing the precise cause of hypopituitarism is helpful in determining treatment and prognosis.

A. Invasive: Space-occupying lesions cause hypopituitarism by destroying the pituitary gland or hypothalamic nuclei or by disrupting the hypothalamic-hypophysial portal venous system. Large pituitary adenomas cause hypopituitarism by these mechanisms, and pituitary function may improve after their removal. Small pituitary tumors—microadenomas (< 10 mm in diameter)—characteristically seen in the hypersecretory states (excess PRL, GH, ACTH) do not directly cause pituitary insufficiency. Craniopharyngioma, the most common tumor of the hypothalamic-pituitary region in children, frequently impairs pituitary function by its compressive effects. Primary central nervous system tumors, including meningioma, chordoma, optic glioma, epidermoid tumors, and dermoid tumors, may decrease hypothalamic-pituitary secretion by their mass effects. Metastatic lesions to this area are common (especially breast carcinoma) but rarely result in clinically obvious hypopituitarism. Anatomic malformations such as basal encephalocele and parasellar aneurysms cause hypothalamic-pituitary dysfunction and may enlarge the sella turcica and mimic pituitary tumors.

B. Infarction: Ischemic damage to the pituitary has long been recognized as a cause of hypopituitarism. In 1914, Simmonds reported pituitary necrosis in a woman with severe puerperal sepsis, and in 1937 Sheehan published his classic description of its occurrence following postpartum hemorrhage and vascular collapse. The mechanism for the ischemia in such cases is not certain. Hypotension along with vasospasm of the hypophysial arteries is currently

Table 5–9. Indications for prolactin measurement.

Galactorrhea
Enlarged sella turcica
Suspected pituitary tumor
Hypogonadotropic hypogonadism
Unexplained amenorrhea
Unexplained male hypogonadism or infertility

believed to compromise arterial perfusion of the anterior pituitary. During pregnancy, the pituitary gland may be more sensitive to hypoxemia because of its increased metabolic needs or more susceptible to vasoconstrictive influences because of the hyperestrogenic state. Some degree of hypopituitarism has been reported in 32% of women with severe postpartum hemorrhage. Other investigators have noted that the hypopituitarism does not always correlate with the degree of hemorrhage but that there is good correlation between the pituitary lesion and severe disturbances of the clotting mechanism (as in patients with placenta previa). Ischemic pituitary necrosis has also been reported to occur with greater frequency in patients with diabetes mellitus.

The extent of pituitary damage determines the rapidity of onset as well as the magnitude of pituitary hypofunction. The gland has a great secretory reserve, and more than 75% must be destroyed before clinical manifestations are evident. The initial clinical feature in postpartum necrosis may be failure to lactate after parturition; failure to resume normal menstrual periods is another clue to the diagnosis. However, the clinical features of hypopituitarism are often subtle, and years may pass before pituitary insufficiency is recognized following an ischemic insult.

Spontaneous hemorrhagic infarction of a pituitary tumor (pituitary apoplexy) frequently results in partial or total pituitary insufficiency. Pituitary apoplexy is often a fulminant clinical syndrome manifested by severe headache, visual impairment, ophthalmoplegias, meningismus, and an altered level of consciousness. Pituitary apoplexy is usually associated with a pituitary tumor; it may also be related to diabetes mellitus, radiotherapy, or open heart surgery. Acute pituitary failure with hypotension may result, and rapid mental deterioration, coma, and death may ensue. Emergency treatment with corticosteroids (see Chapter 9) and transsphenoidal decompression of the intrasellar contents may be lifesaving and may prevent permanent visual loss. Most patients who have survived pituitary apoplexy have developed multiple adenohypophysial deficits, but infarction of the tumor in some patients may cure the hypersecretory pituitary adenoma and its accompanying endocrinopathy. Pituitary infarction may also be a subclinical event (silent pituitary apoplexy), resulting in improvement of pituitary hormone hypersecretion without impairing the secretion of other anterior pituitary hormones.

C. Infiltrative: Hypopituitarism may be the initial clinical manifestation of infiltrative disease processes such as sarcoidosis, hemochromatosis, and histiocytosis X.

1. Sarcoidosis–The most common intracranial sites of involvement of sarcoidosis are the hypothalamus and pituitary gland. At one time, the most common endocrine abnormality in patients with sarcoidosis was thought to be diabetes insipidus; however, many of these patients actually have centrally mediated disordered control of thirst that results in polydipsia and polyuria, which in some cases explains the abnormal water metabolism. Deficiencies of multiple anterior pituitary hormones have been well documented in sarcoidosis and are usually secondary to hypothalamic insufficiency. Granulomatous involvement of the hypothalamic-pituitary unit is occasionally extensive, resulting in visual impairment, and therefore may simulate the clinical presentation of a pituitary or hypothalamic tumor.

2. Hemochromatosis–Hypopituitarism, particularly hypogonadotropic hypogonadism, is a prominent manifestation of iron storage disease—either idiopathic hemochromatosis or transfusional iron overload. Hypogonadism occurs in most such cases and is often the initial clinical feature of iron excess; complete iron studies should be obtained in any male patient presenting with unexplained hypogonadotropic hypogonadism. If the diagnosis is established early, hypogonadism in hemochromatosis may be reversible with iron depletion. Pituitary deficiencies of TSH, GH, and ACTH may occur later in the course of the disease and are not reversible by iron chelation therapy.

3. Histiocytosis X–Histiocytosis X, the infiltration of multiple organs by well-differentiated histiocytes, is often heralded by the onset of diabetes insipidus and anterior pituitary hormone deficiencies. The disorders in this category include Hand-Schüller-Christian disease, Letterer-Siwe disease, and eosinophilic granuloma of bone (eosinophilic infiltration predominates). Most histologic and biochemical studies have indicated that this infiltrative process involves chiefly the hypothalamus, and hypopituitarism occurs only as a result of hypothalamic damage.

D. Injury: Severe head trauma may cause anterior pituitary insufficiency and diabetes insipidus. Posttraumatic anterior hypopituitarism may be due to injury to the anterior pituitary, the pituitary stalk, or the hypothalamus. Pituitary insufficiency with growth retardation has been described in battered children who suffer closed head trauma with subdural hematoma.

E. Immunologic: Lymphocytic hypophysitis resulting in anterior hypopituitarism is a distinct entity, occurring most often in women during pregnancy or in the postpartum period. It may present as a mass lesion of the sella turcica with visual field disturbances simulating pituitary adenoma. An autoimmune process with extensive infiltration of the gland by lymphocytes and plasma cells destroys the anterior pituitary cells. These morphologic features are similar to those of other autoimmune endocrinopathies, eg, thyroiditis, adrenalitis, and oophoritis. About 50% of patients with lymphocytic hypophysitis have other endocrine autoimmune disease, and circulating pituitary autoantibodies have been found in several cases. It is presently uncertain how this disorder should be diagnosed and treated. It must be considered in the differential diagnosis of women with pituitary gland enlargement and hypopituitarism during pregnancy or the postpartum period.

Lymphocytic hypophysitis may result in isolated hormone deficiencies (especially ACTH or prolactin). Consequently, women with this type of hypopituitarism may continue to menstruate while suffering from secondary hypothyroidism or hypoadrenalism.

F. Iatrogenic: Both surgical and radiation therapy to the pituitary gland may compromise its function. The anterior pituitary is quite resilient during transsphenoidal microsurgery, and despite extensive manipulation during the search for microadenomas, anterior pituitary function is usually preserved. The dose of conventional radiation therapy presently employed to treat pituitary tumors is 4500–5000 cGy and results in a 50–60% incidence of hypothalamic and pituitary insufficiency. Such patients most frequently have modest hyperprolactinemia (PRL 30–100 ng/mL [1.3–4.5 nmol/L]) with GH and gonadotropin failure; TSH and ACTH deficiencies are less common. Heavy particle (proton beam) irradiation for pituitary tumors results in a 20–50% incidence of hypopituitarism. Irradiation of tumors of the head and neck (nasopharyngeal cancer, brain tumors) and prophylactic cranial irradiation in leukemia may also cause hypopituitarism. The clinical onset of pituitary failure in such patients is usually insidious and results from both pituitary and hypothalamic injury.

G. Infectious: Although many infectious diseases, including tuberculosis, syphilis, and mycotic infections, have been implicated as causative agents in pituitary hypofunction, anti-infective drugs have now made them rare causes of hypopituitarism.

H. Idiopathic: In some patients with hypopituitarism, no underlying cause is found. These may be isolated (see below) or multiple deficiencies. Familial forms of hypopituitarism characterized by a small, normal, or enlarged sella turcica have been described. Both autosomal recessive and X-linked recessive inheritance patterns have been reported. A variety of complex congenital disorders may include deficiency of one or more pituitary hormones, eg, Prader-Willi syndrome and septo-optic dysplasia. The pathogenesis of these familial disorders is uncertain.

I. Isolated: Isolated (monotropic) deficiencies of the anterior pituitary hormones have been described. Some of these have been associated with mutations in the genes coding for the specific hormones. Others, particularly GH deficiency, have been associated with mutations in genes necessary for normal pituitary development as noted.

1. GH deficiency–In children, congenital monotropic GH deficiency may be sporadic or familial. These children, who may experience fasting hypoglycemia, have a gradual deceleration in growth velocity after 6–12 months of age. Diagnosis must be based on failure of GH responsiveness to provocative stimuli and the demonstration of normal responsiveness of other anterior pituitary hormones. Monotropic GH deficiency and growth retardation have also been observed in children suffering severe emotional deprivation. This disorder is reversed by placing the child in a supportive psychosocial milieu. A more detailed description of GH deficiency and growth failure is provided in Chapter 7.

2. ACTH deficiency–Monotropic ACTH deficiency is rare and is manifested by the signs and symptoms of adrenocortical insufficiency. Lipotropin (LPH) deficiency has also been noted in such patients. The defect in these patients may be due to primary failure of the corticotrophs to release ACTH and its related peptide hormones or may be secondary to impaired secretion of CRH by the hypothalamus. Most acquired cases of monotropic ACTH deficiency are due to lymphocytic hypophysitis.

3. Gonadotropin deficiency–Isolated deficiency of gonadotropins is not uncommon. Kallman's syndrome, an X-linked dominant disorder with incomplete penetrance, is characterized by an isolated defect in GnRH secretion associated with maldevelopment of the olfactory center with hyposmia or anosmia. Sporadic cases occur, and other neurologic defects such as color blindness and nerve deafness have been seen. Since anterior pituitary function is otherwise intact, young men with isolated hypogonadotropic hypogonadism develop a eunuchoid appearance, since testosterone deficiency results in failure of epiphysial closure (see Chapter 12). In women, a state of hypogonadotropic hypogonadism manifested by oligomenorrhea or amenorrhea often accompanies weight loss, emotional or physical stress, and athletic training. Anorexia nervosa and marked obesity both result in hypothalamic dysfunction and impaired gonadotropin secretion. Hypothalamic hypogonadism has also been observed in overtrained male athletes. Sickle cell anemia also causes hypogonadotropic hypogonadism due to hypothalamic dysfunction and results in delayed puberty. Clomiphene treatment has been effective in some cases. Isolated gonadotropin deficiency may also be seen in the polyglandular autoimmune syndrome; this deficiency is related to selective pituitary gonadotrope failure from autoimmune hypophysitis. Other chronic illnesses, eg, poorly controlled diabetes and malnutrition, may result in gonadotropin deficiency. Isolated deficiencies of both LH and FSH without an obvious cause such as those described have been reported but are rare.

4. TSH deficiency–Monotropic TSH deficiency is rare and is caused by a reduction in hypothalamic TRH secretion (tertiary hypothyroidism). Some patients with chronic renal failure appear to have impaired TSH secretion.

5. Prolactin deficiency–PRL deficiency almost always indicates severe intrinsic pituitary damage, and panhypopituitarism is usually present. However, isolated PRL deficiency has been reported after lymphocytic hypophysitis. Deficiencies of TSH and PRL have been noted in patients with pseudohypoparathyroidism.

Clinical Features

The onset of pituitary insufficiency is usually gradual, and the classic course of progressive hypopituitarism is an initial loss of GH and gonadotropin secretion followed by deficiencies of TSH, then ACTH, and finally PRL.

A. Symptoms: Impairment of GH secretion causes decreased growth in children but is, of course, clinically occult in adult patients. Hypogonadism, manifested by amenorrhea in women and decreased libido or impotence in men, may antedate the clinical appearance of a hypothalamic-pituitary lesion.

Hypothyroidism caused by TSH deficiency generally stimulates the clinical changes observed in primary thyroid failure; however, it is usually less severe, and goiter is absent. Cold intolerance, dry skin, mental dullness, bradycardia, constipation, hoarseness, and anemia have all been observed; gross myxedematous changes are uncommon.

ACTH deficiency causes adrenocortical insufficiency, and its clinical features resemble those of primary adrenal failure. Weakness, nausea, vomiting, anorexia, weight loss, fever, and postural hypotension may occur. Since the zona glomerulosa and the renin-angiotensin system is usually intact, the cardiovascular collapse seen in Addison's disease is uncommon. Again, these symptoms are less severe in secondary adrenal insufficiency and, because of their gradual onset, may go undetected for prolonged periods, becoming manifest only during periods of stress. Hypoglycemia aggravated by GH deficiency may occur with fasting and has been the initial presenting feature of some patients with isolated ACTH deficiency. Patients with type I (insulin-dependent) diabetes who develop hypopituitarism often have a reduction in their insulin requirements. In contrast to the hyperpigmentation that occurs during states of ACTH excess (Addison's disease, Nelson's syndrome), depigmentation and diminished tanning have been described as a result of ACTH insufficiency. In addition, lack of ACTH-stimulated adrenal androgen secretion will cause a decrease in body hair if gonadotropin deficiency is also present.

The only symptom of PRL deficiency is failure of postpartum lactation.

B. Signs: Abnormal findings on physical examination may be subtle and require careful observation. Patients with hypopituitarism are not cachectic.

A photograph of a cachectic patient with "Simmonds' syndrome" that appeared in some older textbooks of endocrinology caused confusion. That particular patient probably suffered from anorexia nervosa and was found to have a normal pituitary gland at postmortem examination.

Patients with pituitary failure are usually slightly overweight. The skin is fine, pale, and smooth, with fine wrinkling of the face. Body and pubic hair may be deficient or absent, and atrophy of the genitalia may occur. Postural hypotension, bradycardia, decreased muscle strength, and delayed deep tendon reflexes occur in more severe cases. Neuro-ophthalmologic abnormalities depend on the presence of a large intrasellar or parasellar lesion.

C. Laboratory Findings: These may include anemia (related to thyroid and androgen deficiency and chronic disease), hypoglycemia, hyponatremia (related to hypothyroidism and hypoadrenalism, which cause inappropriate water retention, not sodium loss), and low-voltage bradycardia on ECG. Hyperkalemia, which is common in primary adrenal failure, is not present.

Diagnosis

A. Assessment of Target Gland Function: If endocrine hypofunction is suspected, pituitary hormone deficiencies must be distinguished from primary failure of the thyroid, adrenals, or gonads. Basal determinations of each anterior pituitary hormone are useful only if compared to target gland secretion. Baseline laboratory studies should include thyroid function tests (free T_4) and determination of serum testosterone levels. Testosterone is a sensitive indicator of hypopituitarism in women as well as in men. In women, a substantial decrease in testosterone is commonly observed in pituitary failure related to hypofunction of the two endocrine glands responsible for its production—the ovary and the adrenal. Adrenocortical reserve should initially be evaluated by a rapid ACTH stimulation test.

B. Evaluation of Prolactin: Since hyperprolactinemia (discussed later), regardless of its cause, leads to gonadal dysfunction, serum PRL should be measured early in the evaluation of hypogonadism.

C. Differentiation of Primary and Secondary Hypofunction: Subnormal thyroid function as shown by appropriate tests, a low serum testosterone level, or an impaired cortisol response to the rapid ACTH stimulation test requires measurement of basal levels of specific pituitary hormones. In primary target gland hypofunction (such as polyglandular failure syndrome), TSH, LH, FSH, or ACTH will be elevated. Low or normal values for these pituitary hormones suggest hypothalamic-pituitary dysfunction.

D. Stimulation Tests: Provocative endocrine testing may then be employed to confirm the diagnosis and to assess the extent of hypofunction. At present, these tests are not required in most patients.

Treatment

A. ACTH: Treatment of secondary adrenal insufficiency, like that of primary adrenal failure, must include glucocorticoid support (see Chapter 9). Hydrocortisone (20–30 mg/d orally) or prednisone (5–7.5 mg/d orally) in two or three divided doses provides adequate glucocorticoid replacement for most patients. The minimum effective dosage should be given in order to avoid iatrogenic hypercortisolism. Increased dosage is required during periods of stress such as illness, surgery, or trauma. Patients with only partial ACTH deficiency may need steroid treatment only during stress. A two- to threefold increase in steroid dosage during the stressful situation should be recommended, followed by gradual tapering as the stress resolves. Unlike primary adrenal insufficiency, ACTH deficiency does not usually require mineralocorticoid therapy. Patients with adrenal insufficiency should wear medical alert bracelets so they may receive prompt treatment in case of emergency.

B. TSH: The management of patients with secondary hypothyroidism must be based on clinical grounds and the circulating concentration of serum thyroxine (see Chapter 7). Since some patients with secondary hypothyroidism have a normal TSH response to TRH, basal TSH levels and the TRH test should not be used as guidelines for thyroid replacement. The treatment of secondary and tertiary hypothyroidism is identical to that for primary thyroid failure. Levothyroxine sodium, 0.1–0.15 mg/d orally, is usually adequate. Response to therapy is monitored clinically and with measurement of serum free thyroxine levels.

Caution: Since thyroid hormone replacement in patients with hypopituitarism may aggravate even partial adrenal insufficiency, the adrenal disorder should be treated first.

C. Gonadotropins: The object of treatment of secondary hypogonadism is to replace sex steroids and restore fertility (see Chapters 12 and 13).

1. Estrogens and progesterone–In women, estrogen replacement is essential. Adequate estrogen treatment will maintain secondary sex characteristics (eg, vulvar and vaginal lubrication), prevent osteoporosis, and abolish vasomotor symptoms, with an improvement in sense of well-being. Many estrogen preparations are available, eg, estradiol oral, 1–2 mg daily; conjugated estrogens, 0.3–1.25 mg orally daily; or transdermal estradiol, 0.05–0.1 mg daily. Estrogens should be cycled with a progestin compound (eg, medroxyprogesterone, 5–10 mg orally) to induce withdrawal bleeding and prevent endometrial hyperplasia.

2. Ovulation induction–Ovulation can often be restored in women with hypothalamic-pituitary dysfunction (see Chapter 13). In patients with gonadal failure of hypothalamic origin, clomiphene citrate may cause a surge of gonadotropin secretion resulting in ovulation. Pulsatile subcutaneous injections of GnRH with an infusion pump can also be used to induce ovulation and fertility in women with hypothalamic dysfunction. Combined treatment with FSH (human menopausal gonadotropins; menotropins) and LH (chorionic gonadotropin) can be utilized to provoke ovulation in women with intrinsic pituitary failure. This form of therapy is expensive, and multiple births are a risk.

3. Androgens in women–Because of a deficiency of both ovarian and adrenal androgens, some women with hypopituitarism have diminished libido despite adequate estrogen therapy. Small doses of long-acting androgens (testosterone enanthate, 25–50 mg intramuscularly every 4–8 weeks) may be helpful in restoring sexual activity without causing hirsutism.

4. Androgens in men–In men, testosterone replacement is essential to restore libido and potency, provide adequate beard growth and muscle strength, prevent osteopenia, and improve the sense of well-being. Adequate treatment consists of a long-acting intramuscular preparation such as testosterone enanthate. Three dosage schedules have proved efficacy: 300 mg every 3 weeks, 200 mg every 2 weeks, or 100 mg every week. Side effects, including aggressive sexual behavior, acne, gynecomastia, and fluid retention, are unusual and can be managed by lowering the dosage. Therapy should be withheld in adolescents as long as possible in order to prevent premature epiphysial closure and ensure maximum linear growth. Replacement therapy with oral androgenic preparations should be avoided, since inadequate absorption results in poor androgenization, and serious side effects such as peliosis hepatis (blood-filled cysts within the hepatic parenchyma) may occur. Transdermal testosterone therapy has also been shown to be an effective and acceptable means of administering androgens. (See Chapter 12).

5. Spermatogenesis–Spermatogenesis can be achieved in some patients with the combined use of chorionic gonadotropin and menotropins. If pituitary insufficiency is of recent onset, therapy with chorionic gonadotropin alone may restore both fertility and adequate gonadal steroid production. Pulsatile GnRH infusion pumps have also been used to restore fertility in male patients with secondary hypogonadism.

D. Growth Hormone: (See Chapter 6.) Human growth hormone (hGH) produced by recombinant DNA technology is available for use in children with hypopituitarism. Therapeutic use of human growth hormone in adults with hypopituitarism is under investigation. Some studies indicate improvement in body composition, bone density, psychologic well-being, and functional status. However, the long-term benefits and risks remain to be established.

PITUITARY ADENOMAS

Advances in endocrinologic and neuroradiologic research in recent years have allowed earlier recognition and more successful therapy of pituitary adenomas. Prolactinomas are the most common type, accounting for about 60% of primary pituitary tumors; GH hypersecretion occurs in approximately 20% and ACTH excess in 10%. Hypersecretion of TSH, the gonadotropins, or alpha subunits is unusual. Nonfunctional tumors currently represent only 10% of all pituitary adenomas, and some of these may in fact be gonadotropin-secreting or alpha subunit-secreting adenomas.

Early clinical recognition of the endocrine effects of excessive pituitary secretion, especially the observation that PRL excess causes secondary hypogonadism, has led to early diagnosis of pituitary tumors before the appearance of late manifestations such as sellar enlargement, panhypopituitarism, and suprasellar extension with visual impairment.

Pituitary **microadenomas** are defined as intrasellar adenomas less than 1 cm in diameter that present with manifestations of hormonal excess without sellar enlargement or extrasellar extension. Panhypopituitarism does not occur, and such tumors are very successfully treated.

Pituitary **macroadenomas** are those larger than 1 cm in diameter and cause generalized sellar enlargement. Tumors 1–2 cm in diameter confined to the sella turcica can usually be successfully treated; however, larger tumors—and especially those with suprasellar, sphenoid sinus, or lateral extensions—are much more difficult to manage. Panhypopituitarism and visual loss increase in frequency with tumor size and suprasellar extension.

Insights into the pathogenesis and biologic behavior of pituitary tumors have been gained from studies of pituitary tumor clonality and somatic mutations. Analyses of allelic X inactivation of specific genes has shown that most pituitary adenomas are monoclonal, a finding most consistent with a somatic mutation model of tumorigenesis; polyclonanality of tumors would be expected if tonic stimulation by hypothalamic releasing factors were the mechanism underlying neoplastic transformation. In fact, transgenic animals expressing GRH have exhibited pituitary hyperplasia but not pituitary adenomas. Recently, an animal model system for ACTH-secreting pituitary tumors has been developed involving transgenic mice. One somatic mutation has been found in 30–40% of growth hormone-secreting tumors (but not in leukocytes from the same patients): Point mutations in the alpha subunit of the GTP binding portion of the stimulatory regulator of adenylyl cyclase (G_s protein) results in constitutive (autonomous) activation of pituitary cell growth and function. In studies of anterior pituitary cell ontogeny, Pit-1 is a transcription factor important in pituitary differentiation.

The restriction of its expression to somatotrophs, lactotrophs, and thyrotrophs may account for the plurihormonal expression seen in some tumors.

Treatment

Pituitary adenomas are treated with surgery, irradiation, or drugs to suppress hypersecretion by the adenoma or its growth. The aims of therapy are to correct hypersecretion of anterior pituitary hormones, to preserve normal secretion of other anterior pituitary hormones, and to remove or suppress the adenoma itself. These objectives are currently achievable in most patients with pituitary microadenomas; however, in the case of larger tumors, multiple therapies are frequently required and may be less successful.

A. Surgical: Pituitary surgery is the initial therapy of choice at many centers, and the transsphenoidal microsurgical approach to the sella turcica is the procedure of choice; transfrontal craniotomy is required only in the occasional patient with massive suprasellar extension of the adenoma. In the transsphenoidal procedure, the surgeon approaches the pituitary from the nasal cavity through the sphenoid sinus, removes the anterior-inferior sellar floor, and incises the dura. The adenoma is selectively removed; normal pituitary tissue is identified and preserved. Success rates approach 90% in patients with microadenomas. Major complications, including postoperative hemorrhage, cerebrospinal fluid leak, meningitis, and visual impairment, occur in less than 5% and are most frequent in patients with large or massive tumors. Transient diabetes insipidus lasting a few days to 1–2 weeks occurs in approximately 15%; permanent diabetes insipidus is rare. A transient form of the syndrome of inappropriate secretion of antidiuretic hormone (SIADH) with symptomatic hyponatremia occurs in 10% of patients within 5–14 days of transsphenoidal pituitary microsurgery. Surgical hypopituitarism is rare in patients with microadenomas but approaches 5–10% in patients with larger tumors. The perioperative management of such patients should include glucocorticoid administration in stress doses (see Chapter 9) and postoperative assessment of daily weight, fluid balance, and electrolyte status. Mild diabetes insipidus is managed by giving fluids orally; in more severe cases—urine output greater than 5–6 L/24 h—ADH therapy in the form of desmopressin acetate should be administered (see section on diabetes insipidus). SIADH is managed by fluid restriction; however, in more severe cases, hypertonic saline may be required (See section on SIADH.)

B. Radiologic: Pituitary irradiation is usually reserved for patients with larger tumors who have had incomplete resection of large pituitary adenomas.

1. Conventional irradiation–Conventional irradiation using high energy sources, in total doses of 4000–5000 cGy given in daily doses of 180–200 cGy, is most commonly employed. The response to radiation therapy is slow, and 5–10 years may be required to achieve the full effect (see section on acromegaly). Treatment is ultimately successful in about 80% of acromegalics but only about 55–60% of patients with Cushing's disease. The response rate in prolactinomas is not precisely known, but tumor progression is prevented in most patients. Morbidity during radiotherapy is minimal, though some patients experience malaise and nausea, and serous otitis media may occur. Hypopituitarism is common, and the incidence increases with time following radiotherapy—about 50–60% at 5–10 years. Rare late complications include damage to the optic nerves and chiasm, seizures, and radionecrosis of brain tissue.

2. Heavy particle irradiation–Heavy particle irradiation using alpha particles or protons is also used. Advantages of this technique are the ability to focus the radiation beam precisely; the smaller port allows larger doses (8000–12,000 cGy) to be delivered to the sellar area and limits the radiation exposure of surrounding structures. Disadvantages are the limited availability, and the smaller radiation field which precludes use of this technique in patients with tumors over 1.5 cm in diameter and in those with extrasellar extension. Responses to therapy are more rapid than with conventional irradiation and occur within 2 years in most patients. Successful responses are obtained in a majority of patients with acromegaly or Cushing's disease. Experience with prolactinomas is limited. Neurologic damage and visual impairment are rare complications of heavy particle irradiation, but hypopituitarism occurs in 20–50% and will almost certainly increase with further follow-up.

3. Gamma-knife radiosurgery–This form of radiotherapy utilizes stereotactic CT-guided cobalt-60 gamma radiation to deliver high radiation doses to a narrowly focused area. Limited experience to date has been obtained in patients with acromegaly and Cushing's disease. (See sections following.)

C. Medical: Medical management of pituitary adenomas became feasible with the availability of bromocriptine, a dopamine agonist. This drug is most successful in the treatment of hyperprolactinemia and is also useful in a few patients with acromegaly or Cushing's disease. Octreotide acetate, a somatostatin analog, is useful in the therapy of acromegaly and TSH-secreting adenomas. Specifics of the use of these and other medications are discussed below.

Posttreatment Follow-Up

Patients undergoing transsphenoidal microsurgery should be reevaluated 4–6 weeks postoperatively to document that complete removal of the adenoma and correction of endocrine hypersecretion have been achieved. Prolactinomas are assessed by basal PRL measurements, GH-secreting tumors by glucose suppression testing and IGF-1 levels, and ACTH-secreting adenomas by measurement of urine free cortisol and the response to low-dose dexamethasone suppression (see below). Other anterior pituitary hormones—TSH, ACTH, and LH/FSH—should also be assessed as described above in the section on endocrine evaluation. In patients with successful responses, yearly evaluation should be done to watch for late recurrence; late hypopituitarism does not occur after microsurgery. MRI is not necessary in patients with normal postoperative pituitary function but should be utilized in patients with persisting or recurrent disease.

Follow-up of patients treated by pituitary irradiation is also essential, since the response to therapy may be delayed and the incidence of hypopituitarism increases with time. Yearly endocrinologic assessment of both the hypersecreted hormone and the other pituitary hormones is recommended.

1. PROLACTINOMAS

PRL hypersecretion is the most common endocrine abnormality due to hypothalamic-pituitary disorders, and PRL is the hormone most commonly secreted in excess by pituitary adenomas.

The understanding that PRL hypersecretion causes not only galactorrhea but also gonadal dysfunction and the use of PRL measurements in screening such patients have permitted recognition of these PRL-secreting tumors before the development of sellar enlargement, hypopituitarism, or visual impairment.

Thus, plasma PRL should be measured in patients with galactorrhea, suspected hypothalamic-pituitary dysfunction, or sellar enlargement and in those with unexplained gonadal dysfunction, including amenorrhea, infertility, decreased libido, or impotence (Table 5–10).

Pathology

PRL-secreting pituitary adenomas arise most commonly from the lateral wings of the anterior pituitary, but with progression they fill the sella turcica and compress the normal anterior and posterior lobes. Tumor size varies greatly from microadenomas to large invasive tumors with extrasellar extension. Most patients have microadenomas, ie, tumors less than 1 cm in diameter at diagnosis. Prolactinomas frequently undergo spontaneous partial necrosis, and thus a partially empty sella turcica accompanies the pituitary adenoma in 30–40% of patients.

Prolactinomas usually appear chromophobic on routine histologic study, reflecting the inadequacy of the techniques used. The cells are small and uniform, with round or oval nuclei and scanty cytoplasm, and secretory granules are usually not visible with routine stains. The stroma contains a diffuse capillary network.

Electron microscopic examination shows that prolactinoma cells characteristically contain secretory

Table 5–10. Clinical manifestations of acromegaly in 100 patients.[1]

Manifestations of GH excess	
Acral enlargement	100[2]
Soft tissue overgrowth	100
Hyperhidrosis	88
Lethargy or fatigue	87
Weight gain	73
Paresthesias	70
Joint pain	69
Photophobia	46
Papillomas	45
Hypertrichosis	33
Goiter	32
Acanthosis nigricans	29
Hypertension	24
Cardiomegaly	16
Renal calculi	11
Disturbance of other endocrine functions	
Hyperinsulinemia	70
Glucose intolerance	50
Irregular or absent menses	60
Decreased libido or impotence	46
Hypothyroidism	13
Galactorrhea	13
Gynecomastia	8
Hypoadrenalism	4
Local manifestations	
Enlarged sella	90
Headache	65
Visual deficit	20

[1]Adapted from Tyrrell JB, Wilson CB: Pituitary syndromes. In: *Surgical Endocrinology: Clinical Syndromes.* Friesen SR (editor). Lippincott, 1978.
[2]Percentage of patients in whom these features were present.

granules that usually range from 100 to 500 nm and are spherical. Larger granules (400–500 nm), which are irregular or crescent-shaped, are less commonly seen. The cells show evidence of secretory activity, with a large Golgi area, nucleolar enlargement, and a prominent endoplasmic reticulum. Immunocytochemical studies of these tumors have confirmed that the secretory granules indeed contain PRL.

Clinical Features

The clinical manifestations of PRL excess are the same regardless of the cause (see below). The classic features are galactorrhea and amenorrhea in women and galactorrhea and decreased libido or impotence in men. Although the sex distribution of prolactinomas is approximately equal, microadenomas are much more common in females, presumably because of earlier recognition of the endocrine consequences of PRL excess.

A. Galactorrhea: Galactorrhea occurs in the majority of women with prolactinomas and is less common in men. It is usually not spontaneous, or may be present only transiently or intermittently; careful breast examination is required in most patients to demonstrate galactorrhea. The absence of galactorrhea despite markedly elevated PRL levels is probably due to concomitant deficiency of the go-

nadal hormones required to initiate lactation (see Chapter 16).

B. Gonadal Dysfunction:

1. In women–Amenorrhea, oligomenorrhea with anovulation, or infertility is present in approximately 90% of women with prolactinomas. These menstrual disorders usually present concurrently with galactorrhea if it is present but may either precede or follow it. The amenorrhea is usually secondary and may follow pregnancy or oral contraceptive use. Primary amenorrhea occurs in the minority of patients who have onset of hyperprolactinemia during adolescence. The necessity of measuring PRL in patients with unexplained primary or secondary amenorrhea is emphasized by several studies showing that hyperprolactinemia occurs in as many as 20% of patients with neither galactorrhea nor other manifestations of pituitary dysfunction. A number of these patients have been shown to have prolactinomas.

Gonadal dysfunction in these women is due to interference with the hypothalamic-pituitary-gonadal axis by the hyperprolactinemia and except in patients with large or invasive adenomas is not due to destruction of the gonadotropin-secreting cells. This has been documented by the return of menstrual function following reduction of PRL levels to normal by drug treatment or surgical removal of the tumor. Although basal gonadotropin levels are frequently within the normal range despite reduction of sex steroid levels in hyperprolactinemic patients, PRL inhibits both the normal pulsatile secretion of LH and FSH and the midcycle LH surge, resulting in anovulation. The positive feedback effect of estrogen on gonadotropin secretion is also inhibited; in fact, patients with hyperprolactinemia are usually estrogen-deficient.

Estrogen deficiency in women with prolactinomas may be accompanied by decreased vaginal lubrication, other symptoms of estrogen deficiency, and osteopenia as assessed by bone densitometry. Other symptoms may include weight gain, fluid retention, and irritability. Hirsutism may also occur, accompanied by elevated plasma levels of dehydroepiandrosterone (DHEA) sulfate. Patients with hyperprolactinemia may also suffer from anxiety and depression. Treatment with bromocriptine has been shown to improve psychologic distress in such patients.

2. In men–In men, PRL excess may also occasionally cause galactorrhea; however, the usual manifestations are those of hypogonadism. The initial symptom is decreased libido, which may be dismissed by both the patient and physician as due to psychosocial factors; thus, the recognition of prolactinomas in men is frequently delayed, and marked hyperprolactinemia (PRL > 200 ng/mL [9.1 nmol/L]) and sellar enlargement are usual. Unfortunately, prolactinomas in men are often not diagnosed until late manifestations such as headache, visual impairment, or hypopituitarism appear; virtually all such patients have a history of sexual or gonadal dysfunction. Serum testosterone levels are low, and in the presence of normal or subnormal gonadotropin levels, PRL excess should be suspected as well as other causes of hypothalamic-pituitary-gonadal dysfunction (see section on hypopituitarism). Impotence also occurs in hyperprolactinemic males. Its cause is unclear, since testosterone replacement may not reverse it if hyperprolactinemia is not corrected. Male infertility accompanied by reduction in sperm count is a less common initial complaint.

C. Tumor Progression: In general, the growth of prolactinomas is slow, and several studies have shown that most microadenomas do not progress.

Differential Diagnosis

The many conditions associated with hyperprolactinemia are listed in Table 5–5. Pregnancy, hypothalamic-pituitary disorders, primary hypothyroidism, and drug ingestion are the most common causes.

Hypothalamic lesions frequently cause PRL hypersecretion by decreasing the secretion of dopamine that tonically inhibits PRL release; the lesions may be accompanied by panhypopituitarism. Similarly, traumatic or surgical section of the pituitary stalk leads to hyperprolactinemia and hypopituitarism. The cause and clinical features of hypothalamic lesions are discussed in previous sections.

Pregnancy leads to a physiologic increase in PRL secretion; the levels increase as pregnancy continues and may reach 200 ng/mL (9.1 nmol/L) during the third trimester. Following delivery, basal PRL levels gradually fall to normal over several weeks but increase in response to breast feeding. Hyperprolactinemia persisting for 6–12 months or longer following delivery is an indication for evaluation. PRL levels are also high in normal neonates.

Several systemic disorders lead to hyperprolactinemia. Primary hypothyroidism is a common cause, and measurement of thyroid function, and especially TSH, should be part of the evaluation. In primary hypothyroidism, there is hyperplasia of both thyrotrophs and lactotrophs, presumably due to TRH hypersecretion. This may result in significant pituitary gland enlargement, which may be mistaken for a PRL-secreting pituitary tumor. The PRL response to TRH is usually exaggerated in these patients. PRL may also be increased in liver disease, particularly in patients with severe cirrhosis, and in patients with chronic renal failure.

PRL excess and galactorrhea may also be caused by breast disease, nipple stimulation, disease or injury to the chest wall, and spinal cord lesions. These disorders increase PRL secretion by stimulation of afferent neural pathways. Artifactual elevations in prolactin level may be observed in the presence of anti-prolactin antibodies or of macroprolactinemia. In the latter, a high-molecular-weight complex of prolactin molecules maintains immunologic activity but not bioactivity.

The most common cause of hyperprolactinemia is drug ingestion, and a careful history of drug intake must be obtained. Elevated PRL levels, galactorrhea, and amenorrhea may occur following estrogen therapy or oral contraceptive use, but their persistence should suggest prolactinoma. Many other drugs also cause increased PRL secretion and elevated plasma levels (Table 5–5). PRL levels are usually less than 100 ng/mL (4.5 nmol/L), and the evaluation of these patients is primarily by discontinuance of the drug or medication and reevaluation after several weeks. In patients in whom drug withdrawal is not feasible, neuroradiologic studies, if normal, will usually exclude prolactinoma.

Diagnosis

A. General Evaluation: The evaluation of patients with galactorrhea or unexplained gonadal dysfunction with normal or low plasma gonadotropin levels should first include a history regarding menstrual status, pregnancy, fertility, sexual function, and symptoms of hypothyroidism or hypopituitarism. Current or previous use of medication, drugs, or estrogen therapy should be documented. Basal PRL levels, gonadotropins, thyroid function tests, and TSH levels should be established, as well as serum testosterone in men. Liver and kidney function should be assessed. A pregnancy test should be performed in women with amenorrhea.

Patients with galactorrhea but normal menses may not have hyperprolactinemia and usually do not have prolactinomas. If the PRL level is normal, they may be reassured and followed with sequential PRL measurements. Those with elevated levels require further evaluation as described below.

B. Specific Diagnosis: When other causes of hyperprolactinemia have been excluded, the most likely cause of persisting hyperprolactinemia is a prolactinoma, especially if there is associated hypogonadism. Since currently available suppression and stimulation tests do not distinguish PRL-secreting tumors from other causes of hyperprolactinemia, the diagnosis must be established by the assessment of both basal PRL levels and neuroradiologic studies. Patients with large tumors and marked hyperprolactinemia usually present little difficulty. With very rare exceptions, basal PRL levels greater than 200 ng/mL (9.1 nmol/L) are virtually diagnostic of prolactinoma. In addition, since there is a general correlation between the PRL elevation and the size of the pituitary adenoma, these patients usually have sellar enlargement and obvious macroadenomas. Similarly, if the basal PRL level is between 100 and 200 ng/mL (4.5 and 9.1 nmol/L), the cause is usually prolactinoma. These patients may have either micro- or macroadenomas; however, with basal levels of PRL greater than 100 ng/mL (4.5 nmol/L), the PRL-secreting tumor is usually radiologically evident, and again the diagnosis is generally straightforward. Patients with mild to moderate hyperprolactinemia (20–100 ng/mL [0.9–4.5 nmol/L]) present the greatest difficulty in diagnosis, since both PRL-secreting microadenomas and the many other conditions causing hyperprolactinemia (Table 5–5) cause PRL hypersecretion of this degree. In such patients, MRI should be performed and will frequently demonstrate a definite pituitary microadenoma. Scans showing only minor or equivocal abnormalities should be interpreted with caution, because of the high incidence of false-positive scans in the normal population (see neuroradiologic evaluation, above). Since the diagnosis cannot be either established or excluded in patients with normal or equivocal neuroradiologic studies, they require further evaluation or serial assessment (see below).

Treatment

Satisfactory control of PRL hypersecretion, cessation of galactorrhea, and return of normal gonadal function can be achieved in most patients with PRL-secreting microadenomas, although the choice of primary therapy (surgical or medical) remains controversial. In patients with hyperprolactinemia, ovulation should not be induced without careful assessment of pituitary anatomy, since pregnancy may cause further expansion of these tumors as discussed below. All patients with PRL-secreting macroadenomas should be treated, because of the risks of further tumor expansion, hypopituitarism, and visual impairment. Patients with larger prolactinomas—over 2 cm in diameter, or basal PRL levels over 200 ng/mL (9.1 nmol/L)—may require combined therapy with surgery, radiation, and bromocriptine or long-term suppression with bromocriptine alone.

Treatment for all patients with microadenomas is also recommended to prevent early osteoporosis secondary to persisting hypogonadism and to restore fertility. In addition, surgical or medical therapy is more successful in these patients than in those with larger tumors.

Patients with persisting hyperprolactinemia and hypogonadism and normal neuroradiologic studies—ie, those in whom prolactinoma cannot be definitely established—may be managed by observation if hypogonadism is of short duration. However, in patients whose hypogonadism has persisted for more than 6–12 months, bromocriptine should be used to suppress PRL secretion and restore normal gonadal function. In women with suspected or proved prolactinomas, replacement estrogen therapy is contraindicated because of the risk of tumor growth.

A. Surgical:

1. Transsphenoidal microsurgery–This is the surgical procedure of choice in patients with prolactinomas and is the preferred initial method of therapy in some institutions.

a. Microadenomas–In patients with microadenomas, success, as measured by restitution of normal PRL levels, normal menses, and cessation of galactorrhea, is achieved in 85–90% of cases. Success is most likely in patients with basal PRL levels under 200 ng/mL (9.1 nmol/L) and a duration of amenorrhea of less than 5 years. In these patients, the incidence of surgical complications is less than 5%, and hypopituitarism is a rare complication. Thus, in this group of patients with PRL-secreting microadenomas, PRL hypersecretion can be corrected, gonadal function restored, and secretion of TSH and ACTH preserved. Recurrence rates vary considerably in reported series. In our experience, approximately 85% of patients have had long-term remissions, and 15% have had recurrent hyperprolactinemia.

b. Macroadenomas–Transsphenoidal microsurgery is considerably less successful in restoring normal PRL secretion in patients with macroadenomas; many clinicians would treat these patients with bromocriptine alone. The surgical outcome is directly related to tumor size and the basal PRL level. Thus, in patients with tumors 1–2 cm in diameter without extrasellar extension and with basal PRL levels under 200 ng/mL (9.1 nmol/L), transsphenoidal surgery is successful in about 80% of cases. In patients with higher basal PRL levels and larger or invasive tumors, the success rate—defined as complete tumor resection and restoration of normal basal PRL secretion—is about 25–50%. Although surgical results are relatively poor in this latter group of patients, surgery is recommended at many centers as the primary therapy in order to decompress vital structures such as the optic chiasm and to reduce tumor bulk and PRL hypersecretion. Additional therapy with bromocriptine or radiotherapy is required in the subsequent management of these patients (see below).

2. Transfrontal craniotomy–This procedure should be used only in patients with major suprasellar extension of tumor not accessible via the transsphenoidal route in whom decompression of vital structures is required. It must be followed by bromocriptine or radiation therapy, since residual tumor is virtually always present.

B. Medical:

1. Bromocriptine–Bromocriptine (2-bromo-α-ergocryptine mesylate) is a potent dopamine agonist that stimulates dopamine receptors and has effects at both the hypothalamic and pituitary levels. It is effective therapy for a PRL-secreting pituitary adenoma and directly inhibits PRL secretion by the tumor. The dosage is 2.5–10 mg/d orally in divided doses. Side effects consisting of dizziness, postural hypotension, nausea, and occasionally vomiting are common at onset of therapy but usually resolve with continuation of the medication. They can usually be avoided by starting with a low dose and gradually increasing the dose over days to weeks until the PRL level is suppressed to the normal range. An example would be to give 1.25 mg at bedtime for 2 or 3 days and then increase to 2.5 mg; if tolerated, an additional 2.5 mg can be added in the morning. PRL levels should then be assessed. If they remain elevated, the dosage is gradually increased to a total of 7.5–10 mg/d. With these dosages, hyperprolactinemia is controlled in most patients; further increases in dosage are usually not warranted and are usually accompanied by increased side effects. Most patients tolerate doses of 2.5–10 mg without difficulty; however, in 10–15%, persisting postural hypotension and gastrointestinal side effects necessitate discontinuance of therapy.

a. Microadenomas–In patients with microadenomas, bromocriptine successfully reduces PRL levels to normal in about 80% of cases. About 10% of patients cannot tolerate the drug long-term because of persisting side effects, and another 10% are resistant to the effects of bromocriptine. In addition, correction of hyperprolactinemia allows recovery of normal gonadal function; ovulation and fertility are restored, so that mechanical contraception should be advised if pregnancy is not desired. Bromocriptine induces ovulation in most female patients who wish to become pregnant. In these patients with microadenomas, the risk of major expansion of adenoma during the pregnancy appears to be less than 5%; however, both the patient and the physician must be aware of this potential complication. Current data do not indicate an increased risk of multiple pregnancy, abortion, or fetal malformations in pregnancies occurring in women taking bromocriptine; however, the patient should be instructed to discontinue bromocriptine at the first missed menstrual period and obtain a pregnancy test.

At present, there is no evidence that bromocriptine causes permanent resolution of PRL-secreting microadenomas, and virtually all patients have resumption of hyperprolactinemia following discontinuation of therapy even when it has been continued for several years. Although no late toxicity has yet been reported other than the side effects noted above, questions about possible long-term risk and the indicated duration of therapy in such patients with microadenomas are currently unanswered.

b. Macroadenomas–Bromocriptine is effective in controlling hyperprolactinemia in patients with PRL-secreting macroadenomas even when basal PRL levels are markedly elevated. Bromocriptine may be used either as initial therapy or to control residual hyperprolactinemia in patients unsuccessfully treated with surgery or radiotherapy. Bromocriptine should not be used to induce ovulation and pregnancy in women with untreated macroadenomas, since the risk of tumor expansion and visual deficits in the later part of pregnancy is approximately 15–25%. These patients should be treated with surgery prior to induction of ovulation with bromocriptine or by gonadotropin therapy.

Bromocriptine normalizes PRL secretion in about 60–70% of patients with macroadenomas and also reduces tumor size in about the same number. Reduction of tumor size with bromocriptine may occur within days to weeks following institution of therapy. The drug has been used to restore vision in patients with major suprasellar extension and chiasmal compression. Tumor reduction in response to bromocriptine is sustained only as long as the medication is continued, and reexpansion of the tumor and recurrence of hyperprolactinemia may occur rapidly following discontinuation of therapy.

2. Pergolide–Pergolide mesylate is a long-acting ergot derivative with dopaminergic properties that has been shown to reduce hypersecretion and shrink most PRL-secreting macroadenomas. It is more potent than bromocriptine, requiring doses of 25–300 μg/d to treat hyperprolactinemia. The side effects of pergolide are similar to those of bromocriptine.

3. Other dopamine agonists–Quingolide and cabergoline are non-ergot alkaloid-derived dopamine agonists which are in clinical trials. They normalize PRL values in 70–80% of patients and may have fewer side effects than bromocriptine.

C. Radiotherapy: Conventional radiation therapy is reserved for patients with PRL-secreting macroadenomas who have persisting hyperprolactinemia who have not responded to attempts to control their pituitary adenomas with surgery or bromocriptine. In this group of patients, radiotherapy with 4000–5000 cGy prevents further tumor expansion, though PRL levels usually do not fall into the normal range. Impairment of anterior pituitary function occurs in approximately 50–60% of patients.

Experience with heavy particle irradiation in prolactinomas is limited, as is that with gamma-knife radiosurgery.

Selection of Therapy for Prolactinomas

The selection of therapy for prolactinomas depends on the wishes of the patient, the patient's plans for pregnancy and tolerance of medical therapy, and the availability of a skilled neurosurgeon.

A. Microadenomas: All patients should be treated to prevent tumor progression, and osteopenia and the other effects of prolonged hypogonadism. Medical therapy with bromocriptine effectively restores normal gonadal function and fertility, and pregnancy carries only a small risk of tumor expansion. The major disadvantage is the need for chronic therapy. In contrast, transsphenoidal adenectomy, either initially or after a trial of bromocriptine therapy, carries little risk when performed by an experienced neurosurgeon and offers a high probability of long-term remission.

B. Macroadenomas: Primary surgical therapy in these patients frequently does not result in long-term remission, so medical therapy is being used more often as primary therapy, particularly when the patient's prolactin levels are greater than 200 ng/mL (9.1 nmol/L) and the tumor is larger than 2 cm. Although transsphenoidal microsurgery will rapidly decrease tumor size and decompress the pituitary stalk, the optic chiasm, and the cavernous sinuses, there is usually residual tumor and hyperprolactinemia. Thus, these patients will require additional therapy with bromocriptine or radiation. Although tumor growth and prolactin secretion can be controlled by medical therapy in most patients, therapeutic failure can result from drug intolerance, poor compliance, or resistance. Radiation therapy is reserved for postsurgical patients with residual adenomas who are not controlled with bromocriptine.

2. ACROMEGALY & GIGANTISM

GH-secreting pituitary adenomas are second in frequency to prolactinomas and cause the classic clinical syndromes of acromegaly and gigantism.

The characteristic clinical manifestations are the consequence of chronic GH hypersecretion, which in turn leads to excessive generation of IGF-1 the mediator of most of the effects of GH (see Chapter 6). Although overgrowth of bone is the classic feature, GH excess causes a generalized systemic disorder with deleterious effects and an increased mortality rate, though deaths are rarely due to the space-occupying or destructive effects of pituitary adenoma per se.

Acromegaly and gigantism are virtually always secondary to a pituitary adenoma. Ectopic GRH secretion has been identified as another cause of GH hypersecretion and acromegaly in a few patients with carcinoid or islet cell tumors. Reports of intrapituitary GRH-secreting gangliocytomas in direct contiguity with GH-secreting somatotroph adenomas and a report of a GRH-secreting hypothalamic hamartoma in a patient with acromegaly provide a link between ectopic and eutopic GRH production. Ectopic secretion of GH per se is very rare but has been documented in a few lung tumors.

In adults, GH excess leads to acromegaly, the syndrome characterized by local overgrowth of bone, particularly of the skull and mandible. Linear growth does not occur, because of prior fusion of the epiphyses of long bones. In childhood and adolescence, the onset of chronic GH excess leads to gigantism. Many of these patients have associated hypogonadism, which delays epiphysial closure, and the combination of IGF-1 excess and hypogonadism leads to a striking acceleration of linear growth. Most patients with gigantism also have features of acromegaly if GH hypersecretion persists through adolescence and into adulthood.

Pathology

Pituitary adenomas causing acromegaly are usually over 1 cm in diameter when the diagnosis is established. These tumors arise from the lateral wings of the anterior pituitary; less than 20% are diagnosed as microadenomas.

GH-secreting adenomas are of two histologic types: densely and sparsely granulated. However, there appears to be no difference in the degree of GH secretion or clinical manifestations in these patients. About 15% of GH-secreting tumors also contain lactotrophs, and these tumors thus hypersecrete both GH and PRL.

Densely granulated adenomas are acidophilic by light microscopy using routine stains and are usually strongly positive when stained for GH by immunocytochemical techniques. Electron microscopy demonstrates that the cells are similar to normal somatotrophs; ie, they are spherical or oval, with uniform features, round or oval centrally located nuclei, and abundant cytoplasm. The numerous spherical GH-containing granules are electron-dense, ranging in size from 300 to 600 nm, with the majority measuring 350–450 nm.

The sparsely granulated adenomas are chromophobic by light microscopy, a feature that merely reflects the paucity of stainable secretory granules; they are indistinguishable from other chromophobe adenomas except by the demonstration of GH within them by immunocytochemistry. By electron microscopy, the cells do not resemble normal somatotrophs but have variable shape and size; pleomorphic, frequently crescent-shaped nuclei; and globular fibrous bodies within the cytoplasm. The secretory granules measure 100–250 nm, and fewer are present than in normal somatotrophs or densely granulated adenomas.

Etiology & Pathogenesis

Excessive pituitary GH secretion could be secondary to abnormal hypothalamic function, but in most cases it is a primary pituitary disorder. A mutation in the G_s protein leading to excessive cAMP production has been identified in 40% of GH-secreting adenomas. Pituitary adenomas are present in virtually all patients and are usually greater than 1 cm in diameter; hyperplasia alone is rare, and nonadenomatous anterior pituitary tissue does not exhibit somatotroph hyperplasia when examined histologically. In addition, there is a return of normal GH levels and dynamic control of GH secretion following selective removal of the pituitary adenoma.

Pathophysiology

In acromegaly, GH secretion is increased and its dynamic control is abnormal. Secretion remains episodic; however, the number, duration, and amplitude of secretory episodes are increased, and they occur randomly throughout the 24-hour period. The characteristic nocturnal surge is absent, and there are abnormal responses to suppression and stimulation. Thus, glucose suppressibility is lost (see diagnosis, below), and GH stimulation by hypoglycemia is usually absent. TRH and GnRH may cause GH release, whereas these substances do not normally stimulate GH secretion. Dopamine and dopamine agonists such as bromocriptine and apomorphine, which normally stimulate GH secretion, paradoxically cause GH suppression in about 70–80% of patients with acromegaly.

Most of the deleterious effects of chronic GH hypersecretion are caused by its stimulation of excessive amounts of IGF-1 (see Chapter 6), and plasma levels of this compound are increased in acromegaly. The growth-promoting effects of IGF-1 (DNA, RNA, and protein synthesis) lead to the characteristic proliferation of bone, cartilage, and soft tissues and increase in size of other organs to produce the classic clinical manifestations of acromegaly. The insulin resistance and carbohydrate intolerance seen in acromegaly appear to be direct effects of GH and not due to IGF-1 excess.

Clinical Features

The sex incidence of acromegaly is approximately equal; the mean age at diagnosis is approximately 40 years; and the duration of symptoms is usually 5–10 years before the diagnosis is established.

Acromegaly is a chronic disabling and disfiguring disorder with increased late morbidity and mortality if untreated. Although spontaneous remissions have been described, the course is slowly progressive in the great majority of cases—patients once thought to be "burned out" can almost invariably be shown to have continuing clinical manifestations and GH hypersecretion.

A. Symptoms and Signs: Early manifestations (Table 5–11) include soft tissue proliferation, with enlargement of the hands and feet and coarsening of the facial features. This is usually accompanied by increased sweating, heat intolerance, oiliness of the skin, fatigue, and weight gain.

At diagnosis, virtually all patients have classic manifestations; acral and soft tissue changes are always present. Bone and cartilage changes affect chiefly the face and skull (Figure 5–17). These changes include thickening of the calvarium; increased size of the frontal sinuses, which leads to prominence of the supraorbital ridges; enlargement of the nose; and downward and forward growth of the mandible, which leads to prognathism and widely spaced teeth. Soft tissue growth also contributes to the facial appearance, with coarsening of the features and facial and infraorbital puffiness. The hands and feet are predominantly affected by soft tissue growth; they are large, thickened, and bulky, with blunt, spade-like fingers (Figure 5–18) and toes. A bulky, sweaty handshake frequently suggests the diagnosis, and there are increases in ring, glove, and shoe sizes.

Table 5–11. Actions of vasopressin.

Target Organ	Type of Receptor	Action
Kidney glomerulus:	V_1	Mesangial cell contraction and ↓ glomerular capillary ultrafiltration coefficient.
Vasa recta	V_1	↓ Medullary blood flow.
Cortical and outer medullary collecting tubules	V_2	↑ Water permeability and NaCl reabsorption.
Inner medullary (papillary) collecting tubules	V_2	↑ Water and urea permeability.
Thick ascending limb of loop of Henle	V_2	↑ Na^{2+}, Cl^-, K^+ reabsorption.
Juxtaglomerular cells	V_1	Suppression of renin release.
Cardiovascular system:		
Arterioles	V_1	Constriction.
Blood vessel baroreceptors	V_2 ?	Sensitization of baroreflex via area postrema.
	V_1 ?	Desensitization of baroreflex via vasopressin released in brain.
Liver	V_1	↑ Glyconeogenolysis.
Adenohypophysis	V_1	↑ ACTH release.
Brain	?	Enhances passive avoidance behavior.

There is generalized thickening of the skin, with increased oiliness and sweating. Acne, sebaceous cysts, and fibromata mollusca (skin tags and papillomas) are common, as is acanthosis nigricans of the axillae and neck and hypertrichosis in women.

These bony and soft tissue changes are accompanied by systemic manifestations, which include hyperhidrosis, heat intolerance, lethargy, fatigue, and increased sleep requirement. Moderate weight gain usually occurs. Paresthesias, usually due to carpal tunnel compression, occur in 70%; sensorimotor neuropathies occur uncommonly. Bone and cartilage overgrowth leads to arthralgias and in long-standing cases to degenerative arthritis of the spine, hips, and knees. Photophobia of unknown cause occurs in about half of cases and is most troublesome in bright sunlight and during night driving.

GH excess leads to generalized visceromegaly, clinically evident as thyromegaly and enlargement of the salivary glands. Enlargement of other organs is usually not clinically detectable.

Hypertension of unknown cause occurs in about 25% of patients and cardiomegaly in about 15%. Cardiac enlargement may be secondary to hypertension, atherosclerotic disease, or, rarely, to "acromegalic cardiomyopathy." Renal calculi occur in 11% secondary to the hypercalciuria induced by GH excess.

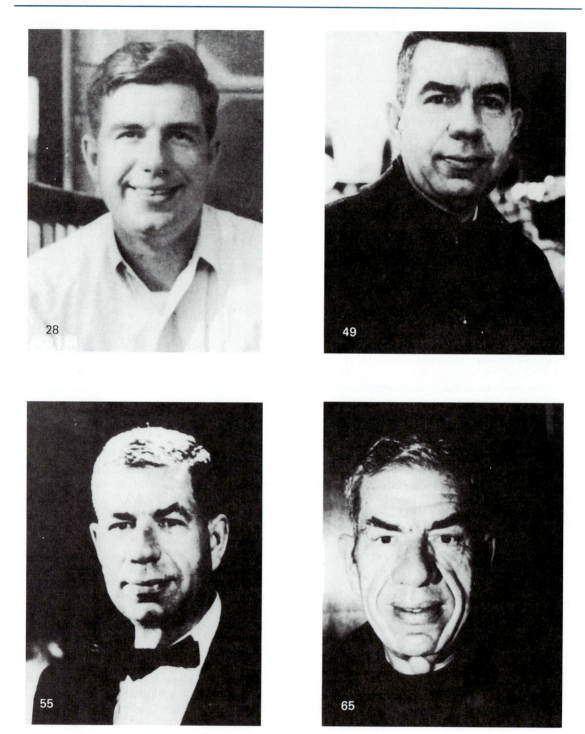

Figure 5–17. Serial photographs of an acromegalic patient at the ages indicated. Note the gradual increase in size of the nose, lips, and skin folds. (Reproduced, with permission, from Reichlin SR: Acromegaly. Med Grand Rounds 1982;1:9.)

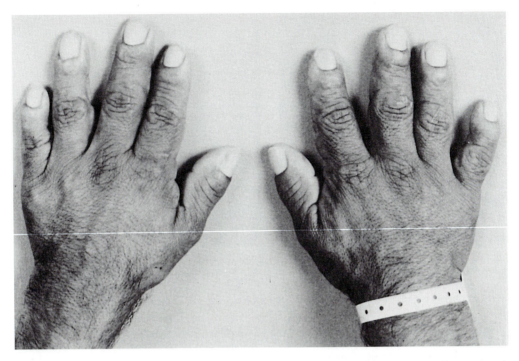

Figure 5–18. Markedly increased soft tissue bulk and blunt fingers in a middle-aged man with acromegaly.

Other endocrine and metabolic abnormalities are common and may be due either to GH excess or to mechanical effects of the pituitary adenoma. Glucose intolerance and hyperinsulinism occur in 50% and 70%, respectively, owing to GH-induced insulin resistance. Overt clinical diabetes occurs in a minority, and diabetic ketoacidosis is rare. Hypogonadism occurs in 60% of female and 46% of male patients and is of multifactorial origin; tumor growth and compression may impair pituitary gonadotropin secretion, and associated hyperprolactinemia (see below) or the PRL-like effect of excessive GH secretion may impair gonadotropin and gonadal function. In men, low total plasma testosterone levels may be due to GH suppression of sex hormone-binding globulin (SHBG) levels; in these cases, plasma free testosterone levels may be normal, with normal gonadal function. With earlier diagnosis, hypothyroidism and hypoadrenalism due to destruction of the normal anterior pituitary are unusual and are present in only 13% and 4% of patients, respectively. Galactorrhea occurs in about 15% and is usually caused by hyperprolactinemia from a pituitary adenoma with a mixed cell population of somatotrophs and lactotrophs. Gynecomastia of unknown cause occurs in about 10% of men. Although acromegaly may be a component of multiple endocrine neoplasia (MEN) type I syndrome, it is distinctly unusual, and concomitant parathyroid hyperfunction or pancreatic islet cell tumors are rare.

When GH hypersecretion is present for many years, late complications occur, including progressive cosmetic deformity and disabling degenerative arthritis (which frequently requires operative treatment). In addition, the mortality rate is increased; after age 45, the death rate in acromegaly from cardiovascular and cerebrovascular atherosclerosis, respiratory diseases, and malignancy is two to four times that of the healthy population. Death rates tend to be higher in patients with hypertension or clinical diabetes mellitus.

Manifestations of the pituitary adenoma are also common in acromegaly; eg, 65% of patients have headache. Although visual impairment was usually present in older series, it now occurs in only 15–20%, since most patients are now diagnosed because of the manifestations of GH excess.

B. Laboratory Findings: Postprandial plasma glucose may be elevated, and serum insulin is increased in 70%. Elevated serum phosphorus (due to increased renal tubular resorption of phosphate) and hypercalciuria appear to be due to direct effects of GH or IGF-1.

C. Imaging Studies: Plain films (Figure 5–19) show sellar enlargement in 90% of cases. Thickening of the calvarium, enlargement of the frontal and maxillary sinuses, and enlargement of the jaw can also be seen. Radiographs of the hand show increased soft tissue bulk, "arrowhead" tufting of the distal phalanges, increased width of intra-articular cartilages,

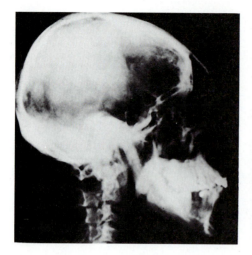
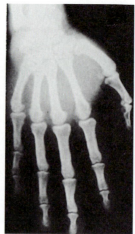
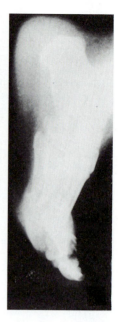

Figure 5–19. Radiologic signs in acromegaly: Left: Skull with enlarged sella turcica and frontal sinuses, thickening of the calvarium, and enlargement of the mandible. Center: Hand with enlarged sesamoid bone and increased soft tissue shadows. Right: Thickened heel pad. (Reproduced, with permission, from Levin SR: Manifestations and treatment of acromegaly. Calif Med [March] 1972;116:57.)

and cystic changes of the carpal bones. Radiographs of the feet show similar changes, and there is increased thickness of the heel pad (normal, < 22 mm).

Diagnosis

Acromegaly is usually clinically obvious and can be readily confirmed by assessment of GH secretion; basal fasting GH levels (normal, 1–5 ng/mL [46–230 pmol/L]) are > 10 ng/mL in over 90% of patients and range from 5 ng/mL (230 pmol/L) to over 500 ng/mL (23,000 pmol/L), with a mean of approximately 50 ng/mL (2300 pmol/L). However, single measurements are not entirely reliable, because GH secretion is episodic in acromegaly and because other conditions may increase GH secretion (see below).

A. Glucose Suppression: Suppression with oral glucose is the simplest and most specific dynamic test for acromegaly. In healthy subjects, oral administration of 100 g of glucose causes a reduction of the GH level to less than 2 ng/mL (93 pmol/L) at 60 minutes. In acromegaly, GH levels may decrease, increase, or show no change; however, they do not decrease to less than 2 ng/mL (93 pmol/L), and this lack of response establishes the diagnosis.

B. IGF-1 Measurement: Measurement of IGF-1 (see Chapter 6) is a useful means of confirming the diagnosis of GH hypersecretion. IGF-1 levels are elevated in virtually all patients with acromegaly (normal ranges vary widely in different laboratories, and some commercial assays are not reliable).

C. Other Tests: Additional procedures that help establish or confirm the diagnosis are (1) GH stimulation with TRH; (2) the absence of a nocturnal GH surge; and (3) the paradoxic suppression of GH by levodopa, dopamine, bromocriptine, or apomorphine. These procedures are usually unnecessary except in patients with mild acromegaly who may have normal or only mildly elevated GH levels and equivocal responses to glucose suppression.

D. Tumor Localization: Radiographic localization of the pituitary adenoma causing acromegaly is usually straightforward (see Neuroradiologic Evaluation, above). In virtually all patients, tumor location and size can be shown by MRI; 90% have tumors over 1 cm in diameter that are readily visualized. In the rare patient with normal neuroradiologic studies, an extrapituitary ectopic source of GH or GRH should be considered. If the scans suggest diffuse pituitary enlargement or hyperplasia, ectopic GRH should also be suspected.

Differential Diagnosis

A. Other Causes of GH Hypersecretion: The presence of clinical features of GH excess, elevated GH and IGF-1 secretion, and abnormal GH dynamics, together with the demonstration of a pituitary tumor by neuroradiologic studies, are diagnostic of acromegaly. However, other conditions associated with GH hypersecretion must be considered in the differential diagnosis. These include anxiety, exercise, acute illness, chronic renal failure, cirrhosis, starvation, protein-calorie malnutrition, anorexia nervosa, and type I (insulin-dependent) diabetes mellitus. Estrogen therapy may increase GH responsiveness to various stimuli. These conditions may be associated with abnormal GH suppressibility by glucose and by abnormal GH responsiveness to TRH; however, patients with these conditions do not have clinical manifestations of GH excess and are thus readily differentiated from patients with acromegaly. In addition, the conditions listed above do not lead to elevation of IGF-1 concentrations.

B. Ectopic GH or GRH Secretion: These rare patients with acromegaly due to ectopic secretion of GH or GRH have typical clinical manifestations of acromegaly. This may occur in lung carcinoma, carcinoid tumors, and pancreatic islet cell tumors. These syndromes should be suspected in patients with a known extrapituitary tumor who have GH excess or in those with clinical and biochemical features of acromegaly who have radiologic procedures that show normal pituitary glands or that suggest diffuse pituitary enlargement or hyperplasia.

Treatment

All patients with acromegaly should undergo therapy to halt progression of the disorder and to prevent late complications and excess mortality outcomes. The objectives of therapy are removal or destruction of the pituitary tumor, reversal of GH hypersecretion, and maintenance of normal anterior and posterior pituitary function. These objectives are currently attainable in most patients, especially those with smaller tumors and only moderate GH hypersecretion. In patients with large tumors who have marked GH hypersecretion, several therapies are usually required to achieve normal GH secretion.

The criteria for an adequate response to therapy continue to evolve. Until recently, many authors used a basal GH level of 5 ng/mL or less to define remission. However, some of these patients continue to have elevated IGF-1 levels, and a recent report described increased late mortality in patients with GH levels greater than 2.5 ng/mL after therapy. The present authors suggest the following criteria for remission: a fasting GH of 2.5 ng/mL or less or glucose-suppressed GH of 2 ng/mL or less accompanied by a normal level of IGF-1.

The initial therapy of choice is transsphenoidal microsurgery because of its high success rate, rapid reduction of GH levels, the low incidence of postoperative hypopituitarism, and the low surgical morbidity rate. Conventional radiotherapy (x-ray radiation) is also successful, though a much longer period is required to reduce GH levels to normal; heavy particle irradiation has limited availability;and there is limited experience with gamma-knife radiosurgery. Octreotide acetate, a long-acting somatostatin analog, is now available for the treatment of acromegaly and

appears to be most useful in patients who have incomplete responses to surgery or irradiation.

A. Surgical Treatment: Transsphenoidal selective adenoma removal is the procedure of choice; craniotomy is necessary in the few patients in whom major suprasellar extension precludes the transsphenoidal approach. Successful reduction of GH levels is achieved in approximately 60–80% of patients. In those with small or moderate-sized tumors (< 2 cm), success is achieved in over 80%, whereas in those with larger tumors and basal GH levels greater than 50 ng/mL (2325 pmol/L)—and particularly in those with major extrasellar extension of the adenoma—successful responses occur in only 30–60%. Recurrence rates in those with a successful initial response are low (about 5% of patients at our institution). Surgical complications (discussed above) occur in less than 5%.

B. Radiotherapy: Conventional supervoltage irradiation in doses of 4500–5000 cGy is successful in 60–80% of patients, though GH levels may not return to normal until years after therapy. Thus, in one series, GH levels were under 10 ng/mL (460 pmol/L) in only 38% of patients at 2 years posttreatment; however, at 5 and 10 years, 73% and 81% had achieved such levels. The incidence of hypopituitarism is appreciable, and in this series hypothyroidism occurred in 19%, hypoadrenalism in 38%, and hypogonadism in approximately 50–60% of patients as a consequence of radiotherapy. Because of the prolonged delay in achieving reduction in GH levels, conventional radiotherapy is generally reserved for patients with persisting GH secretion following pituitary microsurgery.

Heavy particle irradiation is more rapidly effective than conventional irradiation, but because of the limitations of the field size, it can be used only in patients with smaller tumors and those in whom no extrasellar extension is present. About 80% of patients have GH levels under 10 ng/mL (460 pmol/L) at 5 years after irradiation, with most patients having a satisfactory response at 2 years. The incidence of hypopituitarism has been variously reported, but it appears to occur in approximately 40% of patients.

Therapy of acromegaly by radioactive implants within the sella turcica is limited to a few centers. Successful responses are achieved in about 70%; however, there is a significant incidence of hypopituitarism, cerebrospinal fluid rhinorrhea, and meningitis due to local radionecrosis. Because of these complications, the procedure has not gained wide acceptance. Experience with gamma-knife radiosurgery is very limited at present.

C. Medical: Octreotide acetate, a long-acting analog of somatostatin, is effective in the management of acromegaly. It reduces levels of growth hormone to 5 ng/mL or less and IGF-1 to normal in 65% of patients treated, and in some it has even caused tumor shrinkage. Effective doses appear to be in the range of 100–500 µg given by subcutaneous injection three times daily. The drug is expensive, and the need for subcutaneous injection is a disadvantage, since chronic therapy is required. Octreotide is most effective in patients with only mild to moderate GH elevations; therefore, it is probably best utilized in patients who have had incomplete responses to surgery or who are awaiting the effect of radiotherapy. Medical therapy with bromocriptine or other dopamine agonists is successful in only a few patients.

Response to Treatment

In patients with successful reduction in GH hypersecretion, there is cessation of bone overgrowth. In addition, these patients experience considerable clinical improvement, including reduction in soft tissue bulk of the extremities, decreased facial puffiness, increased energy, and cessation of hyperhidrosis, heat intolerance, and oily skin. Headache, carpal tunnel syndrome, arthralgias, and photophobia are also reversible with successful therapy. Glucose intolerance and hyperinsulinemia as well as hypercalciuria are also reversed in most cases.

Posttreatment Follow-Up

Patients undergoing surgery should be seen 4–6 weeks after the operation for assessment of GH secretion and pituitary function. Those with persisting GH hypersecretion should receive further therapy with radiation or octreotide acetate. Patients with postoperative GH levels under 10 ng/mL (460 pmol/L) should have follow-up GH and IGF-1 determinations at 6-month intervals for 2 years and yearly thereafter. Late hypopituitarism after surgery alone does not occur.

Patients treated with radiotherapy should have biannual assessment of GH secretion and annual assessment of anterior pituitary function, since the incidence of late hypopituitarism is appreciable and increases with time following irradiation.

3. ACTH-SECRETING PITUITARY ADENOMAS: CUSHING'S DISEASE

In 1932, Harvey Cushing documented the presence of small basophilic pituitary adenomas in six of eight patients with clinical features of adrenocortical hyperfunction. Years later, ACTH hypersecretion was identified from such tumors and found to be the cause of bilateral adrenal hyperplasia. Pituitary ACTH hypersecretion (Cushing's disease) is now recognized as the most common cause of spontaneous hypercortisolism (Cushing's syndrome) and must be distinguished from the other forms of adrenocorticosteroid excess—ectopic ACTH syndrome and adrenal tumors (see Chapter 9).

Pathology

ACTH-secreting pituitary tumors exist in virtually all patients with Cushing's disease. These tumors are usually benign microadenomas under 10 mm in diameter; 50% are 5 mm or less in diameter, and microadenomas as small as 1 mm have been described. These tumors in Cushing's disease are either basophilic or chromophobe adenomas and may be found anywhere within the anterior pituitary. Rarely, ACTH-secreting tumors are large, with invasive tendencies, and malignant tumors have rarely been reported.

Histologically, the tumors are composed of compact sheets of uniform, well-granulated cells (granule size, 200–700 nm by electron microscopy) with a sinusoidal arrangement and a high content of ACTH and its related peptides (β-LPH, β-endorphin). A zone of perinuclear hyalinization (Crooke's changes) is frequently observed as a result of exposure of the corticotroph cells to prolonged hypercortisolism. A specific ultrastructural finding in these adenomas is the deposition of bundles of perinuclear microfilaments that encircle the nucleus; these are the ultrastructural equivalent of Crooke's hyaline changes seen on light microscopy. In contrast to the adenomas cells, ACTH content in the portion of the anterior pituitary not involved with the tumor is decreased.

Diffuse hyperplasia of anterior pituitary corticotrophs or adenomatous hyperplasia, presumed to result from hypersecretion of corticotropin-releasing hormone (CRH), occurs rarely.

The adrenal glands in Cushing's disease are enlarged, weighing 12–24 g (normal, 8–10 g). Microscopic examination shows a thickened cortex due to hyperplasia of both the zona reticularis and zona fasciculata; the zona glomerulosa is normal. In some cases, ACTH-secreting pituitary adenomas cause bilateral nodular hyperplasia; the adrenals show diffuse bilateral cortical hyperplasia and the presence of one or more nodules that vary from microscopic to several centimeters in diameter, with multiple small nodules being the most common.

Pathogenesis

The weight of current evidence is that Cushing's disease is a primary pituitary disorder and that hypothalamic abnormalities are secondary to hypercortisolism. The endocrine abnormalities in Cushing's disease are as follows: (1) hypersecretion of ACTH, with bilateral adrenocortical hyperplasia and hypercortisolism; (2) absent circadian periodicity of ACTH and cortisol secretion; (3) absent responsiveness of ACTH and cortisol to stress (hypoglycemia or surgery); (4) abnormal negative feedback of ACTH secretion by glucocorticoids; and (5) subnormal responsiveness of GH, TSH, and gonadotropins to stimulation.

Evidence that Cushing's disease is a primary pituitary disorder is based on the high frequency of pituitary adenomas, the response to their removal, and the interpretation of hypothalamic abnormalities as being secondary to hypercortisolism. In addition, molecular studies have found that nearly all corticotroph adenomas are monoclonal. These findings suggest that ACTH hypersecretion arises from a spontaneously developing pituitary adenoma and that the resulting hypercortisolism suppresses the normal hypothalamic-pituitary axis and CRH release and thereby abolishes the hypothalamic regulation of circadian variability and stress responsiveness. There is in vitro evidence that the negative feedback effects of glucocorticoids are exerted directly on the pituitary tumor and that other pharmacologic agents such as vasopressin, cyproheptadine, and bromocriptine directly inhibit the ACTH-secreting adenoma. In addition, the abnormalities of GH, TSH, and gonadotropin secretion are also observed in exogenous Cushing's syndrome and are due to the hypercortisolism per se and not to a primary hypothalamic disorder.

Analysis of the response to therapy by pituitary microsurgery sheds some light on the pathogenesis of Cushing's disease. Selective removal of pituitary microadenomas by transsphenoidal microsurgery corrects ACTH hypersecretion and hypercortisolism in most patients. This suggests that the adenoma—not corticotroph hyperplasia—is responsible for the ACTH excess. Postoperatively, these patients experience transient ACTH deficiency with secondary hypoadrenalism. ACTH response to CRH is blunted immediately after complete removal of these tumors. The secretion of the other anterior pituitary hormones is not only preserved but enhanced once the microadenoma is removed. These findings, which suggest that the normal hypothalamic-pituitary axis is suppressed by the hypercortisolism, are supported by the in vitro demonstration of markedly decreased ACTH content in nonadenomatous pituitary tissue removed from patients with active Cushing's disease. After selective removal of the pituitary adenoma, the following return to normal: the circadian rhythmicity of ACTH and cortisol, the responsiveness of the hypothalamic-pituitary axis to hypoglycemic stress, and the dexamethasone suppressibility of cortisol secretion. Thus, in these patients, there is no evidence for a persisting hypothalamic abnormality.

Clinical Features

Cushing's disease presents with the signs and symptoms of hypercortisolism and adrenal androgen excess (see Chapter 9). The onset of these features is usually insidious, developing over months or years. Obesity (with predominantly central fat distribution), hypertension, glucose intolerance, and gonadal dysfunction (amenorrhea or impotence) are common features. Other common manifestations include moon facies, plethora, osteopenia, proximal muscle weakness, easy bruisability, psychologic distur-

bances, violaceous striae, hirsutism, acne, poor wound healing, and superficial fungal infections. Unlike patients with the classic form of ectopic ACTH syndrome, patients with Cushing's disease rarely have hypokalemia, weight loss, anemia, or hyperpigmentation. Virilization, observed occasionally in patients with adrenal carcinoma, is unusual in Cushing's disease. Clinical symptoms related to the ACTH-secreting primary tumor itself, such as headache or visual impairment, are rare because of the small size of these adenomas.

The usual age range is 20–40 years, but Cushing's disease has been reported in infants and patients over 70. There is a female:male ratio of approximately 8:1. In contrast, the ectopic ACTH syndrome occurs more commonly in men (male:female ratio of 3:1).

Diagnosis

The initial step in the diagnosis of an ACTH-secreting pituitary adenoma is the documentation of endogenous hypercortisolism, which is confirmed by the presence of abnormal cortisol suppressibility to low-dose dexamethasone as well as an increased basal urine free cortisol. The differentiation of an ACTH-secreting pituitary tumor from other causes of hypercortisolism must be based on biochemical studies, including the measurement of basal plasma ACTH levels, the response to high-dose dexamethasone suppression testing, and inferior petrosal sinus sampling to detect a central to peripheral gradient of ACTH levels (see Chapter 9). The diagnosis and differential diagnosis of Cushing's syndrome are presented in Chapter 9.

Treatment

Transsphenoidal microsurgery is the procedure of choice in Cushing's disease. A variety of other therapies—operative, radiologic, pharmacologic—are discussed below.

A. Surgical Treatment: Selective transsphenoidal resection of ACTH-secreting pituitary adenomas is the initial treatment of choice. At operation, meticulous exploration of the intrasellar contents by an experienced neurosurgeon is required. The tumor, which is often found within the anterior lobe tissue, is selectively removed, and normal gland is left intact. If the tumor is too small to locate at surgery, total or hemi-hypophysectomy may be performed in adult patients who are past the age of reproduction and whose biochemical diagnosis has been confirmed with selective venous ACTH sampling.

In about 85% of patients with microadenomas, selective microsurgery is successful in correcting hypercortisolism. Surgical damage to anterior pituitary function is rare, but most patients develop transient secondary adrenocortical insufficiency requiring postoperative glucocorticoid support until the hypothalamic-pituitary-adrenal axis recovers, usually in 6–18 months. Total hypophysectomy is necessary to correct hypercortisolism in another 10% of patients. In the remaining 5% of patients with microadenomas, selective tumor removal is unsuccessful. By contrast, transsphenoidal surgery is successful in only 25% of the 10–15% of patients with Cushing's disease with pituitary macroadenomas or in those with extrasellar extension of tumor.

Transient diabetes insipidus occurs in about 20% of patients, but other surgical complications (eg, hemorrhage, cerebrospinal fluid rhinorrhea, infection, visual impairment, permanent diabetes insipidus) are rare. Hypopituitarism occurs only in patients who undergo total hypophysectomy.

Before the introduction of pituitary microsurgery, bilateral total adrenalectomy was the preferred treatment of Cushing's disease and may still be employed in patients in whom other therapies are unsuccessful. Total adrenalectomy, which can now be performed laparoscopically, corrects hypercortisolism but produces permanent hypoadrenalism, requiring lifelong glucocorticoid and mineralocorticoid therapy. Morbidity is high and relates to poor wound healing, postoperative infection, pancreatic injury, and thromboembolic phenomena. In addition, the ACTH-secreting pituitary adenoma persists and may progress, causing hyperpigmentation and invasive complications (Nelson's syndrome; see below). Persistent hypercortisolism may occasionally follow total adrenalectomy as ACTH hypersection stimulates adrenal remnants or congenital rests.

B. Radiotherapy: There is relatively little recent experience using conventional irradiation in doses of 44500–5000 cGy as primary therapy for Cushing's disease. Reported response rates are 55–60% and require 2–4 years or longer. Because of these low response rates, we do not recommend conventional irradiation as initial therapy. However, conventional radiotherapy is of benefit in patients who have persisting or recurrent disease following pituitary microsurgery. In these patients, reported remission rates are 55–70% at 1–3 years after radiotherapy.

Heavy particle irradiation, also used as initial therapy in patients with no extrasellar tumor extension, is currently available at only one center in the USA. Remissions have been reported in about 80% of patients in 1–2 years, with hypopituitarism reported in about one-third of patients. However, current experience is limited.

Gamma-knife radiosurgery has been reported from one center with remission rates of 75% in adults and 80% in children. However, 55% of the adults developed panhypopituitarism, and each of the children and adolescents were growth hormone-deficient. Therefore, gamma-knife radiosurgery may be best suited for postoperative radiotherapy in patients with unsuccessful responses to pituitary microsurgery.

Implantation of radioactive seeds (gold and yttrium) within the sella turcica has also been used in Cushing's disease. Such techniques have achieved a remission rate of 65%, with an additional 16% improved; however, the frequency of operative complications is high, and panhypopituitarism is common.

C. Medical: Drugs that inhibit adrenal cortisol secretion are useful in Cushing's disease, often as adjunctive therapy (see Chapter 9).

Ketoconazole, an imidazole derivative, has been found to strongly inhibit adrenal steroid biosynthesis. It inhibits the cytochrome P450 enzymes P450scc and P450c11. In daily doses of 600–1200 mg, ketoconazole has been effective in the management of Cushing's syndrome. Hepatotoxicity is common, however, but may be transient. **Aminoglutethimide,** which inhibits P450scc, has also been utilized to reduce cortisol hypersecretion.

These drugs are expensive; their use is accompanied by increased ACTH levels that may overcome the enzyme inhibition; and they cause gastrointestinal side effects that may limit their effectiveness. More effective control of hypercortisolism with fewer side effects is obtained by combined use of these agents. Adequate data are not available on the long-term use of these drugs as the sole treatment of Cushing's disease. Thus, ketoconazole and aminoglutethimide ordinarily are used while awaiting a response to therapy or in the preparation of patients for surgery.

The adrenolytic drug **mitotane** results in adrenal atrophy predominantly of the zonae fasciculata and reticularis. Remission of hypercortisolism is achieved in approximately 80% of patients with Cushing's disease, but most relapse after therapy is discontinued. Mitotane therapy is limited by the delayed response, which may take weeks or months, and by the frequent side effects, including severe nausea, vomiting, diarrhea, somnolence, and skin rash.

Pharmacologic inhibition of ACTH secretion in Cushing's disease has also been attempted with cyproheptadine and bromocriptine. However, only a very few patients have had successful responses, and the use of these agents is not recommended.

4. ACTH-SECRETING PITUITARY TUMORS FOLLOWING ADRENALECTOMY FOR CUSHING'S DISEASE: NELSON'S SYNDROME

The clinical appearance of an ACTH-secreting pituitary adenoma following bilateral adrenalectomy in patients with Cushing's disease was initially described by Nelson et al in 1958.

Pathogenesis

It now seems likely that Nelson's syndrome represents the clinical progression of a preexisting adenoma after the restraint of hypercortisolism on ACTH secretion and tumor growth is removed. That

ACTH secretion in Cushing's disease is restrained by the circulating cortisol levels is demonstrated by its stimulation during therapy with ketoconazole or mifepristone (a glucocorticoid antagonist). Furthermore, the tumors in Nelson's syndrome are dexamethasone-suppressible, although larger doses may be required than with untreated Cushing's disease. Thus, following adrenalectomy, the suppressive effect of cortisol is no longer present, ACTH secretion increases, and the pituitary adenoma may progress.

Incidence

The incidence of Nelson's syndrome ranges from 10% to 78%, depending on what criteria are used for diagnosis (see Chapter 9). Pituitary irradiation before or after adrenalectomy does not prevent the development of this syndrome. Approximately 30% of patients adrenalectomized for Cushing's disease develop classic Nelson's syndrome with progressive hyperpigmentation and an obvious ACTH-secreting tumor; another 50% develop evidence of a microadenoma without marked progression; and about 20% never develop a progressive tumor. The reasons for these differences in clinical behavior are uncertain, and they cannot be predicted prior to adrenal surgery. Continued examination, including plasma ACTH levels, visual fields, and sellar radiology, is required following bilateral adrenalectomy in patients with Cushing's disease.

Clinical Features

The pituitary tumors in patients with classic Nelson's syndrome are among the most aggressive and rapidly growing of all pituitary tumors. These patients present with hyperpigmentation and with manifestations of an expanding intrasellar mass lesion. Visual field defects, headache, cavernous sinus invasion with extraocular muscle palsies, and even malignant changes with local or distant metastases may occur. Pituitary apoplexy may also complicate the course of these tumors.

Diagnosis

Plasma ACTH levels are markedly elevated, usually over 1000 pg/mL (222 pmol/L) and often as high as 10,000 pg/mL (2220 pmol/L). The sella turcica is enlarged on routine radiographs; MRI defines the extent of the tumor.

Treatment

Pituitary surgery, either by the transsphenoidal approach or by transfrontal craniotomy, is the initial mode of treatment. Complete resection is usually not possible, because of the large size of these tumors. Conventional radiotherapy is employed postoperatively in patients with residual tumor or extrasellar extension.

5. THYROTROPIN-SECRETING PITUITARY ADENOMAS

Thyrotropin-secreting pituitary adenomas are rare tumors manifested as hyperthyroidism with goiter in the presence of elevated TSH. Patients with TSH-secreting tumors are often resistant to routine ablative thyroid therapy, requiring large, often multiple doses of ^{131}I and several operations for control of thyrotoxicosis. Histologically, the tumors are chromophobe adenomas. They are often very large and cause visual impairment, which alerts the physician to a pituitary abnormality. Patients with these tumors do not have extrathyroidal systemic manifestations of Graves' disease such as ophthalmopathy or dermopathy. Pituitary TSH hypersecretion in the absence of a demonstrable pituitary tumor has also been reported to cause hyperthyroidism in a few patients.

TSH dynamics are variable; TRH (protirelin) administration rarely stimulates TSH secretion from these tumors, nor do dopamine and bromocriptine suppress TSH as they do the TSH hypersecretion of primary hypothyroidism. The diagnosis is based on findings of hyperthyroidism with elevated serum TSH and alpha subunit, and neuroradiologic studies consistent with pituitary tumor. Differential diagnosis includes those patients with primary hypothyroidism (thyroid failure) who develop major hyperplasia of pituitary thyrotrophs and lactotrophs with sellar enlargement and occasional suprasellar extension.

Treatment should be directed initially at the adenoma via the transsphenoidal microsurgical approach. However, additional therapy is usually required because of the large size of these adenomas.

Octreotide acetate, a long-acting somatostatin analog, normalizes TSH and T_4 levels in more than 70% of these patients when given subcutaneously in doses similar to those used for the treatment of acromegaly (see above). Shrinkage of the tumor has been observed in about 40% of patients.

If tumor growth and TSH hypersecretion cannot be controlled by surgery and octreotide acetate, the next step would be to undertake pituitary irradiation. In addition, such patients may also require ablative therapy of the thyroid with either ^{131}I or surgery to control their thyrotoxicosis.

6. GONADOTROPIN-SECRETING PITUITARY ADENOMAS

Although many pituitary adenomas synthesize gonadotropins (especially FSH) and their subunits, only a minority of these patients have elevated serum levels of FSH or LH. However, the true nature of these tumors can be demonstrated with provocative stimulation tests. The majority of these tumors produce FSH and the alpha subunit, but tumors secreting both

FSH and LH and a tumor secreting only LH have been described.

Gonadotropin-secreting pituitary adenomas are usually large chromophobe adenomas presenting with visual impairment. Most patients have hypogonadism and many have panhypopituitarism. Hormonal evaluation reveals elevated FSH in some patients accompanied by normal LH values. Basal levels of the alpha subunit may also be elevated. The presence of elevation of both FSH and LH should suggest primary hypogonadism. TRH stimulation leads to an increase in FSH secretion in 33% and an increase in LH-β in 66% of patients.

Therapy for gonadotropin-secreting adenomas has been directed at surgical removal. Because of their large size, adequate control of the tumor has not been achieved, and radiotherapy is usually required.

7. ALPHA SUBUNIT-SECRETING PITUITARY ADENOMAS

Excessive quantities of the alpha subunit of the glycoprotein pituitary hormones have been observed in association with the hypersecretion of many anterior pituitary hormones (TSH, GH, PRL, LH, FSH). Recently, however, pure alpha subunit hypersecretion has been identified in several patients with large invasive chromophobe adenomas and partial panhypopituitarism. Thus, the determination of the alpha subunit may be a useful marker in patients with presumed "nonfunctioning" pituitary adenomas.

8. NONFUNCTIONAL PITUITARY ADENOMAS

"Nonfunctional" chromophobe adenomas once represented approximately 80% of all primary pituitary tumors; however, with clinical application of radioimmunoassay of anterior pituitary hormones, these tumors currently account for only about 10% of all pituitary adenomas. Thus, the great majority of these chromophobe adenomas have now been documented to be PRL-secreting; a smaller number secrete TSH or the gonadotropins.

Nonfunctional tumors are usually large when the diagnosis is established; headache and visual field defects are the usual presenting symptoms. However, endocrine manifestations are usually present for months to years before the diagnosis is made, with gonadotropin deficiency being the most common initial symptom. Hypothyroidism and hypoadrenalism are also common, but the symptoms are subtle and may be missed.

Evaluation should include MRI and visual field testing; endocrine studies should include assessment of pituitary hormones and end-organ function to de-

termine whether the adenoma is hypersecreting or whether hormonal replacement is needed.

Since these tumors are generally large, both surgery and radiation therapy are usually required to prevent tumor progression or recurrence. In the absence of an endocrine index of tumor hypersecretion such as PRL excess, serial scans at yearly intervals are required to assess the response to therapy and to detect possible recurrence.

POSTERIOR PITUITARY HORMONES

ANTIDIURETIC HORMONE (ADH; Vasopressin)

ADH acts through two receptors, termed V_1 and V_2, that have different ligand specificities and cellular mechanisms of action (Table 5–12). The V_1 receptors mediate vascular smooth muscle contraction and stimulate prostaglandin synthesis and liver glycogenolysis. Activation of these receptors increases phosphatidylinositol breakdown, thus causing cellular calcium mobilization. The V_2 receptors, which produce the renal actions of vasopressin, activate G proteins and stimulate the generation of cAMP (see Chapter 1).

Renal Actions

The major renal effect of ADH is to increase the water permeability of the luminal membrane of the collecting duct epithelium. In the absence of ADH, permeability of the epithelium is very low and reabsorption of water decreases, leading to polyuria. When ADH is present, epithelial permeability increases markedly, and water is reabsorbed. This ADH effect is caused by ADH binding to the V_2 receptor. Subsequent cellular events that are incompletely understood increase water permeability of the luminal membrane by increasing the number of narrow aqueous channels with radii of about 0.2 nm. Thus, diffusion of water through the membrane is enhanced, as is transcellular flow.

As the collecting ducts traverse the renal medulla,

Table 5–12. Routes of loss of water in an average adult human.

	mL/24 h
Urine	1500
Skin	600
Lungs	400
Feces	100
	2600

the urine passes regions of ever-increasing osmolality up to maximum of 1200 mosm/kg of water at the tip of the papilla. In the presence of ADH, collecting duct fluid equilibrates with this hyperosmotic environment, and urine osmolality approaches that of medullary interstitial fluid. Thus, maximal ADH effect results in low urine flow, and urine osmolality may approximate 1200 mosm/kg; with ADH deficiency, urine flow may be as high as 15–20 mL/min, and urine osmolality is less than 100 mosm/kg.

Cardiovascular Actions

ADH effects on V_1 receptors in peripheral arterioles increase blood pressure. However, ADH blunts this effect by efferent mechanisms such as bradycardia and inhibition of sympathetic nerve activity. These actions may be important during hypovolemia when plasma ADH levels are very high and maintaining tissue perfusion is critical.

OXYTOCIN

Oxytocin primarily affects uterine smooth muscle. It increases both the frequency and the duration of action potentials during uterine contractions. Thus, administration of oxytocin initiates contractions in a quiescent uterus and increases the strength and frequency of muscle contractions in an active uterus. Estrogen enhances the action of oxytocin by reducing the membrane potential of smooth muscle cells, thus lowering the threshold of excitation. Toward the end of pregnancy, as estrogen levels become higher, the membrane potential of uterine smooth muscle cells becomes less negative, rendering the uterus more sensitive to oxytocin. The number of oxytocin receptors in the uterus also increases at this time, and their activation causes cellular calcium to be mobilized through polyphosphatidylinositol hydrolysis.

Female Reproductive System Actions

A. Parturition: As the fetus enters the birth canal, the lower segment of the uterus, the cervix, and then the vagina are dilated, and this causes reflex release of oxytocin. Strong uterine contractions cause further descent of the fetus, further distention, and further release of oxytocin.

B. Lactation: Oxytocin is also involved in lactation. Stimulation of the nipple produces a neurohumoral reflex that causes secretion of oxytocin. In turn, oxytocin causes contraction of the myoepithelial cells of the mammary ducts and the ejection of milk.

Other Actions

A number of stimuli that also release ADH such as increased plasma osmolality and hypovolemia cause oxytocin secretion. Since oxytocin is an effective natriuretic agent—particularly at low rates of urine flow—it may be involved in the regulation of sodium balance.

CONTROL OF WATER BALANCE

Water Requirements

Water balance is precisely controlled by an integrated system that balances water intake via thirst mechanism with water output controlled by ADH. The average individual loses 2.5–3 L of water per day (Table 5–13) and must take in that amount in order to maintain balance. Given free access to water, total human body water rarely varies by more than 1–2%. Approximately 1.2 L of water is taken in food or is provided by oxidative metabolism. The remainder is ingested as water or other fluids.

Concentration of Urine

Renal concentrating mechanism are essential to the maintenance of water balance in order for the kidney to excrete osmotically active solutes derived from the diet.

The average human excretes 1.5 L of urine per day at an osmolality of approximately 600 mosm/kg of water, ie, twice the concentration of plasma (Table 5–13). Without the capacity to concentrate urine, 3 L of water at a concentration of 300 mosm/kg would be excreted and the extra water would have to be ingested. During negative water balance, the urine volume may be reduced to 600 mL/d at a maximum urinary concentration of 1200 mosm/kg. This capacity to concentrate the urine four times more than plasma is of extreme importance, since otherwise it would be necessary to take very large quantities of water in the diet.

Urinary concentration mechanisms can reduce but not completely prevent loss of water in the urine. Even if an individual is maximally concentrating urine, obligatory fluid loss is still considerable. This situation is exacerbated in a warm environment, where many liters of fluid may be lost to maintain a constant temperature via sweating. The only way to bring body fluid levels back to normal is by increasing water intake. It is not surprising that many similarities exist between mechanisms involved in the control of thirst and ADH secretion.

Table 5–13. Causes of neurogenic diabetes insipidus.

Hypophysectomy, complete or partial.
Surgery to remove suprasellar tumors.
Idiopathic.
Familial.
Tumors and cysts (intra- and suprasellar).
Histiocytosis.
Granulomas.
Infections.
Interruption of blood supply.
Autoimmune.

Control of Thirst & ADH Secretion

Cellular and extracellular dehydration are the two major mechanisms involved in the control of thirst and ADH secretion.

A. Cellular Dehydration: Cellular dehydration occurs when extracellular fluid osmolality is increased relative to that of intracellular fluids, leading to the efflux of water from cells. When extracellular fluid osmolality increases, all cells, including the hypothalamic osmoreceptors, become dehydrated, thus providing the signal for secretion of ADH. In humans, an increase of only 1% in plasma osmolality stimulates thirst, water intake, and simultaneously ADH (Figures 5–20 and 5–21).

The relationship between plasma ADH concentration and plasma osmolality in humans in presented in Figure 5–21. The exquisite sensitivity of ADH release to changing plasma osmolality is obvious. Figure 5–21 represents the physiologic range of variations in plasma ADH in humans.

B. Extracellular Fluid Dehydration: Extracellular fluid dehydration—ie, decreased extracellular fluid volume without a change in osmolality—stimulates thirst and ADH secretion. Thus, hemorrhage reduces extracellular fluid volume and results in both thirst and ADH secretion (Figure 5–22). Small decreases in volume have minimal effects on ADH secretion, but reductions larger than 10% cause a

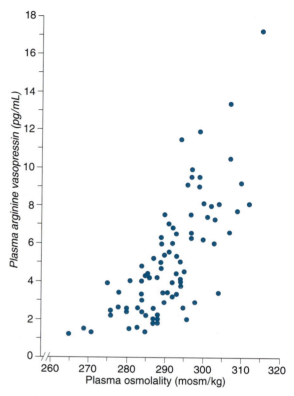

Figure 5–21. Relationship between plasma vasopressin concentration and plasma osmolality in humans during dehydration. (Reproduced, with permission, from Hammer M, Ladefoged J, Olgaard K: Am J Physiol 1980; 238:313.)

marked stimulation of ADH to values > 100 pg/mL (92.5 pmol/L). These high circulating levels of ADH do not further increase water conservation, since maximum urinary concentration is reached at much lower levels. However, the high levels of ADH may support blood pressure via V_1 receptors.

C. Interaction of Osmolality and Volume: Two major mechanisms are involved in hypovolemic stimulation of thirst and ADH secretion. Moderate reductions in blood volume stimulate low-pressure receptors in the left and right atria and in the pulmonary circulation. With more severe hypovolemia, which reduces blood pressure, the arterial baroreceptors are activated. Responses from these baroreceptor areas in the circulation are then transmitted to magnocellular cells in the hypothalamus). In addition, the renin-angiotensin system may be involved, since hypovolemia stimulates renin secretion and angiotensin formation. Angiotensin II also stimulates thirst and ADH secretion. The relative roles of the direct baroreceptor input and angiotensin mechanisms in the responses to extracellular dehydration have yet to be determined.

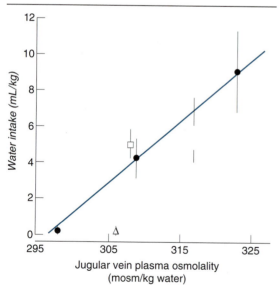

Figure 5–20. Relationship between water intake and jugular vein plasma osmolality. Central osmolality was increased selectively by infusing hypertonic sodium chloride into carotid loops in trained conscious dogs •. Infusion of hypertonic sucrose was equally effective □, whereas hypertonic urea (Δ) did not stimulate drinking. (Data from Wood RJ, Rolls BJ, Ramsay DJ: Am J Physiol 1977;323:88.)

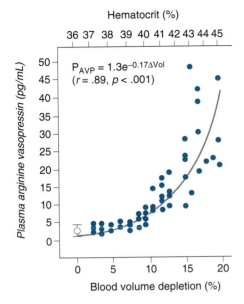

Figure 5–22. Relationship of plasma vasopressin to isosmotic reductions in blood volume in rats. (Reproduced, with permission, from Dunn FL et al: J Clin Invest 1973;52:3212.)

The normal day-to-day regulation of water balance therefore involves interaction between osmotic and volume stimuli. In the case of ADH secretion, the fall in extracellular fluid volume sensitizes the release of ADH to a given osmotic stimulus. Thus, for a given increase in plasma osmolality, the increase in plasma ADH will be greater in hypovolemic than in normovolemic states.

In dehydration, increased plasma osmolality results in withdrawal of fluid from cells. Thus, the reduction in total body water is shared equally between intracellular and extracellular fluid compartments. The increase in plasma osmolality and the reduction of extracellular fluid volume act synergistically to stimulate ADH release. In salt depletion, however, plasma ADH concentrations remain constant or even slightly elevated in spite of a fall in plasma osmolality. Hypovolemia in this situation—as a result of osmotic movements of water from the extracellular into the intracellular fluid space—appears to provide the sensitizing influence.

Thirst mechanisms also involve interactions between extracellular fluid volume and osmolality. During periods of dehydration, increased plasma osmolality provides approximately 70% of the increased thirst drive, and the remaining 30% is due to hypovolemia. In salt depletion, the situation is less clear, but the normal or increased drinking that has been observed in experimental animals has been attributed to the associated hypovolemia.

DIABETES INSIPIDUS

Diabetes insipidus is a disorder resulting from deficient ADH action and is characterized by the passage of copious amounts of very dilute urine. This disorder must be distinguished from other polyuric states such as primary polydipsia (see below) and osmotic diuresis. Central (or neurogenic) diabetes insipidus is due to failure of the posterior pituitary to secrete adequate quantities of ADH; nephrogenic diabetes insipidus results when the kidney fails to respond to circulating ADH. The resulting renal concentrating defect leads to the loss of large volumes of dilute urine, ie, free water. This causes cellular and extracellular dehydration, which stimulate thirst and cause polydipsia.

Classification

A. Central Diabetes Insipidus: The major causes of central diabetes insipidus are shown in Table 5–14.

Many of the disorders discussed above in the section on pituitary and hypothalamic disorders which cause hypopituitarism may also case diabetes insipidus. Primary pituitary adenomas—even those which are large—rarely cause diabetes insipidus, but hypothalamic tumors such as craniopharyngiomas or other primary central nervous system lesions and infiltrative and invasive lesions cause diabetes insipidus more frequently. These lesions cause diabetes insipidus by damage to the pituitary stalk, which interrupts the hypothalamic-neurohypophysial nerve tracts, or by direct damage to the hypothalamic neurons that synthesize ADH. These disorders cause varying degrees of ADH deficiency.

Diabetes insipidus can also be caused by trauma and is common following surgery for hypothalamic or pituitary tumors. Central diabetes insipidus resulting from head trauma frequently follows a triphasic course. The initial phase is followed by a phase of antidiuresis (as ADH is released from damaged axons) and then by persistent diabetes insipidus. How complete the diabetes insipidus is depends upon the extent of the damage. Resection of hypothalamic tu-

Table 5–14. Causes of nephrogenic diabetes insipidus.

Chronic renal disease: Any renal disease that interferes with collecting duct or medullary function, eg, chronic pyelonephritis.
Hypokalemia.
Protein starvation.
Hypercalcemia.
Sickle cell anemia.
Sjögren's syndrome.
Drugs, eg, lithium, fluoride, methoxyflurane anesthesia, demeclocycline, colchicine.
Congenital defect.
Familial.

mors via craniotomy frequently results in permanent diabetes insipidus, which may be complicated by disorders of thirst. Transsphenoidal pituitary microsurgery causes postoperative diabetes insipidus in as many as 20% of patients. This does not appear to be due to destruction of the ADH-secreting neural fibers, since the diabetes insipidus frequently lasts only a few days and rarely longer than 2–3 weeks.

Familial central diabetes insipidus, which is inherited in both recessive or dominant patterns, is rare and has its onset in infancy. The number of ADH-containing fibers in the nuclei, nerve tracts, and posterior pituitary is reduced. Idiopathic diabetes insipidus presents in later childhood or adolescence and in adulthood. It is also associated with a decrease in the number of ADH-containing fibers. As many as 30–40% of these patients have antibodies directed against ADH-secreting hypothalamic neurons. The "posterior pituitary bright spot," which is normally visualized by MRI, is absent in patients with familial or idiopathic diabetes insipidus. An autosomal dominant form of central diabetes insipidus occurs in association with diabetes mellitus, optic atrophy, and deafness (DIDMOAD). Diabetes insipidus with enzymatic destruction of circulating ADH by increased plasma levels of vasopressinase may occur during pregnancy.

B. Nephrogenic Diabetes Insipidus: This group of diseases (Table 5–15) is caused by renal unresponsiveness to the physiologic actions of ADH; thus, ADH levels are normal or elevated. Chronic renal diseases, particularly those affecting the medulla and collecting ducts, can cause nephrogenic diabetes insipidus. Thus, if medullary disease (eg, from pyelonephritis, polycystic disease or medullary cystic disease) prevents formation of a medullary concentration gradient, urine passing through the collecting duct system cannot become concentrated.

The electrolyte disorders hypokalemia and hypercalcemia reduce urinary concentrating capacity. Many drugs have been implicated in the development of nephrogenic diabetes insipidus. For example,

lithium carbonate reduces the sensitivity of the renal tubule to ADH by its inhibitory effect on ADH-sensitive adenylyl cyclase. The ability of demeclocycline to cause nephrogenic diabetes insipidus has been used to advantage in the management of states of ADH excess (see below). Congenital nephrogenic diabetes insipidus is a rare condition caused by a defect in the response of the renal tubule to ADH, with decreased medullary adenylyl cyclase production. It is most common in males with a family history of transmission through apparently healthy females, suggesting X-linked inheritance, though cases have recently been reported in females. Pregnancy may decrease renal responsiveness to ADH.

Primary Polydipsia

Primary polydipsia (psychogenic polydipsia, compulsive water drinking) is a disorder of thirst that is either due to psychogenic causes or to altered osmotic and nonosmotic regulation of thirst, which involves greatly increased drinking, usually in excess of 5 L of water per day, leading to dilution of the extracellular fluid, inhibition of vasopressin secretion, and water diuresis.

Differential Diagnosis

It is important to distinguish both types of diabetes insipidus and primary polydipsia from other common causes of polyuria. In general, other forms of polyuria involve osmotic or solute diuresis. For example, in diabetes mellitus, increased excretion of glucose and other solutes requires excretion of increased volumes of water. In osmotic diuresis, the osmolality of the urine tends toward that of plasma. In sharp contrast, the osmolality of the urine in diabetes insipidus and psychogenic polydipsia is very low when compared with that of plasma. Thus, a urine specific gravity less than 1.005 (osmolality < 200 mosm/kg of water) will generally rule out polyuria due to osmotic diuresis. After a careful history has been taken, focusing on patterns of drinking and urination behavior and the family history, a se-

Table 5–15. Results of diagnostic studies in various types of polyuria.

	Neurogenic Diabetes Insipidus	Nephrogenic Diabetes Insipidus	Psychogenic Polydipsia
Random plasma osmolality	↑	↑	↓
Random urine osmolality	↓	↓	↓
Urine osmolality during mild water deprivation	No change	No change	↑
Urine osmolality during nicotine or hypertonic saline	No change	No change	↑
Urine osmolality following vasopressin intravenously	↑	No change	↑
Plasma vasopressin	Low	Normal or high	Low

ries of investigations should be instituted to distinguish between the two types of diabetes insipidus and primary polydipsia. For unknown reasons patients with idiopathic central diabetes insipidus have a predilection for cold beverages. The physiologic principles are set forth in Table 5–16, and the actual procedures are summarized in Table 5–17.

A. Plasma and Urine Osmolality: The first test is to take plasma and urine samples simultaneously for estimation of osmolality and sodium. Since in both forms of diabetes insipidus the primary problem is inappropriate water diuresis, the urine will be less concentrated than plasma, whereas the plasma osmolality may be higher than normal depending upon the state of hydration. In primary polydipsia, however, dilute plasma is associated with the production of dilute urine. The poor sensitivity of these levels drawn randomly necessitates dynamic testing. Occasionally, even the tests outlined below do not produce a definitive diagnosis, so that a therapeutic trial of desmopressin may be warranted.

B. Water Deprivation: The next step is to examine the effect of water deprivation on urine osmolality under supervision. Supervision is necessary both because the patient with primary polydipsia will go to great lengths to obtain water and because the patient with complete diabetes insipidus may become dangerously dehydrated very rapidly. The patient should be weighed and denied access to water and

Table 5–16. Differential diagnosis of polyuria.

Procedure	Interpretation
Measure plasma and urine osmolality.	A urine osmolality less than that of plasma is consistent with neurogenic or nephrogenic diabetes insipidus; if both urine and plasma are dilute, that is consistent with psychogenic polydipsia.
Dehydration test: If serum osmolality is less than 295 mosm/kg, allow no fluids for 12–18 hours. Measure body weight, urine flow, urine specific gravity, urine and plasma osmolality every 2 hours. Terminate study if body weight falls more than 3%.	A rise in urine osmolality above that of plasma osmolality indicates psychogenic polydipsia. Urine specific gravity less than 1.005 (or 200 mosm/L) indicates either neurogenic or nephrogenic diabetes insipidus.
Measure serum vasopressin at conclusion of dehydration test.	Normal or high vasopressin level usually indicates nephrogenic diabetes insipidus.
Inject 5 units of aqueous vasopressin or 1 μg DDAVP subcutaneously. Measure urine flow and urine and plasma osmolality.	Rise in urine osmolality above that of plasma osmolality indicates neurogenic diabetes insipidus; failure of urine osmolality to rise indicates nephrogenic diabetes insipidus.

Table 5–17. Conditions associated with SIADH.

Malignant lung disease, particularly bronchogenic carcinoma.
Nonmalignant lung disease, eg, tuberculosis.
Tumors at other sites (especially lymphoma, sarcoma), eg, duodenum, pancreas, brain, prostate, thymus.
Central nervous system trauma and infections.
Drugs that stimulate vasopressin release, eg, clofibrate, chlorpropamide, and other drugs such as thiazides, carbamazepine, phenothiazines, vincristine, cyclophosphamide.
Endocrine diseases: adrenal insufficiency, myxedema, anterior pituitary insufficiency.

each voided urine sample measured for specific gravity or osmolality (or both). Whereas the healthy individual will soon reduce urine flow to 0.5 mL/min at a concentration greater than that of plasma, the patient with complete diabetes insipidus will maintain a high urine flow at a specific gravity less than 1.005 (200 mosm/kg of water). The test is continued until urinary osmolality plateaus (an hourly increase of < 30 mosm/kg for 3 successive hours). A period of 18 hours is usually ample to confirm the diagnosis. The test should be terminated if the body weight falls by more than 3%, since serious consequences of dehydration may ensue. Patients with primary polydipsia will always increase urine osmolality to values greater than those of plasma. It may be difficult to distinguish these patients from patients with partial central diabetes insipidus.

C. Vasopressin Test: Once the diagnosis of diabetes insipidus is established, the ADH-insensitive (nephrogenic) disease must be distinguished from the ADH-sensitive (central) form. This is done following water deprivation by injection of aqueous vasopressin or desmopressin acetate. Give 5 units of aqueous vasopressin subcutaneously or 1 μg of desmopressin acetate intravenously, intramuscularly, or subcutaneously, and measure urine osmolality after 1 hour; patients with complete central diabetes insipidus will show an increase of > 50% in urine osmolality, while patients with nephrogenic diabetes insipidus show an increase of < 50%. Patients with partial central diabetes insipidus also show increases of < 50%, and patients with primary polydipsia have responses < 9%. In these cases, measurement of ADH levels is particularly helpful.

D. ADH Radioimmunoassays: Sensitive radioimmunoassays for ADH are available that allow plasma ADH to be measured. Random plasma samples are of little value; levels should be measured as part of dynamic testing, either during water deprivation test or with infusions of hyperosmotic saline. Plasma levels should be interpreted based upon nomograms of their relationship to plasma osmolality. Patients with nephrogenic diabetes insipidus have normal or increased levels of vasopressin following water deprivation, allowing a clear distinction to be made from central forms of diabetes insipidus (Figure 5–23). Patients with partial central diabetes in-

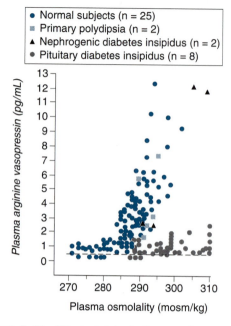

- Normal subjects (n = 25)
- Primary polydipsia (n = 2)
- Nephrogenic diabetes insipidus (n = 2)
- Pituitary diabetes insipidus (n = 8)

Figure 5–23. Effect of dehydration on plasma vasopressin concentration in normal subjects and patients with polyuria. Note that patients with neurogenic (pituitary) diabetes insipidus cannot increase plasma vasopressin concentration with dehydration, in contrast to patients with psychogenic polydipsia and nephrogenic diabetes insipidus. (Reproduced, with permission, from Robertson GL et al: J Clin Invest 1973;52:2346.)

sipidus show a smaller than normal increase in plasma vasopressin concentration following dehydration or infusion of hypertonic saline.

E.   Influence of Endocrine Disease: The diagnosis of central diabetes insipidus is sometimes difficult to make in the presence of anterior pituitary disease. Low or absent levels of glucocorticoids or thyroid hormone reduce the solute load to the kidney and thus reduce urine flow. Patients with normal plasma levels of vasopressin but hyposecretion of adrenal glucocorticoids will retain a water load. Thus, even if diabetes insipidus is present, coincident thyroid or adrenal insufficiency may mask the polyuria.

Treatment

A.   Central Diabetes Insipidus:

1.   Treatment of choice—The drug of choice is desmopressin acetate, a synthetic analog of vasopressin prepared in aqueous solution containing 100 μg/mL. It is administered intranasally as a metered-dose nasal spray that delivers 10 μg (0.1 mL) per spray or via a calibrated plastic catheter in doses of 5–20 μg (0.05–0.2 mL). The frequency of administration varies; patients with mild to moderate diabetes insipidus require one or two doses of 10 μg per 24 hours; Patients with severe diabetes insipidus may

require 10–20 μg two or three times daily. This agent provides excellent control of polyuria and polydipsia in patients with central diabetes insipidus. Serum osmolality and sodium must be monitored at regular intervals (initially every 1–2 weeks, later every 3 months) to be certain that the dose is appropriate. For patients who cannot tolerate intranasal therapy, desmopressin acetate can be given subcutaneously in single doses of 1–2 μg once or twice daily.

2.   Older methods—Lypressin is pure synthetic lysine vasopressin administered by nasal spray. It is effective for only a few hours, so that it must be administered at least every 4–6 hours. Aqueous vasopressin in doses of 5–10 units subcutaneously is also very short-acting (3–6 hours).

B.   Nephrogenic Diabetes Insipidus: The underlying disorder should be treated if possible. It is important to recognize familial disease early, since infants are particularly susceptible to neurologic damage due to dehydration. Diuretics are helpful, along with dietary salt restriction if necessary. Prostaglandin synthesis inhibitors may also be useful. The objective is to maintain the patient in a state of mild sodium depletion and reduce the solute load on the kidney, thus enhancing proximal tubular reabsorption. Reduction in distal tubular flow allows some sodium concentration to take place and minimizes loss of water. Patients with partial sensitivity to vasopressin may be treated with large doses of desmopressin acetate (up to 40 μg/4 h intranasally).

SYNDROME OF INAPPROPRIATE SECRETION OF ANTIDIURETIC HORMONE (SIADH)

A variety of disorders are associated with plasma ADH concentrations that are inappropriately high for the plasma osmolality. Thus, water retention accompanies normal water intake, leading to hyponatremia and hypo-osmolality. The urine is usually more concentrated than plasma but in any case is inappropriately concentrated. Overall sodium balance is essentially normal. It is important to rule out renal and endocrine disorders and drug effects that diminish the kidney's capacity to dilute the urine. The syndrome is termed the syndrome of inappropriate secretion of antidiuretic hormone, or SIADH. The clinical picture can be produced experimentally by giving high doses of vasopressin to a healthy subject receiving normal to high fluid intake. Water restriction in patients suspected of having SIADH will result in plasma osmolality and sodium concentration returning to normal.

The diagnostic criteria for SIADH include (1) hyponatremia with corresponding plasma hypo-osmolality (< 280 mosm/kg); (2) urine less than maximally dilute, ie, inappropriately concentrated (> 100 mosm/kg); (3) euvolemia (including absence of congestive heart failure, cirrhosis, and nephrotic syndrome); and (4) absence of renal, adrenal or thyroid insufficiency. Urinary sodium is usually > 20 mmol/d, probably a consequence of increased atrial natriuretic factor. Dynamic testing and plasma ADH levels are usually unnecessary in diagnosis.

Causes of SIADH

The causes of SIADH are outlined in Table 5–18. A number of malignant neoplasms are associated with ectopic production of vasopressin, leading to high plasma vasopressin levels. Bronchogenic carcinomas are particularly apt to be associated with SIADH. Tumors at other sites such as the pancreas and duodenum have also been shown to produce vasopressin. A number of nonmalignant pulmonary diseases such as tuberculosis and pneumonias are associated with high plasma vasopressin concentrations. Tuberculous lung tissue has been shown to contain assayable levels of vasopressin. However, it is not known whether all types of lung disease causing SIADH do so by producing ectopic vasopressin or by stimulation of pituitary vasopressin.

Many central nervous system disorders are associated with increased vasopressin secretion, leading to the clinical picture of SIADH. Temporary causes of SIADH include surgical trauma, anesthesia, pain, opiates and anxiety. A number of drugs implicated in vasopressin release are listed in Table 5–18. Endocrine disorders such as adrenal insufficiency, myxedema, and anterior pituitary insufficiency may be associated with increased ADH levels and impaired renal excretion of free water. All of these factors—particularly with fluid loading—can lead to hyponatremia and hypo-osmolality. In fact, the majority of hospitalized patients with euvolemic hyponatremia have inappropriately increased ADH levels. The hyponatremia observed in patients with psychosis may reflect a combination of several factors, including inappropriate ADH release and compulsive water drinking.

Types of Osmoregulatory Defects

Serial measurements of serum ADH in patients with SIADH delineate four patterns of osmoregulatory defects in this syndrome. Type A, found in 20% of patients, is characterized by large irregular changes in plasma ADH completely unrelated to serum osmolality. This erratic and irregular secretion

Table 5–18. Conditions associated with SIADH.

Malignant lung disease, particularly bronchogenic carcinoma.
Nonmalignant lung disease, eg, tuberculosis.
Tumors at other sites (especially lymphoma, sarcoma), eg, duodenum, pancreas, brain, prostate, thymus.
Central nervous system trauma and infections.
Drugs that stimulate vasopressin release, eg, clofibrate, chlorpropamide, and other drugs such as thiazides, carbamazepine, phenothiazines, vincristine, cyclophosphamide.
Endocrine diseases: adrenal insufficiency, myxedema, anterior pituitary insufficiency.

of ADH can be associated with both malignant and nonmalignant disease. Type B is found in about 35% of patients and is associated with secretion of ADH that is excessive but proportionate to osmolality. In these patients, the osmotic control of ADH secretion appears to be either set at a low level or abnormally sensitive to changes in serum osmolality. Type C, found in 35% of patients, is characterized by a high basal level of ADH that rises even higher with a rise in serum osmolality. Type D, found in only 10% of patients, represents a different type of problem. ADH is normally suppressed in hypovolemic states and rises normally with increase in osmolality. Thus, SIADH in these patients may be associated with a change in renal sensitivity to serum arginine vasopressin. Thus far, the pattern of arginine vasopressin abnormality cannot be correlated with the pathology of the syndrome.

Treatment

The treatment of SIADH depends upon the underlying cause. A patient with drug-induced SIADH is treated by withholding the drug. The treatment of SIADH in a patient with bronchogenic carcinoma is more complicated, however, and the prognosis is poor. Treatment aims to return plasma osmolality to normal without causing further expansion of the extracellular fluid compartment, as would occur following infusion of hyperosmotic solutions.

A. Fluid Restriction: The simplest form of treatment is fluid restriction, although in the long term the excessive thirst associated with this treatment may be difficult to manage.

B. Diuretics: If plasma osmolality is low and rapid correction is required, diuretics such as furosemide or ethacrynic acid can be employed. These agents prevent the concentration gradient in the medulla from building up and thus decrease the effectiveness of vasopressin. Because diuresis is accompanied by significant urinary losses of potassium, calcium, and magnesium, these electrolytes should be replaced by intravenous infusion.

C. Other Methods: In an emergency situation with severe hyponatremia, hypertonic saline, ie, 3% saline, administered intravenously at a rate of 0.1 mL/kg/min, will increase plasma sodium and osmolarity. However, this must be done with caution, since fluid overload may precipitate heart failure or circulatory collapse, and overly rapid correction may lead to central pontine myelinolysis. Drugs (mentioned earlier in this chapter) that reduce the effect of vasopressin on the kidney may be useful. Demeclocycline, 1–2 g/d orally, causes a reversible form of nephrogenic diabetes insipidus, countering the effect of SIADH. However, it is nephrotoxic, and renal function (blood urea nitrogen and serum creatinine) must be monitored carefully. Lithium carbonate has a similar effect, but therapeutic doses are so close to the toxic dose that this drug is rarely useful.

REFERENCES

General

Frohman LA: Disorders of the anterior pituitary. In: *Endocrinology and Metabolism,* 3rd ed. Felig P, Baxter JD, Frohman LA (editors). McGraw-Hill, 1995.

Hadley ME: *Endocrinology,* 4th ed. Prentice Hall, 1996.

Imura H (editor): *The Pituitary Gland,* 2nd ed. Raven Press, 1995.

Melmed S (editor): *The Pituitary.* Blackwell, 1995.

Molitch ME: Neuroendocrinology. In: *Endocrinology and Metabolism,* 3rd ed. Felig P, Baxter JD, Frohman LA (editors). McGraw-Hill, 1995.

Reeves WB, Andreoli TE: The posterior pituitary and water metabolism. In: *Williams Textbook of Endocrinology,* 8th ed. Wilson JD, Foster DW (editors). Saunders, 1992.

Robertson G: Posterior pituitary. In: *Endocrinology and Metabolism,* 3rd ed. Felig P, Baxter JD, Frohman LA (editors). McGraw-Hill, 1995.

Robertson GL: The endocrine brain and pituitary gland. In: *Principles and Practice of Endocrinology and Metabolism,* Part II. Becker KL (editor). Lippincott, 1994.

Thorner MO et al: The anterior pituitary. In: *Williams Textbook of Endocrinology,* 8th ed. Wilson JD, Foster DW (editors). Saunders, 1992.

Neuroendocrinology

Behan DP et al: Corticotropin-releasing factor-binding protein: A putative peripheral and central modulator of the CRF family of neuropeptides. Ann N Y Acad Sci 1993;697:1.

Chrousos GP: The hypothalamic-pituitary-adrenal axis and immune-mediated inflammation. N Engl J Med 1995;322:1351.

Devesa J, Lima L, Tresguerres JAF: Neuroendocrine control of growth hormone secretion. Trends Endocrinol Metab 1992;3:175.

Dubois PM, El Amraoui A: Embryology of the pituitary gland. Trends Endocrinol Metab 1995;6:1.

Gelato MC: Growth hormone-releasing hormone: Clinical perspectives. The Endocrinologist 1994;4:64.

Haugen BR, Ridgway EC: Transcription factor Pit-1 and its clinical implications: From bench to bedside. The Endocrinologist 1995;5:132.

Hindmarsh PC, Swift PG: An assessment of growth hormone provocation tests. Arch Dis Child 1995;72:362.

Lowry PJ: The corticotropin-releasing factor-binding protein: From artifact to new ligand(s) and axis. J Endocrinol 1995;144:1.

Orth DN: Corticotropin-releasing hormone in humans. Endocr Rev 1992;13:164.

Perez FM, Rose JC, Schwartz J: Anterior pituitary cells: Getting to know their neighbors. Mol Cell Endocrinol 1995;111:C1.

Reichlin S: Neuroendocrine-immune interactions. N Engl J Med 1993;329:1246.

Reyes-Fuentes A, Velduis JD: Neuroendocrine physiology of the normal male gonadal axis. Endocrinol Metab Clin North Am 1993;22:93.

Rosenfeld RG: Circulating growth hormone binding proteins. Horm Res 1994;42:129.

South SA, Yankov VI, Evans WS: Normal reproductive endocrinology in the female. Endocrinol Metab Clin North Am 1993;22:1.

Stevenin B, Lee SL: Hormonal regulation of the thyrotropin releasing hormone (TRH) gene. The Endocrinologist 1995;5:286.

Veldhuis JD: Pulsatile hormone release as a window into the brain's control of the anterior pituitary gland in health and disease: Implications and consequences of pulsatile luteinizing hormone secretion. The Endocrinologist 1994;4:454.

Voss JW, Rosenfeld MG: Anterior pituitary development: Short tales from dwarf mice. Cell 1992;70:527.

Webb SM, Puig-Domingo M: Role of melatonin in health and disease. Clin Endocrinol 1995;42:221.

Pituitary Function Testing and Neuroradiology

Aron DC: Hormone screening in the patients with an incidentally discovered pituitary mass: Current practice and factors in clinical decision making. The Endocrinologist 1995;5:357.

Broide J et al: Low-dose adrenocorticotropin test reveals impaired adrenal function in patients taking inhaled corticosteroids. J Clin Endocrinol Metab 1995;80:1243.

Chong BW et al: Pituitary gland MR: A comparative study of healthy volunteers and patients with microadenomas. Am J Neuroradiol 1994;15:675.

Cianfarani S et al: Is IGF binding protein-3 assessment helpful for the diagnosis of GH deficiency? Clin Endocrinol 1995;43:43.

Elster AD: Modern imaging of the pituitary. Radiology 1993;187:1.

Hall WA et al: Pituitary magnetic resonance imaging in normal human volunteers: Occult adenomas in the general population. Ann Intern Med 1994;120:817.

Johnson MR et al: The evaluation of patients with a suspected pituitary microadenoma: Computer tomography compared to magnetic resonance imaging. Clin Endocrinol 1992;36:335.

Maroldo TV, Dillon WP, Wilson CB: Advances in diagnostic techniques of pituitary tumors and prolactinomas. Curr Opin Oncol 1992;4:105.

Mosely I: Computed tomography and magnetic resonance imaging of pituitary microadenomas. Clin Endocrinol 1992;36:333.

Tordjman K et al: The role of the low dose (1 µg) adrenocorticotropin test in the evaluation of patients with pituitary disease. J Clin Endocrinol Metab 1995;80:1301.

Webb SM et al: Computerized tomography versus magnetic resonance imaging: A comparative study in hypothalamic-pituitary and parasellar pathology. Clin Endocrinol 1992;36:459.

Pituitary Adenomas: General

Aron DC, Tyrrell JB, Wilson CB: Current concepts in diagnosis and management of pituitary tumors. West J Med 1995;162:340.

Aron DC, Ross NS: Pituitary "incidentaloma." Ann Intern Med 1990;113:558.

Donovan LE, Corenblum B: The natural history of the

pituitary incidentaloma. Arch Intern Med 1995; 155:181.

Fagin JA (editor): Pituitary tumors. Baillieres Clin Endocrinol Metab 1995;9:203.

Harris PE et al: Glycoprotein hormone alpha-subunit production in somatotroph adenomas with and without Gs alpha mutations. J Clin Endocrinol Metab 1992;75:918.

Kane LA et al: Pituitary adenomas in childhood and adolescence. J Clin Endocrinol Metab 1994;79:1135.

Karga HJ et al: Ras mutations in human pituitary tumors. J Clin Endocrinol Metab 1992;74:914.

Klibanski A, Zervas NT: Diagnosis and management of hormone-secreting pituitary adenomas. N Engl J Med 1991;324:822.

Mindermann T, Wilson CB: Pediatric pituitary adenomas. Neurosurgery 1995;36:259.

Mindermann T, Wilson CB: Age-related and gender-related occurrence of pituitary adenomas. Clin Endocrinol 1994;41:359.

Molitch ME: Evaluation and treatment of the patient with a pituitary incidentaloma. J Clin Endocrinol Metab 1995;80:3.

Reincke M et al: The "incidentaloma" of the pituitary gland: Is neurosurgery referred? JAMA 1990;263: 2772.

Russell EJ, Molitch ME: The pituitary "incidentaloma." Ann Intern Med 1990;112:925.

ACTH: Cushing's Disease

Aron DC, Tyrrell JB (editors): Cushing's syndrome. Endocrinol Metab Clin North Am 1994;23:451, 925.

Bochicchio D et al: Factors influencing the immediate and late outcome of Cushing's disease treated by transsphenoidal surgery: A retrospective study by the European Cushing's Disease Survey Study Group. J Clin Endocrinol Metab 1995;80:3114.

Helseth A et al: Transgenic mice that develop pituitary tumors: A model for Cushing's disease. Am J Pathol 1992;140:1071.

Lamberts SWJ, van der Lely AJ, de Herder WW: Transsphenoidal selective adenomectomy is the treatment of choice in patients with Cushing's disease: Considerations concerning preoperative medical treatment and the long-term follow-up. J Clin Endocrinol Metab 1995;80:3111.

Magiakow MA et al: Cushing's syndrome in children and adolescents. N Engl J Med 1994;331:752.

McCane DR el al: Assessment of endocrine function after transsphenoidal surgery for Cushing's disease. Clin Endocrinol 1993;38:79.

Stenzel-Poore MP et al: Development of Cushing's syndrome in corticotropin-releasing factor transgenic mice. Endocrinology 1992;130:3378.

Tsigos C, Chrousos GP: Clinical presentation, diagnosis, and treatment of Cushing's syndrome. Curr Opin Endocrinol Diabetes 1995;2:203.

Growth Hormone: Acromegaly

Barzilay J, Heatley GJ, Cushing GW: Benign and malignant tumors in patients with acromegaly. Arch Intern Med 1991;151:1629.

Corpas E, Harman SM, Blackman MR: Human growth hormone and human aging. Endocr Rev 1993;14:20.

de Boer H, Blok G-J, Van der veen EA: Clinical aspects of growth hormone deficiency in adults. Endocr Rev 1995;16:63.

Ezzat S et al: Octreotide treatment of acromegaly: A randomized, multicenter study. Ann Intern Med 1992;117:711.

Fradkin JE: Creutzfeldt-Jakob disease in pituitary growth hormone recipients. The Endocrinologist 1993;3:108.

Ho KY et al: Therapeutic efficacy of the somatostatin analog SMS201-995 (octreotide) in acromegaly: Effects of dose and frequency and long-term safety. Ann Intern Med 1990;112:173.

Melmed S (editor): Acromegaly. Endocrinol Metab Clin North Am 1992;21:483.

Sacca L, Cittadini A, Fazio S: Growth hormone and the heart. Endocr Rev 1994;15:555.

Terzolo M et al: High prevalence of colonic polyps in patients with acromegaly: influence of sex and age. Arch Intern Med 1994;154:1272.

Theill LE, Karin M: Transcriptional control of growth hormone expression and anterior pituitary development. Endocrine Reviews 1993;14:670.

Vance ML, Harris AG: Long-term treatment of 189 acromegalic patients with the somatostatin analog octreotide: Results of the international multicenter acromegaly study group. Arch Intern Med 1991; 151:1573.

PRL: Prolactinoma

Bevan JS et al: Dopamine agonists and pituitary tumor shrinkage. Endocr Rev 1992;13:220.

Biller BMK et al: Progressive trabecular osteopenia in women with hyperprolactinemic amenorrhea. J Clin Endocrinol Metab 1992;75:692.

Cunnah D, Besser M: Management of prolactinomas. Clin Endocrinol 1991;34:231.

Davis JRE, Shepard MC, Heath DA: Giant invasive prolactinoma: A case report and review of nine further cases. Q J Med 1990;74:227.

Lamberts SWJ, Quik RFP: A comparison of the efficacy and safety of pergolide and bromocriptine in the treatment of hyperprolactinemia. J Clin Endocrinol Metab 1991;72:635.

Leite V et al: Characterization of big, big prolactin in patients with hyperprolactinemia. Clin Endocrinol 1992;37:365.

Markoff E, Lee DW: On the nature of serum prolactin in two patients with macroprolactinemia. Fertil Steril 1992;58:78.

Molitch ME: Pathologic hyperprolactinemia. Endocrinol Metab Clin North Am 1992;21:877.

Schlechte J, Walkner L, Kathol M: A longitudinal analysis of premenopausal bone loss in healthy women and women with hyperprolactinemia. J Clin Endocrinol Metab 1992;75:698.

Vance ML et al: Treatment of prolactin-secreting pituitary macroadenomas with the long-acting non-ergot dopamine agonist CV 205-502. Ann Intern Med 1990;112:668.

Webster J et al: Low recurrence rate after partial hypophysectomy for prolactinoma: The predictive value of dynamic prolactin function tests. Clin Endocrinol 1992;33:35.

Gonadotropins (LH/FSH): Gonadotropin-Secreting Pituitary Tumors

Daneshdoost L et al: Identification of gonadotroph adenomas in men with clinically nonfunctioning adenomas by the luteinizing hormone subunit response to thyrotropin-releasing hormone. J Clin Endocrinol Metab 1993;77:1352.

Daneshdoost L et al: Recognition of gonadotroph adenomas in women. N Engl J Med 1991;324:589.

Katznelson L, Alexander JM, Klibanski A: Clinically nonfunctioning pituitary adenomas. J Clin Endocrinol Metab 1993;76:1089.

Molitch ME: Gonadotroph cell pituitary adenomas. N Engl J Med 1991;324:626.

Nobels FRE et al: A comparison between the diagnostic value of gonadotropins, alpha-subunit, and chromogranin-A and their response to thyrotropin-releasing hormone in clinically nonfunctioning, alpha-subunit-secreting, and gonadotroph pituitary adenomas. J Clin Endocrinol Metab 1993;77:784.

Oppenheim DS et al: Prevalence of α-subunit hypersecretion in patients with pituitary tumors: Clinically non-functioning and somatrotroph adenomas. J Clin Endocrinol Metab 1990;70:859.

Petit C: Molecular basis of the X-chromosome-linked Kallmann's syndrome. Trends Endocrinol Metab 1993;4:8.

Wilson CB: Endocrine-inactive pituitary adenomas. Clin Neurosurg 1992;38:10.

TSH: TSH-Secreting Pituitary Tumors

Beckers A et al: Thyrotropin-secreting pituitary adenomas: Report of seven cases. J Clin Endocrinol Metab 1991;72:477.

McCutcheon IE, Weintraub BD, Oldfield EH: Surgical treatment of thyrotropin-secreting pituitary tumors. J Neurosurg 1990;73:674.

Mindermann T, Wilson CB: Thyrotropin-producing pituitary adenomas. J Neurosurg 1993;79:521.

Hypopituitarism and Other Hypothalamic-Pituitary Disorders

Cacciari E et al: Empty sella in children and adolescents with possible hypothalamic-pituitary disorders. J Clin Endocrinol Metab 1994;78:767.

Constine LS, et al: Hypothalamic-pituitary dysfunction after radiation for brain tumors. N Engl J Med 1993;328:87.

Crowley WF Jr, Jameson JL: Gonadotropin-releasing hormone deficiency: Perspectives from clinical investigation. (Clinical Counterpoint.) Endocr Rev 1992;13;13:635.

Freda PU et al: Hypothalamic-pituitary sarcoidosis. Trends Endocrinol Metab 1992;3:321.

Gallardo E et al: The empty sella: Results of treatment in 76 successive cases and high frequency of endocrine and neurological disturbances. Clin Endocrinol 1992;37:529.

Maccagnan P et al: Conservative management of pituitary apoplexy: A prospective study. J Clin Endocrinol Metab 1995;80:2190.

Powrie JK et al: Lymphocytic adenohypophysitis: Magnetic resonance imaging features of two new cases and a review of the literature. Clin Endocrinol 1995;42:315.

Rolih CA, Ober KP: Pituitary apoplexy. Endocrinol Metab Clin North Am 1993;22:291.

Thodou E et al: Lymphocytic hypophysitis: Clinicopathological findings. J Clin Endocrinol Metab 1995;80:2302.

Vance ML: Hypopituitarism. N Engl J Med 1994;330:1651.

Posterior Pituitary

Buonocore CM, Robinson AG: The diagnosis and management of diabetes insipidus during medical emergencies. Endocrinol Metab Clin North Am 1993;22:411.

Maghnie M et al: Correlation between magnetic resonance imaging of posterior pituitary and neurohypophyseal function in children with diabetes insipidus. J Clin Endocrinol Metab 1992;74:795.

Robertson GL: Diabetes insipidus. Endocrinol Metab Clin North Am 1995;24:549.

Thompson CJ, Edwards CR, Baylis PH: Osmotic and non-osmotic regulation of thirst and vasopressin secretion in patients with compulsive water drinking. Clin Endocrinol 1991;35:221.

Verbalis JG: Hyponatremia: Epidemiology, pathophysiology, and therapy. Curr Opinion Nephrol Hypertens 1993;2:636.

Growth

6

Dennis Styne, MD

Assessment of growth in stature is an essential part of the pediatric examination. Growth is an important index of physical and mental health and of the quality of the child's psychosocial environment; chronic problems in any of these areas may be reflected in a decreased growth rate. We will consider influences on normal growth, the normal growth pattern, the measurement of growth, and conditions that lead to disorders of growth.

NORMAL GROWTH

INTRAUTERINE GROWTH

The great changes that take place in the human fetus during intrauterine growth have been summarized by Pierson and Deschamps: From conception to delivery, fetal mass increases 44×10^7 times, compared with a 20-fold increase from birth to adulthood; length increases 3850 times to term, compared with a three- to fourfold increase from birth to adulthood. The determinants of normal prenatal growth are poorly understood, though many factors that lead to abnormal prenatal growth have been identified.

Endocrine Factors

A. Growth Hormone: Although fetal plasma values of growth hormone (GH) are higher than levels reported in most adult acromegalic patients, GH appears to have little influence on length at birth; infants with GH deficiency have normal birth lengths, and even those with anencephaly (who therefore lack hypothalamic releasing factors) have normal body lengths. Remarkably, although GH concentrations are high at birth, IGF-1 concentrations are exceedingly low in normal neonates. Human chorionic somatomammotropin (hCS), a placental hormone similar in structure to GH and prolactin, may not be essential to fetal growth, since mothers lacking the *hCS* gene have given birth to children with normal birth lengths.

<table>
<tr><td colspan="2" align="center">ACRONYMS USED IN THIS CHAPTER</td></tr>
<tr><td>ACTH</td><td>Adrenocorticotropic hormone</td></tr>
<tr><td>cAMP</td><td>Cyclic adenosine monophosphate</td></tr>
<tr><td>DNA</td><td>Deoxyribonucleic acid</td></tr>
<tr><td>GH</td><td>Growth hormone</td></tr>
<tr><td>GHBP</td><td>Growth hormone-binding protein</td></tr>
<tr><td>GnRH</td><td>Gonadotropin-releasing hormone</td></tr>
<tr><td>GRH</td><td>Growth hormone-releasing hormone</td></tr>
<tr><td>hCG</td><td>Human chorionic gonadotropin</td></tr>
<tr><td>hCS</td><td>Human chorionic somatomammotropin</td></tr>
<tr><td>hGH</td><td>Human growth hormone</td></tr>
<tr><td>IGF</td><td>Human insulin-like growth factor (somatomedin)</td></tr>
<tr><td>IGF-1</td><td>Human insulin-like growth factor 1</td></tr>
<tr><td>IGF-2</td><td>Human insulin-like growth factor 2</td></tr>
<tr><td>IGFBP</td><td>Insulin-like growth factor binding protein</td></tr>
<tr><td>IUGR</td><td>Intrauterine growth retardation</td></tr>
<tr><td>LH</td><td>Luteinizing hormone</td></tr>
<tr><td>LS</td><td>Lower segment</td></tr>
<tr><td>NCHS</td><td>National Center for Health Statistics</td></tr>
<tr><td>PTH</td><td>Parathyroid hormone</td></tr>
<tr><td>RTA</td><td>Renal tubular acidosis</td></tr>
<tr><td>RWT</td><td>Roche, Wainer, and Thissen method of height prediction</td></tr>
<tr><td>SS</td><td>Somatostatin</td></tr>
<tr><td>TBG</td><td>Thyroid hormone-binding globulin</td></tr>
<tr><td>TRH</td><td>Thyrotropin-releasing hormone</td></tr>
<tr><td>TSH</td><td>Thyroid-stimulating hormone (thyrotropin)</td></tr>
<tr><td>US</td><td>Upper segment</td></tr>
</table>

B. Thyroid Hormone: The absence of thyroid hormone may have devastating effects on the mental development of a neonate, but hypothyroid newborns have normal length. In fact, perhaps because of the longer duration of pregnancy in hypothyroid fetuses, the hypothyroid newborn may be longer than average.

C. Insulin: Excessive serum insulin concentrations may be associated with increased length in infants of diabetic mothers and in the Beckwith-Wiedemann syndrome, characterized by neonatal hypoglycemia, neonatal gigantism, omphalocele, macroglossia, and hepatomegaly. Inadequate insulin production, found in transient neonatal diabetes mellitus, or insulin resistance, found in the leprechaun syndrome (Donahue syndrome) of inadequate or absent insulin receptor activity, is associated with short newborn length. Genetic defects in the insulin receptor are now described in the leprechaun syndrome.

D. Insulin-Like Growth Factors: (IGF-1, formerly somatomedin C [SMC]; and IGF-2, formerly known as multiplication stimulating activity [MSA] or somatomedin A [SMA].) In rodents, IGF-2 appears to be of significance in producing normal fetal growth, but its role in human fetuses is not clear. IGF-1 is expressed in various tissues of the fetus and is capable of stimulating differentiation. The precise function in fetal growth of IGF-1 is not yet established. Serum IGF-1 values do correlate with newborn weight in normal infants. Laron's dwarfism, characterized by an inability to generate IGF-1 (due to a lack of GH receptors), is associated with short birth length in some case reports.

Genetic, Maternal & Uterine Factors

Maternal factors, often expressed through the uterine environment, exert more influence on birth size than paternal factors. The height of the mother correlates better with fetal size than the height of the father. However there is a genetic component to length at birth that is not sex specific. First-born infants are on the average 100 g heavier than subsequent infants, maternal age over 38 years leads to decreased birth weight, and male infants are heavier than female infants by an average of 150–200 g. Poor maternal nutrition is the most important condition leading to low birth weight and length on a worldwide basis; it also predisposes the infant to other serious health hazards after birth. Chronic maternal disease and eclampsia can also lead to poor fetal growth. Maternal alcohol ingestion has been shown to have severe adverse effects on fetal length and mental development and to predispose to other physical abnormalities such as microcephaly, mental retardation, midfacial hypoplasia, short palpebral fissures, wide-bridged nose, long philtrum, and narrow vermilion border of the lip; affected infants never recover from this loss of length but attain normal growth rate in the postnatal period. Abuse of other substances and chronic use of some medications (eg, phenytoin) can cause intrauterine growth retardation. Cigarette smoking causes not only retarded intrauterine growth but also decreased postnatal growth for as long as 5 years after parturition. Maternal infection—most commonly rubella, toxoplasmosis, and cytomegalovirus infection—leads to many developmental abnormalities as well as short birth length. Congenital HIV infection causes intrauterine growth retardation. In multiple births, the weight of each fetus is usually less than that of the average singleton. Uterine tumors or malformations may decrease fetal growth.

Intrauterine growth retardation (IUGR) is usually defined as a birth weight less than the tenth percentile for gestational age, though it should be clear that 10% of births are not truly abnormal. It is suggested that the third percentile may be more appropriate as a guide to IUGR, while the tenth percentile may characterize the infant small for gestational age (SGA). For term births, 2500 g is the tenth percentile, and this is the lower limit of "normal" or appropriate for gestational age weight. Proportionate IUGR indicates a small head circumference along with a small body; infants with genetic defects, infections, or toxic exposures fall in this classification and usually do not grow well after birth and reach a shorter ultimate stature in adulthood. This is in contrast to premature infants with normal weight for gestational age, who recover to the range of normal height and weight for age by age 2 years. To do this, they must have growth rates that are higher than the average for a period of months. Disproportionate IUGR is heralded by relative sparing of the head circumference, which remains in the range of normal percentiles—in contrast to the small body, which is well below average. This condition most often results from fetal malnutrition, and affected infants may experience catch-up growth after birth. Thus, a key point in assessing the patient with short stature is determining gestational age and relating it to birth weight, length, and head circumference.

Chromosomal Abnormalities & Malformation Syndromes

Many chromosomal abnormalities that lead to malformation syndromes also cause poor fetal growth. Other malformation syndromes associated with a normal karyotype are characterized by intrauterine growth retardation. In most cases, endocrine abnormalities have not been noted. For further discussion of this extensive subject, the reader is referred to other sources listed in the references at the end of this chapter.

POSTNATAL GROWTH

Postnatal growth in stature and weight follows a definite pattern in normal children (Figures 6–1 and 6–2). The highest overall growth rate occurs in the

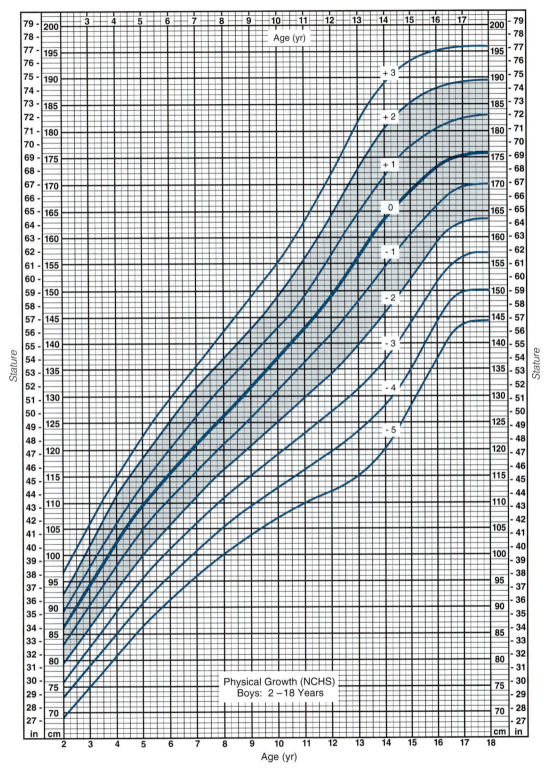

Figure 6–1. Growth chart for boys in the USA. (Redrawn and reprinted with permission of Genentech, Inc. Sources of data: 1976 study of the National Center for Health Statistics [NCHS; Hyattsville, MD]; Hamill PVV et al: Physical growth: National Center for Health Statistics percentiles. Am J Clin Nutr 1979;32:607.)

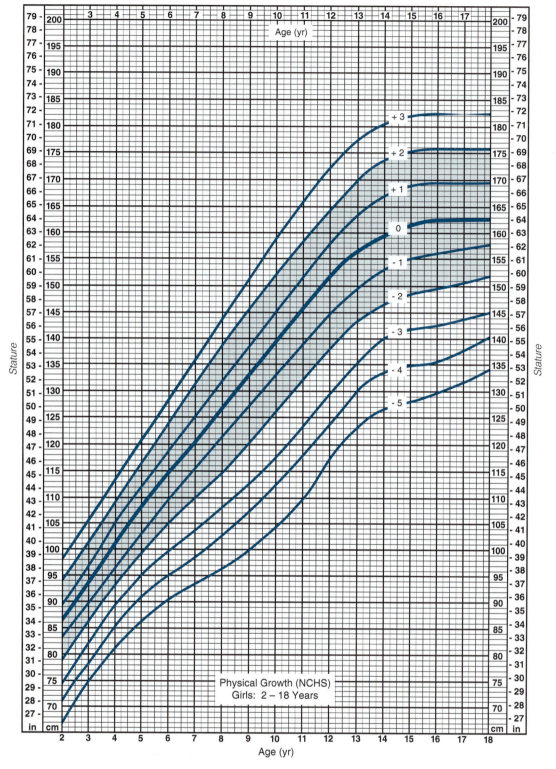

Figure 6–2. Growth chart for girls in the USA. (Redrawn and reprinted with permission of Genentech, Inc. Sources of data: 1976 study of the National Center for Health Statistics [NCHS; Hyattsville, MD]; Hamill PVV et al: Physical growth: National Center for Health Statistics percentiles. Am J Clin Nutr 1979;32:607.)

fetus, the highest postnatal growth rate just after birth, and a slower growth rate follows in mid childhood (Figures 6–3 and 6–4). Several investigators report a growth spurt between 6½ and 7 years in both boys and girls. After another plateau, the striking increase in stature known as the pubertal growth spurt follows, causing a second peak of growth velocity. The final decrease in growth rate then ensues, until the epiphyses of the long bones fuse and growth ceases.

Endocrine Factors

A. Growth Hormone and Insulin-Like Growth Factors:
As discussed in Chapter 5, somatotropin, or growth hormone (GH), is suppressed by hypothalamic growth hormone release-inhibiting factor, somatostatin (SS) and stimulated by growth hormone-releasing hormone (GRH). The gene for GH is located on the long arm of chromosome 17 in a cluster of five genes: *GH-N* codes for human GH, *GH2* codes for a variant GH produced in the placenta, *CSH1* and *CSH2* code for prolactin, and *CSH P1* codes for a variant prolactin molecule. Several families are known with deletions of the *GH-N* gene and profound GH deficiency.

Growth hormone's effects are mainly mediated by the insulin-like growth factors, but GH also has some direct effects. Growth hormone produces insulin resistance and is a diabetogenic substance, increasing blood sugar. Furthermore, growth hormone is lipolytic.

Growth hormone circulates in plasma bound to a protein with a sequence equivalent to that of the extra membrane domain of the growth hormone receptor, the growth hormone-binding protein (GHBP). The physiology of GH-binding protein appears to be of great importance in growth. For example, obese patients have lower plasma GH concentrations but higher GHBP, while starvation raises GH concentrations and lowers GHBP. GHBP may have other physiologic roles in addition to simply reflecting receptor status.

Because of the difficulty in determining true physiologic GH status (as described below), it appeared that measurement of IGFs would improve diagnostic capabilities in growth failure. However, the control of IGF production and secretion is so complex that this promise has not been fully realized. Thus, measurements of serum IGF concentrations assist in the diagnosis of GH deficiency but are not diagnostic.

IGF-1 and IGF-2 have structures similar to the proinsulin molecule but differ from insulin in regulation, receptors, and biologic effects. These factors were first recognized when Salmon and Daughaday demonstrated that GH itself could not cause cartilage growth in vitro but that GH administered in vivo to hypopituitary rodents caused the production of polypeptide factors which themselves stimulated cartilage growth. In the ensuing 35 years, the structure of the factors (originally called sulfation factor and then somatomedin), the genes responsible for their production, and information about their physiology were elucidated.

The single copy gene for prepro-IGF-1 is located on the long arm of chromosome 12. Posttranslational processing produces the 70-amino-acid mature form, and alternative splicing mechanisms produce variants of the molecule in different tissues and developmental stages. The IGF-1 cell membrane receptor (the type I receptor) resembles the insulin receptor in its structure of two α and two β chains. Binding of IGF-1 to type I receptors stimulates tyrosine kinase activity and autophosphorylation of tyrosine molecules, which produce cell differentiation or division (or both). IGF-1 receptors are down-regulated by increased IGF-1 concentrations, while decreased IGF-1 concentrations increase IGF-1 receptors.

IGF molecules bind to a variety of IGF-binding (IGFBP) proteins; at present, information is available about the molecular weights and other properties of six IGFBPs. The IGFBPs were originally thought to inhibit IGF action, but there is increasing evidence that in certain conditions IGFBPs may enhance IGF action. IGFBP-1 is a 25-kDa protein: The serum levels of IGFBP-1 are inversely proportionate to insulin levels, but this protein does not appear to be regulated by GH. IGFBP-2 is a 33-kDa protein, and serum concentrations are inversely proportionate to both GH and insulin concentrations. Most IGF-1 circulates bound to IGFBP-3 in a 150-kDa complex. Serum IGFBP-3 concentrations are directly proportionate to GH concentrations as well as to nutritional status—thus, in malnutrition, IGFBP-3 and IGF-1 fall while GH rises. IGF-1 directly regulates IGFBP-3 as well. IGFBP-3 rises with advancing age in childhood with highest values achieved during puberty, though the pattern of change of IGF-1 at puberty is different from that of IGFBP-3. The molar ratio of IGF-1 to IGFBP-3 also rises at puberty, suggesting that more IGF-1 is free to influence growth during this period.

IGF-1 is produced in most tissues and appears to be exported to neighboring cells to act upon them in a paracrine manner. Thus, serum IGF-1 concentrations may not reflect the most significant actions of this growth factor. The liver is a major site of IGF-1 synthesis, and much of the circulating IGF-1 probably originates in the liver; serum IGF-1 concentrations vary in liver disease with the extent of liver destruction. IGF-1 is a progression factor, so that a cell which has been exposed to a competence factor in stage G_0 of the cell cycle and has transited to G_1 can, with IGF-1 exposure in G_1, undergo division in the S phase of the cell cycle. Besides the stimulatory effects of IGF-1 on cartilage growth, IGF-1 has stimulatory effects upon hematopoiesis, ovarian steroidogenesis, myoblast proliferation and differentiation, and differentiation of the lens.

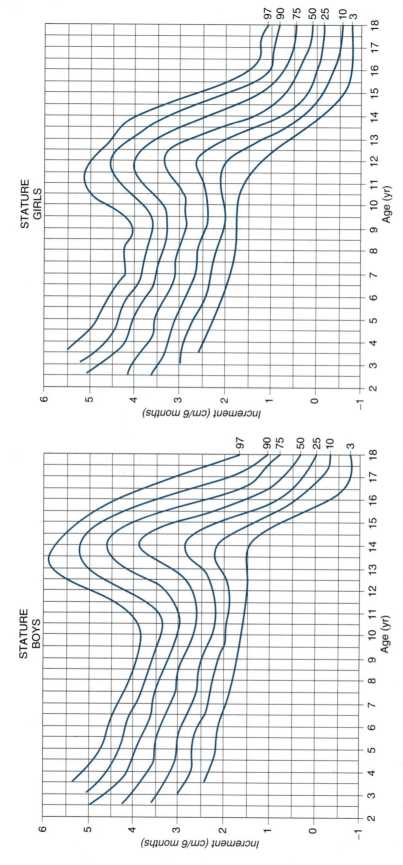

Figures 6–3 and 6–4. Incremental growth charts for boys (Figure 6–3) and girls (Figure 6–4). Height velocity measured over a period of at least 6 months can be compared with the percentiles on the right axis of the charts. (Redrawn and reprinted with permission of Ross Laboratories, Columbus, OH 43216. © 1981 Ross Laboratories. Sources of data: Longitudinal studies of the Fels Research Laboratories [Yellow Springs, OH]; Roche AF, Himes JH: Incremental growth charts. Am J Clin Nutr 1980;33:2041.)

IGF-1 was in short supply until production by recombinant DNA technology became possible. The first clinical studies of IGF-1 administration in human subjects have occurred. IGF-1 administration increases nitrogen retention and decreases BUN—and, in GH-resistant patients (Laron dwarfs), IGF-1 stimulates growth without the presence of GH. Thus, IGF-1 may prove useful in treatment of various clinical conditions from pathologic short stature to catabolic states, including the postoperative period.

IGF-2 is a 67-amino-acid peptide. The gene for prepro-IGF-2 is located on the short arm of chromosome 11, close to the gene for prepro insulin. The type II IGF receptor preferentially binds IGF-2 and is identical to the mannose 6-phosphate receptor, a single-chain transmembrane protein. While most of the effects of IGF-2 appear mediated by its interaction with the type I receptor, independent actions of IGF-2 via the type II receptor are described.

Plasma concentrations of the IGFs vary with age and physiologic condition. IGF-1 concentrations are low at term in neonates and remain low until a peak is reached during puberty, with values rising higher than at any other time in life. IGF-1 then decreases to adult levels, values higher than in childhood but lower than in puberty. With advancing age, serum GH and IGF-1 decrease. IGF-1 concentrations are more highly correlated in monozygotic twins than in same-sex dizygotic twins, indicating a genetic effect upon IGF-1 regulation. In addition, IGF-1 concentrations reflect growth rate better in monozygotic twins than dizygotic twins of unrelated children, further strengthening the relationship between IGF-1 and growth.

GH deficiency leads to lower serum IGF-1 and IGF-2 concentrations, while GH excess leads to elevated IGF-1 but no rise in IGF-2 above normal. Because serum IGF-1 is lower during states of nutritional deficiency, IGF-1 is less useful in the differential diagnosis of conditions of poor growth, which often include impaired nutritional state. IGF-1 suppresses GH secretion, so that patients who lack GH receptors (Laron dwarfs) and are unable to produce IGF-1 have elevated GH concentrations and negligible IGF-1 concentrations.

B. Thyroid Hormone: As noted above, congenital hypothyroid newborns are of normal length, but if untreated they manifest exceedingly poor growth soon after birth. Infants with untreated congenital hypothyroidism will suffer permanent mental retardation. Acquired hypothyroidism leads to a markedly decreased growth rate but no permanent intellectual defects. Bone age advancement is severely delayed in hypothyroidism, usually more so than in GH deficiency. The upper to lower segment ratio (Figure 6–5) is delayed and therefore elevated, owing to poor limb growth.

C. Sex Steroids: Gonadal steroids exert an important influence on the pubertal growth spurt, while

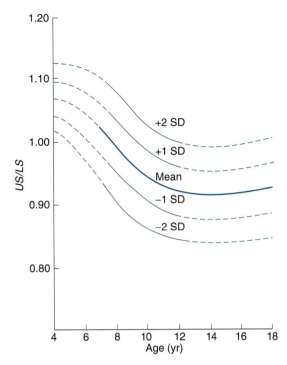

Figure 6–5. Normal upper to lower segment (US:LS) ratios, based on findings in 1015 white children. Values are slightly lower for black children. (Reproduced, with permission, from McKusick V: *Hereditable Disorders of Connective Tissue,* 4th ed. Mosby, 1972.)

absence of these factors is not important in prepubertal growth. Gonadal and adrenal sex steroids in excess can cause a sharp increase in growth rate as well as the premature appearance and progression of secondary sexual features. If unabated, increased sex steroids will cause advancement of skeletal age, premature epiphysial fusion, and short adult stature.

The pubertal rise in gonadal steroids exerts direct and indirect effects upon IGF-1 production. Sex steroids directly stimulate the production of IGF-1 from cartilage as well as increase GH secretion, which stimulates IGF-1 production indirectly. Both actions appear important in the pubertal growth spurt (see Chapter 15).

D. Glucocorticoids: Endogenous or exogenous glucocorticoids in excess will quickly stop growth. The absence of glucocorticoids has little effect on growth if the individual is clinically well in other respects (ie, if hypotension and hypoglycemia are absent).

Other Factors

A. Genetic Factors: Genetic factors influence final height. Good correlation is found between midparental height and the child's height; appropriate charts and tables have been developed to display this phenomenon (Figures 6–6 and 6–7; Tables 6–1 and 6–2). There is a heritable pattern to birth length, postnatal growth in length, and the intrinsic rate of change in growth. These effects are sex-specific. A gene located on the long arm of the Y chromosome is reported to have an influence on postnatal growth.

B. Socioeconomic Factors: Worldwide, the most common cause of short stature is poverty and its effects. Thus, poor nutrition, poor hygiene, and poor health influence growth both before and after birth. In people of the same ethnic group and in the same geographic location, variations in stature are often attributable to these factors. For example, studies have shown that Japanese individuals born and

reared in North America were taller than Japanese-born immigrants to North America. Conversely, when socioeconomic factors are equal, the differences in average height between various ethnic groups are mainly genetic.

C. Nutritional Factors: The influence of malnutrition accounts for much of the socioeconomic discrepancy in height noted above, but malnutrition may occur in the midst of plenty and must always be suspected in disorders of growth. Other factors may be blamed for poor growth when nutritional deficiencies are actually responsible. For example, Sherpas were thought to have short stature because of genetic factors or the effects of altitude on the slopes of

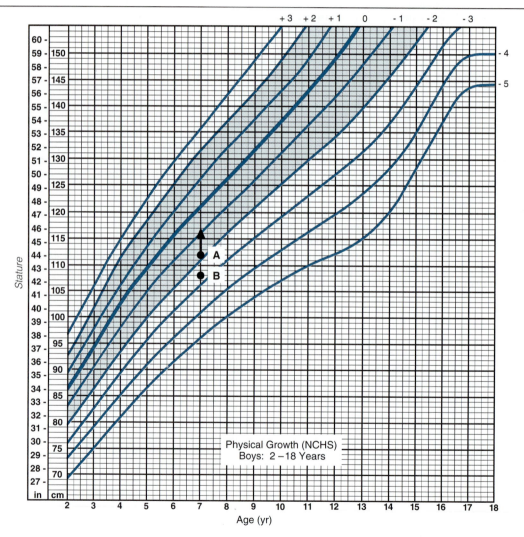

Figure 6–6. Adjustment of height based on midparental stature (Table 6–1). Charts of two boys, each 7 years of age. **A** is 2 SD below the mean, with a height of 112 cm; taking his midparental stature of 158 cm into consideration, his adjusted height of 118 cm **(arrow)** is only 1 SD below the mean, suggesting that he is short because of familial tendency rather than pathology. **B** is almost 3 SD below the mean, with a height of 108 cm; his midparental height of 166 cm causes his adjusted height to rise only 1 cm, suggesting that familial factors may not be the cause of his short stature and he may have a pathologic diagnosis.

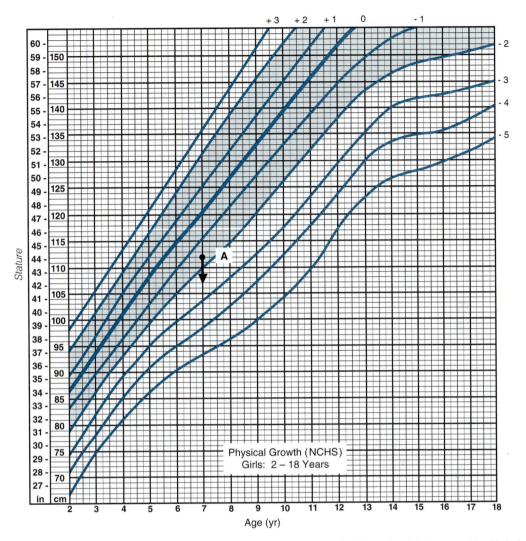

Figure 6–7. Adjustment of height based on midparental stature (Table 6–2). Chart of a girl, 7 years old, with height of 112 cm. She has a midparental stature of 178 cm, causing her adjusted height *(arrow)* to fall 5 cm, suggesting that her short stature is more severe than suspected from the original growth chart and that genetic influences are probably not the cause.

Mount Everest; nutritional supplementation increased stature in this group. The developed world places a premium on appearance, so significant numbers of children, chiefly teenagers, voluntarily decrease their caloric intake even if they are not obese; this factor may account for cases of poor growth. Chronic disease, which hampers adequate nutrition, often leads to short stature. For example, bronchopulmonary dysplasia decreases growth to some degree because it increases metabolic demands, shifting nutrient usage from growth; improved nutrition will increase growth in these patients. Feeding problems in infants, resulting from inexperience of parents or poor child-parent interactions (maternal deprivation), may account for poor growth. Fad diets such as vegan diets that put children at risk of vitamin B_{12} or

iron deficiency as well as dietary manipulation for expected benefit, such a low-fat diet, may place children at risk for deficiency of fat-soluble vitamins; with moderation, such diets may be modified to good effect in childhood. Deliberate starvation of children by caregivers is an extreme form of child abuse that may be first discovered because of poor growth.

There are signifigant endocrine changes associated with malnutrition. Decreased GH receptors or postreceptor defects in GH action, leading to decreased production of IGF-1 and decreased concentration of serum IGF-1 and a decrease in the action of IGF-1, all are notable. The characteristic result in malnutrition is elevation of serum GH and decrease in IGF-1 while obesity is associated with decreased GH with normal IGF-1.

Table 6–1. Parent-specific adjustments (cm) for stature of boys from 3 to 18 years of age.[1]

Age (yr)	Stature (cm)	Mid Parental Stature (cm)																	
		150	152	154	156	158	160	162	164	166	168	170	172	174	176	178	180	182	184
3	86.0– 87.9	7	6	5	5	4	3	2	1	1	0	−1	−2	−3	−3	−4	−5	−6	−7
	88.0– 97.9	8	7	6	5	4	4	3	2	1	0	−1	−1	−2	−3	−4	−5	−5	−6
	98.0–106.9	8	8	7	6	5	4	4	3	2	1	0	0	−1	−2	−3	−4	−4	−5
4	90.0– 93.9	7	6	5	4	4	3	2	1	0	−1	−1	−2	−3	−4	−5	−5	−6	−7
	94.0–103.9	8	7	6	5	4	3	3	2	1	0	−1	−1	−2	−3	−4	−5	−6	−6
	104.0–112.9	8	8	7	6	5	4	3	3	2	1	0	−1	−1	−2	−3	−4	−5	−6
5	96.0–103.9	8	7	6	5	4	3	2	1	0	0	−1	−2	−3	−4	−5	−6	−7	−8
	104.0–113.9	9	8	7	6	5	4	3	2	1	0	0	−1	−2	−3	−4	−5	−6	−7
	114.0–122.9	9	9	8	7	6	5	4	3	2	1	0	0	−1	−2	−3	−4	−5	−6
6	102.0–111.9	8	7	7	6	5	4	3	2	1	0	−1	−2	−3	−4	−5	−6	−7	−8
	112.0–121.9	9	8	7	7	6	5	4	3	2	1	0	−1	−2	−3	−4	−5	−6	−7
	122.0–130.9	10	9	8	7	6	6	5	4	3	2	1	0	−1	−2	−3	−4	−5	−6
7	108.0–117.9	9	8	7	6	5	4	3	2	1	0	−1	−2	−4	−5	−6	−7	−8	−9
	118.0–127.9	10	9	8	7	6	5	4	3	2	1	0	−1	−2	−4	−5	−6	−7	−8
	128.0–136.9	12	10	9	8	7	6	5	4	3	2	1	0	−1	−2	−4	−5	−6	−7
8	114.0–115.9	10	9	8	6	5	4	3	2	1	−1	−2	−3	−4	−5	−6	−8	−9	−10
	116.0–125.9	11	9	8	7	6	5	4	2	1	0	−1	−2	−3	−5	−6	−7	−8	−9
	126.0–135.9	12	10	9	8	7	6	5	3	2	1	0	−1	−2	−4	−5	−6	−7	−8
	136.0–144.9	13	12	10	9	8	7	6	5	3	2	1	0	−1	−2	−4	−5	−6	−7
9	120.0–121.9	11	9	8	7	6	4	3	2	1	0	−2	−3	−4	−5	−7	−8	−9	−10
	122.0–131.9	11	10	9	8	6	5	4	3	1	0	−1	−2	−3	−5	−6	−7	−8	−10
	132.0–141.9	12	11	10	9	7	6	5	4	2	1	0	−1	−2	−4	−5	−6	−7	−9
	142.0–150.9	13	12	11	10	8	7	6	5	4	2	1	0	−1	−3	−4	−5	−6	−7
10	124.0–127.9	11	10	9	7	6	5	3	2	1	−1	−2	−3	−5	−6	−7	−9	−10	−11
	128.0–137.9	12	11	10	8	7	6	4	3	2	0	−1	−2	−4	−5	−6	−8	−9	−10
	138.0–147.9	13	12	11	9	8	7	5	4	3	1	0	−1	−3	−4	−5	−7	−8	−9
	148.0–158.9	14	13	12	11	9	8	7	5	4	3	1	0	−1	−3	−4	−5	−7	−8
11	128.0–133.9	12	10	9	8	6	5	4	2	1	0	−2	−3	−5	−6	−7	−9	−10	−11
	134.0–143.9	12	11	10	8	7	6	4	3	2	0	−1	−2	−4	−5	−6	−8	−9	−10
	144.0–153.9	14	12	11	10	8	7	5	4	3	1	0	−1	−3	−4	−5	−7	−8	−9
	154.0–162.9	15	13	12	11	9	8	7	5	4	3	1	0	−2	−3	−4	−6	−7	−8
12	132.0–141.9	12	10	9	8	6	5	4	2	1	0	−2	−3	−4	−6	−7	−8	−10	−11
	142.0–151.9	13	11	10	9	7	6	5	3	2	1	−1	−2	−3	−5	−6	−7	−9	−10
	152.0–161.9	13	12	11	9	8	7	5	4	3	1	0	−1	−2	−4	−5	−6	−8	−9
	162.0–170.9	14	13	12	10	9	8	6	5	4	2	1	0	−2	−3	−4	−6	−7	−8
13	136.0–139.9	12	10	9	8	6	5	4	2	1	−1	−2	−3	−5	−6	−7	−9	−10	−12
	140.0–149.9	12	11	10	8	7	6	4	3	1	0	−1	−3	−4	−6	−7	−8	−10	−11
	150.0–159.9	13	12	10	9	8	6	5	4	2	1	−1	−2	−3	−5	−6	−7	−9	−10
	160.0–169.9	14	13	11	10	8	7	6	4	3	2	0	−1	−3	−4	−5	−7	−8	−9
	170.0–178.9	15	13	12	11	9	8	6	5	4	2	1	0	−2	−3	−5	−6	−7	−9
14	142.0–145.9	13	11	10	8	7	5	4	2	1	−1	−2	−4	−5	−7	−8	−10	−11	−13
	146.0–155.9	14	12	11	9	8	6	5	3	1	0	−2	−3	−5	−6	−8	−9	−11	−12
	156.0–165.9	15	13	11	10	8	7	5	4	2	1	−1	−2	−4	−5	−7	−8	−10	−11
	166.0–175.9	15	14	12	11	9	8	6	5	3	2	0	−1	−3	−4	−6	−7	−9	−11
	176.0–184.9	16	15	13	12	10	9	7	6	4	3	1	−1	−2	−4	−5	−7	−8	−10
15	148.0–151.9	14	13	11	9	7	6	4	2	0	−1	−3	−5	−7	−8	−10	−12	−14	−15
	152.0–161.9	15	14	12	10	8	7	5	3	1	0	−2	−4	−6	−7	−9	−11	−13	−14
	162.0–171.9	17	15	13	11	10	8	6	4	3	1	−1	−3	−4	−6	−8	−10	−11	−13
	172.0–181.9	18	16	14	13	11	9	7	6	4	2	0	−1	−3	−5	−7	−8	−10	−12
	182.0–190.9	19	17	16	14	12	10	9	7	5	3	2	0	−2	−4	−5	−7	−9	−11
16	156.0–163.9	17	15	13	11	9	7	5	3	1	−1	−3	−5	−7	−9	−11	−13	−16	−18
	164.0–173.9	19	17	15	13	10	8	6	4	2	0	−2	−4	−6	−8	−10	−12	−14	−16
	174.0–183.9	21	19	17	15	12	10	8	6	4	2	0	−2	−4	−6	−8	−10	−12	−14
	184.0–192.9	23	21	19	17	14	12	10	8	6	4	2	0	−2	−4	−6	−8	−10	−12
17	162.0–165.9	17	15	13	11	9	7	4	2	0	−2	−4	−7	−9	−11	−13	−15	−17	−20
	166.0–175.9	20	17	15	13	11	9	6	4	2	0	−2	−4	−7	−9	−11	−13	−15	−18
	176.0–185.9	22	20	18	16	13	11	9	7	5	3	0	−2	−4	−6	−8	−11	−13	−15
	186.0–194.9	25	23	20	18	16	14	12	9	7	5	3	1	−1	−4	−6	−8	−10	−12
18	160.0–165.9	18	16	13	11	9	6	4	2	0	−3	−5	−7	−10	−12	−14	−17	−19	−21
	166.0–175.9	20	18	16	13	11	9	7	4	2	0	−3	−5	−7	−10	−12	−14	−17	−19
	176.0–185.9	23	21	19	16	14	12	9	7	5	3	0	−2	−4	−7	−9	−11	−14	−16
	186.0–194.9	26	24	22	19	17	15	12	10	8	6	3	1	−1	−4	−6	−8	−11	−13

[1]See footnote for Table 6–2.

Table 6–2. Parent-specific adjustments (cm) for stature of girls from 3 to 18 years of age.[1]

Age (yr)	Stature (cm)	Mid Parental Stature (cm)																	
		150	152	154	156	158	160	162	164	166	168	170	172	174	176	178	180	182	184
3	82.0– 83.9	6	5	4	4	3	2	1	1	0	−1	−1	−2	−3	−3	−4	−5	−6	−6
	84.0– 93.9	6	6	5	4	3	3	2	1	1	0	−1	−1	−2	−3	−4	−4	−5	−6
	94.0–102.9	7	7	6	5	4	4	3	2	2	1	0	−1	−1	−2	−3	−3	−4	−5
4	92.0– 93.9	6	6	5	4	3	3	2	1	0	0	−1	−2	−3	−3	−4	−5	−6	−7
	94.0–103.9	7	6	6	5	4	3	2	2	1	0	−1	−1	−2	−3	−4	−4	−5	−6
	104.0–112.9	8	7	7	6	5	4	3	3	2	1	0	0	−1	−2	−3	−3	−4	−5
5	100.0–101.9	8	7	6	5	4	3	2	1	1	0	−1	−2	−3	−4	−5	−5	−6	−7
	102.0–111.9	8	7	6	6	5	4	3	2	1	0	−1	−1	−2	−3	−4	−5	−6	−7
	112.0–120.9	9	8	7	7	6	5	4	3	2	1	1	0	−1	−2	−3	−4	−5	−6
6	106.0–109.9	9	8	7	6	5	4	3	2	1	0	−1	−2	−3	−4	−5	−6	−7	−8
	110.0–119.9	9	9	8	7	6	5	4	3	2	1	0	−1	−2	−3	−4	−5	−6	−7
	120.0–128.9	11	10	9	8	7	6	5	4	3	2	1	0	−1	−2	−3	−4	−5	−6
7	112.0–117.9	9	8	7	6	5	4	3	2	1	0	−1	−2	−3	−4	−5	−6	−7	−8
	118.0–127.9	10	9	8	7	6	5	4	3	2	1	0	−1	−2	−3	−4	−5	−6	−7
	128.0–136.9	11	10	9	8	7	6	5	4	3	2	1	0	−1	−2	−3	−4	−5	−6
8	116.0–123.9	9	8	7	6	5	4	3	2	1	0	−1	−2	−3	−4	−5	−6	−8	−9
	124.0–133.9	10	9	8	7	6	5	4	3	2	1	0	−1	−2	−3	−4	−5	−7	−8
	134.0–142.9	11	10	9	8	7	6	5	4	3	2	1	0	−1	−2	−3	−4	−6	−7
9	122.0–131.9	10	9	8	7	6	5	3	2	1	0	−1	−2	−3	−4	−5	−6	−7	−9
	132.0–141.9	11	10	9	8	7	6	4	3	2	1	0	−1	−2	−3	−4	−5	−7	−8
	142.0–150.9	12	11	10	9	8	6	5	4	3	2	1	0	−1	−2	−3	−5	−6	−7
10	126.0–127.9	10	9	7	6	5	4	3	2	1	0	−1	−2	−3	−5	−6	−7	−8	−9
	128.0–137.9	10	9	8	7	6	5	4	2	1	0	−1	−2	−3	−4	−5	−6	−7	−8
	138.0–147.9	11	10	9	8	6	5	4	3	2	1	0	−1	−2	−3	−4	−5	−7	−8
	148.0–158.9	12	10	9	8	7	6	5	4	3	2	1	0	−1	−3	−4	−5	−6	−7
11	130.0–133.9	10	9	8	6	5	4	3	2	1	0	−1	−2	−3	−4	−6	−7	−8	−9
	134.0–143.9	10	9	8	7	6	5	4	3	1	0	−1	−2	−3	−4	−5	−6	−7	−8
	144.0–153.9	11	10	9	7	6	6	4	3	2	1	0	−1	−2	−3	−5	−6	−7	−8
	154.0–162.9	11	10	9	8	7	6	5	4	3	1	0	−1	−2	−3	−4	−5	−6	−7
12	134.0–139.9	10	9	8	7	6	5	3	2	1	0	−1	−3	−4	−5	−6	−7	−8	−10
	140.0–149.9	11	10	9	7	6	5	4	3	2	0	−1	−2	−3	−4	−6	−7	−8	−9
	150.0–159.9	12	10	9	8	7	6	5	3	2	1	0	−1	−3	−4	−5	−6	−7	−8
	160.0–168.9	12	11	10	9	8	6	5	4	3	2	0	−1	−2	−3	−4	−5	−7	−8
13	140.0–145.9	10	9	8	7	6	4	3	2	1	0	−1	−3	−4	−5	−6	−7	−8	−10
	146.0–155.9	11	10	9	7	6	5	4	3	2	1	0	−1	−2	−3	−4	−6	−7	−9
	156.0–165.9	12	10	9	8	7	6	5	3	2	1	0	−1	−3	−4	−5	−6	−7	−8
	166.0–174.9	12	11	10	9	8	6	5	4	3	2	1	−1	−2	−3	−4	−5	−7	−8
14	146.0–149.9	10	9	8	6	5	4	3	2	1	0	−1	−3	−4	−5	−6	−7	−8	−9
	150.0–159.9	11	9	8	7	6	5	4	3	1	0	−1	−2	−3	−4	−5	−7	−8	−9
	160.0–169.9	11	10	9	8	7	6	5	3	2	1	0	−1	−2	−3	−5	−6	−7	−8
	170.0–178.9	12	11	10	9	8	6	5	4	3	2	1	0	−2	−3	−4	−5	−6	−7
15	146.0–151.9	10	9	8	7	5	4	3	2	1	−1	−2	−3	−4	−5	−6	−8	−9	−10
	152.0–161.9	11	10	9	7	6	5	4	3	1	0	−1	−2	−3	−4	−6	−7	−8	−9
	162.0–171.9	12	11	10	8	7	6	5	4	2	1	0	−1	−2	−4	−5	−6	−7	−8
	172.0–180.9	13	12	11	9	8	7	6	5	3	2	1	0	−1	−3	−4	−5	−6	−7
16	146.0–151.9	11	10	8	7	6	5	3	2	1	−1	−2	−3	−4	−6	−7	−8	−10	−11
	152.0–161.9	12	10	9	8	7	5	4	3	2	0	−1	−2	−4	−5	−6	−7	−9	−10
	162.0–171.9	13	12	10	9	8	6	5	4	3	1	0	−1	−3	−4	−5	−6	−8	−9
	172.0–180.9	14	13	11	10	9	7	6	5	4	2	1	0	−2	−3	−4	−5	−7	−8
17	148.0–153.9	11	10	9	7	6	5	3	2	1	0	−2	−3	−4	−6	−7	−8	−10	−11
	154.0–163.9	12	11	10	8	7	6	4	3	2	0	−1	−2	−4	−5	−6	−8	−9	−10
	164.0–173.9	13	12	11	9	8	7	5	4	3	1	0	−1	−3	−4	−5	−6	−8	−9
	174.0–182.9	14	13	12	10	9	8	6	5	4	2	1	0	−1	−3	−4	−5	−7	−8
18	148.0–149.9	10	9	8	7	5	4	3	2	1	−1	−2	−3	−4	−6	−7	−8	−9	−10
	150.0–159.9	11	10	8	7	6	5	4	2	1	0	−1	−3	−4	−5	−6	−7	−9	−10
	160.0–169.9	12	11	9	8	7	6	4	3	2	1	0	−2	−3	−4	−5	−6	−8	−9
	170.0–178.9	13	11	10	9	8	7	5	4	3	2	1	−1	−2	−3	−4	−5	−7	−8

[1]These figures can be used to adjust measured stature to account for parental heights. The average of the mother's and father's heights (mid parental stature) is calculated, and the column closest to the figure is selected. The intersection of a row containing the child's age and height range with the column showing the mid parental height is noted, and the adjustment figure is read from the chart. If the figure has no sign, it is added to the child's height (cm). If there is a negative sign, the number is subtracted from the measured height (cm). The adjusted height is read from the chart in Figure 6–1 (boys) or Figure 6–2 (girls) to determine in what percentile the adjusted height falls. If the child is short but the height percentile adjusted for mid parental height is closer to the 50th percentile, the child probably has inherited a familial tendency toward short stature. If the adjusted height percentile remains low, the child's height is probably inappropriate for the genetic potential of the family, and diagnostic studies may be indicated for an organic cause of short stature. (Reprinted with permission of Ross Laboratories, Columbus, OH 43216 © 1983 Ross Laboratories. Source of data: Himes JH, Roche AF, Thissen D: *Parent-Specific Adjustments for Assessment of Recumbent Length and Stature.* Vol 13 of: *Monographs in Paediatrics.* Karger, 1981.)

D. Psychologic Factors: Aberrant intrafamilial dynamics, psychologic stress, or psychiatric disease can inhibit growth either by altering endocrine function or by secondary effects on nutrition (psychosocial dwarfism or maternal deprivation). It is essential to differentiate these situations from *bona fide* physiologic disease.

E. Chronic Disease: Even aside from the effects of poor nutrition, many chronic systemic diseases interfere with growth. For example, congestive heart failure and asthma, if uncontrolled, are associated with decreased stature; in some cases, final height is in the normal range because growth continues over a longer period of time. Children of mothers affected with HIV infection are often small at birth and have an increased incidence of poor growth, delayed bone age development, and reduced IGF-1 concentrations; in addition, thyroid dysfunction may develop. Patients born of HIV-infected mothers but without infection themselves exhibit catch-up growth.

Catch-Up Growth

Correction of growth-retarding disorders may be temporarily followed by an abnormally high growth rate as the child approaches normal height for age. This catch-up growth will occur after initiation of therapy for hypothyroidism and GH deficiency, after correction of glucocorticoid excess, and after appropriate treatment of many chronic diseases such as celiac disease. Catch-up growth is usually short-lived and is followed by a more average growth rate.

MEASUREMENT OF GROWTH

Accurate measurement of height is an extremely important aspect of the physical examination of children and adolescents. The onset of a chronic disease may often be determined by an inflection point in the growth chart. In other cases, a detailed growth chart will indicate a normal constant growth rate in a child observed to be short for age. If careful growth records are kept, a diagnosis of constitutional delay in growth and adolescence may be made in such a patient; without previous measurements, the child might be subjected to unnecessary diagnostic testing or months of delay may occur as the child's growth is finally carefully monitored.

Height

The growth charts in most common use in the USA indicate the fifth and 95th percentiles as the outer limits of normal (this equals 2.5 SD above or below the mean). This still leaves 10 out of 100 healthy children outside of these boundaries with 5 out of 100 below the more worrisome "lower limits of normal," and it is both unnecessary and impractical to evaluate 5% of the population. Instead, the examining physician should accurately determine which short children warrant further evaluation and which ones (and their parents) require only reassurance that the child is healthy. When parents see that their child is below the fifth percentile and in a section of the chart colored differently from the "normal area," they assume that there is a serious problem when they may feel less concern if the chart had changed color at, for example, the third percentile or lower. Thus, the format of the chart can dictate parental reaction to height, since all parents want their children to be in the "normal range." Figures 6–1 and 6–2 furnish data necessary to evaluate the height of children at various ages using the standard deviation method (SD) used by the WHO. Standard deviation determination is more useful in extremely short children below the second or first percentile. It has been suggested that a unified chart indicating the four-tenths percentile, which is at 2.67 SD below the mean, would solve the lack of correspondence between charts that impedes communication between countries and colleagues.

Pathologic short stature is usually more than 3.5 SD below the mean, but a diagnosis of pathologic short stature should not usually be based on a single measurement. Serial measurements are required, because they allow determination of growth velocity, which is a more sensitive index of the growth process than a single determination. A very tall child who develops a postnatal growth problem will not fall 2.5 SD below the mean in height for some time but will fall below the mean in growth velocity soon after the onset of the disorder. As Figures 6–3 and 6–4 demonstrate, growth velocity varies at different ages, but as a rough guide, a growth rate of less than 4.5 cm per year between age 4 years and the onset of puberty is abnormal. In children under 4 years of age, normal growth velocity changes more strikingly with age. Healthy term newborns tend to be clustered in length measurements around 21 inches (mostly owing to difficulties in obtaining accurate measurements). In the ensuing 24 months or so, the healthy child's height will enter the channel on the growth chart in which it will continue throughout childhood. Thus, a child with constitutional delay in growth or genetic short stature whose height is at the mean at birth and falls to the tenth percentile at 1 year of age and to the fifth percentile by 2 years of age may in fact be healthy in spite of crossing standard deviation lines in the journey to a growth channel at the fifth percentile. Although the growth rate may decrease during these years, it should not be less than the third percentile for age. A steeper decrease in growth rate is likely be a sign of disease. When a question of abnormal growth arises, previous measurements are always helpful; every physician treating children should record supine length (under 2 years of age) or standing height (after 2 years of age) as well as weight at every office visit. Height and growth velocity should be determined in relation to the standards for the child's age on a graph chart with clear indication of the child's position at measurement (supine or standing).

Patients who cannot be measured in the standing position (eg, because of cerebral palsy) require other approaches: The use of arm span is a possible surrogate for the measurement of height, and there are formulas available for the calculation of height based upon the measurement of upper arm length, tibial length, and knee length (see below).

This discussion presupposes accuracy of measurements, which should be available for children followed by a single physician or group. However, it is reported that screening examinations in the real world fall short of that ideal. Forty-one percent of a presumably normal population screened at a school in England met the criteria for evaluation of abnormal growth (approximately two-thirds grew faster than the normal growth category and one-third were in the slower than normal category), leading to an unreasonable size of a referral population, all due to simple measuring error.

Relation to Midparental Height

There is a positive correlation between midparental height (the average of the heights of both parents) and the stature of a child. This may be taken into account with charts (Tables 6–1 and 6–2), which indicate the number of centimeters to add or subtract from a child's height to adjust for familial tendencies when interpreting the child's height for age on a standard growth chart such as Figures 6–1 and 6–2. An abnormal height may be defined as more than 2 SD below the mean for chronologic age when corrected for midparental height by this chart. Figures 6–6 and 6–7 demonstrate adjustment for midparental height.

Technique of Measurement

Length and height must be measured accurately. Hasty measurements derived from marks made at an infant's foot and head while the infant is squirming on the paper on the examining table are useless. Infants must be measured on a firm horizontal surface with a permanently attached rule, a stationary plate perpendicular to the rule for the head, and a movable perpendicular plate for the feet. One person should hold the head stable while another makes sure the knees are straight and the feet are firm against the movable plate. Children over age 2 are measured standing up but cannot be accurately measured on the measuring rod that projects above the common weight scale; the rod is too flexible, and the scale footplate will in fact drop lower when the patient stands on it. Instead, height should be measured with the child standing back to the wall with heels at the wall, ankles together, and knees and spine straight against a vertical metal rule permanently attached to the wall or an upright board. Height is measured at the top of the head by a sliding perpendicular plate (or square wooden block). A Harpenden stadiometer is a mechanical measuring device capable of such accurate measurement. Standing height is on the average 1.25 cm less than supine length, and it is essential to record the position of measurement each time; shifting from supine height at 2 years to standing height at 2½ years can falsely suggest an inadequate growth rate over that 6-month period. It is preferable to measure in the metric system, since the smaller gradations make measurements more accurate by eliminating the tendency to round off numbers. It is evident that the longer the time between measurements, the more accurate the annualized growth rate will be; the shortest period between measurements in the determination of growth rate should not be less than 3 months, with 1 year obviously giving the most acurate representation. Specialized laser calibrated devices are use to measure tibial length ("kneeometry") which is reported to be accurate for assesment of short-term growth down to weekly intervals; these devices are not generally available outside of research laboratories. The problem of measuring the growth rate of children with orthopedic deformities or contractures is significant, as these patients may have nutritional or endocrine disorders. The measurement of knee height, tibial length, or upper arm length is shown to correlate well with standing height ($r = 0.97$); thus, these measurements may be translated, using linear regression equations provided by the investigators, into total height which is then plotted on standard growth charts.

In addition to height or length, other significant measurements include (1) the frontal occipital head circumference; (2) horizontal arm span (between the outspread middle fingertips with the patient standing against a flat backboard); and (3) the upper segment (US) to lower segment (LS) ratio. For the latter, the LS is measured from the top of the symphysis pubis vertically to the floor with the patient standing straight, and the US is determined by subtracting the LS from the height measurement using the standing height measurement techniques noted above. (Normal standard US:LS ratios are shown in Figure 6–5.) Sitting height is used in some clinical studies of growth.

Height & Growth Rate Summary

In summary, we may consider three criteria for pathologically short stature: (1) height more than 2.5 SD below the mean for chronologic age and preferably below 3.5 SD; (2) growth rate below the third percentile for chronologic age; and (3) height more than 2 SD below the mean for chronologic age when corrected for midparental height.

Weight

The measured weight should be plotted for age on standard graphs developed by the National Center for Health Statistics (NCHS), which are available from various companies producing baby food or growth hormone. Variation in the weights of children in the USA due to differing diets or activity regimens makes it difficult to exactly compare percentiles of height with percentiles of weight. Weight-for-height charts from the NCHS (often included on the charts that show height and weight) provide a better way to determine whether the patient's weight is appropriate. Body mass index (BMI) charts are now available for children and present an excellent way to indicate nutritional status.

SKELETAL (BONE) AGE

Skeletal development is a reflection of physiologic maturation. For example, menarche is better correlated with a skeletal age of 13 years than with a given chronologic age. The prime role of estrogen in advancing skeletal maturation has been emphasized in studies of patients with aromatase deficiency, who cannot make estrogen from testosterone, and in patients with estrogen receptor defects, who cannot respond to estrogen. Skeletal age also affords an indication of remaining growth available to a child and can be used to predict adult height. However, skeletal age is not a definitive diagnostic test of any disease; it can assist in diagnosis only when considered along with other factors.

Bone age is determined by comparing the appearance and stage of fusion of epiphyses or shapes of bones on the patient's radiograph with an atlas demonstrating normal skeletal maturation for various ages. The Greulich and Pyle atlas of radiographs of the left hand and wrist is most commonly used in the USA, but other methods of skeletal age determination such as Tanner and Whitehouse maturity scoring are also used. Any skeletal age more than 2 SD above or below the mean for chronologic age is out of the normal range. For newborn infants, knee and foot radiographs are compared with an appropriate skeletal age atlas; for late pubertal children, just before epiphysial fusion, the knee atlas will reveal whether any further growth can be expected or whether the epiphyses are fused.

Height may be predicted by determining skeletal age and height at the time the radiograph was taken and consulting the Bayley-Pinneau tables in the Greulich and Pyle skeletal atlas of the hand. The Roche, Wainer, and Thissen (RWT) method of height prediction uses patient weight and midparental height—in addition to the variables noted above—to calculate predicted height (Table 6–3). Recently, the method was simplified by eliminating the necessity for a skeletal age assessment in the Khamis-Roche method; results are almost as accurate as the RWT method in white American children. Height prediction by any method becomes more accurate as the child approaches the time of epiphysial fusion.

An easier but less precise method of predicting the expected heights of children within a given family is the calculation of target adult height range using parents' heights and correcting for the sex of the child. For boys, add 5 inches to the mother's height, add the result to the father's height, and divide by 2: this is the target height, and it is expected that sons of these parents will reach a height within 2 SD of this target—or, for simplicity, within 4 inches above and 4 inches below the target height. For girls, subtract 5 inches from the father's height and add the result to the mother's height and divide by 2, leading to the target height. The range for girls will also be within 4 inches above and below this target. This method is only useful in the absence of disease affecting growth.

DISORDERS OF GROWTH

SHORT STATURE DUE TO NONENDOCRINE CAUSES

There are many causes of poor childhood growth and short adult height (Table 6–4). The following discussion covers only the more common conditions, emphasizing those that might be included in an endocrinologic differential diagnosis. Shorter than average stature need not be considered a disease, since variation in stature is a normal feature of the human condition, and a normal child should not be burdened with a misdiagnosis. While the classifications described below may apply to most patients, some will still be resistant to definitive diagnosis.

1. CONSTITUTIONAL SHORT STATURE (or Constitutional Delay in Growth & Adolescence)

Constitutional short stature is not a disease but rather a variation from normal for the population and is considered a disorder of the pace of development. There is usually a delay in pubertal development as well as growth (see Constitutional Delay in Adolescence). It is characterized by moderate short stature (usually not far below the fifth percentile), thin habitus, and retardation of skeletal age. The family history often includes similarly affected members (eg, mother with delayed menarche or father who

Table 6–3. The RWT method for predicting adult stature.[1]

Tables of Multipliers for Boys

Age Yrs	Mos	Recumbent length	Weight	Midparental stature	Skeletal age	Adjustment factor
1	0	0.966	0.199	0.606	-0.673	1.632
1	3	1.032	0.086	0.580	-0.417	-1.841
1	6	1.086	-0.016	0.559	-0.205	-4.892
1	9	1.130	-0.106	0.540	-0.033	-7.528
2	0	1.163	-0.186	0.523	0.104	-9.764
2	3	1.189	-0.256	0.509	0.211	-11.618
2	6	1.207	-0.316	0.496	0.291	-13.114
2	9	1.219	-0.369	0.485	0.349	-14.278
3	0	1.227	-0.413	0.475	0.388	-15.139
3	3	1.230	-0.450	0.466	0.410	-15.729
3	6	1.229	-0.481	0.458	0.419	-16.081
3	9	1.226	-0.505	0.451	0.417	-16.228
4	0	1.221	-0.523	0.444	0.405	-16.201
4	3	1.214	-0.537	0.437	0.387	-16.034
4	6	1.206	-0.546	0.431	0.363	-15.758
4	9	1.197	-0.550	0.424	0.335	-15.400
5	0	1.188	-0.551	0.418	0.303	-14.990
5	3	1.179	-0.548	0.412	0.269	-14.551
5	6	1.169	-0.543	0.406	0.234	-14.106
5	9	1.160	-0.535	0.400	0.198	-13.672
6	0	1.152	-0.524	0.394	0.161	-13.267
6	3	1.143	-0.512	0.389	0.123	-12.901
6	6	1.135	-0.499	0.383	0.085	-12.583
6	9	1.127	-0.484	0.378	0.046	-12.318
7	0	1.120	-0.468	0.373	0.006	-12.107
7	3	1.113	-0.451	0.369	-0.034	-11.948
7	6	1.106	-0.434	0.365	-0.077	-11.834
7	9	1.100	-0.417	0.361	-0.121	-11.756
8	0	1.093	-0.400	0.358	-0.167	-11.701
8	3	1.086	-0.382	0.356	-0.217	-11.652
8	6	1.079	-0.365	0.354	-0.270	-11.592
8	9	1.071	-0.349	0.353	-0.327	-11.498
9	0	1.063	-0.333	0.353	-0.389	-11.349
9	3	1.054	-0.317	0.353	-0.455	-11.118
9	6	1.044	-0.303	0.355	-0.527	-10.779
9	9	1.033	-0.289	0.357	-0.605	-10.306

Tables of Multipliers for Girls

Age Yrs	Mos	Recumbent length	Weight	Midparental stature	Skeletal age	Adjustment factor
1	0	1.087	-0.271	0.386	0.434	21.729
1	3	1.112	-0.369	0.367	0.094	20.684
1	6	1.134	-0.455	0.349	-0.172	19.957
1	9	1.153	-0.530	0.332	-0.374	19.463
2	0	1.170	-0.594	0.316	-0.523	19.131
2	3	1.183	-0.648	0.301	-0.625	18.905
2	6	1.195	-0.693	0.287	-0.690	18.740
2	9	1.204	-0.729	0.274	-0.725	18.604
3	0	1.210	-0.757	0.262	-0.736	18.474
3	3	1.215	-0.777	0.251	-0.729	18.337
3	6	1.217	-0.791	0.241	-0.711	18.187
3	9	1.217	-0.798	0.232	-0.684	18.024
4	0	1.215	-0.800	0.224	-0.655	17.855
4	3	1.212	-0.797	0.217	-0.626	17.691
4	6	1.206	-0.789	0.210	-0.600	17.548
4	9	1.199	-0.777	0.205	-0.582	17.444
5	0	1.190	-0.761	0.200	-0.571	17.398
5	3	1.180	-0.742	0.197	-0.572	17.431
5	6	1.168	-0.721	0.193	-0.584	17.567
5	9	1.155	-0.697	0.191	-0.609	17.826
6	0	1.140	-0.671	0.190	-0.647	18.229
6	3	1.124	-0.644	0.189	-0.700	18.796
6	6	1.107	-0.616	0.188	-0.766	19.544
6	9	1.089	-0.587	0.189	-0.845	20.489
7	0	1.069	-0.557	0.189	-0.938	21.642
7	3	1.049	-0.527	0.191	-1.043	23.011
7	6	1.028	-0.498	0.192	-1.158	24.602
7	9	1.006	-0.468	0.194	-1.284	26.416
8	0	0.938	-0.439	0.196	-1.418	28.448
8	3	0.960	-0.411	0.199	-1.558	30.690
8	6	0.937	-0.384	0.202	-1.704	33.129
8	9	0.914	-0.359	0.204	-1.853	35.747
9	0	0.891	-0.334	0.207	-2.003	38.520
9	3	0.868	-0.311	0.210	-2.154	41.421
9	6	0.845	-0.289	0.212	-2.301	44.415
9	9	0.824	-0.269	0.214	-2.444	47.464

(continued)

Table 6–3. The RWT method for predicting adult stature.[1] (continued)

Tables of Multipliers for Boys

Age Yrs	Mos	Recumbent length	Weight	Midparental stature	Skeletal age	Adjustment factor
10	0	1.021	-0.276	0.360	-0.690	-9.671
10	3	1.008	-0.263	0.363	-0.781	-8.848
10	6	0.993	-0.252	0.368	-0.878	-7.812
10	9	0.977	-0.241	0.373	-0.983	-6.540
11	0	0.960	-0.231	0.378	-1.094	-5.010
11	3	0.942	-0.222	0.384	-1.211	-3.206
11	6	0.923	-0.213	0.390	-1.335	-1.113
11	9	0.902	-0.206	0.397	-1.464	1.273
12	0	0.881	-0.198	0.403	-1.597	3.958
12	3	0.859	-0.191	0.409	-1.735	6.931
12	6	0.837	-0.184	0.414	-1.875	10.181
12	9	0.815	-0.177	0.418	-2.015	13.684
13	0	0.794	-0.170	0.421	-2.156	17.405
13	3	0.773	-0.163	0.422	-2.294	21.297
13	6	0.755	-0.155	0.422	-2.427	25.304
13	9	0.738	-0.146	0.418	-2.553	29.349
14	0	0.724	-0.136	0.412	-2.668	33.345
14	3	0.714	-0.125	0.401	-2.771	37.183
14	6	0.709	-0.112	0.387	-2.856	40.738
14	9	0.709	-0.098	0.367	-2.922	43.869
15	0	0.717	-0.081	0.342	-2.962	46.403
15	3	0.732	-0.062	0.310	-2.973	48.154
15	6	0.756	-0.040	0.271	-2.949	48.898
15	9	0.792	-0.015	0.223	-2.885	48.402
16	0	0.839	-0.014	0.167	-2.776	46.391

The RWT method predicts the height of an individual at 18 years of age; after this age the average total increase in stature is 0.6 cm for girls and 0.8 cm for boys.

Recumbent length is measured in cm (add 1.25 cm to the standing height, without shoes, if that is available). Weight is measured in kg. The *midparental height* is calculated by adding the standing height of each parent in cm (without shoes) and dividing by two; if the parents' heights are unknown, in the USA a height of 174.5 cm can be substituted for the father's height or 162 cm for the mother's height. The skeletal age is determined from an x-ray of the left wrist and hand comparing it to the Greulich and Pyle atlas.

A prediction is made by:

1. Recording the child's data as noted below.
2. Finding the multipliers from the charts on these pages, making sure the positive and negative signs are retained for the calculations.
3. Multiplying the data by the multipliers, taking note of the positive or negative sign.
4. Adding the products to the adjustment factor, taking note of the sign of the factor: the result is a prediction of the height at 18 years of age.

Tables of Multipliers for Girls

Age Yrs	Mos	Recumbent length	Weight	Midparental stature	Skeletal age	Adjustment factor
10	0	0.803	-0.250	0.216	-2.581	50.525
10	3	0.783	-0.233	0.217	-2.710	53.548
10	6	0.766	-0.217	0.217	-2.829	56.481
10	9	0.749	-0.203	0.217	-2.936	59.267
11	0	0.736	-0.190	0.216	-3.029	61.841
11	3	0.724	-0.179	0.214	-3.108	64.123
11	6	0.716	-0.169	0.211	-3.171	66.093
11	9	0.711	-0.159	0.206	-3.217	67.627
12	0	0.710	-0.151	0.201	-3.245	68.670
12	3	0.713	-0.143	0.193	-3.254	69.140
12	6	0.720	-0.136	0.184	-3.244	68.966
12	9	0.733	-0.129	0.173	-3.214	68.061
13	0	0.752	-0.121	0.160	-3.166	66.339
13	3	0.777	-0.113	0.144	-3.100	63.728
13	6	0.810	-0.105	0.127	-3.015	60.150
13	9	0.850	-0.085	0.106	-2.915	55.522
14	0	0.898	-0.083	0.083	-2.800	49.781

The RWT method predicts the height of an individual at 18 years of age; after this age the average total increase in stature is 0.6 cm for girls and 0.8 cm for boys.

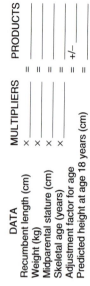

DATA	MULTIPLIERS	PRODUCTS
Recumbent length (cm)	× ____	= ____
Weight (kg)	× ____	= ____
Midparental stature (cm)	× ____	= ____
Skeletal age (years)	× ____	= ____
Adjustment factor for age		= +/- ____
Predicted height at age 18 years (cm)		= ____

[1]Modified and reproduced, with permission, from Roche AF, Wainer H, Thissen D: The RWT method for the prediction of adult stature. *Pediatrics* 1975;56:1026, as modified in Styne DM: Growth Disorders. Page 99 in: *Handbook of Clinical Endocrinology.* Fitzgerald PA (editor). Jones Medical Publications, 1986.

Table 6–4. Causes of abnormalities of growth.

I. CAUSES OF SHORT STATURE

Nonendocrine causes
  Constitutional short stature
  Genetic short stature
  Intrauterine growth retardation
  Syndromes of short stature
    Turner's syndrome and its variants
    Noonan's syndrome (pseudo-Turner's syndrome)
    Prader-Willi syndrome
    Laurence-Moon and Bardet-Biedl syndromes
    Other autosomal abnormalities and dysmorphic
      syndromes
  Chronic disease
    Cardiac disorders
      Left-to-right shunt
      Congestive heart failure
    Pulmonary disorders
      Cystic fibrosis
      Asthma
    Gastrointestinal disorders
      Malabsorption (eg, celiac disease)
      Disorders of swallowing
    Hepatic disorders
    Hematologic disorders
      Sickle cell anemia
      Thalassemia
    Renal disorders
      Renal tubular acidosis
      Chronic uremia
    Immunologic disorders
      Connective tissue disease
      Juvenile rheumatoid arthritis
      Chronic infection
    Central nervous system disorders
    Malnutrition
      Decreased availability of nutrients
      Fad diets
      Voluntary dieting during puberty
      Anorexia nervosa
      Anorexia of cancer chemotherapy

Endocrine disorders
  GH deficiency and variants
    Congenital GH deficiency
      With midline defects
      With other pituitary hormone deficiencies
      Isolated GH deficiency
      Pituitary agenesis
    Acquired GH deficiency
      Hypothalamic-pituitary tumors
      Histiocytosis X
      Central nervous system infections
      Head injuries
      GH deficiency following cranial irradiation
      Central nervous system vascular accidents
      Hydrocephalus
      Empty sella syndrome
    Abnormalities of GH action
      Laron's dwarfism
      Pygmies
  Psychosocial dwarfism
  Hypothyroidism
  Glucocorticoid excess (Cushing's syndrome)
    Endogenous
    Exogenous
  Pseudohypoparathyroidism
  Disorders of vitamin D metabolism
  Diabetes mellitus
  Diabetes insipidus, untreated

II. CAUSES OF TALL STATURE

Nonendocrine causes
  Constitutional tall stature
  Genetic tall stature
  Syndromes of tall stature
    Cerebral gigantism
    Marfan's syndrome
    Homocystinuria
    Beckwith-Wiedemann syndrome
    XYY syndrome
    Klinefelter's syndrome

Endocrine disorders
  Pituitary gigantism
  Sexual precocity
  Thyrotoxicosis
  Infants of diabetic mothers

shaved late and grew past his teenage years). The pubertal aspects of this condition are discussed in Chapter 12.

All other causes of decreased growth must be considered and ruled out before the diagnosis can be made with confidence. The patient may be considered physiologically (but not mentally) delayed in development. Characteristic growth patterns include normal birth length and height, with a gradual decrease in percentiles of height for age by 2 years. Onset of puberty is usually delayed for chronologic age but normal for skeletal age. Adult height is in the normal or low normal range. The final height is often less than the predicted height, because growth is less than expected during puberty (see Figure 6–8).

2. GENETIC SHORT STATURE

Short stature may also occur in a familial pattern without retarded bone age or delay in puberty; this is considered "genetic" short stature. Affected children are closer to the mean on the normal population growth charts after correction for midparental height

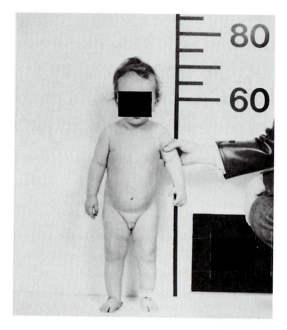

Figure 6–8. A 12-month-old boy with congenital hypopituitarism. He had hypoglycemic seizures at 12 hours of age. At 1 year, he had another hypoglycemic seizure (plasma glucose, 25 mg/dL) associated with an episode of otitis media, and it was noted that his penis was quite small. He was referred for evaluation because of these findings. At 12 months, length was 66.5 cm (–2 SD) and weight was 8.5 kg (–3 SD). The penis was less than 1.5 cm long, and both testes were descended (each 1 cm in diameter). Plasma GH did not rise above 1 ng/mL after arginine and levodopa testing. (No insulin was given because of the history of hypoglycemia.) LH rose only from 8.6 to 11.7 mIU/mL (1 ng of LH [preparation LER 960] = 7.8 mIU) after administration of GnRH (gonadorelin), 100 µg. Serum thyroxine was low (T_4, 6.6 µg/dL; T_4 index, 1.5), and after administration of 200 µg of protirelin (TRH), serum TSH rose with a delayed peak characteristic of tertiary hypothyroidism. Plasma ACTH rose only to 53 pg/mL after metyrapone. Thus, he had GH, ACTH, GnRH, and TRH deficiency. He was given six doses of 2000 units each of chorionic gonadotropin (hCG) intramuscularly over 2 weeks, and plasma testosterone rose to 62 ng/dL. He was then treated with 25 mg of testosterone enanthate every month for 3 months, and his phallus enlarged to 3.5 × 1.2 cm without significant advancement of bone age. With hGH therapy (0.1 unit/kg intramuscularly every other day), he grew at a greater than normal rate for 12 months (catch-up growth), and growth then continued at a normal rate.

(Figures 6–6 and 6–7). Adult height depends on the mother's and father's heights. Patients with the combination of constitutional short stature and genetic short stature are quite noticeably short due to both factors and are the patients most likely to seek evaluation.

3. PREMATURITY & INTRAUTERINE GROWTH RETARDATION

The proportionate IUGR infant will often follow a lifelong pattern of short stature. In comparison, appropriate-for-gestational-age premature infants will usually catch up to the normal range of height and weight by 1–2 years of age. Severe premature infants with birth weights less than 800 g (that are appropriate for gestational age), however, may maintain their growth retardation at least through their third year; only followup studies will determine whether this classification of premature infants reaches reduced adult heights. Bone age, age at onset of puberty, and yearly growth rate are normal in IUGR patients, and the patients are characteristically thin. Within this grouping are many distinctive genetic or sporadically occurring syndromes. The most common example is Russell-Silver dwarfism, characterized by small size at birth, triangular facies, a variable degree of asymmetry of extremities, and clinodactyly of the fifth finger. Intrauterine infections with cytomegalovirus, rubella virus, Toxoplasma gondii, and human immunodeficiency virus are noted to cause IUGR. Furthermore, maternal drug usage, either illicit (eg, cocaine), legal but ill-advised (eg, alcohol during pregnancy), or legally prescribed medication (eg, phenytoin) may cause IUGR. Reports of other syndromes in small-for-gestational-age infants can be found in sources listed in the bibliography.

While IUGR is generally considered to be a non-endocrine cause of short stature, a recent survey indicated a significant incidence of decreased growth hormone secretion and lower serum IGF-1 or IGF-2 concentrations in these conditions. This suggests a renewed necessity for study of the effects of GH treatment in these conditions.

4. SYNDROMES OF SHORT STATURE

Many syndromes have short stature as one of their characteristic features. Some include intrauterine growth retardation and some do not. Common ones are described briefly below. Laurence-Moon (Biedl-Bardet) syndrome, Prader-Willi syndrome, hypothyroidism, glucocorticoid excess, pseudohypoparathyroidism, and GH deficiency combine obesity with short stature. Moderately obese but otherwise normal children without these conditions tend to have slightly advanced bone age and physiologic maturation with increased stature during childhood and early onset of puberty. Thus, short stature in a chubby child must be considered to have an organic cause until proved otherwise.

Turner's Syndrome & Its Variants

While classic Turner's syndrome of 45,XO gonadal dysgenesis (see Chapter 14) is often correctly diagnosed, it is not always appreciated that any phenotypic female with short stature may have a variant of Turner's syndrome. Thus, a karyotype determination should be done for every short girl if no other cause for short stature is found (see Chapters 13, 14, and 15).

Noonan's Syndrome (Pseudo-Turner's Syndrome)

This syndrome shares several phenotypic characteristics of Turner's syndrome, but the karyotype is 46,XX in the female or 46,XY in the male with Noonan's syndrome, and other features clearly differentiate it from Turner's syndrome; pseudo-Turner's syndrome is an autosomal dominant disorder (see Chapters 12 and 15).

Prader-Willi Syndrome

This condition is characterized by infantile hypotonia, acromicria (small hands and feet), mental retardation, almond-shaped eyes, and extreme obesity. Glucose intolerance and delayed puberty are characteristic. This syndrome is associated with abnormalities of chromosome 15 in approximately 50% of affected cases and genetic probes are now available for diagnosis (see Chapter 15).

Laurence-Moon and Biedl-Bardet Syndromes

The Biedl-Bardet syndrome of developmental delay, retinitis pigmentosa, polydactly, and obesity, and the Laurence-Moon syndrome of developmental delay, retinitis pigmentosa, delayed puberty and spastic paraplegia, are also associated with poor growth. They are inherited as an autosomal recessive disorder (see Chapter 15).

Autosomal Karyotypic Disorders & Syndromes

Numerous autosomal karyotypic disorders and syndromes of dysmorphic children with or without mental retardation are characterized by short stature. Often the key to diagnosis is the presence of several major or minor physical abnormalities that indicate the need for karyotype determination. Other abnormalities may include unusual body proportions, such as short extremities, leading to aberrant US:LS ratios, and arm spans quite discrepant from stature. Some conditions, such as trisomy 21 (Down's syndrome), are quite common, while others are rare. Details of these syndromes can be found in the references listed at the end of the chapter.

Skeletal Dysplasias

There are more than 100 known types of genetic skeletal dysplasias (osteochondrodysplasias). Often they are noted at birth because of the presence of short limbs or trunk, but some are only diagnosed after a period of growth. The most common condition is autosomal dominant achondroplasia. This condition is char-

acterized by short extremities, a relatively large head with a prominent forehead and a depressed nasal bridge, and lumbar lordosis in later life. Adult height is quite short, with a mean of 132 cm for males and 123 cm for females. Limb lengthening operations have been used to improve stature in a few centers. Children with achondroplasia have received GH and some demonstrated improved growth; however one experienced atlanto-occipital dislocation and the abnormal brain growth and its relationship to abberant skull shape mandates the caution that GH is not an established therapy for this condition and may have severe side effects. Hypochondroplasia is manifested on a continuum from severe short limb dwarfism to apparent normal development until puberty, when there is an attenuated or absent pubertal growth spurt, leading to short adult stature. Growth hormone is reported to increase growth rate in short-term studies of this condition but it is too early to draw strong conclusions about such a course of therapy.

5. CHRONIC DISEASE

Severe chronic disease involving any organ system can cause poor growth in childhood and adolescence. In many cases, there will be adequate physical findings by the time of consultation to permit diagnosis; in some cases, however—most notably celiac disease and regional enteritis—short stature and decreased growth may precede obvious signs of malnutrition or gastrointestinal disease. In some cases, growth is only delayed. In others, growth can be increased by improved nutrition; patients with gastrointestinal disease, kidney disease, or cancer may benefit from nocturnal parenteral nutritional infusions. Cystic fibrosis combines several causes of growth failure: lung disease impairs oxygenation and predisposes to chronic infections, gastrointestinal disease decreases nutrient availability, and late-developing abnormalities of the endocrine pancreas cause symptoms of diabetes mellitus. Children with cystic fibrosis experience decreased growth rates after one year of age following a normal birth size. The pubertal growth spurt is often decreased in amount of growth and delayed in its timing: secondary sexual development may be delayed especially in those with impaired pulmonary function. Study of growth in these patients allowed development of a cystic fibrosis specific growth chart and indicates that a reasonable outcome is an adult height in the 25th percentile. Children with congestive heart failure due to a variety of congenital heart diseases or acquired myocarditis grow poorly unless successfully treated with medications or surgery; patients with cyanotic heart disease experience less deficit in growth.

Celiac disease may present initially with growth failure. Early diagnosis can be made by determination of antigliadin or antiendomesial antibodies. On a gluten-free diet, patients experience catch-up growth which is strongest in the first year of therapy but continues for several more. Adult height may still be impaired, depending upon the period without treatment. Untreated patients with celiac disease have decreased serum IGF-1 concentrations, presumably due to malnutrition while IGF-1 concentrations rise with dietary therapy; thus serum IGF-1 in this condition as in many with nutrtional deficiencies is not a reliable indicator of GH secretory status. Crohns disease is associated with poor growth and decreased serum, IGF-1 concentrations. On an elemental diet growth rate increases and with glucocorticiod therapy, growth rate improves even though serum IGF-1 decreases.

Patients with chronic hematologic diseases, such as sickle cell anemia or thalassemia, often have poor growth, delayed puberty, and short adult stature. Juvenile rheumatoid arthritis may compromise growth before or after therapy with glucocorticoids. There is only 1 year of data that suggests GH treatment may be used to increase the growth rate of these children; thus, it is too early to draw conclusions about the efficacy of such therapy in juvenile rheumatoid arthritis.

Chronic renal disease is known to interfere with growth. Hypophosphatemic vitamin D-resistant rickets will usually lead to short adult stature, but treatment with 1,25-dihydroxyvitamin D_3 (cholecalciferol) and oral phosphate in most cases will lead to normal adult stature. Children with chronic renal failure are reported to have increased growth rate with GH therapy and improved nutrition in several studies.

The two forms of renal tubular acidosis, proximal and distal, may both cause short stature. Proximal renal tubular acidosis causes bicarbonate wasting at normal or low plasma bicarbonate concentrations; patients have hypokalemia, alkaline urine pH, severe bicarbonaturia, and, later, acidemia. The condition may be inherited, sporadic, or secondary to many metabolic or medication-induced disorders. Distal renal tubular acidosis is caused by inability to acidify the urine; it may occur in sporadic or familial patterns or be acquired as a result of metabolic disorders or medication therapy. Distal renal tubular acidosis is characterized by hypokalemia, hypercalciuria, and occasional hypocalcemia. The administration of bicarbonate is the primary therapy for either type of renal tubular acidosis, and proper treatment can substantially improve growth rate.

Obstructive sleep apnea is associated with poor growth. The amount of energy expended during sleep in children with sleep apnea appears to limit weight and length gain, a pattern which reverses with the resolution of the obstruction.

Hemoglobin, white blood cell count, erythrocyte sedimentation rate, serum carotene and folate levels, antigliadin or antiendomesial antibodies, plasma bicarbonate levels, and liver and kidney function should be assessed in short but otherwise apparently healthy children before endocrine screening tests are done. Urinalysis should be performed, with attention to specific gravity (to rule out diabetes insipidus) and ability to acidify urine (to evaluate possible renal tubular acidosis). All short girls without a diagnosis should undergo karyotype testing to rule out Turner's syndrome. A list of chronic diseases causing short stature is presented in Table 6–4.

6. MALNUTRITION (Other Than That Associated With Chronic Disease)

Malnutrition is the most common cause of short stature worldwide. Diagnosis in the developed world is based on historical and physical findings, particularly the dietary history. Food faddism and anorexia nervosa—as well as voluntary dieting can cause poor growth. Infection with parasites such as Ascaris lumbricoides or Giardia can decrease growth. Specific nutritional deficiencies can have particular effects upon growth. For example, severe iron deficiency can cause a thin habitus as well as growth retardation. Zinc deficiency (though probably invoked too often as a cause of growth retardation) can cause anorexia, decreased growth, and delayed puberty, usually in the presence of chronic systemic disease or infection. There are no simple laboratory tests for diagnosis of malnutrition, though serum IGF-1 concentrations are low in malnutrition, as they are in GH deficiency.

7. DRUGS

Children with hyperactivity disorders (or those incorrectly diagnosed as such) are frequently managed with chronic dextroamphetamine or methylphenidate administration. In larger doses, these agents can decrease weight gain—probably because of their effects on appetite—and growth rate. Discontinuing therapy temporarily, usually during vacations from school, allows some catch-up growth in weight and height, but it is controversial whether the height deficit is completely repaired. These drugs must be used in moderation and only in children who definitely need them.

Exogenous glucocorticoids are a potent cause of poor growth (see below).

SHORT STATURE DUE TO ENDOCRINE DISORDERS

1. GROWTH HORMONE DEFICIENCY & ITS VARIANTS (Table 6–5)

Current concepts of endocrine regulation of growth propose that GH stimulates growth through

Table 6–5. Postulated disorders of hGH release and action.

Site of Defect	Clinical Condition
Hypothalamus	Idiopathic GH deficiency due to decreased GRH secretion; hypothalamic tumors.
Pituitary gland	Dysplasia, trauma, surgery, or tumor of the pituitary gland.
Sites of IGF production	Laron's dwarfism with high GH and low IGF concentrations (GH receptor defect). Pygmies with normal GH, low IGF-1, and normal IGF-2 concentrations.
Cartilage	Glucocorticoid-induced growth failure. Resistance to IGF-1.

intermediary substances, the insulin-like growth factors (see above).

The incidence of GH deficiency is estimated to be between 1:4000 and 1:3500 in Utah and in the Scottish population, so the disorder should not be considered rare. Using the conservative criteria of height less than the third percentile and growth velocity less than 5 cm per year, the incidence of endocrine disease in 114,881 Utah children was 5%, with a higher incidence in boys than girls by a ratio of over 2.5:1. In this population, 48% of the children with Turner's syndrome or growth hormone deficiency were not diagnosed prior to the careful evaluation afforded by this study. Most patients with idiopathic GH deficiency apparently lack GRH. One who suffered an accident and came to autopsy had adequate numbers of pituitary somatotrophs that had considerable GH stores; the pituitary gland produced growth hormone, but there was no way to stimulate its secretion. Long-term treatment of these patients with GRH can cause GH release and improve growth. Patients with pituitary tumors or those rare patients with congenital absence of the pituitary gland lack somatotrophs. Several kindreds have been described that lack various regions of the GH gene responsible for producing GH.

Before 1986, the only clinical method of treatment for GH deficiency was replacement therapy with human GH (hGH) derived from cadaver donors. In 1985 and thereafter, Creutzfeldt-Jakob disease, a degenerative neurologic disease rare in patients so young, was diagnosed in patients who had received natural hGH 10–15 years before. Because of the possibility that prions contaminating donor pituitary glands were transmitted to the GH-deficient patients and caused their death, natural growth hormone from all sources was removed from distribution. Recombinant DNA technology now accounts for the world's current supply of growth hormone.

Commercial growth hormone is currently available in the 191-amino-acid natural-sequence form (somatropin) and the 192-amino-acid methionyl form (somatrem). There is no convincing evidence that either form is clinically superior to the other, but the direction of therapy is turning toward somatropin. GH is now available in virtually unlimited amounts, allowing innovative treatment regimens not previously possible owing to scarce supplies; however, the potential for abuse of GH in athletes or in children of normal size whose parents wish them to be taller than average must now be addressed.

GRH was first isolated from pancreatic GH-releasing tumor, sequenced, and synthesized, but hypothalamic GRH has the same structure as GRH from the pancreatic tumors. GRH has potential in the diagnosis and treatment of GH deficiency; GH-deficient patients have demonstrated lower or absent GH secretion after administration of GRH. Furthermore, episodic doses of GRH have restored GH secretion, insulin-like growth hormone production, and growth in children with idiopathic GH deficiency. The ability of GRH administration to cause pituitary GH secretion further supports the concept that idiopathic GH deficiency is primarily a disease of the hypothalamus, not of the pituitary gland.

IGF-1 (previously called somatomedin C) is now produced by recombinant DNA technology. Although no long-term human treatment program has yet been reported, initial studies suggest that IGF-1 may be a useful treatment for short stature, particularly in Laron dwarfism (and perhaps African pygmies) where no other treatment is possible. Growth disturbances due to disorders of GH release or action are shown in Table 6–5. Earlier theories suggested the liver as the sole source of plasma IGF-1 that affects cartilage, but it is clear that many organs produce IGF-1, although the liver still seems to be the greatest source. IGF-1 is an autocrine or paracrine factor that influences its own cell of origin or neighboring cells rather than solely an endocrine agent that acts at a distance via blood-borne transport. This complicates the measurement and interpretation of serum IGF-1 concentrations. Recombinant DNA technology has increased the supply of IGF-1, and it is used to determine the direct effects of the insulin-like growth factors.

Congenital Growth Hormone Deficiency

Congenital GH deficiency presents with normal birth length but decreased growth rate soon after birth. The disorder is identified by careful measurement in the first year and becomes more obvious by 1–2 years of age. Patients with classic GH deficiency have short stature, obesity with immature facial appearance, immature high-pitched voice, and some delay in skeletal maturation. Less severe forms of partial GH deficiency are described. Growth hormone deficient patients lack the lipolytic effects of growth hormone. There is a higher incidence of hyperlipidemia with elevated total cholesterol and apoprotein C-III in GH deficiency and longitudinal studies demonstrate further elevation of apoprotein C-III with GH treatment. Males with GH deficiency may have microphallus, especially if the condition is accompanied by gonadotropin-releasing hormone (GnRH) deficiency (Figure 6–8). GH deficiency in the neonate or child can also lead to symptomatic hypoglycemia and seizures; if ACTH deficiency is also present, hypoglycemia is usually more severe. The differential diagnosis of neonatal hypoglycemia in a full-term infant who has not sustained birth trauma must include neonatal hypopituitarism. If microphallus (in a male subject), optic hypoplasia, or some other midline facial or central nervous system defect is noted, the diagnosis of congenital GH deficiency is likely. Congenital GH deficiency is also statistically correlated with breech delivery. Intelligence is normal in GH deficiency unless repeated or severe hypoglycemia has compromised brain development. When thyrotropin-releasing hormone (TRH) deficiency is also present, there may be additional signs of hypothyroidism. Secondary or tertiary congenital hypothyroidism is not usually associated with mental retardation as is congenital primary hypothyroidism, but a few cases of isolated TRH deficiency and severe mental retardation have been reported.

Congenital GH deficiency may present with midline anatomic defects. Optic hypoplasia with visual defects ranging from nystagmus to blindness is found with variable hypothalamic deficiency, including diabetes insipidus; about half of patients with optic hypoplasia have absence of the septum pellucidum on CT scan or MRI, leading to the diagnosis of septo-optic dysplasia. Cleft palate or other forms of oral dysraphism are associated with GH deficiency in about 7% of cases; thus, such children may need more than nutritional support to improve their growth. An unusual midline defect associated with GH deficiency has been described in children with a single maxillary incision.

Congenital absence of the pituitary, which has been found in an autosomal recessive pattern, leads to severe hypopituitarism, including hypoglycemia and hypopituitarism; affected patients have shallow development or absence of the sella turcica. This defect is quite rare.

Hereditary GH deficiency is described in several kindreds. Recent biochemical techniques have defined various genetic defects in affected families. Patients with absent or abnormal GH genes do initially respond to exogenous hGH administration, but some soon develop high antibody titers that terminate the effect of therapy; one reported kindred had a heterogeneous response as one sibling continued to grow and did not develop blocking antibodies while the opposite effect occured in two other siblings in the same family. Type IA GH deficiency is inherited in an autosomal recessive pattern, and patients have defects in the GH genome; unlike those with classic sporadic GH deficiency, some of these children have been described with short birth lengths. Type IB patients have autosomal recessive GH deficiency but no such gene deletion; type II patients have autosomal dominant GH deficiency; and type III patients have X-linked GH deficiency. Those patients who cannot secrete growth hormone will develop blocking antibodies when treated with exogenous growth hormone. Those with high titers of blocking antibodies are reported to benefit from IGF-1 therapy in place of GH therapy.

Acquired Growth Hormone Deficiency

Onset of GH deficiency in late childhood or adolescence, particularly if accompanied by other pituitary hormone deficiencies, is ominous and may be due to a hypothalamic-pituitary tumor. The development of posterior pituitary deficiency in addition to anterior pituitary deficiency makes a tumor even more likely. Conditions that cause acquired GH deficiency—craniopharyngiomas, germinomas, gliomas, Histiocytosis X, etc—are described in Chapters 5 and 15.

The empty sella syndrome is more frequently associated with hypothalamic-pituitary abnormalities in childhood than in adulthood; thus, GH deficiency may be found in affected patients. Some patients—chiefly boys—with constitutional delay in growth and adolescence may have transient GH deficiency on testing before the actual onset of puberty; when serum testosterone concentrations begin to increase in these patients, GH secretion and growth rate also increase.

Cranial irradiation of the hypothalamic-pituitary region to treat head tumors or acute lymphoblastic leukemia may result in GH deficiency approximately 12–18 months later, owing to radiation-induced hypothalamic (or perhaps pituitary) damage. Higher doses of irradiation such as the 2400 cGy previously routinely used for the treatment of central nervous system leukemia have greater effect (final height was −1.7 SD in a recent study) than the 1800 cGy used more routinely now; girls treated at an early age still appear to be at risk for growth failure. All children must be carefully observed for growth failure after irradiation. If these patients receive spinal irradiation, upper body growth may also be impaired, causing a lower US:LS ratio. Abdominal irradiation for Wilms' tumor may lead to decreased spinal growth with an estimated loss of height from megavoltage therapy of 10 cm for treatment at 1 year of age, and 7 cm from treatment at 5 years of age. Others receiving gonadal irradiation (or chemotherapy) have impaired gonadal function and lack onset or progression of puberty and the pubertal growth spurt.

Other Types of Growth Hormone Dysfunction or Deficiency

Other disorders of GH production or action are not manifested in the classic manner of GH deficiency.

Laron's dwarfism is characterized by high plasma GH and low plasma IGF-1 concentrations. Growth rate does not increase and IGF-1 values do not rise when exogenous hGH is administered. However, IGF-1 administration raises growth rate and suppresses GH concentrations. The basic defect is an inability to produce IGF-1 in response to growth hormone because of impaired or absent GH receptors due to abnormal genetic expression of the growth hormone receptor. GHBP is absent in the serum of most but not all patients. Numerous defects in the gene are described from families throughout the world, including nonsense mutations, deletions, RNA processing defects, and translational stop codons. Birth weight is normal; about one-third have hypoglycemia, half of the boys have microphallus. Laron dwarfism is inherited as an autosomal recessive disorder.

Very short, poorly growing children with delayed skeletal maturation, normal GH and IGF-1 values, and no signs of organic disease have responded to GH therapy with increased growth rates equal to those of patients with *bona fide* GH deficiency. These patients may have a variation of constitutional delay in growth or genetic short stature, but a subtle abnormality of GH secretion or action is possible.

What is the reason that certain normal children, perhaps within a short family, have stature significantly lower than the mean? There is no overall answer to this long-standing question, but some patients are demonstrated to have decreased serum GHBP concentrations which suggests a decrease in GH receptors in these children. A recent study confirms that a minority of short, poorly growing children have definable genetic abnormalities of their GH receptors; more patients may have other, yet to be defined abnormalities. Another recent study claims that serum IGF-1 and IGFBP-3 are lower in normal but short children than in those of normal height. It appears that many routes of investigation will ultimately answer this presently unanswered question; it is likely that short stature is the final common pathway of numerous biochemical abnormalities.

In this era of plentiful GH supplies, there is increasing pressure to treat more children—usually boys—who are not severely short and are not growing extremely slowly and do not have greatly delayed bone ages. While some controlled studies of treatment of such children are under way the results of studies to date are contradictory about the final height that can be achieved with such treatment.

Pygmies are reported to have normal serum GH, low IGF-1, and normal IGF-2 concentrations. They would not respond to exogenous GH with improved growth rate or a rise in IGF-1. They have a congenital inability to produce IGF-1, which is of greater importance in stimulating growth than is IGF-2. Pygmy children are reported to lack a pubertal growth spurt,

suggesting that IGF-1 is essential to attain a normal peak growth velocity. Efe pygmies, the shortest of the pygmies, are significantly smaller at birth than neighboring Africans and their growth is slower throughout childhood, leading to statures of progressively more standard deviations below the mean. Presumably, IGF-1 therapy would increase growth rates in this population during childhood and puberty, but such therapy has not yet been reported.

Adults who had growth hormone deficiency in childhood or adolescence have decreased bone mass compared to normals even when bone mass is corrected for their smaller size. These patients were treated with growth hormone for various periods, but it appears that growth hormone therapy may not reverse the effects of growth hormone deficiency on skeletal density.

Diagnosis of Growth Hormone Deficiency

Because basal values of serum GH are low in normal children and GH-deficient patients alike, the diagnosis of GH deficiency has rested upon demonstration of an inadequate rise of serum GH after provocative stimuli. This process is complicated because different radioimmunoassay systems vary widely in their measurements of GH in the same blood sample; a result may be above 10 ng/mL in one assay but only 6 ng/mL in another. The physician must be aware of the standards of the laboratory being used.

The very concept of growth hormone testing provides a further complication. Growth hormone is released in episodic pulses. Originally GH secretion appeared highly correlated with the state of entering stage III-IV sleep (usually 90 minutes after onset of sleep). However, recent studies have cast doubt on the relationship between GH secretion and deep sleep in short normal children and others. While a patient who does not secrete GH in response to standard challenges is generally considered to be GH-deficient, a normal GH response to these tests may not rule out GH deficiency. Except for sleep studies, testing should occur after an overnight fast; carbohydrate ingestion will suppress GH response. Obesity suppresses GH secretion, and a chubby child may falsely appear to have GH deficiency. Because 10% or more of healthy children will not have an adequate rise in GH with one test of GH reserve, at least two methods of assessing GH reserve are necessary before the diagnosis of classic GH deficiency is assigned. Serum GH values should rise after 10 minutes of vigorous exercise. After an overnight fast, GH levels should also rise in response to arginine infusion (0.5 g/kg body weight [up to 20 g] over 30 minutes), oral levodopa (125 mg for up to 15 kg body weight, 250 mg for up to 35 kg, or 500 mg for over 35 kg), or clonidine (0.10–0.15 mg/m^2 orally). Side effects of levodopa include nausea; those of clonidine include some drop in blood pressure and drowsiness.

GH levels also rise after acute hypoglycemia due to insulin administration; this test carries a risk of seizure if the blood glucose level drops excessively. An insulin tolerance test may be performed if a 10–25% dextrose infusion is available for emergency administration in the face of hypoglycemic coma or seizure, if the patient can be continuously observed by a physician, and if the patient has no history of hypoglycemic seizures. The patient must have a normal glucose concentration at the beginning of the test. Regular insulin, 0.075–0.1 unit/kg in saline, may be given as an intravenous bolus. In 20–40 minutes, a 50% drop in blood glucose will occur and a rise in serum GH and cortisol should follow. Glucose should be monitored, and an intravenous line must be maintained for emergency dextrose infusion in case the patient becomes unconscious or has a hypoglycemic seizure. If dextrose infusion is necessary, it is imperative that blood glucose not be raised far above the normal range, since hyperosmolality has been reported from overzealous glucose replacement. (See Chapter 5.)

A new family of penta- and hexapepetides, growth hormone releasing peptides (GHRPs) are described which stimulate GH secretion in normals and growth hormone-deficient subjects and may become available for clincal use in testing and treatment of growth disorders.

Patients who respond to pharmacologic stimuli (eg, levodopa, clonidine, or insulin) but not to physiologic stimuli such as exercise or sleep were said to have neurosecretory dysfunction; these patients may have decreased 24-hour secretion of hGH (or integrated concentrations of hGH) compared with healthy subjects, patterns similar to those observed in GH-deficient patients. The true status of such patients and the role of 24-hour GH monitoring are still controversial. This long discussion of the interpretation of GH after secretagogue testing brings into question the very standard for the diagnosis of GH deficiency. It is clear that pharmacologic testing cannot always determine which patients truly need GH therapy and some suggest we abandon such testing.

Serum IGF-1 values will be low in most GH-deficient subjects, but, as noted above, short patients with normal serum IGF-1 concentrations are reported who require GH treatment for improvement of growth rate. In addition, starvation will lower IGF-1 values in healthy children and incorrectly suggest GH deficiency. Children with psychosocial dwarfism—who need family therapy or foster home placement rather than GH therapy—have low GH and IGF-1 concentrations and may falsely appear to have growth hormone deficiency. Likewise, patients with constitutional delay in adolescence will have low IGF-1 values for chronologic age but normal values for skeletal age and may have temporarily decreased GH response to secretagogues. Thus, IGF-1 determinations are not infallible in the diagnosis of GH deficiency. They must be interpreted with regard to nutrition, psychosocial status, and skeletal ages.

Alternative determinations are used to improve the diagnosis of GH deficiency. Low serum IGF-2 in addition to low IGF-1 levels improve the prediction of GH deficiency. Acid extraction of serum on a Sephadex column to separate IGF from its binding protein yields IGF-1 concentrations more closely related to growth rate and stature than are IGF-1 determinations done by direct radioimmunoassay, as was frequently done in the past. Still, IGF-1 concentrations do not reliably indicate all patients with growth hormone deficiency. IGFBP-3 is GH-dependent and if low is said to be more indicative than IGF-1 determinations of GH deficiency, although IGFBP-3 concentrations vary with body mass index while IGF-1 concentrations do not. Serum IGF II and IGFBP-2 do not increase with puberty and IGFBP-1 decreases with pubertal development. Many combinations of measurements of IGFs and IGFBPs were attempted to increase the accuracy of the diagnosis of GH deficiency but, to date, none has proved to be foolproof.

Although pharmacologic tests of GH secretion and serum IGF-1 values will usually indicate who has classic GH deficiency, the diagnosis will remain in doubt in some cases. This should not lead to the conclusion that all short children should receive GH therapy. Only very short children (height well below the fifth percentile or > 2.5–3.5 SD below the mean) who grow very slowly (growth velocity below the fifth percentile for age) with delayed bone ages meticulously studied in research protocols were shown to benefit from hGH therapy in the absence of classic GH deficiency in about 50% of cases. Patients with Turner's syndrome and renal failure derived some benefit in careful studies. However, children meeting less stringent criteria have been treated with GH in controlled trials, producing some increase in growth rate; it is not yet clear whether this treatment increases adult height. Thus, in the absence of classic GH deficiency, no clearly recognized measurement can predict which short child is likely to respond to GH therapy before it is instituted. A 3- to 6-month therapeutic trial is needed in some cases.

Treatment of Growth Hormone Deficiency

A. Hormonal Replacement: GH-deficient children require biosynthetic somatropin (natural sequence GH) at a dose of 0.18–0.3 mg/kg/wk or somatrem (methionyl GH) at a dose of 0.3 mg/kg/wk administered in one dose per day six or seven times per week during the period of active growth before epiphysial fusion. The increase in growth rate (Figures 6–9, 6–10, and 6–11) is most marked during the first year of therapy. Older children do not respond as well and may require larger doses. GH will not in-

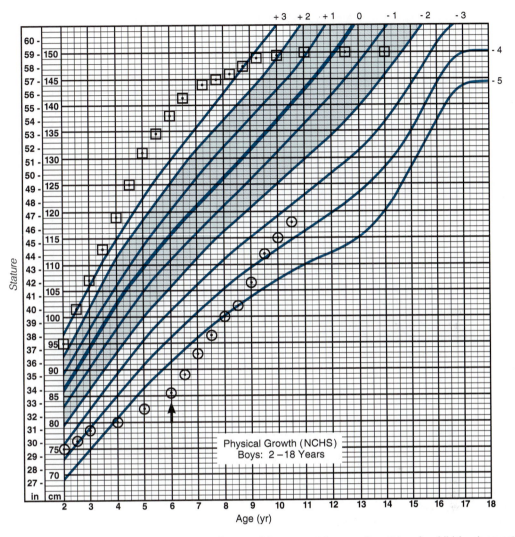

Figure 6–9. Examples of abnormal growth charts. Squares (□) represent the growth pattern of a child (such as patient A in Figure 6–11) with precocious sexual development and early excessive growth leading to premature closure of the epiphyses and cessation of growth. Circles (○) represent growth of a boy (such as patient B in Figure 6–11) with GH deficiency who showed progressively poorer growth until 6 years of age, when he was treated with hGH *(arrow),* after which catch-up growth occurred.

crease growth rate without adequate nutrition and euthyroid status.

Antibodies to GH are present in measurable quantities in the serum of children receiving GH. While antibodies are more frequent in those treated with somatrem than somatropin, a high titer of blocking antibodies with significant binding capacity is rare and only a few patients are reported to have temporarily ceased growing on somatrem therapy.

GH exerts anti-insulin effects. Although clinical diabetes is not a likely result of GH therapy, the long-term effects of a small rise in glucose in an otherwise healthy child are unknown. Another potential risk is the rare tendency to develop slipped capital femoral epiphyses which occurs in thinner children,

usually of younger age, with growth hormone therapy than in the general population; slipped capital femoral epiphyses, if associated with endocrinopathies, is most common in treated hypothyroid patients (50% one series of 80 episodes of slipped capital femoral epiphyses) and next most common in treated growth hormone deficienct patients (25% of the series). This condition may occur bilaterally as high as 62–100% in this treated group and prophylactic treatement of the nonaffected side is recommended by several authorities. Organomegaly and skeletal changes like those found in acromegaly are other potential side effects of excessive GH therapy. Further, cases of prepubertal gynecomastia are reported with growth hormone therapy. The discovery

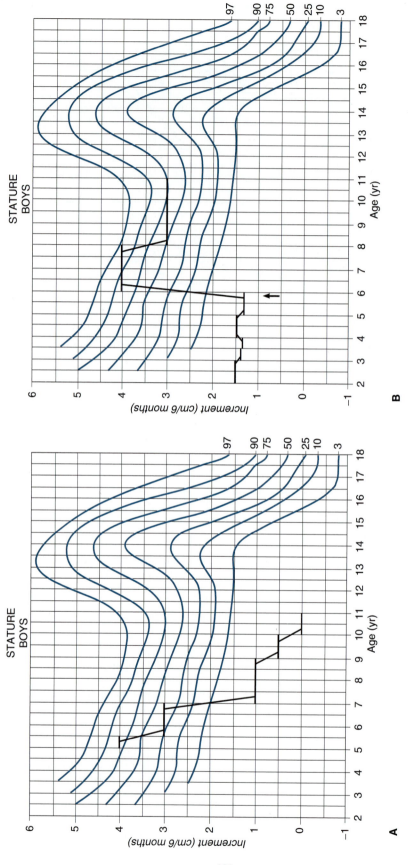

Figure 6–10. Two examples of abnormal growth plotted on a height velocity chart. **A:** The plot is taken from the data recorded as squares in Figure 6–9, describing a patient with precocious puberty, premature epiphysial closure, and cessation of growth. **B:** The plot is taken from the data recorded as circles in Figure 6–9, describing a patient with GH deficiency who was treated with hGH (**arrow**) at age 6. Initial catch-up growth is noted for 2 years, with a lower (but normal) velocity of growth following.

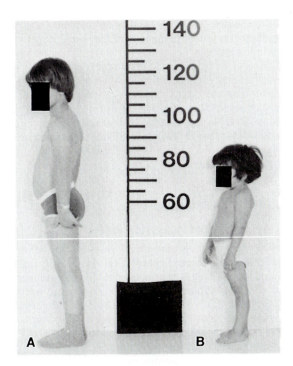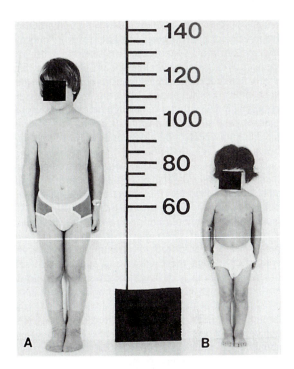

Figure 6–11. Two boys demonstrating extremes of growth. The boy at left in each photograph **(A)** has precocious puberty due to a central nervous system lesion. At 4½ years, he was 125.1 cm tall, which is 5 SD above the mean. (The mean height for a 4-year-old is 101.5 cm.) His testes measured 2 × 3.5 cm each, his penis 9.8 × 2.8 cm. He was muscular and had acne and a deep voice. His bone age was 10 years, the testosterone level was 480 ng/dL, and the LH rose after 100 μg of GnRH (gonadorelin) to 23.4 mIU/mL, which is a pubertal response. His brain CT scan revealed a hamartoma of the tuber cinereum. The boy at right **(B)** at 4½ years was 85 cm tall, which is 4.5 SD below the mean. He had the classic physical and historical characteristics of idiopathic GH deficiency, including early growth failure and a cherubic appearance. His plasma GH values did not rise after provocative testing.

of cases of leukemia in young adults previously treated with growth hormone was worrisome, but at present no cause and effect relationship is proved. GH does not increase the recurrence rate of tumors existing before therapy; thus, patients with craniopharyngiomas, for example, may receive GH, if indicated, after the disease is clinically stable, without significant worry that the GH will precipitate a recurrence. Clinicians usually wait 1 year after completion of tumor therapy before starting tumor patients on GH therapy.

Treatment with GH has been studied in chronic renal disease in childhood. GH increases growth rate above the untreated state without excessive advancement in bone age, according to several studies. However, until a large cohort is studied until final height it cannot be stated with certainty that final height is improved with such therapy.

Monitoring of growth hormone replacement is mainly accomplished by measuring growth rate and reguarly assesing bone age advancement. Serum IGF-1 and IGFBP-3 will rise with successful therapy while GHBP will not change appreciably. Serum bone alkaline phosphatase rises with successful ther-

apy. Urinary hydroxyproline, deoxypyridinolone and galactosyl-hydroxylysine reflect growth rate and are used in clinical studies to reflect increased growth rate with therapy.

Alternative therapies include recombinant derived IGF-1 for patients with GH resistance (Laron dwarfs), and several years of data now indicate its efficacy. GRH is used for the diagnosis of growth hormone deficiency and may ultimately prove useful in the therapy of growth disorders.

Other effects of growth hormone are under investigation. Growth hormone appears to improve the rate of wound healing and shortens the length of hospital stay. The use of growth hormone in adult growth hormone deficiency or in adults who had GH deficiency in childhood is now an approved indication, but the results of long term studies must appear before routine administration is indicated.

B. Psychologic Management and Outcome: Research into the psychologic outcome of patients with short stature is flawed by lack of consistent methods of investigation and lack of controlled studies, but some results are of interest. Studies vary in concluding whether short stature is harmful in a child's psychologic development or not and whether, by inference, growth hormone is helpful in improving the child's psychologic functioning. Children with growth hormone deficiency are the most extensively studied; earlier investigations suggest that they have more passive personality traits than do healthy children. Such patients may have delayed emotional maturity and suffer from infantilization from parents, teachers, and peers. Their academic achievement has been generally substandard even if intelligence is normal; this was attributed to delayed emotional maturity or poor body image, both fostered by short stature. However, many of these children have been held back in school because of their size without regard to their academic abilities. Some patients retain a body image of short stature even after normal height has been achieved with treatment. More recent studies challenge these views and suggest that self image in children with height below the 5% who do not have growth hormone deficiency is closely comparable to a population of children with normal height. This, then, suggests that short stature itself is not cause for grave psychologic concern and surely should not mandate growth hormone therapy because of psychologic reasons. Nonetheless, we do find in certain cases that depression and suicidal behavior can occur in affected adolescents because of the psychologic stress of short stature and delayed development. We cannot avoid the fact that our "heightist" society values physical stature and equates it with the potential for success, a perception that is not lost on the children with short stature and their parents. A supportive environment in which they are not allowed to act younger than their age nor to occupy a "privileged place" in the family is recommended for children with short stature. Psychologic help is indicated in severe cases of depression or maladjustment.

2. PSYCHOSOCIAL DWARFISM
(Figure 6–12)

Children with psychosocial dwarfism present with poor growth, potbellied immature appearance, and bizarre eating and drinking habits. Parents may report that the affected child begs for food from neighbors, forages in garbage cans, and drinks from toilet bowls. As a rule, this tragic condition occurs in only one of several children in a family. Careful questioning and observation reveal a disordered family structure in which the child is either ignored or severely disciplined. Caloric deprivation or physical battering may or may not be a feature of the history. These children have functional hypopituitarism. Testing will often reveal GH deficiency at first, but after the child is removed from the home, GH function quickly returns to normal. Diagnosis rests upon improvement in behavior or catch-up growth in the hospital or in a foster home. Separation from the family

is therapeutic, but the prognosis is guarded. Family psychotherapy may be beneficial, but long-term follow-up is lacking.

Growth disorder due to abnormal parent-child interaction in a younger infant is called maternal deprivation. Caloric deprivation due to parental neglect may be of greater significance in this younger age group. Even in the absence of nutritional restriction or full-blown psychosocial dwarfism, constant negative interactions within a family may inhibit the growth of a child.

3. HYPOTHYROIDISM

Thyroid hormone deficiency decreases growth rate and skeletal development and, if onset is at or before birth, leads to mental retardation. Screening programs for the diagnosis of congenital hypothyroidism have been instituted all over the world, and early treatment following diagnosis in the neonatal period markedly reduces growth failure and mental retardation caused by severe primary congenital hypothyroidism. Indeed early treated congenital hypothyroid patients demonstrate normal growth in later infancy. Acquired hypothyroidism in older children, such as lymphocytic thyroiditis, may lead to growth failure. Characteristics of hypothyroidism are decreased growth rate and short stature, retarded bone age, and an increased US:LS ratio for chronologic age. Patients are apathetic and sluggish and have constipation, bradycardia, coarsening of features and hair, hoarseness, and delayed pubertal development (Figure 7–35). Intelligence is unaffected in late-onset hypothyroidism, but the apathy and lethargy may make it seem otherwise.

Hypothyroidism cannot be diagnosed solely on the basis of a low plasma total T_4 value; an indication of a low free T_4 value or low free T_4 index is necessary to rule out the relatively frequent occurrence (1:10,000) of thyroid hormone-binding globulin (TBG) deficiency, which will artifactually lower total T_4 values into the hypothyroid range without affecting the more important free T_4 values or euthyroid status. If a free T_4 determination or if a test of TBG levels (such as a resin T_3 uptake or plasma TBG concentration) is obtained along with the total T_4, this diagnostic trap can be avoided. Since the majority of cases of hypothyroidism are of the primary classification, elevated TSH levels will confirm the diagnosis of *bona fide* hypothyroidism. Positive antimicrosomal or antithyroglobulin antibodies will indicate Hashimoto's (lymphocytic) thyroiditis. Low values of TSH on the newer sensitive assays may suggest secondary (pituitary) or tertiary (hypothalamic) hypothyroidism; such diagnoses must precipitate a search for other hypothalamic-pituitary endocrine deficiencies and central nervous system pathology (see Chapter 7).

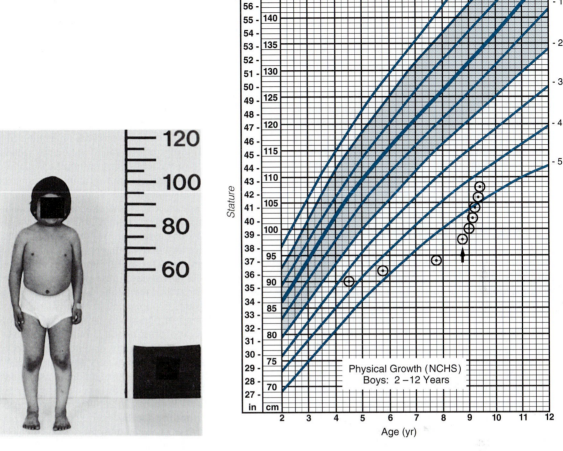

Figure 6–12. Photograph and growth chart of a 9½-year-old boy with psychosocial dwarfism. He had a long history of poor growth (< 3 cm/yr). The social history revealed that he was given less attention and punished more frequently than his 7 sibs. He ate from garbage cans and begged for food, though he was not completely deprived of food at home. When the photograph was taken, he was 99 cm tall (−7 SD) and weighed 14.7 kg (−3 SD). His bone age was 5 years, with growth arrest lines visible. Serum thyroxine was 7.8 μg/dL. Peak serum GH varied from nondetectable to 8 ng/mL on different provocative tests between age 6 years and 8½ years. He was placed in a hospital chronic care facility **(arrow)** for a 6-month period and grew 9 cm, which projects to a yearly growth velocity of 18 cm. On repeat testing, the peak serum GH was 28 ng/mL

4. CUSHING'S SYNDROME

Excess glucocorticoids (either exogenous or endogenous) will lead to decreased growth before obesity and other signs of Cushing's syndrome develop. The underlying disease may be bilateral adrenal hyperplasia due to abnormal ACTH-cortisol regulation in Cushing's disease, autonomous adrenal adenomas, or adrenal carcinoma. The appropriate diagnosis may be missed if urinary cortisol and 17-hydroxycorticosteroid determinations are not interpreted on the basis of the child's body size or if inappropriate doses of dexamethasone are used for testing (appropriate doses are 20 mg/kg/d for the low-dose and 80 mg/kg/d for the high-dose dexamethasone suppres-

sion test) (see Chapter 9). Furthermore, daily variations in cortisol production necessitate several urinary or plasma cortisol determinations before Cushing's disease can be appropriately diagnosed or ruled out. Techniques for inferior petrosal sinus sampling are not routinely available in children, but are reported to be of great utility in the differential diagnosis of Cushing' disease versus alternative causes of Cushing' syndrome. CRH testing is not routinely available outside of clinical trials, but is also of use in differential diagnosis. The accuracy of various methods are: high dose dexamethasone test was positive in 68% of a recent series of children, CRH test in 80%, MRI of the pituitary in only 52% while the maximal central to peripheral ratio of plasma ACTH with inferior petrosal sampling was 100% accurate. Transsphenoidal microadenomectomy is the treatment of choice in Cushing's disease.

Exogenous glucocorticoids that suppress growth may be oral corticosteroids used to treat asthma or even overzealous use of topical corticosteroid ointments or creams. These iatrogenic cases of Cushing's syndrome, if resolved early, may allow catch-up growth and so may not affect final height. Thus, an accurate history of prior medications is important in diagnosis. Treatment of the underlying disorder (eg, transsphenoidal microadenomectomy for Cushing's disease) will restore growth rate to normal (catch-up growth may occur initially) if epiphysial fusion has not occurred, but final height will depend upon the length of the period of growth suppression.

5. PSEUDOHYPOPARATHYROIDISM

Pseudohypoparathyroidism is a rare disorder consisting of a characteristic phenotype and chemical signs of hypoparathyroidism (low serum Ca^{2+} and high serum PO_4^-), though circulating PTH levels are elevated and target tissues fail to respond to exogenous PTH administration. Children with pseudohypoparathyroidism are short and chubby, with characteristic round facies, short fourth and fifth metacarpals, and often developmental delay. A defect in the guanylyl nucleotide-sensitive regulatory protein that couples PTH-occupied receptors to adenylyl cyclase is the cause. Remarkably, this defect occurs in the same regulatory protein system affected in McCune-Albright syndrome, in which hyperactive endocrine events result (see Chapter 15). Thus, administration of PTH fails to induce a rise in nephrogenous cAMP or an increase in urinary phosphorus. A rarer variant of this disorder (pseudohypoparathyroidism type II), in which administration of PTH produces a rise in nephrogenous cAMP but fails to induce an increase in phosphorus excretion, appears to have a defect distal to the receptor-adenylyl cyclase complex. Treatment with high-dose vitamin D or physiologic replacement with 1,25-dihydroxyvitamin D_3 (calcitriol) and calcium-binding as well as phosphate-binding agents will correct the biochemical defects and control hypocalcemic seizures but will not improve stature or mentation.

Children with the pseudohypoparathyroid phenotype but with normal circulating levels of calcium, phosphate, and PTH have pseudopseudohypoparathyroidism. They require no calcium or vitamin D therapy. (See Chapter 8.) Two remarkable patients are reported with pseudohypoparathyroidism and premature Leydig cell maturation, both due to abnormalities in the same G protein. Because the abnormality was heat-sensitive, there was decreased activity in the kidneys and bones where the body temperature 36.7 °C while there was increased activity in the testes which were cooler due to the location in the scrotum.

6. DISORDERS OF VITAMIN D METABOLISM

Short stature and poor growth are features of rickets in its obvious or more subtle forms. The cause may be vitamin D deficiency due to inadequate oral intake, fat malabsorption, inadequate sunlight exposure, anticonvulsant therapy, or renal or hepatic disease. Classic findings of vitamin D deficiency rickets include bowing of the legs, chest deformities (rachitic rosary), and characteristic radiographic findings of the extremities associated with decreased serum calcium and phosphate levels and elevated serum alkaline phosphatase levels. Vitamin D dependency due to abnormalities of the receptor for vitamin D leading to decreased activity may be diagnosed when vitamin D is required in doses far higher than necessary to resolve vitamin D deficiency. Presently the most common cause of rickets in the US is X-linked hypophosphatemic rickets, a dominant genetic disorder of renal reabsorption of phosphate associated with short stature, severe and progressive bowing of the legs (but no changes in the wrists or chest), normal or slightly elevated serum Ca^{2+}, very low serum PO_4^- and urinary PO_4^- wasting. Short stature is associated with rickets in other renal disorders with hypophosphatemia due to a defect in renal reabsorption of phosphate; examples are Fanconi's syndrome (including cystinosis and other inborn errors of metabolism) and renal tubular acidosis.

When treatment is effective in these disorders (eg, vitamin D for vitamin D deficiency or alkali therapy for appropriate types of renal tubular acidosis), growth rate will improve. Vitamin D therapy and phosphate replacement is appropriate therapy for vitamin D resistant rickets which improves the bowing of the legs and leads to improved growth although there is a risk of nephrocalcinosis.

In the Williams syndrome of infantile hypercalcemia, elfin facies, supravalvular aortic stenosis, and mental retardation with gregarious personality, patients have intrauterine growth retardation and greatly reduced height in childhood and as adults; this disorder is no longer considered a disorder of vitamin D as a genetic defect at 7q11.23 occurs in most (see Chapters 8 and 15).

7. DIABETES MELLITUS

Growth in insulin-dependent diabetes mellitus depends on the efficacy of therapy; well-controlled diabetes mellitus is compatible with normal growth, while poorly controlled diabetes often causes slow growth. Another factor that may decrease growth rate in children with diabetes mellitus is the increased incidence of Hashimoto's thyroiditis; yearly thyroid function screening is advisable as the peripubertal period approaches. Liver and spleen enlargement in a poorly controlled short diabetic child is Mauriac's syndrome, rarely seen now owing to improved diabetic care. Growth hormone concentrations are higher in children with diabetes, and this factor may play a role in the development of complications of diabetes mellitus. IGF-1 concentrations tend to be normal or low, depending upon glucose control, but judging from the elevated GH, the stimulation of IGF-1 by GH is blocked in these children. (See Chapter 18.)

8. DIABETES INSIPIDUS

Polyuria and polydipsia due to inadequate vasopressin (neurogenic diabetes insipidus) or inability of the kidney to respond to vasopressin (nephrogenic diabetes insipidus) leads to poor caloric intake and decreased growth. With appropriate treatment (see Chapter 5), the growth rate should return to normal. Acquired neurogenic diabetes insipidus may herald a hypothalamic-pituitary tumor, and growth failure may be due to associated GH deficiency.

THE DIAGNOSIS OF SHORT STATURE

As previously stated, an initial decision must be made about whether a child is pathologically short or simply distressed because his or her height is not as close to the 50th percentile as desired by the patient or the parents. Performing unnecessary tests is expensive and may be a source of long-term concern to the parents—a concern that could have been avoided by appropriate reassurance. Alternatively, missing a diagnosis of pathologic poor growth may cause the patient to lose inches of final height.

If a patient's stature, growth rate, or height adjusted for midparental height is sufficiently decreased to warrant evaluation, an orderly approach to diagnosis will eliminate unnecessary laboratory testing. The medical history will provide invaluable information regarding intrauterine course and toxin exposure, birth size and the possibility of birth trauma, mental and physical development, symptoms of systemic diseases (Table 6–4), abnormal diet, and family heights and ages at which pubertal maturation occurred. Evaluation of psychosocial factors affecting the family and the relationship of parents and child can be carried out during the history-taking encounter. Often the diagnosis can be made at this point.

On physical examination, present height—measured without shoes on an accurate measuring device—and weight should be plotted and compared with any previous data available. If no past heights

are available, a history of lack of change in clothing and shoe sizes or failure to lengthen skirts or pants may reflect poor growth. Questions about how the child's stature compares with that of his or her peers and whether the child's height has always had the same relationship to that of classmates are useful. One of the most important features of the evaluation process is to determine height velocity and compare the child's growth rate with the normal growth rate for age. Adjustment for midparental height is calculated and nutritional status determined. Arm span, head circumference, and US:LS ratio are measured. Physical stigmas of syndromes or systemic diseases are evaluated. Neurologic examination is essential.

If no specific diagnosis emerges from the physical examination, a set of laboratory evaluations may prove useful. Complete blood count, urinalysis, and serum chemistry screening with electrolyte measurements may reveal anemia, abnormalities of hepatic or renal disease (including concentration defects), glucose intolerance, acidosis, calcium disorder, or other electrolyte disturbances. Age-adjusted values must be used, since the normal ranges of serum alkaline phosphatase and phosphorus values are higher in children than in adults. A sedimentation rate, serum carotene, or antigliadin antiendomesial, or antireticulin antibody determination may indicate connective tissue disease, Crohn's disease, or malabsorption. Determination of TSH, and free T_4 are important. Skeletal age evaluation will not make a diagnosis; however, if the study shows delayed bone age, the possibility of constitutional delay in growth, hypothyroidism, or GH deficiency must be considered. The tests used for the diagnosis of GH deficiency are detailed above. If serum IGF-1 is normal for age, classic GH deficiency or malnutrition is unlikely; if serum IGF-1 is low, it must be considered in relation to skeletal age, nutritional status, and general health status before interpretation of the value can be made. Serum IGFBP-3 may add to the evaluation of short stature. Serum gonadotropin and sex steroid determinations are performed if puberty is delayed. Serum prolactin may be elevated in cases of hypothalamic disorder. Karyotyping for Turner's syndrome is obtained in any short girl without another diagnosis, especially if puberty is delayed or gonadotropins are elevated. If Turner syndrome is diagnosed, evaluation of thyroid function and determination of thyroid antibodies is important. Elevated 24-hour urinary 17-hydroxycorticoids (normal, < 4.5 mg/m^2/24 h [12.4 mmol/m^2/24 h]) and urinary free cortisol (normal, < 60 mg/m^2/24 h [0.166 mmol/m^2]/24 h) signify Cushing's syndrome. If GH deficiency or impairment is found or if there is another hypothalamic-pituitary defect, an MRI is indicated with particular attention to the hypothalamic-pituitary area to rule out a congenital defect or neoplasm of the area. These noninvasive techniques are used more frequently than the previously utilized, invasive pneumoencephalograms. Ectopic location of the posterior pituitary is now shown to be relatively frequent in congenital GH deficiency, as is a decreased pituitary volume on MRI.

If no diagnosis is apparent after all of the above have been considered and evaluated, more detailed procedures, such as provocative testing for GH deficiency, are indicated. It must be emphasized that a long and expensive evaluation is not necessary until it is likely that psychologic or nutritional factors are not at fault. Likewise, if a healthy-appearing child presents with borderline short stature, normal growth rate, and short familial stature, a period of observation may be more appropriate than laboratory tests.

TALL STATURE DUE TO NONENDOCRINE CAUSES

1. CONSTITUTIONAL TALL STATURE

A subject who has been taller than his or her peers through most of childhood, is growing at a velocity within the normal range with a moderately advanced bone age, and has no signs of the disorders listed below may be considered to be constitutionally advanced. Predicted final height will usually be in the normal adult range for the family.

Exogenous obesity in an otherwise healthy child will usually lead to moderate advancement of bone age, slightly increased growth rate, and tall stature in childhood. Puberty will begin in the early range of normal, and adult stature will conform to genetic influences.

2. GENETIC TALL STATURE

Children with exceptionally tall parents have a genetic tendency to reach a height above the normal range. The child will be tall for age, will grow at a high normal rate, and the bone age will be close to chronologic age, leading to a tall height prediction. Children with tall stature have been noted to have growth hormone secretory patterns similar to those associated with acromegaly—eg, GH levels increase after TRH administration.

Occasionally, children will be concerned about being too tall as adults. These worries are more common in girls and will often be of greater concern to the parents than to the patient. Final height can be limited by promoting early epiphysial closure with estrogen in girls or testosterone in boys but such therapy should not be undertaken without careful consideration of the risks involved. Testosterone therapy decreases HDL cholesterol levels. Acne fulminans may be caused by testosterone therapy and progression may occur, even after therapy has been withdrawn. Estrogen carries the theoretic risk of causing

thrombosis, ovarian cysts, and galactorrhea, but few complications have been reported. High-dose estrogen therapy is estimated to decrease predicted final height by as much as 4.5–7 cm. Such therapy will be more effective if started 3–4 years before epiphysial fusion. Some studies suggest that bromocriptine will decrease growth rate in children with tall stature, but other studies have not confirmed this observation. No therapy to limit stature is warranted until a careful assessment of the parents' and the child's expectations and reasons for seeking therapy is performed. Counseling and reassurance are usually more appropriate than endocrine therapy. Height limiting therapy is extremely rarely invoked in the present era.

3. SYNDROMES OF TALL STATURE

Cerebral Gigantism

The sporadic syndrome of rapid growth in infancy, prominent forehead, high-arched palate, sharp chin, and hypertelorism (Sotos syndrome) is not associated with GH excess. Mentation is usually impaired. The growth rate decreases to normal in later childhood, but stature remains tall.

Marfan's Syndrome

Marfan's syndrome is an autosomal dominant abnormality of connective tissue exhibiting variable penetrance. This condition may be diagnosed by characteristic physical manifestations of tall stature, long thin fingers (arachnodactyly), hyperextension of joints, and superior lens subluxation. Pectus excavatum and scoliosis may be noted. Furthermore, aortic or mitral regurgitation or aortic root dilation may be present, and aortic dissection or rupture may ultimately occur. In patients with this syndrome, arm span exceeds height, and the US:LS ratio is quite low owing to long legs.

Homocystinuria

Patients with homocystinuria have an autosomal recessive deficiency of cystathionine β-synthetase and phenotypes similar to those of patients with Marfan's syndrome. Additional features of homocystinuria include mental retardation, increased incidence of seizures, osteoporosis, inferior lens dislocation, and increased urinary excretion of homocystine with increased plasma homocystine and methionine but low plasma cystine. Thromboembolic phenomena may precipitate a fatal complication. This disease is treated by restricting dietary methionine and, in responsive patients, administering pyridoxine.

Beckwith-Wiedemann Syndrome

A recent review of a large cohort of patients with Beckwith-Wiedemann syndrome indicated overweight (> 90th percentile) in 88%, increased postnatal growth, omphalocele in 80%, macroglossia in

97%, and hypoglycemia due to the hyperinsulinism of pancreatic hyperplasia in 63%. Other reported features include fetal adrenocortical cytomegaly, and large kidneys with medullary dysplasia. The majority of patients occur in a sporadic pattern, but analysis of pedegree suggest the possibilty of familial patterns.

XYY Syndrome

Patients with one (47,XYY) or more (48,XYYY) extra Y chromosomes achieve greater than average adult heights. They have normal birth lengths but higher than normal growth rates. Excess GH secretion has not been documented (see Chapter 14).

Klinefelter's Syndrome

Patients with Klinefelter's syndrome (see Chapter 15) tend toward tall stature, but this is not a constant feature.

TALL STATURE DUE TO ENDOCRINE DISORDERS

1. PITUITARY GIGANTISM

If a GH-secreting pituitary adenoma occurs before epiphysial fusion, the result will be excessive linear growth rather than just the acral overgrowth characteristic of acromegaly. Height velocity will be abnormally rapid, and other somatic signs that occur in acromegaly may be found in addition to increased stature (see Chapter 5). Elevated fasting serum GH and IGF-1 concentrations are diagnostic.

2. SEXUAL PRECOCITY

Early onset of secretion of estrogens or androgens will lead to abnormally increased height velocity. Because bone age is advanced, there will be the paradox of the tall child who, because of early epiphysial closure, is short as an adult. The conditions include complete and incomplete sexual precocity (including virilizing congenital adrenal hyperplasia) (Figures 6–9, 6–10, and 6–11).

3. THYROTOXICOSIS

Excessive thyroid hormone due to endogenous overproduction or overtreatment with exogenous thyroxine will lead to increased growth, advanced bone age, and, if occurring in early life, craniosynostosis. If the condition remains untreated, final height will be reduced.

4. INFANTS OF DIABETIC MOTHERS

Birth weight and size in infants of moderately diabetic mothers will be quite high, although severely diabetic women who have poor control may have babies with intrauterine growth retardation. Severe hypoglycemia and hypocalcemia will be evident in the babies soon after birth. The appearance and size of such babies is so striking that women have been diagnosed as having gestational diabetes as a result of giving birth to affected infants.

REFERENCES

Normal Growth

Hamill PVV et al: Physical growth: National Center for Health Statistics percentiles. Am J Clin Nutr 1979; 32:607.

Himes JH, Roche AF, Thissen D: *Parent-Specific Adjustments for Assessment of Recumbent Length and Stature.* Vol 13 of: *Monographs in Paediatrics.* Karger, 1981.

Juul A et al: Serum levels of insulin-like growth factor (IGF)-binding protein-3 (IGFBP-3) in healthy infants, children, and adolescents: The relation to IGF-I, IGF-II, IGFBP-1, IGFBP-2, age, sex, body mass index, and pubertal maturation. J Clin Endocrinol Metab 1995;80:2534.

Khamis HJ, Roche AF: Predicting adult stature without using skeletal age: The Khamis-Roche method. Pediatrics 1994;94:504.

Pierson M, Deschamps J-P: Growth. In: *Pediatric Endocrinology.* Job J-C, Pierson M (editors). Wiley, 1981.

Roche AF, Himes JH: Incremental growth charts. Am J Clin Nutr 1980;33:2041.

Roche AF, Wainer H, Thissen D: The RWT method for the prediction of adult stature. Pediatrics 1975;56: 1027.

Salo P et al: Deletion mapping of stature determinants on the long arm of the Y chromosome. Hum Genet 1995;95:283.

Styne DM: Growth. In: *Pediatric Endocrinology for the House Officer.* Williams & Wilkins, 1988.

Tanner JM, Whitehouse RH: Clinical longitudinal standards for height, weight, height velocity, weight velocity, and stages of puberty. Arch Dis Child 1976; 51: 170.

Thakrar A, Taylor EM, Wales JK: Height velocity screening: The real world. J Pub Health Med 1994; 16:200-204.

US Department of Health, Education, and Welfare, Public Health Service: NCHS Growth Curves for Children: Birth–18 Years, United States. Publication No. (PHS) 78–1650. Series 11, No. 165, 1977.

Short Stature

Appan S et al: Growth and growth hormone therapy in hypochondroplasia. Acta Paediatr Scand 1990;79:796.

Balsan S, Tieder M: Linear growth in patients with hypophosphatemic vitamin D-resistant rickets: Influence of treatment regimen and parental height. J Pediatr 1990;116:365.

Berg MA et al: Diverse growth hormone receptor gene mutations in Laron syndrome. Am J Hum Genet 1993;52:998.

Bosio L et al: Growth acceleration and final height after treatment for delayed diagnosis of celiac disease. J Pediatr Gastroenterol Nutr 1990;11:324.

Braga S et al: Familial growth hormone deficiency resulting from a 7.6 kb deletion within the growth hormone gene cluster. Am J Med Genet 1986;25:443.

Bridges N A, Brook CG:. Progress report: growth hormone in skeletal dysplasia. Horm Res 1994;42:231.

Brown P: Human growth hormone therapy and Creutzfeldt-Jakob disease: A drama in three acts. Pediatrics 1988;81:85.

Buzi F et al: Overnight growth hormone secretion in short children: independence of the sleep pattern. J Clin Endocrinol Metab 1993;77:1495.

Byard PJ: The adolescent growth spurt in children with cystic fibrosis. Ann Hum Biol 1994;21:229.

Carlsson LM: Reduced concentration of serum growth hormone-binding protein in children with idiopathic short stature. National Cooperative Growth Study. J Clin Endocrinol Metab 1994;78:1325.

Clarren SK, Smith DW: The fetal alcohol syndrome. N Engl J Med 1978;298:1063.

Cole TJ: Do growth chart centiles need a face lift? BMJ 1994;308:641.

Davies UM et al: Treatment of growth retardation in juvenile chronic arthritis with recombinant human growth hormone. J Rheumatol 1994;21:153.

de Muinck K et al: Dose-response study of biosynthetic human growth hormone (GH) in GH-deficient children: Effects on auxological and biochemical parameters. Dutch Growth Hormone Working Group. J Clin Endocrinol Metab 1992;74:898.

Favier AE: Hormonal effects of zinc on growth in children. Biol Trace Elem Res 1992;32:383.

Fine RN et al: Growth after recombinant human growth hormone treatment in children with chronic renal failure: report of a multicenter randomized double-blind placebo-controlled study. Genentech Cooperative Study Group. J Pediatr 1994;124:374.

Griffiths AM et al: Growth and clinical course of children with Crohn's disease. Gut 1993;34:939.

Harris DA et al: Somatomedin-C in normal puberty and in true precocious puberty before and after treatment with a potent luteinizing hormone-releasing hormone agonist. J Clin Endocrinol Metab 1985;61:152.

Jones KL: *Smith's Recognizable Patterns of Human Malformation,* 4th ed. Saunders, 1988.

Kao PC, Matheny AP, Lang CA: Insulin-like growth factor-I comparisons in healthy twin children. J Clin Endocrinol Metab 1994;78:310.

Kaplan SL: Normal growth. In: *Rudolph's Pediatrics,* 20th ed. Rudolph AM, Hoffman JIE, Rudolph CD (editors). Appleton & Lange, 1996.

Karlberg J, Kjellmer I, Kristiansson B: Linear growth in children with cystic fibrosis. I. Birth to 8 years of age. Acta Paediatr Scand 1991;80:508.

Klein GL, Dungy CI, Galant SP: Growth and the nutritional status of nonsteroid-dependent asthmatic children. Ann Allergy 1991;67:80.

Klein RG, Mannuzza S: Hyperactive boys almost grown up: III. Methylphenidate effects on ultimate height. Arch Gen Psychiatry 1988;45:1131.

Laron Z et al: Effects of insulin-like growth factor on linear growth, head circumference, and body fat in patients with Laron-type dwarfism. Lancet 1992;339:1258.

Laron Z et al: Growth hormone releasing activity by intranasal administration of a synthetic hexapeptide (hexarelin). Clin Endocrinol (Oxf) 1994;41:539.

Levitsky LL: Growth and pubertal pattern in insulin-dependent diabetes mellitus. Semin Adolesc Med 1987;3:233.

Lindsay RM et al: Utah Growth Study: Growth standards and the prevalence of growth hormone deficiency. J Pediatr 1994;125:29.

Loder RT, Wittenberg B, DeSilva G: Slipped capital femoral epiphysis associated with endocrine disorders. J Pediatr Orthop 1995;15:349.

Longo N et al: Two mutations in the insulin receptor gene of a patient with leprechaunism: Application to prenatal diagnosis. J Clin Endocrinol Metab 1995;80:1496.

Magiakou MA et al: Cushing's syndrome in children and adolescents. Presentation, diagnosis, and therapy. N Engl J Med 1994;331:629.

Mandel S et al: Changes in insulin-like growth factor-I (IGF-I), IGF-binding protein-3, growth hormone (GH)-binding protein, erythrocyte IGF-I receptors, and growth rate during GH treatment. J Clin Endocrinol Metab 1995;80:190.

Matarazzo P et al: Growth impairment, IGF I hyposecretion and thyroid dysfunction in children with perinatal HIV-1 infection. Acta Paediatr 1994;83:1029.

Nishi Y et al: Treatment of isolated growth hormone deficiency type IA due to *GH-I* gene deletion with recombinant human insulin-like growth factor I. Acta Paediatr 1993;82:983.

Oberger E, Engstrom I, Karlberg J: Long-term treatment with glucocorticoids/ACTH in asthmatic children: III. Effects on growth and adult height. Acta Paediatr Scand 1990;79:77.

Okabe T et al: Growth-promoting effect of human growth hormone on patients with achondroplasia. Acta Paediatr Jpn 1991;33:357.

Roe F, Kaufman FR: Review of slipped capital femoral epiphysis associated with endocrine disease. J Pediatr Orthop 13:610.

Rosenfeld RG, Rosenbloom AL, Guevara Aguirre J: Growth hormone (GH) insensitivity due to primary GH receptor deficiency. Endocrine Reviews, 1994;15:369.

Rosenfeld RG et al. Six year results of a randomized, prospective trial of human growth hormone and oxandrolone in Turner syndrome. J Pediatr 1992;121:49.

Saavedra JM et al: Longitudinal assessment of growth in children born to mothers with human immunodeficiency virus infection. Arch Pediatr Adolesc Med 1995;149:497.

Sandberg DE, Brook AE, Campos SP: Short stature: a psychosocial burden requiring growth hormone therapy? Pediatrics 1994;94:832.

Sanders JE et al: Growth and development following marrow transplantation for leukemia. Blood 1986; 68:1129.

Schaefer GB et al: Lipids and apolipoproteins in growth hormone-deficient children during treatment. Metabolism 1994;43:1457.

Sklar C et al: Final height after treatment for childhood acute lymphoblastic leukemia: Comparison of no cranial irradiation with 1800 and 2400 centigrays of cranial irradiation. J Pediatr 1993;123:59.

Smith WJ et al: Use of insulin-like growth factor-binding protein-2 (IGFBP-2), IGFBP-3, and IGF-I for assessing growth hormone status in short children. J Clin Endocrinol Metab 1993;77:1294.

Stevenson RD: Use of segmental measures to estimate stature in children with cerebral palsy. Arch Pediatr Adolesc Med 1995;149:658.

Styne DM et al: Treatment of Cushing's disease in childhood and adolescence by transsphenoidal microadenomectomy. N Engl J Med 1984;310:889.

Tanner JM, Lejarraga H, Cameron N: The natural history of the Silver-Russell syndrome: A longitudinal study of thirty-nine cases. Pediatr Res 1975; 9:611.

Thomas AG et al: Insulin like growth factor-I, insulin like growth factor binding protein-1, and insulin in childhood Crohn's disease. Gut 1993;34:944-947.

Towne B et al: Genetic analysis of patterns of growth in infant recumbent length. Hum Biol 1993;65:977.

Underwood LE, Van Wyk JJ: Normal and aberrant growth. In: *Williams Textbook of Endocrinology,* 8th ed. Wilson JD, Foster DW (editors). Saunders, 1992.

Tall Stature

Conte FA, Grumbach MM: Epidemiological aspects of estrogen use: Estrogen use in children and adolescents: A survey. Pediatrics 1978;62(Suppl):1091.

Costin G, Fefferman RA, Kogut MD: Hypothalamic gigantism. J Pediatr 1973;83:419.

Elliott MR et al: Clinical features and natural history of Beckwith-Wiedemann syndrome: presentation of 74 new cases. Clin Genet 1994;46:168.

Karlberg J, Wit JM: Linear growth in Sotos syndrome. Acta Paediatr Scand 1991;80:956.

7

The Thyroid Gland

Francis S. Greenspan, MD

The thyroid gland is the largest organ specialized for endocrine function in the human body. Its function is to secrete a sufficient amount of thyroid hormones, primarily 3,5,3′,5′-*l*-tetraiodothyronine (T_4), and a lesser quantity of 3,5,3′-*l*-triiodothyronine (T_3). Thyroid hormones promote normal growth and development and regulate a number of homeostatic functions, including energy and heat production. In addition, the parafollicular cells of the human thyroid gland secrete calcitonin, which is important in calcium homeostasis (Chapter 8).

ANATOMY & HISTOLOGY

The thyroid gland originates as an outpouching in the floor of the pharynx, which grows downward anterior to the trachea, bifurcates, and forms a series of cellular cords. These form tiny balls or follicles and develop into the two lateral lobes of the thyroid connected by a thin isthmus. The origin of the gland at the base of the tongue is evident as the foramen cecum. The course of its downward migration is marked by the **thyroglossal duct,** remnants of which may persist in adult life as thyroglossal duct cysts. These are mucus-filled cysts, lined with squamous epithelium, and are usually found in the anterior neck between the thyroid cartilage and the base of the tongue. A remnant of the caudal end of the thyroglossal duct is found in the pyramidal lobe, attached to the isthmus of the gland (Figure 7–1).

The isthmus of the thyroid gland is located just below the cricoid cartilage, midway between the apex of the thyroid cartilage ("Adam's apple") and the suprasternal notch. Each lobe is pear-shaped and measures about 2.5–4 cm in length, 1.5–2 cm in width, and 1–1.5 cm in thickness. The weight of the gland in the normal individual, as determined by ultrasonic examination, varies depending on dietary iodine intake, age, and body weight, but in adults is approximately 10–20 g. Upward growth of the thyroid

ACRONYMS USED IN THIS CHAPTER	
DIT	Diiodotyrosine
ELISA	Enzyme linked immunoassay
FNAB	Fine-needle aspiration biopsy
FT_4	Free thyroxine
FT_4I	Free thyroxine index
GRTH	Generalized resistance to thyroid hormone
hTg	Human thyroglobulin
hTR	Human thyroid hormone receptor
IP_3	Inositol 1,4,5-trisphosphate
LATS	Long-acting thyroid stimulator (TSH-R Ab [stim])
MIT	Monoiodotyrosine
PBI	Protein-bound iodine
PIP_2	Phosphatidylinositol 4,5-bisphosphate
PRTH	Pituitary resistance to thyroid hormone
RAIU	Radioactive iodide uptake
RER	Rough endoplasmic reticulum
RIA	Radioimmunoassay
rT_3	Reverse T_3; 3,3′,5′-triiodothyronine
T_4	Tetraiodothyronine, levothyroxine
T_3	3,5,3′-Triiodothyronine, liothyronine
T_2	Diiodothyronine
TRH	Thyrotropin-releasing hormone
TBG	Thyroxine-binding globulin
TBP	Thyroxine-binding protein
TBPA	Thyroxine-binding prealbumin; transthyretin
TBII	Thyrotropin binding inhibiting immune globulin
THBR	Thyroid hormone binding ratio
Tg	Thyroglobulin
TPO	Thyroid peroxidase
TRE	Thyroid hormone response element
TSH	Thyroid-stimulating hormone, thyrotropin
TSH-R	TSH receptor
TSH-R Ab [stim]	TSH receptor-stimulating antibody
TSH-R Ab [block]	TSH receptor-blocking antibody

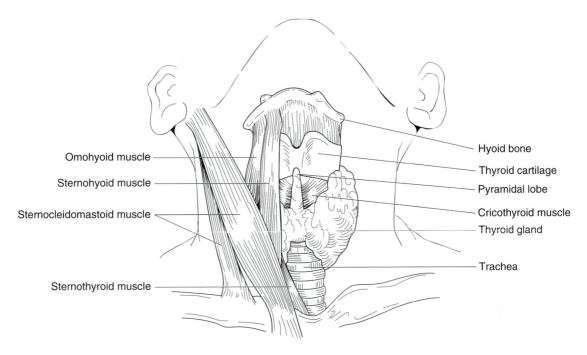

Figure 7–1. Gross anatomy of the human thyroid gland (anterior view).

gland is limited by the attachment of the sternothyroid muscle to the thyroid cartilage; however, posterior and downward growth is unhampered, so that thyroid enlargement, or goiter, will frequently extend posteriorly and inferiorly, or even substernally.

Transverse section of the neck at the level of the thyroid isthmus shows the relationships of the thyroid gland to the trachea, esophagus, carotid artery, and jugular vein (Figure 7–2). Ultrasonography, CT scans, or MRI reveal these relationships in vivo.

The thyroid gland has a rich blood supply (Figure 7–3). The superior thyroid artery arises from the common or external carotid artery, the inferior thyroid artery from the thyrocervical trunk of the subclavian artery, and the small thyroid ima artery from the brachiocephalic artery at the aortic arch. Venous

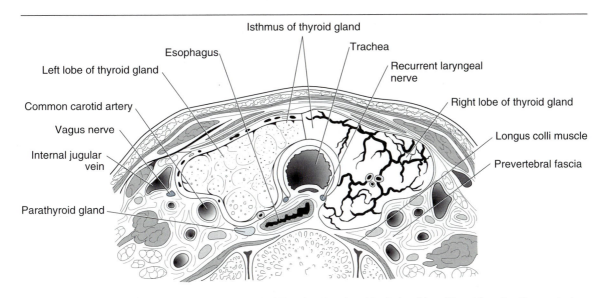

Figure 7–2. Cross section of the neck at the level of T1, showing thyroid relationships. (Reproduced, with permission, from Lindner HH: *Clinical Anatomy.* Appleton & Lange, 1989.)

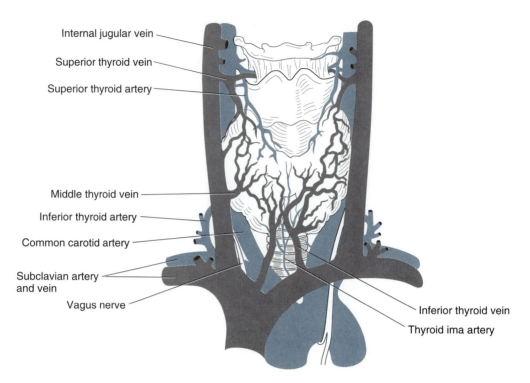

Figure 7–3. Arteries and veins related to the thyroid gland. (Reproduced, with permission, from Lindner HH: *Clinical Anatomy.* Appleton & Lange, 1989.)

drainage is via multiple surface veins coalescing into superior, lateral, and inferior thyroid veins. The blood flow to the thyroid gland is about 5 mL/g/min; in hyperthyroidism, the blood flow to the gland is markedly increased, and a whistling sound, or bruit, may be heard over the lower poles of the gland and may even be felt in the same areas as a vibration, or thrill. Other important anatomic considerations include the two pairs of parathyroid glands that usually lie behind the upper and middle thyroid lobes and the recurrent laryngeal nerves, which course along the trachea behind the thyroid gland.

On microscopic examination, the thyroid gland is found to consist of a series of follicles of varying sizes. The follicles contain a pink-staining material (with hematoxylin-eosin stain) called "colloid" and are surrounded by a single layer of thyroid epithelium. Tissue culture studies suggest that each follicle may represent an individual clone of cells. These cells become columnar when stimulated by TSH and flattened when resting (Figure 7–4). The follicle cells synthesize thyroglobulin, which is extruded into the lumen of the follicle. The biosynthesis of T_4 and T_3 occurs within thyroglobulin at the cell-colloid interface. Numerous microvilli project from the surface of the follicle into the lumen; these are involved in endocytosis of thyroglobulin, which is then hydrolyzed in the cell to release thyroid hormones (Figure 7–5).

PHYSIOLOGY

STRUCTURE OF THYROID HORMONES

Thyroid hormones are unique in that they contain 59–65% of the trace element iodine. The structures of the thyroid hormones, T_4 and T_3, are shown in Figure 7–6. The iodinated thyronines are derived from iodination of the phenolic rings of tyrosine residues in thyroglobulin to form mono- or diiodotyrosine, which are coupled to form T_3 or T_4 (see below).

IODINE METABOLISM

Iodine* enters the body in food or water in the form of iodide or iodate ion, the iodate ion being converted to iodide in the stomach. In the course of millenia, iodine has been leached from the soil and washed down into the oceans, so that in mountainous

---

*In this chapter, the words "iodine" and "iodide" are used interchangeably.

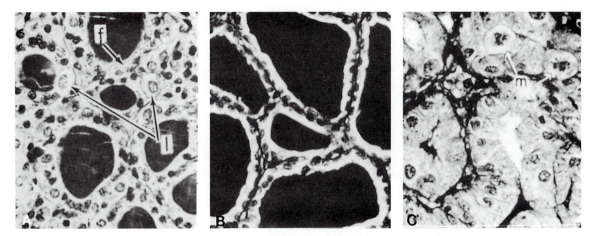

Figure 7–4. **A:** Normal rat thyroid. A single layer of cuboidal epithelial cells surrounds PAS-positive material in the follicular space (colloid). The larger, lighter-staining cells indicated by the arrows (l) are C cells that produce calcitonin. (F, follicular cells.) **B:** Inactive rat thyroid several weeks after hypophysectomy. The follicular lumens are larger and the follicular cells flatter. **C:** Rat thyroid under intensive TSH stimulation. The animal was fed an iodine-deficient diet and injected with propylthiouracil for several weeks. Little colloid is visible. The follicular cells are tall and columnar. Several mitoses (m) are visible. (Reproduced, with permission, from Halmi NS in: *Histology.* Greep R0, Weiss L [editors]. McGraw-Hill, 1973.)

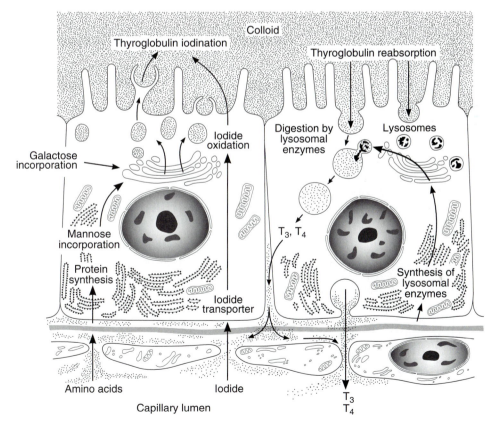

Figure 7–5. Processes of synthesis and iodination of thyroglobulin (left) and its reabsorption and digestion (right). These events occur in the same cell. (Reproduced, with permission, from Junqueira LC, Carneiro J, Kelley R: *Basic Histology,* 7th ed. Appleton & Lange, 1992.)

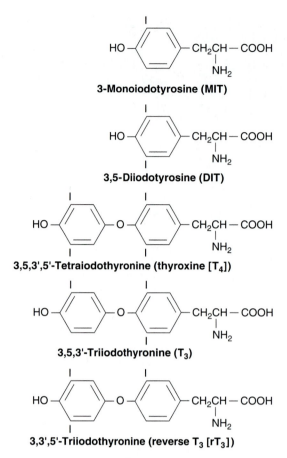

Figure 7–6. Structure of thyroid hormones and related compounds. (Reproduced, with permission, from Murray RK et al: *Harper's Biochemistry*, 24th ed, Appleton & Lange, 1996.)

tric, and breast secretions. Although the concentration of inorganic iodide in the extracellular fluid pool will vary directly with iodide intake, extracellular fluid I^- is usually quite low because of the rapid clearance of iodide from extracellular fluid by thyroidal uptake and renal clearance. In the example shown, the I^- concentration in extracellular fluid is 0.6 µg/dL, or a total of 150 µg of I^- in an extracellular pool of 25 L. In the thyroid gland, there is active transport of I^- from the serum across the basement membrane of the thyroid cell (see below). The thyroid takes up about 115 µg of I^- per 24 hours; about 75 µg of I^- is utilized for hormone synthesis and stored in thyroglobulin; the remainder leaks back into the extracellular fluid pool. The thyroid pool of organified iodine is very large, averaging 8–10 mg, and represents a store of hormone and iodinated tyrosines protecting the organism against a period of iodine lack. From this storage pool, about 75 µg of hormonal iodide is released into the circulation daily. This hormonal iodide is mostly bound to serum thyroxine-binding proteins, forming a circulating pool of about 600 µg of hormonal I^- (as T_3 and T_4). From this pool, about 75 µg of I^- as T_3 and T_4 is taken up and metabolized by tissues. About 60 µg of I^- is returned to the iodide pool and about 15 µg of hormonal I^- is conjugated with glucuronide or sulfate in the liver and excreted into the stool. Since most of the dietary iodide is excreted in the urine, 24-hour urinary iodide is an excellent index of dietary intake. The 24-hour radioactive iodine uptake (RAIU) by the thyroid gland is inversely proportionate to the size of the inorganic iodide pool and directly proportionate to thyroidal activity. Typical RAIU curves are shown in Figure 7–8. In the USA, the 24-hour thyroidal radioiodine uptake has decreased from about 40–50% in the 1960s to about 8–30% in the 1990s because of increased dietary iodide intake.

THYROID HORMONE SYNTHESIS & SECRETION

The synthesis of T_4 and T_3 by the thyroid gland involves six major steps: (1) active transport of I^- across the basement membrane into the thyroid cell (trapping of iodide); (2) oxidation of iodide and iodination of tyrosyl residues in thyroglobulin; (3) coupling of iodotyrosine molecules within thyroglobulin to form T_3 and T_4; (4) proteolysis of thyroglobulin, with release of free iodothyronines and iodotyrosines; (5) deiodination of iodotyrosines within the thyroid cell, with conservation and reuse of the liberated iodide, and (6) under certain circumstances, intrathyroidal 5'-deiodination of T_4 to T_3.

Thyroid hormone synthesis involves a unique glycoprotein, thyroglobulin, and an essential enzyme, thyroid peroxidase (TPO). This process is summarized in Figure 7–9.

and inland areas the supply of iodine may be quite limited, whereas the element is plentiful in coastal areas. The thyroid gland concentrates and traps iodide and synthesizes and stores thyroid hormones in thyroglobulin, which compensates for the scarcity of iodine.

The recommended intake of iodine is 150 µg/d; if intake is below 50 µg/d, the gland is unable to maintain adequate hormonal secretion, and thyroid hypertrophy (goiter) and hypothyroidism result. In the United States, the average daily intake of iodine increased from a range of 100–200 µg/d in the 1960s to 240–740 µg/d in the 1980s, largely owing to the introduction of iodate as a bread preservative. Other sources of dietary iodine include iodized salt, vitamin preparations, iodine-containing medications, and iodinated contrast media. An approximation of iodine turnover in subjects on this high-iodine diet is depicted in Figure 7–7. Iodide, like chloride, is rapidly absorbed from the gastrointestinal tract and distributed in extracellular fluids as well as in salivary, gas-

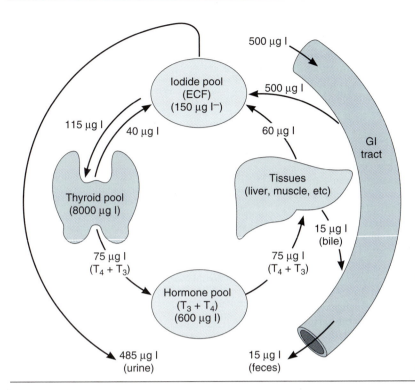

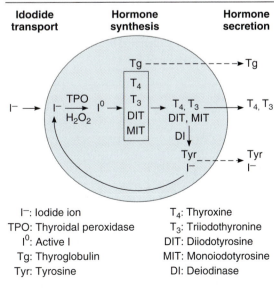

Figure 7–7. Iodine metabolism. The values indicated are representative of those that might be found in a healthy subject ingesting 500 μg of iodine a day. The actual iodine intake varies considerably among different individuals.

Thyroglobulin

Thyroglobulin is a large glycoprotein molecule containing 5496 amino acids, with a molecular weight of about 660,000 and a sedimentation coefficient of 19S. It contains about 140 tyrosyl residues and about 10% carbohydrate in the form of mannose, N-acetylglucosamine, galactose, fucose, sialic acid, and chondroitin sulfate. The 19S thyroglobulin compound is a dimer of two identical 12S subunits, but small amounts of the 12S monomer and a 27S tetramer are often present. The iodine content of the molecule can vary from 0.1% to 1% by weight. In thyroglobulin containing 0.5% iodine (26 atoms of iodine per 660-kDa molecule), there would be 5 mol-

ecules of monoiodotyrosine (MIT), 4.5 molecules of diiodotyrosine (DIT), 2.5 molecules of thyroxine (T_4), and 0.7 molecules of triiodothyronine (T_3). About 75% of the thyroglobulin monomer consists of repetitive domains with no hormonogenic sites. There are four tyrosyl sites for hormonogenesis on the thyroglobulin molecule: One site is located at the

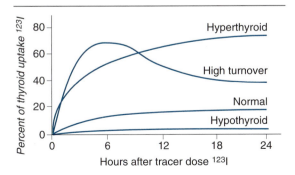

Figure 7–8. Typical curves of 24-hour radioiodine uptake in normal subjects and in patients with thyroid disease.

Iodide transport	Hormone synthesis	Hormone secretion

I⁻: Iodide ion
TPO: Thyroidal peroxidase
I⁰: Active I
Tg: Thyroglobulin
Tyr: Tyrosine

T_4: Thyroxine
T_3: Triiodothyronine
DIT: Diiodotyrosine
MIT: Monoiodotyrosine
DI: Deiodinase

Figure 7–9. Thyroid hormone synthesis in a thyroid follicle.

amino-terminal end of the molecule, and the other three are located in a sequence of 600 amino acids at the carboxyl terminal end. There is a surprising homology between this area of the thyroglobulin molecule and the structure of acetylcholinesterase, suggesting conservation in the evolution of these proteins.

The human thyroglobulin (*hTg*) gene lies on the long arm of chromosome 8 distal to the c-*myc* oncogene. TSH stimulates the transcription of the thyroglobulin gene, and hypophysectomy or T_3 therapy decreases its transcription. The thyroglobulin gene contains about 8500 nucleotides, which encode the prethyroglobulin (pre-Tg) monomer. The pre-thyroglobulin monomer contains a 19-amino-acid signal peptide, followed by a 2750-amino-acid chain that constitutes the thyroglobulin monomer. The mRNA is translated in the rough endoplasmic reticulum, and thyroglobulin chains are glycosylated during transport to the Golgi apparatus (Figure 7–5). In the Golgi apparatus, the thyroglobulin dimers are incorporated into exocytotic vesicles that fuse with the basement membrane and release the thyroglobulin into the follicular lumen. There, at the apical-colloid border, tyrosinases within thyroglobulin are iodinated and stored in colloid (Figure 7–10).

Thyroidal Peroxidase

Thyroidal peroxidase is a membrane-bound glycoprotein with a molecular weight of about 102,000 and a heme compound as the prosthetic group of the enzyme. This enzyme mediates both the oxidation of iodide ions and the incorporation of iodine into tyrosine residues of thyroglobulin. Thyroidal peroxidase is synthesized in the rough endoplasmic reticulum (RER). After insertion into the membrane of its cisternae, it is transferred to the apical cell surface by Golgi elements and exocytic vesicles. Here, at the cell colloid interface, it is available for iodination and hormonogenesis in thyroglobulin. Thyroidal peroxidase biosynthesis is stimulated by TSH.

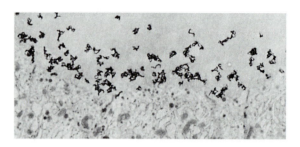

Figure 7–10. Evidence that iodination of thyroglobulin occurs at or near the apical (follicular) border of the thyroid cell. The figure depicts electronmicroscopic autoradiography of part of a rat thyroid cell 30–40 seconds after administration of sodium ^{125}I to the animal in vivo. The radioactive iodine is represented on a photographic emulsion layer by the silver grains. Few radioactive iodine molecules are localized over the thyroid cell itself, but there are many at the junction of the thyroid cell and the follicular colloid. (× 7000.) (Reproduced, with permission, from Ekholm R: *Endocrinology.* DeGroot LJ et al [editors]. Grune & Stratton, 1979.)

Iodide Transport (the Iodide Trap)

I^- is transported across the basement membrane of the thyroid cell by an intrinsic membrane protein called the Na^+/I^- symporter. The energy released by the inward movement of sodium drives the I^- transport process; this energy is generated by the activation of the Na^+-K^+ ATPase (Figure 7–11). This active transport system allows the human thyroid gland to maintain a concentration of free iodide 30–40 times that in plasma. The thyroiodide trap is markedly stimulated by TSH and by TSH receptor stimulating antibody (TSH-R Ab [stim]) found in Graves' disease. It is saturable with large amounts of I^- and inhibited by ions such as ClO_4^-, SCN^-, NO_3^-, and TcO_4^-. Some of these ions have clinical utility. Potassium perchlorate has been used clinically with ^{123}I to demonstrate

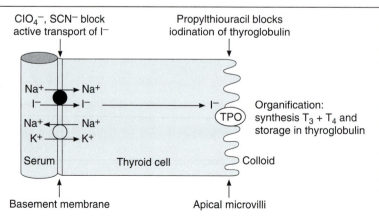

Figure 7–11. The iodide transporter in the thyroid cell. The large solid circle represents the Na^+/I^- symporter actively transporting I^- into the cell; the large open circle represents Na^+-K^+ ATPase supplying the energy for the reaction while transporting Na^+ out of the cell. I^- diffuses across the cell to the apical microvilli, where organification and hormone synthesis take place in the colloid at the colloid-apical membrane, catalyzed by thyroidal peroxidase (TPO).

organification defects in the thyroid gland; it will displace and allow the discharge of nonorganified I^- from the iodide trap (Figure 7–12). Potassium perchlorate and potassium thiocyanate have been used to treat iodide-induced hyperthyroidism; both discharge I^- from the trap and prevent further I^- uptake. Sodium pertechnetate Tc 99m, which has a 6-hour half-life and a 140-keV gamma emission, is used for rapid visualization of the thyroid for size and functioning nodules. Although I^- is concentrated by salivary, gastric, and breast tissue, these tissues do not organify or store I^- and are not stimulated by TSH.

Iodination of Tyrosyl in Thyroglobulin

Within the thyroid cell, at the cell-colloid interface, iodide is rapidly oxidized by H_2O_2, catalyzed by thyroperoxidase, and converted to an active intermediate which is incorporated into tyrosyl residues in thyroglobulin. H_2O_2 is probably generated by a dihydronicotinamide adenine dinucleotide phosphate (NADPH) oxidase in the presence of Ca^{2+}; this process is stimulated by TSH. The iodinating intermediate may be iodinium ion (I^+), hypoiodate, or an iodine-free radical. The site of iodination at the apical (colloid) border of the thyroid cell can be demonstrated by autoradiography (Figure 7–10).

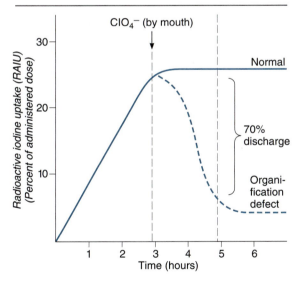

Figure 7–12. Perchlorate discharge of thyroidal inorganic iodine. Two to 3 hours after administration of a tracer dose of radioactive iodide, perchlorate is administered orally, blocking further active transport of iodide into the thyroid cell. In the normal subject (solid line), no significant decrease in radioactivity is detectable over the thyroid gland. In the representative example shown by the dashed line, there is a significant discharge of thyroidal iodide, indicating that iodide organification has been incomplete. (ClO_4^-, perchlorate.)

Thyroidal peroxidase will catalyze iodination of tyrosyl molecules in proteins other than thyroglobulin, such as albumin or thyroglobulin fragments. However, no thyroactive hormones are formed in these proteins. The metabolically inactive protein may be released into the circulation, draining thyroidal iodide reserves.

Coupling of Iodotyrosyl Residues in Thyroglobulin

The coupling of iodotyrosyl residues in thyroglobulin is also catalyzed by thyroidal peroxidase. It is thought that this is an intramolecular mechanism involving three steps: (1) oxidation of iodotyrosyl residues to an activated form by thyroidal peroxidase; (2) coupling of activated iodotyrosyl residues within the same thyroglobulin molecule to form a quinol ether intermediate; and (3) splitting of the quinol ether to form iodothyronine, with conversion of the alanine side chain of the donor iodotyrosine to dehydroalanine (Figure 7–13). For this process to occur, the dimeric structure of thyroglobulin is essential: Within the thyroglobulin molecule, two molecules of DIT may couple to form T_4, and an MIT and a DIT molecule may couple to form T_3. Thiocarbamide drugs—particularly propylthiouracil, methimazole, and carbimazole—are potent inhibitors of thyroidal peroxidase and will block thyroid hormone synthesis (Figure 7–14). These drugs are clinically useful in the management of hyperthyroidism.

Proteolysis of Thyroglobulin & Thyroid Hormone Secretion

The pattern of proteolysis of thyroglobulin and secretion of thyroid hormones is illustrated in Figure 7–5. Lysosomal enzymes are synthesized by the rough endoplasmic reticulum and packaged by the Golgi apparatus into lysosomes. These structures, surrounded by membrane, have an acidic interior and are filled with proteolytic enzymes, including proteases, endopeptidases, glycoside hydrolyases, phosphatases, and other enzymes. At the cell-colloid interface, colloid is engulfed into a colloid vesicle by a process of macropinocytosis or micropinocytosis and is absorbed into the thyroid cell. The lysosomes then fuse with the colloid vesicle and hydrolysis of thyroglobulin occurs, releasing T_4, T_3, DIT, MIT, peptide fragments, and amino acids. T_3 and T_4 are released into the circulation, while DIT and MIT are deiodinated and the I^- is conserved. Thyroglobulin with a low iodine content is hydrolyzed more rapidly than thyroglobulin with a high iodine content, which may be beneficial in geographic areas where natural iodine intake is low. The mechanism of transport of T_3 and T_4 through the thyroid cell is not known, but it may involve a specific hormone carrier. Thyroid hormone secretion is stimulated by TSH, which activates adenylyl cyclase, and by the cAMP analog

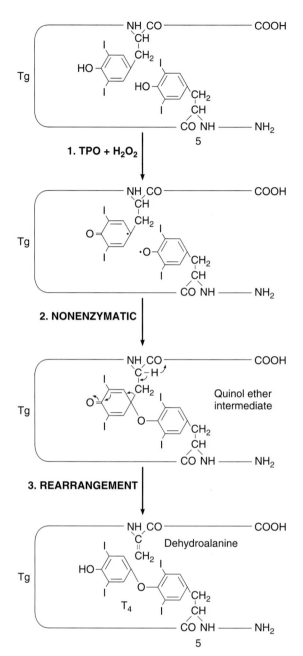

Figure 7–13. Hypothetical coupling scheme for intramolecular formation of T_4 within the thyroglobulin molecule. The major hormonogenic site at tyrosyl residue 5 is indicated. (Reproduced, with permission, from Taurog A: Thyroid hormone synthesis. Thyroid iodine metabolism. In: *Werner and Ingbar's The Thyroid,* 6th ed. Braverman LE, Utiger RD [editors]. Lippincott, 1991.)

(Bu)$_2$cAMP, suggesting that it is cAMP-dependent. Thyroglobulin proteolysis is inhibited by excess iodide (see below) and by lithium, which, as lithium carbonate, is used for the treatment of bipolar disorders. A small amount of unhydrolyzed thyroglobulin is also released from the thyroid cell; this is markedly increased in certain situations such as subacute thyroiditis, hyperthyroidism, or TSH-induced goiter (Figure 7–9). Thyroglobulin (perhaps modified) may also be synthesized and released by certain thyroid malignancies such as papillary or follicular thyroid cancer and may be useful as a marker for metastatic disease.

Intrathyroidal Deiodination

MIT and DIT formed during the synthesis of thyroid hormone are deiodinated by intrathyroidal deiodinase (Figure 7–9). This enzyme is a an NADPH-dependent flavoprotein found in mitochondria and microsomes. It acts on MIT and DIT but not on T_3 and T_4. The iodide released is mostly reutilized for hormone synthesis; a small amount leaks out of the thyroid into the body pool (Figure 7–7). The 5′-deiodinase that converts T_4 to T_3 in peripheral tissues is also found in the thyroid gland. In situations of iodide deficiency, the activity of this enzyme may increase the amount of T_3 secreted by the thyroid gland, increasing the metabolic efficiency of hormone synthesis.

ABNORMALITIES IN THYROID HORMONE SYNTHESIS & RELEASE

Inherited Metabolic Defects (Dyshormonogenesis)

Inherited metabolic defects may involve any phase of hormonal biosynthesis. These result in "dyshormonogenesis," or impaired hormonal synthesis. Patients present with thyroid enlargement, or goiter, mild to severe hypothyroidism, low serum T_3 and T_4, and elevated serum TSH. The defects are described in more detail in the section on nontoxic goiter, below.

Effect of Iodide Deficiency on Hormone Biosynthesis

A diet very low in iodine reduces intrathyroidal iodine content, increases the intrathyroidal ratio of MIT to DIT, increases the ratio of T_3 to T_4, decreases the secretion of T_4, and increases serum TSH. In the adult, this results in goiter, with a high iodine uptake and mild to severe hypothyroidism; in the neonate, it may result in cretinism (see below). The adaptations that occur involve the increased synthesis of T_3 relative to T_4 and the increased intrathyroidal 5′-deiodination of T_4 to T_3 to produce a more active hormone mixture.

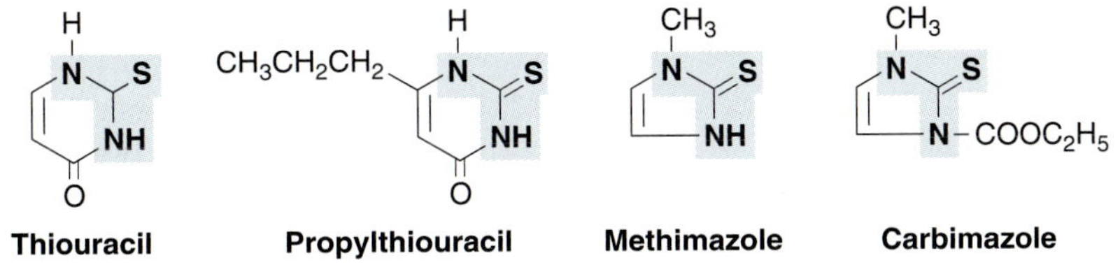

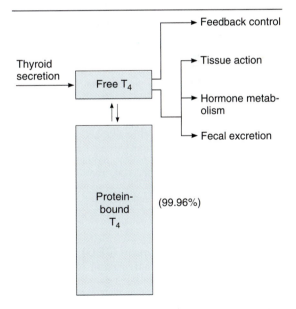

Figure 7–14. Thiocarbamide inhibitors of thyroidal iodide organification.

Effect of Iodine Excess on Hormone Biosynthesis

Increasing doses of iodide given to iodide-deficient rats initially induce increased iodide organification and hormone formation until a critical level is reached. At that point, inhibition of organification occurs and hormonogenesis decreases. This **Wolff-Chaikoff effect** (Figure 7–15) is probably due to inhibition of H_2O_2 generation by the high intrathyroidal I^- content. The most striking observation was that the effect is transient and that the normal thyroid gland "escapes" from the I^- effect. This is due to inhibition of the trapping of I^- with reduction in intrathyroidal iodide, allowing hormonogenesis to proceed. If the gland is unable to make this adaptation—as may occur in patients with autoimmune thyroiditis or in some patients with dyshormonogenesis—iodide-induced hypothyroidism will ensue. In some patients, an iodide load will induce hyperthyroidism ("jodbasedow" effect). This may develop in patients with latent Graves' disease, in those with multinodular goiters, or occasionally in those with previously normal thyroid glands.

THYROID HORMONE TRANSPORT

Thyroid hormones are transported in serum bound to carrier proteins. Although only 0.04% of T_4 and 0.4% of T_3 are "free," it is the free fraction that is responsible for hormonal activity (Figure 7–16). There are three major thyroid hormone transport proteins: thyroxine-binding globulin (TBG); thyroxine-binding prealbumin (TBPA), or transthyretin; and albumin (Figure 7–17).

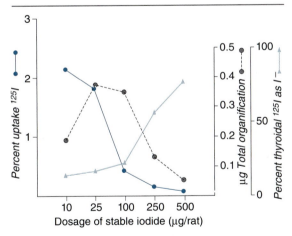

Figure 7–15. The Wolff-Chaikoff block. As increasing doses of iodide are administered to rats, there is an initial increase in iodide organification. At a critical concentration, however, higher doses of iodide given to the animals block iodide organification. The effect of increasing doses of iodide on thyroid hormone synthesis is therefore biphasic. Concomitantly with the increase in the organification block, the intracellular inorganic iodide concentration rises. As the amount of stable iodide injected is increased, there is a decrease in thyroidal uptake of radioactive iodide. (Reproduced, with permission, from DeGroot LJ, Stanbury JB: *The Thyroid and Its Diseases,* 4th ed. Wiley, 1975.)

Figure 7–16. Representation of free T_4 (and free T_3) as the biologically active hormone at the level of the pituitary and the peripheral tissues. Most of the thyroid hormones circulating in plasma are protein-bound and have no biologic activity. This pool of bound hormone is in equilibrium with the free hormone pool. (Reproduced, with permission, from DeGroot LJ, Stanbury JB: *The Thyroid and Its Diseases,* 4th ed. Wiley, 1975.)

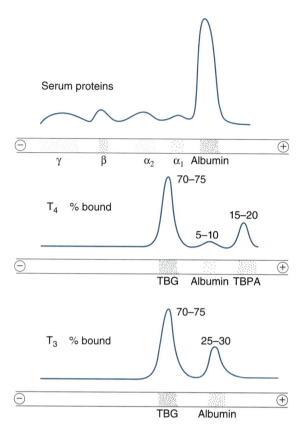

Figure 7–17. Diagrammatic representation of the distribution of radioactive T_4 and T_3 among serum thyroid hormone-binding proteins. ***Top:*** Paper electrophoretic pattern of serum proteins. ***Middle:*** Radioactive T_4 was added to serum and was then subjected to paper electrophoresis. The peaks represent the mobility of radioactive T_4 bound to different serum proteins. (TBG, thyroid hormone-binding globulin; TBPA, thyroxine-binding prealbumin.) ***Bottom:*** Radioactive T_3 was added to serum and subjected to paper electrophoresis. The peaks indicate the relative distribution of protein-bound radioactive T_3. The figures above each peak indicate the relative hormone distribution among the binding proteins in a normal adult. (Reproduced, with permission, from Rosenfield RL et al: *Pediatric Nuclear Medicine.* James AE Jr, Wagner HN Jr, Cooke RE [editors]. Saunders, 1974.)

Thyroxine-Binding Globulin (TBG)

TBG, a single 54-kDa polypeptide chain, is synthesized in the liver. It contains four carbohydrate chains, representing 23% of the molecule by weight, and has homology with α_1-antichymotrypsin and α_1-antitrypsin. Normally, there are about ten sialic acid residues per molecule. Pregnancy or estrogen therapy increases the sialic acid content of the molecule, resulting in decreased metabolic clearance and elevated serum levels of TBG. Each molecule of TBG has a single binding site for T_4 or T_3. The serum concentration of TBG is 15–30 μg/mL, or 280–560 nmol/L.

The affinity constant (K_a) for T_4 is 1×10^{10} M^{-1}, and for T_3 it is 5×10^8 M^{-1}. The high affinity for T_3 and T_4 allows TBG to carry about 70% of the circulating thyroid hormones. When fully saturated, TBG can carry about 20 μg of T_4 per deciliter.

Congenital TBG deficiency is an X-linked trait with a frequency of 1:2500 live births. One variant occurs in African Pygmies, Panamanians, African blacks, Micronesians, and Indonesians. Another variant occurs in 40% of Australian aborigines. Despite the low circulating T_4 and T_3 levels, the free hormone levels are normal and the patients are not hypothyroid. Congenital TBG deficiency is often associated with congenital CBG deficiency (Chapter 9). Congenital TBG excess is rare; it presents with elevated total T_4 and T_3 concentrations but normal free hormone levels and normal TSH.

Androgenic steroids and glucocorticoids lower TBG levels, as does major systemic illness (Table 7–1). Drugs such as salicylates, phenytoin, phenylbutazone, and diazepam may bind to TBG, displacing T_4 and T_3, in effect producing a low-TBG state. Heparin stimulates lipoprotein lipase, releasing free fatty acids, which displace T_3 and T_4 from TBG. This can occur in vivo and also in vitro, where even minute quantities of heparin will increase the measured levels of free T_4 and T_3.

Thyroxine-Binding Prealbumin

Transthyretin, or thyroxine-binding prealbumin (TBPA), is a 55-kDa globular polypeptide consisting of four identical subunits, each containing 127 amino acids. It binds about 10% of circulating T_4. Its affinity for T_3 is about tenfold lower than for T_4, so that it mostly carries T_4. The dissociation of T_4 and T_3 from TBPA is very rapid, so that TBPA is a source of rapidly available T_4. There are binding sites on TBPA for retinol-binding protein, but the transport of

Table 7–1. Factors influencing the concentration of protein-bound thyroid hormones in serum.

A. Increased TBG concentration
1. Congenital
2. Hyperestrogenic states: pregnancy, estrogen therapy
3. Diseases: acute infectious hepatitis, hypothyroidism

B. Decreased TBG concentration
1. Congenital
2. Drugs: androgenic steroids, glucocorticoids
3. Major systemic illness: Protein malnutrition, nephrotic syndrome, cirrhosis, hyperthyroidism

C. Drugs affecting thyroid hormone binding to normal concentrations of binding protein
1. Phenytoin
2. Salicylates
3. Phenylbutazone
4. Mitotane (Lysodren)
5. Diazepam
6. FFA released by heparin stimulation of lipoprotein lipase

T_4 is independent of the transport of retinol-binding protein. The concentration of TBPA in serum is 120–240 mg/L, or 2250–4300 nmol/L.

Increased levels of TBPA may be familial and may occur in patients with glucagonoma or pancreatic islet cell carcinoma. These patients have an elevated total T_4 but a normal free T_4. Abnormal TBPA has been described in familial amyloidotic polyneuropathy, associated with a low total T_4 but normal free hormone levels.

Albumin

Albumin has one strong binding site for T_4 and T_3 and several weaker ones. Because of its high concentration in serum, albumin carries about 15% of circulating T_4 and T_3. The rapid dissociation rates of T_4 and T_3 from albumin make this carrier a major source of free hormone to tissues. Hypoalbuminemia, as occurs in nephrosis or in cirrhosis of the liver, is associated with a low total T_4 and T_3, but the free hormone levels are normal.

Familial dysalbuminemic hyperthyroxinemia is an autosomal dominant inherited disorder in which 25% of the albumin exhibits high-affinity T_4 binding, resulting in an elevated total T_4 level, but normal free T_4 and euthyroidism. Affinity for T_3 may be elevated but is usually normal.

Kinetics of Thyroid Hormone Binding to Transport Proteins

The kinetics of thyroid hormone binding to the thyroid binding proteins can be expressed by conventional equilibration equations. Thus, for T_4:

$$(T_4) + (TBG) \rightleftharpoons (TBG\text{-}T_4)$$

where (T_4) represents free (unbound) hormone, (TBG) is TBG not containing T_4, and $(TBG\text{-}T_4)$ is TBG-bound T_4. This can be expressed by the mass action relationship:

$$kT_4 = \frac{(TBG\text{-}T_4)}{(T_4)(TBG)}$$

where k is the equilibrium constant for the interaction. Rearranging:

$$(T_4) = \frac{(TBG\text{-}T_4)}{kT_4(TBG)}$$

From this equation, it can be seen that T_4 exists in plasma in both free and bound forms, and the free hormone level is inversely proportionate to the free binding sites on TBG and the binding affinity for the hormone. The same relationships exist for the other thyroid hormone-binding proteins.

The effect of a change in the concentration of thyroid hormone-binding protein is shown in Figure 7–18. The levels of free thyroid hormone are normal

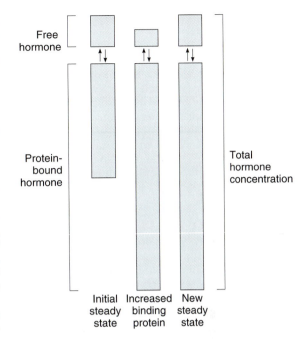

Figure 7–18. The effect of an increase in thyroid hormone-binding protein concentration on the free and protein-bound hormone concentrations. The initial increase in binding protein concentration (as may occur with estrogen administration) increases the amount of bound hormone and transiently decreases the free hormone concentration. There follows a transient increase in thyroid hormone secretion under the stimulus of TSH to replenish the free hormone pool. Another contributing factor is a transient decrease in the metabolic clearance rate of thyroid hormone. A new steady state is attained in which the free hormone secretion, metabolism, and plasma concentration are the same as initially except that the free hormone is now in equilibrium with a larger pool of bound hormone. In subjects receiving thyroid hormone medication, the same daily dose of thyroid hormone is necessary to maintain euthyroidism irrespective of the size of the bound hormone pool.

in states where there are primary or secondary changes in plasma binding, because TSH release is controlled by the free thyroid hormone level and adjusts to normalize it irrespective of how much hormone is bound by the plasma proteins.

There has been much speculation on the role of the thyroid hormone transport proteins. The three major hypotheses are as follows: (1) they form a storage pool of readily available free hormone; 2) they allow the delivery of T_3 and T_4 to all tissues because the tiny free hormone pool is continually replenished as the hormones are absorbed by tissues; and (3) they protect tissues from massive hormone release. Thus, although the transport proteins are not essential for thyroid hormone activity, they may make the system more efficient.

METABOLISM OF THYROID HORMONES

The daily secretion of the normal thyroid gland is about 100 nmol of T_4, about 5 nmol of T_3, and less than 5 nmol of metabolically inactive reverse T_3 (rT_3) (Figure 7–19). Most of the plasma pool of T_3 is derived from peripheral metabolism (5′-deiodination) of T_4. The biologic activity of thyroid hormones is greatly dependent on the location of the iodine atoms (Table 7–2). Deiodination of the *outer ring* of T_4 (5′-deiodination) produces 3,5,3′-triiodothyronine (T_3), which is three to eight times more potent than T_4. On the other hand, deiodination of the *inner ring* of T_4 (5-deiodination) produces 3,3′,5′-triiodothyronine (reverse T_3, or rT_3), which is metabolically inert. The deiodinative pathways of thyroxine metabolism are presented in Figure 7–20. Monodeiodination of the outer ring of thyroxine is a "step up" process, increasing the metabolic activity of the resultant compound, while monodeiodination of the inner ring is a "step down" or inactivation process. Further deiodination of the molecule abolishes hormonal activity.

At least three enzymes catalyze these monodeiodination reactions: type 1, 5′-deiodinase; type 2, 5′-deiodinase; and type 3, tyrosyl ring deiodinase, or 5-deiodinase. They differ in tissue localization, substrate specificity, and effect of disease. The properties of these deiodinases are summarized in Table 7–3.

Type 1 5′-deiodinase is the most abundant deiodinase and is found largely in liver and kidney and in lesser quantity in the thyroid gland, skeletal muscle, heart muscle, and other tissues. Molecular cloning of type 1 5′-deiodinase has revealed that it contains selenocysteine and that this is probably the active deiodinating site. The major function of type 1 5′-deiodinase is to provide T_3 to the plasma. It is increased in hyperthyroidism and decreased in hypothyroidism. The increased activity in hyperthyroidism accounts in part for the high T_3 levels in this syndrome. The enzyme is inhibited by propylthiouracil but not methimazole, which explains why propylthiouracil is more effective than methimazole in reducing T_3 levels in severe hyperthyroidism. Inhibition of type 1 5′-deiodinase activity results in impaired conversion of T_4 to T_3. Some conditions associated with decreased conversion of T_4 to T_3 are listed in Table 7–4. Note that only propylthiouracil, amiodarone, and ipodate impair intracellular conversion of T_4 to T_3; the other conditions may modify the ratio of T_4 to T_3 in serum, requiring interpretation of thyroid tests (see below), but they do not change intracellular T_3 production. Dietary deficiency of selenium also impairs conversion of T_4 to T_3. In the presence of iodine deficiency, repletion of selenium causes increased type 1 5′-deiodinase activity, an acceleration of T_4 metabolism, and a worsening of hypothyroidism, since the iodine-deficient gland cannot compensate for the increased T_4 metabolism.

Type 2 5′-deiodinase is found largely in the brain and pituitary gland. It is resistant to propylthiouracil but very sensitive to circulating T_4. The major effect of the enzyme is to maintain a constant level of intracellular T_3 in the central nervous system. Reduction in circulating T_4 results in a rapid increase in the amount of the enzyme in brain and pituitary cells, probably by altering the rate of enzyme degradation and inactivation, maintaining the level of intracellular T_3 and cellular function. High levels of serum T_4 reduce type 2 5′-deiodinase, protecting brain cells from excessive T_3. This may be the mechanism whereby the hypothalamus and pituitary monitor the levels of circulating T_4. Other metabolic products of T_4 metabolism such as rT_3 can also modify the levels of type 2 5′-deiodinase in the brain and the pituitary gland, and alpha-adrenergic compounds stimulate type 2 5′-deiodinase in brown fat. The physiologic significance of these reactions is not clear.

Type 3 5-deiodinase, or tyrosyl ring deiodinase, is found in placental chorionic membranes and glial cells in the central nervous system. It inactivates T_4 by converting it to rT_3 and T_3 by converting it to 3,3′-diiodothyronine (3,3′-T_2) (Figure 7–20). It is elevated in hyperthyroidism and decreased in hypothyroidism. Thus, it may help to protect the fetus and the brain from excess or deficiency of T_4.

About 80% of T_4 is metabolized by deiodination, 35% to T_3 and 45% to rT_3 (Figure 7–19). The remainder is inactivated mostly by glucuronidation in the liver and secretion into bile, or to a lesser extent

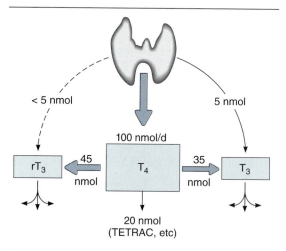

Figure 7–19. Major pathways of thyroxine metabolism in normal adult humans. Rates are expressed in nmol/24 h and are approximations based upon available data. 100 nmol of T_4 is equivalent to approximately 75 μg. (rT_3, reverse T_3; TETRAC, tetraiodothyroacetic acid.) (Reproduced, with permission, from Cavalieri RR, Rapoport B: Impaired peripheral conversion of thyroxine to triiodothyronine. Ann Rev Med 1977;28:5765.)

Table 7–2. Chemical structures and biologic activity of thyroid hormones.

Hormone	Common Name	Biologic Activity
L-3,5,3′,5′-Tetraiodothyronine	L-Thyroxine; T_4	100
L-3,5,3′-Triiodothyronine	T_3	300–800
L-3,3′,5′-Triiodothyronine	Reverse T_3; rT_3	< 1
DL-3,3′-Diiodothyronine	$3,3′-T_2$	< 1–3
DL-3,5-Diiodothyronine	$3,5-T_2$	7–11
DL-3′,5′-Diiodothyronine	$3′5′-T_2$	0
L-3,5,3′,5′-Tetraiodothyroacetic acid	Tetrac	? 10–50
L-3,5,3′-Triiodothyroacetic acid	Triac	? 25–35

by sulfonation and deiodination in the liver or kidney. Other metabolic reactions include deamination of the alanine side chain, forming thyroacetic acid derivatives of low biologic activity (Table 7–2); or decarboxylation or cleavage of the ether bridge, forming inactive compounds.

Representative iodothyronine kinetic values are summarized in Table 7–5. The volume of distribution is the quantity of plasma that would contain the equivalent of the total extrathyroidal pool of the compound. Thus, for T_4, the serum concentration is about 100 nmol/L, the volume of distribution is about

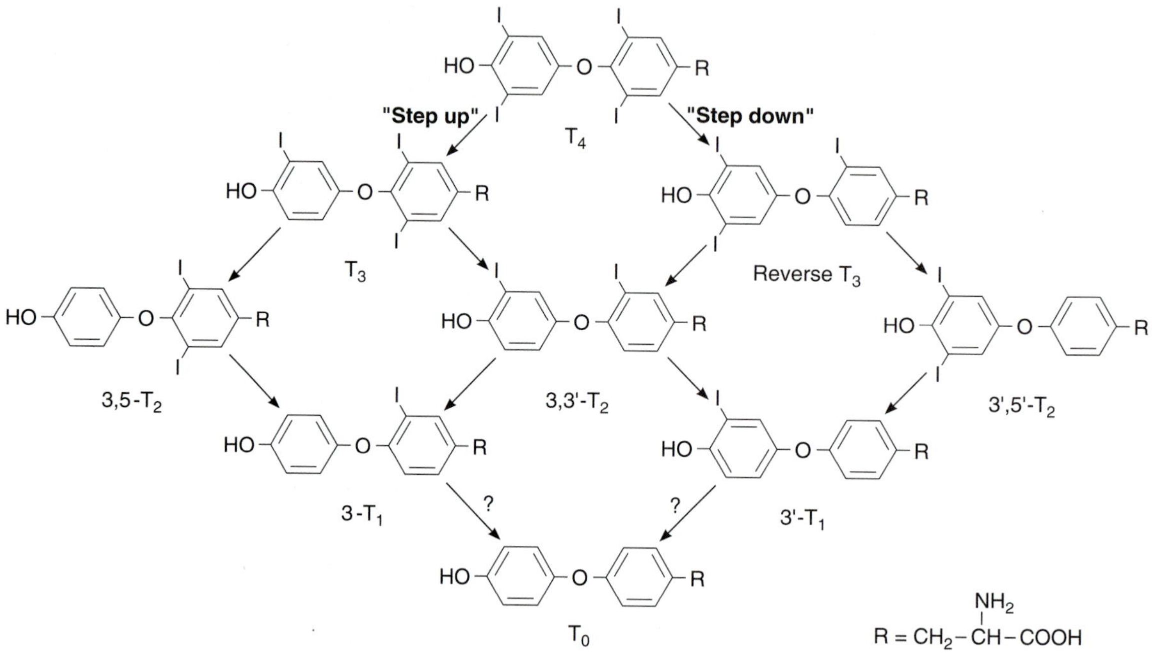

Figure 7–20. The deiodinative pathway of thyroxine metabolism. The monodeiodination of T_4 to T_3 represents a "step up" in biologic potency, whereas the monodeiodination of T_4 to reverse T_3 has the opposite effect. Further deiodination of T_3 essentially abolishes hormonal activity.

10 L, and the body pool is about 1000 nmol. The metabolic clearance rate for T_4 is only about 10% per day (100 nmol), and the half-life of T_4 in plasma is about 7 days. The body pool of T_3 is much smaller and the turnover more rapid, with a plasma half-life of 1 day. The total body pool of rT_3 is about the same size as that of T_3, but it has a much more rapid turnover, with a plasma half-life of only 0.2 day. The rapid clearance of T_3 and rT_3 is due to lower binding affinity for thyroid binding proteins.

Table 7–3. Iodothyronine deiodinases.[1]

Parameter	Type 1 (5')	Type 2 (5')	Type 3 (5)
Physiologic role	Provide T_3 to plasma	Provide intracellular T_3	Inactivate T_3 and T_4
Tissue location	Liver, kidney, muscle, thyroid	CNS, pituitary, brown fat, placenta	Placenta, CNS, skin, fetal liver
Substrate	$rT_3 \gg T_4 > T_3$	$T_4 = rT_3$	$T_3 > T_4$
K_m for T^4	1×10^{-6} M	1×10^{-9} M	6×10^{-9} M (T_3), 37×10^{-9} M (T_4)
Deiodination site	Outer and inner ring	Outer ring	Inner ring
Kinetic mechanism	Ping-pong	Sequential	Sequential
Dithiothreitol	Stimulates	Stimulates	Stimulates
K for PTU	5×10^{-7} M sensitive	4×10^{-3} M resistant	?($> 10^{-3}$ M) resistant
Active site	Selenocysteine	Selenocysteine	Selenocysteine
Ipanoic acid	Inhibits	Inhibits	Inhibits
Hypothyroidism	Decrease	Increase	Decrease
Hyperthyroidism	Increase	Decrease	Increase

[1]Adapted and modified, with permission, from Larsen PR, Ingbar SH. The thyroid gland. In: *Williams Textbook of Endocrinology,* 8th ed. Wilson JW, Foster DW (editors). Saunders, 1992.

Table 7–4. Conditions or factors associated with decreased conversion of T_4 to T_3.

1. Fetal life.
2. Caloric restriction.
3. Hepatic disease.
4. Major systemic illness.
5. Drugs:
    Propylthiouracil
    Glucocorticoids
    Propranolol (mild effect)
    Iodinated x-ray contrast agents (iopanoic acid, ipodate sodium)
    Amiodarone
6. Selenium deficiency

Table 7–5. Representative iodothyronine kinetic values in a euthyroid human.

	T_4	T_3	rT_3
Serum levels			
Total, µg/dL (nmol/L)	8 (103)	0.12 (1.84)	0.04 (0.51)
Free, ng/dL (pmol/L)	1.5 (19)	0.28 (4.3)	0.24 (3.69)
Body pool, µg (nmol)	800 (1023)	46 (70.7)	40 (61.5)
Distribution volume (L)	10	38	98
Metabolic clearance rate (MCR) (L/d)	1	22	90
Production (disposal) rate. MCRX serum concentration, µg/d (nmol/d)	80 (103)	26 (34)	36 (46)
Half-life in plasma ($t_{1/2}$) (days)	7	1	0.2

(***Note:*** T_4 µg/dL × 12.87 = nmol/L; T_3 µg/dL × 15.38 = nmol/L)

CONTROL OF THYROID FUNCTION

The growth and function of the thyroid gland is controlled by at least four mechanisms: (1) the classic hypothalamic-pituitary-thyroid axis (Figure 7–21), in which hypothalamic thyrotropin-releasing hormone (TRH) stimulates the synthesis and release of anterior pituitary thyroid-stimulating hormone (TSH), which in turn stimulates growth and hormone secretion by the thyroid gland; (2) the pituitary and peripheral deiodinases, which modify the effects of T_4 and T_3; (3) autoregulation of hormone synthesis by the thyroid gland itself in relationship to its iodine supply; and (4) stimulation or inhibition of thyroid function by TSH receptor autoantibodies.

Thyrotropin-Releasing Hormone

Thyrotropin-releasing hormone (TRH) is a tripeptide, pyroglutamyl-histidyl-prolineamide, synthesized by neurons in the supraoptic and supraventricu-lar nuclei of the hypothalamus (Figure 7–22). It is stored in the median eminence of the hypothalamus and then transported via the pituitary portal venous system down the pituitary stalk to the anterior pituitary gland, where it controls synthesis and release of TSH. TRH is also found in other portions of the hypothalamus, the brain, and the spinal cord, where it may function as a neurotransmitter. The gene for human preproTRH, located on chromosome 3, contains a 3.3-kb transcription unit that encodes six TRH molecules. The gene also encodes other neuropeptides that may be biologically significant. In the anterior pituitary gland, TRH binds to specific membrane receptors on thyrotrophs and prolactin-secreting cells, stimulating synthesis and release of both TSH and prolactin. Thyroid hormones cause a slow depletion of pituitary TRH receptors, diminishing TRH response; estrogen increases TRH receptors, increasing pituitary sensitivity to TRH.

The response of the pituitary thyrotroph to TRH is bimodal: First, it stimulates release of stored hormone; and second, it stimulates gene activity, which increases hormone synthesis. The TRH receptor (TRH-R) is a member of the seven-transmembrane-spanning, GTP-binding, protein-coupled receptor family (Table 3–1; Figure 3–2). The *TRH-R* gene is

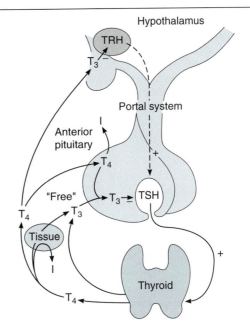

Figure 7–21. The hypothalamic-hypophysial-thyroid axis. TRH produced in the hypothalamus reaches the thyrotropes in the anterior pituitary by the hypothalamic-hypophysial-portal system and stimulates the synthesis and release of TSH. In both the hypothalamus and the pituitary, it is primarily T_3 that inhibits TRH and TSH secretion. T_4 undergoes monodeiodination to T_3 in neural and pituitary as well as in peripheral tissues.

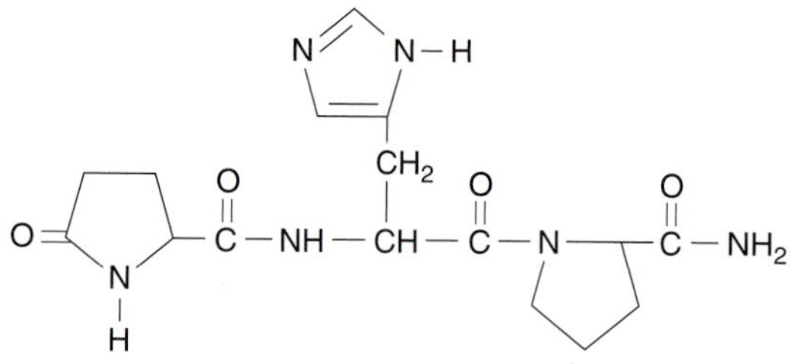

(pyro)Glu-His-Pro-(NH₂)

Figure 7–22. Chemical structure of thyrotropin-releasing hormone (TRH).

Table 7–6. Factors controlling the secretion of thyroid hormones.

1. HYPOTHALAMIC: Synthesis and release of TRH
   Stimulatory:
       Decreased serum T_4 and T_3, and intraneuronal T_3
       Neurogenic: Pulsatile secretion and circadian rhythm
       Exposure to cold (animals and human newborn)
       Alpha-adrenergic catecholamines
       Arginine vasopressin
   Inhibitory:
       Increased serum T_4 and T_3, and intraneuronal T_3
       Alpha-adrenergic blockers
       Hypothalamic tumors
2. ANTERIOR PITUITARY: Synthesis and release of TSH
   Stimulatory:
       TRH
       Decreased serum T_4 and T_3, and intrathyrotrope T_3
       Decreased activity Type 2 5′-deiodinase
       Estrogen: increased TRH binding sites
   Inhibitory:
       Increased serum T_4 and T_3, and intrathyrotrope T_3
       Increased activity Type 2 5′-deiodinase
       Somatostatin
       Dopamine, dopamine agonists: bromocriptine
       Glucocorticoids
       Chronic illness
       Pituitary tumors
3. THYROID: Synthesis and release of thyroid hormones
   Stimulatory:
       TSH
       TSH-R stimulating antibodies
   Inhibitory:
       TSH-R blocking antibodies
       Iodide excess
       Lithium therapy

located on chromosome 8. Large glycoprotein hormones such as TSH and LH bind to the extracellular portions of their receptors, but TRH, a small peptide, binds to the transmembrane helix 3 of the TRH-R. After binding to its receptor on the thyrotroph, TRH activates a G protein, which in turn activates phospholipase c to hydrolyze phosphatidylinositol 4,5-bisphosphate (PIP_2) to inositol 1,4,5-trisphosphate (IP_3). IP_3 stimulates the release of intracellular Ca^{2+}, which causes the first burst response of hormone release. Simultaneously, there is generation of 1,2-diacylglycerol (1,2-DG), which activates protein kinase C, thought to be responsible for the second and sustained phase of hormone secretion. The increases in intracellular Ca^{2+} and in protein kinase C may be involved in increased transcription. TRH also stimulates the glycosylation of TSH, which is necessary for full biologic activity of the hormone. Thus, patients with hypothalamic tumors and hypothyroidism may have measurable TSH, which is biologically inactive.

Elegant studies in vitro and in vivo demonstrated that T_3 directly inhibits the transcription of prepro-TRH gene and thus the synthesis of TRH in the hypothalamus. Since T_4 is converted to T_3 within peptidergic neurons, it is also an effective inhibitor of TRH synthesis and secretion (Table 7–6).

TRH is rapidly metabolized, with a half-life of intravenously administered hormone of about 5 minutes. Plasma TRH levels in normal subjects are very low, ranging from 25 to 100 pg/mL.

TRH-stimulated TSH secretion occurs in a pulsatile fashion throughout the 24 hours (Figure 7–23). Normal subjects have a mean TSH pulse amplitude of about 0.6 μU/mL and an average frequency of one pulse every 1.8 hours. In addition, normal subjects show a circadian rhythm, with a peak serum TSH at night, usually between midnight and 4 AM. This peak is unrelated to sleep, eating, or the secretion of other pituitary hormones. This rhythm is presumably controlled by a hypothalamic neuronal "pulse generator" driving TRH synthesis in the supraoptic and supraventricular nuclei. In hypothyroid patients, the amplitude of the pulses and the nocturnal surge are much larger than normal, and in patients with hyperthyroidism both the pulses and the nocturnal surge are markedly suppressed.

In experimental animals and in the newborn human, exposure to cold increases TRH and TSH secretion, but this is not noted in the adult human.

Certain hormones and drugs may modify TRH synthesis and release. TRH secretion is stimulated by decreased serum T_4 or T_3 (with decreased intraneuronal T_3), by alpha-adrenergic agonists, and by arginine vasopressin. Conversely, TRH secretion is inhibited by increased serum T_4 or T_3 (with increased intraneuronal T_3) and alpha-adrenergic blockade (Table 7–6).

TRH administered intravenously to humans in a bolus dose of 200–500 μg results in a rapid rise in serum TSH, peaking at about 30 minutes and lasting for 2–3 hours. Typical responses to TRH in various clinical conditions are presented in Figures 7–24 and 7–25. Note the exaggerated response of pituitary TSH to TRH in patients with primary hypothyroidism and the suppressed response in patients with hyperthyroidism, nodular goiter with autonomously functioning nodules, or pituitary hypothyroidism. TRH and its dipeptide metabolite cyclo(HisPro) are also found in the islet cells of the pancreas, the gastrointestinal tract, the placenta, the heart, and in the

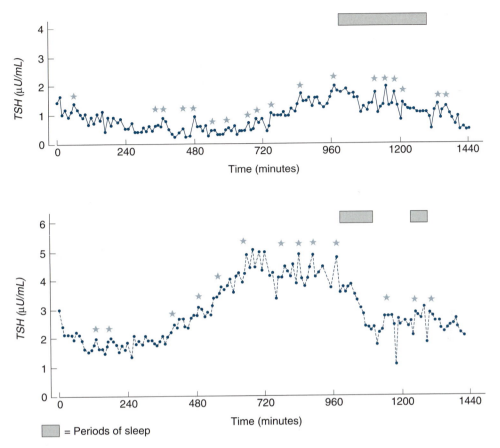

Figure 7–23. Serum TSH in two normal subjects demonstrating spontaneous pulses and the circadian rhythm of TSH secretion. (0 time is 0900; Stars indicate significant pulses.) (Reproduced, with permission, from Greenspan SL et al: Pulsatile secretion of TSH in man. J Clin Endocrinol Metabol 1986;63:664. Copyright © 1986 by The Endocrine Society.)

prostate, testes, and ovaries. TRH mRNA in these peripheral tissues is not inhibited by T_3, and the role of TRH in these tissues has not yet been determined.

Thyrotropin

Thyroid-stimulating hormone, or thyrotropin (TSH), is a glycoprotein synthesized and secreted by the thyrotropes of the anterior pituitary gland. It has a molecular weight of about 28,000 and is composed of two noncovalently linked subunits, α and β. The α subunit is common to the two other pituitary glycoproteins, FSH and LH, and also to the placental hormone hCG; the β subunit is different for each glycoprotein hormone and confers specific binding properties and biologic activity. The human α subunit has an apoprotein core of 92 amino acids and contains two oligosaccharide chains; the TSH β subunit has an apoprotein core of 112 amino acids and contains one oligosaccharide chain. Glycosylation takes place in the rough endoplasmic reticulum and the Golgi of the thyrotroph, where glucose, mannose, and fucose residues and terminal sulfate or sialic acid residues are linked to the apoprotein core. The function of these carbohydrate residues is not entirely clear, but it is likely that they enhance TSH biologic activity and modify its metabolic clearance rate. For example, deglycosylated TSH will bind to its receptor, but its biologic activity is markedly decreased and its metabolic clearance rate is markedly increased.

The gene for the human α subunit is located on chromosome 6 and the gene for the human β subunit on chromosome 1. A schematic representation of the α and β subunit genes is presented in Figure 7–26. Several kindreds have been reported with a point mutation in the TSH β gene, resulting in a TSH-β subunit that did not combine with the α subunit to produce biologically active TSH. The disorders were autosomal recessive, and the clinical picture was that of nongoitrous hypothyroidism.

TSH is the primary factor controlling thyroid cell growth and thyroid hormone synthesis and secretion. It achieves this effect by binding to a specific **TSH receptor** (TSH-R) on the thyroid cell membrane and

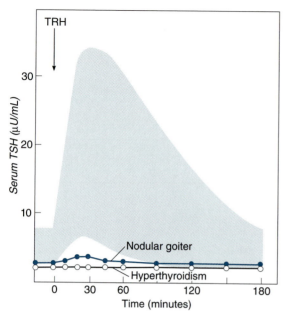

Figure 7–24. Typical serum TSH responses to TRH in patients with hyperthyroidism or toxic nodular goiter. The shaded area indicates normal range. (Reproduced, with permission, from Utiger RD: *The Thyroid,* 4th ed. Werner SC, Ingbar SH [editors]. Harper & Row, 1978.)

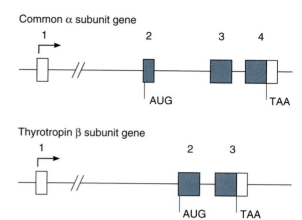

Figure 7–26. Schematic representation of the human TSH subunit genes. The human common α subunit gene (on chromosome 6) and the TSH β subunit gene (on chromosome 1) have four and three exons, respectively, represented by boxes separated by introns (thin lines). Point mutations in the TSH β subunit gene have been found in patients with nongoitrous hypothyroidism. (Reproduced, with permission, from Wondisford FE et al: Chemistry and biosynthesis of thyrotropin. In: *Werner and Ingbar's The Thyroid,* 6th ed. Braverman LE, Utiger RD [editors]. Lippincott, 1991.)

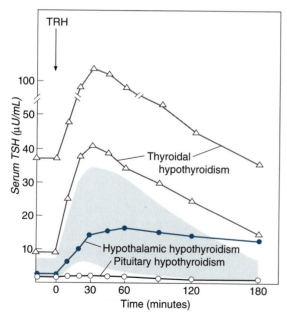

Figure 7–25. Typical serum TSH responses to TRH in patients with thyroid (primary), pituitary (secondary), and hypothalamic (tertiary) hypothyroidism. The shaded area indicates the normal range. (Reproduced, with permission, from Utiger RD: *The Thyroid,* 4th ed. Werner SC, Ingbar SH [editors]. Harper & Row, 1978.)

activating both the G protein-adenylyl cyclase-cAMP and the phospholipase C signaling systems. The TSH receptor (TSH-R) has been cloned and is a single-chain glycoprotein containing 744 amino acids. Like the TRH receptor of the anterior pituitary, the TSH-R in the thyroid follicular cell is a member of the seven-transmembrane-spanning, GTP-binding, protein-coupled receptor family. The human TSH-R gene is located on chromosome 14q31. The TSH-R is unique in that it has binding sites not only for TSH but also for TSH receptor–stimulating autoantibodies (TSH-R Ab [stim]), which are found in patients with autoimmune hyperthyroidism (Graves' disease), and also for autoantibodies that bind to the TSH receptor and block the action of TSH (TSH-R Ab [block]); these latter antibodies are found in severe hypothyroidism due to atrophic thyroiditis (see below). The binding sites for these factors lie in the extracellular portion of the receptor. A hypothetical model of the structure of the TSH-R is presented in Figure 7–27. It is thought that TSH-R Ab [block] binds to residues 295–302 and 385–395, whereas TSH-R Ab [stim] binds to residues 30–56; TSH binds to both areas. The difference in binding site of the autoantibodies may account for the marked difference in the clinical syndromes of Graves' disease and atrophic thyroiditis with myxedema. TSH up-regulates TSH-R mRNA, increasing the number of TSH receptors on the thyroid cell membrane.

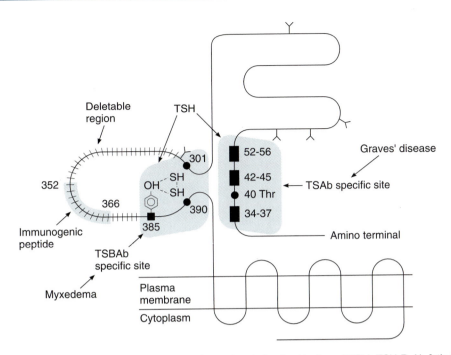

Figure 7–27. Model of the TSH-R with approximate determinants for the binding of TSH, TSH-R Ab [stim] (TSAb specific site), and TSH-R Ab [block] (TSBAb specific site). The former are implicated in patients with Graves' disease and neonatal hyperthyroidism, the latter in patients with idiopathic myxedema and neonatal hypothyroidism. They are presumed to comprise the TSH-R site based on competitive antagonism or agonism of TSH with monoclonal stimulating or inhibitory receptor antibodies. (TR, thyroid hormone receptor.) (Reproduced, with permission, from Kosugi S, Ban T, Kohn LD: Identification of the thyroid stimulating antibody specific interaction sites in the N-terminal region of the thyrotropin receptor. Molecular Endocrinology 1993; 7:114.)

Mutations in the TSH-R have been associated with either spontaneous activation of the receptor and clinical hyperthyroidism or with resistance to TSH. Activating mutations involving the intracellular portion of the TSH-R have been found in some toxic adenomas and in rare cases of sporadic familial hyperthyroidism. Resistance to TSH due to mutations in the extracellular portion of the receptor is associated with elevated serum TSH levels and euthyroidism.

Effects of TSH on the Thyroid Cell

TSH has many actions on the thyroid cell. Most of its actions are mediated through the G protein-adenylyl cyclase-cAMP system, but activation of the phosphatidylinositol (PIP2) system with increase in intracellular calcium may also be involved. The major actions of TSH include the following:

A. Changes in Thyroid Cell Morphology: TSH rapidly induces pseudopods at the cell-colloid border, accelerating thyroglobulin resorption. Colloid content is diminished. Intracellular colloid droplets are formed and lysosome formation is stimulated, increasing thyroglobulin hydrolysis (Figure 7–5).

B. Cell Growth: Individual thyroid cells increase in size (Figure 7–4); vascularity is increased; and, over a period of time, thyroid enlargement, or goiter, develops.

C. Iodine Metabolism: TSH stimulates all phases of iodide metabolism, from increased iodide uptake and transport to increased iodination of thyroglobulin and increased secretion of thyroid hormones. The increase in cAMP mediates increased iodide transport, while PIP2 hydrolysis and increased intracellular Ca^{2+} stimulate the iodination of thyroglobulin. The TSH effect on iodide transport is biphasic: Initially, it is depressed (iodide efflux); and then, after a lag of several hours, iodide uptake is increased. The efflux of iodide may be due to the rapid increase in hydrolysis of thyroglobulin with release of hormone and leakage of iodide out of the gland.

D. Increase in mRNA for thyroglobulin and thyroidal peroxidase, with an increase in incorporation of I⁻ into MIT, DIT, T_3 and T_4.

E. Increased lysosomal activity, with increased secretion of T_4 and T_3 from the gland. There is also increased activity of type 1 5'-deiodinase, conserving intrathyroidal iodine.

F. TSH has many other effects on the thyroid gland, including stimulation of glucose uptake, oxygen consumption, CO_2 production, and an increase in glucose oxidation via the hexosemonophosphate pathway and the Krebs cycle. There is accelerated turnover of phospholipids and stimulation of synthesis of purine and pyrimidine precursors, with increased synthesis of DNA and RNA.

Serum TSH

Normally, only α subunit and intact TSH are present in the serum. The level of α subunit is about 0.5–2.0 μg/L; it is elevated in postmenopausal women and in patients with TSH-secreting pituitary tumors (see below). The serum level of TSH is about 0.5–5 mU/L; it is increased in hypothyroidism and decreased in hyperthyroidism, whether endogenous or from excessive oral intake of thyroid hormones. The plasma half-life of TSH is about 30 minutes, and the daily production rate is about 40–150 mU/d.

Control of Pituitary TSH Secretion

The two major factors controlling the synthesis and release of TSH are the level of intrathyrotroph T_3, which controls mRNA for TSH synthesis and release, and TRH, which controls glycosylation, activation, and release of TSH (Table 7–6).

TSH synthesis and release are inhibited by high serum levels of T_4 and T_3 (hyperthyroidism) and stimulated by low levels of thyroid hormone (hypothyroidism). In addition, certain hormones and drugs inhibit TSH secretion. These include somatostatin, dopamine, dopamine agonists such as bromocriptine, and glucocorticoids. Acute or chronic disease may cause inhibition of TSH secretion during active illness, and there may be a rebound rise in TSH as the patient recovers. The magnitude of these effects is variable; thus, the drugs mentioned above will suppress serum TSH, but it will usually be detectable. In contrast, hyperthyroidism will turn off TSH secretion entirely. These observations are important clinically in interpreting serum TSH levels in patients receiving these medications.

Destructive lesions or tumors of the hypothalamus or anterior pituitary gland may impair TRH and TSH secretion by destruction of secretory cells. This will result in "secondary hypothyroidism" due to pituitary thyrotroph destruction or "tertiary hypothyroidism" due to destruction of TRH-secreting neurons. Differential diagnosis of these lesions is discussed below (see Thyroid Tests).

Other Thyroid Stimulators & Inhibitors

The thyroid follicle has a rich supply of capillaries that carry noradrenergic nerve fibers from the superior cervical ganglion and acetylcholine esterase-positive nerve fibers derived from the vagal nodose and thyroid ganglia. The parafollicular "C" cells secrete both calcitonin and calcitonin gene-related peptide (CGRP). In experimental animals, these and other neuropeptides modify thyroid blood flow and hormone secretion. In addition, growth factors such as insulin, IGF-1, and EGF and the autocrine actions of prostaglandins and cytokines may modify thyroid cell growth and hormone production. However, it is not yet clear how important these effects are in clinical situations.

Role of Pituitary & Peripheral Deiodinases

Pituitary type 2 5′-deiodinase converts T_4 to T_3 in the brain and pituitary, providing the main source of intracellular T_3. Its increased activity in hypothyroidism helps to maintain intracellular T_3 in the presence of falling serum T_4 concentrations. In hyperthyroidism, the decrease in its activity helps to prevent overloading of pituitary and neural cells with thyroid hormone. In contrast, type 1 5′-deiodinase is decreased in hypothyroidism, conserving T_4, and increased in hyperthyroidism, accelerating T_4 metabolism (Table 7–3).

Thyroidal Autoregulation

Autoregulation may be defined as the capacity of the thyroid gland to modify its function to adapt to changes in the availability of iodine, independent of pituitary TSH. Thus, humans can maintain normal thyroid hormone secretion with iodide intakes varying from 50 μg to several milligrams per day. Some of the effects of iodide deficiency or excess are discussed above. The major adaptation to low iodide intake is the preferential synthesis of T_3 rather than T_4, increasing the metabolic effectiveness of the secreted hormone. Iodide excess, on the other hand, inhibits many thyroidal functions, including I^- transport, cAMP formation, H_2O_2 generation, hormone synthesis and secretion, and the binding of TSH and TSH-R Ab to the TSH receptor. Some of these effects may be mediated by the formation of intrathyroidal iodinated fatty acids. The ability of the normal thyroid to "escape" from these inhibitory effects (Wolff-Chaikoff effect) allows the gland to continue to secrete hormone despite a high dietary iodide intake. It is important to note that this is different from the therapeutic effect of iodide in the treatment of Graves' disease. Here, the high levels of iodide inhibit thyroglobulin endocytosis and lysosomal activity, decreasing thyroid hormone release and lowering circulating hormone levels. In addition, the inhibition of TSH-R Ab [stim] activity reduces the vascularity of the gland, with beneficial consequences during surgery. This effect is also transient, lasting about 10 days to 2 weeks.

Autoimmune Regulation

The ability of B lymphocytes to synthesize TSH receptor antibodies that can either block the action of TSH or mimic TSH activity by binding to different areas on the TSH receptor provides a form of thyroid regulation by the immune system.

Thus, the synthesis and secretion of thyroid hormones are controlled at three different levels: (1) the level of the hypothalamus, by modifying TRH secretion; (2) the pituitary level, by inhibition or stimulation of TSH secretion; and (3) the level of the thyroid, by autoregulation and blockade or stimulation of the TSH receptor (Table 7–6).

THE ACTION OF THYROID HORMONES

1. THE THYROID HORMONE RECEPTOR

Thyroid hormones, T_3 and T_4, circulate in plasma largely bound to protein but in equilibrium with the free hormone. It is the free hormone that is transported either by passive diffusion or by specific carriers through the cell membrane, through the cell cytoplasm, to bind to a specific receptor in the cell nucleus. Within the cell, T_4 is converted to T_3 by 5′ deiodinase, suggesting that T_4 is a prohormone and T_3 the active form of the hormone. The nuclear receptor for T_3 has been cloned. It is one of a "family" of receptors, all similar to the receptor for the retrovirus that causes erythroblastosis in chickens, v-*erb* A, and to the nuclear receptors for glucocorticoids, mineralocorticoids, estrogens, progestins, vitamin D_3, and retinoic acid (Figure 3–13).

In the human, there are two genes for the thyroid hormone receptor, alpha and beta. TRα is located on chromosome 17 and TRβ on chromosome 3. Each gene produces at least two products, TRβ 1 and 2. The structure and characteristics of these products are portrayed in Figure 7–28. Each has three domains: a ligand-independent domain at the amino terminal, a centrally located DNA binding area with two cysteine-zinc "fingers," and a ligand-binding domain at the carboxyl terminal (Figures 3–12 and 3–13). Note that TRα2 does not bind T_3 and may actually inhibit T_3 action. The concentration of these receptors in tissue varies with the stage of development and the tissue. For example, the brain contains mostly TRα, the liver mostly TRβ, and cardiac muscle contains both. The binding affinity of T_3 analogs is directly proportionate to the biologic activity of the analog. Point mutations in the ligand-binding domain of the TRβ gene are responsible for the syndrome of resistance to thyroid hormone (Refetoff's syndrome; see below).

The thyroid hormone receptors may bind to the specific thyroid hormone response element (TRE) sites on DNA even in the absence of T_3 (Figure 7–29)—unlike the steroid hormone receptors). The TREs are located near, generally upstream with respect to the start of transcription, to the promoters where transcription of specific thyroid hormone responsive genes is initiated. T_3 binding to the receptors results in stimulation, or in some cases inhibition, of the transcription of these genes with consequent changes in the levels of the mRNAs transcribed from them. The changes in mRNA levels alter the levels of the protein product of these genes. These proteins then mediate the thyroid hormone response. These receptors often function as heterodimers with other transcription factors such as the retinoic X receptor and the retinoic acid receptor.

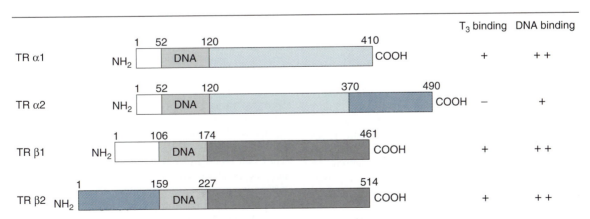

Figure 7–28. Deduced protein structure of the thyroid hormone receptor α and β gene products. The receptor protein has three domains: a DNA-binding domain with a high degree of similarity among the different types of receptors, a carboxyl terminal triiodothyronine (T_3) binding domain, and an amino terminal domain that is not required for full function. The numbers above the structures represent amino acid numbers. The properties of the receptors with respect to their ability to bind T_3 and bind to a T_3-response element of DNA are shown on the right. Identical shading of receptor domains indicates identical amino acid sequences. (TR, thyroid hormone receptor.) (Reproduced, with permission, from Brent GA: The molecular basis of thyroid hormone action. N Engl J Med 1994;331:847.)

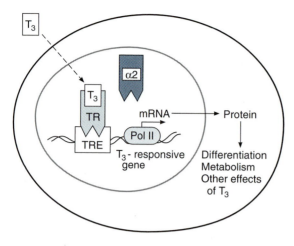

Figure 7–29. Model of the mediation of T_3 action by nuclear thyroid hormone receptors. T_3 either enters the cell (as depicted) or is derived from intracellular deiodination of T_4. Nuclear interaction between a T_3-bound TR and a thyroid hormone-responsive element (TRE) results in increased or decreased activity of RNA polymerase II (pol II) on a T_3-responsive gene. The TRE is indicated as containing two half-sites, and the TR may bind as a dimer. Effects on mRNA levels are translated into increased or decreased cellular concentrations of proteins so as to promote differentiation, metabolic processes, and other cell-specific effects of T_3. In the absence of T_3, the TRE-bound TR may repress basal transcription. c-$erbA_a$2 ("a2"), the non-T_3-binding splice variant, can inhibit the effects of T_3-bound TRs by a mechanism that has not yet been established, probably involving heterodimer formation or competition for the TRE. A similar mechanism is likely to explain the dominant negative effect of the v-erbA oncoprotein and mutated TRs, as in the syndromes of generalized resistance to T_3. (Reproduced, with permission, from Lazar MA, Chin WW: Nuclear thyroid hormone receptors. J Clin Invest 1990;86:1777. © 1990 by The American Society for Clinical Investigation.)

2. PHYSIOLOGIC EFFECTS OF THYROID HORMONES

The transcriptional effects of T_3 characteristically demonstrate a lag time of hours or days to achieve full effect. These genomic actions result in a number of effects, including those on tissue growth, brain maturation, and increased heat production and oxygen consumption due in part to increased activity of Na^+-K^+ ATPase, production of increased beta-adrenergic receptors. Some actions of T_3 are not genomic, such as reduction of pituitary type 2 5′-deiodinase and increase in glucose and amino acid transport. Some specific effects of thyroid hormones are summarized in what follows.

Effects on Fetal Development

The thyroid and the anterior pituitary TSH system begin to function in the human fetus at about 11

weeks. Prior to this time, the fetal thyroid does not concentrate ^{123}I. Because of the high placental content of type 3 5-deiodinase, most maternal T_3 and T_4 are inactivated in the placenta, and very little free hormone reaches the fetal circulation. This small amount of free hormone from the mother may be important for early fetal brain development. However, after 11 weeks' gestation, the fetus is largely dependent on its own thyroidal secretion. Although some fetal growth occurs in the absence of fetal thyroid hormone secretion, brain development and skeletal maturation are markedly impaired, resulting in cretinism (mental retardation and dwarfism).

Effects on Oxygen Consumption, Heat Production, & Free Radical Formation

T_3 increases O_2 consumption and heat production in part by stimulation of Na^+-K^+ ATPase in all tissues except the brain, spleen, and testis. This contributes to the increased basal metabolic rate (O_2 consumption by the whole animal at rest) and the increased sensitivity to heat in hyperthyroidism, and the converse in hypothyroidism. Thyroid hormones also decrease superoxide dismutase levels, resulting in increased superoxide anion free radical formation. This may contribute to the deleterious effects of chronic hyperthyroidism.

Cardiovascular Effects

T_3 stimulates transcription of myosin heavy chain α and inhibits myosin heavy chain β, improving cardiac muscle contractility. T_3 also increases transcription of Ca^{2+} ATPase in the sarcoplasmic reticulum, increasing diastolic contraction of the heart; alters isoforms of Na^+-K^+ ATPase genes; and increases beta-adrenergic receptors and the concentration of G proteins. Thus, thyroid hormones have marked positive inotropic and chronotropic effects on the heart. This accounts for the increased cardiac output and marked increase in heart rate in hyperthyroidism and the reverse in hypothyroidism.

Sympathetic Effects

As noted above, thyroid hormones increase the number of beta-adrenergic receptors in heart muscle, skeletal muscle, adipose tissue, and lymphocytes. They also decrease myocardial alpha-adrenergic receptors. In addition, they may amplify catecholamine action at a postreceptor site. Thus, sensitivity to catecholamines is markedly increased in hyperthyroidism, and therapy with beta-adrenergic blocking agents may be very helpful in controlling tachycardia and arrhythmias.

Pulmonary Effects

Thyroid hormones maintain normal hypoxic and hypercapnic drive in the respiratory center. In severe hypothyroidism, hypoventilation occurs, occasionally requiring assisted ventilation.

Hematopoietic Effects

The increased cellular demand for O_2 in hyperthyroidism leads to increased production of erythropoietin and increased erythropoiesis. However, blood volume is usually not increased because of hemodilution and increased red cell turnover. Thyroid hormones increase the 2,3-diphosphoglycerate content of erythrocytes, allowing increased O_2 dissociation from hemoglobin and increasing O_2 availability to tissues. The reverse occurs in hypothyroidism.

Gastrointestinal Effects

Thyroid hormones stimulate gut motility, which can result in increased motility and diarrhea in hyperthyroidism and slowed bowel transit and constipation in hypothyroidism. This may also contribute to the modest weight loss in hyperthyroidism and weight gain in hypothyroidism.

Skeletal Effects

Thyroid hormones stimulate increased bone turnover, increasing bone resorption and, to a lesser degree, bone formation. Thus, chronic hyperthyroidism may result in significant osteopenia and, in severe cases, modest hypercalcemia, hypercalciuria, and increased excretion of urinary hydroxyproline and pyridinium cross-links.

Neuromuscular Effects

Although thyroid hormones stimulate increased synthesis of many structural proteins, in hyperthyroidism there is increased protein turnover and loss of muscle tissue, or myopathy. This may be associated with spontaneous creatinuria. There is also an increase in the speed of muscle contraction and relaxation, noted clinically in the hyperreflexia of hyperthyroidism—or the reverse in hypothyroidism. As noted above, thyroid hormones are essential for normal development, and function of the central nervous system, and failure of fetal thyroid function results in severe mental retardation. In the adult, hyperactivity in hyperthyroidism and sluggishness in hypothyroidism can be striking.

Effects on Lipid & Carbohydrate Metabolism

Hyperthyroidism increases hepatic gluconeogenesis and glycogenolysis as well as intestinal glucose absorption. Thus, hyperthyroidism will exacerbate underlying diabetes mellitus. Cholesterol synthesis and degradation are both increased by thyroid hormones. The latter effect is due largely to an increase in the hepatic low-density lipoprotein (LDL) receptors, so that cholesterol levels decline with thyroid overactivity. Lipolysis is also increased, releasing fatty acids and glycerol. Conversely, cholesterol levels are elevated in hypothyroidism.

Endocrine Effects

Thyroid hormones increase the metabolic turnover of many hormones and pharmacologic agents. For example, the half-life of cortisol is about 100 minutes in the normal individual, about 50 minutes in a hyperthyroid patient, and about 150 minutes in a hypothyroid patient. The production rate of cortisol will increase in the hyperthyroid patient with normal adrenal function, thus maintaining a normal circulating hormone level. However, in a patient with adrenal insufficiency, the development of hyperthyroidism or thyroid hormone treatment of hypothyroidism may unmask the adrenal disease. Ovulation may be impaired in both hyperthyroidism and hypothyroidism, resulting in infertility, which will be corrected by restoration of the euthyroid state. Serum prolactin levels are increased in about 40% of patients with hypothyroidism, presumably a manifestation of increased TRH release; this will revert to normal with T_4 therapy. Other endocrine effects will be discussed in appropriate sections elsewhere in this chapter.

PHYSIOLOGIC CHANGES IN THYROID FUNCTION

Thyroid Function in the Fetus

Prior to the development of independent fetal thyroid function, the fetus is dependent on maternal thyroid hormones for early neural development. However, by the 11th week of gestation, the hypophysial portal system has developed, and measurable TSH and TRH are present. At about the same time, the fetal thyroid begins to trap iodine. The secretion of thyroid hormone probably begins in mid gestation (18–20 weeks). TSH increases rapidly to peak levels at 24–28 weeks, and T_4 levels peak at 35–40 weeks. T_3 levels remain low during gestation; T_4 is converted to rT_3 by type 3 5-deiodinase during fetal development. At birth, there is a sudden marked rise in TSH, a rise in T_4, a rise in T_3, and a fall in rT_3 (Chapter 16). These parameters gradually return to normal over the first month of life.

Thyroid Function in Pregnancy

The striking change in thyroid parameters during pregnancy is the rise in TBG and consequent rise in total T_4 and total T_3 in the serum. The rise in TBG is due to estrogen-induced hepatic glycosylation of TBG with N-acetylgalactosamine, which prolongs the metabolic clearance rate of TBG. There is usually no change in thyroxine-binding prealbumin and little change in albumin. Although total T_4 and T_3 are increased, a new equilibrium develops between free and bound thyronines, and the levels of free T_4 and free T_3 are normal. Other changes in pregnancy include an increase in iodide clearance, which, in areas of low iodine intake, may result in impaired hormone synthesis and a fall in T_4, a rise in TSH, and thyroid enlargement. hCG, which peaks near the end of the first trimester, has a weak TSH agonist activity and may be responsible for the slight thyroid enlargement that occurs at that time. Maternal I^- crosses the placenta and supplies the fetal requirement; in large amounts, I^- can inhibit fetal thyroid function. Maternal TSH-R Ab [stim] and TSH-R Ab [block] can also cross the placenta and may be responsible for thyroid dysfunction in the fetus. As noted above, most maternal T_3 and T_4 are deiodinated by placental type 3 5-deiodinase and do not reach the fetus. However, antithyroid drugs such as propylthiouracil and methimazole do cross the placenta and in large doses will block fetal thyroid function.

Changes in Thyroid Function With Aging

Thyroxine turnover is highest in infants and children, and gradually falls to adult levels after puberty. The T_4 turnover rate is then stable until after age 60, when it again drops slightly. Thus, replacement doses of levothyroxine will vary with age and other factors, and patients taking the drug must be monitored regularly (see below and Chapter 25).

Effects of Acute & Chronic Illness on Thyroid Function (Euthyroid Sick Syndrome)

Acute or chronic illness may have striking effects on circulating thyroid hormone levels by modifying the peripheral metabolism of T_4 or by interference with T_4 binding to TBG. These effects can be classified as (1) the low T_3 syndrome or (2) the low T_3-T_4 syndrome.

The peripheral metabolism of T_4 is diagrammed in Figure 7–20. Inhibition of outer ring type 1 5'-deiodinase or activation of type 3 5-deiodinase accelerates conversion of T_4 to rT_3 and conversion of T_3 to 3,3'-T_2. These reactions will markedly lower the circulating level of T_3, resulting in the low T_3 syndrome. This occurs physiologically in the fetus and pathologically in circumstances of carbohydrate restriction, as in malnutrition, starvation, anorexia nervosa, and diabetes mellitus, and in patients with hepatic disease or major acute or chronic systemic illnesses (Table 7–4). Drugs that inhibit type 1 5'-deiodinase also lower the circulating levels of T_3; corticosteroids, amiodarone, and iodinated dyes are the most effective, and propylthiouracil and propranolol are relatively weak. The pathogenesis of the low T_3 syndrome when associated with acute or chronic illness is thought to involve cytokines such as tumor necrosis factor, secreted by inflammatory cells, which inhibit type 1 5'-deiodinase, accelerating inner ring deiodination of T_4.

Serum thyroid hormone levels in the low T_3 syndrome are presented diagrammatically in Figure 7–30. T_3 levels are low; total T_4 levels are normal or slightly elevated; free T_4 (by dialysis) often is slightly elevated; and rT_3 is elevated. TSH is normal. True hypothyroidism can be ruled out by the normal T_4, FT_4, and TSH and by the elevated rT_3.

Patients with the low T_3-T_4 syndrome are usually much sicker, and indeed the mortality rate in this group of patients may approach 50%. Serum T_3 and T_4 levels are both low; FT_4 (by dialysis) is usually normal; and rT_3 is elevated. TSH is usually normal, though it may be low if the patient is receiving dopamine or corticosteroids, which suppress TSH. The pathogenesis of this syndrome is thought to involve the liberation of unsaturated fatty acids, such as oleic acid, from anoxic or injured tissue, which inhibits the binding of T_4 to TBG. The syndrome can be differentiated from true hypothyroidism by the normal levels of free T_4 and TSH.

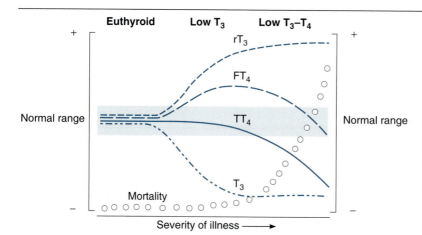

Figure 7–30. A schematic representation of the changes in serum thyroid hormone values with increasing severity of nonthyroidal illness. A rapidly rising mortality rate accompanies the fall in serum total T_4 (TT_4) and free T_4 (FT_4) values. (Reproduced, with permission, from Nicoloff JT: Abnormal measurements in nonendocrine illness. In: *Medicine for the Practicing Physician,* 2nd ed. Hurst JW [editor]. Butterworth-Heinemann, 1991.)

These abnormalities subside when the patient recovers. Recovery is frequently accompanied by a transient elevation of the serum TSH that may be misinterpreted as hypothyroidism. In this setting, in the absence of clinically apparent hypothyroidism, it is best to avoid thyroid hormone therapy and to reevaluate at a later time following recovery. It is possible that intracellular hypothyroidism exists in these patients, but administration of T_3 or T_4 does not benefit the patient and may worsen the situation. Thus, these changes may represent a protective adaptation on the part of the organism to severe illness. For example, one effect would be to reduce oxygen and other metabolic demands.

THYROID AUTOIMMUNITY

Autoimmune mechanisms are involved in the pathogenesis of many thyroid diseases, including the hyperthyroidism, ophthalmopathy, and dermopathy associated with Graves' disease; the nontoxic goiter or atrophic hypothyroidism associated with Hashimoto's thyroiditis; neonatal Graves' disease and some forms of neonatal hypothyroidism; and postpartum hyperthyroidism or hypothyroidism. Thus, it is important that we understand how the immune system works and how thyroid disease develops. Excellent reviews are available (Kendall-Taylor, 1995).

Immunologic defense against foreign substances and neoplastic cells involves macrophages that ingest and digest the foreign material and present peptide fragments on the cell surface in association with a class II protein coded by the HLA-DR region of the MHC gene complex. This complex is recognized by a T cell receptor on a CD4 "helper" T cell, which stimulates the release of cytokines such as interleukin 2 (IL-2). These cytokines amplify the response by inducing T cell activation and division, induction of "killer cell activity" in CD8 suppressor cells, and stimulation of antibody formation against the foreign antigen by B lymphocytes. Eventually, the activation process is muted by the action of the CD8 suppressor cells.

In 1956, three major observations suggested the possibility that immunologic reactions could develop involving the thyroid gland: (1) Rose and Witebsky produced thyroiditis in one lobe of a rabbit thyroid by immunization of the animal with a suspension of the other lobe in Freund's adjuvant; (2) Roitt and Doniach demonstrated the presence of precipitating human thyroglobulin antibodies in the serum of patients with thyroiditis; and (3) Adams and Purves demonstrated the presence of a long-acting thyroid stimulator (later proved to be an antibody to the TSH receptor) in the serum of patients with Graves' disease. Thus, the concept of autoimmune thyroid disease was born.

There are three major thyroidal autoantigens: thyroglobulin (Tg), thyroidal peroxidase (TPO), and the TSH receptor (TSH-R). In addition, a 64-kDa protein expressed on thyroid membranes and on orbital cell membranes may account for the involvement of both the orbital contents and the thyroid in patients with Graves' disease. The properties of some of these antigens are summarized in Table 7–7. Autoantibodies to these antigens are useful as markers for the presence of autoimmune thyroid disease. However, the pathogenesis of the thyroid disease probably involves lymphocyte sensitization to these and possibly other thyroidal antigens. Thyroid cells have the capacity to ingest antigen (eg, thyroglobulin) and, when stimulated by cytokines such as gamma interferon, will express cell surface class II molecules (eg, DR4) to present these antigens to T lymphocytes. Whereas the presence of both the antigen and the class II molecule may be required for autoimmune thyroid disease to develop, other unknown factors also are critical. Active inquiry is under way into whether the process is initiated or promoted either by external antigens that lead to antibody and cellular immune responses through cross-reactivity with thyroid gland antigens or by primary or secondary immunologic imbalances—or by both mechanisms. Clues to the pathogenesis may come from understanding the roles

Table 7–7. Thyroid autoantigens.[1]

Antigen	Molecular Weight (kD$_a$)	Structure	Function	Comment
Thyroglobulin (Tg)	660	5496-amino acid dimer	Prothyroid hormone	Major colloid component.
Thyroid peroxidase (TPO)	102	926 amino acids	Catalyzes T_3 and T_4 synthesis	Membrane-bound.
TSH receptor (TSH-R)	100	744 amino acids	Transduction of TSH message	Antibodies can stimulate or block.
64-kDa antigen	64	Unknown	Unknown	Antigen common to thyroid and orbital membranes.

[1]Adapted and modified, with permission, from Mariotti S, Pinchera P: Role of the immune system in the control of thyroid function. In: *The Thyroid Gland.* Greer MA (editor). Raven, 1990.

of both genetic and environmental factors now known to be associated with autoimmune thyroid disease.

Genetic factors play a large role in the autoimmune process. HLA typing in patients with Graves' disease reveals a high incidence of HLA-B8 and HLA-DR3 in Caucasians, HLA-Bw46 and HLA-B5 in Chinese, and HLA-B17 in blacks. In Caucasians, atrophic thyroiditis has been associated with HLA-B8 and goitrous Hashimoto's thyroiditis with HLA-DR5. These associations are of limited diagnostic or prognostic value but illustrate the genetic predisposition to autoimmune thyroid disease. Volpé has suggested that a genetically induced antigen-specific defect in suppressor T lymphocytes may be the basis for autoimmune thyroid disease.

Environmental factors may also play a role in the pathogenesis of autoimmune thyroid disease. Viruses infecting human thyroid cell cultures induce the expression of DR4 on the follicle cell surface, probably as an effect of a cytokine such as alpha interferon. The increased incidence of autoimmune thyroid disease in postpubertal and premenopausal women, as well as the occurrence of postpartum thyroiditis, implies a role for sex hormones in the pathogenesis of autoimmune thyroid disease. The gram-negative bacillus *Yersinia enterocolitica,* which can cause chronic enterocolitis in humans, has a saturable binding site for mammalian thyrotropin as well antigens that cross-react with human thyroid antigens. It has been postulated that antibodies against *Y enterocolitica* could cross-react with the TSH-R on the thyroid cell membrane and trigger an episode of Graves' disease. A high iodine intake may result in more highly iodinated thyroglobulin, which is more immunogenic and would favor the development of autoimmune thyroid disease. Therapeutic doses of lithium, used for the treatment of manic-depressive psychoses, can interfere with suppressor cell function and precipitate autoimmune thyroid disease. Thus, there are a number of environmental and genetic factors that could contribute to the development of this disorder (see Chapter 4).

TESTS OF THYROID FUNCTION

The function of the thyroid gland may be evaluated in many different ways: (1) tests of thyroid hormones in blood, (2) evaluation of the hypothalamic-pituitary-thyroid axis, (3) assessment of iodine metabolism, (4) estimation of gland size, (5) thyroid biopsy, (6) observation of the effects of thyroid hormones on peripheral tissues, and (7) measurement of thyroid autoantibodies.

TESTS OF THYROID HORMONES IN BLOOD

The total serum T_4 and total serum T_3 are measured by radioimmunoassay or immunofluorescent assay. If the concentration of serum thyroid hormone binding proteins is normal, these measurements provide a reasonably reliable index of thyroid gland activity. However, changes in serum concentration of thyroid-binding proteins or the presence of drugs that modify the binding of T_4 or T_3 to TBP (Table 7–1) will modify the total T_4 and T_3 but not the amount of free hormone. Thus, further tests must be performed to assess the *free* hormone level that determines biologic activity (Figure 7–16).

The free T_4 level can be estimated using the **free thyroxine index** (FT_4I), or it can be measured directly by dialysis (free thyroxine by dialysis; FT_4D) or by radioimmunoassay. These tests are reliable in patients with normal thyroxine-binding proteins (TBPs) but may not be reliable in the presence of a marked abnormality in TBP or in the presence of severe illness (euthyroid sick syndrome) or in patients taking drugs that modify the quantity or binding capacity of TBP (Table 7–1).

FT_4I is the product of the total T_4 multiplied by the percentage of labeled T_4 taken up by a resin, charcoal, or antibody added to the serum. Thus, if the range of total serum T_4 is 5–12 µg/dL (64–154 nmol/L) and resin T_4 uptake (RT_4U) is 25–35%, the normal range of the calculated FT_4I ($T_4 \times RT_4U$) will be 1.3–4.2 in arbitrary units (16–54 in arbitrary SI units). The method can be improved by using the ratio of counts taken up by the resin divided by counts remaining in the serum (free:bound ratio); this is called the **thyroid hormone-binding ratio** (THBR). The patient's THBR is "normalized" by dividing it by the THBR of a normal or reference serum. The patient's total T_4 is then multiplied by this ratio, producing an "adjusted FT_4I," in which the total T_4 is adjusted downward if TBG is high and upward if TBG is low. The normal range for the FT_4I as calculated by this method will then be the same as the normal range for total T_4 in a patient with normal TBP, ie, 5–12 (USA units) or 64–154 (SI units).

Although the FT_4I has been very useful as an estimate of the free T_4 level, a direct measure of the free hormone would be much more precise. Analogs of T_4 and T_3 have been prepared which theoretically bind to specific antibodies but not to TBG—and thus could be used to measure, by displacement, the binding of FT_4 to a T_4 antibody. Unfortunately, some of these analogs will bind to serum albumin, limiting the reliability of the test. However, a reliable microdialysis method for determination of FT_4 is available. The levels of free T_4 in normal adults are 0.9–2 ng/dL (12–26 pmol/L).

The FT_4I is valid for most patients except those with marked dysproteinemia or severe illness. In patients with very high or very low thyroid-binding proteins, the THBR may not completely correct for the abnormal binding protein, and in severely ill patients there may be factors that interfere with T_4 binding to thyroid-binding proteins or to the resin or charcoal matrix. In these situations, FT_4D is more reliable. Both FT_4I and FT_4D will be inappropriately low in patients receiving replacement therapy with liothyronine or in patients with early Graves' disease or toxic nodular goiter, in whom hyperthyroidism is associated with overproduction of T_3 rather than T_4 (T_3 toxicosis). Antiepileptic drugs such as phenytoin and carbamazepine and the antituberculosis drug rifampin increase hepatic metabolism of T_4, resulting in a low total T_4, a low free T_4, and a low FT_4I. However, serum T_3 and serum TSH levels are normal, indicating that patients receiving these drugs are euthyroid. As noted above, T_4 and FT_4I may be low in severe illness, but FT_4D and TSH are usually normal, which will distinguish these very ill patients from patients who are hypothyroid.

At times, FT_4I and FT_4D will be inappropriately elevated. For example, drugs such as iodinated contrast media, amiodarone, glucocorticoids, and propranolol (Table 7–4) inhibit type 1 5'-deiodinase and the conversion of T_4 to T_3 in peripheral tissues, resulting in elevation of total T_4, FT_4I, and FT_4D and depression of T_3. Hyperthyroidism is ruled out by the low T_3 and normal TSH. FT_4I and FT_4D are inappropriately elevated in the rare syndrome of generalized resistance to thyroid hormone (see below). The presence of heparin in serum, even in the tiny amounts that would be found in a patient with a "heparin lock" indwelling intravenous catheter, will cause a spurious increase in FT_4D. This occurs in the test tube, since heparin activates lipoprotein lipase, releasing free fatty acids that displace T_4 from TBG.

Total T_3 can be measured in serum by immunoassay with specific T_3 antisera. The normal range in adults is 95–190 ng/dL (1.5–2.9 nmol/L). The measurement of total T_3 is most useful in the differential diagnosis of hyperthyroidism, because T_3 is preferentially secreted in early Graves' disease or toxic nodular goiter. For example, the normal ratio of serum T_3 in ng/dL to T_4 in μg/dL is less than 20 (eg, T_3 120 ng/dL, T_4 8 μg/dL: ratio = 15). In hyperthyroidism, this ratio will usually be well over 20, and it will be even higher in T_3 thyrotoxicosis. T_3 levels are often maintained in the normal range in hypothyroidism because TSH stimulation increases the relative secretion of T_3; thus, serum T_3 is not a good test for hypothyroidism.

T_3 is bound to TBG, and the total T_3 concentration in serum will vary with the level of TBG (Table 7–1). Serum free T_3 (FT_3) can be measured by equilibrium dialysis; the normal adult FT_3 is 0.2–0.52 ng/dL (3–8 pmol/L). However, this method is technically difficult, and for clinical purposes FT_3 is best estimated by a free T_3 index (FT_3I). This is obtained

by multiplying the normalized THBR by the total T_3 as measured by immunoassay. The adjusted FT_3I in the normal adult is the same as the total T_3.

Reverse T_3 (rT_3) can be measured by radioimmunoassay. The serum concentration of rT_3 in adults is about one-third of the total T_3 concentration, with a range of 25–75 ng/dL (0.39–1.15 nmol/L). RT_3 can be used to differentiate chronic illness from hypothyroidism because rT_3 levels are elevated in chronic illness and low in hypothyroidism. However, this differential diagnosis can be made by determination of TSH (see below), so that it is rarely necessary to measure rT_3.

Thyroglobulin (Tg) can be measured in serum by double antibody radioimmunoassay. The normal range will vary with method and laboratory, but generally the normal range is less than 40 ng/mL (< 40 μg/L) in the euthyroid individual and less than 5 ng/mL (< 5 μg/L) in a thyroidectomized individual. The major problem with the test is that endogenous thyroglobulin antibodies interfere with the assay procedure and, depending on the method, may result in spuriously low or spuriously high values. Serum thyroglobulin is elevated in situations of thyroid overactivity such as Graves' disease and toxic multinodular goiter; in subacute or chronic thyroiditis, where it is released as a consequence of tissue damage; and in patients with large goiters, in whom the thyroglobulin level is proportionate to the size of the gland. Serum thyroglobulin determinations have been most useful in the management of patients with papillary or follicular thyroid carcinoma. Following thyroidectomy and ^{131}I therapy, thyroglobulin levels should be very low. In such a patient, serum thyroglobulin greater than 10 ng/dL (> 10 μg/L) indicates the presence of metastatic disease, and a rise in serum thyroglobulin in a patient with known metastases indicates progression of the disease.

EVALUATION OF THE HYPOTHALAMIC-PITUITARY-THYROID AXIS

The hypothalamic-pituitary-thyroid axis is illustrated in Figure 7–21. It has not been clinically feasible to measure TRH in the peripheral circulation in humans. However, very sensitive methods for the measurement of TSH have been developed using monoclonal antibodies against human TSH. The general principle is this: One monoclonal TSH antibody is fixed to a solid matrix to bind serum TSH, and a second monoclonal TSH antibody labeled with isotope or enzyme or fluorescent tag will bind to a separate epitope on the TSH molecule. The quantity of TSH in the serum is thus proportionate to the quantity of bound second antibody. The earlier TSH radioimmunoassays, which could detect about 1 μU of TSH/mL, were adequate for the diagnosis of elevated

TSH in hypothyroidism but could not detect suppressed TSH levels in hyperthyroidism. The "second generation" of "sensitive" TSH assays, using monoclonal antibodies, can detect about 0.1 μU/mL, and the "third generation" of "supersensitive" assays are sufficiently sensitive to detect about 0.01 μU/mL. This has allowed measurement of TSH well below the normal range of 0.5–5 μU/mL (0.5–5 mU/L) and has enabled the clinician to detect partially and totally suppressed serum TSH levels. The level of FT_4 is inversely related to the logarithm of the TSH concentration (Figure 7–31A). Thus, a small change in FT_4 may result in a large change in TSH. The relationship; between TSH and FT_4 in various situations is demonstrated in Figure 7–31A and 7–31B. Serum TSH below 0.1 μU/mL (0.1 mU/L) and an elevated FT_4D or FT_4I is indicative of hyperthyroidism. This may be due to Graves' disease, toxic nodular goiter, or high-dose thyroxine therapy. In the rare case of hyperthyroidism due to a TSH-secreting pituitary tumor, FT_4I or FT_4D will be elevated and TSH will not be suppressed but will actually be normal or slightly elevated. An elevated TSH (> 10 μU/mL; 10 mU/L) and a low FT_4D or FT_4I is diagnostic of hypothyroidism. In patients with hypothyroidism due to a pituitary or hypothalamic tumor (central hypothyroidism), FT_4I or FT_4D will be low and TSH will not be elevated. This diagnosis can be confirmed by demonstrating the failure of serum TSH to increase following an injection of TRH (TRH test; Figure 7–25). Note that corticosteroids and dopamine inhibit TSH secretion (Table 7–6), which will modify the interpretation of serum TSH levels in patients taking these drugs.

Serum TSH levels reflect the anterior pituitary gland sensing the level of circulating FT_4. High FT_4 levels suppress TSH and low FT_4 increases TSH release. Thus, the ultrasensitive measurement of TSH has become the most sensitive, most convenient, and most specific test for the diagnosis of both hyperthyroidism and hypothyroidism. Indeed, a suppressed TSH correlates so well with impaired pituitary response to TRH that the simple measurement of serum TSH has replaced the TRH test in the diagnosis of hyperthyroidism.

IODINE METABOLISM & BIOSYNTHETIC ACTIVITY

Radioactive iodine allows assessment of the turnover of iodine by the thyroid gland in vivo. Iodine-123 is the ideal isotope for this purpose: It has a half-life of 13.3 hours and releases a 28-keV x-ray and a 159-keV gamma photon but no beta emissions. Thus, it is easily measured and causes little tissue damage. It is usually administered orally in a dose of 100–200 μCi, and radioactivity over the thyroid area is measured with a scintillation counter at 4 or 6

hours and again at 24 hours (Figure 7–8). The normal **radioactive iodine uptake** (RAIU) will vary with the iodide intake. In areas of low iodide intake and endemic goiter, the 24-hour RAIU may be as high as 60–90%. In the USA—a country with a relatively high iodide intake—the normal uptake at 6 hours is 5–15% and at 24 hours 8–30%. In thyrotoxicosis due to Graves' disease or toxic nodular goiter, 24-hour RAIU is markedly elevated, although if the iodide turnover is very rapid, the 5-hour uptake may be even higher than the 24-hour uptake (Figure 7–8). Thyrotoxicosis with a very low thyroidal RAIU occurs in the following situations: (1) in subacute thyroiditis; (2) during the active phase of Hashimoto's thyroiditis, with release of preformed hormone, causing "spontaneously resolving thyrotoxicosis"; (3) in thyrotoxicosis factitia due to oral ingestion of a large amount of thyroid hormone; (4) as a result of excess iodide intake (eg, amiodarone therapy), inducing thyrotoxicosis in a patient with latent Graves' disease or multinodular goiter, the low uptake being due to the huge iodide pool; (5) in struma ovarii; and (6) in ectopic functioning metastatic thyroid carcinoma after total thyroidectomy.

In normal individuals, administration of 75–100 μg of T_3 in divided doses daily for 5 days will reduce the 24-hour RAIU by more than 50% (suppression test). Failure of the thyroid to suppress on this treatment indicates autonomous thyroid function, as in Graves' disease, or autonomously functioning thyroid nodules.

The efficiency of the thyroid organification process may be tested with the "perchlorate discharge test." As noted above, $KClO_4$ will displace I^- from the iodide trap. Thus, oral administration of 0.5 g $KClO_4$ to a normal individual will block further uptake of ^{123}I, but not more than 5% of the previously accumulated radioiodine will be released. Conversely, if there is an organification defect, not only is further uptake blocked but I^- diffuses out of the gland or is "discharged" (Figure 7–12). Positive tests are seen in some patients with congenital iodide organification defects, Hashimoto's thyroiditis, Graves' disease after ^{131}I therapy, or patients receiving inhibitors of iodide organification such as methimazole or propylthiouracil. The perchlorate discharge test is rarely used clinically, but it can be very helpful in understanding the pathophysiology of some of the above illnesses.

THYROID IMAGING

1. RADIONUCLIDE IMAGING

^{123}I or technetium Tc 99m pertechnetate (^{99m}Tc as TcO_4) is useful for determining the *functional* activity of the thyroid gland. ^{123}I is administered orally in

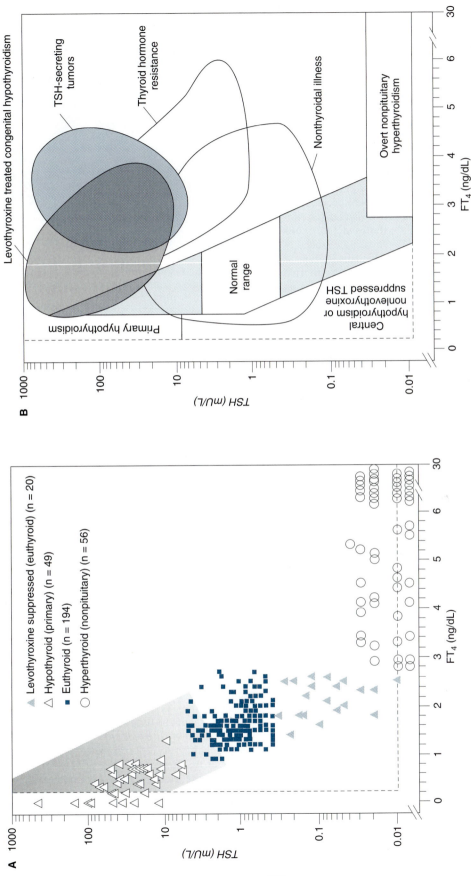

Figure 7–31. A: Relationship between serum free thyroxine by dialysis (FT₄) ng/dL and log₁₀ TSH in euthyroid, hyperthyroid, hypothyroid, and L-T₄-suppressed euthyroid individuals. Note that for each unit change in T₄ there is a logarithmic change in TSH. **B:** Relationship between FT₄ by dialysis and log₁₀ TSH in normal subjects and subjects with various illnesses including primary hypothyroidism, central hypothyroidism and non-levothyroxine-suppressed TSH, levothyroxine-treated congenital hypothyroidism, TSH-secreting tumors, thyroid hormone resistance, nonthyroidal illness, and nonpituitary hyperthyroidism. (Reproduced, with permission, from Kaptein EM: Clinical applications of free thyroxine determinations. Clin Lab Med 1993;13:654.)

a dose of 200–300 μCi, and a scan of the thyroid is obtained at 8–24 hours. $^{99m}TcO_4$ is administered intravenously in a dose of 1–10 mCi, and the scan is obtained at 30–60 minutes. Images can be obtained with either a rectilinear scanner or a gamma camera. The rectilinear scanner moves back and forth over the area of interest; it produces a life-size picture, and special areas, such as nodules, can be marked directly on the scan (Figure 7–32). The gamma camera has a pinhole collimator, and the scan is obtained on a fluorescent screen and recorded on Polaroid film. The camera has greater resolution, but special areas must be identified with a radioactive marker for clinical correlation (Figure 7–33). Radionuclide scans provide information about both the size and shape of the thyroid gland and the geographic distribution of functional activity in the gland. Functioning thyroid nodules are called "hot" nodules, and nonfunctioning ones are called "cold" nodules. The incidence of malignancy in hot nodules is about 1%, but they may become toxic, producing enough hormone to suppress the rest of the gland and induce thyrotoxicosis. About 16% of surgically removed cold nodules have been malignant. Occasionally, a nodule will be hot with $^{99m}TcO_4$ and cold with ^{123}I, and a few of these nodules have been malignant. For large substernal goiters or for distant metastases from a thyroid cancer, ^{131}I is the preferred isotope because of its long half-life (8 days) and its 0.72 MeV gamma emission.

Fluorescent Scanning

The iodine content and an image of the thyroid gland can be obtained by fluorescent scanning without administration of a radioisotope. An external source of Americium-241 is beamed at the thyroid gland, and the resulting emission of 28.5 keV x-ray from iodide ions is recorded, producing an image of

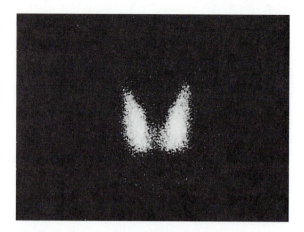

Figure 7–33. Scintiphoto (pinhole collimator) thyroid scan performed 6 hours after the ingestion of 100 μCi of sodium ^{123}I. (Courtesy of RR Cavalieri.)

the thyroid gland similar to that obtained with ^{123}I (Figure 7–32). The advantage of this procedure is that the patient receives no radioisotope and the gland can be imaged even when it is loaded with iodine—as, for example, after intravenous contrast media. The disadvantage of this study is that it requires specialized equipment that may not be generally available.

THYROID ULTRASONOGRAPHY OR MAGNETIC RESONANCE IMAGING

A rough estimate of thyroid size and nodularity can be obtained from radionuclide scanning, but much better detail can be obtained by thyroid ultrasonography or MRI.

Thyroid ultrasonography is particularly useful for measuring the size of the gland or individual nodules and for evaluating the results of therapy. It is useful also for differentiating solid from cystic lesions and to guide the operator to a deep nodule during fine-needle thyroid aspiration biopsy (see below). Thyroid ultrasonography is limited to thyroid tissue in the neck, ie, it cannot be used for substernal lesions.

MRI provides an excellent image of the thyroid gland, including posterior or substernal extension of a goiter or malignancy. Both transverse and coronal images of the gland can be obtained, and lymph nodes as small as 1 cm can be visualized. MRI is invaluable for the demonstration of tracheal compression from a large goiter, tracheal invasion or local extension of a thyroid malignancy, or metastases to local or mediastinal lymph nodes.

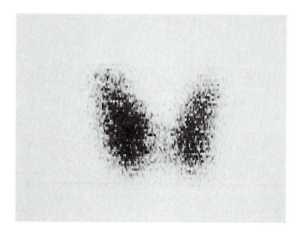

Figure 7–32. Rectilinear sodium ^{123}I scan performed 6 hours after the ingestion of 100 μCi of sodium ^{123}I. (Courtesy of RR Cavalieri.)

THYROID BIOPSY

Fine-needle aspiration biopsy of a thyroid nodule has proved to be the best method for differentiation of benign from malignant thyroid disease. It is performed as an outpatient procedure and requires no preparation. The skin over the nodule is cleansed with alcohol, and, if desired, a small amount of 1% lidocaine can be injected intracutaneously for local anesthesia. A No. 25 1½-inch needle is then inserted into the nodule and moved in and out until a small amount of bloody material is seen in the hub of the needle; the needle is then removed, and with a syringe, the contents of the needle are expressed onto a clean slide. A second clean slide is placed on top of the first slide, and a thin smear is obtained by drawing the slides apart quickly. Alternatively, a 10 mL or 20 mL syringe in an appropriate syringe holder can be used with a No. 23 1-inch needle to sample the nodule or to evacuate cystic contents.

The slides are fixed—either dry and stained with Wright's or Giemsa's stain, or fixed in alcohol and stained with Papanicolaou's stain. The sensitivity (true-positive results divided by total cases of disease) is about 95%, and the specificity (true-negative results divided by total cases of no disease) is also about 95%. For best results, fine-needle aspiration biopsy requires an adequate tissue sample and a specially trained cytologist to interpret it.

EFFECTS OF THYROID HORMONES ON PERIPHERAL TISSUES

The definitive test of thyroid function would be a test of the effect of thyroid hormones on body tissues. Thyroid hormones increase heat production and oxygen consumption. A measurement of this basal oxygen in the intact organism became one of the first tests of thyroid function, the **basal metabolic rate** (BMR). However, this test is nonspecific and insensitive and is rarely used today. The speed of muscle contraction and relaxation is increased in hyperthyroidism and decreased in hypothyroidism. The contraction and relaxation time of the Achilles tendon has been standardized and measured by an instrument called the **photomotogram.** However, there is considerable overlap between normal subjects and patients with thyroid dysfunction, limiting the usefulness of this procedure.

Cardiac muscle contractility can also be measured as an index of thyroid hormone action. With echocardiography, it is relatively easy to measure such indices as the preejection period (PEP), the time from onset of the QRS complex to the opening of the aortic valve; or the left ventricular ejection time (LVET). These are prolonged in hypothyroidism and shortened in hyperthyroidism. Although these measurements are modified by coexistent cardiac disease, they may be the best objective tests for measuring the peripheral effects of thyroid hormone action.

Thyroid hormones influence the concentration of a number of enzymes and blood constituents. For example, serum cholesterol is usually lowered in hyperthyroidism and elevated in hypothyroidism. Serum creatine kinase and lactic dehydrogenase, probably of skeletal muscle origin, are elevated in hypothyroidism—and indeed, isoenzyme determination may be required to differentiate the enzyme changes occurring in myocardial infarction from those occurring in myxedema.

Sex hormone-binding globulin (SHBG) and angiotensin-converting enzyme are also increased in hyperthyroidism and decreased in hypothyroidism. However, none of these biochemical or enzyme changes are sensitive or specific enough for diagnostic use.

MEASUREMENT OF THYROID AUTOANTIBODIES

Thyroid autoantibodies include (1) thyroglobulin antibody (Tg Ab); (2) thyroid peroxidase antibody (TPO Ab), formerly called microsomal antibody; and (3) TSH receptor antibody, either stimulating (TSH-R Ab [stim]) or blocking (TSH-R Ab [block]). Tg Ab and TPO Ab have been measured by hemagglutination, enzyme-linked immunoassay (ELISA), or radioimmunoassay (RIA). The hemagglutination technique is much less sensitive than the ELISA or RIA methods. For example, in the Whickham study of a normal population in northeastern England, TPO antibodies were found in about 8% of young women (aged 18–24) and 13.7% of older women (aged 45–54). In a similar study of normal blood donors and using radioimmunoassay, TPO antibodies were found in 10.6% of younger and in 30.3% of older women. The incidence of positive TPO antibodies in normal men (by hemagglutination) was low—about 2%—and did not increase with age. On the other hand, high Tg Ab and TPO Ab titers by RIA are found in 97% of patients with Graves' disease or Hashimoto's thyroiditis. Thyroglobulin antibodies are often high early in the course of Hashimoto's thyroiditis and decrease with time; TPO antibodies are usually measurable for the life of the patient. The titers of both Tg and TPO antibodies will decrease with time following institution of T_4 therapy in Hashimoto's thyroiditis or with antithyroid therapy in Graves' disease. A strongly positive test for either of these antibodies is an indication of the presence of autoimmune thyroid disease but is not specific for the type of disease, ie, hyperthyroidism, hypothyroidism, or goiter.

The thyroid receptor stimulating antibody (TSH-R

Ab [stim]) is characteristic of Graves' disease (see above). It was originally measured by demonstrating prolonged discharge of radioiodine from the thyroid gland of the mouse after injection of serum from a patient with Graves' disease; it was then called long-acting thyroid stimulator (LATS). This laborious assay has been replaced by a bioassay using human thyroid cells in culture and measuring the increase in thyroid cAMP following incubation with serum or IgG. The test is positive in 90% of patients with Graves' disease and undetectable in healthy subjects or patients with Hashimoto's thyroiditis (without ophthalmopathy), nontoxic goiter, or toxic nodular goiter. It is most useful for the diagnosis of Graves' disease in patients with euthyroid ophthalmopathy or in predicting neonatal Graves' disease in the newborn of a mother with active or past Graves' disease.

The same type of assay can be used to detect TSH receptor-blocking antibody (TSH-R Ab [block]). In this assay, the increase in cAMP induced by TSH added to a human thyroid cell culture is blocked by concurrent incubation with the patient's serum. The TSH-binding inhibition assay (TBII) measures the ability of serum IgG to inhibit the binding of labeled TSH to a thyroid cell membrane preparation containing the TSH receptor. This technique is not as satisfactory as the bioassay because there are a variety of nonspecific interfering substances, such as thyroglobulin, which inhibit TSH binding. However, a modification of the TSH-binding inhibition assay using recombinant human TSH receptor has proved to be more reliable. Detection of a TSH receptor-blocking antibody in maternal serum may be very helpful in predicting the occurrence of congenital hypothyroidism in newborns of mothers with autoimmune thyroid disease.

SUMMARY: CLINICAL USE OF THYROID FUNCTION TESTS

The diagnosis of thyroid disease has been greatly simplified by the development of sensitive assays for TSH and free thyroxine. The estimate of free thyroxine, either FT_4I or FT_4D, and a sensitive TSH determination are used both for the diagnosis of thyroid disease and for following patients receiving T_4 replacement or antithyroid drug therapy. An elevated TSH and low free thyroxine establish the diagnosis of hypothyroidism, and a suppressed TSH and elevated FT_4 establish the diagnosis of hyperthyroidism.

Other tests are available for special uses. In hypothyroidism, Tg Ab or TPO Ab tests will clarify the etiology of the illness, and in hyperthyroidism elevation of free T_3, abnormal radioiodine uptake and scan, and a positive test for TSH-R Ab [stim] may be useful. In patients with nodules or goiter, fine-needle aspiration biopsy will rule out malignancy; radioiodine scan may help to determine function; and thy-

roid ultrasound or MRI may be helpful in following the size or growth of the goiter. Patients with known thyroid cancer are followed with serial thyroglobulin determinations, and ^{131}I scan or MRI may be useful for detection of metastatic disease.

DISORDERS OF THE THYROID

Patients with thyroid disease will usually complain of (1) thyroid enlargement, which may be diffuse or nodular; (2) symptoms of thyroid deficiency, or hypothyroidism; (3) symptoms of thyroid hormone excess, or hyperthyroidism; or (4) complications of a specific form of hyperthyroidism—Graves' disease—which may present with striking prominence of the eyes (exophthalmos) or, rarely, thickening of the skin over the lower legs (thyroid dermopathy).

History

The history should include evaluation of symptoms related to the above complaints, discussed in more detail below. Exposure to ionizing radiation in childhood has been associated with an increased incidence of thyroid disease, including cancer. Iodide ingestion in the form of kelp or iodide-containing cough preparations may induce goiter, hypothyroidism, or hyperthyroidism. Lithium carbonate, used in the treatment of manic-depressive psychiatric disorder, can also induce hypothyroidism and goiter or hyperthyroidism. Residence in an area of low dietary iodide is associated with iodine deficiency goiter ("endemic goiter"). Although dietary iodide is generally adequate in developed countries, there are still areas low in natural iodine (ie, developing countries in Africa, Asia, South America, and inland mountainous areas). Finally, the family history should be explored with particular reference to goiter, hyperthyroidism, or hypothyroidism as well as immunologic disorders such as diabetes, rheumatoid disease, pernicious anemia, alopecia, vitiligo, or myasthenia gravis, which may be associated with an increased incidence of autoimmune thyroid disease. Multiple endocrine neoplasia type IIa (Sipple's syndrome) with medullary carcinoma of the thyroid gland is an autosomal dominant condition.

Physical Examination

Physical examination of the thyroid gland is illustrated in Figure 7–34. The thyroid is firmly attached to the anterior trachea midway between the sternal notch and the thyroid cartilage; it is often easy to see and to palpate. The patient should have a glass of water for comfortable swallowing. There are three maneuvers: (1) With a good light coming from behind

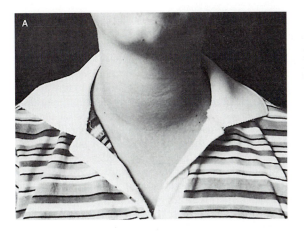
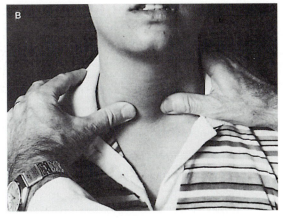
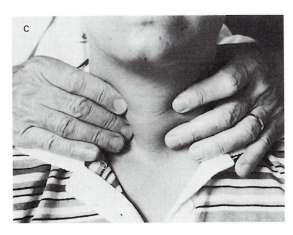
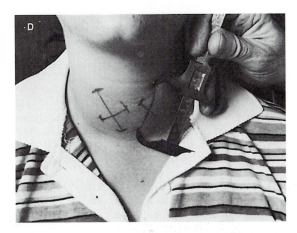

Figure 7–34. Examination of the thyroid gland. *A:* Observe the neck, especially as the patient swallows. *B:* Examine from the front, rotating the gland slightly with one thumb while palpating the other lobe with the other thumb. *C:* Examine from behind, using three fingers and the same technique. *D:* The size of each lobe or of thyroid nodules can be measured by first drawing an outline on the skin.

the examiner, the patient is instructed to swallow a sip of water. Observe the gland as it moves up and down. Enlargement and nodularity can often be noted. (2) Palpate the gland anteriorly. Gently press down with one thumb on one side of the gland to rotate the other lobe forward, and palpate as the patient swallows. (3) Palpate the gland from behind the patient with the middle three fingers on each lobe while the patient swallows. An outline of the gland can be traced on the skin of the neck and measured (Figure 7–34D). Nodules can be measured in a similar way. Thus, changes in the size of the gland or in nodules can easily be followed.

On physical examination, the palpable bulbous portion of each lobe of the normal thyroid gland measures about 2 cm in vertical dimension and about 1 cm in horizontal dimension above the isthmus. An enlarged thyroid gland is called **goiter.** Generalized enlargement is termed diffuse goiter; irregular or lumpy enlargement is called nodular goiter.

HYPOTHYROIDISM

Hypothyroidism is a clinical syndrome resulting from a deficiency of thyroid hormones, which in turn results in a generalized slowing down of metabolic processes. Hypothyroidism in infants and children results in marked slowing of growth and development, with serious permanent consequences including mental retardation. Hypothyroidism with onset in adulthood causes a generalized slowing down of the organism, with deposition of glycosaminoglycans in intracellular spaces, particularly in skin and muscle, producing the clinical picture of **myxedema.** The symptoms of hypothyroidism in adults are largely reversible with therapy.

Etiology & Incidence (Table 7–8)

Hypothyroidism may be classified as (1) primary (thyroid failure), (2) secondary (to pituitary TSH

Table 7–8. Etiology of hypothyroidism.

Primary:
1. Hashimoto's thyroiditis:
   a. With goiter.
   b. "Idiopathic" thyroid atrophy, presumably end-stage autoimmune thyroid disease, following either Hashimoto's thyroiditis or Graves' disease.
   c. Neonatal hypothyroidism due to placental transmission of TSH-R blocking antibodies.
2. Radioactive iodine therapy for Graves' disease.
3. Subtotal thyroidectomy for Graves' disease or nodular goiter.
4. Excessive iodide intake (kelp, radiocontrast dyes).
5. Subacute thyroiditis.
6. Rare causes in the USA:
   a. Iodide deficiency.
   b. Other goitrogens such as lithium; antithyroid drug therapy.
   c. Inborn errors of thyroid hormone synthesis.

Secondary: Hypopituitarism due to pituitary adenoma, pituitary ablative therapy, or pituitary destruction.

Tertiary: Hypothalamic dysfunction (rare).

Peripheral resistance to the action of thyroid hormone.

deficit), or (3) tertiary (due to hypothalamic deficiency of TRH)—or may be due to (4) peripheral resistance to the action of thyroid hormones. Hypothyroidism can also be classified as goitrous or nongoitrous, but this classification is probably unsatisfactory, since Hashimoto's thyroiditis may produce hypothyroidism with or without goiter.

The incidence of various causes of hypothyroidism will vary depending on geographic and environmental factors such as dietary iodide and goitrogen intake, the genetic characteristics of the population, and the age distribution of the population (pediatric or adult). The causes of hypothyroidism, listed in approximate order of frequency in the USA, are presented in Table 7–8. Hashimoto's thyroiditis is probably the most common cause of hypothyroidism. In younger patients, it is more likely to be associated with goiter; in older patients, the gland may be totally destroyed by the immunologic process, and the only trace of the disease will be a persistently positive test for TPO (thyroid microsomal) autoantibodies. Similarly, the end stage of Graves' disease may be hypothyroidism. This is accelerated by destructive therapy such as administration of radioactive iodine or subtotal thyroidectomy. Thyroid glands involved in autoimmune disease are particularly susceptible to excessive iodide intake (eg, ingestion of kelp tablets, iodide-containing cough preparations, or the antiarrhythmic drug amiodarone) or administration of iodide-containing radiographic contrast media. The large amounts of iodide block thyroid hormone synthesis, producing hypothyroidism with goiter in the patient with an abnormal thyroid gland; the normal gland usually "escapes" from the iodide block (see above). Although the process may be temporarily reversed by withdrawal of iodide, the underlying disease will often

progress, and permanent hypothyroidism will usually supervene. Hypothyroidism may occur during the late phase of subacute thyroiditis; this is usually transient, but it is permanent in about 10% of patients. Iodide deficiency is rarely a cause of hypothyroidism in the USA but may be more common in developing countries. Certain drugs can block hormone synthesis and produce hypothyroidism with goiter; at present, the most common pharmacologic causes of hypothyroidism (other than iodide) are lithium carbonate, used for the treatment of manic-depressive states, and amiodarone. Chronic therapy with the antithyroid drugs propylthiouracil and methimazole will do the same. Inborn errors of thyroid hormone synthesis result in severe hypothyroidism if the block in hormone synthesis is complete, or mild hypothyroidism if the block is partial. Pituitary and hypothalamic deficiencies as causes of hypothyroidism are quite rare and are usually associated with other symptoms and signs of pituitary insufficiency (Chapter 5). Peripheral resistance to thyroid hormones is discussed below.

Pathogenesis

Thyroid hormone deficiency affects every tissue in the body, so that the symptoms are multiple. Pathologically, the most characteristic finding is the accumulation of glycosaminoglycans—mostly hyaluronic acid—in interstitial tissues. Accumulation of this hydrophilic substance and increased capillary permeability to albumin account for the interstitial edema that is particularly evident in the skin, heart muscle, and striated muscle. The accumulation is due not to excessive synthesis but to decreased destruction of glycosaminoglycans.

Clinical Presentations & Findings

A. Newborn Infants (Cretinism): The term cretinism was originally applied to infants—in areas of low iodide intake and endemic goiter—with mental retardation, short stature, a characteristic puffy appearance of the face and hands, and (frequently) deaf mutism and neurologic signs of pyramidal and extrapyramidal tract abnormalities (Figure 7–35). In the USA, neonatal screening programs have revealed that in the white population the incidence of neonatal hypothyroidism is 1:5000, while in the black population the incidence is only 1:32,000. Neonatal hypothyroidism may result from failure of the thyroid to descend during embryonic development from its origin at the base of the tongue to its usual site in the lower anterior neck, which results in an "ectopic thyroid" gland that functions poorly. Placental transfer to the embryo of TSH-R Ab [block] from a mother with Hashimoto's thyroiditis, may result in agenesis of the thyroid gland and "athyreotic cretinism." Inherited defects in thyroid hormone biosynthesis induce neonatal hypothyroidism and goiter. Rare causes of neonatal hypothyroidism include adminis-

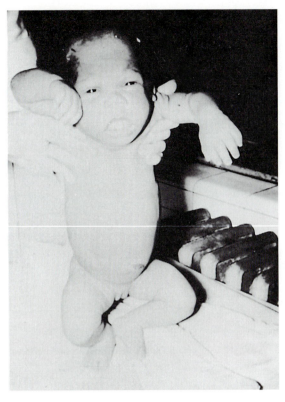

Figure 7–35. A 9-month-old infant with hypothyroidism (cretinism). Note the puffy face, protuberant abdomen, umbilical hernia, and muscle weakness (infant cannot sit up unassisted).

tration during pregnancy of iodides, antithyroid drugs, or radioactive iodine for thyrotoxicosis.

The symptoms of hypothyroidism in newborns include respiratory difficulty, cyanosis, jaundice, poor feeding, hoarse cry, umbilical hernia, and marked retardation of bone maturation. The proximal tibial epiphysis and distal femoral epiphysis are present in almost all full-term infants with a body weight of over 2500 g. Absence of these epiphyses strongly suggests hypothyroidism. The introduction of routine screening of newborns for TSH or T_4 has been a major achievement in the early diagnosis of neonatal hypothyroidism. A serum T_4 under 6 μg/dL or a serum TSH over 30 μU/mL is indicative of neonatal hypothyroidism. The diagnosis can then be confirmed by radiologic evidence of retarded bone age.

B. Children: Hypothyroidism in children is characterized by retarded growth and evidence of mental retardation. In the adolescent, precocious puberty may occur, and there may be enlargement of the sella turcica in addition to short stature. This is not due to pituitary tumor but probably to pituitary hypertrophy associated with excessive TSH production.

C. Adults: In adults, the common features of hypothyroidism include easy fatigability, coldness, weight gain, constipation, menstrual irregularities, and muscle cramps. Physical findings include a cool, rough, dry skin, puffy face and hands, a hoarse, husky voice, and slow reflexes (Figure 7–36). Reduced conversion of carotene to vitamin A and increased blood levels of carotene may give the skin a yellowish color.

1. Cardiovascular signs–Hypothyroidism is manifested by impaired muscular contraction, bradycardia, and diminished cardiac output. The ECG reveals low voltage of QRS complexes and P and T waves, with improvement in response to therapy. Cardiac enlargement may occur, due in part to interstitial edema, nonspecific myofibrillary swelling, and left ventricular dilation but often to pericardial effusion (Figure 7–37). The degree of pericardial effusion can easily be determined by echocardiography. Although cardiac output is reduced, congestive heart failure and pulmonary edema are rarely noted. There is controversy about whether myxedema induces coronary artery disease, but coronary artery disease is more common in patients with hypothyroidism, particularly in older patients. In patients with angina pectoris, hypothyroidism may protect the heart from ischemic stress, and replacement therapy may aggravate the angina.

2. Pulmonary function–In the adult, hypothyroidism is characterized by shallow, slow respirations

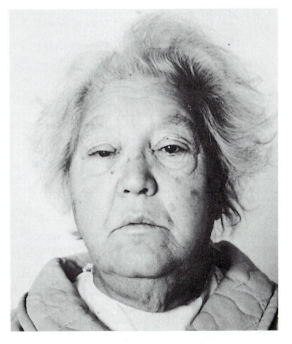

Figure 7–36. Hypothyroidism in adult (myxedema). Note puffy face, puffy eyes, frowsy hair, and dull and apathetic appearance.

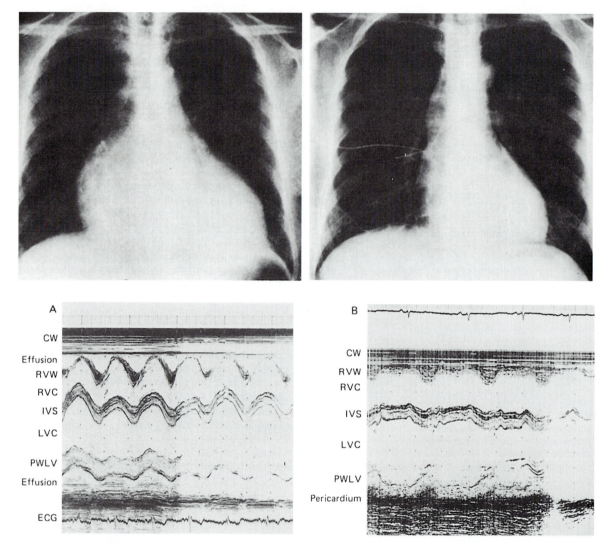

Figure 7–37. *Top:* Chest x-ray studies of patient with hypothyroid cardiomyopathy. *Left:* Before therapy, showing pronounced cardiomegaly. *Right:* Six months after institution of thyroxine therapy, the heart size has returned to normal (Reproduced, with permission, from Reza MJ, Abbasi AS: Congestive cardiomyopathy in hypothyroidism. West J Med 1975;123:228). *Bottom:* Echocardiogram of a 29-year-old woman with hypothyroidism *(A)* before and *(B)* after 2 months of therapy with levothyroxine sodium. (CW, chest wall; RVW, right ventricular wall; RVC, right ventricular cavity; IVS, interventricular septum; LVC, left ventricular cavity; PWLV, posterior wall left ventricle.) Note disappearance of pericardial effusion following levothyroxine therapy. (Reproduced, with permission, from Sokolow M, Mcilroy MB: *Clinical Cardiology,* 4th ed. Lange, 1986.)

and impaired ventilatory responses to hypercapnia or hypoxia. Respiratory failure is a major problem in patients with myxedema coma.

3. Intestinal peristalsis is markedly slowed, resulting in chronic constipation and occasionally severe fecal impaction or ileus.

4. Renal function is impaired, with decreased glomerular filtration rate and impaired ability to excrete a water load. This predisposes the myxedematous patient to water intoxication if excessive free water is administered.

5. Anemia–There are at least four mechanisms that may contribute to **anemia** in patients with hypothyroidism: (1) impaired hemoglobin synthesis as a result of thyroxine deficiency; (2) iron deficiency from increased iron loss with menorrhagia, as well as impaired intestinal absorption of iron; (3) folate deficiency from impaired intestinal absorption of folic acid; and (4) pernicious anemia, with vitamin B_{12}-deficient megaloblastic anemia. The pernicious anemia is often part of a spectrum of autoimmune diseases, including myxedema due to chronic thyroiditis associated with thyroid autoantibodies, pernicious anemia associated with parietal cell autoantibodies, diabetes mellitus associated with islet cell autoantibodies, and adrenal insufficiency associated with adrenal autoantibodies (Schmidt's syndrome; see Chapter 24).

6. Neuromuscular system–Many patients complain of symptoms referable to the neuromuscular system, eg, severe muscle cramps, paresthesias, and muscle weakness.

7. Central nervous system symptoms may include chronic fatigue, lethargy, and inability to concentrate. Hypothyroidism impairs the conversion of estrogen precursors to estrogens, resulting in altered FSH and LH secretion and in anovulatory cycles and infertility. This may also be associated with severe menorrhagia. Patients with myxedema are usually quite placid but can be severely depressed or even extremely agitated ("myxedema madness").

Diagnosis

The combination of a low serum FT_4 or FT_4I and an elevated serum TSH is diagnostic of primary hypothyroidism (Figure 7–38). Serum T_3 levels are variable and may be within the normal range. A positive test for thyroid autoantibodies suggests underlying Hashimoto's thyroiditis. In patients with pituitary myxedema, the FT_4I or FT_4 will be low but serum TSH will not be elevated. It may then be necessary to differentiate pituitary from hypothalamic disease, and for this the TRH test is most helpful (Figure 7–25). Absence of TSH response to TRH indicates pituitary deficiency. A partial or "normal" type response indicates that pituitary function is intact but

that a defect exists in hypothalamic secretion of TRH. The patient may be taking thyroid medication (levothyroxine or desiccated thyroid tablets) when first seen. A palpable or enlarged thyroid gland and a positive test for thyroid autoantibodies would suggest underlying Hashimoto's thyroiditis, in which case the medication should be continued. If antibodies are absent, the medication should be withdrawn for 6 weeks and determinations made for FT_4I or FT_4 and for TSH. The 6-week period of withdrawal is necessary because of the long half-life of thyroxine (7 days) and to allow the pituitary gland to recover after a long period of suppression. The pattern of recovery of thyroid function after withdrawal of T_4 is noted in Figure 7–39. In hypothyroid individuals, TSH becomes markedly elevated at 5–6 weeks and T_4 remains subnormal, whereas both are normal after 6 weeks in euthyroid controls.

The clinical picture of fully developed myxedema is usually quite clear, but the symptoms and signs of mild hypothyroidism may be very subtle. Patients with hypothyroidism will at times present with unusual features: neurasthenia with symptoms of muscle cramps, paresthesias, and weakness; refractory anemia; disturbances in reproductive function, including infertility, delayed puberty, or menorrhagia; idiopathic edema or pleuropericardial effusions; retarded growth; obstipation; chronic rhinitis or hoarseness due to edema of nasal mucosa or vocal cords; and severe depression progressing to emotional instability or even frank paranoid psychosis. In the elderly, hypothyroidism may present with apathy and withdrawal, often attributed to senility (Chapter 25). In such cases, the diagnostic studies outlined above

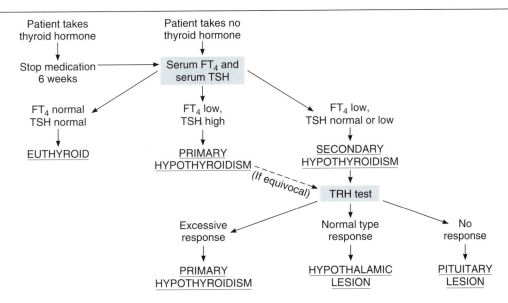

Figure 7–38. Diagnosis of hypothyroidism. Either free thyroxine (FT_4) or free thyroxine index (FT_4I) may be used with TSH for evaluation.

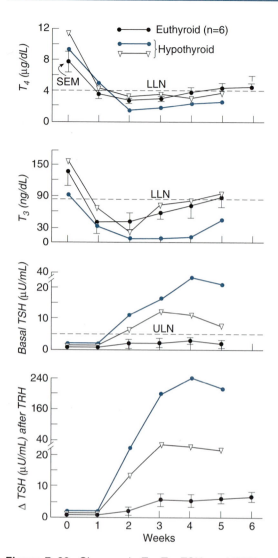

Figure 7–39. Changes in T_4, T_3, TSH, and TRH response following abrupt withdrawal of suppressive thyroxine therapy. Note that in euthyroid individuals the T_4 may not return to normal until 6 weeks after withdrawal of therapy and that serum TSH is never elevated. In hypothyroid patients, TSH may be elevated as early as 2 weeks after withdrawal of therapy, and TRH response is exaggerated. (LLN, lower limit of normal; ULN, upper limit of normal.) (Reproduced, with permission, from Wood LC: Controversial questions in thyroid disease. Workshop in the Thyroid, American Thyroid Association, Nov 1979, as adapted from Vagenakis AG et al: Recovery of pituitary thyrotropic function after withdrawal of prolonged thyroid suppression therapy. N Engl J Med 1975;293:681.)

will confirm or rule out hypothyroidism as a contributing factor.

Complications

A. Myxedema Coma: Myxedema coma is the end stage of untreated hypothyroidism. It is characterized by progressive weakness, stupor, hypothermia, hypoventilation, hypoglycemia, hyponatremia, water intoxication, shock, and death. Although rare now, in the future it may occur more frequently in association with the increasing use of radioiodine for the treatment of Graves' disease, with resulting permanent hypothyroidism. Since it occurs most frequently in older patients with underlying pulmonary and vascular disease, the mortality rate is extremely high.

The patient (or a family member if the patient is comatose) may recall previous thyroid disease, radioiodine therapy, or thyroidectomy. The medical history is of gradual onset of lethargy progressing to stupor or coma. Examination reveals bradycardia and marked hypothermia, with body temperature as low as 24 °C (75 °F). The patient is usually an obese elderly woman with yellowish skin, a hoarse voice, a large tongue, thin hair, puffy eyes, ileus, and slow reflexes. There may be signs of other illnesses such as pneumonia, myocardial infarction, cerebral thrombosis, or gastrointestinal bleeding. Laboratory clues to the diagnosis of myxedema coma include lactescent serum, high serum carotene, elevated serum cholesterol, and increased cerebrospinal fluid protein. Pleural, pericardial, or abdominal effusions with high protein content may be present. Serum tests will reveal a low FT_4 and a markedly elevated TSH. Thyroidal radioactive iodine uptake is low, and thyroid autoantibodies are usually strongly positive, indicating underlying chronic thyroiditis. The ECG shows sinus bradycardia and low voltage. If laboratory studies are not readily available, which is frequently the case, the diagnosis must be made clinically.

The pathophysiology of myxedema coma involves three major aspects: (1) CO_2 retention and hypoxia, (2) fluid and electrolyte imbalance, and (3) hypothermia. CO_2 retention and hypoxia are probably due in large part to a marked depression in the ventilatory responses to hypoxia and hypercapnia, though factors such as obesity, heart failure, ileus, immobilization, pneumonia, pleural or peritoneal effusions, central nervous system depression, and weak chest muscles may also contribute. The failure of the myxedema patient to respond to hypoxia or hypercapnia may be due to the hypothermia. Impairment of ventilatory drive is often severe, and assisted respiration is almost always necessary in patients with myxedema coma. Thyroid hormone therapy in patients with myxedema corrects the hypothermia and markedly improves the ventilatory response to hypoxia. The major fluid and electrolyte disturbance is water intoxication due to the syndrome of inappropriate secretion of vasopressin (SIADH). This presents as hyponatremia and is managed by water restriction. Hypothermia is frequently not recognized, because the ordinary clinical thermometer only goes down to about 34 °C (93 °F); a laboratory type thermometer that registers a broader scale must be used to obtain accurate body temperature readings. Active rewarming of the body is contraindicated, because it may induce vasodilation and vascular collapse. A rise in body temperature is a useful indication of therapeutic effectiveness of thyroxine.

Disorders that may precipitate myxedema coma include heart failure, pneumonia, pulmonary edema, pleural or peritoneal effusions, ileus, excessive fluid administration, or administration of sedative or narcotic drugs to a patient with severe hypothyroidism. Adrenal insufficiency occurs occasionally in association with myxedema coma, but it is relatively rare and usually associated with either pituitary myxedema or concurrent autoimmune adrenal insufficiency (Schmidt's syndrome). Seizures, bleeding episodes, hypocalcemia, or hypercalcemia may be present. It is important to differentiate *pituitary* myxedema from *primary* myxedema. In pituitary myxedema, glucocorticoid replacement is essential. Clinical clues to the presence of pituitary myxedema include the following: a history of amenorrhea or impotence; scanty pubic or axillary hair; and normal serum cholesterol and normal or low TSH levels. CT scan or MRI may reveal an enlarged sella turcica. The treatment of myxedema coma is discussed below.

B. Myxedema and Heart Disease: In the past, treatment of patients with myxedema and heart disease, particularly coronary artery disease, was very difficult, because levothyroxine replacement was frequently associated with exacerbation of angina, heart failure, or myocardial infarction. Now that coronary angioplasty and coronary artery bypass surgery are available, patients with myxedema and coronary artery disease can be treated surgically first, and more rapid thyroxine replacement therapy will then be tolerated.

C. Hypothyroidism and Neuropsychiatric Disease: Hypothyroidism is often associated with depression, which may be quite severe. More rarely, myxedematous patients may become confused, paranoid, or even manic ("myxedema madness"). Screening of psychiatric admissions with FT_4 and TSH is an efficient way to find these patients, who will frequently respond to levothyroxine therapy alone or in combination with psychopharmacologic agents. The effectiveness of levothyroxine therapy in disturbed hypothyroid patients has given rise to the hypothesis that the addition of T_3 or T_4 to psychotherapeutic regimens for depressed patients may be helpful in patients without demonstrable thyroid disease. Further work needs to be done to establish this concept as standard treatment.

Treatment

A. Treatment of Hypothyroidism: Hypothyroidism is treated with levothyroxine (T_4), which is available in pure form and is stable and inexpensive. Intracellularly, levothyroxine is converted to T_3, so that both hormones become available even though only one is administered. Desiccated thyroid is unsatisfactory because of its variable hormone content, and triiodothyronine (as liothyronine) is unsatisfactory because of its rapid absorption, short half-life, and transient effects. The half-life of levothyroxine is about 7 days, so it need be given only once daily. It is well absorbed, and blood levels are easily monitored by following FT_4I or FT_4 and serum TSH levels. There is a rise in T_4 or FT_4I of about 1–2 μg/dL (13–26 nmol/L) and a concomitant fall in TSH of 1–2 μU/mL (1–2 mU/L) beginning about 2 hours and lasting about 8–10 hours after an oral dose of 0.1–0.15 mg of levothyroxine (Figure 7–40). It is best, therefore, to take the daily dose of levothyroxine in the morning to avoid symptoms such as insomnia if the medication is taken at bedtime. In addition, when monitoring serum thyroxine levels, it is important that blood be drawn fasting or before the daily dose of the hormone in order to obtain consistent data.

Dosage of levothyroxine: Replacement doses of levothyroxine in adults range from 0.05 to 0.2 mg/d, with a mean of 0.125 mg/d. The dose of levothyroxine varies according to the patient's age and body weight (Table 7–9). Young children require a surprisingly high dose of levothyroxine compared

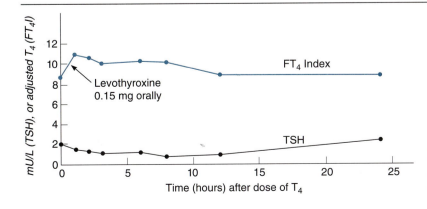

Figure 7–40. Rise in serum free thyroxine index (FT_4I) and fall in serum TSH following an oral dose of 0.15 mg levothyroxine.

Table 7–9. Replacement doses of levothyroxine.[1]

Age	Dose of Levothyroxine (μg/kg/d)
0–6 mo	8–10
7–11 mo	6–8
1–5 yr	5–6
6–10 yr	3–4
11–20 yr	2–3
Adult	1–2

[1]Adapted and modified, with permission, from Dussault J, Fisher DE: Hypothyroidism in infants and children. In: *Werner and Ingbar's The Thyroid,* 6th ed. Braverman LE, Utiger RD (editors). Lippincott, 1991.

with adults. In adults, the mean replacement dose of T_4 is about 1.7 μg/kg/d, or about 0.8 μg/lb/d. In older adults, the replacement dose is lower, about 1.6 μg/kg/d, or about 0.7 μg/lb/d. For TSH suppression in patients with nodular goiters or cancers of the thyroid gland, the average dose of levothyroxine is about 2.2 μg/kg/d (1 μg/lb/d). Malabsorptive states or concurrent administration of aluminum preparations or cholestyramine will modify T_4 absorption, and in these patients larger doses of T_4 may be necessary. Levothyroxine has a sufficiently long half-life (7 days) so that if the patient is unable to take medications by mouth for a few days, omitting levothyroxine therapy will not be detrimental. However, if the patient is being managed by sustained parenteral therapy, the parenteral dose of T_4 is about 75–80% of the usual oral dose.

B. Treatment of Myxedema Coma: Myxedema coma is an acute medical emergency and should be treated in the intensive care unit. Blood gases must be monitored regularly, and the patient usually requires intubation and mechanical ventilation. Associated illnesses such as infections or heart failure must be sought and treated by appropriate therapy. Intravenous fluids should be administered with caution, and excessive free water intake must be avoided. Because patients with myxedema coma absorb all drugs poorly, it is imperative to give levothyroxine intravenously. These patients have marked depletion of serum thyroxine with a large number of empty binding sites on thyroxine-binding globulin and therefore should receive an initial loading dose of thyroxine intravenously, followed by a small daily intravenous dose. An initial dose of 300–400 μg of levothyroxine is administered intravenously, followed by 50 μg of levothyroxine intravenously daily. The clinical guides to improvement are a rise in body temperature and the return of normal cerebral and respiratory function. If the patient is known to have had normal adrenal function before the coma, adrenal support is probably not necessary. If, however, no data are available, the possibility of concomitant adrenal insufficiency (due to autoimmune adrenal disease or pituitary insufficiency) does exist. In this case, the plasma cortisol should be measured or, if time permits (30 minutes), a cosyntropin stimulation test should performed (Chapter 9). Then, full adrenal support should be administered, eg, hydrocortisone hemisuccinate, 100 mg intravenously, followed by 50 mg intravenously every 6 hours, tapering the dose over 7 days. Adrenal support can be withdrawn sooner if the pretreatment plasma cortisol is 20 μg/dL or greater or results of a cosyntropin stimulation test are within normal limits. When giving levothyroxine intravenously in large doses, there is an inherent risk of precipitating angina, heart failure, or arrhythmias in older patients with underlying coronary artery disease. Thus, this type of therapy is not recommended for ambulatory patients with myxedema; in these patients, it is better to start slowly and build up the dose as noted below.

C. Myxedema With Heart Disease: In long-standing hypothyroidism or in older patients—particularly those with known cardiovascular disease—it is imperative to start treatment slowly. Levothyroxine is given in a dosage of 0.025 mg/d for 2 weeks, increasing by 0.025 mg every 2 weeks until a daily dose of 0.1 mg or 0.125 mg is reached. It usually takes about 2 months for a patient to come into equilibrium on full dosage. In these patients, the heart is very sensitive to the level of circulating thyroxine, and if angina pectoris or cardiac arrhythmia develops, it is essential to reduce the dose of thyroxine immediately. In younger patients or those with mild disease, full replacement may be started immediately.

Toxic Effects of Levothyroxine Therapy

There are no reported instances of allergy to pure levothyroxine, though it is possible that a patient may develop an allergy to the coloring dye or some component of the tablet. The major toxic reactions to levothyroxine overdosage are symptoms of hyperthyroidism—particularly cardiac symptoms—and osteoporosis. The most common thyrotoxic cardiac symptom is arrhythmia, particularly paroxysmal atrial tachycardia or fibrillation. Insomnia, tremor, restlessness, and excessive warmth may also be troublesome. Simply omitting the daily dose of levothyroxine for 3 days and then reducing the dosage will correct the problem.

Increased bone resorption and severe osteoporosis have been associated with long-standing hyperthyroidism and will develop in patients chronically overtreated with levothyroxine. This can be prevented by regular monitoring and by maintaining normal serum FT_4 and TSH in patients receiving long-term replacement therapy. In patients receiving TSH-suppressive therapy for nodular goiter or thyroid cancer, if FT_4I or FT_4 is kept in the upper range of normal—even if TSH is suppressed—the adverse effects of T_4 therapy on bone will be minimal (Chapter 25).

Course & Prognosis

The course of untreated myxedema is one of slow deterioration, leading eventually to myxedema coma and death. With appropriate treatment, however, the long-term prognosis is excellent. Because of the long half-life (7 days) of thyroxine, it takes time to establish equilibrium on a fixed dose. Therefore, it is important to monitor the FT_4I or FT_4 and the serum TSH every 4–6 weeks until equilibrium is reached. Thereafter, FT_4 and TSH can be monitored once a year. The dose of T_4 must be increased about 25% during pregnancy and lactation. Older patients metabolize T_4 more slowly, and the dose will gradually decrease with age (Chapter 25).

The mortality rate of myxedema coma was about 80% at one time. The prognosis has been vastly improved as a result of recognition of the importance of mechanically assisted respiration and the use of intravenous levothyroxine. At present, the outcome probably depends upon how well the underlying disease problems can be managed.

HYPERTHYROIDISM & THYROTOXICOSIS

Thyrotoxicosis is the clinical syndrome that results when tissues are exposed to high levels of circulating thyroid hormone. In most instances, thyrotoxicosis is due to hyperactivity of the thyroid gland, or hyperthyroidism. Occasionally, thyrotoxicosis may be due to other causes such as excessive ingestion of thyroid hormone or excessive secretion of thyroid hormone from ectopic sites. The various forms of thyrotoxicosis are listed in Table 7–10. These syndromes will be discussed individually below.

1. DIFFUSE TOXIC GOITER (Graves' Disease)

Graves' disease is the most common form of thyrotoxicosis and may occur at any age, more commonly in females than in males. The syndrome consists of one or more of the following features: (1) thyrotoxicosis, (2) goiter, (3) ophthalmopathy (exophthalmos), and (4) dermopathy (pretibial myxedema).

Table 7–10. Conditions associated with thyrotoxicosis.

1. Diffuse toxic goiter (Graves' disease)
2. Toxic adenoma (Plummer's disease)
3. Toxic multinodular goiter
4. Subacute thyroiditis
5. Hyperthyroid phase of Hashimoto's thyroiditis
6. Thyrotoxicosis factitia
7. Rare forms of thyrotoxicosis: ovarian struma, metastatic thyroid carcinoma (follicular), hydatiform mole, "hamburger thyrotoxicosis," TSH-secreting pituitary tumor, pituitary resistance to T_3 and T_4

Etiology

Graves' disease is currently viewed as an autoimmune disease of unknown cause. There is a strong familial predisposition in that about 15% of patients with Graves' disease have a close relative with the same disorder, and about 50% of relatives of patients with Graves' disease have circulating thyroid autoantibodies. Females are involved about five times more commonly than males. The disease may occur at any age, with a peak incidence in the 20- to 40-year age group. (See section on thyroid autoimmunity, above.)

Pathogenesis

In Graves' disease, T lymphocytes become sensitized to antigens within the thyroid gland and stimulate B lymphocytes to synthesize antibodies to these antigens (see section on thyroid autoimmunity, above, and Figure 7–41). One such antibody is directed against the TSH receptor site in the thyroid

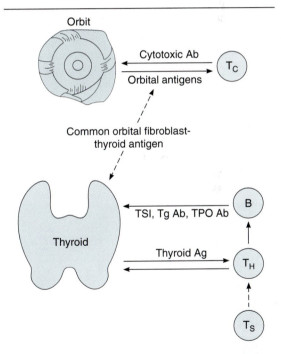

Figure 7–41. One theory of the pathogenesis of Graves' disease. There is a defect in suppressor T lymphocytes (T_s) that allows helper T lymphocytes (T_H) to stimulate B lymphocytes (B) to synthesize thyroid autoantibodies. The thyroid-stimulating immunoglobulin (TSI, or TSH-R Ab[stim]) is the driving force for thyrotoxicosis. The inflammatory process in the orbital muscles may be due to sensitization of cytotoxic T lymphocytes (T_C), or killer cells, to orbital antigens in association with cytotoxic antibodies. The thyroid and the eye may be linked by a common antigen in thyroid and orbital fibroblasts. It is not yet clear what triggers this immunologic cascade. (Tg Ab, thyroglobulin antibody; TPO Ab, thyroperoxidase or microsomal antibody; Ag, antigen; Ab, antibody.)

cell membrane and has the capacity to stimulate the thyroid cell to increased growth and function (TSH-R Ab [stim]; see Table 7–7). The presence of this circulating antibody is positively correlated with active disease and with relapse of the disease. There is an underlying genetic predisposition, but it is not clear what "triggers" the acute episode. Some factors that may incite the immune response of Graves' disease are (1) pregnancy, particularly the postpartum period; (2) iodide excess, particularly in geographic areas of iodide deficiency, where the lack of iodide may hold latent Graves' disease in check; (3) lithium therapy, perhaps by modifying immune responsiveness; (4) viral or bacterial infections; and (5) glucocorticoid withdrawal. It has been postulated that "stress" may trigger an episode of Graves' disease, but there is no evidence to support this hypothesis. The pathogenesis of ophthalmopathy may involve cytotoxic lymphocytes (killer cells) and cytotoxic antibodies sensitized to a common antigen (perhaps a 64-kDa antigen related to thyroglobulin or the TSH-R itself) in orbital fibroblasts, orbital muscle, and thyroid tissue (Figure 7–41). Cytokines from these sensitized lymphocytes would cause inflammation of orbital fibroblasts and orbital myositis, resulting in swollen orbital muscles, proptosis of the globes, and diplopia as well as redness, congestion, and conjunctival and periorbital edema (thyroid ophthalmopathy; Figures 7–42 and 7–43). The pathogenesis of thyroid dermopathy (pretibial myxedema) (Figure 7–44) and the rare subperiosteal inflammation on the phalanges of the hands and feet (thyroid osteopathy) (Figure 7–45) may also involve lymphocyte cytokine stimulation of fibroblasts in these locations.

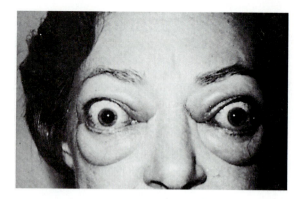

Figure 7–43. Severe ophthalmopathy of Graves' disease. Note marked periorbital edema, injection of corneal blood vessels, and proptosis. There was also striking limitation of upward and lateral eye movements and reduced visual acuity. ***Classification*** (Table 7–11): class 1, severe; class 2, severe; class 3, severe; class 4, severe; class 5, none; class 6, mild.

Many symptoms of thyrotoxicosis suggest a state of catecholamine excess, including tachycardia, tremor, sweating, lid lag, and stare. Circulating levels of epinephrine are normal; thus, in Graves' disease, the body appears to be hyperreactive to catecholamines. This may be due in part to a thyroid hormone-mediated increase in cardiac catecholamine receptors.

Clinical Features

A. Symptoms and Signs: In younger individuals, common manifestations include palpitations, ner-

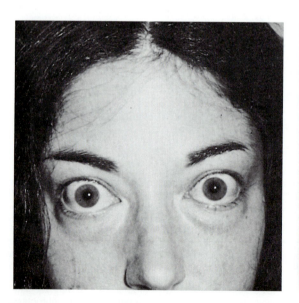
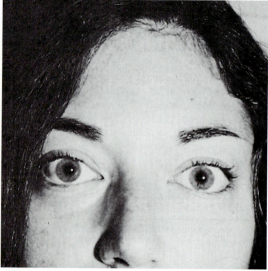

Figure 7–42. Patient with mild ophthalmopathy of Graves' disease. ***Left:*** Before radioactive iodine therapy. Note white sclera visible above and below the iris as well as mild periorbital edema. Classification (Table 7–11): class 1, mild; class 2, mild: class 3, mild. ***Right:*** After radioactive iodine therapy. Marked improvement is noted.

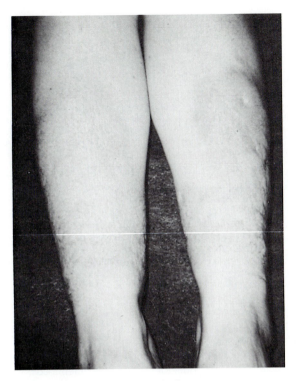

Figure 7–44. Dermopathy of Graves' disease. Marked thickening of the skin is noted, usually over the pretibial area. Thickening will occasionally extend downward over the ankle and the dorsal aspect of the foot but almost never above the knee.

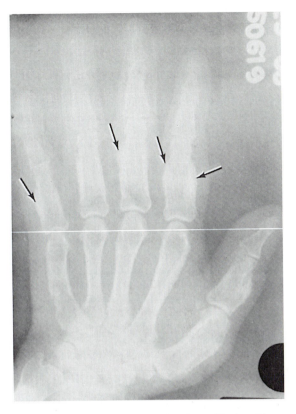

Figure 7–45. X-ray of hand of patient with thyroid osteopathy. Note marked periosteal thickening of the proximal phalanges.

vousness, easy fatigability, hyperkinesia, diarrhea, excessive sweating, intolerance to heat, and preference for cold. There is often marked weight loss without loss of appetite. Thyroid enlargement, thyrotoxic eye signs (see below), and mild tachycardia commonly occur. Muscle weakness and loss of muscle mass may be so severe that the patient cannot rise from a chair without assistance. In children, rapid growth with accelerated bone maturation occurs. In patients over age 60, cardiovascular and myopathic manifestations predominate; the most common presenting complaints are palpitation, dyspnea on exertion, tremor, nervousness, and weight loss (Chapter 25).

The eye signs of Graves' disease have been classified by the American Thyroid Association as set forth in Table 7–11. This classification is useful in describing the extent of the eye involvement, though it is not helpful in following the progress of the illness since one class does not always progress into the next. The first letters of each class form the mnemonic "NO SPECS." Class 1 involves spasm of the upper lids associated with active thyrotoxicosis and usually resolves spontaneously when the thyrotoxicosis is adequately controlled. Classes 2–6 represent true infiltrative disease involving orbital muscles and orbital tissues (Figures 7–42 and 7–43). Class 2 is characterized by soft tissue involvement with periorbital edema, congestion or redness of the conjunctiva, and swelling of the conjunctiva (chemosis). Class 3 consists of proptosis as measured by the Hertel exophthalmometer. This instrument consists of

Table 7–11. Classification of eye changes in Graves' disease.[1]

Class	Definition
0	*No* signs or symptoms.
1	*Only* signs, no symptoms. (Signs limited to upper lid retraction, stare, lid lag.)
2	*Soft* tissue involvement (symptoms and signs).
3	*Proptosis* (measured with Hertel exophthalmometer).[2]
4	*Extraocular* muscle involvement.
5	*Corneal* involvement.
6	*Sight* loss (optic nerve involvement).

[1]Reproduced, with permission, from Werner, SC: Classification of the eye changes of Graves' disease. J Clin Endocrinol Metab 1969;29:782 and 1977;44:203.
[2]Upper limits of normal according to race: Oriental, 18mm; white, 20 mm; black, 22 mm. Increase in proptosis of 3–4 mm is mild involvement; 5–7 mm, moderate involvement; and over 8 mm, severe involvement. Other classes can be similarly graded as mild, moderate, or severe.

two prisms with a scale mounted on a bar. The prisms are placed on the lateral orbital ridges, and the distance from the orbital ridge to the anterior cornea is measured on the scale (Figure 7–46). The upper limits of normal according to race are listed in the footnote to Table 7–11. Class 4 consists of muscle involvement. The muscle most commonly involved in the infiltrative process is the inferior rectus, limiting upward gaze. The muscle next most commonly involved is the medial rectus, impairing lateral gaze. Class 5 is characterized by corneal involvement (keratitis) and class 6 loss of vision from optic nerve involvement. As noted above, thyroid ophthalmopathy is due to infiltration of the extraocular muscles with lymphocytes and edema fluid in an acute inflammatory reaction. The orbit is a cone enclosed by bone, and swelling of the extraocular muscles within this closed space causes proptosis of the globe and impaired muscle movement, resulting in diplopia. Ocular muscle enlargement can be demonstrated by orbital CT scanning or MRI (Figure 7–47). When muscle swelling occurs posteriorly, toward the apex of the orbital cone, the optic nerve is compressed, which may cause loss of vision.

Thyroid dermopathy consists of thickening of the skin, particularly over the lower tibia, due to accumulation of glycosaminoglycans (Figure 7–44). It is relatively rare, occurring in about 2–3% of patients with Graves' disease. It is usually associated with ophthalmopathy and with a very high serum titer of TSH-R Ab [stim]. The skin is markedly thickened and cannot be picked up between the fingers. Sometimes the dermopathy involves the entire lower leg and may extend onto the feet. Bony involvement (os-

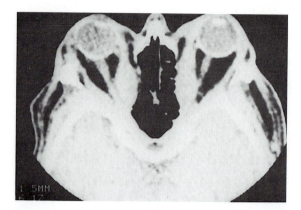

Figure 7–47. Orbital CT scan in a patient with severe ophthalmopathy and visual failure. Note the marked enlargement of extraocular muscles posteriorly, with compression of the optic nerve at the apex of the orbital cone.

teopathy), with subperiosteal bone formation and swelling, is particularly evident in the metacarpal bones (Figure 7–45). This too is a relatively rare finding. A more common finding in Graves' disease is separation of the fingernails from their beds, or onycholysis (Figure 7–48).

B. Laboratory Findings: The laboratory findings in hyperthyroidism are summarized in Figure 7–49. Essentially, the combination of an elevated FT_4 and a suppressed TSH makes the diagnosis of hyperthyroidism. If eye signs are present, the diagnosis of Graves' disease can be made without further tests. If eye signs are absent and the patient is hyper-

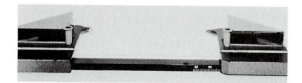

A

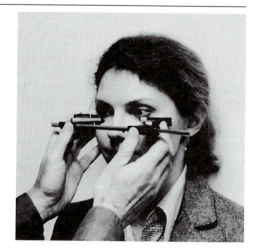

B

Figure 7–46. A: Hertel exophthalmometer. **B:** Proper use of the exophthalmometer. The edges of the instrument are placed on the lateral orbital ridges, and the distance from the orbital bone to the anterior cornea is read on the scale contained within the prisms.

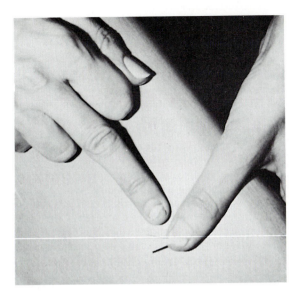

Figure 7–48. Onycholysis (separation of the nail from its bed) in Graves' disease usually resolves spontaneously as the patient improves.

thyroid with or without a goiter, a radioiodine uptake test should be done. An elevated uptake is diagnostic of Graves' disease or toxic nodular goiter. A low uptake is seen in patients with spontaneously resolving hyperthyroidism, as in subacute thyroiditis or a flare-up of Hashimoto's thyroiditis. Low uptakes will also be found in patients who are iodine-loaded, or are on

T_4 therapy, or, rarely, in association with a struma ovarii. If both FT_4 and TSH are elevated, consider a TSH-secreting pituitary tumor or generalized or pituitary resistance syndromes. If FT_4 is normal and TSH is suppressed, check FT_3. FT_3 will be elevated in early Graves' disease or in T_3-secreting toxic nodules. Low FT_3 will be found in the euthyroid sick syndrome or in patients receiving corticoids or dopamine.

Thyroid autoantibodies, Tg Ab and TPO Ab, are usually present in both Graves' disease and Hashimoto's thyroiditis, but TSH-R Ab [stim] is specific for Graves' disease. This may be a useful diagnostic test in the "apathetic" hyperthyroid patient or in the patient who presents with unilateral exophthalmos without obvious signs or laboratory manifestations of Graves' disease. The ^{123}I or technetium scan is useful to evaluate the size of the gland or the presence of "hot" or "cold" nodules. Since the ultrasensitive TSH test will detect TSH suppression, TRH and TSH suppression tests (see above) are rarely indicated. CT and MRI scans of the orbit have revealed muscle enlargement in most patients with Graves' disease even when there is no clinical evidence of ophthalmopathy. In patients with ophthalmopathy, orbital muscle enlargement may be striking (Figure 7–47).

Differential Diagnosis

Graves' disease occasionally presents in an unusual or atypical fashion, in which case the diagnosis may not be obvious. Marked muscle atrophy may suggest severe myopathy that must be differentiated

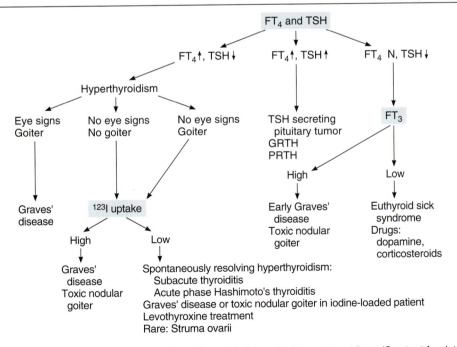

Figure 7–49. Laboratory tests useful in the differential diagnosis of hyperthyroidism. (See text for details.)

from primary neurologic disorder. **Thyrotoxic periodic paralysis** usually occurs in Asian males and presents with a sudden attack of flaccid paralysis and hypokalemia. The paralysis usually subsides spontaneously and can be prevented by K^+ supplementation and beta-adrenergic blockade. The illness is cured by appropriate treatment of the thyrotoxicosis. Patients with **thyrocardiac disease** present primarily with symptoms of heart involvement—especially refractory atrial fibrillation insensitive to digoxin—or with high-output heart failure. About 50% of these patients have no evidence of underlying heart disease, and the cardiac problems are cured by treatment of the thyrotoxicosis. Some older patients will present with weight loss, small goiter, slow atrial fibrillation, and severe depression, with none of the clinical features of increased catecholamine reactivity. These placid patients have **"apathetic hyperthyroidism."** Finally, some young women may present with amenorrhea or infertility as the primary symptom. In all of these instances, the diagnosis of hyperthyroidism can usually be made on the basis of the clinical and laboratory studies described above.

In the syndrome called **"familial dysalbuminemic hyperthyroxinemia"** (see above), an abnormal albumin-like protein is present in serum that preferentially binds T_4 but not T_3. This results in elevation of serum T_4 and FT_4I, but free T_4, T_3, and TSH are normal. It is important to differentiate this euthyroid state from hyperthyroidism. In addition to the absence of clinical features of hyperthyroidism, a normal serum T_3 and a normal TSH level will rule out hyperthyroidism.

Complications

Thyrotoxic crisis ("thyroid storm") is the acute exacerbation of all of the symptoms of thyrotoxicosis, often presenting as a syndrome that may be of life-threatening severity. Occasionally, thyroid storm may be mild and present simply as an unexplained febrile reaction after thyroid surgery in a patient who has been inadequately prepared. More commonly, it occurs in a more severe form after surgery, radioactive iodine therapy, or parturition in a patient with inadequately controlled thyrotoxicosis or during a severe, stressful illness or disorder such as uncontrolled diabetes, trauma, acute infection, severe drug reaction, or myocardial infarction. The clinical manifestations of thyroid storm are marked hypermetabolism and excessive adrenergic response. Fever ranges from 38 to 41 °C and is associated with flushing and sweating. There is marked tachycardia, often with atrial fibrillation and high pulse pressure and occasionally with heart failure. Central nervous system symptoms include marked agitation, restlessness, delirium, and coma. Gastrointestinal symptoms include nausea, vomiting, diarrhea, and jaundice. A fatal outcome will be associated with heart failure and shock.

At one time it was thought that thyroid storm was due to sudden release or "dumping" of stored thyroxine and triiodothyronine from the thyrotoxic gland. Careful studies have revealed, however, that the serum levels of T_4 and T_3 in patients with thyroid storm are not higher than in thyrotoxic patients without this condition. There is no evidence that thyroid storm is due to excessive production of triiodothyronine. There is evidence that in thyrotoxicosis the number of binding sites for catecholamines increases, so that heart and nerve tissues have increased sensitivity to circulating catecholamines. In addition, there is decreased binding to TBG, with elevation of free T_3 and T_4. The present theory is that in this setting, with increased binding sites available for catecholamines, an acute illness, infection, or surgical stress triggers an outpouring of catecholamines which, in association with high levels of free T_4 and T_3, precipitates the acute problem.

The most striking clinical diagnostic feature of thyrotoxic crisis is hyperpyrexia out of proportion to other findings. Laboratory findings include elevated serum T_4, FT_4, and T_3 as well as a suppressed TSH.

Treatment of Graves' Disease

Although autoimmune mechanisms are responsible for the syndrome of Graves' disease, management has been largely directed toward controlling the hyperthyroidism. Three good methods are available: (1) antithyroid drug therapy, (2) surgery, and (3) radioactive iodine therapy.

A. Antithyroid Drug Therapy: In general, antithyroid drug therapy is most useful in young patients with small glands and mild disease. The drugs (propylthiouracil or methimazole) are given until the disease undergoes spontaneous remission. This occurs in 20–40% of patients treated for 6 months to 15 years. Although this is the only therapy that leaves an intact thyroid gland, it does require a long period of observation, and the incidence of relapse is high, perhaps 60–80% even in selected patients. The relapse rate may be decreased using the regimen of total thyroid block described below. Antithyroid drug therapy is generally started with large divided doses; when the patient becomes clinically euthyroid, maintenance therapy may be achieved with a lower single morning dose. A common regimen consists of giving propylthiouracil, 100–150 mg every 6 hours initially, and then in 4–8 weeks reducing the dose to 50–200 mg once or twice daily. Propylthiouracil has one advantage over methimazole in that it partially inhibits the conversion of T_4 to T_3, so that it is effective in bringing down the levels of activated thyroid hormone more quickly. However, methimazole has a longer duration of action and is more useful if a single daily dose is desirable. A typical program would start with a 40-mg dose of methimazole each morning for 1–2 months; this dose would then be reduced to 5–20 mg each morning for maintenance therapy.

The laboratory tests of most value in monitoring the course of therapy are serum FT_4 and TSH.

An alternative method of therapy utilizes the concept of a total block of thyroid activity. The patient is treated with methimazole until euthyroid (about 3–6 months), but instead of continuing to taper the dose of methimazole, at this point levothyroxine is added in a dose of about 0.1 mg/d. The patient then continues to receive the combination of methimazole 10 mg/d and levothyroxine 0.1 mg/d for another 12–24 months. At the end of this time, or when the size of the gland has returned to normal, methimazole is discontinued and levothyroxine continued for another year. With this therapy, the fall in antithyroid antibody titer is striking, and long-term remissions occur in 40–50% of treated patients.

1. Duration of therapy—The duration of therapy with antithyroid drugs in Graves' disease is quite variable and can range from 6 months to 20 years or more. A sustained remission may be predicted in about 80% of treated patients in the following circumstances: (1) if the thyroid gland returns to normal size; (2) if the disease can be controlled with a relatively small dose of antithyroid drugs; (3) if TSH-R Ab [stim] is no longer detectable in the serum; and (4) if the thyroid gland becomes normally suppressible following the administration of liothyronine.

2. Reactions to antithyroid drugs—Allergic reactions to antithyroid drugs involve either a rash (about 5% of patients) or agranulocytosis (about 0.5% of patients). The rash can be managed by simply administering antihistamines, and unless it is severe it is not an indication for discontinuing the medication. Agranulocytosis requires immediate cessation of all antithyroid drug therapy, institution of appropriate antibiotic therapy, and shifting to an alternative therapy, usually radioactive iodine. Agranulocytosis is usually heralded by sore throat and fever. Thus, all patients receiving antithyroid drugs are instructed that if sore throat or fever develops, they should stop the drug, obtain a white blood cell and differential count, and see their physician. If the white blood cell count is normal, the antithyroid drug can be resumed. Cholestatic jaundice, angioneurotic edema, hepatocellular toxicity, and acute arthralgia are serious but rare side effects that also require cessation of drug therapy.

B. Surgical Treatment: Subtotal thyroidectomy is the treatment of choice for patients with very large glands or multinodular goiters. The patient is prepared with antithyroid drugs until euthyroid (about 6 weeks). In addition, starting 2 weeks before the day of operation, the patient is given saturated solution of potassium iodide, 5 drops twice daily. This regimen has been shown empirically to diminish the vascularity of the gland and to simplify surgery. There is disagreement about how much thyroid tissue should be removed. Total thyroidectomy is usually not necessary unless the patient has severe progressive ophthalmopathy (see below). However, if too much thyroid tissue is left behind, the disease will relapse. Most surgeons leave 2–3 g of thyroid tissue on either side of the neck. Many patients, however, require thyroid supplementation following thyroidectomy for Graves' disease.

Hypoparathyroidism and recurrent laryngeal nerve injury occur as complications of surgery in about 1% of cases.

C. Radioactive Iodine Therapy: In the USA, sodium iodide I 131 is the preferred treatment for most patients over age 21. In many patients without underlying heart disease, radioactive iodine may be given immediately in a dosage of 80–120 μCi/g of thyroid weight estimated on the basis of physical examination and sodium ^{123}I rectilinear scan. The dosage is corrected for iodine uptake according to the following formula:

$$^{131}I(\mu Ci/g) \times \begin{array}{c} \text{Estimated} \\ \text{thyroid} \\ \text{weight (g)} \end{array} \times \frac{100}{\begin{array}{c} 24\text{-hour} \\ \text{RAI uptake} \end{array}} = \begin{array}{c} \text{Therapeutic} \\ \text{dose of } ^{131}I \\ \text{in } \mu Ci \end{array}$$

In patients with underlying heart disease, severe thyrotoxicosis, or large glands (> 100 g), it is desirable to achieve a euthyroid state before radioactive iodine is started. These patients are treated with antithyroid drugs (as above) until they are euthyroid; medication is then stopped for 5–7 days; radioactive iodine uptake and scan are done; and a dose of 100–150 μCi/g of estimated thyroid weight is calculated on the basis of this uptake. A slightly larger dose is necessary in patients previously treated with antithyroid drugs. Following the administration of radioactive iodine, the gland will shrink, and the patient will usually become euthyroid over a period of 6–12 weeks.

The major complication of radioactive iodine therapy is hypothyroidism, which ultimately develops in 80% or more of patients who are adequately treated. However, this complication may indeed be the best assurance that the patient will not have a recurrence of hyperthyroidism. Serum FT_4 and TSH levels should be followed, and when hypothyroidism develops, prompt replacement therapy with levothyroxine, 0.05–0.2 mg daily, is instituted.

Hypothyroidism may occur after any type of therapy for Graves' disease—even after antithyroid drug therapy; in some patients, "burned-out" Graves' disease may be an end result of autoimmune thyroid disease. Accordingly, all patients with Graves' disease require lifetime follow-up to be certain that they remain euthyroid.

D. Other Medical Measures: During the acute phase of thyrotoxicosis, beta-adrenergic blocking agents are extremely helpful. Propranolol, 10–40 mg every 6 hours, will control tachycardia, hypertension, and atrial fibrillation. This drug is gradually withdrawn as serum thyroxine levels return to normal. Adequate nutrition, including multivitamin supplements, is essential. Barbiturates accelerate T_4 metabolism, and phenobarbital may be helpful both for its sedative effect and to lower T_4 levels. Ipodate sodium or iopanoic acid has been shown to inhibit both thyroid hormone synthesis and release as well as peripheral conversion of T_4 to T_3. Thus, in a dosage of 1 g daily, this drug may help to rapidly restore the euthyroid state. It leaves the gland saturated with iodide, so it should not be used before ^{131}I therapy or antithyroid drug therapy with propylthiouracil or methimazole. Cholestyramine, 4 gm tid p.o. will lower serum T_4 by binding it in the gut. In a patient with a large toxic goiter and a severe allergic reaction to antithyroid drugs, ipodate sodium and beta blockade can be used effectively as preparation for surgery.

Choice of Therapy

Choice of therapy will vary with the nature and severity of the illness and prevailing customs. For example, in the USA, radioiodine therapy has been the preferred treatment for the average patient, whereas in Europe and Asia, antithyroid drug therapy is preferred. In the opinion of this author, most patients should be treated with antithyroid drugs until euthyroid. If there is a prompt response and the gland begins to shrink, the option of long-term antithyroid drug therapy with or without simultaneous levothyroxine therapy should be considered. If large doses of antithyroid drugs are required for control and the gland does not shrink in response to therapy, radioiodine would be the treatment of choice. If the gland is very large (> 150 g) or multinodular—or if the patient wishes to become pregnant very soon—thyroidectomy is a reasonable option. A serious allergic reaction to an antithyroid drug is an indication for radioiodine therapy.

Treatment of Complications

A. Thyrotoxic Crisis: Thyrotoxic crisis (thyroid storm) requires vigorous management. Propranolol, 1–2 mg slowly intravenously or 40–80 mg every 6 hours orally, is helpful in controlling arrhythmias. In the presence of severe heart failure or asthma and arrhythmia, cautious intravenous administration of verapamil in a dose of 5–10 mg may be effective. Hormone synthesis is blocked by the administration of propylthiouracil, 250 mg every 6 hours. If the patient is unable to take medication by mouth, methimazole in a dose of 25 mg every 6 hours can be given by rectal suppository or enema. After administration of an antithyroid drug, hormone release is retarded by the administration of sodium iodide, 1 g intravenously over a 24-hour period, or saturated solution of potassium iodide, 10 drops twice daily. Ipodate sodium, 1 g daily given intravenously or orally, may be used instead of sodium iodide, but this will block the definitive use of ra-

dioiodine therapy for 3–6 months. The conversion of T_4 to T_3 is partially blocked by the combination of propranolol and propylthiouracil, but the administration of hydrocortisone hemisuccinate, 50 mg intravenously every 6 hours, is additive. Supportive therapy includes a cooling blanket and acetaminophen to help control fever. Aspirin is probably contraindicated because of its tendency to bind to TBG and displace thyroxine, rendering more thyroxine available in the free state. Fluids, electrolytes, and nutrition are important. For sedation, phenobarbital is probably best because it accelerates the peripheral metabolism and inactivation of thyroxine and triiodothyronine, ultimately bringing these levels down. Oxygen, diuretics, and digitalis are indicated for heart failure. Finally, it is essential to treat the underlying disease process that may have precipitated the acute exacerbation. Thus, antibiotics, anti-allergy drugs, and postoperative care are indicated for management of these problems. As an extreme measure (rarely needed) to control thyrotoxic crisis, plasmapheresis or peritoneal dialysis may be used to remove high levels of circulating thyronines.

B. Ophthalmopathy: Management of ophthalmopathy due to Graves' disease involves close cooperation between the endocrinologist and the ophthalmologist. The thyroid disease may be managed as outlined above, but in the opinion of this author, total surgical excision of the thyroid gland or total ablation of the thyroid gland with radioactive iodine is indicated. Although there is controversy over the need for total ablation, removal or destruction of the thyroid gland certainly prevents exacerbations and relapses of thyrotoxicosis, which may reactivate residual ophthalmopathy. A course of prednisone following radioactive iodine therapy will prevent the transitory rise in thyroid antibodies following radioiodine ablation of the gland. Keeping the patient's head elevated at night will diminish periorbital edema. For the severe acute inflammatory reaction, a short course of corticosteroid therapy is frequently effective, eg, prednisone, 100 mg daily orally in divided doses for 7–14 days, then every other day in gradually diminishing dosage for 6–12 weeks. If corticosteroid therapy is not effective, external x-ray therapy to the retrobulbar area may be helpful. The dose is usually 2000 cGy in ten fractions given over a period of 2 weeks. The lens and anterior chamber structures must be shielded.

In very severe cases where vision is threatened, orbital decompression can be used. One type of orbital decompression involves a transantral approach through the maxillary sinus, removing the floor and the lateral walls of the orbit. In the alternative anterior approach, the orbit is entered under the globe, and portions of the floor and the walls of the orbit are removed. Both approaches have been extremely effective, and exophthalmos can be reduced by 5–7 mm in each eye by these techniques. After the acute process has subsided, the patient is frequently left with double vision or lid abnormalities owing to muscle fibrosis and contracture. These can be corrected by cosmetic lid surgery or eye muscle surgery.

C. Thyrotoxicosis and Pregnancy: Thyrotoxicosis during pregnancy presents a special problem. Radioactive iodine is contraindicated because it crosses the placenta freely and may injure the fetal thyroid. Two good alternatives are available. If the disease is detected during the first trimester, the patient can be prepared with propylthiouracil, and subtotal thyroidectomy can be performed safely during the mid trimester. It is essential to provide thyroid supplementation during the balance of the pregnancy. Alternatively, the patient can be treated with antithyroid drugs throughout the pregnancy, postponing the decision regarding long-term management until after delivery. The dosage of antithyroid drugs must be kept to the minimum necessary to control symptoms, because these drugs cross the placenta and may affect the function of the fetal thyroid gland. If the disease can be controlled by initial doses of propylthiouracil of 300 mg or less and maintenance doses of 50–150 mg/d, the likelihood of fetal hypothyroidism is extremely small. The FT_4I or FT_4 should be maintained in the upper range of normal by appropriately reducing the propylthiouracil dosage. Supplemental thyroxine is not necessary. Breast feeding is not contraindicated, because propylthiouracil is not concentrated in the milk.

Graves' disease may occur in the newborn infant **(neonatal Graves' disease).** There seem to be two forms of the disease. In both types, the mother has a current or recent history of Graves' disease. In the first type, the child is born small, with weak muscles, tachycardia, fever, and frequently respiratory distress or neonatal jaundice. Examination reveals an enlarged thyroid gland and occasionally prominent, puffy eyes. The heart rate is rapid, temperature is elevated, and heart failure may ensue. Laboratory studies reveal an elevated FT_4I or FT_4, a markedly elevated T_3, and usually a low TSH—in contrast to normal infants, who have elevated TSH at birth. Bone age may be accelerated. TSH-R Ab [stim] is usually found in the serum of both the infant and the mother. The pathogenesis of this syndrome is thought to involve transplacental transfer of TSH-R Ab [stim] from mother to fetus, with subsequent development of thyrotoxicosis. The disease is self-limited and subsides over a period of 4–12 weeks, coinciding with the fall in the child's TSH-R Ab [stim]. Therapy for the infant includes propylthiouracil in a dose of 5–10 mg/kg/d (in divided doses at 8-hour intervals); strong iodine (Lugol's) solution, 1 drop (8 mg potassium iodide) every 8 hours; and propranolol, 2 mg/kg/d in divided doses. In addition, adequate nutrition, antibiotics for infection if present, sedatives if necessary, and supportive therapy are indicated. If the child is very toxic, corticosteroid therapy (prednisone, 2 mg/kg/d) will partially block conversion of T_4 to T_3 and may be helpful in the acute phase. The above medications are gradually reduced as the child improves and can usually be discontinued by 6–12 weeks.

A second form of neonatal Graves' disease occurs in children from families with a high incidence of that disorder. Symptoms develop more slowly and may not be noted until the child is 3–6 months old. This syndrome is thought to be a true genetic inheritance of defective lymphocyte immunoregulation. It is much more severe, with a 20% mortality rate and evidence of persistent brain dysfunction even after successful treatment. The hyperthyroidism may persist for months or years and requires prolonged therapy.

Maternal sera may contain TSH-R blocking antibodies that can cross the placenta and produce transient hypothyroidism in the infant. This condition may need to be treated with T_4 supplementation for a short time.

Course & Prognosis

In general, the course of Graves' disease is one of remissions and exacerbations over a protracted period of time unless the gland is destroyed by surgery or radioactive iodine. Although some patients may remain euthyroid for long periods after treatment, many eventually develop hypothyroidism. Lifetime follow-up is therefore indicated for all patients with Graves' disease.

2. OTHER FORMS OF THYROTOXICOSIS

Toxic Adenoma (Plummer's Disease)

A functioning adenoma hypersecreting T_3 and T_4 will cause hyperthyroidism. These lesions start out as a "hot nodule" on the thyroid scan, slowly increase in size, and gradually suppress the other lobe of the gland (Figure 7–50). The typical patient is an older individual (usually over 40) who has noted recent growth of a long-standing thyroid nodule. Symptoms of weight loss, weakness, shortness of breath, palpitation, tachycardia, and heat intolerance are noted. Infiltrative ophthalmopathy is never present. Physical examination reveals a definite nodule on one side, with very little thyroid tissue on the other side. Laboratory studies usually reveal suppressed TSH and marked elevation in serum T_3 levels, often with only borderline elevation of thyroxine levels. The scan reveals that the nodule is "hot." Toxic adenomas are almost always follicular adenomas and almost never malignant. They are easily managed by administration of antithyroid drugs such as propylthiouracil, 100 mg every 6 hours, or methimazole, 10 mg every 6 hours, followed by treatment with radioactive iodine or unilateral lobectomy. Sodium ^{131}I in doses of 20–30 mCi

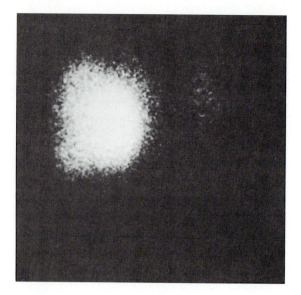

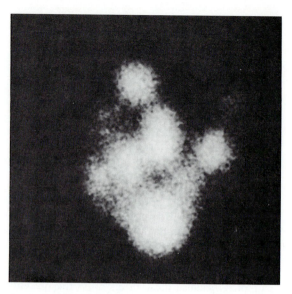

Figure 7–50. Toxic multinodular goiter as it appears on **99m**Tc pertechnetate scan. Note multiple functioning thyroid nodules. (Courtesy of JM Lowenstein.)

Figure 7–51. Multinodular goiter at the time of surgery. The asymmetric enlargement and the nodularity are apparent, as is the rightward deviation of the trachea resulting from marked enlargement of the lobe.

is usually required to destroy the benign neoplasm. Radioactive iodine is preferable for smaller toxic nodules, but larger ones are best managed surgically.

Toxic Multinodular Goiter

This disorder usually occurs in older patients with long-standing multinodular goiter. Ophthalmopathy is extremely rare. Clinically, the patient presents with tachycardia, heart failure, or arrhythmia and sometimes weight loss, nervousness, weakness, tremors, and sweats. Physical examination reveals a multinodular goiter that may be small or quite large and may even extend substernally. Laboratory studies reveal a suppressed TSH and striking elevation in serum T_3 levels, with less striking elevation of serum T_4. Radioiodine scan reveals multiple functioning nodules in the gland or occasionally an irregular, patchy distribution of radioactive iodine (Figure 7–51).

Hyperthyroidism in patients with multinodular goiters can often be precipitated by the administration of iodides ("jodbasedow" effect, or iodide-induced hyperthyroidism). Some thyroid adenomas do not develop the Wolff-Chaikoff effect (see above) and cannot adapt to an iodide load. Thus, they are driven to excess hormone production by a high level of circulating iodide. This is the mechanism for the development of hyperthyroidism after administration of the antiarrhythmic drug amiodarone (see below).

The management of toxic nodular goiter is difficult. Control of the hyperthyroid state with antithyroid drugs followed by subtotal thyroidectomy would seem to be the therapy of choice, but often these pa-

tients are elderly and have other illnesses that make them poor candidates for surgery. The toxic nodules can be destroyed with ^{131}I, but the multinodular goiter will remain, and other nodules may become toxic, requiring repeated doses of ^{131}I.

Amiodarone is an antiarrhythmic drug that contains 37.3% iodine. In the body, it is stored in fat, myocardium, liver and lung and has a half-life of about 50 days. About 2% of patients treated with amiodarone develop iodine-induced thyrotoxicosis. This presents a most difficult problem. Patients taking amiodarone have serious underlying heart disease, and in many cases the amiodarone cannot be discontinued. If the thyrotoxicosis is mild, it can often be controlled with methimazole, 40–60 mg daily, while amiodarone therapy continues. If the disease is severe, $KClO_4$ in a dose of 250 mg every 6 hours may be added to saturate the iodide trap and prevent further uptake of iodide. Long-term $KClO_4$ has been associated with aplastic anemia and requires monitoring. The only way to eliminate the large store of intrathyroidal hormone would be to surgically remove the goiter. This would be feasible only if the patient could withstand the stress of thyroidectomy.

Subacute or Chronic Thyroiditis

These entities will be discussed in a separate section, but it should be mentioned here that thyroiditis, either subacute or chronic, may present with an acute release of T_4 and T_3, producing symptoms of mild to severe thyrotoxicosis. These illnesses can be differentiated from other forms of thyrotoxicosis in that the radioiodine uptake is markedly suppressed, and the symptoms usually subside spontaneously over a period of weeks or months.

Thyrotoxicosis Factitia

This is a psychoneurotic disturbance in which the patient ingests excessive amounts of thyroxine or thyroid hormone, usually for purposes of weight control. The individual is often someone connected with the field of medicine who can easily obtain thyroid medication. Features of thyrotoxicosis, including weight loss, nervousness, palpitation, tachycardia, and tremor, may be present, but no goiter or eye signs. Characteristically, TSH is suppressed, serum T_4 and T_3 levels are elevated, serum thyroglobulin in low, and radioactive iodine uptake is nil. Management requires careful discussion of the hazards of long-term thyroxine therapy, particularly cardiovascular damage, muscle wasting, and osteoporosis. Formal psychotherapy may be necessary.

Rare Forms of Thyrotoxicosis

A. Struma Ovarii: In this syndrome, a teratoma of the ovary contains thyroid tissue that becomes hyperactive. Mild features of thyrotoxicosis result, such as weight loss and tachycardia, but there is no evidence of goiter or eye signs. Serum FT_4 and T_3 are mildly elevated, serum TSH is suppressed, and radioiodine uptake in the neck is nil. Body scan reveals uptake of radioiodine in the pelvis. The disease is curable by removal of the teratoma.

B. Thyroid Carcinoma: Carcinoma of the thyroid, particularly follicular carcinoma, may concentrate radioactive iodine, but only rarely does it retain the ability to convert this iodide into active hormone. Only a few cases of metastatic thyroid cancer have presented with hyperthyroidism. The clinical picture consists of weakness, weight loss, palpitation, and a thyroid nodule but no ophthalmopathy. Body scan with ^{131}I reveals areas of uptake usually distant from the thyroid, eg, bone or lung. Treatment with large doses of radioactive iodine may destroy the metastatic deposits.

C. Hydatidiform Mole: Hydatidiform moles produce chorionic gonadotropin, which has intrinsic TSH-like activity. This may induce thyroid hyperplasia, increased iodine turnover, suppressed TSH, and mild elevation of serum T_4 and T_3 levels. It is rarely associated with overt thyrotoxicosis and is totally curable by removal of the mole.

D. "Hamburger Thyrotoxicosis": An epidemic of thyrotoxicosis in midwestern United States was traced to hamburger made from "neck trim," the strap muscles from the necks of slaughtered cattle that contained beef thyroid tissue. The United States Department of Agriculture has now prohibited the use of this material for human consumption.

E. Syndrome of Inappropriate TSH Secretion: A group of patients have been reported with elevated serum free thyroxine concentrations in association with elevated serum immunoreactive TSH. This has been called the "syndrome of inappropriate TSH secretion." Two types of problems are found: (1) TSH-secreting pituitary adenoma and (2) nonneoplastic pituitary hypersecretion of TSH.

Patients with **TSH-secreting pituitary adenomas** usually present with mild thyrotoxicosis and goiter, often with evidence of gonadotropic hormone deficiency such as amenorrhea or impotence. There are no eye signs of Graves' disease. Study reveals elevated total and free serum T_4 and T_3. Serum TSH, usually undetectable in Graves' disease, is within the normal range or even elevated. The TSH α subunit secretion from these tumors is markedly elevated; a molar ratio of α subunit:TSH greater than 1 is usually diagnostic of the presence of a TSH-secreting pituitary adenoma. In addition, there is no hormonal response to TRH, and the increased radioactive iodine uptake is not suppressible with exogenous thyroid hormone. Visual field examination may reveal temporal defects, and CT or MRI of the sella usually reveals a pituitary tumor. Management usually involves control of the thyrotoxicosis with antithyroid drugs and removal of the pituitary tumor via transsphenoidal hypophysectomy. These tumors are often quite aggressive and may extend widely out of the sella. If the tumor cannot be completely removed, it may be necessary to treat residual tumor with radiation therapy and to control thyrotoxicosis with radioactive iodine. Long-acting somatostatin (octreotide) will suppress TSH secretion in many of these patients and may even inhibit tumor growth in some.

Nonneoplastic pituitary hypersecretion of TSH is essentially a form of pituitary (and occasionally peripheral) resistance to T_3 and T_4. This is discussed below.

THYROID HORMONE RESISTANCE SYNDROMES

Several forms of resistance to thyroid hormones have been reported: (1) generalized resistance to thyroid hormones (GRTH), (2) selective pituitary resistance to thyroid hormones (PRTH), and possibly (3) a selective peripheral resistance to thyroid hormones (perRTH).

Generalized resistance to thyroid hormones was first described in 1967 by Refetoff et al as a familial syndrome of deaf mutism, stippled epiphyses, goiter, and abnormally high thyroid hormone levels with normal TSH. The clinical presentation in the more than 200 families that have been reported has been variable; while most patients are euthyroid, many present with goiter, stunted growth, delayed maturation, attention deficits, hyperactivity disorders, and resting tachycardia. Inheritance is usually autosomal dominant, though it was recessive in 10% of the families studied. Laboratory tests reveal elevated T_4, FT_4, T_3, and normal or elevated TSH. Dynamic tests to distinguish generalized resistance to thyroid hormones from TSH-secreting adenomas usually reveal an increase in TSH after administration of TRH, a fall in TSH with T_3 suppression, and a molar ratio of α subunit:TSH of less than 1. In addition, in patients with GRTH, pituitary MRI fails to demonstrate a microadenoma. Molecular studies have revealed point mutations in the carboxyl terminal ligand-binding portion of the human thyroid receptor beta gene (hTR-β), which produces a defective thyroid hormone receptor (TR) that fails to bind T_3 (Figure 7–28). Although this is a recessive mutation, the abnormal receptor may partially block the action of normal receptors, so that it appears to be inherited in an autosomal dominant mode (a "dominant recessive mutation"). Different point mutations in different families may account in part for the differences in clinical expression of the syndrome. Furthermore, identification of the mutation may allow the use of molecular screening methods for the diagnosis of the syndrome in some families.

In most patients with generalized resistance to thyroid hormones, the increased levels of T_3 and T_4 will compensate in part for the receptor defect, and treatment is not necessary. In some children, administration of thyroid hormone may be necessary to correct defects in growth or mental development.

Selective pituitary resistance to thyroid hormones is less common and usually presents with symptoms of mild hyperthyroidism, goiter, elevated serum T_4 and T_3, and normal or elevated serum TSH. In this syndrome, T_3 receptors in peripheral tissues are normal, but there is a failure of T_3 to inhibit pituitary TSH secretion, resulting in inappropriate TSH secretion and TSH-induced hyperthyroidism. Differentiation from TSH-secreting pituitary adenoma can be made using the dynamic tests and MRI of the pituitary as outlined above.

This syndrome may be due in part to some abnormality in the pituitary type 2 5'-deiodinase with failure to convert intrapituitary T_4 to T_3, leading to PTHR. Ablation of the thyroid gland with ^{131}I or treatment with antithyroid drugs may lead to pituitary hyperplasia. However, administration of T_3 or triiodothyroacetic acid (TRIAC) has been reported to suppress TSH, reduce the size of the goiter, lower serum T_4, and correct the hyperthyroidism.

Only one case of suspected selective peripheral resistance to T_3 has been reported, and it is not yet clear that this is a distinct entity.

TSH Receptor Gene Mutations

Mutations in the TSH receptor gene can produce a variety of clinical syndromes. Mutations in the 7 transmembrane loop of the TSH-R may activate the receptor, producing hyperfunctioning adenomas or, more rarely, congenital hyperthyroidism in the newborn. Mutations in the extracellular amino terminal of the TSH-R produce resistance to TSH. The patient reported by Refetoff had normal FT_4 and FT_3 and normal growth and development but persistently elevated serum TSH. The patients reported by Medeiros-Neto were severely hypothyroid (cretinoid), with low FT_4 levels, elevated TSH, and no response to exogenous TSH. In this group, the defect may be in the coupling of TSH-R and the G_s protein necessary for activation of adenylyl cyclase.

NONTOXIC GOITER

Etiology

Nontoxic goiter usually represents enlargement of the thyroid gland from TSH stimulation, which in turn results from inadequate thyroid hormone synthesis. Table 7–12 lists some of the causes of nontoxic goiter.

Iodine deficiency was the most common cause of nontoxic goiter or "endemic goiter"; with the widespread use of iodized salt and the introduction of iodides into fertilizers, animal feeds, and food preservatives, iodide deficiency in developed countries is relatively rare. It does not exist in the USA. However, there are large areas such as central Africa, the mountainous areas of central Asia, the Andes of central South America, and Indonesia (particularly New Guinea), where iodine intake is still markedly deficient. Optimal iodine requirements for adults are in the range of 150–300 µg/d. In endemic goiter areas, the daily intake (and urinary excretion) of iodine falls below 50 µg/d; in areas where iodine is extremely scarce, excretion falls below 20 µg/d. It is in these areas that 90% of the population will have goiters, and 5–15% of infants will be born with myxedematous or neurologic changes of cretinism. The variability in the extent of goiter in these areas may be related to the presence of other, unidentified goitrogens.

Dietary goitrogens are a rare cause of goiter, and of these the most common is iodide itself. Large amounts of iodide, as in amiodarone or kelp tablets, may in susceptible individuals produce goiter and hypothyroidism (see above). Withdrawal of iodide reverses the process. Other goitrogens include lithium carbonate and some vegetable foodstuffs such as goitrin, found in certain roots and seeds; and cyan-

Table 7–12. Etiology of nontoxic goiter.

1. Iodine deficiency.
2. Goitrogen in the diet.
3. Hashimoto's thyroiditis.
4. Subacute thyroiditis.
5. Inadequate hormone synthesis due to inherited defect in thyroidal enzymes necessary for T_4 and T_3 biosynthesis.
6. Generalized resistance to thyroid hormone (rare).
7. Neoplasm, benign or malignant.

ogenic glycosides, found in cassava and cabbage, that release thiocyanates which may cause goiter, particularly in the presence of iodide deficiency. In addition, compounds such as phenols, phthalates, pyridines, and polyaromatic hydrocarbons found in industrial waste water are weakly goitrogenic. The role of these vegetable and pollutant goitrogens in the production of goiter is not clearly established.

The most common cause of thyroid enlargement in developed countries is chronic thyroiditis (Hashimoto's thyroiditis; see below). Subacute thyroiditis causes thyroid enlargement with exquisite tenderness (see below).

Nontoxic goiter may be due to impaired hormone synthesis resulting from genetic deficiencies in enzymes necessary for hormone biosynthesis (thyroid dyshormonogenesis, or familial goiter). These effects may be complete, resulting in a syndrome of cretinism with goiter; or partial, resulting in nontoxic goiter with mild hypothyroidism. At least five separate biosynthetic abnormalities have been reported: (1) impaired transport of iodine; (2) deficient peroxidase with impaired oxidation of iodide to iodine and failure to incorporate iodine into thyroglobulin; (3) impaired coupling of iodinated tyrosines to triiodothyronine or tetraiodothyronine; (4) absence or deficiency of iodotyrosine deiodinase, so that iodine is not conserved within the gland; and (5) excessive production of metabolically inactive iodoprotein by the thyroid gland (Figure 7–9). The latter may involve impaired or abnormal thyroglobulin synthesis. In all of these syndromes, impaired production of thyroid hormones presumably results in TSH release and goiter formation.

Finally, thyroid enlargement can be due to a benign lesion, such as adenoma, or to a malignant one such as carcinoma.

Pathogenesis

The development of nontoxic goiter in patients with dyshormonogenesis or severe iodine deficiency involves impaired hormone synthesis and, secondarily, an increase in TSH secretion. TSH induces diffuse thyroid hyperplasia, followed by focal hyperplasia with necrosis and hemorrhage, and finally the development of new areas of focal hyperplasia. Focal or nodular hyperplasia usually involves a clone of cells that may or may not be able to pick up iodine or synthesize thyroglobulin. Thus, the nodules will vary from "hot" nodules that can concentrate iodine to "cold" ones that cannot, and from colloid nodules that can synthesize thyroglobulin to microfollicular ones that cannot. Initially, the hyperplasia is TSH-dependent, but later the nodules become TSH-independent, or autonomous. Thus, a diffuse nontoxic TSH-dependent goiter progresses over a period of time to a multinodular toxic or nontoxic TSH-independent goiter.

The mechanism for the development of au-

tonomous growth and function of thyroid nodules may involve mutations that occur with TSH-induced cell division in an oncogene that activates the G_s protein in the cell membrane. Mutations of this oncogene, called the *gsp* oncogene, have been found in a high proportion of nodules from patients with multinodular goiter. Chronic activation of the G_s protein would result in thyroid cell proliferation and hyperfunction even when TSH is suppressed.

Clinical Features

A. Symptoms and Signs: Patients with nontoxic goiter usually present with thyroid enlargement, which, as noted above, may be diffuse or multinodular. The gland may be relatively firm but is often extremely soft. Over a period of time, the gland becomes progressively larger, so that in long-standing multinodular goiter, huge goiters may develop and extend inferiorly to present as substernal goiter. The patient may complain of pressure symptoms in the neck, particularly on moving the head upward or downward, and of difficulty in swallowing. Vocal cord paralysis due to recurrent laryngeal nerve involvement is rare. There may be symptoms of mild hypothyroidism, but most of these patients are euthyroid. Thyroid enlargement probably represents compensated hypothyroidism.

B. Laboratory Findings: Laboratory studies will reveal a low or normal free thyroxine and, usually, normal levels of TSH. The increased mass of thyroid tissue compensates for inefficient synthesis of hormone. In patients with dyshormonogenesis due to abnormal iodoprotein synthesis, PBI and serum thyroglobulin may be elevated out of proportion to serum T_4, because of secretion of nonhormonal organic iodide compounds. Radioiodine uptake may be high, normal, or low, depending upon the iodide pool and the TSH drive.

C. Imaging Studies: Isotope scanning usually reveals a patchy uptake, frequently with focal areas of increased uptake corresponding to "hot" nodules and areas of decreased uptake corresponding to "cold" nodules. Radioactive iodine uptake of the "hot" nodules may not be suppressible on administration of thyroid hormones such as liothyronine. Thyroid ultrasound is a simple way to follow the growth of the goiter and in addition may reveal cystic changes in one or more of the nodules, representing previous hemorrhage and necrosis.

Differential Diagnosis

The major problem in differential diagnosis is to rule out cancer. This will be discussed in the section on thyroid carcinoma.

Treatment

With the exception of those due to neoplasm, the current management of nontoxic goiters consists simply of giving thyroid hormones until TSH is completely suppressed. Levothyroxine in doses of 0.1–0.2 mg (approximately 2.2 µg/kg, or 1 µg/lb) daily to suppress pituitary TSH will correct hypothyroidism and often result in slow regression of the goiter. Long-standing goiters may have areas of necrosis, hemorrhage, and scarring as well as autonomously functioning nodules that will not regress on thyroxine therapy. However, the lesions will usually grow more slowly while the patient is taking thyroxine. In older patients with multinodular goiters, administration of levothyroxine must be done very cautiously since the "hot" nodules are usually autonomous and the combination of endogenous and exogenous hormone will rapidly produce toxic symptoms.

Surgery is indicated for goiters that continue to grow despite TSH suppression with T_4 or those that produce obstructive symptoms. Substernal extension of a goiter is usually an indication for surgical removal. The gross appearance of a multinodular goiter at the time of surgery is presented in Figure 7–52. Note that the left lobe of the gland extends downward from the middle of the thyroid cartilage to just above the clavicle. The pressure of this enlargement has caused deviation of the trachea to the right. The surface of the gland is irregular, with many large and small nodules. Although these multinodular goiters are rarely malignant, the size of the mass with resulting pressure symptoms requires subtotal thyroidectomy.

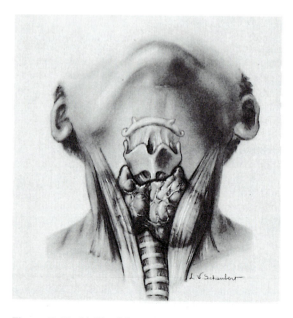

Figure 7–52. Multinodular goiter at the time of surgery. The asymmetric enlargement and the nodularity are apparent, as is the rightward deviation of the trachea resulting from marked enlargement of the lobe.

Course & Prognosis

Patients with nontoxic goiter must usually take levothyroxine for life. They should avoid iodides, which may induce either hyperthyroidism or, in the absence of thyroxine therapy, hypothyroidism. Occasionally, single adenomas or several adenomas will become hyperfunctional, producing a toxic nodular goiter (discussed above). Nontoxic goiter is often familial, and other members of the family should be examined and observed for the possible development of goiter.

THYROIDITIS

1. SUBACUTE THYROIDITIS

Subacute thyroiditis (De Quervain's thyroiditis, or granulomatous thyroiditis) is an acute inflammatory disorder of the thyroid gland most likely due to viral infection. A number of viruses, including mumps virus, coxsackievirus, and adenoviruses, have been implicated, either by finding the virus in biopsy specimens taken from the gland or by demonstration of rising titers of viral antibodies in the blood during the course of the infection. Pathologic examination reveals moderate thyroid enlargement and a mild inflammatory reaction involving the capsule. Histologic features include destruction of thyroid parenchyma and the presence of many large phagocytic cells, including giant cells.

Clinical Features

A. Symptoms and Signs: Subacute thyroiditis usually presents with fever, malaise, and soreness in the neck, which may extend up to the angle of the jaw or toward the ear lobes on one or both sides of the neck. Initially, the patient may have symptoms of hyperthyroidism, with palpitations, agitation, and sweats. There is no ophthalmopathy. On physical examination, the gland is exquisitely tender, so that the patient will object to pressure upon it. There are no signs of local redness or heat suggestive of abscess formation. Clinical signs of toxicity, including tachycardia, tremor, and hyperreflexia, may be present.

B. Laboratory Findings: Laboratory studies will vary with the course of the disease (Figure 7–53). Initially, T_4 and T_3 are elevated, whereas serum TSH and thyroid radioactive iodine uptake are extremely low. The erythrocyte sedimentation rate is markedly elevated, sometimes as high as 100 mm/h by the Westergren scale. Thyroid autoantibodies are usually not detectable in serum. As the disease progresses, T_4 and T_3 will drop, TSH will rise, and symptoms of hypothyroidism are noted. Later, radioactive iodine uptake will rise, reflecting recovery of the gland from the acute insult.

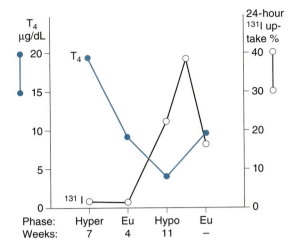

Figure 7–53. Changes in serum T$_4$ and radioactive iodine uptake in patients with subacute thyroiditis. In the initial phase, serum T$_4$ is elevated and the patient may have symptoms of thyrotoxicosis, but radioactive iodine uptake is markedly suppressed. The illness may pass through phases of euthyroidism and hypothyroidism before remission. (Data adapted, with permission, from Woolf PD, Daly R: Thyrotoxicosis with painless thyroiditis. Am J Med 1976;60:73.)

Differential Diagnosis

Subacute thyroiditis can be differentiated from other viral illnesses by the involvement of the thyroid gland. It is differentiated from Graves' disease by the presence of low thyroid radioiodine uptake associated with elevated serum T$_3$ and T$_4$ and suppressed serum TSH and by the absence of thyroid antibodies.

Treatment

In most cases, only symptomatic treatment is necessary, eg, acetaminophen, 0.5 g four times daily. If pain, fever, and malaise are disabling, a short course of a nonsteroidal anti-inflammatory drug or a glucocorticoid such as prednisone, 20 mg three times daily for 7–10 days, may be necessary to reduce the inflammation. Levothyroxine, 0.1–0.15 mg once daily, is indicated during the hypothyroid phase of the illness in order to prevent reexacerbation of the disease induced by the rising TSH levels. In about 10% of patients, permanent hypothyroidism ensues and long-term levothyroxine therapy is necessary.

Course & Prognosis

Subacute thyroiditis usually resolves completely and spontaneously over weeks or months. Occasionally, the disease may begin to resolve and then suddenly get worse, sometimes involving first one lobe of the thyroid gland and then the other (migrating thyroiditis). Exacerbations often occur when the T$_4$ levels have fallen, TSH has risen, and the gland is starting to recover function. Rarely, the course may extend over several years, with repeated bouts of inflammatory disease.

2 . CHRONIC THYROIDITIS

Chronic thyroiditis (Hashimoto's thyroiditis, lymphocytic thyroiditis) is probably the most common cause of hypothyroidism and goiter in the USA. It is certainly the major cause of goiter in children and young adults and is probably the major cause of "idiopathic myxedema," which represents an end stage of Hashimoto's thyroiditis, with total destruction of the gland. **Riedel's struma** is probably a variant of Hashimoto's thyroiditis, with extensive fibrosis extending outside the gland and involving overlying muscle and surrounding tissues. Riedel's struma presents as a stony-hard mass that must be differentiated from thyroid cancer.

Etiology & Pathogenesis

Hashimoto's thyroiditis is thought to be an immunologic disorder in which lymphocytes become sensitized to thyroidal antigens and autoantibodies are formed that react with these antigens (see thyroid autoimmunity, above). In Hashimoto's thyroiditis, the three most important thyroid autoantibodies are thyroglobulin antibody (Tg Ab), thyroid peroxidase antibody (TPO Ab), formerly called microsomal antibody, and TSH receptor blocking antibody (TSH-R Ab [block]) (Table 7–7). During the early phases of Hashimoto's thyroiditis, Tg Ab is markedly elevated and TPO Ab is slightly elevated. Later, Tg Ab may disappear, but TPO Ab will be present for many years. TSH-R Ab [block] is found in patients with **atrophic thyroiditis** and myxedema and in mothers giving birth to infants with no detectable thyroid tissue **(athyreotic cretins).** The pathology of Hashimoto's thyroiditis involves a heavy infiltration of lymphocytes totally destroying normal thyroidal architecture. Lymphoid follicles and germinal centers may be formed. The follicular epithelial cells are frequently enlarged and contain a basophilic cytoplasm (Hurthle cells). Destruction of the gland results in a fall in serum T$_3$ and T$_4$ and a rise in TSH. Initially, TSH may maintain adequate hormonal synthesis by the development of thyroid enlargement or goiter, but often the gland fails, and hypothyroidism with or without goiter ensues.

Hashimoto's thyroiditis is part of a spectrum of thyroid diseases that includes Graves' disease at one end and idiopathic myxedema at the other (Figure 7–54). It is familial and may be associated with other autoimmune diseases such as pernicious anemia, adrenocortical insufficiency, idiopathic hypoparathyroidism, myasthenia gravis, and vitiligo. **Schmidt's syndrome** consists of Hashimoto's thyroiditis, idio-

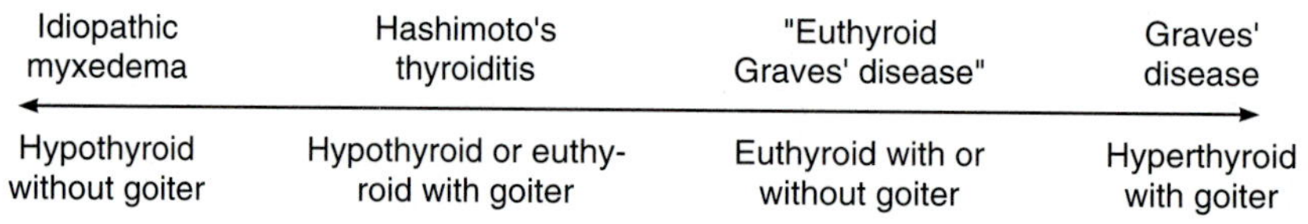

Idiopathic myxedema	Hashimoto's thyroiditis	"Euthyroid Graves' disease"	Graves' disease
Hypothyroid without goiter	Hypothyroid or euthyroid with goiter	Euthyroid with or without goiter	Hyperthyroid with goiter

Figure 7–54. Spectrum of autoimmune disease of the thyroid gland. The clinical manifestations of autoimmune disease of the thyroid gland range from idiopathic myxedema, through nontoxic goiter, to diffuse toxic goiter, or Graves' disease. Progression of autoimmune disease from one form to another in the same patient can occasionally occur.

pathic adrenal insufficiency, hypoparathyroidism, diabetes mellitus, ovarian insufficiency, and (rarely) candidal infections. Schmidt's syndrome represents destruction of multiple endocrine glands on an autoimmune basis (Chapter 24).

Clinical Features

A. Symptoms and Signs: Hashimoto's thyroiditis usually presents with goiter in a patient who is euthyroid or has mild hypothyroidism. The sex distribution is about four females to one male. The process is painless, and the patient may be unaware of the goiter unless it becomes very large. Older patients may present with severe hypothyroidism with only a small, firm atrophic thyroid gland (idiopathic myxedema).

B. Laboratory Findings: There are multiple defects in iodine metabolism. Peroxidase activity is decreased, so that organification of iodine is impaired. This can be demonstrated by a positive perchlorate discharge test (Figure 7–12). In addition, iodination of metabolically inactive protein material occurs, so that there will be a disproportionately high serum PBI and serum globulin compared to serum T_4. Radioiodine uptake may be high, normal, or low. Circulating thyroid hormone levels are usually normal or low, and if low, TSH will be elevated.

The most striking laboratory finding is the high titer of autoantibodies to thyroidal antigens in the serum. Serum tests for either Tg Ab or TPO Ab are positive in most patients with Hashimoto's thyroiditis. Another diagnostic test that may be helpful is the fine-needle aspiration biopsy, which reveals a large infiltration of lymphocytes as well as the presence of Hurthle cells.

Differential Diagnosis

Hashimoto's thyroiditis can be differentiated from other causes of nontoxic goiter by serum antibody studies and if necessary by fine-needle aspiration biopsy.

Complications & Sequelae

The major complication of Hashimoto's thyroiditis is progressive hypothyroidism. Although only 10–15% of young patients presenting with goiter and hypothyroidism seem to progress to permanent hypothyroidism, the high incidence of permanent hypothyroidism in older patients with positive antibody tests and elevated TSH levels suggests that long-term treatment is desirable. Rarely, a patient with Hashimoto's thyroiditis may develop lymphoma of the thyroid gland, but whether the two conditions are causally related is not clear. Thyroid lymphoma is characterized by rapid growth of the gland despite continued thyroid hormone therapy; the diagnosis of lymphoma must be made by surgical biopsy (see below).

There is no evidence that adenocarcinoma of the thyroid gland occurs more frequently in patients with Hashimoto's thyroiditis, but the two diseases—chronic thyroiditis and carcinoma—can coexist in the same gland. Cancer must be suspected when a solitary nodule or thyroid mass grows or fails to regress while the patient is receiving maximal tolerated doses of thyroxine. Fine-needle aspiration biopsy is helpful in this differential diagnosis.

Treatment

The indications for treatment of Hashimoto's thyroiditis are goiter or hypothyroidism; a positive thyroid antibody test does not require therapy. Sufficient levothyroxine is given to suppress TSH and allow regression of the goiter. Surgery is rarely indicated.

Course & Prognosis

Without treatment, Hashimoto's thyroiditis will usually progress from goiter and hypothyroidism to myxedema. The goiter and the myxedema are totally corrected by adequate thyroxine therapy. Hashimoto's thyroiditis may go through periods of activity when large amounts of T_4 and T_3 are released or "dumped," resulting in transient symptoms of thyrotoxicosis. This syndrome, which has been called **spontaneously resolving hyperthyroidism,** is characterized by low radioiodine uptake. However, it can be differentiated from subacute thyroiditis in that the gland is not tender, the erythrocyte sedimentation rate is not elevated, autoantibodies to thyroidal antigens are strongly positive, and fine-needle aspiration biopsy reveals lymphocytes and Hurthle cells. Therapy is symptomatic, usually requiring only propranolol, until symptoms subside; T_4 supplementation may then be necessary.

Because Hashimoto's thyroiditis may be part of a

syndrome of multiple autoimmune diseases (Chapter 24), the patient should be monitored for other autoimmune diseases such as pernicious anemia, adrenal insufficiency, hypothyroidism, or diabetes mellitus. Patients with Hashimoto's thyroiditis may also develop true Graves' disease, occasionally with severe ophthalmopathy or dermopathy (Figure 7–54). The chronic thyroiditis may blunt the severity of the thyrotoxicosis, so that the patient may present with eye or skin complications of Graves' disease without marked thyrotoxicosis, a syndrome often called euthyroid Graves' disease. The thyroid gland will invariably be nonsuppressible, and this, plus the presence of thyroid autoantibodies, will help to make the diagnosis. The ophthalmopathy and dermopathy are treated as if thyrotoxic Graves' disease were present.

3. OTHER FORMS OF THYROIDITIS

The thyroid gland may be subject to acute abscess formation in patients with septicemia or acute infective endocarditis. Abscesses cause symptoms of pyogenic infection, with local pain and tenderness, swelling, and warmth and redness of the overlying skin. Needle aspiration will confirm the diagnosis and identify the organism. Treatment includes antibiotic therapy and occasionally incision and drainage. A thyroglossal duct cyst may become infected and present as acute suppurative thyroiditis. This too will respond to antibiotic therapy and occasionally incision and drainage.

EFFECTS OF IONIZING RADIATION ON THE THYROID GLAND

Ionizing radiation can induce both acute and chronic thyroiditis. Thyroiditis may occur acutely in patients treated with large doses of radioiodine and may be associated with release of thyroid hormones and an acute thyrotoxic crisis. Such an occurrence is extremely rare, however, and pretreatment with antithyroid drugs to bring the patient to a euthyroid state prior to ^{131}I therapy will completely prevent this type of radiation thyroiditis.

External radiation was used many years ago for the treatment of respiratory problems in the newborn, thought to be due to thymic hyperplasia, and for the treatment of benign conditions such as severe acne and chronic tonsillitis or adenoiditis. This treatment was often associated with the later development of nodular goiter, hypothyroidism, or thyroid cancer. Another source of radiation exposure is fallout from atomic bomb testing or a nuclear reactor accident.

The incidence of thyroid lesions after irradiation is summarized in Table 7–13. As little as 6.5 cGy (1 cGy = 1 rad) to the thyroid gland received during the radiation treatment of tinea capitis has been reported to cause cancer in 0.11% of exposed children; the incidence of thyroid cancer in sibling controls was 0.02%. Radiation therapy to the thymus delivered to the thyroid dosages of 100–400 cGy, and the incidence of thyroid cancer attributed to this source ranged from 0.5% to 5%. X-ray therapy to the neck and chest given to children or adolescents for acne or chronic upper respiratory infections delivered thyroid doses ranging from 200 cGy to 1500 cGy, resulting in the development of nodular goiter in about 27% and thyroid cancer in 5–7% of the patients so treated. These tumors developed 10–40 years after radiation was administered, with a peak incidence at 20–30 years. Radiation fallout with a thyroid dose of 700–1400 cGy has produced nodular goiter in approximately 40% of exposed victims and thyroid cancer in about 6%. However, radioiodine therapy, which exposes the thyroid to a dosage of around 10,000 cGy, was rarely associated with the development of thyroid cancer, presumably because the thyroid gland is largely destroyed by these doses of radioiodine, so that—although the inci-

Table 7–13. Thyroid lesions after irradiation.

Areas Treated	Estimated Dose to Thyroid (cGy)	Incidence (%)		Source
		Nodular Goiter	Cancer	
Scalp	6.5	. . .	0.11	Modan et al (1974)
Thymus Total group	119	1.8	0.8	Hemplemann et al (1975)
Subgroup	399	7.6	5.0	
Neck, chest	807 180–1500	27.2 26.2	5.7 6.8	Favus et al (1975) Refetoff et al (1975)
Radiation fallout	< 50 > 50 175 (γ) and 700–1400 (β)	. . . . . . 39.6	0.4 6.7 5.7	Parker et al (1974) Sampson et al (1969) Conrad et al (1970)
^{131}I therapy	≈10,000	0.17	0.08	Dobyns et al (1974)

dence of postradiation hypothyroidism is high—the incidence of thyroid cancer is extremely low. Ninety percent of patients with radiation-induced thyroid cancer develop papillary carcinoma; the remainder develop follicular carcinoma. Medullary carcinoma and anaplastic carcinomas have been rare following radiation exposure. Although the overall incidence of thyroid carcinoma in irradiated patients is low, data from several large series suggest that the incidence of cancer in a patient who presents with a solitary cold nodule of the thyroid gland and a history of therapeutic radiation of the head, neck, or chest is around 50%. The most recent episode of radiation-induced thyroid neoplasia was the Chernobyl disaster in April 1986, at which time huge amounts of radioactive material, especially radioiodine, were released. As early as 4 years later, a striking increase in the incidence of thyroid nodules and thyroid cancer was noted in children in Gomel, an area in the Republic of Belarus, close to Chernobyl and heavily contaminated. A high proportion of the cancers arose in young children and developed after a very short latency period. The sex distribution was equal. Most of the cancers were papillary carcinomas and were very aggressive, with intraglandular, capsular, local, and lymph node invasion.

Patients who have been exposed to ionizing radiation should be followed carefully for life. Annual studies should include physical examination of the neck for goiter or nodules, and FT_4 or TSH to rule out hypothyroidism. Periodic thyroid ultrasound may detect nodules that are not palpable. If a nodule is found, it should be scanned with ^{123}I, and if cold, fine-needle aspiration biopsy should be done. If the nodule is malignant, the patient should have total thyroidectomy; if benign, the patient should be treated with levothyroxine in a dose sufficient to suppress TSH. If the nodule persists or grows while T_4 therapy is being given, the thyroid gland should be surgically removed.

THYROID NODULES & THYROID CANCER

In 95% of cases, thyroid cancer presents as a nodule or lump in the thyroid. In occasional instances, particularly in children, enlarged cervical lymph nodes are the first sign of the disease, though on careful examination a small primary focus in the form of a thyroid nodule can often be felt. Rarely, distant metastasis in lung or bone is the first sign of thyroid cancer. Thyroid nodules are extremely common, particularly among women. The prevalence in the USA has been estimated to be about 4% of the adult population, with a female:male ratio of 4:1. In young children, the incidence is less than 1%; in persons aged 11–18 years, about 1.5%; and in persons over age 60, about 5%.

In contrast to thyroid nodules, thyroid cancer is a rare condition, with an incidence of 0.004% per year according to the Third National Cancer Survey. Thus, most thyroid nodules are benign, and it is important to identify those that are likely to be malignant.

1. BENIGN THYROID NODULES

Etiology

Benign conditions that can produce nodularity in the thyroid gland are listed in Table 7–14. They include focal areas of chronic thyroiditis, a dominant portion of a multinodular goiter, a cyst involving thyroid tissue, parathyroid tissue, or thyroglossal duct remnants, and agenesis of one lobe of the thyroid, with hypertrophy of the other lobe presenting as a mass in the neck. It is usually the left lobe of the thyroid that fails to develop, and the hypertrophy occurs in the right lobe. Scarring in the gland following surgery—or regrowth of the gland after surgery or radioiodine therapy—can present with nodularity. Finally, benign neoplasms in the thyroid include follicular adenomas such as colloid or macrofollicular adenomas, fetal adenomas, embryonal adenomas, and Hurthle cell or oxyphil adenomas. Rare types of benign lesions include teratomas, lipomas, and hemangiomas. Except for thyroid hyperplasia of the right lobe of the gland in the presence of agenesis of the left lobe—and some follicular adenomas—all of the above lesions present as "cold" nodules on isotope scanning.

Differentiation of Benign & Malignant Lesions

Risk factors that predispose to benign or malignant disease are set forth in Table 7–15 and discussed below.

A. History: A family history of goiter suggests benign disease, as does residence in an area of endemic goiter. However, a family history of medullary carcinoma or a history of recent thyroid growth, hoarseness, dysphagia, or obstruction strongly suggests cancer. The significance of exposure to ionizing radiation is discussed above.

Table 7–14. Etiology of benign thyroid nodules.

1. Focal thyroiditis
2. Dominant portion of multinodular goiter
3. Thyroid, parathyroid, or thyroglossal cysts
4. Agenesis of a thyroid lobe
5. Postsurgical remnant hyperplasia or scarring
6. Postradioiodine remnant hyperplasia
7. Benign adenomas:
   a. Follicular:
      Colloid or macrofollicular
      Fetal
      Embryonal
      Hurthle cell
   b. Rare: Teratoma, lipoma, hemangioma

Table 7–15. Risk factors useful in distinguishing benign from malignant thyroid lesions.

	More Likely Benign	More Likely Malignant
History	Family history of benign goiter Residence in endemic goiter area	Family history of medullary cancer of thyroid Previous therapeutic irradiation of head or neck Recent growth of nodule Hoarseness, dysphagia, or obstruction
Physical characteristics	Older woman Soft nodule Multinodular goiter	Child, young adult, male Solitary, firm nodule clearly different from rest of gland ("dominant nodule") Vocal cord paralysis, firm lymph nodes, distant metastases
Serum factors	High titer of thyroid autoantibodies	Elevated serum calcitonin
Scanning techniques ^{123}I or $^{99m}TcO_4$	"Hot nodule"	"Cold nodule"
Echo scan	Cyst (pure)	Solid or semicystic
Biopsy (needle)	Benign appearance on cytologic examination	Malignant or suggestion of malignancy
Levothyroxine therapy (TSH suppression for 3–6 months)	Regression	No regression

B. Physical Characteristics: Physical characteristics associated with a low risk for thyroid cancer include older age, female sex, soft thyroid nodules, and the presence of a multinodular goiter. Individuals at higher risk for thyroid cancer include children, young adults, and males. A solitary firm or dominant nodule that is clearly different from the rest of the gland signifies an increased risk of malignancy. Vocal cord paralysis, enlarged lymph nodes, and suspected metastases are strongly suggestive of malignancy.

C. Serum Factors: A high titer of thyroid autoantibodies in serum suggests chronic thyroiditis as the cause of thyroid enlargement but does not rule out an associated malignancy. However, an elevated serum calcitonin, particularly in patients with a family history of medullary carcinoma, strongly suggests the presence of thyroid cancer. Elevated serum thyroglobulin following total thyroidectomy for papillary or follicular thyroid cancer usually indicate metastatic disease, but serum thyroglobulin is not usually helpful in determining the nature of a thyroid nodule.

D. Imaging Studies: Scanning procedures can be used to identify "hot" or "cold" nodules, ie, those that take up more or less radioactive iodine than surrounding tissue. Hot nodules are almost never malignant, whereas cold ones may be. Scintillation camera photographs with ^{99m}Tc pertechnetate give the best resolution (Figure 7–55). Thyroid ultrasound can distinguish cystic from solid lesions. A pure cyst is almost never malignant. Cystic lesions that have internal septa or solid lesions on ultrasound may be benign or malignant. CT scanning or MRI may be helpful in defining substernal extension or deep thyroid nodules in the neck.

E. Needle Biopsy: The major advance in management of the thyroid nodule in recent years has been the fine-needle aspiration biopsy (see above). Large-needle core aspiration biopsies of thyroid nodules have been available since about 1930, but they are limited to large nodules and are relatively traumatic. Söderström in 1952 introduced the technique of fine-needle aspiration biopsy, which is simple, safe, reliable, and well-tolerated. Fine-needle aspiration biopsy separates thyroid nodules into three groups: (1) Malignant thyroid nodules: The technique is diagnostic in about 95% of all types of thyroid malignancies. (2) Follicular neoplasms: About 15% of these lesions are malignant and about 85% are benign, but these two groups cannot be distinguished by cytology. Thus, a diagnosis of follicular neoplasm is always suspicious for malignancy. On isotope scan, a "hot" follicular neoplasm is benign, and a "cold" follicular neoplasm may be benign or malignant. (3) Benign thyroid nodules (Figure 7–56). About 5% of fine-needle aspiration readings are false-positives and about 5% false-negatives. Thus, results are accurate in about 90% of cases, as demonstrated by subsequent surgery or long-term follow-up of patients with lesions originally reported to be benign. The results of the biopsy study must be interpreted by the clinician but are extremely useful for the diagnosis of malignancy in thyroid nodules.

F. Suppressive Therapy: Benign lesions may undergo spontaneous involution and regression, and some may be sufficiently TSH-dependent to shrink on thyroxine therapy. Some studies have shown no regression of solitary nodules on T_4 therapy, while others have shown a 20–30% reduction in size, particularly in multinodular goiters. However, malignant

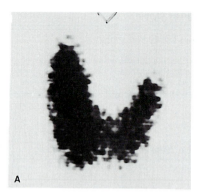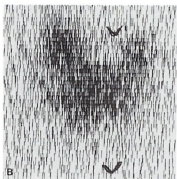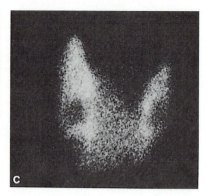

Figure 7–55. Demonstration of resolution obtained utilizing different scanning techniques: **A:** ^{123}I scintiscan with rectilinear scanner. **B:** Fluorescent scan with rectilinear scanner. **C:** ^{99m}Tc pertechnetate scan with the pinhole collimated gamma camera. Note the presence of two "cold" nodules, one in each lobe of the thyroid, easily detected in **C** but not clearly delineated in the other two scans. The lesion in the right lobe was palpable, about 1 cm in diameter, and was shown to be follicular carcinoma on needle biopsy. The lesion in the left lobe was either a metastatic tumor or a second primary follicular carcinoma. (Courtesy of MD Okerlund.)

lesions are unlikely to regress either spontaneously or on T_4 therapy.

Management of Thyroid Nodules

A decision matrix for management of a thyroid nodule is presented in Figure 7–56. A patient with a thyroid nodule should have fine-needle aspiration biopsy as the initial screening test for a thyroid mass. If the nodule is malignant, the patient is referred directly to the surgeon. If the cytologic report shows that the nodule is benign, the patient is given thyroxine, and if the lesion regresses, the patient is maintained on thyroxine indefinitely at a dose sufficient to suppress serum TSH. If there is no regression, the lesion is biopsied again—or, if it grows or changes in consistency, it may be excised. In patients who are reported to have follicular neoplasms, radionuclide scan is obtained. If the scan reveals the nodule to be hot, the patient is simply observed, with or without thyroxine therapy. If the lesion is cold and there is an increased chance of malignancy (large lesion over 2 cm in diameter, firm nodule, young patient), the patient might be referred directly to the surgeon. If the risk is low (small lesion 1 cm or less in diameter, soft nodule, older patient), the patient is given thyroxine. If thyroxine does not induce regression in the latter case, the lesion should probably be excised.

There are two groups that represent special problems: patients with thyroid cysts and patients who have received radiation therapy. Although thyroid cysts are almost always benign, cancer is occasionally found in the wall of the cyst. For this reason, recurrent cysts should be studied with ultrasonography, and if there is evidence of a septate lesion or growth in the wall of the lesion, surgical removal is indicated. In patients who have received radiation therapy, there may be multiple lesions, some benign and some malignant. Therefore, the presence of a cold

nodule in a patient who has had radiation exposure is an indication for surgical removal.

If this protocol is followed, there will be a marked reduction in surgery for benign thyroid nodules, and the incidence of malignancy at the time of surgery will be about 40%. The cost savings is enormous, since unnecessary surgery is eliminated and the cost of the thyroid nodule workup is cut in half. In addition, there is no delay in making the diagnosis and referring the patient with thyroid cancer for appropriate therapy.

2. THYROID CANCER

Pathology

The types and approximate frequency of malignant thyroid tumors are listed in Table 7–16.

A. Papillary Carcinoma: Papillary carcinoma of the thyroid gland usually presents as a nodule that is firm, solitary, "cold" on isotope scan, solid on thyroid ultrasound, and clearly different from the rest of the gland. In multinodular goiter, the cancer will usually be a "dominant nodule"—larger, firmer, and (again) clearly different from the rest of the gland. About 10% of papillary carcinomas, especially in children, present with enlarged cervical nodes, but careful examination will often reveal a "cold" nodule in the thyroid. Rarely, there will be hemorrhage, necrosis, and cyst formation in the malignant nodule, but on thyroid ultrasound of these lesions, clearly defined internal echoes will differentiate the semicystic malignant lesion from the nonmalignant "pure cyst." Finally, papillary carcinoma may be found incidentally as a microscopic focus of cancer in the middle of a gland removed for other reasons such as Graves' disease or multinodular goiter.

Microscopically, the tumor consists of single lay-

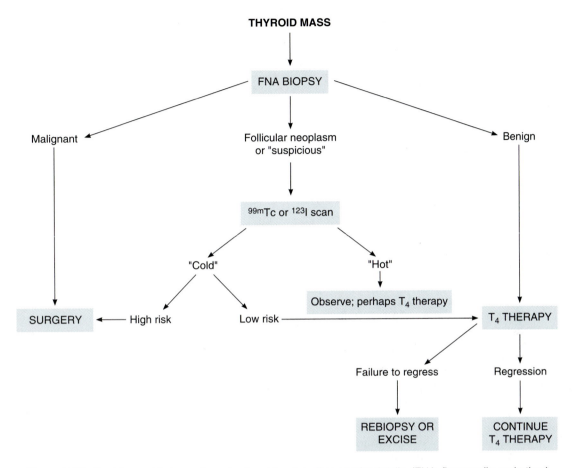

Figure 7–56. Decision matrix for workup of a thyroid nodule. See text for details. (FNA, fine-needle aspiration.)

ers of thyroid cells arranged in vascular stalks, with papillary projections extending into microscopic cyst-like spaces. The nuclei of the cells are large and pale and frequently contain clear, glassy intranuclear inclusion bodies. About 40% of papillary carcinomas form laminated calcified spheres—often at the tip of a papillary projection—called "psammoma bodies," which are usually diagnostic of papillary carcinoma. These cancers usually extend by intraglandular metastasis and by local lymph node invasion. They grow very slowly and remain confined to the thyroid gland and local lymph nodes for many years. In older

patients, they may become more aggressive and invade locally into muscles and trachea. In later stages, they can spread to the lung. Death is usually due to local disease, with invasion of deep tissues in the neck; less commonly, death may be due to extensive pulmonary metastases. In some older patients, a long-standing, slowly growing papillary carcinoma will begin to grow rapidly and convert to undifferentiated or anaplastic carcinoma. This "late anaplastic shift" is another cause of death from papillary carcinoma. Many papillary carcinomas secrete thyroglobulin, which can be used as a marker for recurrence or metastasis of the cancer.

B. Follicular Carcinoma: Follicular carcinoma is characterized by the presence of small follicles, though colloid formation is poor. Indeed, follicular carcinoma may be indistinguishable from follicular adenoma except by capsular or vascular invasion. The tumor is somewhat more aggressive than papillary carcinoma and can spread either by local invasion of lymph nodes or by blood vessel invasion with distant metastases to bone or lung. Microscopically, the cells are cuboidal, with large nuclei, arranged

Table 7–16. Approximate frequency of malignant thyroid tumors.

Pipillary carcinoma (including mixed papillary and follicular)	75%
Follicular carcinoma	16%
Medullary carcinoma	5%
Undifferentiated carcinomas	3%
Miscellaneous (including lymphoma, fibrosarcoma, squamous cell carcinoma, malignant hemangioendothelioma, teratomas, and metastatic carcinomas)	1%

around follicles that frequently contain dense colloid. These tumors often retain the ability to concentrate radioactive iodine, to form thyroglobulin, and, rarely, to synthesize T_3 and T_4. Thus, the rare "functioning thyroid cancer" is almost always a follicular carcinoma. This characteristic makes these tumors more likely to respond to radioactive iodine therapy. In untreated patients, death is due to local extension or to distant bloodstream metastasis with extensive involvement of bone, lungs, and viscera.

A variant of follicular carcinoma is the "Hurthle cell" carcinoma, characterized by large individual cells with pink-staining cytoplasm filled with mitochondria. They behave like follicular cancer except that they rarely take up radioiodine. Mixed papillary and follicular carcinomas behave more like papillary carcinoma. Thyroglobulin secretion by follicular carcinomas can be used to follow the course of disease.

C. Medullary Carcinoma: Medullary cancer is a disease of the C cells (parafollicular cells) derived from the ultimobranchial body and capable of secreting calcitonin, histaminase, prostaglandins, serotonin, and other peptides. Microscopically, the tumor consists of sheets of cells separated by a pink-staining substance that has characteristics of amyloid. This material stains with Congo red. Amyloid consists of chains of calcitonin laid down in a fibrillary pattern—in contrast to other forms of amyloid, which may have immunoglobulin light chains or other proteins deposited in a fibrillary pattern.

Medullary carcinoma is somewhat more aggressive than papillary or follicular carcinoma but not as aggressive as undifferentiated thyroid cancer. It extends locally into lymph nodes and into surrounding muscle and trachea. It may invade lymphatics and blood vessels and metastasize to lungs and viscera. Calcitonin and carcinoembryonic antigen (CEA) secreted by the tumor are clinically useful markers for diagnosis and follow-up. About one-third of medullary carcinomas are familial, involving multiple endocrine glands (multiple endocrine neoplasia, type II (MEN II; Sipple's syndrome) (Chapter 24). MEN IIa is characterized by medullary carcinoma, pheochromocytoma, and parathyroid adenomas; and MEN IIb is characterized by medullary carcinoma, pheochromocytomas, and multiple neuromas of the tongue, lip, and bowel. About one-third of medullary carcinomas are familial medullary thyroid cancer (FMTC), involving only the thyroid cancer, and about one-third are isolated instances of the malignancy. If medullary carcinoma is diagnosed by fine-needle aspiration biopsy or at surgery, it is essential that the patient be screened for the other endocrine abnormalities found in MEN II and that family members be screened for medullary carcinoma and MEN II as well. Screening involves measurement of serum calcitonin after pentagastrin or calcium infusion in patients who have demonstrated mutations in the RET protooncogene on DNA analysis (see below).

Pentagastrin is administered intravenously in a bolus of 0.5 μg/kg, and venous blood specimens are drawn at 1, 3, 5, and 10 minutes. An abnormal rise in serum calcitonin at 3 or 5 minutes is indicative of the presence of the malignancy (Chapter 8).

D. Undifferentiated (Anaplastic) Carcinoma: Undifferentiated thyroid gland tumors include small cell, giant cell, and spindle cell carcinomas. They usually occur in older patients with a long history of goiter in whom the gland suddenly—over weeks or months—begins to enlarge and produce pressure symptoms, dysphagia, or vocal cord paralysis. Death from massive local extension usually occurs within 6–36 months. These tumors are very resistant to therapy.

E. Miscellaneous Types:

1. Lymphoma–The only type of rapidly growing thyroid cancer that is responsive to therapy is the lymphoma, which may develop as part of a generalized lymphoma or may be primary in the thyroid gland. Thyroid lymphoma occasionally develops in a patient with long-standing Hashimoto's thyroiditis and may be difficult to distinguish from chronic thyroiditis. It is characterized by lymphocyte invasion of thyroid follicles and blood vessel walls, which helps to differentiate thyroid lymphoma from chronic thyroiditis. If there is no systemic involvement, the tumor may respond dramatically to radiation therapy.

2. Cancer metastatic to the thyroid–Systemic cancers that may metastasize to the thyroid gland include cancers of the breast and kidney, bronchogenic carcinoma, and malignant melanoma. The primary site of involvement is usually obvious. Occasionally, the diagnosis is made by needle biopsy or open biopsy of a rapidly enlarging cold thyroid nodule. The prognosis is that of the primary tumor.

3. Molecular biology of thyroid neoplasms– Extensive studies have revealed evidence of gene mutations in both benign and malignant thyroid neoplasms (Figure 7–57). Activating mutations in the Gsp oncogene in the thyroid follicular cell have been associated with increased growth and function in the "hot" or "toxic" thyroid nodule. Aberrant DNA methylation, activation of the RAS oncogene and mutation of the MEN I gene 11q13 are associated with benign follicular adenomas. Loss of the 3P suppressor gene may then result in the development of follicular carcinoma, and further loss of suppressor gene P53 may allow progression to an anaplastic carcinoma. Mutations in the RET and TRK oncogenes are associated with the development of papillary carcinomas—and again, loss of P53 suppressor gene may allow progression to anaplastic carcinoma. This hypothesis suggests a progression of benign to malignant lesions and from differentiated to undifferentiated carcinoma. Indeed in pathology specimens from older patients with long-standing goiters and recent rapid enlargement, we may see a transition from papillary or follicular thyroid carcinoma to anaplastic

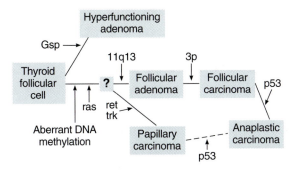

Fig 7–57: Molecular defects associated with development and progression of human thyroid neoplasms. The hypothetical role of specific mutational events in thyroid tumorigenesis is inferred from their prevalence in the various thyroid tumor phenotypes. (Reproduced, with permission, from Fagin JA: Genetic basis of endocrine disease 3: Molecular defects in thyroid gland neoplasia. J Clin Endocrinol Metabol 75:1398, 1992.)

carcinoma, a phenomenon termed "late anaplastic shift."

As noted above, activating mutations of the RET protooncogene on chromosome 10 have been shown to be associated with MEN IIa, MEN IIb, and famil-

ial medullary thyroid carcinoma (FMTC). The RET oncogene encodes a receptor-like tyrosine kinase. About 85–90% of the mutations found in MEN IIa and FMTC occur in exons 10 and 11, whereas about 95% of the mutations associated with MEN IIb are found in exon 16 of the RET oncogene. These mutations can be demonstrated in DNA from peripheral white blood cells utilizing the polymerase chain reaction (PCR) and restriction fragment length polymorphism (RFLP). In patients with MEN II or FMTC who do not demonstrate a mutation in the RET oncogene, family unit linkage analysis may demonstrate an oncogene mutation. Thus, families can be screened for the carrier state, and early diagnosis and treatment can be instituted (Figure 7–58).

Management of Thyroid Cancer (Figure 7–59)

A. Papillary and Follicular Carcinoma: Lobectomy is satisfactory for small (< 2 cm) papillary and follicular thyroid carcinomas, but total thyroidectomy is required for larger lesions or for cancers with evidence of intrathyroidal or extrathyroidal extension. Modified neck dissection is indicated if there is evidence of lymph node metastases. Prophylactic neck dissections are not recommended. Postoperative radioiodine scan and therapy are indicated for

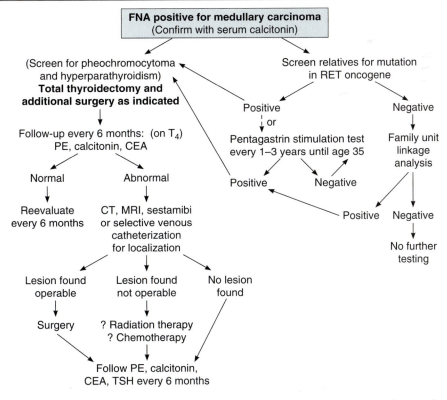

Figure 7–58. Decision matrix for the management of patients with medullary carcinoma. See text for details.

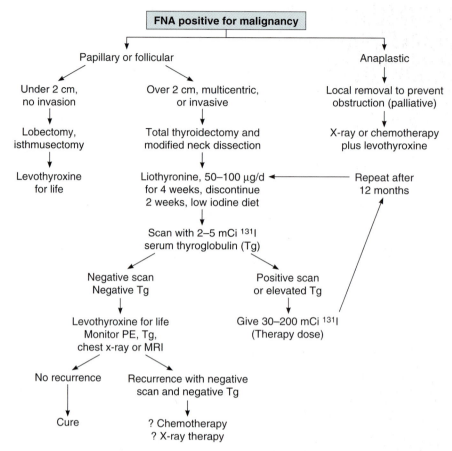

Figure 7–59: Decision matrix for the management of papillary, follicular, or anaplastic thyroid carcinoma. See text for details.

patients with large papillary or follicular carcinomas (> 2 cm) or with evidence of intra- or extrathyroidal extension. After recovery from surgery, the patient receives liothyronine, 50–100 µg daily in divided doses for 4 weeks; the medication is then stopped for 2 weeks, and the patient is placed on a low-iodine diet. The patient is scanned at 24 and 72 hours after a dose of 2–5 mCi of ^{131}I. Liothyronine is used for replacement therapy because it is cleared from the blood rapidly; after 2 weeks off therapy, serum TSH is usually over 50 mU/L, which is necessary for good scanning studies. If there is evidence of residual radioactive iodine uptake in the neck or elsewhere, radioactive iodine (^{131}I) is effective treatment. The scan is repeated at intervals of 12 months until no further uptake is observed; the patient is then maintained on maximum replacement therapy with levothyroxine, 0.15–0.3 mg daily, to suppress serum TSH to undetectable levels. The availability of injectable recombinant human TSH (rHTSH) would allow postoperative diagnostic scans to be performed without the withdrawal of thyroid hormone therapy, thus avoiding the discomfort of transient hypothy-

roidism. It may be possible to use rHTSH for the treatment phase as well.

Follow-up at intervals of 6–12 months should include careful examination of the neck for recurrent masses. If a lump is noted, needle biopsy examination is indicated to confirm or rule out cancer. Serum thyroglobulin will usually be less than 5 ng/mL (5 µg/L) after total thyroidectomy and levothyroxine therapy. A rise in serum thyroglobulin to more than 10 ng/mL (10 µg/L) suggests recurrence of thyroid cancer. Chest x-ray, thyroid ultrasound, or MRI every 2–3 years may reveal local or pulmonary metastases, though a rising serum thyroglobulin concentration is a more sensitive indicator. If the patient does develop a mass in the neck, a rise in serum thyroglobulin, or a mass on chest x-ray, thyroid ultrasound, or MRI, ^{131}I scan should be repeated following the technique outlined above. If the lesions concentrate ^{131}I, the patient can be treated with the isotope; if they do not, local excision or local x-ray therapy may be useful. For recurrences that cannot be managed by these modalities, chemotherapy should be considered.

B. Medullary Carcinoma: Patients with medullary carcinoma should be followed in a similar way, except that the marker for recurrent medullary cancer is serum calcitonin or carcinoembryonic antigen (CEA). Family members should be screened for RET oncogene mutations as noted above (Figure 7–58). Histaminase and other peptides are also secreted by these tumors, but assays for these substances are not generally available. If a patient has a persistently elevated serum calcitonin concentration after total thyroidectomy and regional node dissection, MRI of the neck and chest or selective venous catheterization and sampling for serum calcitonin may reveal the location of the metastases. If this fails to localize the lesion (as is often the case), the patient must be followed until the metastatic lesion shows itself as a palpable mass or a shadow on chest x-ray or MRI. Metastatic medullary carcinoma cannot be treated with ^{131}I; therefore, initial thorough surgical excision and postoperative levothyroxine therapy are essential. Chemotherapy for medullary carcinoma has not been effective.

C. Anaplastic Carcinoma: Anaplastic carcinoma of the thyroid has a very poor prognosis. Treatment consists of isthmusectomy (to confirm the diagnosis and to prevent tracheal compression) and palliative x-ray therapy (Figure 7–59). Thyroid lymphomas are quite responsive to x-ray therapy; giant cell, squamous cell, spindle cell, and anaplastic carcinomas are unresponsive. Chemotherapy is not very effective for anaplastic carcinomas. Doxorubicin, 75 mg/m^2 as a single injection or divided into three consecutive daily injections repeated at 3-week intervals, has been useful in some patients with disseminated thyroid cancer unresponsive to surgery, TSH suppression, or radiation therapy. This drug is quite toxic; side effects include cardiotoxicity, myelosuppression, alopecia, and gastrointestinal symptoms.

D. X-Ray Therapy: Local x-ray therapy has been useful in the treatment of solitary metastatic lesions, particularly follicular or papillary tumors, that do not concentrate radioactive iodine. It is particularly effective in isolated nonfunctional bone metastases.

Course & Prognosis

The staging of cancer has been a useful method for the prediction of the outcome of therapy. The International Union Against Cancer (UICC) and the American Joint Committee on Cancer (AJCC) have proposed the TNM (Tumor, Nodes, Metastases) system for staging thyroid cancer (Table 7–17).

In this system, papillary and follicular thyroid carcinomas are grouped together and the staging is directly related to the age of the patient at the time of the diagnosis. The cause-specific 5-year mortality rates in a group of 1500 patients studied by Hay were as follows: stage 1, 0%; stage 2, 0.6%; stage 3, 5.3%; and stage 4, 77%. Similarly, DeGroot et al demon-

Table 7–17. Tumor (T), lymph node (N), and distant metastasis (M) classification and staging of thyroid cancer.[1]

DEFINITIONS

Primary Tumor (T)
All categories may be subdivided: (a) solitary; (b) multifocal—measure the largest for classification.
TX   Primary tumor cannot be assessed
T0   No evidence of primary tumor
T1   Tumor 1 cm or less in greatest dimension limited to the thyroid
T2   Tumor more than 1 cm but not more than 4 cm
T3   Tumor more than 4 cm in greatest dimension limited to the thyroid
T4   Tumor of any size extending beyond the thyroid capsule

Lymph Node (N)
Regional nodes are the cervical and upper mediastinal lymph nodes
NX   Regional lymph nodes cannot be assessed
N0   No regional lymph node metastasis
N1   Regional lymph node metastasis
   N1a   Metastasis in ipsilateral cervical lymph nodes
   N1b   Metastasis in bilateral, midline, or contralateral cervical or mediastinal lymph nodes

Distant Metastasis (M)
MX   Presence of distant metastasis cannot be assessed
M0   No distant metastasis
M1   Distant metastasis

STAGE GROUPING
Separate stage groupings are recommended for papillary and follicular, medullary, and undifferentiated

Papillary or follicular
Under 45 Years
Stage I   Any T, Any N, M0
Stage II   Any T, Any M, M1

45 Years and Older
Stage I   T1, N0, M0
Stage II   T2, N0, M0
            T3, N0, M0
Stage III   T4, N0, M0
            Any T, N1, M0
Stage IV   Any T, Any N, M1

Medullary

Stage I	T1	N0	M0
Stage II	T2	N0	M0
	T3	N0	M0
	T4	N0	M0
Stage III	Any T	N1	M0
Stage IV	Any T	Any N	M1

Undifferentiated
All cases are Stage IV
Stage IV   Any T   Any N   Any M

[1]Reproduced, with permission, from Beahrs OH, Myers MH: *Manual for Staging of Cancer,* 4th ed. Lippincott, 1992.

strated 80–90% survival for stage 1 and stage 2 patients followed for up to 38 years; about 50% survival for stage 3 patients followed for 20 years; and 0% survival for stage 4 patients followed for 10 years. The TNM system may underestimate the risk of recurrence and death in younger patients with aggressive disease. This is particularly true for patients under age 7 with local invasion or distant metastases, who should probably be grouped in stage 3 or stage

4. However, the system recognizes that for most younger patients, papillary and follicular thyroid carcinomas are relatively indolent and thus can be classified as stage 1 or stage 2.

Outcome is also dependent upon adequate therapy. There has been controversy over the extent of initial surgery for papillary and follicular thyroid cancer. Lesions under 1 cm with no evidence of local or distant metastases (T1, N0, M0) can probably be treated with lobectomy alone. However, in all other groups, total thyroidectomy and modified regional neck dissection (if gross evidence of spread is noted at the time of surgery) is indicated for two reasons: (1) it removes all local disease, and (2) it sets the stage for ^{131}I therapy and follow-up utilizing serum thyroglobulin measurements. Total or near-total thyroidectomy must be performed by an experienced thyroid surgeon to minimize the complications of surgery. The improvement in outcome following total thyroidectomy is presented in Figure 7–60.

A second factor in survival is the use of radioiodine for ablation of residual thyroid tissue after thyroidectomy and the treatment of residual or recurrent disease. Low doses of 30–50 mCi ^{131}I are used to ablate residual thyroid tissue, but larger doses of 100–200 mCi are necessary for the treatment of metastatic disease. Acute adverse effects of the larger doses include radiation sickness, sialitis, gastritis, and transient oligospermia. Cumulative doses of ^{131}I above 500 mCi may be associated with infertility in the female and azoospermia in the male, pancytopenia in about 4%, and leukemia in about 0.3% of patients. Radiation pneumonitis may occur in patients with diffuse pulmonary metastases, but this is minimized by utilization of high-dose treatment no more than once a year. The effectiveness of ^{131}I therapy in reducing cancer mortality is presented in Figure 7–61.

A third factor in survival is the adequate use of TSH suppression therapy. T_4 in a dose of 2.2 μg/kg/d (1 μg/lb/d) will usually suppress TSH to 0.1 mU/L or less, which removes a major growth factor for papillary or follicular thyroid cancer. However, high-dose T_4 therapy is not without risk: angina, tachycardia, or heart failure in older patients or tachycardia and nervousness in younger patients. In addition, there is an increased risk of osteoporosis in postmenopausal women. Estrogen or bisphosphonate therapy may prevent bone loss in these patients, but the treatment program must be individualized.

Medullary carcinoma is more aggressive. It is most aggressive in patients with MEN IIb, less in the sporadic type, and least virulent in MEN IIa and FMTC. Early and adequate initial surgery is the best therapy; once the disease has started to metastasize, it is very difficult to control, although the more favorable types often progress very slowly. Anaplastic thyroid carcinomas have a very poor prognosis, with death to be anticipated within 3 years.

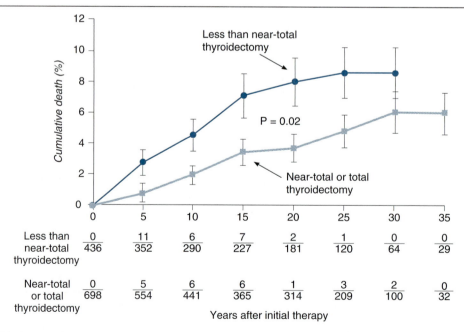

Figure 7–60: Improved survival in patients with papillary or follicular thyroid carcinoma following total or near-total thyroidectomy compared to less than near total thyroidectomy. (Reproduced, with permission, from Mazzaferri EL, Jhiang SM: Long term impact of initial surgical and medical therapy on papillary and follicular thyroid cancer. Am J Med 1994;97:418.)

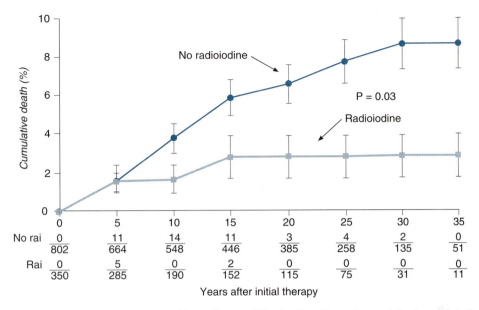

Figure 7–61. Improved survival in patients with papillary or follicular thyroid carcinoma following radioiodine therapy compared to those receiving no radioiodine. (Reproduced, with permission, from Mazzaferri EL: Presented at the Endocrine Society Meeting June 15, 1994.)

REFERENCES

General

Braverman LE, Utiger RD (editors): *Werner and Ingbar's The Thyroid: A Fundamental and Clinical Text,* 7th ed. Lippincott, 1996.

Burrow FN: The thyroid: nodules and neoplasms. In: *Endocrinology and Metabolism,* 3rd ed. Felig P, Baxter JD, Frohman LA (editors). McGraw-Hill, 1995.

Greenspan FS (editor): Thyroid diseases. Med Clin North Am 1991;75:1.

Greer MA (editor): *The Thyroid Gland.* Comprehensive Endocrinology Series. Martini L (editor). Raven Press, 1990.

Larsen PR, Ingbar SH: The thyroid gland. In: *Williams Textbook of Endocrinology,* 8th ed. Wilson JD, Foster DW. Saunders, 1992.

Medeiros-Neto G, Stanbury JB: *Inherited Disorders of the Thyroid System.* CRC Press. 1994.

Utiger RD: The thyroid: physiology, thyrotoxicosis, hypothyroidism and the painful thyroid. In: *Endocrinology and Metabolism,* 3rd ed. Felig P, Baxter JD, Frohman LA (editors). McGraw-Hill, 1995.

Wartofsky L (editor): The thyroid gland. In: *Principles and Practice of Endocrinology and Metabolism,* 2nd ed. Becker KL (editor). Lippincott, 1995.

Weintraub BD (editor): *Molecular Endocrinology: Basic Concepts and Clinical Correlations.* Raven Press, 1995.

Wheeler MH, Lazarus JH: *Diseases of the Thyroid: Pathophysiology and Management.* Chapman & Hall, 1994.

Anatomy

Fujita H: Functional morphology of the thyroid. Int Rev Cytol 113:145,1988.

Hegedus L: Thyroid size determined by ultrasound: Influence of physiological factors and non-thyroidal disease. Dan Med Bull 1990;37:249.

Lindner HH: The thyroid gland. In: *Clinical Anatomy.* Appleton & Lange, 1989.

Siminowski S: The rational clinical examination: Does this patient have a goiter? JAMA 1995;273:813.

Physiology

Bartalena L, Robbins J: Thyroid hormone transport proteins. Clin Lab Med 1993;13:583.

Beckett GJ, Arthur JR: The iodothyronine deiodinases and 5′ deiodination. Baillieres Clin Endocrinol Metab 1994;8:285.

Berry MJ, Larsen PR: The role of selenium in thyroid hormone action. Endocr Rev 1992;13:207.

Brabant G, von zur Muhlen A: Physiological regulation and biological function of thyrotropin. Supplement Series No. 23 In: *Hormone and Metabolic Research.* Pfeiffer EF, Reaven GM (editors). Thieme, 1990.

Brent GA: The molecular basis of thyroid hormone action. N Engl J Med 1994;331:847.

Carrasco N: Iodide transport in the thyroid gland. Biochim Biophys Acta 1993;1154:65.

Delange F: The disorders induced by iodine deficiency. Thyroid. 1994;4:107.

Dunn JT: Thyroglobulin: Chemistry and biosynthesis.

In: *Werner and Ingbar's The Thyroid: A fundamental and Clinical Text,* 6th ed. Braverman LE, Utiger RD (editors). Lippincott, 1991.

Eckholm R. Biosynthesis of thyroid hormones. Int Rev Cytol 1990;120:243.

Glinoer D et al: Regulation of maternal thyroid during pregnancy. J Clin Endocrinol Metab 1990;71:276.

Goldberg Y et al: Thyroid hormone action and the *erb*A oncogene family. Biochimie 1989;71:279.

Henneman G, Doctor R: Plasma transport proteins and their role in tissue delivery of thyroid hormone. In: *The Thyroid Gland.* Greer MA (editor). Comprehensive Endocrinology Series. Martini L (editor), Raven Press, 1990.

Hinuma S et al: Molecular cloning and functional expression of a human thyrotropin-releasing hormone (TRH) receptor gene. Biochim Biophys Acta 1994; 1219:251.

Kendall-Taylor P: Autoimmune endocrine disease. Baillieres Clin Endocrinol Metab 1995;9:1.

Kohn LD et al: Cloning and regulation of glycoprotein hormone receptor genes. In: Molecular Endocrinology: Basic Concepts & Clinical Correlations. Weintraub BD (editor). Raven Press, 1995.

Lazar MA, Chin WW. Nuclear thyroid hormone receptors. J Clin Invest 1990;86:1777.

Ludgate ME, Vassart G: The thyrotropin receptor as a model to illustrate receptor and receptor antibody diseases. Baillieres Clin Endocrinol Metab 1995;9:95.

Magner JA: Thyroid-stimulating hormone: Biosynthesis, cell biology and bioactivity. Endocr Rev 1990; 11:354.

Magnusson RP: Thyroid peroxidase. In: *Peroxidases in Chemistry and Biology,* vol 1. Everse J, Grisham MB (editors). CRC Press 1990.

Malthiery Y et al: Thyroglobulin structure and function: Recent advances. Biochimie 1989;71:195.

McLachlan SM, Rapaport B: The molecular biology of thyroid peroxidase: Cloning, expression and role as autoantigen in autoimmune thyroid disease. Endocr Rev 1992;13:1992.

Metcalf G, Jackson IMD (editors): Thyrotropin-releasing hormone: Biomedical significance. Ann N Y Acad Sci 1989;553:1.

Pisarev MA: Thyroid autoregulation. J Endocrinol Invest 1985;8:475.

Rapaport B, Nagayama Y: The thyrotropin receptor 25 years after its discovery: New insights after molecular cloning. Mol Endocrinol 1992;6:145.

Ribeiro RCJ, Kushner PJ, Baxter JD: The nuclear hormone receptor gene superfamily. Ann Rev Med 1995;46:443.

Schwartz HL, Strait KA, Oppenheimer JH: Molecular mechanisms of thyroid hormone action: A physiologic perspective. Clin Lab Med 1993;13:543.

Shupnik MA, Ridgeway EC, Chin WW: Molecular biology of thyrotropin. Endocr Rev 1989;4:459.

Stevenin B, Lee SL: Hormonal regulation of the thyrotropin releasing hormone (TRH) gene. Endocrinologist 1995;5:286.

Surks MI et al: Normal free thyroxine in critical nonthyroidal illnesses measured by ultrafiltration of undiluted serum and equilibrium dialysis. J Clin Endocrinol Metab 1988;67:1031.

Taurog A: Hormone synthesis: Thyroid iodine metabolism. In: *Werner and Ingbar's The Thyroid: A Fundamental and Clinical Text,* 6th ed. Braverman LE, Utiger RD (editors). Lippincott, 1991.

Tibaldi JM, Surks MI: Effects of nonthyroidal illness on thyroid function. Med Clin North Am 1985;69:899.

Utiger RD: Thyrotropin-receptor mutations and thyroid dysfunction. N Engl J Med 1995;332:183.

Volpé R: Autoimmunity causing thyroid dysfunction. Endocrinol Metab Clin North Am 1991;20:565.

Weetman AP, McGregor AM: Autoimmune thyroid disease: Further developments in our understanding. Endocr Rev 1994;15:788.

Weinberger C et al: The c-erb-A gene encodes a thyroid hormone receptor. Nature 1986;324:641.

Wolff J. Excess iodide inhibits the thyroid gland by multiple mechanisms. In: *Control of the Thyroid Gland.* Eckholm R, Kohn LD, Wollman SH (editors), Plenum, 1989.

Wolff J: Iodide transport: Anion selectivity and the iodide "trap." In: *Diminished Thyroid Hormone Formation.* Reinwein D, Klein E (editors). Schattauer, 1982.

Xue-Yi C et al: Timing of vulnerability of the brain to iodine deficiency in endemic cretinism. N Engl J Med 1994;331:1739.

Tests of Thyroid Function

Bartalena L, Bogazzi F, Pinchera A: Thyroid function tests and diagnostic protocols for investigation of thyroid dysfunction. Ann Inst Super Sanita 1991;27:531.

Bayer MF: Effective laboratory evaluation of thyroid status. Med Clin North Am 1991;75:1.

Cavalieri RR: The effects of nonthyroid disease and drugs on thyroid function. Med Clin North Am 1991; 75:27.

Davies PH, Franklyn JA: The effect of drugs on tests of thyroid function. Eur J Clin Pharmacol 1991;40:439.

Ekins R: Analytic measurements of free thyroxine. Clin Lab Med 1993;13:599.

Hay ID et al: American Thyroid Association assessment of current free thyroid hormone and thyrotropin measurements and guidelines for future clinical assays. Clin Chem 1991;37:2002.

Kaptein EM: Clinical application of free thyroxine determinations. Clin Lab Med 1993;13:654.

Klee GG, Hay ID: Role of thyrotropin measurements in the diagnosis and management of thyroid disease. Clin Lab Med 1993;13:673.

Liewendahl K: Assessment of thyroid status by laboratory methods: Developments and perspectives. Scand J Clin Lab Invest 1990;201(Suppl):83.

Prentice LM et al: Geographical distribution of subclinical autoimmune thyroid disease in Britain: A study using highly sensitive direct assays for autoantibodies to thyroglobulin and thyroid peroxidase. Acta Endocrinol (Copenh) 1990;123:493.

Rees Smith B, McLachlan SM, Furmaniak J: Autoantibodies to the thyrotropin receptor. Endocr Rev 1988; 9:106.

Sapin R et al: Determination of free triiodothyronine by six different methods in patients with nonthyroidal illness and in patients treated with amiodarone. Ann Clin Biochem 1995;32:314.

Surks MI et al: American Thyroid Association guidelines for use of laboratory tests in thyroid disorders. JAMA 1990;263:1529.

Tunbridge WMG et al: The spectrum of thyroid disease in a community: The Whickham survey. Clin Endocrinol (Oxf) 1977;7:481.

Hypothyroidism

Dussault JH: Neonatal screening for congenital hypothyroidism. Clin Lab Med 1993;13:645.

Fisher DA: Management of congenital hypothyroidism. Clinical review 19. J Clin Endocrinol Metab 1991; 72:523.

Greenspan SL et al: Skeletal integrity in premenopausal and postmenopausal women receiving long-term l-thyroxine therapy. Am J Med 1991;91:5.

Jordan RM: Myxedema coma: Pathophysiology, therapy and factors affecting prognosis. Med Clin North Am 1995;79:185.

Lazarus JH, Hall R (editors): Hypothyroidism and goiter. Baillieres Clin Endocrinol Metab 1988;2:531.

Mandel SJ et al: Increased need for thyroxine during pregnancy in women with primary hypothyroidism. N Eng J Med 1990;323:91.

Martino E et al: Amiodarone iodine-induced hypothyroidism: Risk factors and follow-up in 28 cases. Clin Endocrinol 1987;26:227.

Nicoloff JT, LoPresti JS: Myxedema coma, a form of decompensated hypothyroidism. Endocrinol Metab Clin North Am 1993;22:279.

Ross DS: Subclinical Hyperthyroidism: Possible danger of overzealous thyroxine replacement therapy. Mayo Clin Proc 1988;63:1223.

Singer PA et al: Treatment guidelines for patients with hyperthyroidism and hypothyroidism. JAMA 1995; 273:808.

Toft AD: Thyroxine therapy. N Engl J Med 1994;331: 174.

Hyperthyroidism

Aronow WS: The heart and thyroid disease. Clin Geriatr Med 1995;11:219.

Bahn RS et al: Diagnosis and management of Graves' ophthalmopathy. Clinical review 13. J Clin Endocrinol Metab 1990;71:559.

Becks GP, Burrow GN: Thyroid disease and pregnancy. Med Clin North Am 1991;75:121.

Bradley EL III et al: Modified subtotal thyroidectomy in the management of Graves' disease. Surgery 1980; 7:623.

Carter JA, Utiger RD: The ophthalmopathy of Graves' disease. Ann Rev Med 1992;43:487.

Char DH: *Thyroid Eye Disease,* 2nd ed. Churchill Livingston, 1990.

DeGroot LJ et al: Therapeutic controversies: Radiation and Graves' ophthalmopathy. J Clin Endocrinol Metab 1995;80:339.

Farrar JJ, Toft AD: Iodine-131 treatment of hyperthyroidism: Current issues. Clin Endocrinol 1991; 35:207.

Feldt-Rasmussen U: Reassessment of antithyroid drug therapy of Graves' disease. Ann Rev Med 1993; 44:323.

Franklyn JA: The management of hyperthyroidism. N Engl J Med 1994;330:1731.

Hashizume K et al: Administration of thyroxine in treated Graves' disease: Effects on the level of antibodies to thyroid stimulating hormone receptors and on the risk of recurrence of hyperthyroidism. N Eng J Med 1991;324:947.

Heufelder AE: Pathogenesis of Graves' ophthalmopathy: Recent controversies and progress. Eur J Endocrinol 1995;132:532.

McDougall IR: Graves' disease: Current concepts. Med Clin North Am 1991;75:79.

Nabil N et al: Methimazole: An alternative route of administration. J Clin Endocrinol Metab 1982;54:180.

Nademanee K et al: Amiodarone and thyroid function. Prog Cardiovasc Dis 1989;21:427.

Sills IN: Hyperthyroidism. Pediatr Rev 1994;15:417.

Tietgens ST, Leinung MC: Thyroid storm. Med Clin North Am 1995;79:169.

Thyroid Hormone Resistance Syndromes

Franklyn JA: Syndromes of thyroid hormone resistance. Clin Endocrinol 1991;34:237.

Jameson JL: Mechanisms by which thyroid hormone receptor mutations cause clinical syndromes of resistance to thyroid hormone. Thyroid 1994;4:485.

Refetoff S, Weiss RE, Usala SJ: The syndromes of resistance to thyroid hormones. Endocr Rev 1993;14:348.

Refetoff S: The syndrome of generalized resistance to thyroid hormone (GRTH). Endocr Res 1989;15:717.

Usala SJ, Weintraub BD: Thyroid hormone resistance syndromes. Trends Endocrinol Metab 1991;2:140.

Syndrome of Inappropriate TSH Secretion

Beckers A et al: Thyrotropin-secreting pituitary adenomas: Report of seven cases. J Clin Endocrinol Metab 1991;72:477.

Chayen SD et al: TSH producing pituitary tumor: Biochemical diagnosis and long-term management with octreotide. Horm Metabol Res 1992;24:34.

Gesundheit N et al: Thyrotropin-secreting pituitary adenomas: Clinical and biochemical heterogeneity. Ann Int Med 1989;111:827.

Hermus A et al: Hyperthyroidism due to inappropriate secretion of thyroid stimulating hormone: Diagnosis and management. Neth J Med 1991;38:193.

Kopp P et al: Brief Report: Congenital hyperthyroidism caused by a mutation in the thyrotropin-receptor gene. N Engl J Med 1995;332:150.

Sunthornthepvarakul T et al: Brief Report: Resistance to thyrotropin caused by mutations in the thyrotropin-receptor gene. N Engl J Med 1995;332:155.

Nontoxic Goiter

Foley TP Jr: Goiter in adolescents. Endocrinol Metab Clin North Am 1993;22:593.

Gaitan E, Nelson NC, Poole GV: Endemic goiter and endemic thyroid disorders. World J Surg 1991;15:205.

Greenspan FS: The problem of the nodular goiter. Med Clin North Am 1991;75:195.

Lamberg BA: Endemic goiter-iodine deficiency disorders. Ann Med 1991;23:367.

Studer H, Derwahl M: Mechanisms of nonneoplastic endocrine hyperplasia—a changing concept: A review focused on the thyroid gland. Endocr Rev 1995;16: 411.

Thyroiditis

Amino N: Autoimmunity and hypothyroidism. Baillieres Clin Endocrinol Metab 1988;2:591.

LiVolsi VA: The pathology of autoimmune thyroid disease: A review. Thyroid 1994;4:333.

Nagataki S, Mori T, Torizuma K: 80 years of Hashimoto's disease. Excerpta Medica 1993; International Congress Series 1028.

Rapoport B: Pathophysiology of Hashimoto's thyroiditis and hypothyroidism. Ann Rev Med 1991;42:91.

Roti E, Emerson CH: Postpartum thyroiditis. Clinical review 29. J Clin Endocrinol Metab 1992;74:3.

Tomer Y, Davies TF: Infection, thyroid disease and autoimmunity. Endocr Rev 1993;14:107.

Volpé R: The management of subacute (De Quervain's) thyroiditis. Thyroid 1993;3:253.

Radiation Exposure

DeGroot LJ: Effects of irradiation on the thyroid gland. Endocrinol Metab Clin North Am 1993;22:607.

Hancock SL, McDougall IR, Constine LS: Thyroid abnormalities after therapeutic external radiation. Int J Radiat Oncol Biol Phys 1995;31:1165.

Sako K: Head and neck irradiation in childhood: Increased risk of developing thyroid disease. Semin Surg Oncol 1991;7:112.

Williams ED Pacini F, Pinchera A: Thyroid cancer following Chernobyl. J Endocrinol Invest 1995;18:144.

Thyroid Nodules & Thyroid Cancer

Cady B: Papillary carcinoma of the thyroid. Semin Surg Oncol 1991;7:81.

DeGroot LJ et al: Does the method of management of papillary carcinoma make a difference in outcome? World J Surg 1994;18:123.

Fagin JA: Genetic basis of endocrine disease 3: Molecular defects in thyroid gland neoplasia. J Clin Endocrinol Metab 1992;75:1398.

Gagel RF et al: Clinical Review 44. Medullary thyroid cancer: Recent progress. J Clin Endocrinol Metab 1993;76:809.

Gupta KL: Neoplasms of the thyroid gland. Clin Geriatr Med 1995;11:271.

Hay ID: Papillary thyroid carcinoma. Endocrinol Metab Clin North Am 1990;19:545.

Mazzaferri EL, Jhiang SM: Long term impact of initial surgical and medical therapy on papillary and follicular thyroid cancer. Am J Med 1994;97:418.

Ridgway EC: Clinician's evaluation of a solitary thyroid nodule. Clinical review 30. J Clin Endocrinol Metabol 1992;74:231.

Robbins J: Prognostic factors in the management of thyroid cancer. J Endocrinol Invest 1995;18:159.

Robbins J: Treatment of thyroid cancer in childhood. Proceedings of a workshop held September 10–11, 1992, at the NIH, Bethesda, Md. US Dept Commerce, National Technical Information Service, 1993.

Samaan NA: The results of various modalities of treatment of well differentiated thyroid carcinoma: A retrospective review of 1599 patients. J Clin Endocrinol Metab 1992;75:714.

Simpson WJ: Radioiodine and radiotherapy in the management of thyroid cancer. Otolaryngol Clin North Am 1990;23:509.

Thomas CG Jr: Role of thyroid stimulating hormone suppression in the management of thyroid cancer. Semin Surg Oncol 1991;7:115.

Wynford-Thomas D.: Molecular genetics of thyroid cancer. Tr Endocrinol Metab 1993;4:224.

Mineral Metabolism & Metabolic Bone Disease

8

Gordon J. Strewler, MD

CELLULAR & EXTRACELLULAR CALCIUM METABOLISM

In virtually all organisms, the divalent cation calcium serves a central role in cellular physiology and metabolic regulation. **Extracellular** calcium levels in humans are tightly regulated within a narrow physiologic range to provide for proper functioning of many tissues: excitation-contraction coupling in the heart and other muscles, synaptic transmission and other functions of the nervous system, platelet aggregation, coagulation, and secretion of hormones and other regulators by exocytosis. The level of **intracellular** calcium is also tightly controlled, at levels about 10,000-fold lower than extracellular calcium, in order for calcium to serve as an intracellular second messenger in the regulation of cell division, muscle contractility, cell motility, membrane trafficking, and secretion.

It is the concentration of ionized calcium ($[Ca^{2+}]$) that is regulated in the extracellular fluid. The ionized calcium concentration averages 1.25 ± 0.07 mmol/L (Table 8–1). However, only about 50% of the total calcium in serum and other extracellular fluids is present in the ionized form. The remainder is bound to albumin (about 40%) or complexed with anions such as phosphate and citrate (about 10%). The protein-bound and complexed fractions of serum calcium are metabolically inert and are not regulated by hormones; only the $[Ca^{2+}]$ serves a regulatory role, and only this fraction is itself regulated by the calciotropic hormones parathyroid hormone (PTH) and vitamin D. However, large increases in the serum concentrations of phosphate or citrate can, by mass action, markedly increase the complexed fraction of calcium. For example, massive transfusions of blood, in which citrate is used as an anticoagulant, can reduce the $[Ca^{2+}]$ enough to produce tetany. In addition, because calcium and phosphate circulate at concentrations close to saturation, a substantial rise in the serum concentration of either calcium or phosphate can lead to the precipitation of calcium phosphate salts in tissues, and this is a source of major clinical problems in patients with severe hypercal-

cemia (eg, malignant tumors) and in those with severe hyperphosphatemia (eg, in renal failure or rhabdomyolysis).

What is remarkable about calcium metabolism is that the extracellular fluid $[Ca^{2+}]$, which represents a tiny fraction of the total body calcium, can be so tightly regulated in the face of the rapid fluxes of calcium through it that take place during the course of calcium metabolism (Figure 8–1). The total calcium in extracellular fluid amounts to about 1% of total body calcium, with most of the remainder sequestered in bone. Yet from the extracellular fluid compartment, which contains about 900 mg of calcium, 10,000 mg/d is filtered at the glomerulus and 500 mg/d is added to a labile pool in bone; and to the extracellular fluid compartment are added about 200 mg absorbed from the diet, 9800 mg reabsorbed by the renal tubule, and 500 mg from bone.

The challenge of the calcium homeostatic system, then, is to maintain a constant level of $[Ca^{2+}]$ in the

Table 8–1. Calcium concentrations in body fluids.

Total serum calcium	8.5–10.5 mg/dL	(2.1–2.6 mmol/L)
Ionized calcium	4.4–5.2 mg/dL	(1.1–1.3 mmol/L)
Protein-bound calcium	4.0–4.6 mg/dL	(0.9–1.1 mmol/L)
Complexed calcium	0.7 mg/dL	(0.18 mmol/L)
Intracellular free calcium	0.00018 mmol/L	(180 nmol/L)

extracellular fluid, simultaneously providing adequate amounts of calcium to cells, to bone, and for renal excretion—and all the while compensating, on an hourly basis, for changes in daily intake of calcium, bone metabolism, and renal function. It is scarcely surprising that this homeostatic task requires two hormones, PTH and vitamin D, or that the secretion of each hormone is exquisitely sensitive to small changes in the serum calcium, or that each hormone is able to regulate calcium exchange across all three interfaces of the extracellular fluid: the gut, the bone, and the renal tubule. We will reexamine the integrated roles of PTH and vitamin D in calcium homeostasis after their actions and secretory control have been described.

The challenge of the cellular calcium economy is to maintain a cytosolic $[Ca^{2+}]$, or $[Ca^{2+}]_i$, of about 0.1 μmol/L, about 10,000-fold less than what is present outside cells, providing for rapid fluxes through the intracellular compartment as required for regulation while maintaining a large gradient across the cell membrane. The calcium gradient across the cell membrane is maintained by ATP-dependent calcium pumps and by a Na^+-Ca^{2+} exchanger. Calcium can enter cells through several calcium channels, some of which are voltage-operated or receptor-operated, to provide for rapid influx in response to depolarization or receptor stimulation. The cell also maintains large

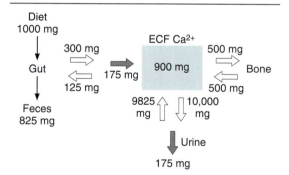

Figure 8–1. Calcium fluxes in a normal individual in a state of zero external mineral balance. The open arrows denote unidirectional calcium fluxes; the solid arrows denote net fluxes. (Reproduced, with permission, from Felig P, Baxter JD, Broadus AE, Frohman LA [editors], Endocrinology and Metabolism, 2nd ed, McGraw-Hill, 1987.)

stores of calcium in microsomal and mitochondrial pools, from which calcium can be released rapidly by cellular signals such as 1,4,5-inositol trisphosphate. Reuptake mechanisms are also present, so that cytosolic calcium transients can be rapidly terminated by returning calcium to storage pools.

PARATHYROID HORMONE

Anatomy & Embryology of the Parathyroid Glands

Parathyroid hormone is secreted from four glands located adjacent to the thyroid gland in the neck. The glands weigh an average of 40 mg each. The two superior glands are usually found near the posterior aspect of the thyroid capsule; the inferior glands are most often located near the inferior thyroid margin. However, the exact location of the glands is variable, and 12–15% of normal persons have a fifth parathyroid gland. The parathyroid glands arise from the third and fourth branchial pouches. The inferior glands are actually those derived from the third branchial pouches. Beginning cephalad to the other pair, they migrate further caudad, and one of them sometimes follows the thymus gland into the superior mediastinum. The small size of the parathyroids and the vagaries of their location and number make parathyroid surgery a challenging enterprise for all but the expert surgeon.

The parathyroid glands are composed of epithelial cells and stromal fat. The predominant epithelial cell is the chief cell. The chief cell is distinguished by its clear cytoplasm from the oxyphil cell, which is slightly larger and has eosinophilic granular cytoplasm. Both cell types contain PTH, and it is not known whether their secretory regulation differs.

Secretion of Parathyroid Hormone

In order to carry out its function to regulate the extracellular calcium concentration, PTH must be under exquisite control by the serum calcium concentration. Thus, the negative feedback relationship of PTH with serum $[Ca^{2+}]$ is steeply sigmoidal, with the steep portion of the curve corresponding exactly to the normal range of serum calcium—precisely the relationship to create a high "gain" controller and assure maintenance of the normal serum calcium concentration by PTH (Figure 8–2).

To sense the concentration of extracellular $[Ca^{2+}]$ and thereby regulate the secretion of PTH, the parathyroid cell relies on a sensor of extracellular calcium. This calcium sensor has recently been identified as a 120-kDa G protein-coupled receptor, with the canonical structure of the seven-transmembrane-domain receptors of this class (Figure 3–2). The large first extracellular domain of the parathyroid calcium receptor has sequence homologies to the metabotropic glutamate receptors of the brain; these in turn are ho-

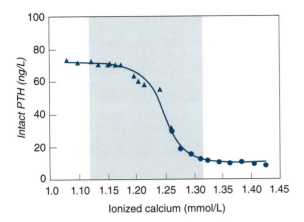

Figure 8–2. The relations between the serum ionized calcium level and the simultaneous serum concentration of intact PTH in normal humans. The serum calcium concentration was altered by the infusion of calcium (closed circles) or citrate (closed triangles). Parathyroid sensitivity to changes in serum calcium is maximal within the normal range (the shaded area). Low concentrations of PTH persist in the face of hypercalcemia (Modified from Conlin PR et al: Hysteresis in the relationship between serum ionized calcium and intact parathyroid hormone during recovery from induced hyper- and hypocalcemia in normal humans. J Clin Endocrinol Metab 1989;69:593. By permission of the Journal of Clinical Endocrinology and Metabolism.)

mologous to a class of bacterial membrane proteins involved in ion recognition, and it is likely that calcium binds directly to this domain. Like other G protein-coupled receptors, the calcium receptor has seven serpentine membrane-spanning domains. The intracellular loops that connect these domains are directly involved in coupling the receptor to a G protein, probably G_q. Thus, the overall architecture of the calcium receptor marries an ancient ion-sensing motif (the "fly trap") to a canonical structure which is necessary to link the receptor to an intracellular messenger system—"the marriage of the fly trap to the serpent."

The identification of the receptor immediately provided a molecular explanation for a familial form of hypercalcemia, familial benign hypocalciuric hypercalcemia, a disorder of calcium sensing caused by a mutation in the parathyroid calcium receptor. The calcium receptor is not unique to the parathyroids. The same receptor regulates the responses to calcium in several other tissues, including the thyroid C cells, which secrete calcitonin in response to high extracellular calcium, and the distal nephron of the kidney, where the receptor regulates calcium excretion. It is possible that the calcium receptor also controls the response of many other body tissues to extracellular calcium.

The primary cellular signal by which increased ex-

tracellular calcium inhibits the secretion of PTH is an increase in $[Ca^{2+}]_i$. The calcium receptor is directly coupled by G_q to the enzyme phospholipase C, which hydrolyses the phospholipid phosphatidylinositol 4,5- bisphosphate (PIP_2) to liberate the intracellular messengers 1,4,5-inositol trisphosphate (IP_3) and diacylglycerol (see Figure 3–5). IP_3 binds to a receptor in endoplasmic reticulum that releases calcium from membrane stores. The release of stored calcium raises the $[Ca^{2+}]_i$ within seconds and is followed by a sustained influx of extracellular calcium, probably through channels that are operated by the receptor, to produce a sustained plateau in $[Ca^{2+}]_i$. Increased intracellular calcium is probably sufficient for inhibition of PTH release, but it is unclear whether calcium release from intracellular stores or sustained calcium influx from the cell exterior is most important. The other product of phospholipase C action is the lipid diacylglycerol, an activator of the calcium- and phospholipid-sensitive protein kinase, protein kinase C. The effects of protein kinase C on the release of PTH from the gland are complex.

The primary effect of high extracellular calcium is to inhibit the secretion of preformed PTH from storage granules in the gland by blocking the fusion of storage granules with the cell membrane and release of their contents. In most cells, stimulation of exocytosis ("stimulus-secretion coupling") is a calcium-requiring process, which is inhibited by depletion of calcium. The parathyroid cell is necessarily an exception to this rule, because this cell must increase secretion of PTH when the calcium level is low. In the parathyroids, intracellular magnesium appears to serve the role in stimulus-secretion coupling that calcium does in other cells. As discussed below in the section on hypoparathyroidism, depletion of magnesium stores can paralyze the secretion of PTH, leading to reversible hypoparathyroidism.

Besides calcium, there are several other secretagogues for PTH. Hypermagnesemia inhibits PTH secretion. During treatment of premature labor with infusions of magnesium sulfate, a reduction in the PTH level and occasionally hypocalcemia are observed. Conversely, moderate hypomagnesemia can stimulate PTH secretion, even though prolonged depletion of magnesium will paralyze it. On a molar basis, magnesium is a less potent secretagogue than calcium. Catecholamines, acting through β-adrenergic receptors and cAMP, also stimulate the secretion of PTH. This effect does not appear to be clinically significant. The hypercalcemia sometimes observed in patients with pheochromocytoma usually has another basis, secretion of parathyroid hormone-related protein (PTHrP) by the tumor.

Not only do changes in serum calcium regulate the secretion of PTH—they also regulate the synthesis of PTH at the level of gene transcription. It is estimated that glandular stores of PTH are sufficient to maintain maximal rates of secretion for no more than 1.5

hours, so increased synthesis is required to meet sustained hypocalcemic challenges.

Transcription is also regulated by vitamin D: high levels of 1,25-dihydroxyvitamin D inhibit PTH gene transcription. This is one of many ways that the calciotropic hormones are intertwined in regulation of calcium homeostasis, and it has therapeutic implications. Vitamin D analogs can be used to prevent secondary hyperparathyroidism in dialysis patients with renal osteodystrophy.

Synthesis and Processing of Parathyroid Hormone

PTH is an 84-amino-acid peptide with a molecular weight of 9300. Its gene is located on chromosome 11. The gene encodes a precursor called preproPTH with a 29-amino-acid extension added at the amino terminal of the mature PTH peptide (Figure 8–3). This extension includes a 23-amino-acid signal sequence (the "pre" sequence) and a six-residue prohormone sequence. The signal sequence in pre-

proPTH functions precisely as it does in most other secreted protein molecules, to allow recognition of the peptide by a signal recognition particle, which binds to nascent peptide chains as they emerge from the ribosome and guides them to the endoplasmic reticulum, where they are inserted through the membrane into the lumen (Figure 8–4). The process is discussed in detail in Chapter 2.

In the lumen of the endoplasmic reticulum, a signal peptidase cleaves the signal sequence from preproPTH to leave proPTH, which exits the endoplasmic reticulum and travels to the Golgi apparatus, where the "pro" sequence is cleaved from PTH by an enzyme called furin (Chapter 2). While preproPTH is evanescent, proPTH has a life span of about 15 minutes. The processing of proPTH is quite efficient, and proPTH, unlike other prohormones (eg, proinsulin), is not secreted. As it leaves the Golgi apparatus, PTH is repackaged into dense neuroendocrine-type secretory granules, where it is stored to await secretion.

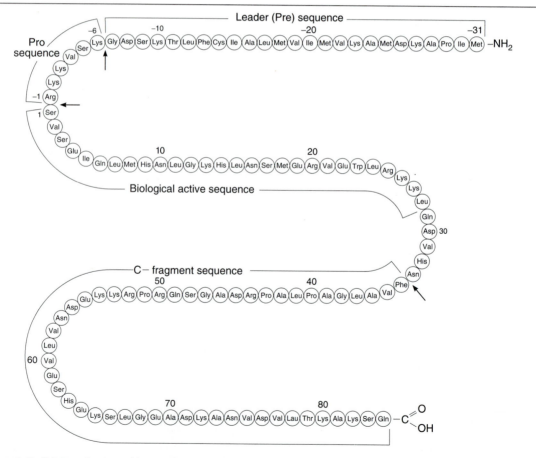

Figure 8–3. Primary structure of human preparathyroid hormone. The arrows indicate sites of specific cleavages which occur in the sequence of biosynthesis and peripheral metabolism of the hormone. The biologically active sequence is enclosed in the center of the molecule. (Reproduced, with permission, from Felig P, Baxter JD, Frohman LA [editors]: *Endocrinology and Metabolism*, 3rd ed, McGraw-Hill, 1995.)

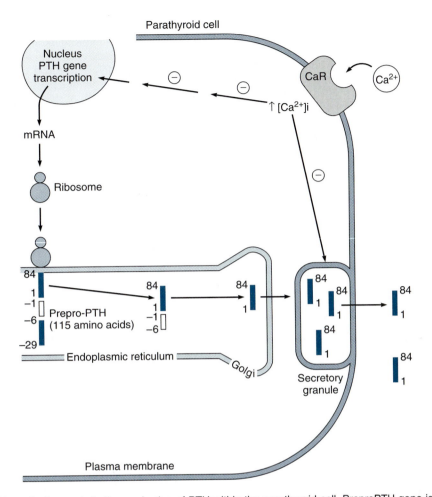

Figure 8–4. Biosynthetic events in the production of PTH within the parathyroid cell. PreproPTH gene is transcribed to its mRNA, which is translated on the ribosomes to preproPTH (amino acids −29 to +84). The pre- sequence is removed within the endoplasmic reticulum, yielding proPTH (−6 to +84). Mature PTH(1−84) released from the Golgi is packaged in secretory granules and released into the circulation in the presence of hypocalcemia. The calcium receptor is proposed to sense changes in extracellular calcium that affect both the release of PTH and the transcription of the preproPTH gene. (Reproduced, with permission, from McPhee SJ et al [editors]: *Pathophysiology of Disease: An Introduction to Clinical Medicine.* Appleton & Lange, 1995.)

Clearance & Metabolism of PTH

PTH secreted by the gland has a circulating half-life of 2–4 minutes. Intact PTH(1–84) is predominantly cleared in the liver and kidney. There, PTH is cleaved at the 33–34 and 36–37 positions to produce an amino terminal fragment and a carboxyl terminal fragment. The amino terminal fragment is not demonstrable in blood, but carboxyl terminal fragments are. Carboxyl terminal fragments are cleared from blood by filtration at the kidney, and they accumulate in chronic renal failure. Although all the classic activities of PTH are encoded in the amino terminal, carboxyl terminal fragments may not be metabolically inert. Recent evidence suggests that they have their own receptor, and they may yet be shown to have a distinct set of biologic actions.

Assay of PTH

Modern assays of intact PTH(1–84) employ two-site immunoradiometric assay (IRMA) or immuno-chemiluminescent assay (ICMA) techniques, in which the normal range for PTH is 10–60 pg/mL (1–6 pmol/L). By utilizing antibodies to two determinants, one near the amino terminal of PTH and the other near the carboxyl terminal, these assays are designed to measure the intact, biologically active hormone specifically (Figure 8–5). In practice, such assays have sufficient sensitivity and specificity not only to detect increased levels of PTH in hyperparathyroid disorders but also to detect suppressed levels of PTH in patients with nonparathyroid hypercalcemia. The ability to detect suppression of PTH makes these assays powerful tools for the differential

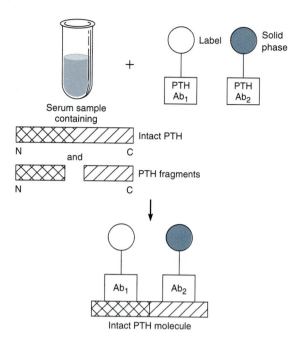

Figure 8–5. Schematic representation of the principle of the two-site assay for intact PTH. The label may be a luminescent probe or ^{125}I in the immunochemiluminescent or immunoradiometric assay, respectively. Two different region-specific antibodies are used (Ab1 and Ab2). Only the hormone species containing both immunodeterminants is counted in the assay. (Reproduced, with permission, from McPhee SJ et al [editors]: *Pathophysiology of Disease: An Introduction to Clinical Medicine.* Appleton & Lange, 1995.)

diagnosis of hypercalcemia: If hypercalcemia results from some form of hyperparathyroidism, then the serum PTH level will be high; if hypercalcemia has a nonparathyroid basis, then PTH will be suppressed. For this reason, two-site assays of intact PTH have largely replaced earlier techniques, many of which measured inert carboxyl terminal fragments. Assays for carboxyl terminal fragments could not detect suppression of PTH in nonparathyroid disorders, and this produced considerable diagnostic confusion. In addition, the levels of carboxyl terminal fragments are greatly increased in renal failure, because their main site of clearance is the kidney.

Biologic Effects of PTH

The function of PTH is to regulate serum calcium levels by concerted effects on three principal target organs: bone, intestinal mucosa, and kidney. The effect of PTH on intestinal calcium absorption is indirect, resulting from increased renal production of the intestinally active vitamin D metabolite 1,25-dihydroxyvitamin D. By its integrated effects on the kidney, gut, and bone, PTH acts to increase the inflow of calcium into the extracellular fluid and thus de-

fend against hypocalcemia. Removal of the parathyroid glands results in profound hypocalcemia and ultimately in tetany and death.

In the kidney, PTH has direct effects on the tubular reabsorption of calcium, phosphate, and bicarbonate. Although the bulk of calcium is resorbed from tubule fluid together with sodium in the proximal convoluted tubule, the fine tuning of calcium excretion occurs in the distal nephron. There, PTH markedly increases the reabsorption of calcium, predominantly in the distal convoluted tubule. Although calcium is actively transported against an electrochemical gradient, the precise nature of the calcium transport process that is regulated by PTH is controversial. However, from a physiologic standpoint, the ability to limit renal losses of calcium is one important means by which PTH protects the serum calcium level.

PTH inhibits the reabsorption of phosphate in the renal proximal tubule. In this nephron segment, phosphate is transported across the apical membrane of the tubule cell by a specific sodium-phosphate cotransporter, with phosphate influx driven by the energy of the sodium gradient. The transport protein has recently been identified by molecular cloning. It is suspected that PTH may inhibit sodium-phosphate reabsorption by reducing the rate of insertion of transporters from a sequestered cytoplasmic pool into the apical membrane. In any case, the phosphaturic effect of PTH is profound. It is best quantified by calculating the tubule reabsorption of phosphate (TRP) from the clearances of phosphate and creatinine (TRP = $1 - C_P/C_{creat}$, normal range 80–97%), or by calculating the renal phosphate threshold (TmP/GFR) from a standard nomogram. Because it is primarily the renal phosphate threshold that sets the level of serum phosphorus, the phosphaturic effect of PTH is mirrored in the serum phosphorus level, eg, hypophosphatemia in hyperparathyroidism. Hyperparathyroid states may also be characterized by impaired bicarbonate reabsorption and a mild hyperchloremic metabolic acidosis, because of inhibition of Na^+-H^+ antiporter activity by PTH.

Though the hypocalciuric effect of PTH is readily understood as part of the concerted actions of the hormone to protect the serum calcium level, the utility of the phosphaturic effect of PTH is less obvious. One consideration is that the phosphaturic effect tends to prevent an increase in serum phosphate, which would otherwise result from the obligatory release of phosphate with calcium during bone resorption and would tend to dampen the homeostatic increase in serum calcium by complexing calcium in blood. An example is renal osteodystrophy. When phosphate clearance is impaired by renal failure, the hypocalcemic effect of phosphate released during bone remodeling is an important contributor to progressive secondary hyperparathyroidism as part of a positive feedback loop—the more that bone resorption is stimulated and phosphate released, the more hyperparathyroidism is induced.

Mechanism of Action of Parathyroid Hormone

The parathyroid hormone receptor in kidney and bone is an 80,000-MW glycoprotein member of the G protein receptor superfamily. It has the canonical architecture of such receptors, with a large first extracellular domain, seven consecutive membrane-spanning domains, and a cytoplasmic tail (see Figure 3–2). PTH probably binds to the large extracellular domain of the receptor. The hormone-bound form of the receptor then activates associated G proteins via several determinants in the intracellular loops. The PTH receptor is only remotely related in sequence to most other G protein coupled receptors, but it is closely related to a small subfamily of peptide hormone receptors, which includes those for secretin, VIP, ACTH, and calcitonin.

PTH itself has a close structural resemblance to a sister protein, PTHrP, and also resembles the peptides secretin, VIP, calcitonin, and ACTH. As noted above, the receptors for these related ligands are themselves members of a special family. The peptide hormones themselves are characterized by an amino terminal α-helical domain, thought to be directly involved in receptor activation, and an adjacent α-helical domain which seems to be the primary receptor-binding domain. In the case of PTH, residues 1–6 are required for activation of the receptor; truncated analogs without these residues (eg, PTH[7–34]) can bind the receptor but cannot efficiently activate it and thus serve as competitive antagonists of PTH action. The primary receptor-binding domain consists of PTH(18–34). Although the intact form of PTH is an 84-amino-acid peptide, PTH(35–84) does not seem to have any important role in binding to the bone-kidney receptor. However, a separate PTH(35–84) receptor may exist; the carboxyl terminal PTH receptor could mediate an entirely new set of actions of PTH.

The classic PTH receptor in kidney and bone binds PTH and its sister hormone PTHrP with equivalent affinity and is therefore designated the PTH/PTHrP receptor. Inheritance of a constitutively active form of the receptor produces lifelong hypercalcemia as part of a rare heritable disorder called Jansen-type metaphysial chondrodysplasia. Activation of the receptor by binding of either PTH or PTHrP induces the active, GTP-bound state of two receptor-associated G proteins. G_s couples the receptor to the effector adenylyl cyclase and thereby to the generation of cAMP as a cellular second messenger. G_q couples the receptor to a separate effector system, phospholipase C, and thereby to an increase in $[Ca^{2+}]i$ and to activation of protein kinase C (Figure 3–5). Although it is not clear which of the cellular messengers, cAMP or intracellular calcium, is re-

sponsible for each of the various cellular effects of PTH, there is evidence from an experiment of nature that cAMP is the intracellular second messenger for calcium homeostasis and renal phosphate excretion. The experiment is pseudohypoparathyroidism, in which null mutations in the stimulatory G protein subunit $G_s\alpha$ cause hypocalcemia and unresponsiveness of renal phosphate excretion to PTH.

PTHrP

When secreted in abundance by malignant tumors, PTHrP produces severe hypercalcemia by activating the PTH/PTHrP receptor. However, the physiologic role of PTHrP is quite different from that of PTH. PTHrP is produced in many fetal and adult tissues. Based on gene knockout experiments and overexpression of PTHrP in individual tissues, we now know that PTHrP is required for normal development as a regulator of the proliferation and mineralization of cartilage cells and as a regulator of placental calcium transport. In postnatal life, PTHrP appears to regulate the epithelial-mesenchymal interactions that are critical for development of the mammary gland, skin, and hair follicle. In most physiologic circumstances, PTHrP carries out local rather than systemic actions. PTHrP is discussed more fully in Chapter 23.

CALCITONIN

Calcitonin is a 32-amino-acid peptide whose principal function is to inhibit osteoclast-mediated bone resorption. Calcitonin is secreted by parafollicular C cells of the thyroid. These are neuroendocrine cells derived developmentally from the ultimobranchial body, which fuses with the fetal thyroid to distribute C cells throughout the gland. C cells make up only about 0.1% of the mass of the thyroid.

The secretion of calcitonin is under the control of the serum $[Ca^{2+}]$. The C cell uses the same calcium receptor as the parathyroid cell to sense changes in the ambient calcium concentration, but the C cell increases secretion of calcitonin in response to hypercalcemia and shuts off hormone secretion during hypocalcemia.

The calcitonin gene is composed of six exons, and, through alternative exon splicing, it encodes two entirely different peptide products (Figure 8–6). In the thyroid C cell, the predominant splicing choice generates mature calcitonin (Figure 8–7), which is incorporated within a 141-amino-acid precursor. In other tissues, especially neurons of the central nervous system, a peptide called calcitonin gene-related peptide (CGRP) is produced from a 128-amino-acid precursor. CGRP is a 37-amino-acid peptide with considerable homology to calcitonin. The amino terminal of both peptides incorporates a seven-member disulfide-bonded ring (Figure 8–7). Acting through its own receptor, CGRP is among the most potent vasodilator

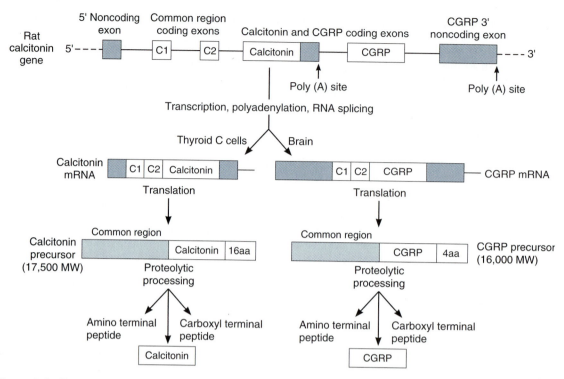

Figure 8–6. Alternative processing of the human calcitonin gene. Calcitonin is produced by thyroid C cells; CGRP is produced in the brain. (Modified and reproduced, with permission, from Rosenfeld MG et al: Production of a novel neuropeptide encoded by the calcitonin gene via tissue-specific RNA processing. Nature 1983;304:129.)

substances known. CGRP can probably also act as a neurotransmitter, with effects on food intake in rodents. Finally, CGRP is recognized, albeit weakly, by the calcitonin receptor and thereby has calcitonin-like effects to inhibit osteoclasts. The details of RNA splicing of the calcitonin gene have been widely studied as the classic example of tissue-specific RNA processing.

When administered intravenously, calcitonin produces a rapid and dramatic decline in levels of serum calcium and phosphorus, primarily through actions on bone. The major effect of the hormone is to inhibit osteoclastic bone resorption. After exposure to calcitonin, the morphology of the osteoclast changes rapidly. Within minutes, the cell withdraws its processes, shrinks in size, and retracts the ruffled border, the organelle of bone resorption, from the bone surface. Osteoclasts and cells of the proximal renal tubule express a calcitonin receptor. Like the PTH receptor, this is a serpentine G protein-coupled recep-

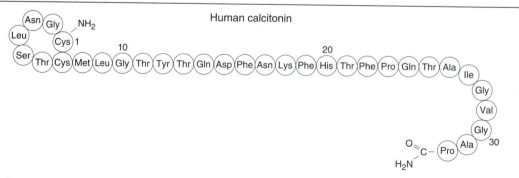

Figure 8–7. Amino acid sequence of human calcitonin, demonstrating its biochemical features, including an amino terminal disulfide bridge and carboxyl terminal prolinamide (Reproduced, with permission, from McPhee SJ et al [editors]: *Pathophysiology of Disease: An Introduction to Clinical Medicine*. Appleton & Lange, 1995.)

tor with seven membrane-spanning regions which is coupled by G_s to adenylyl cyclase and thereby to the generation of cAMP in target cells. Indeed, the PTH and calcitonin receptors are family members which are related in amino acid sequence, though their ligands are not. Calcitonin also has renal effects. At the kidney, calcitonin inhibits the reabsorption of phosphate, thus promoting renal phosphate excretion. Calcitonin also induces a mild natriuresis and increases the renal excretion of calcium. The renal effects of calcitonin are not essential for its acute effect on serum calcium levels, which results from blockade of bone resorption.

Although its secretory control by calcium and its antiresorptive actions enable calcitonin to counter PTH in the control of calcium homeostasis, thus engendering bihormonal regulation, it is actually unlikely that calcitonin plays an essential physiologic role in humans and other terrestrial animals. This surprising conclusion is supported by two lines of evidence. First, removal of the thyroid gland—the only known source of calcitonin in mammals—has no perceptible impact on calcium handling or bone metabolism. Second, secretion of extremely high calcitonin levels by medullary thyroid carcinoma, a malignancy of the C cell, likewise has no apparent effect on mineral homeostasis. Thus, in humans, calcitonin is a hormone in search of a function. It plays a much more obvious homeostatic role in salt-water fish, in which the major challenge is maintenance of blood calcium levels in the sea, where the ambient calcium concentration is very high.

Calcitonin is of clinical interest for two reasons. First, calcitonin is important as a tumor marker in medullary thyroid carcinoma, a malignancy of thyroid C cells. Second, calcitonin has found several therapeutic uses as an inhibitor of osteoclastic bone resorption. Calcitonin can be administered either parenterally or as a nasal spray and is used in the treatment of Paget's disease of bone, hypercalcemic crisis, and osteoporosis.

VITAMIN D

Biosynthesis, Chemistry, & Activation of Vitamin D

Vitamin D is really a sterol hormone. The endogenous form of vitamin D, cholecalciferol (vitamin D_3), is synthesized in the skin from the cholesterol metabolite 7-dehydrocholesterol by breakage of the A ring of 7-dehydrocholesterol, a steroid, to produce a sterol (Figure 8–8). Synthesis of cholecalciferol is nonenzymatic and is driven by tanning rays of ultraviolet light of 290–310 nm. There is actually no significant natural dietary source of vitamin D. Vitamin D_2 (ergocalciferol), which is used to fortify dairy products with vitamin D, is produced by ultraviolet irradiation of the plant sterol ergosterol. Vitamin D_2

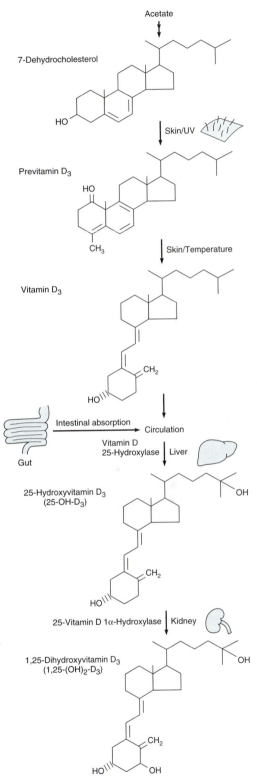

Figure 8–8. The synthesis and activation of vitamin D (Reproduced, with permission, from McPhee SJ et al [editors]: *Pathophysiology of Disease: An Introduction to Clinical Medicine.* Appleton & Lange, 1995.)

and vitamin D_3 are equipotent (1 μg = 40 IU), and their metabolism is identical, so in this chapter we will generally refer to vitamin D generically. (Although the sterol is not really a vitamin at all, that usage is too firmly entrenched to be disregarded.)

Vitamin D requires further metabolism to achieve an active form. It is carried to the liver by a specific vitamin D-binding protein—it requires a carrier protein because it is extremely lipophilic. In the liver to vitamin D is hydroxylated to produce 25-hydroxyvitamin D (Figure 8–8). This process is enzymatic, involving microsomal and mitochondrial P450, but it is very loosely regulated. After metabolism in the liver, 25-hydroxyvitamin D is transported on the vitamin D-binding protein to stores in body fat, where it is the principal storage form of vitamin D. For this reason, the serum level of 25-hydroxyvitamin D is the best available measure of body vitamin D stores in individuals who are suspected of vitamin D deficiency.

The final synthetic step in the activation of vitamin D takes place in the proximal tubule of the kidney. There, 25-hydroxyvitamin D is further hydroxylated to produce 1,25-dihydroxyvitamin D [$1,25(OH)_2D$], the most active form of the hormone. In humans whose diet is supplemented with ergocalciferol (vitamin D_2), the $1,25(OH)_2D$ formed in the kidney will be a mixture of $1,25(OH)_2D_2$ and $1,25(OH)_2D_3$, which are equipotent of the receptor. In this chapter, we shall refer to the two forms generically as $1,25(OH)_2D$. The synthetic enzyme, 25-hydroxyvitamin D 1α-hydroxylase, is a mitochondrial cytochrome P450 mixed-function oxidase that requires reduced NADP and molecular oxygen. Although the amino acid sequence of the enzyme is unknown, it appears to function similarly to steroidogenic enzymes of the adrenal cortex.

Unlike previous steps in vitamin D metabolism, this final step is under exquisite metabolic control, thus integrating vitamin D tightly into the concerted regulation of calcium homeostasis. Some of the important factors that regulate the activity of the synthetic enzyme, 1α-hydroxylase, are shown in Table 8–2. Of these, the most important are PTH, the dietary intake of phosphorus, the serum calcium, and the serum level of $1,25(OH)_2D$ itself.

PTH stimulates renal synthesis of $1,25(OH)_2D$. In the integrated control of calcium homeostasis, this serves to link the vitamin D endocrine system directly to the serum calcium level. In addition, by reg-

ulating the synthesis of $1,25(OH)_2D$, PTH gains the ability, via vitamin D, to regulate the intestinal absorption of calcium. The production of $1,25(OH)_2D$ is also regulated by the dietary phosphate intake. Changes in the dietary phosphate intake have a powerful influence on $1,25(OH)_2D$ production and can sometimes override PTH. For example, oral phosphate treatment will decrease $1,25(OH)_2D$ production in the face of rising PTH levels; conversely, phosphate restriction in moderate renal insufficiency increases the serum concentration of $1,25(OH)_2D$ as PTH levels fall. It is not clear how changes in dietary phosphate intake are sensed, but dietary phosphate intake tightly regulates the reabsorption of phosphate. Thus, the proximal tubule cell may sense changes in phosphate intake as the flux of phosphate through the cell.

Renal 1α-hydroxylase activity is markedly increased in vitamin D deficiency, serving to protect the $1,25(OH)_2D$ level from variations in nutritional intake and endogenous production. Conversely, the serum level of $1,25(OH)_2D$ is often normal in vitamin D intoxication. In this circumstance, many of the toxic effects of vitamin D are actually exerted by other metabolites, notably 25-hydroxyvitamin D. Because of this remarkably tight regulation of the synthesis of $1,25(OH)_2D$, the serum level of $1,25(OH)_2D$ is a poor measure of vitamin D status in states of vitamin D deficiency or excess; in both cases, it is preferable to measure the 25-hydroxyvitamin D level in serum (see discussion below on assay of vitamin D).

Other Vitamin D Metabolites

The kidney metabolizes 25-hydroxyvitamin D either to $1,25(OH)_2D$ or to 24,25-dihydroxyvitamin D. Quantitatively, 24,25-dihydroxyvitamin D is the principal circulating metabolite of 25-hydroxyvitamin D, with a serum concentration of 2–4 ng/mL (5–10 nmol/L), 100-fold higher than the concentration of $1,25(OH)_2D$. Ordinarily, the renal synthesis of $1,25(OH)_2D$ and 24,25-dihydroxyvitamin D are regulated reciprocally. Despite its abundance, the biologic role of 24,25-dihydroxyvitamin D is obscure. Although many reports suggest that this metabolite has actions distinct from those of $1,25(OH)_2D$, it appears that vitamin D deficiency can be cured with $1,25(OH)_2D$ analogs that are incapable of conversion to 24,25-dihydroxyvitamin D.

Vitamin D and its metabolites are disposed of by several pathways, including conjugation to glucuronides or sulfates and oxidation of the side chain. $1,25(OH)_2D$ increases its own metabolic clearance rate and those of other metabolites, probably by inducing several degradative enzymes.

Vitamin D Nutrition

In much of the world, the requirement for vitamin D is satisfied by endogenous synthesis. For example,

Table 8–2. Regulators of 1α-hydroxylase.

Parathyroid hormone
Phosphate
$1,25(OH)_2D_3$
Serum calcium
Growth hormone
Prolactin
Glucocorticoids

exposure of Caucasians to a whole-body dose of sunlight sufficient to produce minimal erythema generates about 2000 IU of vitamin D, or 10 times the recommended daily allowance. However, in temperate zones, seasonal variations in vitamin D stores are profound, with a substantial fraction of a healthy population in the northern United States having borderline low serum 25-hydroxyvitamin D levels at their nadir, which occurs in the spring. The diet in the United States is supplemented with vitamin D. Dairy products are supplemented with the equivalent of 400 IU of vitamin D per quart (as either cholecalciferol or ergocalciferol). Consequently, dietary vitamin D deficiency is quite uncommon in the United States, However, vitamin D deficiency can occur as a consequence of malabsorption of this fat-soluble vitamin in celiac disease, pancreatic insufficiency, etc.

The recommended daily allowance (RDA) of vitamin D for adults is 200 IU (5 μg); for infants, children, and pregnant and lactating women it is 400 IU (10 μg). Recent studies have shown that in the winter months in New England, many of the elderly not only have borderline insufficient serum levels of 25-hydroxyvitamin D but also have secondary hyperparathyroidism, indicating a significant impact of the low supply of vitamin D on calcium homeostasis. Consequently, many authorities believe that the elderly should be supplemented with 400–800 IU. The dose of vitamin D in most multivitamin preparations is 400 IU per capsule.

Assay of Vitamin D Metabolites

The two clinically relevant metabolites of vitamin D are 25-hydroxyvitamin D and 1,25(OH)$_2$D. As discussed above, the best test for vitamin D sufficiency is assay of the serum level of 25-hydroxyvitamin D. The normal range is 10–50 ng/mL (25–125 nmol/L). Most assays employ competitive binding to the serum 25-hydroxyvitamin D-binding protein after chromatography to remove other metabolites that also bind to the protein. The serum level of 25-hydroxyvitamin D is reduced not only with nutritional vitamin D deficiency but also in disorders where the level of the binding protein is reduced—liver disease and the nephrotic syndrome. The level of 25-hydroxyvitamin D is increased in states of vitamin D intoxication and in hyperestrogenemic states, where the level of the binding protein is increased.

Despite its central role in calcium homeostasis, there are only a few clinical indications for determination of 1,25(OH)$_2$D in serum. Its production is too tightly regulated for its serum level to reflect the intake or nutritional status, and the primary indication for its determination is in the differential diagnosis of hypercalcemia. Sarcoidosis, lymphoma, and other granulomatous disorders may produce hypercalcemia through the extrarenal synthesis of 1,25(OH)$_2$D. Most methods for assay of 1,25(OH)$_2$D now use the vitamin D receptor as a binding protein. Other vitamin D metabolites also bind to the receptor and must be removed prior to assay by chromatography of serum (HPLC or through a C-18-OH cartridge). The normal serum concentration of 1,25(OH)$_2$D is 20–60 pg/mL (50–150 pmol/L).

Vitamin D Action

A. Cellular Basis of Vitamin D Action: Vitamin D regulates gene transcription from genomic DNA by binding to a nuclear receptor, the vitamin D receptor (VDR). The VDR is a member of the large nuclear hormone receptor superfamily, which now has more than 150 known members. The VDR has a central DNA-binding domain, which is highly conserved throughout the family, and a carboxyl terminal hormone-binding domain (see Figure 3–13). The hormone-binding domain can be thought of as a switch that, upon binding a vitamin D metabolite, shifts the receptor to a transcriptionally active state. The receptor binds many vitamin D metabolites, with affinities that generally mirror their antirachitic potencies for correction of vitamin D deficiency. For example, 25-hydroxyvitamin D has an affinity for the VDR about one-thousandth that of 1,25(OH)$_2$D, the most potent vitamin D metabolite.

The VDR regulates transcription by binding to target genes as a heterodimer with RXR, a retinoic acid receptor specific for 9-*cis*-retinoic acid. RXR is a "silent partner" in the heterodimer, because heterodimer formation actually prevents RXR from binding its own ligand. The binding site of the heterodimer on DNA is a direct repeat of the sequence XGXTCA, with a spacing of three, four, or five nucleotides between the repeats. Many genes have such motifs in their promoter regions and are thus targets for regulation by vitamin D (see below).

B. Intestinal Calcium Absorption: The most important target for vitamin D is the gut, where vitamin D increases intestinal calcium absorption, primarily in the jejunum and ileum. Its primary cellular effect is to increase the uptake of calcium through the brush border membrane of the enterocyte. Vitamin D induces two calcium binding proteins, the calbindins, which may ferry calcium across the cell, and it may also accelerate the efflux of calcium from the basolateral side of the cell into the blood. The exit step is carried out by a vitamin D-sensitive pump, driven by ATP, and also by a Na^+-Ca^{2+} exchanger, which is driven by the sodium gradient. The initial effects of vitamin D on intestinal calcium absorption occur within minutes—too rapidly to be readily explained by effects on gene transcription—and do not appear to require new protein synthesis. It has therefore been suggested that the actions of vitamin D on intestinal calcium transport may be mediated by a nongenomic receptor, which is distinct from the genomic vitamin D receptor described above. In this regard, it is notable that impaired calcium absorption and severe rickets are seen in individuals with mutations that disrupt the function of the genomic vitamin D receptors. Thus, at least some of the important effects of vitamin D on intestinal calcium transport require the genomic receptor.

C. Actions of Vitamin D on Bone: Vitamin D has a multitude of effects upon the metabolism and function of bone cells, both osteoblasts and osteoclasts. The osteoblast is a primary target cell for vitamin D. Both mature osteoblasts and their progenitor cells have vitamin D receptors, and vitamin D affects the transcription of a variety of osteoblast-derived matrix proteins. Transcription of the bone matrix protein osteocalcin is stimulated by vitamin D, and bidirectional effects are seen on several other matrix proteins, including type I collagen and alkaline phosphatase. However, vitamin D is also an important bone-resorbing hormone. Vitamin D accelerates the formation of osteoclasts by enhancing the maturation of their monocytic precursors (see Bone Anatomy and Remodeling, below) and also activates bone resorption by mature osteoclasts. It is thought that the effect of vitamin D on mature osteoclasts is indirect, requiring a signal from another bone cell, as mature osteoclasts, surprisingly, appear to lack vitamin D receptors. In individuals with sarcoidosis or vitamin D intoxication, increased bone resorption can produce frank hypercalcemia.

The ultimate consequence of vitamin D deficiency with regard to bone is the development of osteomalacia, a severe impairment of mineralization of bone matrix by the osteoblast (see Osteomalacia, below). Despite the multitudinous direct effects of vitamin D on bone cell function, it appears that the proximate cause of osteomalacia is impaired intestinal calcium absorption rather than a direct effect of the hormone on bone. The evidence for this conclusion comes from patients with inherited absence of the vitamin D receptor. These individuals have severe osteomalacia that can be healed completely by a series of intravenous calcium infusions. What, then, is the biologic significance of the many biochemical effects of vitamin D on bone? This question cannot presently be answered.

D. Actions of Vitamin D on the Kidney: Vitamin D regulates renal ion transport. It is likely that the direct effects of $1,25(OH)_2D$ on the kidney include stimulation of proximal phosphate reabsorption and maintenance of normal calcium reabsorption. However, the details of these effects at the level of the tubule cell are poorly understood.

E. Actions of Vitamin D in Other Tissues: Vitamin D receptors are present in many tissues. In vitro, vitamin D stimulates the maturation of cells in the macrocyte series, and $1,25(OH)_2D$ inhibits the proliferation of activated T lymphocytes. However, no major immune defect is apparent in individuals who lack vitamin D receptors. Vitamin D also inhibits proliferation and stimulates the maturation of epidermal keratinocytes. The antiproliferative effect

of vitamin D is being used therapeutically. Analogs of $1,25(OH)_2D$ are in use in Europe for the treatment of psoriasis, a hyperproliferative skin disorder. In addition, many (but not all) persons who lack vitamin D receptors have lifelong alopecia totalis, indicating that vitamin D also plays a role in the maturation of the hair follicle.

INTEGRATED CONTROL OF MINERAL HOMEOSTASIS

Consider a person who switches from a high normal to a low normal intake of calcium and phosphate—from 1200 per day to 300 mg per day of calcium (the equivalent of leaving three glasses of milk out of the daily diet). The net absorption of calcium falls sharply, causing a transient decrease in the serum calcium level. The homeostatic response to this transient hypocalcemia is led by an increase in PTH, which stimulates the release of calcium and phosphate from bone and the retention of calcium by the kidney. The phosphaturic effect of PTH allows elimination of phosphate, which is resorbed from bone together with calcium. In addition, the increase in PTH, along with the fall in serum calcium and serum phosphorus, activates renal $1,25(OH)_2D$ synthesis. In its turn, $1,25(OH)_2D$ increases the fractional absorption of calcium and further increases bone resorption. External calcium balance is thus restored by increased fractional absorption of calcium and increased bone resorption at the expense of increased steady state levels of PTH and $1,25(OH)_2D$.

MEDULLARY THYROID CARCINOMA

Medullary carcinoma, a neoplasm of thyroidal C cells, accounts for about 5% of all thyroid malignancies. Approximately 80% of medullary carcinomas are sporadic. The remaining 20% are familial, and they are associated with one of three heritable syndromes: familial isolated medullary carcinoma; multiple endocrine neoplasia 2a (MEN 2a), consisting of medullary carcinoma, pheochromocytoma, and primary hyperparathyroidism; or multiple endocrine neoplasia 2b (MEN 2b), consisting of medullary carcinoma, pheochromocytoma, and multiple mucosal neuromas (Table 8–3). The MEN syndromes are more extensively discussed in Chapter 24.

Our understanding of the pathogenesis of medullary carcinoma has been greatly enhanced by the identification of causative mutations in the *RET* protooncogene. The *RET* gene encodes a tyrosine ki-

Table 8–3. Clinical features of multiple endocrine neoplasia syndromes.

MEN 1
  Parathyroid hyperplasia (very common)
  Pancreatic tumors (benign or malignant)
    Gastrinoma
    Insulinoma
    Glucagonoma, VIPoma (both rare)
  Pituitary tumor
    Growth hormone-secreting
    Prolactin-secreting
    ACTH-secreting
  Other tumors: lipomas, carcinoids, adrenal and thyroid
    adenomas

MEN 2a
  Medullary carcinoma of the thyroid
  Pheochromocytoma (benign or malignant)
  Parathyroid hyperplasia

MEN 2b
  Medullary carcinoma of the thyroid
  Pheochromocytoma
  Mucosal neuromas, ganglioneuromas
  Marfanoid habitus
  Hyperparathyroidism (very rare)

nase receptor for an unknown growth factor. This receptor is expressed developmentally in migrating neural crest cells that will give rise to hormone-secreting neuroendocrine cells and to the parasympathetic and sympathetic ganglia of the peripheral nervous system. Remarkably, different mutations in RET can produce five distinct diseases. Inheritance of activating mutations is responsible for MEN 2a and familial medullary thyroid carcinoma. Inheritance of a different set of activating mutations causes MEN 2b. In over half of sporadic medullary thyroid carcinomas, the tumor has a clonal somatic mutation (present in the tumor but not in genomic DNA), which is identical to one of the mutations that is responsible for the familial forms of medullary carcinoma. Almost certainly, such somatic mutations cause sporadic medullary carcinoma. In addition to its role in medullary carcinoma, where the RET gene product is activated by point mutations, the RET gene is sometimes rearranged in papillary carcinoma, and recent transgenic experiments indicate that the rearranged RET gene is sufficient to cause papillary thyroid carcinoma. Finally, mutations that inactivate the RET gene produce Hirschsprung's disease, a congenital absence of the enteric parasympathetic ganglia, in which intestinal motility is disturbed, resulting in megacolon.

Medullary carcinoma is usually located in the middle or upper portions of the thyroid lobes. It is typically unilateral in sporadic cases but often multicentric and bilateral in familial forms of medullary carcinoma. Pathologically, medullary thyroid carcinoma was originally distinguished from other thyroid cancers by the presence of amyloid, eosinophilic material which stains with Congo red. Molecular studies have shown that amyloid consists of dense fibrillar deposits of protein in a β-pleated sheet structure. In the case of medullary carcinoma, the protein deposited as amyloid is procalcitonin or calcitonin itself. Thus, the pathologic diagnosis of medullary carcinoma can now be made by immunohistochemical staining for calcitonin.

The natural history of medullary carcinoma is variable. Sporadic tumors may be quite aggressive or very indolent; the mean five-year survival rate is about 50%. The behavior of familial forms varies among syndromes. MEN 2b has the most aggressive form of medullary carcinoma, with a 2-year survival of about 50%; MEN 2a has a course similar to that of sporadic medullary carcinoma, and familial medullary carcinoma has the most indolent course of all. The tumor may spread to regional lymph nodes or undergo hematogenous spread to the lungs and other viscera. When metastatic, medullary thyroid carcinoma is sometimes associated with a chronic diarrhea syndrome. The pathogenesis of the diarrhea is unclear. In addition to calcitonin, these tumors secrete a variety of other bioactive products, including prostaglandins, serotonin, histaminase, and peptide hormones (ACTH, somatostatin, CRH). In some cases the associated diarrhea responds dramatically to treatment with long-acting somatostatin analogs such as octreotide, which block secretion of these bioactive products.

Calcitonin is a tumor marker for medullary thyroid carcinoma. It is most sensitive for this purpose when secretion is stimulated with provocative agents. The standard provocative tests use pentagastrin (0.5 μg/kg intravenously over 5 seconds) or a rapid infusion of calcium gluconate (2 mg calcium/kg over 1 minute). Blood samples are obtained at baseline and 1, 2, and 5 minutes after the stimulus. Some authorities believe that for maximal sensitivity the two tests should be combined, with the calcium infusion immediately followed by administration of pentagastrin. Commercially available assays for calcitonin vary in their sensitivity and specificity for epitopes in the calcitonin molecule. For provocative testing, it is important to use an assay with validated normative data on the response of calcitonin to stimulation.

Although basal calcitonin levels are often normal in early tumors, calcitonin levels may be many times higher than normal in patients with disseminated medullary carcinoma, yet the patients are uniformly normocalcemic. Although tumors secrete large forms of calcitonin with decreased biologic activity, monomeric calcitonin levels are often high as well. The lack of hypocalcemia is taken as evidence that calcitonin may not be critical to mineral homeostasis in humans.

Families that carry RET mutations must be screened for medullary thyroid carcinoma and for the associated tumors which occur in MEN 2a and MEN 2b (Chapter 24). The classic screening technique has been determination of stimulated calcitonin levels after administration of pentagastrin or calcium. In the familial forms of medullary carcinoma, an exaggerated calcitonin response to provocative testing can identify small, curable intrathyroidal tumors in asymptomatic individuals and can also identify a premalignant state termed C cell hyperplasia. Removal of the thyroid at this point can be lifesaving. However, If the initial test is normal, repetitive testing at approximately yearly intervals up to age 30 is required. In addition, both false-positive and false-negative responses to provocative testing have been recorded, and in MEN 2b testing must be carried out at a very young age to identify the aggressive neoplasms that occur in the syndrome.

Molecular genetic diagnosis of medullary thyroid carcinoma is now possible. In a kindred with a known *RET* mutation, children can be screened at birth using genomic DNA. Early thyroidectomy can be carried out in carriers of the trait, and further testing can be abandoned in genetically normal family members. It is controversial whether thyroidectomy should always be carried out immediately after a positive genetic diagnosis or whether subsequent calcitonin testing should be used to decide upon the timing of surgery. In addition, genetic testing currently presents its own difficulties: It must be accessible and reliable, and it has legal and ethical implications which are not fully resolved.

Apparently sporadic medullary thyroid carcinoma also calls for family studies, since up to 25% of new cases may actually be probands of families who harbor one of the familial syndromes. As in known familial cases, screening can be accomplished by provocative testing of the calcitonin response in first-degree relatives. Alternatively, tumor and genomic DNA from the patient may be screened for *RET* mutations. Identification of a mutation only in tumor tissue would establish that the mutation is somatic and the tumor therefore a sporadic one. Identification of the same *RET* mutation in tumor and genomic DNA would make the diagnosis of a familial form of the disorder and would mandate careful screening of the family.

HYPERCALCEMIA

Clinical Features

A number of symptoms and signs accompany the hypercalcemic state: central nervous system effects such as lethargy, depression, psychosis, ataxia, stupor, and coma; neuromuscular effects such as weakness, proximal myopathy, and hypertonia; cardiovascular effects such as hypertension, bradycardia (and

eventually asystole), and a shortened QT interval; renal effects such as stones, decreased glomerular filtration, polyuria, hyperchloremic acidosis, and nephrocalcinosis; gastrointestinal effects such as nausea, vomiting, constipation, and anorexia; eye findings such as band keratopathy; and systemic metastatic calcification. This constellation of clinical findings has led to the mnemonic for recalling the signs and symptoms of hypercalcemia: "stones, bones, abdominal groans, and psychic moans" (Figure 8–9).

Mechanisms

Although many disorders are associated with hypercalcemia (Table 8–4), they can produce hypercalcemia through only a limited number of mechanisms: (1) increased bone resorption, (2) increased gastrointestinal absorption of calcium, or (3) decreased renal excretion of calcium. While any of these mechanisms can be involved in a given patient, the common feature of virtually all hypercalcemic disorders is accelerated bone resorption. The only recognized hypercalcemic disorder in which bone resorption does not play a part is the milk-alkali syndrome.

The central feature of the defense against hyper-

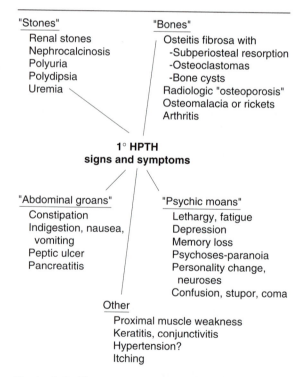

Figure 8–9. Mnemonic used for categorizing the signs and symptoms of hyperparathyroidism. (Reproduced, with permission, from Felig P, Baxter JD, Frohman LA [editors]: *Endocrinology and Metabolism,* 3rd ed. McGraw-Hill, 1995.)

Table 8–4. Causes of hypercalcemia.

Primary hyperparathyroidism
    Sporadic
    Associated with MEN 1 or MEN 2a
    Familial
    After renal transplantation

Variant forms of hyperparathyroidism
    Familial benign hypocalciuric hypercalcemia
    Lithium therapy
    Tertiary hyperparathyroidism in chronic renal failure

Malignancies
    Humoral hypercalcemia of malignancy
        Caused by PTHrP (solid tumors, adult T cell leukemia
            syndrome)
        Caused by $1,25(OH)_2D$ (lymphomas)
        Caused by ectopic secretion of PTH (rare)
    Local osteolytic hypercalcemia (multiple myeloma,
        leukemia, lymphoma)

Sarcoidosis or other granulomatous diseases

Endocrinopathies
    Thyrotoxicosis
    Adrenal insufficiency
    Pheochromocytoma
    VIPoma
    Acromegaly

Drug-induced
    Vitamin A intoxication
    Vitamin D intoxication
    Thiazide diuretics
    Lithium
    Milk-alkali syndrome
    Estrogens, androgens, tamoxifen (in breast carcinoma)

Immobilization

Acute renal failure

Idiopathic hypercalcemia of infancy

In ICU patients

Serum protein disorders

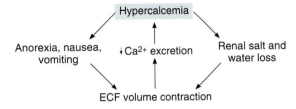

Figure 8–10. Once established, hypercalcemia can be maintained or aggravated as depicted. (Reproduced, with permission, from Felig P, Baxter JD, Frohman LA [editors]: *Endocrinology and Metabolism,* 3rd ed. McGraw-Hill, 1995.)

calcemia is suppression of PTH secretion. This reduces bone resorption; reduces renal production of $1,25(OH)_2D$, and thereby inhibits calcium absorption; and increases urinary calcium losses. The kidney plays a key role in the adaptive response to hypercalcemia as the only route of net calcium elimination, and the level of renal calcium excretion is markedly increased by the combined effects of an increased filtered load of calcium and the suppression of PTH. However, the patient who relies on the kidneys to excrete an increased calcium load is in precarious balance: Glomerular filtration is impaired by hypercalcemia; the urinary concentrating ability is diminished, predisposing to dehydration; poor mentation may interfere with access to fluids; and nausea and vomiting may further predispose to dehydration and renal azotemia. Renal insufficiency in turn compromises calcium clearance, leading to a downward spiral (Figure 8–10). Thus, once established, many hypercalcemic states are self-perpetuating or aggravated through the "vicious cycle of hypercalcemia."

The only alternative to the renal route for elimination of calcium from the extracellular fluid is deposition as calcium phosphate and other salts in bone and soft tissues. Soft tissue calcification is observed with massive calcium loads, with massive phosphate loads (as in crush injuries and compartment syndromes), and when renal function is markedly impaired.

Differential Diagnosis

The differential diagnosis is set forth in Table 8–4. As a practical matter, the categories can be divided into primary hyperparathyroidism and everything else. Hyperparathyroidism is by far the commonest cause of hypercalcemia and has distinctive pathophysiologic features. Thus, the first step in the differential diagnosis is determination of PTH, using an assay for intact PTH (Figure 8–11). If the PTH level is high and thus inappropriate for hypercalcemia, little further workup is required except to consider the variant forms of hyperparathyroidism which are discussed below. If the PTH level is suppressed, then a search for other entities must be conducted. Most other entities in Table 8–4 are readily diagnosed by their distinctive features, as discussed below.

DISORDERS CAUSING HYPERCALCEMIA

1. PRIMARY HYPERPARATHYROIDISM

Primary hyperparathyroidism is a hypercalcemic disorder that results from excessive secretion of PTH. With the advent of multiphasic screening of serum chemistries, we have come to recognize that primary hyperparathyroidism is a common and usually asymptomatic disorder. Its incidence is approximately 42 per 100,000, and its prevalence is up to 4 per 1000 in women over age 60. Primary hyperparathyroidism is approximately two to three times as common in women as in men. In many ways, its clinical features define the manifestations of hypercalcemia.

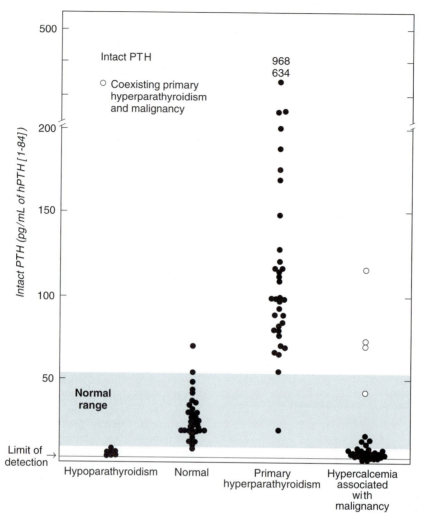

Figure 8–11. Clinical utility of immunoradiometric assay for intact PTH. (Reproduced, with permission, from Endres DB et al: Measurement of parathyroid hormone. Endocrinol Metab Clin North Am 1989;18:611.)

Etiology & Pathogenesis

Primary hyperparathyroidism is caused by a single parathyroid adenoma in about 80% of cases and by primary hyperplasia of the parathyroids in about 15%. Parathyroid carcinoma is a rare cause of hyperparathyroidism, accounting for 1–2% of cases. Parathyroid carcinoma is often recognizable preoperatively because it presents with severe hypercalcemia or a palpable neck mass. Primary hyperparathyroidism can occur as part of at least three different familial endocrinopathies. All of them are autosomal dominant traits, and all of them cause four-gland parathyroid hyperplasia. They include MEN 1, MEN 2A, and isolated familial hyperparathyroidism.

Parathyroid adenomas have a clonal origin, indicating that they can be traced back to an oncogenic mutation in a single progenitor cell. A few of these mutations are identified or can tentatively be assigned a genomic locus. About 25% of sporadic parathyroid adenomas have chromosomal deletions involving chromosome 11q12–13 that are thought to eliminate a tumor suppressor gene. As reviewed below and in Chapter 24, loss of a tumor suppressor gene at this locus is the cause of parathyroid, pituitary, and pancreatic tumors in the MEN I syndrome. An additional 40% of parathyroid adenomas display allelic loss on chromosome 1p (1p32-pter).

A rarer but interesting mutation is a chromosomal rearrangement that, by inversion of a piece of chromosome 11, brings the *PRAD1* cell cycle regulatory gene under the control of the PTH gene promoter. This rearrangement results in marked overexpression of *PRAD1* in the parathyroid. The *PRAD1* gene encodes a cell cycle regulatory protein, cyclin D, which is normally expressed at high levels in the G_1 phase of the cell cycle and permits entry of cells into the mitotic phase of the cycle. Thus, a parathyroid-specific disorder of cell cycle regulation leads to abnormal proliferation. It is estimated that the *PRAD1* mutation accounts for about 4% of sporadic parathyroid adenomas.

Parathyroid hyperplasia occurs spontaneously, accounting for 12–15% of cases of primary hyperparathyroidism and as part of three forms of familial hyperparathyroidism: MEN 1, MEN 2a, and isolated familial hyperparathyroidism. Parathyroid hyperplasia was traditionally viewed as an example of true hyperplasia, a polyclonal expansion of cell number. This occurs in other endocrine tissues when a trophic hormone is present in excess, eg, ACTH excess produces bilateral adrenal hyperplasia. Molecular analysis has revised this view. In MEN 1, it is thought that there is an inherited absence of one allele of a tumor suppressor gene and that somatic mutations that result in loss of the other allele would then produce tumors in endocrine tissues where the gene is expressed. In this view, separate somatic mutations would account for the occurrence of four-gland hyperparathyroidism. In MEN 2, the occurrence of parathyroid hyperplasia is presumably a consequence of expression of activating mutations of the *RET* gene, a putative growth factor receptor, in the four glands. Surprisingly, it has recently been shown that the majority of glands in spontaneous parathyroid hyperplasia are monoclonal, implying that they arose from a single progenitor cell, presumably as the result of a somatic mutation. Perhaps there is a parathyroid trophic hormone, eg, the *RET* receptor ligand, in some cases of parathyroid hyperplasia, and the increased mitotic rate in hyperplastic glands predisposes to clonal oncogenic mutations.

Parathyroid carcinomas frequently display loss of the retinoblastoma tumor-suppressor gene *RB*, another cell cycle regulator. Certain parathyroid carcinomas show loss of another tumor-suppressor, the *p53* gene. The *p53* and *RB* mutations do not commonly occur in parathyroid adenomas, whereas loss of one or both of these tumor suppressors is prevalent in many other kinds of carcinoma. It is thus likely that these abnormalities in parathyroid carcinoma account for its aggressiveness.

Several candidate parathyroid oncogenes appear to have been eliminated by molecular study. Familial benign hypocalciuric hypocalcemia is caused by an inactivating mutation of one allele of the parathyroid calcium sensor. Somatic mutations of the parathyroid calcium sensor could theoretically produce isolated primary hyperparathyroidism, but such mutations appear to be very uncommon. Similarly, despite the occurrence of parathyroid hyperplasia in MEN II, the *RET* mutations that cause MEN II are quite uncommon in sporadic parathyroid tumors.

Clinical Features

A. Symptoms and Signs: The typical clinical presentation of primary hyperparathyroidism has evolved considerably over the past two decades. As the disease is detected increasingly by multiphasic screening that includes determination of serum calcium levels, there has been a marked reduction in the frequency of the classic signs and symptoms of primary hyperparathyroidism, renal disease—renal stones, decreased renal function, and occasionally nephrocalcinosis—and the classic hyperparathyroid bone disease osteitis fibrosa cystica. In fact, about 85% of patients presenting today have neither bony nor renal manifestations of hyperparathyroidism and are regarded as asymptomatic or minimally symptomatic. At the same time, we have begun to recognize more subtle manifestations of hyperparathyroidism in some patients. This has presented a number of questions about the role of parathyroid surgery in primary hyperparathyroidism, which are discussed below (see Treatment).

1. Hyperparathyroid bone disease—The classic bone disease of hyperparathyroidism is osteitis fibrosa cystica. Formerly common, this disorder now occurs in less than 10% of patients. Clinically, osteitis fibrosa cystica causes bone pain and sometimes pathologic fractures. The most common laboratory finding is an elevation of the alkaline phosphatase level, reflecting high bone turnover. Histologically, there is an increase in the number of bone-resorbing osteoclasts, marrow fibrosis, and cystic lesions that may contain fibrous tissue (brown tumors) or cyst fluid. The most sensitive and specific radiologic finding of osteitis fibrosa cystica is subperiosteal resorption of cortical bone, best seen in high-resolution films of the phalanges (Figure 8–12A). A similar process in the skull leads to a salt-and-pepper appearance (Figure 8–12B). Bone cysts or brown tumors may be evident as osteolytic lesions. Dental films may disclose loss of the lamina dura of the teeth, but this is a nonspecific finding also seen in periodontal disease.

The other important form of hyperparathyroid bone disease is osteoporosis. Unlike other osteoporotic disorders, hyperparathyroidism typically results in predominant loss of cortical bone (Figure 8–13). In general, both the mass and the mechanical strength of trabecular bone are relatively well maintained. Patients who are followed medically for primary hyperparathyroidism often do not experience progressive bone loss even when they are osteoporotic at diagnosis. Under certain circumstances, PTH has an obvious anabolic effect to increase bone mass. Once-daily subcutaneous administration of the active PTH fragment PTH(1–34) is being actively explored as an anabolic treatment of osteoporosis. Although osteoporosis is generally considered to be an indication for surgical treatment of primary hyperparathyroidism, its real impact on morbidity is presently hard to assess (see Treatment of Hypercalcemia).

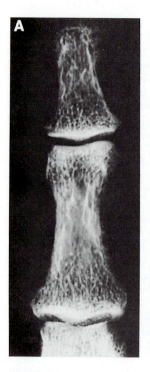
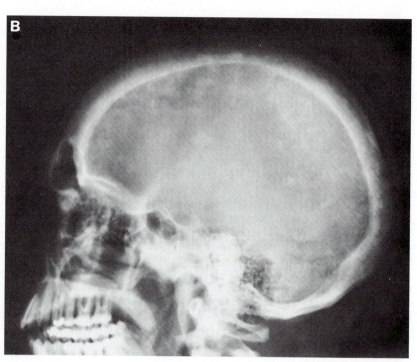

Figure 8–12. A: Magnified x-ray of index finger on fine-grain industrial film showing classic subperiosteal resorption in a patient with severe primary hyperparathyroidism. Note the left (radial) surface of the distal phalanx, where the cortex is almost completely resorbed, leaving only fine wisps of cortical bone. **B:** Skull x-ray from a patient with severe secondary hyperparathyroidism due to end-stage renal disease. Extensive areas of demineralization alternate with areas of increased bone density, resulting in the "salt and pepper" skull x-ray. (Both films courtesy of H Genant.)

2. Hyperparathyroid kidney disease—Once common in primary hyperparathyroidism, kidney stones now occur in less than 15% of cases. These are usually calcium oxalate stones. From the perspective of a stone clinic, only about 7% of calcium stone formers will prove to have primary hyperparathyroidism. They are difficult to manage medically, and stones constitute one of the agreed indications for parathyroidectomy. Clinically evident nephrocalcinosis rarely occurs, but a gradual loss of renal function is not uncommon. Renal function is stabilized after a successful parathyroidectomy, and otherwise unexplained renal insufficiency in the setting of primary hyperparathyroidism is also considered to be an indication for surgery because of the risk of progression. Chronic hypercalcemia can also compromise the renal concentrating ability, giving rise to polydipsia and polyuria.

3. Nonspecific features of primary hyperparathyroidism—Although stupor and coma occur in severe hypercalcemia, the degree to which milder impairments of central nervous system function affect the typical patient with primary hyperparathyroidism is unclear. Lethargy, fatigue, depression, difficulty in concentrating, and personality changes occur and in some patients appear to benefit from parathyroidectomy. Frank psychosis will also respond to surgery on occasion. Muscle weakness with characteristic electromyographic changes is also seen, and there is good evidence from controlled clinical trials that surgery can improve muscle strength. It was formerly thought that the incidence

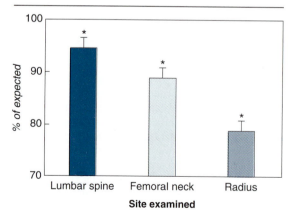

Figure 8–13. Bone density at several sites in primary hyperparathyroidism. (Reproduced, with permission, from Silverberg SJ, Shane E, Jacobs TP et al: Nephrolithiasis and bone involvement in primary hyperparathyroidism. Am J Med 1990;89:327.)

of hypertension was increased in primary hyperparathyroidism, but more recent evidence suggests that the appreciable incidence in this patient group is probably no greater than in age-matched controls, and parathyroidectomy appears to be of no benefit. Dyspepsia, nausea, and constipation all occur, probably as a consequence of hypercalcemia, but there is probably no increase in the incidence of peptic ulcer disease. The articular manifestations of primary hyperparathyroidism are several. Chondrocalcinosis occurs in up to 5% of patients, but acute attacks of pseudogout are less frequent. There may be an increased occurrence of gouty arthritis as well.

B. Laboratory Findings: Hypercalcemia is virtually universal in primary hyperparathyroidism, though the serum calcium sometimes fluctuates into the upper normal range. In patients with subtle hyperparathyroidism, repeated serum calcium measurements over a period of time may be required to establish the pattern of intermittent hypercalcemia. Both total and ionized calcium are elevated, and in most clinical instances there is no advantage to measuring the ionized calcium level. The rare patient with normocalcemic primary hyperparathyroidism usually has some specific comorbid disorder that prevents hypercalcemia, most commonly vitamin D deficiency. The serum phosphorus level is low-normal (< 3.5 mg/dL) or low (< 2.5 mg/dL) because of the phosphaturic effect of PTH. A mild hyperchloremic metabolic acidosis may be manifest as hyperchloremia.

The diagnosis of primary hyperparathyroidism in a hypercalcemic patient can be made by determining the intact PTH level with a two-site assay. As shown in Figure 8–11, an elevated or even upper-normal level of PTH is clearly inappropriate in a hypercalcemic patient and makes the diagnosis of hyperparathyroidism (or one of its variants: familial benign hypercalciuric hypercalcemia, lithium-induced hypercalcemia, or renal osteodystrophy). The reliability of the modern PTH assay allows the diagnostic evaluation of primary hyperparathyroidism to be curtailed markedly. In a patient with a high PTH level, there is no need to screen for metastatic malignancy, sarcoidosis, etc. Determinations of renal function and a plain abdominal radiograph for renal stones are often obtained for prognostic reasons. A determination of urinary calcium may be obtained to exclude the variant syndrome called familial benign hypocalciuric hypercalcemia.

Treatment

The definitive treatment of primary hyperparathyroidism is surgical parathyroidectomy. The surgical strategy depends upon the cause of hyperparathyroidism as determined intraoperatively by the surgeon. If exploration of the four parathyroid glands discloses an enlarged gland, the gland can be removed and the remaining parathyroid glands visualized and biopsied. If the remaining glands are small, then the likely diagnosis is parathyroid adenoma. If multiple enlarged glands are found, the likely diagnosis is parathyroid hyperplasia, and the preferred operation is a 3½-gland parathyroidectomy, leaving a remnant sufficient to prevent hypocalcemia. Double parathyroid adenomas are found in some patients. The pathologist is of little help in distinguishing among normal tissue, parathyroid adenoma, and parathyroid hyperplasia: these in essence are surgical diagnoses, based on the size and appearance of the glands. The recurrence rate of hypercalcemia is high in patients who have parathyroid hyperplasia—particularly in those with one of the MEN syndromes, because of the inherited propensity for tumor growth. In such cases, the parathyroid remnant can be removed from the neck and implanted in pieces in forearm muscles to allow for easy subsequent removal of some additional parathyroid tissue if hypercalcemia recurs.

In competent hands, the cure rate of parathyroid adenoma is over 95%. The success rate in primary parathyroid hyperplasia is somewhat lower, because of missed glands and recurrent hyperparathyroidism in patients with MEN syndromes. There is a 20% incidence of persistent or recurrent hypercalcemia. However, parathyroidectomy is difficult surgery: the normal parathyroid gland weighs only about 40 mg and may be located throughout the neck or upper mediastinum. It is mandatory not only to locate a parathyroid adenoma but to find the other glands and determine whether they are normal. Complications of surgery include damage to the recurrent laryngeal nerve, which passes close to the posterior thyroid capsule, and inadvertent removal or devitalization of all parathyroid tissue, producing permanent hypoparathyroidism. In skilled hands, the incidence of these complications is less than 1%. It is critical that parathyroid surgery be performed by someone with specialized skill.

There is probably no value in preoperative studies to localize parathyroid tumors: as Doppman has quipped, "The only localization study needed in a patient with hyperparathyroidism is to locate an experienced parathyroid surgeon." However, localization studies are very useful in reoperative parathyroid surgery, in which some parathyroid tissue has been removed and the anatomy of the neck has been distorted. The most successful procedures are ultrasonography, ^{99m}Tc-sestamibi scanning, computed tomography, and MRI. Individually, each has a sensitivity of 60–80% in experienced hands. Used in combination, they are successful in at least 80% of reoperated cases. Invasive studies, such as angiography and venous sampling, are rarely performed.

There is no definitive medical therapy for hyperparathyroidism. In postmenopausal women, estrogen replacement therapy in high doses (1.25 mg of conjugated estrogens or 30–50 µg of ethinyl estradiol) will produce an average decrease of 0.5–1 mg/dL in the serum calcium, but the effect of estrogen treatment is on the bone response to PTH, and PTH levels do not fall.

The relatively asymptomatic state of most patients today presents a dilemma: Which of them should be subjected to surgery? To answer this question definitively, it would be necessary to know more than we presently to about the natural history of untreated primary hyperparathyroidism. However, in observational studies over as many as 10 years, it is clear that most patients are stable with regard to serum calcium, stone disease, and renal function. Recent data also indicate that osteoporosis, when present, is usually nonprogressive. On the other hand, surgery is usually curative. In experienced hands, surgery has a low morbidity rate. Although parathyroid surgery is expensive, it may have a long-term cost benefit compared with a lifetime of medical follow-up. Moreover, there is a marked improvement in bone density after surgery (Figure 8–14), with sustained increases over at least 5 years postoperatively. Some surgeons also argue that the nonspecific symptoms often present may improve with surgery, but no controlled trial has excluded the placebo effect of surgery as a possible explanation for these results.

A 1990 Consensus Development Conference at NIH considered the issue of surgery in primary hyperparathyroidism and arrived at the following recommendations: Surgery should be recommended (1) if the serum calcium is markedly elevated (above 11.4–12 mg/dL [2.8–3 mmol/L]); (2) if there has been a previous episode of life-threatening hypercalcemia; (3) if the creatinine clearance is reduced below 70% of normal; (4) if a kidney stone is present; (5) if the urinary calcium is markedly elevated (> 400 mg/24 h); (6) if bone mass is substantially reduced (less than 2 SD below normal for age, sex, and race, ie, two Z-scores below normal); or (7) if the patient is young (under 50 years of age, particularly premenopausal women). In addition, medical surveillance is not considered suitable for patients who request surgery, patients who are unlikely to comply with long-term follow-up schedules, or patients with a coexisting illness complicating their management. These recommendations should be regarded as provisional. They will require modification as the natural history of primary hyperparathyroidism and the results of surgery are clarified. For example, the surgical benefits to bone density were found in patients who met NIH criteria for surgery; it will be important to determine whether similar benefits accrue when parathyroidectomy is performed in milder cases.

Variants of Primary Hyperparathyroidism

A. Familial Benign Hypocalciuric Hypercalcemia (FBHH): Inherited as an autosomal dominant trait, this disorder is responsible for lifelong asymp-

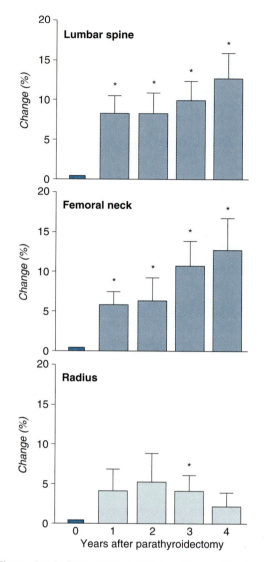

Figure 8–14. Bone mineral density after parathyroidectomy. Cumulative percentage change in bone mineral density after parathyroidectomy by site. *, change from year 0 baseline at $P \ll 0.05$. (Reproduced, with permission, from Silverberg SJ, Gartenberg F, Jacobs TP et al: Increased bone mineral density after parathyroidectomy in primary hyperparathyroidism. J Clin Endocrinol Metab 1995;80:729.)

tomatic hypercalcemia, first detectable in cord blood. Hypercalcemia is usually mild (10.5–12 mg/dL [2.7–3 mmol/L]) and is often accompanied by mild hypophosphatemia and hypermagnesemia. The PTH level is normal or slightly elevated, indicating that this is a PTH-dependent form of hypercalcemia. The parathyroid glands are normal in size or slightly enlarged, . The most celebrated laboratory feature of the disorder is hypocalciuria. The urinary calcium level is usually less than 50 mg/24 h, and the calcium/creatinine clearance ratio is less than 0.10. Hypocalciuria is an intrinsic renal trait, as it persists even in patients who have undergone total parathyroidectomy.

Since FBHH is an asymptomatic trait, the most important role of diagnosis is to distinguish it from primary hyperparathyroidism and avoid an unnecessary parathyroidectomy. If a subtotal parathyroidectomy is performed, the serum calcium invariably returns shortly to preoperative levels; these persons resist attempts to lower their serum calcium. Unfortunate patients with this variant who have undergone total parathyroidectomy are rendered hypoparathyroid and are dependent on calcium and vitamin D.

The diagnosis must be considered in patients with asymptomatic mild hypercalcemia who are relatively hypocalciuric. However, an unequivocal diagnosis of FBHH cannot be made biochemically because the serum and urinary calcium and PTH levels all overlap with typical primary hyperparathyroidism. Family studies are necessary to make the diagnosis. The penetrance of the phenotype is 100%, and affected family members are hypercalcemic throughout life, so if the proband has FBHH, each first-degree relative who is screened will have a 50% chance of being hypercalcemic.

FBHH is caused by loss-of-function mutations in the parathyroid calcium receptor. Loss of one functional receptor allele shifts the set-point for inhibition of PTH release to the right, producing hypercalcemia. The same receptor is expressed in the distal renal nephron, and given the FBHH phenotype of hypocalciuria, the renal calcium receptor must regulate calcium excretion. A large number of different point mutations in the calcium receptor produce the FBHH phenotype. Hence, molecular genetic diagnosis is impractical at present.

Children of two parents with FBHH may inherit a mutant allele from each parent, producing a disorder called neonatal severe hypercalcemia. This is a life-threatening disorder in which failure to sense extracellular calcium produces severe hyperparathyroidism, requiring total parathyroidectomy soon after birth.

B. MEN Syndromes: As noted above, primary hyperparathyroidism is a feature of both MEN 1 and MEN 2a. The penetrance of primary hyperparathyroidism in MEN 1 is over 90% by age 40. Patients with the MEN I syndrome are thought to inherit a loss-of-function mutation of a tumor suppressor gene on chromosome 11q12–13. A chromosomal deletion during mitosis of a parathyroid cell that resulted in loss of the remaining allele in that cell would abrogate the cell's growth control mechanism and permit clonal expansion of its progeny to make up the parathyroid tumor. A similar mechanism may well exist in sporadic parathyroid adenomas with 11q12–13 deletions.

The penetrance of primary hyperparathyroidism in MEN 2A is about 30%. As discussed under in the section on medullary thyroid carcinoma, the disorder is caused by activating mutations in the *RET* oncogene, which encodes a tyrosine kinase receptor for an unknown ligand. Evidently, the *RET* gene product is less important for growth of the parathyroids than for thyroid C cells, since the penetrance of primary hyperparathyroidism is fairly low and since in MEN 2b a separate class of activating *RET* mutations produces medullary carcinoma and pheochromocytoma without primary hyperparathyroidism. The treatment for parathyroid hyperplasia in MEN 1 or MEN 2 is subtotal parathyroidectomy. The recurrence rate is higher than in sporadic parathyroid hyperplasia and approaches 50% in MEN 1. For this reason, transplantation of the parathyroid remnant to the forearm has been advocated in MEN patients because of the relative ease with which additional parathyroid tissue can be removed in patients with recurrent hyperparathyroidism.

C. Lithium Therapy: Both in patients and in isolated parathyroid cells, exposure to extracellular lithium shifts the set-point for inhibition of PTH secretion to the right. Clinically, this results in hypercalcemia and a detectable or elevated level of PTH. Lithium treatment also produces hypocalciuria and is thus a virtual phenocopy of FBHH. Most patients with therapeutic lithium levels for bipolar affective disorder will have a slight increase in the serum calcium level, and up to 10% become mildly hypercalcemic, with PTH levels that are high normal or slightly elevated. Lithium treatment can also unmask underlying primary hyperparathyroidism. It is difficult to diagnose primary hyperparathyroidism in a lithium-treated patient, particularly when temporary cessation of lithium therapy is deemed dangerous. However, the likelihood of underlying primary hyperparathyroidism is high when the serum calcium is greater than 11.5 mg/dL, and the decision to undertake surgery must be based on such clinical criteria. Unfortunately, surgical cure of hyperparathyroidism rarely ameliorates the underlying psychiatric condition.

2. MALIGNANCY-ASSOCIATED HYPERCALCEMIA

Malignancy-associated hypercalcemia is the second most common form of hypercalcemia, with an incidence of 15 cases per 100,000 per year—about one-half the incidence of primary hyperparathyroidism. It is, however, much less prevalent than primary hyperparathyroidism, because most patients have a very limited survival. Nonetheless, malignancy-associated hypercalcemia is the commonest cause of hypercalcemia in hospitalized patients. The clinical features and pathogenesis of malignancy-associated hypercalcemia are presented in Chapter 23. The treatment of nonparathyroid hypercalcemia is presented below.

3. SARCOIDOSIS & OTHER GRANULOMATOUS DISORDERS

Hypercalcemia is seen in up to 10% of patients with sarcoidosis and hypercalciuria in at least one-third. Hypercalcemia in sarcoidosis is caused by extrarenal conversion of 25-hydroxyvitamin D to its active form, $1,25(OH)_2D$, by the enzyme 25-hydroxyvitamin D 1α-hydroxylase in macrophages of sarcoid tissue. Even alveolar macrophages isolated from normocalcemic sarcoid patients are capable of this metabolic conversion, and provocative testing by administration of vitamin D suggests that most sarcoidosis patients have abnormal vitamin D metabolism. Thus, normocalcemic patients with sarcoidosis have markedly increased $1,25(OH)_2D$ levels after administration of vitamin D, demonstrating that the normal regulation of its synthesis has been abrogated. High $1,25(OH)_2D$ levels stimulate both intestinal calcium absorption and bone resorption. However, normocalcemia can persist, at the expense of hypercalciuria, as long as the kidneys are able to excrete an increased calcium load. In chronically hypercalciuric patients, hypercalcemia can be induced by increased substrate availability, such as high endogenous production of vitamin D in the summer months, or by events that interfere with the renal excretion of calcium.

The diagnosis of sarcoidosis should be considered in hypercalcemic patients in whom the level of PTH is suppressed. The finding of an elevated $1,25(OH)_2D$ level supports the diagnosis, particularly since $1,25(OH)_2D$, like PTH, should normally be suppressed by hypercalcemia. The treatment is administration of glucocorticoids, and a short course of hydrocortisone (40 mg three times daily for 10 days) can also be used as a trial of treatment to confirm the diagnosis.

Hypercalcemia occurs by the same mechanism in a variety of other granulomatous disorders. Mild hypercalcemia is present in up to 28% of patients with untreated pulmonary tuberculosis. Hypercalcemia also occurs in berylliosis, disseminated coccidioidomycosis, histoplasmosis, leprosy, and pulmonary eosinophilic granulomatosis.

4. ENDOCRINOPATHIES

Thyrotoxicosis

Mild hypercalcemia is found in about one-fourth of patients with thyrotoxicosis. The PTH is suppressed and the serum phosphorus is in the upper normal range. The serum alkaline phosphatase and urinary hydroxyproline may be mildly increased. Significant hypercalcemia is seen only in patients with severe thyrotoxicosis, particularly if they are temporarily immobilized. Thyroid hormone has direct bone-resorbing properties, and bone in thyrotoxicosis is in a high-turnover state, which often produces mild osteoporosis.

Adrenal Insufficiency

Hypercalcemia can be a feature of acute adrenal crisis and responds rapidly to glucocorticoid therapy. Animal studies suggest that hemoconcentration is a critical factor, and in experimental adrenal insufficiency $[Ca^{2+}]$ is normal.

5. ENDOCRINE TUMORS

Hypercalcemia in patients with pheochromocytoma is most often a manifestation of the MEN 2a syndrome, but hypercalcemia is found occasionally in uncomplicated pheochromocytoma, where it appears to result from secretion of PTHrP by the tumor. About 40% of tumors secreting vasoactive intestinal peptide (VIPomas) are associated with hypercalcemia. The cause is unknown. It is known, however, that at high levels VIP may activate the PTH/PTHrP receptor.

6. THIAZIDE DIURETICS

The administration of thiazides and related diuretics such as chlorthalidone, metolazone, and indapamide can produce an increase in the serum calcium which is not fully accounted for by hemoconcentration. Hypercalcemia is mild and usually transient, lasting for days or weeks, but occasionally it persists. Thiazide administration can also exacerbate the effects of underlying primary hyperparathyroidism; in fact, thiazide administration was formerly used as a provocative test for hyperparathyroidism in patients with borderline hypercalcemia. Most patients with persistent hypercalcemia while receiving thiazides will prove to have primary hyperparathyroidism.

7. VITAMIN D & VITAMIN A

Hypercalcemia occurs in patients taking large doses of vitamin D, usually at least 50,000 IU daily. Calcium absorption and bone resorption are increased; severe hypercalciuria is present; and patients are prone to calcium urolithiasis. The PTH level is suppressed. In patients who are intoxicated with cholecalciferol (vitamin D_3), ergocalciferol (vitamin D_2), or calcifediol (25-hydroxyvitamin D_3), the diagnosis may be established by determining serum 25-hydroxyvitamin D levels, which are often five to ten times normal. The serum level of $1,25(OH)_2D$ may be normal or slightly raised, a tribute to the tight control of its synthetic rate in the face of massive levels of its precursor. Thus, hypercalcemia probably results from direct effects of 25-hydroxyvitamin D, whose affinity for the vitamin D receptor is about one-thousandth that of $1,25(OH)_2D$. Treatment consists of withdrawal of vitamin D and administration of glucocorticoids.

Vitamin A intoxication requires large doses of vitamin A (50,000–200,000 IU daily) and produces a syndrome of lassitude, headache, anorexia, cheilitis, glossitis, a scaly pruritic rash, hepatomegaly, and bone pain and tenderness. The serum level of vitamin A is increased. In hypercalcemic patients, the serum phosphorus is normal and the serum alkaline phosphatase may be increased. Hypercalcemia probably results from direct bone-resorbing effects of vitamin A and responds to glucocorticoids.

8. MILK-ALKALI SYNDROME

The ingestion of large quantities of calcium together with an absorbable alkali can produce hypercalcemia with alkalosis, renal impairment, and often nephrocalcinosis. The syndrome was more common when absorbable antacids were the standard treatment for peptic ulcer disease, but it is still seen occasionally. This is the only recognized example of pure absorptive hypercalcemia. The details of its pathogenesis are poorly understood.

9. MISCELLANEOUS CONDITIONS

Immobilization

In immobilized patients there is a marked increase in bone resorption, which often produces hypercalciuria, and is powerful enough to cause hypercalcemia mainly in individuals in a preexisting high bone turnover state, such as adolescents and patients with thyrotoxicosis or Paget's disease. The disorder remits with the restoration of activity. If acute treatment is required, bisphosphonates appear to be the treatment of choice.

Acute Renal Failure

Hypercalcemia is often seen when renal failure is precipitated by rhabdomyolysis and usually occurs during the early recovery stage. It resolves over a few weeks. The pathogenesis is uncertain.

TREATMENT OF HYPERCALCEMIA

Initial management of hypercalcemia consists of assessing the hydration state of the patient and rehydrating as necessary with saline. The first goal is to restore renal function, which is often impaired in hypercalcemia because of reduced glomerular filtration and dehydration. Hypercalcemia impairs the urinary concentrating ability, leading to polyuria, and at the same time impairs the sensorium, diminishing the sense of thirst. Once renal function is restored, renal excretion of calcium can be further enhanced by inducing a saline diuresis. Because most of the filtered calcium is reabsorbed by bulk flow in the proximal tubule along with sodium chloride, a saline diuresis will markedly increase calcium excretion. However, a vigorous saline diuresis will also induce substantial urinary losses of potassium and magnesium, and these must be monitored and replaced as necessary.

After these initial steps, attention should be given to finding a suitable chronic therapy. It is important to start chronic therapy soon after hospitalization, as several of the most useful agents take up to 5 days to have their full effect. The drug of first choice for most patients is pamidronate disodium. This is a bisphosphonate drug that acts by inhibiting osteoclastic bone resorption. The initial dose is 60–90 mg by intravenous infusion over 4–24 hours. Over 90% of patients with malignancy-associated hypercalcemia will normalize the serum calcium after a 90 mg infusion of pamidronate. However, the nadir of serum calcium does not occur until 4–5 days after administration. The hypocalcemic effect of pamidronate may persist for 1–6 weeks, and re-treatment can then be carried out. Transient fever and myalgia occur in 20% of patients. Increased serum creatinine (≥ 0.5 mg/dL) occurs in about 15% of patients. Pamidronate should be used cautiously and at reduced doses when the baseline serum creatinine exceeds 2.5 mg/dL.

In patients with severe hypercalcemia and those with renal insufficiency that is refractory to rehydration, it may be necessary to use a second antiresorptive agent for a few days while awaiting the full therapeutic effect of pamidronate. For this purpose, synthetic salmon calcitonin may be administered at a dose of 4–8 IU/kg subcutaneously every 12 hours. This is a useful adjunct acutely, but most patients become totally refractory to calcitonin within a few days, so it is not suitable for chronic use. Another agent that may be used acutely is plicamycin, which is discussed below.

The use of an antiresorptive agent together with saline diuresis provides for a two-pronged approach to hypercalcemia, and several agents besides pamidronate are available. Of these, the most useful is plicamycin (formerly mithramycin). This cytotoxic antibiotic has a tropism for the osteoclast and is a potent inhibitor of bone resorption. It is administered intravenously in doses up to 25 μg/kg. The serum calcium is reduced within 24 hours, with a nadir at 48–72 hours. Treatment may then be repeated at weekly intervals as necessary, but the use of plicamycin is limited by its hepatic, renal, and bone marrow toxicity, which will eventually necessitate reducing the dose or delaying treatment. For this reason, one should use plicamycin acutely for severe hypercalcemia and reserve chronic plicamycin treatment for patients who fail pamidronate.

Other antiresorptive agents that are available for treatment of hypercalcemia include the bisphosphonate etidronate disodium and gallium nitrate. Both of these agents require repeated intravenous administration for 3–5 days and neither has the efficacy of pamidronate, so they are little used at present.

Glucocorticoid administration is first-line treatment for hypercalcemia in patients with multiple myeloma, lymphoma, sarcoidosis, or intoxication with vitamin D or vitamin A. Glucocorticoids are also beneficial in some patients with breast carcinoma. However, they are of little use in most other patients with solid tumors and hypercalcemia.

HYPOCALCEMIA

Classification

Both PTH and $1,25(OH)_2D$ function to maintain a normal serum calcium and are thus central to the defense against hypocalcemia. Hypocalcemic disorders are best understood as failures of the adaptive response. Thus, chronic hypocalcemia can result from a failure to secrete PTH, a failure to respond to PTH, a deficiency of vitamin D, or a failure to respond to vitamin D. Acute hypocalcemia is most often the consequence of an overwhelming challenge to the adaptive response such as rhabdomyolysis, in which a flood of phosphate from injured skeletal muscle inundates the extracellular fluid (Table 8–5).

Clinical Features

Most of the symptoms and signs of hypocalcemia occur because of increased neuromuscular excitability (tetany, paresthesias, seizures, organic brain syndrome) or because of deposition of calcium in soft tissues (cataract, calcification of basal ganglia).

A. Neuromuscular Manifestations: Clinically, the hallmark of severe hypocalcemia is tetany. Tetany is a state of spontaneous tonic muscular contraction. Overt tetany is often heralded by tingling paresthesias in the fingers and about the mouth, but the classic muscular component of tetany is carpopedal spasm. This begins with adduction of the thumb, followed by flexion of the metacarpophalangeal joints, extension of the interphalangeal joints, and flexion of the wrists to produce the *main d'accoucheur* posture (Figure 8–15). These involuntary muscle contractions are painful. Although the hands are most typically involved, tetany can involve other muscle groups, including life-threatening spasm of laryngeal muscles. Electromyographically, tetany is typified by repetitive motor neuron action potentials, usually grouped as doublets. Tetany is not specific for hypocalcemia. It also occurs with hypomagnesemia and metabolic alkalosis, and the most common cause of tetany is respiratory alkalosis from hyperventilation.

Lesser degrees of neuromuscular excitability (eg, serum calcium 7–9 mg/dL) produce latent tetany,

Table 8–5. Causes of hypocalcemia.

Hypoparathyroidism
  Surgical
  Idiopathic
  Neonatal
  Familial
  Deposition of metals (iron, copper, aluminum)
  Postradiation
  Infiltrative
  Functional (in hypomagnesemia)
Resistance to PTH action
  Pseudohypoparathyroidism
  Renal insufficiency
  Medications that block osteoclastic bone resorption
    Plicamycin
    Calcitonin
    Bisphosphonates
Failure to produce $1,25(OH)_2D_3$ normally
  Vitamin D deficiency
  Hereditary vitamin D-dependent rickets, type 1 (renal 25-OH-vitamin D 1α-hydroxylase deficiency)
Resistance to $1,25(OH)_2D_3$ action
  Hereditary vitamin D-dependent rickets, type 2 (defective VDR)
Acute complexation or deposition of calcium
  Acute hyperphosphatemia
    Crush injury with myonecrosis
    Rapid tumor lysis
    Parenteral phosphate administration
    Excessive enteral phosphate
      Oral (phosphate-containing antacids)
      Phosphate-containing enemas
  Acute pancreatitis
  Citrated blood transfusion
  Rapid, excessive skeletal mineralization
    Hungry bones syndrome
    Osteoblastic metastasis
    Vitamin D therapy for vitamin D deficiency

which can be elicited by testing for Chvostek's and Trousseau's signs. Chvostek's sign is elicited by tapping the facial nerve about 2 cm anterior to the earlobe, just below the zygoma. The response is a contraction of facial muscles ranging from twitching of the angle of the mouth to hemifacial contractions.

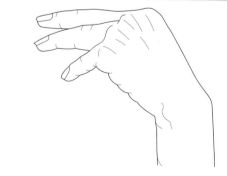

Figure 8–15. Position of fingers in carpal spasm due to hypocalcemic tetany (Reproduced, with permission, from Ganong WF: Review of Medical Physiology, 16th ed. Appleton & Lange, 1993.)

The specificity of the test is low; about 25% of normal individuals have a mild Chvostek sign. Trousseau's sign is elicited by inflating a blood pressure cuff to about 20 mm Hg above systolic pressure for 3 minutes. A positive response is carpal spasm. Trousseau's sign is more specific than Chvostek's, but 1–4% of normals have positive Trousseau signs.

Hypocalcemia predisposes to focal or generalized seizures. Other central nervous system effects of hypocalcemia include pseudotumor cerebri, papilledema, and confusion, lassitude, and organic brain syndrome. Twenty percent of children with chronic hypocalcemia develop mental retardation. The basal ganglia are often calcified in patients with long-standing hypoparathyroidism or pseudohypoparathyroidism. This is usually asymptomatic but can produce a variety of movement disorders.

B. Other Manifestations of Hypocalcemia:

1. Cardiac effects–Repolarization is delayed, with prolongation of the QT interval. Excitation-contraction coupling may be impaired, and refractory congestive heart failure is sometimes observed, particularly in patients with underlying cardiac disease.

2. Ophthalmologic effects–Subcapsular cataract is common in chronic hypocalcemia, and its severity is correlated with the duration and level of hypocalcemia.

3. Dermatologic effects–The skin is often dry and flaky and the nails brittle. A dermatitis known as impetigo herpetiformis or pustular psoriasis is peculiar to hypocalcemia.

CAUSES OF HYPOCALCEMIA

1. HYPOPARATHYROIDISM

Hypoparathyroidism may be surgical, autoimmune, familial, or idiopathic. The signs and symptoms are those of chronic hypocalcemia. Biochemically, the hallmarks of hypoparathyroidism are hypocalcemia, hyperphosphatemia (because the phosphaturic effect of PTH is lost), and an inappropriately low or undetectable PTH level.

Surgical Hypoparathyroidism

The most common cause of hypoparathyroidism is surgery on the neck, with removal or destruction of the parathyroid glands. The operations most often associated with hypoparathyroidism are cancer surgery, total thyroidectomy, and parathyroidectomy, but the skill and experience of the surgeon are more important predictors than the nature of the operation. Tetany ensues 1 or 2 days postoperatively, but about half of patients with postoperative tetany will recover sufficiently not to require long-term replacement therapy. In these cases, a devitalized parathyroid remnant has recovered its blood supply and resumes secretion of PTH. In some patients, hypocalcemia

may not become evident until years after the procedure. Surgical hypoparathyroidism is the presumptive diagnosis for hypocalcemia in any patient with a surgical scar on the neck.

In patients with severe hyperparathyroid bone disease preoperatively, a syndrome of postoperative hypoparathyroidism can follow successful parathyroidectomy. This is the "hungry bones syndrome," which results from such avid uptake of calcium and phosphate by the bones that the parathyroids, though intact, cannot compensate. The syndrome is usually seen in patients with an elevated preoperative serum alkaline phosphatase. It can usually be distinguished from surgical hypoparathyroidism by the serum phosphorus, which is low in the hungry bones syndrome because of skeletal avidity for phosphate, and high in hypoparathyroidism.

Idiopathic Hypoparathyroidism

Acquired hypoparathyroidism is sometimes seen in the setting of polyglandular endocrinopathies. Most commonly, it is associated with primary adrenal insufficiency and mucocutaneous candidiasis in the syndrome of pluriglandular autoimmune endocrinopathy, or type I polyglandular autoimmune syndrome (Chapter 24). The age at onset of hypoparathyroidism is 5–9 years. A similar form of hypoparathyroidism can occur as an isolated finding. The age at onset of idiopathic hypoparathyroidism is 2–10 years, and there is a preponderance of female cases. Circulating parathyroid antibodies are common in both the polyglandular and isolated forms, and the hypoparathyroidism is assumed to have an autoimmune basis. Up to one-third of patients have antibodies that recognize the parathyroid calcium sensor, though the pathogenetic role of these autoantibodies is not yet clarified.

Familial Hypoparathyroidism

Hypoparathyroidism can rarely present in a familial form, which may be transmitted as an autosomal dominant or an autosomal recessive trait. Two families with PTH gene mutations that interfere with the normal processing of PTH have been reported. A recently described mutation in the parathyroid calcium receptor gene produces a mild form of hypoparathyroidism in which affected individuals are hypocalcemic but do not require replacement therapy. This is an activating mutation of the calcium receptor, which enhances its sensitivity to calcium, shifting the set-point for calcium suppression of PTH secretion to the right and thereby producing a syndrome that is the mirror image of familial benign hypocalciuric hypercalcemia.

Other Causes of Hypoparathyroidism

Neonatal hypoparathyroidism can be part of the **DiGeorge syndrome** (dysgenesis of the thymus and parathyroids); rarely, isolated **congenital aplasia of** the parathyroids also occurs. Transfusion-dependent individuals with thalassemia or red cell aplasia who survive into the third decade of life are susceptible to hypoparathyroidism as the result of **iron deposition** in the glands. **Copper deposition** can cause hypoparathyroidism in Wilson's disease. **Aluminum deposition** in dialysis patients blunts the parathyroid reserve. Infiltration with metastatic carcinoma is a rare cause of hypoparathyroidism.

Severe **magnesium depletion** temporarily paralyzes the parathyroid glands, preventing secretion of PTH. The clinical settings of the disorder include gastrointestinal losses, renal wasting, and alcoholism. Serum magnesium levels in hypoparathyroid patients are below 1 mg/dL (0.4 mmol/L). The syndrome responds immediately to infusion of magnesium. As discussed above in the section on regulation of parathyroid hormone secretion, magnesium is probably required for stimulus-secretion coupling in the parathyroids, fulfilling the role of calcium in other glands.

2. PSEUDOHYPOPARATHYROIDISM

Pseudohypoparathyroidism is a heritable disorder of target-organ unresponsiveness to parathyroid hormone. Biochemically, it mimics hormone-deficient forms of hypoparathyroidism, with hypocalcemia and hyperphosphatemia, but the PTH level is elevated and there is a markedly blunted response to the administration of PTH (see Diagnosis, below).

Clinical Features

Two distinct forms of pseudohypoparathyroidism are recognized. Pseudohypoparathyroidism type 1B is a disorder of isolated resistance to PTH, which presents with the biochemical features of hypocalcemia, hyperphosphatemia and secondary hyperparathyroidism. Pseudohypoparathyroidism type 1A has, in addition to these biochemical features, a characteristic somatic phenotype known as Albright's hereditary osteodystrophy. This consists of short stature, a round face, short neck, brachydactyly (short digits), and subcutaneous ossifications. Because of shortening of the metacarpal bones—most often the fourth and fifth metacarpals—affected digits have a dimple, instead of a knuckle, when a fist is made (Figure 8–16). In addition, primary hypothyroidism occurs commonly, and many patients have abnormalities of reproductive function—oligomenorrhea in females and infertility in males. Interestingly, some individuals in families with pseudohypoparathyroidism inherit the somatic phenotype of Albright's hereditary osteodystrophy without any disorder of calcium metabolism; this state, which mimics pseudohypoparathyroidism, is called **pseudopseudohypoparathyroidism.**

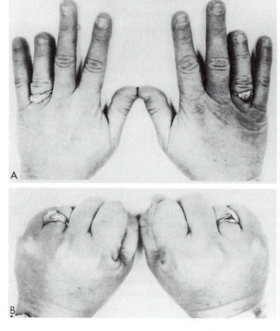
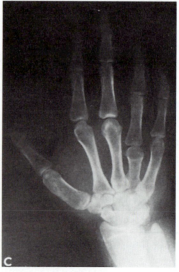

Figure 8–16. Hands of a patient with pseudohypoparathyroidism. *A:* Note the short fourth finger. *B:* Note the "absent" fourth knuckle. *C:* Film shows the short fourth metacarpal. (Reproduced, with permission, from Potts JT: Pseudohypoparathyroidism: Clinical features; signs and symptoms; diagnosis and differential diagnosis. In: *The Metabolic Basis of Inherited Disease,* 4th ed, Stanbury JB, Wyngaarden JB, Fredrickson DS [editors]. McGraw-Hill, 1978.)

Pathophysiology

Pseudohypoparathyroidism type 1A is caused by loss of one functional allele of the gene encoding the G protein subunit $G_s\alpha$, which leads to a 50% deficiency of the heterotrimer G_s, which couples the PTH receptor to adenylyl cyclase. Thus, patients with pseudohypoparathyroidism type 1A have a markedly blunted response of urinary cAMP to administration of PTH. Since G_s also couples many other receptors to adenylyl cyclase, the expected result of this mutation would be a generalized disorder of hormonal unresponsiveness. The high prevalence of primary hypothyroidism and primary hypogonadism indicates that in fact resistance to TSH, LH, and FSH are commonly present, but the response to other hormones (eg, ACTH, glucagon) is fairly normal. Thus, a 50% loss of G_s produces resistance to some hormones but not others. G_s is also deficient in individuals with pseudopseudohypoparathyroidism, who have Albright's hereditary osteodystrophy but normal responsiveness to PTH. Thus, the G_s mutation invariably produces Albright's hereditary osteodystrophy but only sometimes produces resistance to PTH, suggesting that the occurrence of resistance may be determined by a nonallelic modifier gene (Table 8–6).

In pseudohypoparathyroidism type 1B, where there is resistance to PTH but no somatic phenotype, G_s is normal. Pseudohypoparathyroidism Type 1B is not linked genetically to the PTH receptor, and the molecular basis of this disorder of isolated PTH resistance is unknown.

Genetics

Pseudohypoparathyroidism type 1A is inherited as an autosomal dominant trait. Few cases of male-to-male transmission are recognized, but this is probably because of male infertility in affected individuals. Individuals who have acquired the trait from their fathers almost always present with pseudopseudohypoparathyroidism and lack hormone resistance. When inheritance is from the mother, pseudohypoparathyroidism with hormone resistance is almost always present. These features suggest genomic imprinting, where the maternal allele is preferentially

Table 8–6. Features of pseudohypoparathyroidism (PHP).

	PHP 1A	PPHP[1]	PHP 1B
Hypocalcemia	Yes	No	Yes
Response to PTH	No	Yes	No
Albright's hereditary osteodystrophy	Yes	Yes	No
G_s mutation	Yes	Yes	No
Generalized unresponsiveness	Yes	No	No

[1]Pseudopseudohypoparathyroidism.

expressed in the kidney. The inheritance of pseudohypoparathyroidism 1B is unclear.

Diagnosis

Several disorders present with hypocalcemia and secondary hyperparathyroidism (eg, vitamin D deficiency), but when these features occur together with hypophosphatemia or Albright's hereditary osteodystrophy, this suggests the diagnosis of pseudohypoparathyroidism. To confirm that resistance to PTH is present, the patient is challenged with PTH (the Ellsworth-Howard test). For this purpose, synthetic human PTH(1–34) (teriparatide acetate, 3 IU/kg body weight) is infused intravenously over 10 minutes during a water diuresis, and urine is collected (–60 to 0 minutes, 0–30 minutes, 30–60 minutes, and 60–120 minutes) and assayed for cAMP and creatinine. Data are expressed as nanomoles of cAMP per liter of glomerular filtrate, based on creatinine measurements. Normally, there is an increase in urinary cAMP of > 300 nmol/L glomerular filtrate after administration of PTH. The use of the urinary phosphate response as a gauge of PTH responsiveness is much less reliable.

3. OTHER HYPOCALCEMIC DISORDERS

Hypoalbuminemia produces a low total serum calcium concentration because of a reduction in the bound fraction of calcium, but the ionized calcium is normal. The ionized calcium level can be determined directly, or the effect of hypoalbuminemia can be roughly corrected using the following formula:

Corrected serum calcium = Measured serum calcium + (0.8)(4 − Measured serum albumin)

Thus, in a patient with a serum calcium of 7.8 mg/dL and a serum albumin of 2 mg/dL, the corrected serum calcium is 7.8 + (0.8)(4–2) = 9.4 mg/dL.

Several disorders produce acute hypocalcemia despite intact homeostasis, simply because they overwhelm the adaptive mechanisms. Acute hyperphosphatemia that results from rhabdomyolysis or tumor lysis, often in the setting of renal insufficiency, may produce severe symptomatic hypocalcemia. Transfusion of citrated blood causes acute hypocalcemia by complexation of calcium as calcium citrate. In acute pancreatitis, hypocalcemia is an ominous prognostic sign. The mechanism of hypocalcemia is sequestration of calcium by saponification with fatty acids, which are produced in the retroperitoneum by the action of pancreatic lipases. Skeletal mineralization, when very rapid, can cause hypocalcemia. This is seen in the "hungry bones syndrome," which was discussed above under in the section on surgical hypoparathyroidism, and occasionally with widespread osteoblastic metastases from prostatic carcinoma.

TREATMENT OF HYPOCALCEMIA

Acute Hypocalcemia

Patients with tetany should receive intravenous calcium as calcium chloride (272 mg calcium per 10 mL), calcium gluconate (90 mg calcium per 10 mL), or calcium gluceptate (90 mg calcium per 10 mL). Approximately 200 mg of elemental calcium can be given over several minutes. The patient must be observed for stridor and the airway secured if necessary. Oral calcium and a rapidly acting preparation of vitamin D should be started. If necessary, calcium can be infused in doses of 400–1000 mg/24 h until oral therapy has taken effect. Intravenous calcium is irritating to the veins. Caution must be exercised in patients taking digitalis, since they are predisposed to toxicity by infusion of calcium.

Chronic Hypocalcemia

The objective of chronic therapy is to keep the patient free of symptoms and to maintain a serum calcium of approximately 8.5–9.2 mg/dL. With lower serum calcium levels, the patient may not only experience symptoms but may be predisposed over time to cataracts. With serum calcium concentrations in the upper normal range, there may be marked hypercalciuria, which occurs because the hypocalciuric effect of PTH has been lost. This may predispose to nephrolithiasis, nephrocalcinosis, and chronic renal insufficiency. In addition, the patient with a borderline elevated calcium is at increased risk of overshooting the therapeutic goal, with symptomatic hypercalcemia.

The mainstays of treatment are calcium and vitamin D. Oral calcium can be given in a dose of 1.5–3 g of elemental calcium per day. These large doses of calcium reduce the necessary dose of vitamin D and allow for rapid normalization of calcium if vitamin D intoxication subsequently occurs. Numerous preparations of

calcium are available. Both short-acting preparations of vitamin D, such as $1,25(OH)_2D_3$ (calcitriol) and the synthetic analog dihydrotachysterol, and very long-acting preparations such as vitamin D_2 (ergocalciferol) are available (Table 8–7). By far the most inexpensive regimens are those that use ergocalciferol. In addition to economy, they have the advantage of rather easy maintenance in most patients. The disadvantage is that ergocalciferol can slowly accumulate and produce delayed and prolonged vitamin D intoxication. Caution must be exercised in the introduction of other drugs that influence calcium metabolism. For example, thiazide diuretics have a hypocalciuric effect. By reducing urinary calcium excretion in treated patients, whose other adaptive mechanisms, PTH and $1,25(OH)_2D$, are nonoperative and who are thus absolutely dependent on renal excretion of calcium to maintain the serum calcium level, thiazides may produce severe hypercalcemia. In a similar way, intercurrent illnesses that compromise renal function may produce dangerous hypercalcemia in the patient who is maintained on large doses of vitamin D. Short-acting preparations are less prone to some of these effects but may require more frequent titration and are much more expensive than vitamin D_2.

BONE ANATOMY & REMODELING

FUNCTIONS OF BONE

Bone has three major functions: (1) It provides rigid support to extremities and body cavities containing vital organs. In disease situations in which bone is weak or defective, erect posture may be impossible, and vi-

Table 8–7. Pharmacology of vitamin D and its analogs.[1]

Characteristic	Ergocalciferol (Vitamin D_2)	Calcifediol (25[OH]D_3)	Dihydrotachysterol (DHT)	Calcitriol (1α,25[OH]$_2D_3$)	Alfacalcidol (1α-Hydroxy-cholecalciferol)[2]
Need for 25-hydroxylation	+	−	+	−	−
Need for 1-hydroxylation	+	+	−	−	−
Time for normocalcemia[3]	4–8 weeks	2–4 weeks	1–2 weeks	0.5–1 weeks	1–2 weeks
Persistence after cessation	6–8 weeks	4–12 weeks	1–3 weeks	0.5–1 weeks	1–2 weeks
Approximate daily dose	1000–3000 IU (40,000–120,000 IU)[4]	74–255 µg	300–1000 µg	0.75–2.25 µg	1–3 µg
Dosage forms	50,000 IU[4]	20 and 50 µg	0.125, 0.2, and 0.4 mg	0.25 and 0.5 µg	−

[1]Modified from Parfitt AM: Surgical, idiopathic, and other varieties of parathyroid hormone-deficient hypoparathyroidism. In: DeGroot LR (editor): *Endocrinology*. Saunders, 1989.
[2]Not available in the United States.
[3]Can be decreased by use of loading dose.
[4]40,000 IU = 1 mg.

tal organ function may be compromised. (An example is the cardiopulmonary dysfunction that occurs in patients with severe kyphosis due to vertebral collapse.) (2) Bones are crucial to locomotion in that they provide efficient levers and sites of attachment for muscles. With bony deformity, these levers become defective, and severe abnormalities of gait develop. (3) Finally, bone provides a large reservoir of ions, such as calcium, phosphorus, magnesium, and sodium, that are critical for life and can be mobilized when the external environment fails to provide them.

STRUCTURE OF BONE

Bone is not only rigid and resists forces that would ordinarily break brittle materials but is also light enough to be moved by the muscle contractions. Cortical bone, composed of densely packed layers of mineralized collagen, provides rigidity and is the major component of tubular bones (Figure 8–17). Trabecular (cancellous) bone is spongy in appearance, provides strength and elasticity, and constitutes the major portion of the axial skeleton. Disorders in

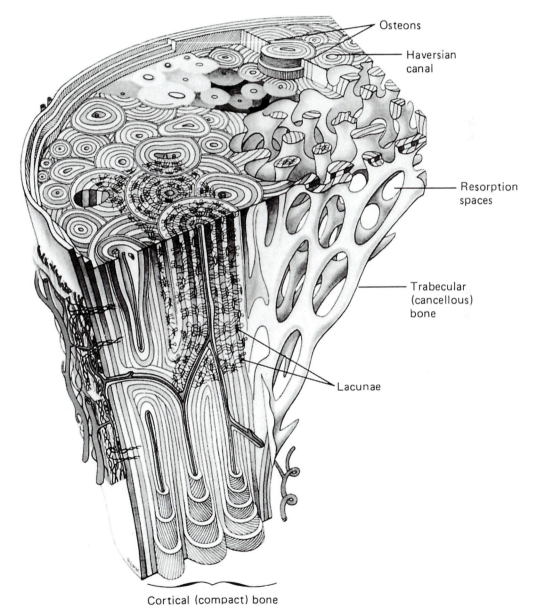

Figure 8–17. Diagram of some of the measures of the microstructure of mature bone seen in both transverse (top) and longitudinal section. Areas of cortical (compact) and trabecular (cancellous) bone are included. (Reproduced, with permission, from *Gray's Anatomy,* 35th ed. Warwick R, Williams PL [editors]. Longman, 1973.)

which cortical bone is defective or scanty lead to fractures of the long bones, whereas disorders in which trabecular bone is defective or scanty lead preferentially to vertebral fractures. Fractures of long bones may also occur because normal trabecular bone reinforcement is lost.

Two-thirds of the weight of bone is due to mineral; the remainder is due to water and type I collagen. Minor organic components such as proteoglycans, lipids, acidic proteins containing γ-carboxyglutamic acid, osteonectin, osteopontin, and growth factors are probably important, but their functions are poorly understood.

Bone Mineral

The mineral of bone is present in two forms. The major form consists of hydroxyapatite in crystals of varying maturity. The remainder is amorphous calcium phosphate, which lacks a coherent x-ray diffraction pattern, has a lower calcium-to-phosphate ratio than pure hydroxyapatite, occurs in regions of active bone formation, and is present in larger quantities in young bone.

Bone Cells

Bone is composed of three types of cells: the osteoblast, the osteocyte, and the osteoclast.

A. The Osteoblast: The osteoblast is the principal bone-forming cell. It arises from a pool of mesenchymal precursor cells in the bone marrow which, as they differentiate, acquire a set of characteristics including PTH and vitamin D receptors; surface expression of alkaline phosphatase; and expression of bone matrix protein genes—type I collagen, osteocalcin, etc. Differentiated osteoblasts are directed to the bone surface, where they line regions of new bone formation, laying down bone matrix (osteoid) in orderly lamellae and inducing its mineralization (Figure 8–18). In the mineralization process, hydroxyapatite crystals are deposited on the collagen layers to produce lamellar bone. Mineralization requires an adequate supply of extracellular calcium and phosphate as well as the enzyme alkaline phosphatase, which is secreted in large amounts by active osteoblasts. The fate of senescent osteoblasts is not well defined. Some probably become flattened, inactive lining cells on trabecular bone surfaces, and some are buried in cortical bone as osteocytes.

B. The Osteocyte: Osteoblasts that are trapped in cortical bone during the remodeling process become osteocytes. Protein synthetic activity decreases markedly, and the cells develop multiple processes that reach out through lacunae in bone tissue to communicate with nutrient capillaries, with processes of other osteocytes within a unit of bone (osteon) and also with the cell processes of surface osteoblasts (Figure 8–17). The physiologic importance of osteocytes is controversial, but they are believed to act as a cellular syncytium that permits translocation of

1. Osteoclast recruitment and activation

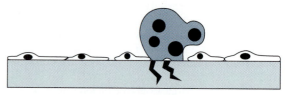

2. Resorption and osteoblast recruitment

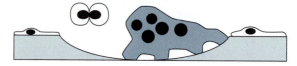

3. Osteoblastic bone formation

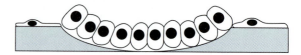

4. Completed remodelling cycle

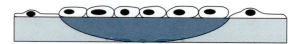

Figure 8–18. Sequential steps in remodeling of trabecular bone. (Reproduced, with permission, from Felig P, Baxter JD, Frohman LA [editors]: *Endocrinology and Metabolism,* 3rd ed. McGraw-Hill, 1995.)

mineral in and out of regions of bone removed from surfaces.

C. The Osteoclast: The osteoclast is a multinucleated giant cell that is specialized for resorption of bone. Osteoclasts are terminally differentiated cells that arise continuously from hematopoietic precursors in the monocyte lineage and do not divide. In a process that requires hematopoietic growth factors such as macrophage colony-stimulating factor (M-CSF, also called CSF-1) and is accelerated by cytokines such as interleukin-6 and by the systemic calciotropic hormones PTH and vitamin D, osteoclast precursors gradually mature, acquire the capacity to produce osteoclast-specific enzymes, and finally fuse to produce the mature multinucleate cell (Figure 8–19).

To resorb bone, the motile osteoclast alights on a bone surface and seals off an area by forming an adhesive ring. Having isolated an area of bone surface, the osteoclast develops above the surface an elaborately invaginated plasma membrane structure called the **ruffled border** (Figure 8–20). The ruffled border is a distinctive organelle, but it acts essentially as a huge lysosome, which dissolves bone mineral by secreting acid onto the isolated bone surface and simultaneously breaks down bone matrix by secretion of

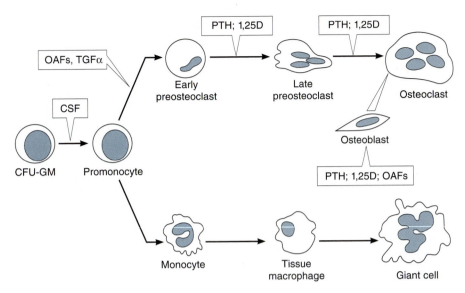

Figure 8–19. Working model of cells in the osteoclast lineage and the sites of action of various growth and differentiation factors. (Reproduced, with permission, from Favus MJ [editor]: *Primer on the Metabolic Bone Diseases and Disorders of Mineral Metabolism,* 2nd ed, Raven Press, 1993.)

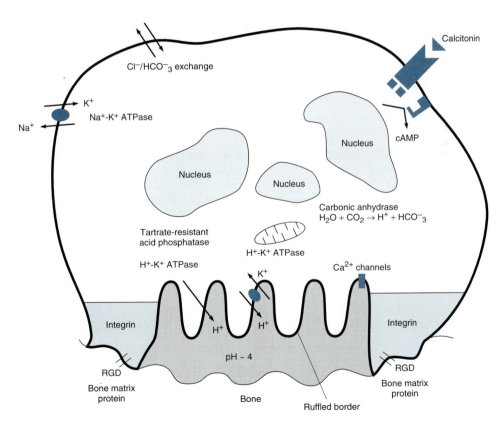

Figure 8–20. Osteoclast-mediated bone resorption. The osteoclast attaches to the bone surface via integrin-mediated binding to bone matrix bone proteins. When enough integrin binding has occurred, the osteoclast is anchored and a sealed space if formed. The repeatedly folded plasma membrane creates a "ruffled" border. Secreted into the sealed space are acid and enzymes forming an extracellular "lysosome." (Reproduced, with permission, from Felig P, Baxter JD, Frohman LA [editors]: *Endocrinology and Metabolism,* 3rd ed. McGraw-Hill, 1995.)

cathptic proteases. The resulting collagen peptides have pyridinoline structures that can be assayed in urine as a measure of bone resorption rates. Bone resorption can be controlled in two ways: by regulating the formation of osteoclasts to change their number or by regulating the activity of the mature osteoclast. The mature osteoclast has receptors for calcitonin but does not appear to have PTH or vitamin D receptors.

Bone Remodeling

Bone is constantly renewing itself by the process of bone remodeling. Bone remodeling occurs in an orderly cycle in which old bone is first resorbed and new bone then deposited. Cortical bone is remodeled from within by cutting cones, groups of osteoclasts that cut tunnels through the compact bone (Figure 8–21). They are followed by trailing osteoblasts, lining the tunnels and laying down a cylinder of new bone on their walls, so that the tunnels are progressively narrowed until all that remains are the tiny Haversian canals, by which the cells which are left behind as resident osteocytes are fed. The packet of new bone formed by a single cutting cone is called an osteon (Figure 8–17).

In trabecular bone, the remodeling process occurs on the surface. Osteoclasts first excavate a pit, and the pit is then filled in with new bone by osteoblasts (Figure 8–18). In a normal adult, this cycle takes 200 days. At each remodeling site, bone resorption and new bone formation are coupled, so that in a state of zero net bone balance, the amount of new bone

formed is precisely equivalent to the amount of old bone resorbed. This state of perfection is only briefly maintained, however. Until the age of 20–30, bone mass increases as we consolidate the gains in bone growth that were achieved during adolescence. After age 30, we begin to lose bone slowly. However, the rates of bone gain and bone loss during adulthood are too slow to be evident from the perspective of an individual bone remodeling unit.

Thus, in both cortical and cancellous compartments, bone is remodeled in packets or quanta by a multicellular unit, termed the "basic multicellular unit" (BMU). The duration of the remodeling cycle in cortical and cancellous bone is similar (Table 8–8). However, because of its large surface-to-volume ratio, the birthrate of BMUs is higher in cancellous bone than in cortical bone (Table 8–8). Consequently, the turnover rate of cancellous bone (26% per year) is also higher than the rate in cortical bone (3% per year). Because of its higher turnover rate, cancellous bone is lost more rapidly in osteoporosis than is cortical bone.

How do osteoclasts and osteoblasts communicate to achieve the coupling that ensures perfect (or near-perfect) bone balance? It appears that the important signals are local, not systemic, but they have not been identified. The process of bone remodeling does not absolutely require systemic hormones except to maintain intestinal absorption of minerals and thus ensure an adequate supply of calcium and phosphorus. For example, bone is quite normal, aside from low turnover, in patients with hypoparathyroidism. However, systemic hormones use the bone pool as a source of minerals for regulation of extracellular calcium homeostasis. When they do, the coupling mechanism ensures that bone is replenished. For example, when bone resorption is activated by PTH to provide calcium to correct hypocalcemia, bone formation will also increase, tending to replenish lost bone. One probable mechanism of coupling has to do with the apparent absence of PTH receptors and the VDR on osteoclasts. This means that other bone cells that have receptors for these hormones, such as osteoblasts, must receive the hormonal signal and pass it along to the osteoclast. This would allow for bone

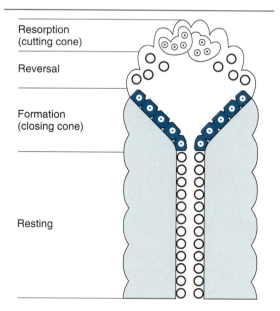

Figure 8–21. Schematic representation of the four principal stages involved in the formation of a new basic structural unit in cortical bone. (Reproduced, with permission, from Felig P, Baxter JD, Frohman LA [editors]: *Endocrinology and Metabolism,* 3rd ed. McGraw-Hill, 1995.)

Resorption (cutting cone)

Reversal

Formation (closing cone)

Resting

Table 8–8. Remodeling rates in the human skeleton.

Factor	Cortical Bone	Cancellous Bone
Mineral apposition rate	0.8 μm/d	0.6 μm/d
Duration of resorption period	24 days	21 days
Duration of formation period	124 days	91 days
Total birth rate of basic multicellular units	180/h	720/h
Bone turnover rate	3% per year	26% per year

formation to be activated along with bone resorption. The coupling factor responsible for activating osteoclasts has not been identified.

OSTEOPOROSIS

Osteoporosis is the loss of bone mass. It is the most common of all metabolic bone diseases, responsible for immense morbidity and considerable mortality. Osteoporosis is not a single entity, but rather a pathologic state with many causes.

Epidemiology

About 1.3 million fractures per year in the United States are attributable to osteoporosis, accounting for a social cost of about $20 billion. The three classic sites of osteoporotic fractures are the vertebral body, the forearm (Colles' fracture), and the hip. The risk of osteoporotic fractures depends upon gender, race, and age. For example, the lifetime risk of hip fracture is 17% in white women and 6% in white men (Table 8–9), but blacks and Hispanics are relatively protected from hip fractures: the lifetime risk of hip fracture has been estimated at about 6% for black women and 3% for black men. Age is a powerful determinant of fracture incidence, depending on the site of fracture. In women aged 50–70 years, the incidence of vertebral and wrist fractures is higher than the incidence of hip fracture. However, the incidence of hip fracture rises geometrically with advanced age in both men and women, so that after age 75 the hip is the commonest site of an osteoporotic fracture (Figure 8–22).

Etiology

A. Aging: The most common form of osteoporosis results from age-related bone loss. During

Table 8–9. Estimated lifetime fracture risk (%) in 50-year-old white women and men.[1]

	Women (95% CI)	Men (95% CI)
Proximal femoral fracture	17.5 (16.8, 18.2)	6.0 (5.6, 6.5)
Vertebral fracture[2]	15.6 (14.8, 16.3)	5.0 (4.6, 5.4)
Distal forearm fracture	16.0 (15.2, 16.7)	2.5 (2.2, 3.1)
Any of the three	39.7 (38.7, 40.6)	13.1 (12.4, 13.7)

CI = confidence interval
[1]Age 50 years was chosen because this is about the average age at menopause.
[2]Using incidence of clinically diagnosed fractures only.

our lifetimes, bone mass changes in three phases. The first phase is attainment of peak bone mass (Figure 8–23) as a result of bone growth and the subsequent consolidation of bone mass during the postpubertal years. This consolidation is completed between the ages of 20 and 30. Factors that determine the peak bone mass are gender, race, heredity, nutrition, and physical activity. Men have a significantly higher peak bone mass than women, which is partly determined by their greater body mass. Blacks have a higher peak bone mass than whites or Asians. Heredity is also a determinant of peak bone density within a given ethnic group. Among white women, for example, over one-half of the variance in peak bone mass appears to be accounted for by genetic factors. The intake of calcium during the period of peak bone growth is important. It is known from twin studies, for example, that calcium supplementation during adolescence produces a significant increment in bone mass.

The second phase in the life of the skeleton commences at age 30–40 and consists of slow, age-dependent bone loss. This persists throughout life at a similar rate in men and women, and similar amounts of cortical and trabecular bone are lost—about 25%

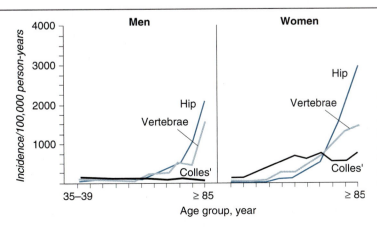

Figure 8–22. Incidence rates for the three common osteoporotic fractures (Colles', hip, and vertebral) in men and women, plotted as a function of age at the time of the fracture. (Reproduced, with permission, from Cooper C, Melton LJ III: Epidemiology of osteoporosis. Trends Endocrinol Metab 1992;314:224).

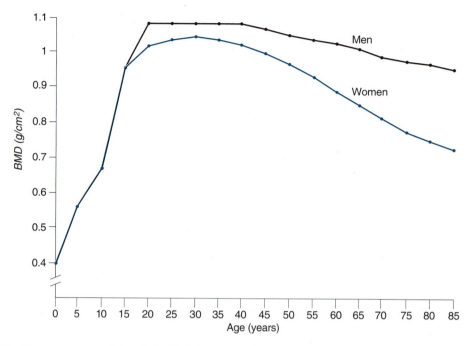

Figure 8–23. Mean bone mineral density by DXA in white males (upper curve) and females (lower curve) aged 5–85 years. The data are from Southard RN et al: Bone mass in healthy children: Measurement with quantitative DXA. Radiology 1991;179:735; and from Kelly TL: Bone mineral reference databases for American men and women. J Bone Miner Res 1990;5[Suppl 2]:702. Courtesy of Hologic, Inc.)

of the bone in each compartment over a lifetime. Enough bone is lost with aging to put the skeleton at considerably increased risk of fracture, particularly in those individuals who did not attain a high peak bone mass. Age-related bone loss occurs at a grossly similar rate in blacks, whites, and Asians.

B. Sex Hormone Deficiency: The third phase in the life of the skeleton is ordinarily confined to women, who experience rapid bone loss in the postmenopausal years because of estrogen deficiency. Estrogen deficiency is associated with bone loss regardless of age or the cause of the estrogen-deficient state. Thus, amenorrheic female athletes, hyperprolactinemic women, women who have undergone oophorectomy, and women with endometriosis in whom an "artificial menopause" is induced with luteinizing hormone-releasing hormone agonists will all experience accelerated bone loss. Accelerated postmenopausal bone loss, in conjunction with their reduced peak bone mass, puts women at substantially higher risk of osteoporotic fractures than men. and early menopause increases the risk. Postmenopausal bone loss is disproportionately from the trabecular compartment, where approximately 25% of bone is lost, compared with about 10% of cortical bone. The disproportionate loss of trabecular bone in the postmenopausal years may explain the earlier appearance of vertebral than of hip fractures in women, as the vertebral body is a site of mainly trabecular bone.

Hypogonadal men also undergo bone loss, which responds to replacement with testosterone. With regard to bone, testosterone would thus appear to subserve the same role in men that estrogen does in women. However, epiphysial closure is delayed and peak bone mass is markedly reduced in rare cases of impaired estrogen action in males, arising either from a deficiency of aromatase, the last enzyme in estrogen synthesis, or from a deficiency of estrogen receptors. This indicates that even in men with normal levels of testosterone, estrogen is important for cartilage and bone and suggests that gonadal failure is more a multifactorial insult to bone than had been appreciated.

A variety of factors can modify the mass of the skeleton and the risk of osteoporotic fractures. These include hereditary factors, constitutional factors, lifestyle, habits, and nutrition. In addition, a number of other disorders can cause secondary osteoporosis, including several heritable disorders affecting bone, hormonal disorders, and medications (Table 8–10).

C. Heredity: About 60–80% of the variance in bone density is genetically determined, based on twin studies and mother-daughter comparisons. A woman's risk of hip fracture is doubled by a maternal history of hip fracture. Although the inheritance of bone density is undoubtedly polygenic, studies of an Australian population have suggested that up to 75% of the genetic effect can be accounted for by inheritance of polymorphic alleles of the vitamin D receptor

Table 8–10. Causes of osteoporosis.

Primary osteoporosis
   Aging (senile or involutional)
   Juvenile
   Idiopathic (young adults)

Connective tissue diseases
   Osteogenesis imperfecta
   Homocystinuria
   Ehlers-Danlos syndrome
   Marfan's syndrome
   Menkes' syndrome
   Lysinuric protein intolerance

Drug-induced
   Corticosteroids
   Alcohol
   Thyroid hormone
   Chronic heparin
   Anticonvulsants

Hematologic
   Multiple myeloma
   Systemic mastocytosis

Immobilization

Endocrine
   Hypogonadism
   Hypercortisolism
   Hyperthyroidism
   Hyperparathyroidism
   Diabetes mellitus

Gastrointestinal disorders
   Subtotal gastrectomy
   Malabsorption syndromes
   Obstructive jaundice
   Biliary cirrhosis

gene. It is not known whether these polymorphisms in the gene affect the function of the vitamin D receptor, and it is controversial whether the Australian findings apply to other populations.

D. Constitutional Factors: Body mass is one of the most important determinants of peak bone mass. Although it is obvious that large people would have large bones, body weight is a more important factor than stature per se. Changes in body weight are also a powerful determinant of hip fracture incidence: postmenopausal women whose body weight has gone up by more than 50% since age 25 have a sixfold lower incidence of hip fracture than women who have not become heavy with increasing age.

E. Lifestyle and Habits: Exercise is clearly beneficial to the skeleton. Both premenopausal and postmenopausal women who exercise regularly have more bone mass than their sedentary counterparts, and the benefits of exercise in postmenopausal women have been confirmed in short-term trials. Regular exercise also decreases hip fracture risk, but this benefit is not completely explained by greater bone density. Undoubtedly, some of the value of exercise in fracture prevention has to do with maintaining strength, balance, and agility and thus avoiding falls.

Alcohol abuse is associated with a low-turnover state of bone and a reduction in trabecular bone vol-

ume. In the Framingham study, long-term alcohol use substantially increased the risk of hip fracture in men and women. However, moderate alcohol use in postmenopausal women is not a strong risk factor for osteoporosis, particularly after adjustment for poorer self-reported health.

Cigarette smoking has an adverse influence on bone mineral density and on the rate of bone loss in both women and men. Women who smoke metabolize exogenous estrogen more rapidly than women who do not, but there is no evidence that smoking affects the production or metabolism of endogenous estrogen. However, smoking has not emerged as an independent risk factor for hip fracture.

A high caffeine intake has been associated with decreased bone mass, and caffeine use does increase hip fracture risk independently of bone density.

F. Nutrition: In adolescents and young adults, increasing calcium intake enhances the accretion of bone mineral, indicating that an adequate calcium intake is required to attain one's genetically determined peak bone mass. A high-calcium intake is also required to maintain positive calcium balance in the elderly and prevent postmenopausal bone loss. Thus, a recent NIH consensus conference has proposed a 1200- to 1500-mg calcium intake as optimal in adolescents and young adults, 1000 mg calcium in adults, and 1500 mg in those over 65 years of age (Table 8–11). Estimated calcium intakes in the USA are far lower than optimal in adolescents and the aged, with one-third of postmenopausal women having intakes under 400 mg. Calcium supplementation slows the rate of bone loss in the elderly, most effectively in those with a low calcium intake at baseline. However, most epidemiologic studies have failed to show an influence of self-reported calcium intake on fracture risk. Thus, the long-term benefits of calcium supplementation are not well defined.

It is believed that, in general, Americans have adequate supplies of vitamin D, which is required for as-

Table 8–11. Calcium nutrition and osteoporosis.

Optimal daily calcium intakes	
(NIH Consensus Statement, 1994)	
Children	
1–5 years	800 mg
6–10 years	800–1200 mg
Adolescents	1200–1500 mg
Adults 25–50 years	1000 mg
Women	
Pregnant or lactating	1200 mg
Postmenopausal, on estrogen	1000 mg
Postmenopausal, not on estrogen	1500 mg
Elderly (age > 65)	1500 mg
Actual daily calcium intake	550 mg
(avg in women aged 65)	
Calcium sources	
Dairy product-free diet	400 mg
Cow's milk (8 oz)	300 mg
Calcium carbonate (500 mg)	200 mg

similation of dietary calcium. However, the ability to synthesize and absorb vitamin D declines with age, and at high latitudes synthesis in the skin is markedly attenuated in the winter. Elderly women in the northern United States manifest secondary hyperparathyroidism in the late winter months, when serum 25-hydroxyvitamin D levels are low, indicating the presence of a subclinical vitamin D deficiency state. In Europe, where the dietary intake of vitamin D is lower than in the United States, supplementation of the elderly with 1.2 g of calcium and 800 IU of vitamin D_3 reduced the rate of hip fracture. Thus, a case can be made that, in conjunction with calcium supplementation, the elderly should probably be supplemented beyond the current RDA of 200 IU of vitamin D to an intake of 400–800 IU

G. Secondary osteoporosis:

1. Glucocorticoid-induced osteoporosis–Osteoporosis is a feature both of Cushing's syndrome and of exogenous glucocorticoid administration. It is estimated that one-third to one-half of patients treated chronically with glucocorticoids develop osteoporosis. The disorder has a strong predilection for trabecular bone in the axial skeleton. Vertebral fractures are common, but there is no marked increase in the risk of hip fracture. Histologically, bone formation is decreased and bone resorption is increased, both disorders probably resulting from direct effects of glucocorticoids on bone. Thus, glucocorticoid-induced osteoporosis is an example of an uncoupled bone state; perhaps this accounts for the rapid bone loss often seen with high-dose glucocorticoid treatment. In addition to these direct skeletal effects, glucocorticoids in high doses also inhibit the intestinal absorption of calcium, increase the renal excretion of calcium (perhaps owing to increased bone resorption as well as direct tubule effects), and tend to impair gonadal function, with oligomenorrhea in women and reduced testosterone levels in men. The extraskeletal effects of glucocorticoids are probably important in the pathogenesis of osteoporosis. Thus, supplementation with calcium and vitamin D and replacement of gonadal steroids are important facets of the treatment of glucocorticoid-induced osteoporosis. Recent reports indicate that bone mass recovers considerably after successful treatment of Cushing's syndrome, but little is known about the reversibility of osteoporosis after the cessation of exogenous glucocorticoid administration.

2. Hyperthyroidism–Hyperthyroidism is a high-turnover bone state, which is probably caused by direct stimulation of bone resorption by thyroid hormone. The levels of bone formation markers in serum and of bone resorption markers in urine are increased. Although osteoporosis is common in hyperthyroidism, fractures are unusual, perhaps because hyperthyroidism is typically treated promptly, and most of the skeletal effects of hyperthyroidism are reversible. However, in postmenopausal women a history of hyperthyroidism does impose a significant risk of subsequent hip fracture. Whether thyroid suppression therapy is also a risk factor for osteoporosis is controversial. Initial reports indicated a high incidence of osteoporosis in individuals taking thyroid hormone in whom the TSH level was suppressed, an issue of particular concern in patients with a past history of thyroid carcinoma, in whom suppression of TSH is the goal of therapy. However, more recent reports suggest that the risk of thyroid suppressive therapy is relatively low.

3. Diabetes mellitus–Moderate osteopenia of cortical bone is common in insulin-dependent diabetes, but epidemiologic studies have not disclosed an increased likelihood of fractures. In contrast, bone mass is normal or even high in patients with type II diabetes, perhaps reflecting the effects of obesity.

4. Immobilization–Osteoporosis is a major problem in patients confined to chronic bed rest because of spinal cord injury or neuromuscular disorders. Rapid bone loss has also been noted during space flight. Immobilization causes a marked increase in bone resorption, with hypercalciuria and even hypercalcemia, in young patients with high preexisting bone turnover.

5. Connective tissue disorders–A variety of heritable disorders that affect the synthesis of bone matrix eventuate in osteoporosis. These include osteogenesis imperfecta, Ehlers-Danlos syndrome, homocystinuria, Menkes' syndrome, and Marfan's syndrome. Osteogenesis imperfecta is caused by mutations in the type I collagen gene, which codes for the principal structural protein of bone matrix. Hundreds of mutations have been reported, with phenotypes ranging from embryonic lethality to postmenopausal osteoporosis. The diagnosis of osteogenesis imperfecta should be considered in a postmenopausal woman with blue scleras, joint laxity, or a history of multiple childhood fractures; the diagnosis is made by collagen phenotyping of skin fibroblasts.

Clinical Features

A. Symptoms and Signs: Osteoporosis is an insidious disorder that evolves for many years without clinical symptoms. The initial symptoms are usually due to a fracture. A spinal compression fracture may be heralded by acute back pain, which is exacerbated by weight bearing and relieved by bed rest, and often persists for 1–2 months. The pain may remit after healing of the fracture occurs. Persistent back pain after a spinal fracture often reflects spasm of the paraspinus muscles, a consequence of biomechanical alterations induced by spinal collapse. Spinal fractures may also be painless, and individuals with multiple spinal compression fractures sometimes present with height loss and a characteristic dorsal kyphosis, often called the "dowager's hump." Anterior kyphosis occurs because osteoporotic fractures are often wedged anteriorly. The characteristic sites of appendicular osteoporotic fractures are the femoral neck and distal radius. Osteoporosis does not produce deformities of the extremities unless fractures occur.

B. Laboratory Findings: The serum chemistry values are typically normal in osteoporosis, though alkaline phosphatase may be elevated during healing of osteoporotic fractures. The serum PTH level is significantly higher in the aged than in younger subjects, and this finding reflects a true state of hyperparathyroidism, as discussed below under Pathogenesis, but it does not appear that the extent of hyperparathyroidism differs between osteoporotic subjects and age-matched controls. Similarly, the serum level of 1,25(OH)$_2$D may decrease slightly with age, primarily as a consequence of diminished renal mass, but the level of 1,25(OH)$_2$D is also poorly correlated with bone density or fracture risk. There is a progressive age-dependent increase in the levels of markers of bone turnover, and superimposed on this gradient is a rapid increase in bone

turnover at the time of menopause in women. Markers of bone formation, such as osteocalcin and bone-specific alkaline phosphatase, and markers of bone resorption, such as urinary pyridinolines or urinary *N*-telopeptide, are increased in parallel. These findings suggest that both postmenopausal and age-related osteoporosis occur in the setting of high bone turnover, as discussed below under Pathogenesis.

C. Imaging Studies: A decrease in bone mass may be apparent radiographically as osteopenia, but 30–50% of bone mass must be lost before osteoporosis is apparent radiologically. Not only is the radiograph insensitive—it is also lacking in specificity, because an overpenetrated film a normal spine may appear markedly osteopenic. Thus one must rely on more specific features for the radiologic assessment of osteoporosis. In the spine, horizontal trabeculae are lost preferentially, leaving a pattern of vertical trabeculation (Figure 8–24A). Preferential loss of trabecular over cortical bone may give a "picture-

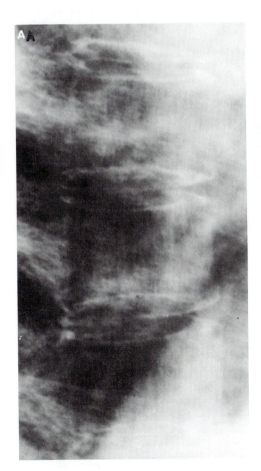

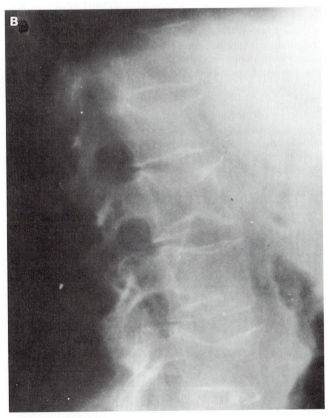

Figure 8–24. *A:* Magnified x-rays of thoracic vertebrae from a woman with osteoporosis. Note the relative prominence of vertical trabeculae and the absence of horizontal trabeculae. *B:* Lateral x-ray of the lumbar spine of a woman with postmenopausal osteoporosis. Note the increased density of the superior and inferior cortical margins of vertebrae, the marked demineralization of vertebral bodies, and the central compression of articular surfaces of vertebral bodies by intervertebral disks. (Courtesy of G Gordan.)

frame" vertebra. Localized herniations of the nucleus pulposus of the intervertebral disk, or "Schmorl's nodes," are also seen (Figure 8–24B). In addition, fractures of the vertebral bodies lead to loss of their height and anterior wedging. Fractures of the posterior elements of the vertebrae are quite uncommon in osteoporosis and suggest the presence of metastatic bone disease. In general, osteoporosis of the hip and distal forearm is difficult to diagnose radiologically. The loss of trabecular bone in the hip may be graded on x-rays (the "Singh index"), but the radiographic findings are poorly correlated with measurements of bone density.

D. Bone Densitometry: The most reliable diagnosis of osteoporosis is made by a direct measurement of bone density. The preferable technique for most purposes is dual-energy x-ray absorptiometry. This procedure measures absorption of a beam of photons generated by an x-ray source to determine areal bone density (g/cm^2) and can measure total body calcium or bone density at the spine, the hip, or the wrist. The measurement is rapid and precise (precision error 1–2%) and delivers a radiation dose of 1–3 mrem, a small fraction of the radiation dose delivered by a chest x-ray. Other bone density techniques include single photon absorptiometry of the wrist and quantitative computed tomography (QCT). Quantitative computed tomography provides a measurement of trabecular bone density in the spine, but this means of measurement is inherently less precise and less accurate than dual-energy x-ray absorptiometry.

The World Health Organization defines osteoporosis as a bone density > 2.5 SD below the young normal mean. Because bone loss is virtually universal with aging, a substantial portion of the elderly population are osteoporotic (Figure 8–25). For example, up to 30% of postmenopausal women meet the WHO definition of osteoporosis. To be of use for prognosis, however, bone density measurements must be able to predict the risk of fracture. It has recently been determined that the risk of hip fracture is increased two- to threefold for each standard deviation of bone density below the mean for age. That is, a 70-year-old woman with a bone density 2 SD below the mean for her age would have a four- to sixfold increase in the risk of subsequent hip fracture. Because osteoporosis is a systemic problem, reduced bone density at any of the standard skeletal sites is predictive of hip fracture, but the greatest predictive value comes from measurements at the hip. Thus, bone density measurements can be used to diagnose osteoporosis; to assess the risk of subsequent fractures and thus guide the choice of treatment; or to follow the response to specific therapy.

Pathogenesis

Estrogen deficiency is the form of osteoporosis whose pathogenesis is best understood. Estrogen lack induces an increase in bone resorption, with increased resorption surfaces and an increased activation frequency of basic multicellular units on bone biopsy, an increase in urinary excretion of calcium and collagen metabolites (pyridinolines and *N*-telopeptide), and a mild suppression of the PTH level. Because coupling is maintained, bone formation rates are also increased in estrogen deficiency, with an increase in the serum alkaline phosphatase, bone-specific alkaline phosphatase, and osteocalcin. The levels of the markers of bone remodeling are increased by 30–100% in postmenopausal women, indicating that estrogen lack is a high-turnover state.

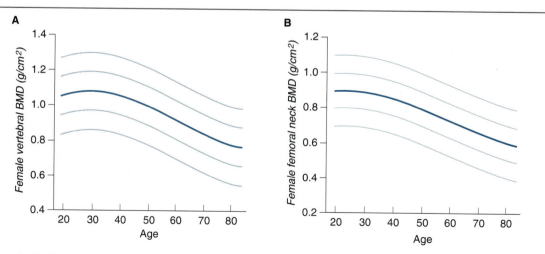

Figure 8–25. Bone density of **(A)** the lumbar spine (L2–4) and **(B)** femoral neck. The bold line represents the mean of 650 women with no overt bone disease; dotted lines represent 1 SD and 2 SD above and below the mean. (Courtesy of Hologic, Inc.)

The cellular basis for the effects of estrogen deficiency on bone may involve the derepression of bone-resorbing cytokines. Both interleukin-1 and interleukin-6 are stimulators of osteoclastic bone resorption, and there is evidence for increased production of these cytokines in estrogen deficiency, both from circulating monocytes and from osteoblasts and marrow stromal cells in bone. Increased production of cytokines is reversible with estrogen replacement. However, a causal relationship between these cytokines and bone loss has yet to be demonstrated.

The pathogenesis of age-related bone loss is less certain. It was formerly thought that both low-turnover and high-turnover forms of osteoporosis were prevalent in the elderly, but the measurement of biochemical markers of bone turnover has shown that the high levels of bone turnover in postmenopausal women persist until old age. One obvious factor is calcium deficiency. The dietary calcium requirement to maintain calcium balance increases with age, because of reduced intestinal calcium absorption in the elderly. The reduction in calcium absorption is explained by effects of estrogen deficiency on the gastrointestinal tract, by a modest reduction in the serum level of $1,25(OH)_2D$ because of declining renal mass, and by resistance to vitamin D in the aging intestine—there is a significant reduction in the VDR content of duodenal mucosa in aged women. As discussed above, most elderly subjects do not increase their dietary calcium to counter this impairment in calcium absorption and are thus in negative calcium balance.

The serum level of biologically active PTH rises with aging. This is partly an adaptive response to calcium deficiency. There is also evidence that the set-point for regulation of PTH secretion by calcium is shifted to the right in aged subjects—ie, that the sensitivity of the parathyroid gland to calcium is reduced. Hyperparathyroidism would be expected to induce bone resorption and could thus account for bone loss in the aged. However, neither the level of calcium intake nor the level of PTH is strongly correlated with bone mass, indicating that other factors are also involved in the pathogenesis of osteoporosis. Calcium replacement appears to reduce the rate of bone loss by approximately 50%. This suggests that other aspects of aging must account for at least half of the decline in bone mass.

Diagnosis

The diagnosis of osteoporosis is made by determining bone mass, usually by dual-energy x-ray absorptiometry. Although osteoporosis is defined by the World Health Organization as a bone density > 2.5 SD below the young normal mean for age and race, bone density is a continuous variable, and lesser degrees of bone loss may also be significant. The differential diagnosis of reduced bone density includes osteomalacia, renal tubular acidosis, and multiple myeloma. Osteomalacia often presents with diffuse bone pain and tenderness; in addition to osteopenia, characteristic pseudofractures are sometimes present on x-ray. Biochemically, the serum phosphorus and serum calcium are often depressed, and the alkaline phosphatase level is increased. Vitamin D-deficient osteomalacia can be excluded by determination of 25-hydroxyvitamin D in serum. Frank renal tubular acidosis is usually obvious, but incomplete renal tubular acidosis presents without metabolic acidosis. The urinary pH is > 6.0, marked hypercalciuria is present, and nephrocalcinosis is common. In 30% of patients, multiple myeloma presents as diffuse osteoporosis without the characteristic punched-out osteolytic lesions. Anemia is usually present. Multiple myeloma can be excluded by serum and urinary protein electrophoresis.

As a practical matter, the evaluation of an osteoporotic patient should include a history and physical examination, including a careful measurement of height. Evidence of hyperthyroidism, Cushing's syndrome, or osteogenesis imperfecta should be sought. Screening laboratory studies should include serum calcium, phosphorus, alkaline phosphatase, electrolytes and creatinine, TSH, a compete blood count, serum protein electrophoresis, and urinalysis. A urinary pH < 6.0 effectively excludes renal tubular acidosis, and normal individuals have a urinary pH < 6.0 on a first morning voided urine. Radiographic assessment should include lateral films of the thoracic and lumbar spine. Bone density at the lumbar spine and hip should be determined by dual-energy x-ray absorptiometry.

Treatment

A. General Measures: Most osteoporotic individuals have a suboptimal intake of calcium. The dietary calcium intake can be estimated from a dietary history, by adding the calcium content of a diet free of dairy products (300–400 mg/d) to the average daily intake of dairy products (Table 8–11). The diet can then be supplemented to the recommended intake of 1500 mg, using dairy products or various calcium preparations. The most useful calcium preparations consist of calcium carbonate, which contains 40% elemental calcium by weight, or calcium citrate, which contains 21% elemental calcium (Table 8–12). The absorption of calcium from calcium carbonate preparations may be reduced in achlorhydria, which is common in the elderly. To avoid this problem, calcium carbonate is taken with meals. To assure an adequate intake of vitamin D, 400–800 IU of vitamin D are prescribed, usually in the form of multivitamins. These measures are useful in all forms of osteoporosis and by themselves can reduce the rate of bone loss by up to 50%. Supplementation with calcium and vitamin D is not indicated in patients with a history of calcium urolithiasis and should be used with caution in chronic renal failure. However, calcium

Table 8–12. Calcium preparations in common use.

Trade Name	Form of Salt	Elemental Calcium per Tablet (mg)	Cost per Day for 1500 mg
Os-Cal[1]	Carbonate	250	$0.54
Os-Cal 500	Carbonate	500	$0.44
Generic oyster shell calcium	Carbonate	500	$0.15
Tums	Carbonate	200	$0.29
Posture	Phosphate	600	$0.38
Citracal	Citrate	200	$0.70
PhosLo	Acetate	169	$1.46

[1]Contains 125 IU cholecalciferol.

supplementation does not appear to increase the risk of calcium stone disease in individuals without a history of stones.

Acute back pain responds to analgesia, heat, and massage. A brief period of bed rest is sometimes necessary. Chronic back pain is usually the consequence of the musculoskeletal effects of spinal deformity. It is difficult to relieve completely, but many patients will benefit from back exercises devised to improve the function and tone of the paraspinus and abdominal muscles. A back brace is occasionally beneficial. Exercise should be encouraged.

Measures to prevent falling should be instituted in patients at risk of osteoporotic fractures. Risk factors for falling include muscle weakness, poor vision, poor hearing, impaired balance, use of sedatives, and postural hypotension. Environmental factors include loose rugs, waxed floors, and unsafe stairs. Intervention strategies targeted at these risk factors have been shown to reduce the incidence of falls. The use of padded hip protectors has been reported to reduce occurrences of hip fracture in a nursing home population.

B. Estrogens: Estrogen replacement has conclusively been shown to reduce the loss of bone mass in postmenopausal women, and case-control studies suggest that the incidence of hip fracture is reduced by as much as 50% in postmenopausal estrogen users. Although it was once believed that to be effective, estrogen replacement should be started within 10 years after menopause, more recent studies have shown benefit in women up to 65 years of age. Estrogen replacement therapy also prevents vasomotor symptoms of menopause ("hot flushes") and may reduce the loss of skin collagen. Retrospective studies suggest that the incidence of coronary heart disease may be reduced by 35–45%, and prospective studies are under way to examine this issue. If the cardioprotective effects of estrogens can be confirmed in prospective studies, the enormous benefits would far outweigh the considerations of risk/benefit ratios for osteoporosis treatment that are discussed below.

Although conjugated estrogens (0.625 mg/d) re-

main the most popular regimen for replacement therapy, a variety of other estrogen preparations are also effective, including ethinyl estradiol, 0.02 mg/d, micronized estradiol, 1–2 mg/d, and transdermal estradiol, 0.05 mg patch twice a week. The occurrence of endometrial carcinoma is sharply increased by the use of unopposed estrogen. To prevent the development of endometrial hyperplasia and eventual endometrial carcinoma, women with an intact uterus should be given estrogen in combination with a progestin. The progestin can be administered cyclically (eg, medroxyprogesterone, 10 mg daily for 10–14 days per month) or continuously (eg, medroxyprogesterone, 2.5 mg daily). The cyclic regimen produces sustained withdrawal bleeding in a large fraction of women. The continuous regimen often produces irregular spotting for the first year of treatment but infrequent uterine bleeding thereafter. Although many women object to the prospect of continued monthly uterine bleeding, the irregular bleeding on continuous regimens, albeit infrequent, results in a higher likelihood of repeated evaluations for dysfunctional bleeding. An increasingly popular noninvasive approach to evaluation of dysfunctional uterine bleeding is the use of transvaginal ultrasound. If the endometrial thickness by ultrasound is less than 4 mm, a neoplasm is highly unlikely, and endometrial sampling can be avoided.

Although the risk of uterine carcinoma can be minimized by combined estrogen-progestin therapy, routine pelvic examinations, and thorough evaluation of dysfunctional bleeding, estrogen replacement therapy also carries a risk of developing breast carcinoma. Current estimates are that the breast cancer risk is increased about 30% by chronic estrogen use. The preponderance of risk is in chronic estrogen users, particularly those with more than 5–10 years of estrogen use, in whom the relative risk of breast cancer is about 1.7. Concomitant progestin therapy does not appear to alter the risk of breast cancer in estrogen users.

The decision for estrogen replacement must be individualized. Some women find the decision easy; for others, a careful weighing of risks and benefits is useful in their decision making. Bone densitometry is of use in advising undecided women (Figure 8–26). Since women whose bone density is in the lower range of normal have a substantially increased risk of future fractures—eg, a two- to threefold greater risk than average if the bone density is 1 SD below the average for age—they can be encouraged to consider replacement therapy. Conversely, women whose bone density is in the upper normal range can be encouraged to make their decision based on other issues—the cosmetic and possible cardiovascular benefits of estrogen versus the relatively small increment in risk of breast cancer.

C. Bisphosphonates: The bisphosphonate drug alendronate disodium was recently approved for treatment of osteoporosis. Like other bisphosphonates, alendronate is an inhibitor of bone resorption. Bisphosphonates are analogs of pyrophosphate in which the oxygen in the pyrophosphate core ($HO_3P-O-PO_3H$) has been replaced by a carbon ($RO_3P-C-PO_3R'$), rendering the bisphosphonates extremely stable. Administered orally or intravenously, these drugs bind to hydroxyapatite crystals in bone, as does pyrophosphate, and inhibit osteoclastic bone resorption with a long duration of action. Treatment with oral alendronate (10 mg daily) for 3 years produces an 8% increase in bone density at the spine and the trochanter and a 50% decrease in new vertebral fractures. Although the data have not yet been published, it is also clear that the risk of hip fracture is also reduced by about 50% by 3 years of alendronate treatment. Alendronate thus offers an alternative to estrogen in menopausal women, and is also suitable for the treatment of osteoporosis in

older women and potentially in men. It is poorly absorbed and should be administered fasting; its absorption is markedly impaired by concomitant administration of calcium preparations. The principal side effect is esophageal and gastric irritation.

The older (first-generation) bisphosphonate etidronate disodium may also be useful in treatment of osteoporosis. Etidronate is administered at a dose of 400 mg daily for the first 2 weeks of a 3-month period. Available data suggest that the rate of new vertebral fractures is reduced by treatment with etidronate, but the evidence is less impressive than the data on alendronate.

D. Calcitonin: Calcitonin is an antiresorptive hormone whose biochemistry and mechanism of action were discussed above. The preparation of the hormone that is used in osteoporosis is synthetic salmon calcitonin, which, curiously, is more potent in humans than human calcitonin. Calcitonin may be administered either subcutaneously or as a nasal spray. The dose for subcutaneous administration is 50–100 IU, either daily or every other day. The nasal spray is administered at a dose of 200 IU daily because of poor absorption by the nasal route. Calcitonin increases bone density, and several small studies suggest that the incidence of vertebral fractures may be diminished by calcitonin therapy. In addition, well-controlled clinical trials have shown that calcitonin administration has a mild analgesic effect, which may be useful in patients with symptomatic fractures. Calcitonin treatment is safe, and transient flushing and nausea are the principal side effects, both of which occur shortly after administration in about 10% of patients.

E. Anabolic Agents: All the available agents for osteoporosis treatment are inhibitors of bone re-

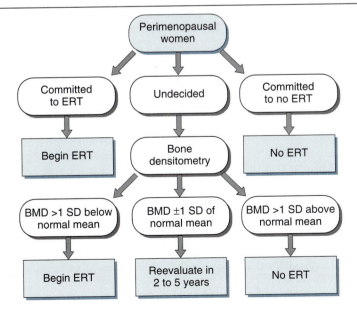

Figure 8–26. Algorithm for making decisions about the use of estrogen replacement therapy to prevent osteoporosis in postmenopausal women. (Reproduced, with permission, from Riggs BL, Melton LJ III: The prevention and treatment of osteoporosis. N Engl J Med 1992;327: 620.)

sorption. Although they increase bone mass over 1–3 years, their long-term ability to restore lost bone mass is probably limited by the physiologic coupling of bone resorption and bone formation, since bone formation rates eventually slow to match the new, lower rate of bone resorption. There are two experimental agents that can increase bone formation. Sodium fluoride was the first agent other than estrogen to be used for specific treatment of osteoporosis. Although controlled clinical trials showed no benefit of sodium fluoride at a dose of 75 mg daily, more recent data support the use of a lower dose of sodium fluoride (50 mg daily) administered as a sustained-release preparation . Parathyroid hormone is also anabolic when administered subcutaneously as a single daily dose. Both of these drugs hold promise for restoration of lost bone, and they may eventually be useful agents in the treatment of established osteoporosis.

F. Treatment of Glucocorticoid-Induced Osteoporosis: The most important measure to prevent glucocorticoid-induced osteoporosis is to minimize the dose and duration of steroid therapy. Prophylactic measures to prevent the extraskeletal effects of glucocorticoids should be introduced at the onset of steroid therapy. These should include provision of an adequate intake of calcium (1500 mg daily) and vitamin D (400 IU) and treatment of sex hormone deficiency with estrogen in women and testosterone in men. Some authorities believe that reducing urinary calcium losses with thiazide diuretics may also be of benefit. Bone density should be determined by dual-energy x-ray absorptiometry at the outset of steroid use and again at 6–12 months; in individuals with a reduced bone density at baseline or a rapid rate of loss (> 5% per year), specific therapy should be considered. Cyclic etidronate therapy (400 mg daily for the first 2 weeks of each 3-month period) has been shown to reduce bone loss in glucocorticoid-induced osteoporosis. Alendronate also holds promise for this indication but has not yet been well studied. Calcitonin has also been reported to improve bone density in steroid-treated patients.

OSTEOMALACIA

Osteomalacia is defined as a defect in the mineralization of bone matrix. Early in the industrial revolution, it was endemic in cities as a manifestation of vitamin D deficiency. Osteomalacia is now less common, but it still occurs in vitamin D deficiency or because of lack of other components critical for the normal mineralization of bone matrix. In children with osteomalacia, the mineralization of bone at the growth plate is impaired, producing widening and disorganization of the growth plate (epiphysial dysplasia), retardation of longitudinal bone growth, and a variety of skeletal deformities. This complex is known as **rickets.**

Pathology

In rickets, the growth plate is widened because cartilage cells in the growth plate proliferate abundantly but fail to mineralize the surrounding matrix. In osteomalacia, the characteristic pathologic changes involve bone remodeling. Impaired mineralization of bone matrix, or osteoid, results in the accumulation of large surfaces of unmineralized osteoid in thick seams. Overlying the osteoid seams are numerous active osteoblasts. It must be emphasized that osteomalacia is quite difficult to diagnose in a routine bone biopsy because unmineralized osteoid cannot be distinguished from mineralized bone after decalcification of the specimen for sectioning and staining. Thus, specialized bone biopsy techniques must be used for the diagnosis. The bone biopsy specimen is embedded without decalcification, and sections are cut with a special microtome. Tetracycline can be administered before obtaining the biopsy to label the mineralizing bone surface. If two tetracycline labels are administered 2 weeks apart, they can be visualized as a pair of fluorescent lines at sites of bone formation, and the distance between the lines is a measure of the amount of bone that was mineralized in the interval between the two labels. In osteomalacia, undecalcified bone sections will have thickened osteoid seams, greatly increased coverage of the bone surface by osteoid, reduced tetracycline labeling, and a reduction in the mineralization rate as measured by double tetracycline labeling. When osteomalacia is caused by vitamin D deficiency, associated findings of secondary hyperparathyroidism may be present, such as large numbers of osteoclasts and fibrosis of the bone marrow.

Pathophysiology

Normal mineralization of bone requires several components. There must be an adequate supply of the minerals calcium and phosphate; bone cells must be capable of synthesizing the enzyme alkaline phosphatase, which is required for bone mineralization; and toxic factors must be absent. The causes of osteomalacia can be grouped into categories as shown in Table 8–13). The largest group consists of disorders of vitamin D availability, synthesis, or action. These disorders produce osteomalacia, in large part at least because reduced intestinal absorption of calcium and phosphate leads to an inadequate supply of these minerals at the mineralizing surface. Rachitic cartilage will mineralize in vitro in the presence of normal concentrations of calcium and phosphate. Loss of the many direct effects of vitamin D on the osteoblast is thought to be of secondary importance

Table 8–13. Causes of osteomalacia and rickets.

Vitamin D abnormalities
  Nutritional deficiency (rare)
  Malabsorption
  Impaired activation
    Hereditary vitamin D-dependent rickets type 1 (renal
      25-OH-vitamin D 1α-hydroxylase deficiency)
  End-organ resistance
    Hereditary vitamin D-dependent rickets type II (absent or
      defective vitamin D receptor)

Phosphate deficiency
  Renal phosphate wasting
    X-linked hypophosphatemic rickets
    Autosomal recessive hypophosphatemic rickets
    X-linked recessive hypophosphatemic rickets
    Fanconi's syndrome
    Renal tubular acidosis (type II)
    Oncogenous osteomalacia (acquired, associated with
      mesenchymal tumors)
  Malabsorption
    Phosphate-binding antacids

**Deficient alkaline phosphatase: hereditary
  hypophosphatasia**

Toxic
  Fluoride
  Aluminum (chronic renal failure)
  Etidronate disodium therapy
  Phosphate-binding antacids

Chronic renal failure

Fibrogenesis imperfecta ossium

in osteomalacia because experimental osteomalacia can be healed by the provision of calcium and phosphate and because osteomalacia in patients with hereditary resistance to vitamin D can also be healed by chronic infusions of calcium. A second group consists of disorders that produce hypophosphatemia, thus limiting the availability of phosphate for mineralization of bone. A third type of osteomalacia is caused by inherited defects in the synthesis of alkaline phosphatase. Finally, certain drugs, including the bisphosphonate etidronate and the anabolic agent sodium fluoride, are toxic to the mineralizing osteoblast.

Clinical Features

A. Symptoms and Signs: The manifestations of osteomalacia depend not only upon the severity and duration of the disorder but also on the patient's age. The symptoms of osteomalacia are bone pain and sometimes bone tenderness. In vitamin D-deficient osteomalacia, proximal muscle weakness can also be a prominent feature, producing a characteristic waddling gait. Proximal myopathy is uncommon in other forms of osteomalacia, eg, hypophosphatemic osteomalacia. Rickets produces short stature because of impaired growth plate function in growing long bones and produces deformities of bone that include frontal bossing of the cranium, bulging of the costochondral junctions (the "rachitic rosary"), lateral indentation of the chest wall at the diaphragmatic insertion (Harrison's groove), bowing of the long bones, and varus or valgus deformities of the knee. In adults with osteomalacia, skeletal deformities are very uncommon.

B. Laboratory Findings: The laboratory features of osteomalacia depend upon the cause. In vitamin D deficiency, the 25-hydroxyvitamin D level is low. Nearly all of the other laboratory abnormalities can be related to progressive secondary hyperparathyroidism. Progressive hypophosphatemia occurs because of reduced absorption as well as secondary hyperparathyroidism. The serum calcium level may be normal in earlier stages of osteomalacia, reflecting the relative success of secondary hyperparathyroidism in maintaining calcium homeostasis in the extracellular fluid, but it is also reduced in the late stages of the disease. The serum alkaline phosphatase is usually high. The concentration of PTH is elevated. The serum $1,25(OH)_2D$ is often normal, though a "normal" level is inappropriate in the face of hypophosphatemia, hypocalcemia, and secondary hyperparathyroidism. The excretion of calcium in a 24-hour urine specimen is very low, and urinary calcium can be virtually undetectable. Other urinary findings include a lowered renal tubular threshold for phosphate, signifying secondary hyperparathyroidism, and generalized aminoaciduria, which is also thought to be related to secondary hyperparathyroidism. In hypophosphatemic rickets, the renal phosphate threshold is usually decreased, indicating the presence of a primary renal phosphate wasting state. The alkaline phosphatase is high. The level of serum calcium and the concentration of PTH are both normal in untreated patients, though mild secondary hyperparathyroidism is seen in patients treated with large doses of oral phosphate. The urinary calcium may be low but seldom as low as it can be in vitamin D deficiency.

C. Imaging Studies: Advanced rickets gives rise to widening of the epiphyses, fraying of the epiphysial ends, and widening and cupping of the metaphyses, all manifestations of epiphysial dysplasia and delayed mineralization at the growth plate. In adults with osteomalacia, the skeleton is demineralized and the cortices are thin. These changes, however, are indistinguishable radiologically from osteoporosis. The pathognomonic feature of osteomalacia is the presence of pseudofractures, also known as Looser's zones or Milkman's syndrome. These are discrete zones of bone rarefaction that have the appearance of nondisplaced fractures and most often occur at sites where arteries cross the bones. Pseudofractures are often bilaterally symmetric, and the most common locations are the femoral neck and shaft, the pubic and ischial rami, the clavicles, ribs, and scapulae, and the radius and ulna (Figure 8–27). Their cause is unknown, but they heal promptly with treatment of osteomalacia. In addition to bone rarefaction and pseudofractures, vitamin D-deficient osteomalacia may

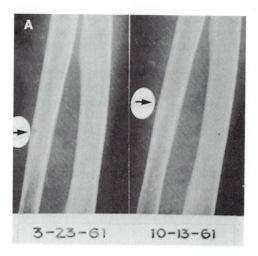
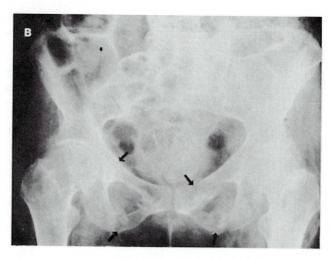

Figure 8–27. ***A:*** X-rays of the radius and ulna of a patient with severe osteomalacia, showing healing of a pseudofracture (arrows) during seven months of treatment with ergocalciferol. ***B:*** X-ray of the pelvis, showing pseudofractures (Looser's zones, or Milkman's fractures) in a woman with severe osteomalacia. (Courtesy of G Gordan.)

also evidence signs of hyperparathyroidism, such as subperiosteal bone resorption.

Specific Disorders

A. Vitamin D Abnormalities: Osteomalacia is a feature of nutritional vitamin D deficiency, malabsorption of vitamin D, abnormal metabolism of vitamin D, and peripheral resistance to vitamin D.

1. Nutritional vitamin D deficiency–Formerly common, nutritional deficiency of vitamin D is now very uncommon in the USA because of supplementation of foods with the vitamin. It can develop only when both the diet and exposure to ultraviolet light are inadequate. This occasionally occurs in vegans not given vitamin D supplementation. Three stages of the development of rickets can be distinguished: In stage I, hypocalcemia is the only significant biochemical abnormality. In stage II, the serum calcium concentration returns to normal but hypophosphatemia appears because of the development of secondary hyperparathyroidism. Stage III encompasses symptomatic rickets, worsening hypophosphatemia, and the recurrence of hypocalcemia, reflecting the failure of PTH to resorb sufficient calcium from severely osteomalacic bone.

2. Malabsorption of vitamin D–A fat-soluble substance, vitamin D depends upon the action of pancreatic lipases and bile salts for its absorption. Malabsorption of vitamin D may be a complication of pancreatic insufficiency, the loss of bile salts, or diffuse disorders of the intestinal mucosa, such as celiac disease. It would appear that in the sunlight-exposed patient, endogenous synthesis of vitamin D should compensate for impaired absorption, but there is evidence of active enterohepatic recirculation of 25-hydroxyvitamin D, suggesting that endogenously syn-

thesized vitamin D metabolites may be lost in malabsorption syndromes. The bone disease associated with malabsorption syndromes is complex; many patients present with diffuse osteoporosis rather than osteomalacia.

3. Abnormal vitamin D metabolism–Abnormalities in the conversion of vitamin D to its 25-hydroxy metabolite in the liver are rarely associated with significant osteomalacia. Osteomalacia does not occur in severe liver disease, and in the United States osteomalacia is uncommon in patients treated with anticonvulsant drugs that enhance the oxidation of vitamin D in the liver, shunting metabolism away from 25-hydroxyvitamin D. The conversion of 25-hydroxyvitamin D to $1,25(OH)_2D$ is severely impaired in chronic renal failure, and this contributes significantly to the pathogenesis of renal osteodystrophy. However, pure osteomalacia is seen only rarely in this setting.

Vitamin D-dependent rickets type I is a rare autosomal recessive trait which is thought to be due to deficiency of the renal 25-hydroxyvitamin D 1α-hydroxylase. Patients present with severe rickets, hypocalcemia, and low circulating $1,25(OH)_2D$ levels, and their bone disease is healed by provision of physiologic doses of $1,25(OH)_2D$.

4. Peripheral resistance to vitamin D–Vitamin D-dependent rickets type II is a rare disorder caused by mutations in the vitamin D receptor that impair the transcriptional response to vitamin D. This autosomal recessive trait is characterized by severe rickets, hypocalcemia, normal levels of 25-hydroxyvitamin D, and elevated circulating levels of $1,25(OH)_2D$. In some patients the disorder is associated with alopecia totalis. Several mutations of the VDR have been identified in the syndrome. Some impair vitamin D binding; others prevent binding of the receptor to DNA. A few patients have shown dramatic healing of their bone disease with chronic intravenous infusions of calcium, demonstrating that healing of rickets does not require a functional vitamin D receptor in bone and thus suggesting that the critical function of vitamin D is to provide sufficient calcium to mineralizing bone and cartilage surfaces, presumably by stimulating the intestinal absorption of calcium.

B. Hypophosphatemic Disorders: The hypophosphatemic conditions most commonly associated with rickets are hereditary and acquired disorders of renal phosphate wasting. The classic form is familial X-linked hypophosphatemic rickets. Although uncommon, this disorder is the predominant cause of childhood rickets. Affected males are severely rachitic; the penetrance of bone disease is variable in female carriers. The serum phosphorus is very low because of renal phosphate wasting. The concentration of $1,25(OH)_2D$ in serum is often in the lower range of normal—inappropriately low for a hypophosphatemic individual. The serum calcium and parathyroid hormone concentrations are normal. The bone disease responds to aggressive phosphate supplementation, with the addition of $1,25(OH)_2D$ to prevent secondary hyperparathyroidism (see Treatment, below). It has long been debated whether X-linked hypophosphatemic rickets is caused by an intrinsic defect in the Na^+-HPO_4^- cotransporter in the renal proximal tubule or by a defect extrinsic to the kidney. In a mouse model, the *hyp* mouse, renal phosphate wasting is attributable to an extrinsic lesion because transplantation of a normal kidney into a *hyp* mouse does not cure the disorder and, conversely, transplantation of a *hyp* kidney into a normal mouse does not induce phosphate wasting. The locus of X-linked hypophosphatemia in humans has recently been identified by positional cloning. Surprisingly, the candidate gene on the X chromosome encodes for an endopeptidase, whose tissue distribution and whose role in the pathogenesis of phosphate wasting remain to be clarified.

Several other renal phosphate wasting conditions also produce hypophosphatemic osteomalacia. Heritable disorders include **autosomal recessive hypophosphatemic rickets,** which is associated with osteosclerosis; and **X-linked recessive hypophosphatemic rickets,** which has recently been associated with mutations in a renal chloride channel—a channel which is also mutated in hypercalciuric nephrolithiasis (Dent's disease) and X-linked recessive nephrolithiasis. Rickets and osteomalacia also occur in **Fanconi's syndrome,** a generalized renal transport disorder. **Oncogenous osteomalacia** is an acquired disorder of renal phosphate wasting and osteomalacia that is caused by benign or malignant tumors—usually mesenchymal tumors—or by fibrous dysplasia. Such tumors must secrete a humoral factor that induces phosphaturia, since the syndrome can be cured by resection of the tumor. It is further discussed in Chapter 23.

C. Hypophosphatasia: Hypophosphatasia is a rare cause of rickets and osteomalacia. It may be inherited as an autosomal recessive or an autosomal dominant trait, and in some cases a mutation in the gene for the liver-kidney-bone form of alkaline phosphatase has been identified. The biochemical features of the disorders are low alkaline phosphatase activity, high serum and urinary levels of inorganic pyrophosphate and phosphoryl ethanolamine, and hypercalcemia in children. It is assumed that the bone disease reflects an essential role of alkaline phosphatase in the mineralization process.

D. Drug-Induced Osteomalacia: Fluoride is a potent inhibitor of mineralization and may cause severe rickets or osteomalacia in areas of endemic fluorosis or in patients treated with pharmacologic doses of sodium fluoride, usually more than 40 mg/d. The bisphosphonate etidronate disodium also produces osteomalacia, uncommonly at the usual dose of 5 mg/kg/d but more commonly at doses of 10–20 mg/kg/d, which have been used for treatment of Paget's disease. The newer bisphosphonates have a considerably reduced propensity to cause osteomalacia, but a few cases of mild osteomalacia have been reported with repeated intravenous administration of pamidronate disodium.

Diagnosis

The diagnosis of osteomalacia is straightforward when the features of rickets are present or when radiologic examination in a patient with bone pain discloses pseudofractures. In some patients the biochemical features of severe vitamin D deficiency or renal phosphate wasting lead to a presumptive diagnosis of osteomalacia and the institution of therapy. However, the milder forms of the disorder may be difficult to diagnose biochemically. In vitamin D deficiency, cases of osteomalacia are seen in which the serum concentrations of calcium and phosphorus are normal or the alkaline phosphatase is normal. Bone biopsy with tetracycline labeling and quantitative histomorphometry of undecalcified sections is required in these instances to make a definitive diagnosis, and several laboratories offer quantitative histomorphometry as a service.

Treatment

Vitamin D-deficient osteomalacia may be treated with replacement doses of vitamin D (400 IU) but will heal more rapidly if treated with higher doses. Patients with malabsorption may require as much as 50,000–100,000 IU of ergocalciferol (vitamin D_2), and in this instance calcifediol ($25(OH)D_3$) offers the benefits of precise formulation and better absorption (Table 8–7); if the response is poor in either case, the blood level of $25(OH)D_3$ can be monitored. Even with large doses, the likelihood of vitamin D intoxication is minimized by the tight regulation of renal activation of vitamin D. An adequate supply of calcium and phosphate should be provided; the diet is often adequate, but particularly in cases of malabsorption, the diet should be supplemented with 1000 mg of elemental calcium (Table 8–12). The initial response is an increase in the serum $1,25(OH)_2D$ levels; thereafter, the serum phosphorus concentration will be normalized within 4–8 days. In severe cases, the serum calcium concentration may initially fall and the alkaline phosphatase rise as bone is rapidly mineralized, but even in these cases the serum calcium concentration will be normalized within weeks. Bone pain and muscle weakness improve within weeks, but full restoration of muscle strength may require many months.

The treatment of rickets caused by phosphate-wasting disorders consists of supplying enough phosphate to compensate for renal losses. Phosphate is provided as frequent doses (eg, 3–5 g daily, administered every 4 hours). Coadministration of calcitriol (0.25–1 μg daily) is necessary to prevent hypocalcemia as a result of large oral phosphate doses and to optimize bone healing. The provision of an active vitamin D metabolite has been shown to increase the mature height attained in children treated with oral phosphate supplementation. Careful monitoring is required to maintain a normal serum calcium, and urinary calcium excretion should also be measured, as there is a high incidence of medullary nephrocalcinosis with this regimen, as determined by renal sonography. It is not clear whether there is substantial benefit to adults from this kind of aggressive treatment regimen.

PAGET'S DISEASE OF BONE
(Osteitis Deformans)

Paget's disease is a focal disorder of bone remodeling that leads to greatly accelerated rates of bone turnover, disruption of the normal architecture of bone, and sometimes to gross deformities of bone. As a focal disorder it is not, strictly speaking, a metabolic bone disease. Paget's disease is highly prevalent in northern Europe, particularly in England and Germany, where up to 4% of people over age 40 are affected. It is also common in the United States but is unusual in Africa and Asia.

Etiology

It has long been thought that Paget's disease, with its late onset and spotty involvement of the skeleton, might be due to a chronic slow virus infection of

bone. Inclusion bodies that resemble paramyxovirus inclusions have been identified in pagetic osteoclasts, and the presence of measles virus DNA has recently been detected by molecular cloning. However, considerably more work would be required to prove the infectious etiology of Paget's disease. There are also familial clusters of the disease, with up to 20% of patients in some studies having afflicted first-degree relatives.

Pathology

At the microscopic level, the disorder is characterized by highly vascular and cellular bone, consistent with its high metabolic activity. The osteoclasts are sometimes huge and bizarre, with up to 100 nuclei per cell. Because pagetic ostoclasts initiate the bone remodeling cycle in a chaotic fashion, the end result of remodeling is a mosaic pattern of lamellar bone. Paget's disease (and other high turnover states) can also produce woven bone—bone that is laid down rapidly and in a disorganized fashion, without the normal lamellar architecture.

Pathogenesis

Abnormal osteoclastic bone resorption is the probable initiating event in Paget's disease. Not only are the osteoclasts very abnormal histologically and prone to unruly behavior, but some forms of the disease are marked by an early resorptive phase in which pure osteolysis occurs without an osteoblastic response. Additionally, Paget's disease responds dramatically to inhibitors of osteoclastic bone resorption.

The rate of bone resorption is often increased by as much as 10- to 20-fold, and this is reflected in biochemical indices of bone resorption, including urinary excretion of collagen metabolites like hydroxyproline and pyridinoline cross-linked peptides of collagen. Over the skeleton as a whole, osteoblastic new bone formation responds appropriately to this challenge. Even though local disparities in remodeling may result in areas with the radiographic appearance of osteolysis or dense new bone, there is a linear relationship between biochemical markers of bone resorption (eg, urinary hydroxyproline) and biochemical markers of bone formation (eg, alkaline phosphatase). Because this tight coupling is maintained in Paget's disease in the face of enormously increased skeletal turnover rates, systemic mineral homeostasis is usually unperturbed. The serum calcium is normal, and calcium balance is maintained. (When patients with extensive Paget's disease are immobilized, they may become hypercalciuric or even hypercalcemic, as do immobilized patients in other high turnover states, but this is rare.)

Clinical Features

A. Symptoms and Signs: Paget's disease may affect any of the bones, but the most common sites are the sacrum and spine (50% of patients), the femur

(46%), the skull (28%), and the pelvis (22%). The clinical features of Paget's disease are pain, fractures, deformity, or manifestations of the neurologic, rheumatologic or metabolic complications of the disease. However, at least two-thirds of patients are asymptomatic. Thus, Paget's disease is often discovered as an incidental radiologic finding or during the investigation of an elevated alkaline phosphatase level. On physical examination, enlargement of the skull, frontal bossing, or deafness may be evident. Involvement of the weight-bearing long bones of the lower extremity often results in bowing. The femur and tibia bow anteriorly and laterally, but the fibula is almost never affected by Paget's disease. Cutaneous erythema and warmth, as well as bone tenderness, may be evident over affected areas of the skeleton, reflecting greatly increased blood flow through pagetic bone. The findings of pain, warmth, and erythema led to the appellation osteitis deformans, though Paget's disease is not truly an inflammatory disorder. The most common fractures in Paget's disease are vertebral crush fractures and incomplete "fissure" fractures through the cortex, usually on the convex surface of the tibia or femur. Affected bones may fracture completely; when they do, healing is usually rapid and complete—the increased metabolic activity of pagetic bone seems to favor fracture healing.

B. Laboratory Findings: The serum alkaline phosphatase and urinary hydroxyproline are usually increased, sometimes to very high levels. Levels of the newer biochemical markers of bone turnover are also high, but it is not clear that their determination offers any special benefit. The serum osteocalcin level is usually increased less than the alkaline phosphatase. The serum calcium and phosphorus and the urinary calcium are normal.

C. Imaging Studies: The early stages of Paget's disease are often osteolytic. Examples are erosion of the temporal bone of the skull, osteoporosis circumscripta, and pagetic lesions in the extremities, which begin in the metaphysis and migrate down the shaft as a V-shaped resorptive front (Figure 8–28). Over years, or even decades, the typical mixed picture of late Paget's disease evolves. Trabeculae are thickened and coarse. The bone may be enlarged or bowed. In the pelvis, the iliopectineal line or pelvic brim is often thickened (Figure 8–29). In the spine, osteoblastic lesions of the vertebral bodies may present a "picture-frame" appearance or a homogeneously increased density, the "ivory vertebra." Associated osteoarthritis may present with narrowing of the joint space (Figure 8–29). Osteosarcoma may present with cortical destruction or a soft tissue mass (Figure 8–29). Radionuclide bone scanning with technetium-labeled bisphosphonates or other bone-seeking agents is uniformly positive in active Paget's disease and is useful for surveying the skeleton when a focus of Paget's disease has been found radiographically (Figure 8–30).

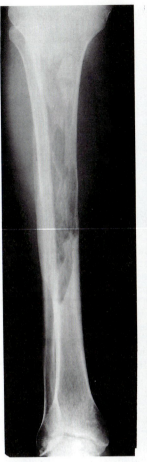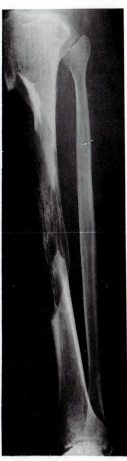

Figure 8–28. Lytic Paget's disease in the tibia before (left) and after (right) immobilization in a cast. The lytic area has a flame- or V-shaped leading edge (left). (Reproduced, with permission, from Strewler GJ: Paget's disease of bone. West J Med 1984;140:763.)

Complications

Complications of Paget's disease may be neurologic, rheumatologic, neoplastic, or cardiac (Table 8–14).

A. Neurologic: The brain, spinal cord, and peripheral nerves are all at risk. Sensorineural deafness occurs in up to 50% of patients in whom the skull is involved, and compression of the other cranial nerves can also occur. At the base of the skull, Paget's disease can produce platybasia and basilar impression of the brain stem, with symptoms of brain stem compression, obstructive hydrocephalus, or vertebrobasilar insufficiency. Spinal stenosis is common in vertebral Paget's disease, in part because the pagetic vertebra can be enlarged, and may spread posteriorly when collapse occurs, but spinal stenosis responds well to medical treatment of the disease. Peripheral nerve entrapment syndromes include carpal and tarsal tunnel syndromes.

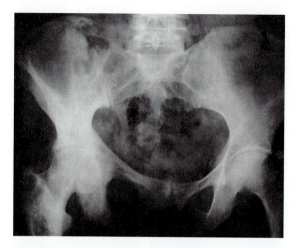

Figure 8–29. Paget's disease of the right femur and pelvis. The right femur displays cortical thickening and coarse trabeculation. The right ischium is enlarged, with sclerosis of ischial and pubic rami and the right ilium. Two complications of Paget's disease are present. There is concentric bilateral narrowing of the hip joint space, signifying osteoarthritis. The destructive lesion interrupting the cortex of the right ilium is an osteosarcoma. (Reproduced, with permission, from Strewler GJ: Paget's disease of bone. West J Med 1984;140:763.)

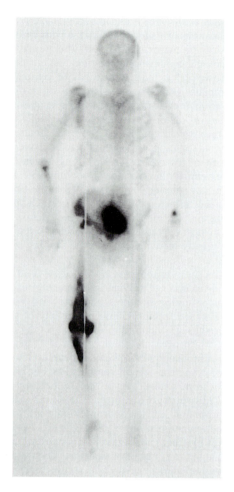

Figure 8–30. Bone scan of a patient with Paget's disease of the skull, spine, pelvis, right femur, and acetabulum. Note localization of bone-seeking isotope (^{99m}Tc-labeled bisphosphonate) in these areas.

B. Rheumatologic: Osteoarthritis is common in Paget's disease. It may be an unrelated finding in elderly patients with the disorder, or it may result directly from pagetic deformities and their effects on wear and tear in the joints. Arthritis presents a conundrum to the clinician attempting to relieve pain, as it may be difficult to determine whether the pain originates in pagetic bone or in the nearby joint. An association of osteitis deformans and gout was first noted by James Paget himself, and asymptomatic hyperuricemia is also common.

C. Neoplastic: The most terrible complication of Paget's disease is development of bone sarcoma. The tumor arises in pagetic bone, typically in individuals with polyostotic involvement, and may present with soft tissue swelling, increased pain, or a rapidly increasing alkaline phosphatase. Osteosarcoma, chondrosarcoma, and giant cell tumors all occur in Paget's disease, with a combined incidence of about 1%. Because osteosarcoma is otherwise uncommon in the elderly, fully 30% of elderly patients with osteosarcoma have underlying Paget's disease.

D. Cardiac: High-output congestive heart failure occurs rarely and is due to markedly increased blood flow to bone, usually in patients with more than 50% involvement of the skeleton.

Treatment

Bone pain in a pagetic patient that is unresponsive to nonsteroidal anti-inflammatory agents deserves a trial of specific therapy. As noted above, it may not be easy to differentiate pagetic bone pain from associated osteoarthritis. The other indications for treatment of Paget's disease are controversial. Treatment has been advocated for neurologic compression syndromes, as preparation for surgery, and to prevent deformities. Neurologic deficits often respond to medical treatment, and a trial of treatment is often warranted. Pretreatment for 2–3 months before orthopedic surgery will prevent excessive bleeding and postoperative hypercalcemia, but satisfactory bone healing usually occurs without medical treatment. Paget's disease is sometimes treated in the hope of arresting the progress of deformities, eg, bowing of the extremities and resultant osteoarthritis, but it is not certain whether medical treatment can achieve this aim or whether it will arrest the progression of deafness in patients with skull involvement.

Three classes of agents are used in the treatment of

Table 8–14. Complications of Paget's disease.

Rheumatologic
  Osteoarthritis
  Gout
  Calcific periarthritis
  Rheumatoid arthritis

Neurologic
  Basilar impression
  Cranial nerve dysfunction (especially deafness)
  Spinal cord and root compression
  Peripheral nerve entrapment (carpal and tarsal tunnel
    syndromes)

Metabolic
  Immobilization hypercalciuria-hypercalcemia
  Urolithiasis

Neoplastic
  Bone sarcoma
  Giant cell tumor

Paget's disease: the calcitonins, the bisphosphonates, and plicamycin. All are inhibitors of osteoclastic bone resorption.

A. Salmon Calcitonin: Salmon calcitonin is administered initially at a dose of 50–100 IU daily until symptoms are improved; thereafter, many patients can be maintained on 50 units three times a week. Improvement in pain is usually evident within 2–6 weeks. On average, the alkaline phosphatase and urinary hydroxyproline will fall by 50% within 3–6 months, with the alkaline phosphatase lagging slightly behind the hydroxyproline. Many patients will have a sustained response to treatment extending over years, and the biochemical parameters are often suppressed for 6 months to 1 year after treatment is discontinued. Up to 20% of patients receiving chronic calcitonin treatment will develop late resistance to calcitonin, which may be antibody-mediated. Human calcitonin therapy has been uniformly effective in these patients. Salmon calcitonin nasal spray has recently become available, but data on its efficacy in Paget's disease are limited.

B. Bisphosphonates: The bisphosphonate etidronate disodium has long been available for treatment of Paget's disease and is clearly beneficial in controlled clinical trials. It is administered in a dose of 5 mg/kg/d for 6 months, and about 60% of patients will respond biochemically. However, some patients will experience worsening of bone pain or lytic bone lesions, and etidronate can impair bone mineralization, particularly at higher doses.

Two newer bisphosphonates appear to be superior to etidronate. Alendronate disodium may be administered orally in a dose of 40 mg daily for 6 months. On average, alkaline phosphatase is suppressed 80%. Biochemical remissions are often prolonged for more than 1 year after the drug is stopped. The main side effect is significant gastrointestinal upset, requiring discontinuation of therapy in about 6% of patients. It may be more convenient or more timely to administer

an equivalent dose of bisphosphonate intravenously. Pamidronate disodium, a bisphosphonate closely related to alendronate, has been used for this purpose, though in the United States it is approved only for treatment of hypercalcemia. Administered in one to four intravenous infusions of 60 mg, pamidronate produces a high remission rate and a durable response. The principal side effect observed with intravenous administration is an acute phase response, including fever and myalgia, that occurs in about 20% of patients and may last for several days after a dose.

C. Plicamycin: Plicamycin is a cytotoxic antibiotic that has been used as a "last resort" in Paget's disease unresponsive to less toxic agents. With the advent of the newer bisphosphonates, there will be few indications for treatment with plicamycin.

RENAL OSTEODYSTROPHY

Bone disease is an almost universal feature of chronic renal failure and requires special measures for prophylaxis and treatment. The best-understood form of renal osteodystrophy is secondary hyperparathyroidism, which occurs in renal insufficiency because of inadequate renal synthesis of $1,25(OH)_2D$ and because of retention of phosphate by the failing kidney. However, as measures to control secondary hyperparathyroidism have improved, a second form of renal osteodystrophy, adynamic renal osteodystrophy, has also emerged.

Pathogenesis

A. Secondary Hyperparathyroidism: An increase in the serum level of PTH is first seen when the creatinine clearance drops below 40 mL/min, and secondary hyperparathyroidism is virtually universal with a creatinine clearance less than 20 mL/min. The precipitating event is probably a defect in renal $1,25(OH)_2D$ synthesis, with reduced intestinal absorption of calcium and a secondary increase in the secretion of PTH to protect the serum calcium level (Figure 8–31). This initial defect in activation of vitamin D is related to altered renal handling of phosphate. With reduced nephron number, the remaining nephrons must handle more phosphate per nephron to maintain external phosphate balance. The best evidence that altered phosphate handling leads to early renal osteodystrophy is that $1,25(OH)_2D$ levels rise and PTH levels fall when phosphate intake is restricted in early renal failure.

At least two factors exacerbate secondary hyperparathyroidism in patients being maintained on chronic dialysis (Figure 8–31). The first is retention of phosphate. Dialytic treatments cannot clear phos-

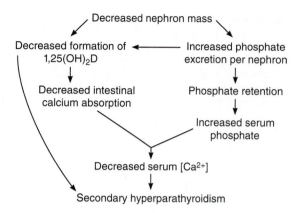

Figure 8–31. Schema for the pathogenesis of renal osteodystrophy.

phate as efficiently as the kidney, and phosphate retention in chronic dialysis is a major challenge to calcium homeostasis. As the product of serum calcium and serum phosphorus rises to 60–70 (eg, serum calcium 10 mg/dL, serum phosphorus 6–7 mg/dL), the solubility product of calcium × phosphate is exceeded, and amorphous deposits of calcium phosphate are laid down in soft tissues and bone. Increased bone resorption is induced by PTH to compensate for the efflux of calcium from the extracellular fluid, but the compensatory rise in bone resorption releases phosphate as well as calcium from bone, thus setting up a vicious circle in which each increment in bone resorption necessitates a further increase in the PTH level. Management of the dietary intake of phosphate is an important control measure. Coupling of bone turnover is maintained in renal osteodystrophy, and the markedly increased bone resorption in the hyperparathyroid form of renal osteodystrophy is coupled with similar increases in bone resorption; thus, this form of renal osteodystrophy is a high-turnover state of bone.

A second mechanism that perpetuates secondary hyperparathyroidism acts at the parathyroid gland itself, where low $1,25(OH)_2D$ levels release the gland from the normal tonic inhibition of PTH release, permitting higher levels of PTH to be secreted. This stimulus to hyperparathyroidism can be controlled by providing adequate amounts of $1,25(OH)_2D$ or another active form of the vitamin.

Rarely, frank hypercalcemia occurs in renal failure because of severe secondary hyperparathyroidism or "tertiary hyperparathyroidism" (Figure 8–31). The preferred management of the hypercalcemic patient is subtotal parathyroidectomy. Although it is theoretically possible to achieve hypercalcemia because of a large mass of hyperplastic but otherwise normal parathyroid tissue under normal secretory control (severe secondary hyperparathyroidism), the glands removed at surgery from such patients are often

monoclonal, indicating that their cells all arose from a single progenitor cell, and are thus indistinguishable from parathyroid adenomas (tertiary hyperparathyroidism). It is likely that hyperplastic parathyroid tissue is susceptible to oncogenic mutations because of its increased mitotic rate.

B. Adynamic Renal Osteodystrophy: The pathogenesis of adynamic bone disease in renal failure is much less well understood than the pathogenesis of secondary hyperparathyroidism. Adynamic renal osteodystrophy was once uncommon, but with the increased success of measures to control secondary hyperparathyroidism, it has emerged as a significant problem and now accounts for 20–60% of cases of renal osteodystrophy, depending on the population. In the adynamic variant, bone is hypocellular and bone turnover is very low. Low bone turnover was initially attributed to deposition of aluminum at bone-forming surfaces. Bone can be exposed to high tissue levels of aluminum because it is poorly dialyzed and because of the intake of high levels of aluminum in inadequately demineralized dialysate or in the form of aluminum-containing antacids, which are sometimes administered in large amounts to bind phosphate in the gastrointestinal tract. However, it has become clear that adynamic bone disease is also common in dialysis patients who were never exposed to excessive amounts of aluminum and have not accumulated stainable aluminum in bone matrix. Risk factors for adynamic bone disease include the use of peritoneal dialysis with supraphysiologic calcium concentrations, use of calcium carbonate, and diabetes mellitus, as well as aluminum use. All of these circumstances will tend to reduce secretion of PTH, and the PTH level is markedly lower in patients with adynamic bone disease than in other forms of renal osteodystrophy. Secondary hyperparathyroidism, by inducing a high-turnover state, may protect bone from other insults of the uremic environment which, when unmasked, eventuate in hypocellular bone with low rates of turnover.

Clinical Features

A. Symptoms and Signs: Patients with mild renal osteodystrophy are often asymptomatic, but more severe cases have bone pain and tenderness, pathologic fractures, and muscle weakness. In the hyperparathyroid form of renal osteodystrophy, extraskeletal calcium deposition also occurs, with vascular calcification, periarticular calcification, cutaneous calcification with uremic pruritus, and sometimes a syndrome called calciphylaxis, consisting of digital gangrene. Both uremic itching and calciphylaxis may respond dramatically to parathyroidectomy.

B. Laboratory Findings: The biochemical features of renal osteodystrophy are variable. In the early stages of the hyperparathyroid form, the serum calcium and phosphorus are normal. With the progression of renal failure to dialysis, the serum phosphorus rises, sometimes to high levels; the serum calcium may be normal or low, depending on how successfully the syndrome is managed with calcium and vitamin D supplementation. In the most severe form of the disease, hypercalcemia and a high alkaline phosphatase level occur, and the serum phosphorus is high and very difficult to manage. All of these alterations reflect greatly increased bone turnover.

C. Imaging Studies: Radiographically, renal osteodystrophy may display signs of hyperparathyroidism, such as subperiosteal bone resorption and cortical tunneling (Figure 8–32); or evidence of osteosclerosis, often occurring near the end plates of adjacent vertebrae to produce a striped appearance—the "rugger jersey spine." Osteoporosis is uncommon. Vascular calcification may be evident. The bone scan shows diffusely increased uptake, and extraskeletal calcification is sometimes evident as uptake of the tracer in the stomach, lungs, or heart.

Treatment

Measures to control secondary hyperparathyroidism should be instituted in the predialysis period, when the creatinine clearance reaches 20–40 mL/min. These measures should include supplementation with oral calcium and a moderate dietary phosphate restriction. If the PTH level does not fall with these measures, a vitamin D preparation may be added (Table 8–7). The most useful in renal failure are those that do not require renal activation, such as calcitriol ($1,25[OH]_2D_3$) or the analog dihydrotachysterol. When phosphate retention occurs, it is necessary to restrict dietary phosphate further and to introduce agents to bind dietary phosphate in the gastrointestinal tract and prevent its absorption. The first choice for this purpose is oral calcium, which for this purpose is often administered as calcium acetate (Table 8–12). The calcium intake can be pushed to 5–10 g/d so long as hypercalcemia is avoided. Compared with calcium carbonate, calcium acetate seems to provide equivalent phosphate binding at about one-half the calcium intake. If necessary, aluminum hydroxide preparations can be added to improve phosphate binding. However, these are second-line agents that should be used in moderation because of the recognized toxicities of aluminum.

If, despite these measures, significant hyperpara-

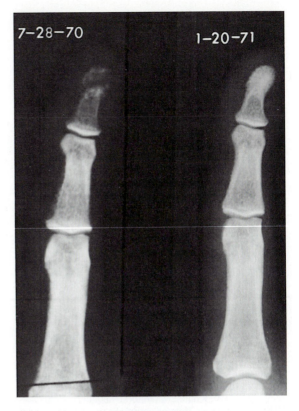

Figure 8–32. X-rays of index finger of a patient before (left) and after (right) plasma phosphate was reduced to normal with aluminum hydroxide gel and dialysis against a high calcium bath (reproduced, with permission, from Vosik WM et al: Successful medical management of osteitis fibrosa due to tertiary hyperparathyroidism. Mayo Clin Proc 1972;47:110.)

thyroidism has been established, calcitriol can be given intravenously (0.5–3 μg) three times weekly. The use of intravenous calcitriol often permits aggressive suppression of PTH secretion without hypercalcemia. It is thought that the pharmacokinetics of intravenous calcitriol, with its relatively short half-life, favor parathyroid suppression over stimulation of calcium absorption, and this accounts for the efficacy of the intravenous route. Patients who are frankly hypercalcemic or who have uremic pruritus or calciphylaxis may require subtotal parathyroidectomy.

REFERENCES

Calcium Metabolism

Berridge MJ: Inositol trisphosphate and calcium signaling. Nature 1993;361:315.

Strewler, GJ, Rosenblatt M: Mineral metabolism. In: *Endocrinology and Metabolism,* 3rd ed. Felig P, Baxter JD, Frohman LA (editors). McGraw-Hill, 1995.

Parathyroid Hormone

Bilezikian JP et al: *The Parathyroids.* Raven Press, 1994.

Bringhurst FR et al: Peripheral metabolism of PTH: Fate of biologically active amino terminus in vivo. Am J Physiol 1988;255:E886.

Brown EM et al: The cloning of extracellular Ca^{2+}-sensing receptors from parathyroid and kidney: Molecular mechanisms of extracellular Ca^{2+}-sensing. J Nutr 1995;125(7 Suppl):1965S.

Brown EM: Homeostatic mechanism regulating extracellular and intracellular calcium metabolism. In: *The Parathyroids.* Bilezikian JP et al (editors), Raven Press, 1994.

Jüppner H: Functional properties of the PTH/PTHrP receptor. Bone 1995;(2 Suppl):39S.

Kronenberg HM et al: Parathyroid hormone biosynthesis and metabolism. In: *The Parathyroids.* Bilezikian JP et al (editors) Raven Press, 1994.

LiVolsi VA: Embryology, anatomy, and pathology of the parathyroids. In: *The Parathyroids.* Bilezikian JP et al (editors). Raven Press, 1994.

Nussbaum SR, Potts JT Jr: Advances in immunoassays for parathyroid hormone. In: *The Parathyroids.* Bilezikian JP et al (editors). Raven Press, 1994.

Segre GV: Receptors for parathyroid hormone and parathyroid hormone-related protein. In: *The Parathyroids.* Bilezikian JP et al (editors) Raven Press, 1994.

Spiegel AM, Weinstein LS: G proteins as transducers of parathyroid hormone action. In: *The Parathyroids.* Bilezikian JP et al (editors), Raven Press, 1994.

Calcitonin

Martin TJ, Moseley JM: Calcitonin. In: *Metabolic Bone Disease and Clinically Related Disorders,* 2nd ed. Avioli LV, Krane SM (editors). Saunders, 1990.

Martin TJ, et al: Heterogeneity of the calcitonin receptor: Functional aspects in osteoclasts and other sites. J Nutr 1995;125:2009S.

Vitamin D

Bikle DD, Pillai S: Vitamin D, calcium, and epidermal differentiation. Endocr Rev 1993;14:3.

Bikle DD: Clinical Counterpoint—Vitamin D: New actions, new analogs, new therapeutic potential. Endocr Rev 1992;13:765.

Bouillon R et al: Structure-function relationships in the vitamin D endocrine system. Endocr Rev 1995;16:200.

Haussler MR et al: New understanding of the molecular mechanism of receptor-mediated genomic actions of the vitamin D hormone. Bone 1995;17:33S.

Holick MF, Adams JS: Vitamin D metabolism and biological function. In: *Metabolic Bone Disease and Clinically Related Disorders.* 2nd ed. Avioli LV, Krane SM (editors). Saunders, 1990.

Kumar R: Metabolism of 1,25-dihydroxyvitamin D_3. Physiol Rev 1984;64:478.

Mangelsdorf DJ et al: The nuclear receptor superfamily: The second decade. Cell 1995;83:835.

Okuda K et al: Recent progress in enzymology and molecular biology of enzymes involved in vitamin D metabolism. J Lipid Res 1995;36:1641.

Stern PH: Vitamin D and bone. Kidney Int 1990;38:S17.

Suda T et al: Role of vitamin D in bone resorption. J Cell Biochem 1992;49:53.

Medullary Thyroid Carcinoma

Ledger GA et al: Genetic testing in the diagnosis and management of multiple endocrine neoplasia type II. Ann Intern Med 1995;122:118.

Lips CJ et al: Clinical screening as compared with DNA analysis in families with multiple endocrine neoplasia type 2A. N Engl J Med 1994;331:828.

Moley JF: Medullary thyroid cancer. Surg Clin North Am 1995;75:405.

Mulligan LM, Ponder BA: Genetic basis of endocrine disease: Multiple endocrine neoplasia type 2. J Clin Endocrinol Metab 1995;80:1989.

Snow KJ, Boyd AE 3rd: Management of individual tumor syndromes: Medullary thyroid carcinoma and hyperparathyroidism. Endocrinol Metab Clin North Am 1994;23:157.

Hypercalcemic Disorders

Arnold A et al: Monoclonality of parathyroid tumors in chronic renal failure and in primary parathyroid hyperplasia. J Clin Invest 1995;95:2047.

Arnold A: Molecular mechanisms of parathyroid neoplasia. Endocrinol Metab Clin North Am 1994;23:93.

Bilezikian JP: Management of acute hypercalcemia. N Engl J Med 1992;326:1196.

Cryns VL et al: Loss of the retinoblastoma tumor-suppressor gene in parathyroid carcinoma. N Engl J Med 1994;330:757.

Heath H 3rd: Familial benign hypercalcemia: From clinical description to molecular genetics. West J Med 1994;160:554.

Joborn C et al: Maximal isokinetic muscle strength in patients with primary hyperparathyroidism before and after parathyroid surgery. Br J Surg 1988;75:77.

Joborn C et al: Primary hyperparathyroidism in patients with organic brain syndrome. Acta Med Scand 1986; 219:91.

Joborn C et al: Self-rated psychiatric symptoms in patients operated on because of primary hyperparathyroidism and in patients with long-standing mild hypercalcemia. Surgery 1989;105:72.

Kapsner P et al: Milk-alkali syndrome in patients treated with calcium carbonate after cardiac surgery. Arch Int Med 1986;146:1965.

Mallette LE: Pseudohypoparathyroidism. Curr Ther Endocrinol Metab 1994;5:532.

Melton LJ 3d et al: Risk of age-related fractures in patients with primary hyperparathyroidism. Arch Intern Med 1992;152:2269.

Mitchell BK et al: Primary hyperparathyroidism: Preoperative localization using technetium-sestamibi scanning. (Editorial.) J Clin Endocrinol Metab 1995;80:7.

NIH Consensus Development Conference: Diagnosis and management of asymptomatic primary hyperparathyroidism. Ann Intern Med 1991;114:593.

Nussbaum SR: Pathophysiology and management of severe hypercalcemia. Endocrinol Metab Clin North Am 1993;22:343.

Palmer M et al: Survival and renal function in untreated hypercalcemia. Lancet 1987;1:59.

Potts JT Jr (editor): Proceedings of the NIH consensus development conference on diagnosis and management of asymptomatic primary hyperparathyroidism. J Bone Miner Res 1991;6(Suppl 2):1.

Rao DS et al: Lack of biochemical progression or continuation of accelerated bone loss in mild asymptomatic primary hyperparathyroidism: Evidence of biphasic disease course. J Clin Endocrinol Metab 1988;67:1294.

Shane E, Bilezikian JP: Parathyroid carcinoma: A review of 62 patients. Endocr Rev 1982;3:218.

Silverberg SJ et al: Longitudinal measurements of bone density and biochemical indices in untreated primary hyperparathyroidism. J Clin Endocrinol Metab 1995; 80:723.

Silverberg SJ et al: Increased bone mineral density after parathyroidectomy in primary hyperparathyroidism. J Clin Endocrinol Metab 1995;80:729.

Stern PH, De Olazabal J, Bell NH: Evidence for abnormal regulation of circulating 1α,25-dihydroxyvitamin D in patients with sarcoidosis and normal calcium metabolism. J Clin Invest 1980;66:852.

Strewler GJ: Indications for surgery in patients with minimally symptomatic hyperparathyroidism. Surg Clin North Am 1995;75:439.

Hypocalcemic Disorders

Bassett JH, Thakker RV: Molecular genetics of disorders of calcium homeostasis. Baillieres Clin Endocrinol Metab 1995;9:581.

Brasier AR, Nussbaum SR: Hungry bone syndrome: Clinical and biochemical predictors of its occurrence after parathyroid surgery. Am J Med 1988;84:654.

Levine MA et al: Pseudohypoparathyroidism. In: *The Parathyroids.* Bilezikian JP et al (editors). Raven Press, 1994.

Li Y et al: Autoantibodies to the extracellular domain of the calcium sensing receptor in patients with acquired hypoparathyroidism. J Clin Invest 1996;97:910.

Weinstein LS, Shenker A: G protein mutations in human disease. Clin Biochem 1993;26:333.

Whyte MP: Autoimmune aspects of hypoparathyroidism. In: *The Parathyroids.* Bilezikian JP et al (editors). Raven Press, 1994.

Bone Anatomy and Remodeling

Aubin JE et al: Osteoblast and chondroblast differentiation. Bone 1995;17:77S.

Delmas PD: Biochemical markers of bone turnover. J Bone Miner Res 1993;8:S549.

Suda T et al: Modulation of osteoclast differentiation by local factors. Bone 1995;17:87S.

Suda T et al: Modulation of osteoclast differentiation. Endocr Rev 1992;13:66.

Osteoporosis

Cummings SR, Black D: Bone mass measurements and risk of fracture in Caucasian women: A review of findings from prospective studies. Am J Med 1995; 98:24S.

Cummings SR et al: Bone density at various sites for prediction of hip fractures. Lancet 1993;341:72.

Cummings SR et al: Risk factors for hip fracture in white women. Study of Osteoporotic Fractures Research Group. N Engl J Med 1995;332:767.

Dawson-Hughes B et al: A controlled trial of the effect of calcium supplementation on bone density in postmenopausal women. N Engl J Med 1990;323:878.

Dawson-Hughes B et al: Effect of vitamin D supplementation on wintertime and overall bone loss in healthy postmenopausal women. Ann Intern Med 1991;115: 505.

Delmas PD: Diagnostic procedures for osteoporosis in the elderly. Horm Res 1995;43:80.

Eisman JA: Vitamin D receptor gene alleles and osteoporosis: An affirmative view. (Editorial.) J Bone Miner Res 1995;10:1289.

Finkelstein JS et al: Parathyroid hormone for the prevention of bone loss induced by estrogen deficiency. N Engl J Med 1994;331:1618.

Grady D et al: Hormone therapy to prevent disease and prolong life in postmenopausal women. Ann Intern Med 1992;117:1016.

Grampp S et al: Radiologic diagnosis of osteoporosis: Current methods and perspectives. Radiol Clin North Am 1993;31:1133.

Johnston CC Jr, Slemenda CW: Pathogenesis of osteoporosis. Bone 1995;17:19S.

Johnston CC Jr et al: Calcium supplementation and increases in bone mineral density in children. N Engl J Med 1992;327:82.

Johnston CC Jr et al: Clinical use of bone densitometry. N Engl J Med 1991;324:1105.

Kelepouris N et al: Severe osteoporosis in men. Ann Intern Med 1995;123:452.

Liberman UA et al: Effect of oral alendronate on bone mineral density and the incidence of fractures in postmenopausal osteoporosis. N Engl J Med 1995;333:1437.

Lukert BP, Raisz LG: Glucocorticoid-induced osteoporosis. Rheum Dis Clin North Am 1994;20:629.

Norman AW, Collins ED: Correlation between vitamin D receptor allele and bone mineral density. Nutr Rev 1994;52:147.

Pak CY et al: Treatment of postmenopausal osteoporosis with slow-release sodium fluoride: Final report of a randomized controlled trial. Ann Intern Med 1995; 12:401.

Riggs BL, Melton LJ 3d: *Osteoporosis: Etiology, Diagnosis, and Management,* 2nd ed. Lippincott-Raven, 1995.

Riggs BL, Melton LJ 3d: The prevention and treatment of osteoporosis. N Engl J Med 1992;327:620.

Sowers M: Epidemiology of calcium and vitamin D in bone loss. J Nutr 1993;123:413.

Tinetti ME et al: A multifactorial intervention to reduce the risk of falling among elderly people living in the community. N Engl J Med 1994;331:821.

Watts NB et al: Intermittent cyclical etidronate treatment of postmenopausal osteoporosis. N Engl J Med 1990; 323:73.

Osteomalacia

Hutchison FN, Bell NH: Osteomalacia and rickets. Semin Nephrol 1992;12:127.

The HYP Consortium: A gene *(PEX)* with homologies to endopeptidases is mutated in patients with X-linked hypophosphatemic rickets. Nat Genet 1995;11:130.

Lloyd SE et al: A common molecular basis for three inherited kidney stone diseases. Nature 1996;379:445.

Parfitt AM: Osteomalacia and related disorders. In: *Metabolic Bone Disease and Clinically Related Disorders,* 2nd ed. Avioli LV, Krane SM (editors) Saunders, 1990.

Tovey FI et al: A review of postgastrectomy bone disease. J Gastroenterol Hepatol 1992;7:639.

Paget's Disease

Hamdy RC: Clinical features and pharmacologic treatment of Paget's disease. Endocrinol Metab Clin North Am 1995;24:421.

Klein RM, Norman A: Diagnostic procedures for Paget's disease: Radiologic, pathologic, and laboratory testing. Endocrinol Metab Clin North Am 1995; 24:437.

Mirra JM et al: Paget's disease of bone: Review with emphasis on radiologic features. Part I. Skeletal Radiol 1995;24:163.

Mirra JM et al: Paget's disease of bone: Review with emphasis on radiologic features. Part II. Skeletal Radiol 1995;24:173-184.

Singer FR, Minoofar PN: Bisphosphonates in the treatment of disorders of mineral metabolism. Adv Endocrinol Metab 1995;6:259.

Siris E et al: Comparative study of alendronate versus etidronate for the treatment of Paget's disease of bone. J Clin Endocrinol Metab 1996;81:961.

Strewler GH: Paget's disease of bone. West J Med 1984; 140:763

Renal Osteodystrophy

Delmez JA et al: Calcium acetate as a phosphorus binder in hemodialysis patients. J Am Soc Nephrol 1992; 3:96.

Goodman WG et al: Calcium-regulated parathyroid hormone release in patients with mild or advanced secondary hyperparathyroidism. Kidney Int 1995;48:1553.

Pei Y et al: Risk factors for renal osteodystrophy: A multivariant analysis. J Bone Miner Res 1995;10:149.

Portale AA et al: Physiologic regulation of the serum concentration of 1,25-dihydroxyvitamin D by phosphorus in normal men. J Clin Invest 1989;83:1494.

Sherrard DJ et al: The spectrum of bone disease in end-stage renal failure—an evolving disorder. Kidney Int 1993;43:436.

Slatopolsky E, Delmez JA: Pathogenesis of secondary hyperparathyroidism. Miner Electrolyte Metab 1995; 21:91.

Glucocorticoids & Adrenal Androgens

9

James W. Findling, MD, David C. Aron, MD, MS, & J. Blake Tyrrell, MD

The adrenal cortex produces many steroid hormones of which the most important are cortisol, aldosterone, and the adrenal androgens. Disorders of the adrenal glands lead to classic endocrinopathies such as Cushing's syndrome, Addison's disease, hyperaldosteronism, and the syndromes of congenital adrenal hyperplasia. This chapter describes the physiology and disorders of the glucocorticoids and the adrenal androgens. Disorders of aldosterone secretion are discussed in Chapter 10 and congenital defects in adrenal hormone biosynthesis in Chapters 10 and 14. Hirsutism and virilization (which reflect excess androgen action) are discussed in Chapter 13.

Advances in diagnostic procedures have simplified the evaluation of adrenocortical disorders; in particular, the assay of plasma glucocorticoids, androgens, and ACTH has allowed more rapid and precise diagnosis. In addition, advances in surgical and medical treatment have improved the outlook for patients with these disorders.

EMBRYOLOGY & ANATOMY

Embryology

The adrenal cortex is of mesodermal origin and is identifiable as a separate organ in the 2-month-old fetus. At 2 months' gestation, the cortex is composed of a **fetal zone** and a **definitive zone** similar to the adult adrenal cortex. The adrenal cortex then increases rapidly in size; at mid gestation it is considerably larger than the kidney and much larger than the adult gland in relation to total body mass. The fetal zone makes up the bulk of the weight of the adrenal cortex at this time. Factors other than ACTH, such as insulin-like growth factor II, may be involved in the development of the fetal adrenal cortex.

The fetal adrenal is under the control of ACTH by mid pregnancy, but the fetal zone is deficient in the activity of 3β-hydroxysteroid dehydrogenase (see section on biosynthesis of cortisol and adrenal androgens, below) and thus produces mainly dehydroepiandrosterone (DHEA) and DHEA sulfate, which serve as precursors of maternal-placental estrogen

ACRONYMS USED IN THIS CHAPTER	
ACTH	Adrenocorticotropic hormone
ADH	Antidiuretic hormone (vasopressin)
cAMP	Cyclic adenosine monophosphate
CBG	Corticosteroid-binding globulin
CRH	Corticotropin-releasing hormone
DHEA	Dehydroepiandrosterone
DNA	Deoxyribonucleic acid
DOC	Deoxycorticosterone
GH	Growth hormone
GIP	Gastrointestinal inhibitory polypeptide
GnRH	Gonadotropin-releasing hormone
HLA	Human leukocyte antigen
HPLC	High-performance liquid chromatography
IPSS	Inferior petrosal sinus sampling
LH	Luteinizing hormone
LPH	Lipotropin
mRNA	Messenger ribonucleic acid
NADPH	Dihydronicotinamide adenine dinucleotide phosphate
P450scc	Side-chain cleavage enzyme
PMN	Polymorphonuclear neutrophil
PPNAD	Primary pigmented nodular adrenocortical disease
PRA	Plasma renin activity
PRL	Prolactin
PTH	Parathyroid hormone
REM	Rapid eye movement
RNA	Ribonucleic acid
SHBG	Sex hormone-binding globulin
TRH	Thyrotropin-releasing hormone
TSH	Thyroid-stimulating hormone (thyrotropin)
VLCFA	Very long chain fatty acids

production after conversion in the liver to 16α-hydroxylated derivatives. The definitive zone synthesizes a number of steroids and is the major site of fetal cortisol synthesis.

Anatomy

The anatomic relationship of the fetal and definitive zones is maintained until birth, at which time the fetal zone gradually disappears, with a consequent decrease in adrenocortical weight in the 3 months following delivery. During the next 3 years, the adult adrenal cortex develops from cells of the outer layer of the cortex and differentiates into the three adult zones: glomerulosa, fasciculata, and reticularis.

The adult adrenal glands, with a combined weight of 8–10 g, lie in the retroperitoneum above or medial to the upper poles of the kidneys (Figure 9–1). A fibrous capsule surrounds the gland; the yellowish outer cortex comprises 90% of the adrenal weight, the inner medulla about 10%.

The adrenal cortex is richly vascularized and receives its main arterial supply from branches of the inferior phrenic artery, the renal arteries, and the aorta. These small arteries form an arterial plexus beneath the capsule and then enter a sinusoidal system that penetrates the cortex and medulla, draining into a single central vein in each gland. The right adrenal vein drains directly into the posterior aspect of the vena cava; the left adrenal vein enters the left renal vein. These anatomic features account for the fact that it is relatively easier to catheterize the left adrenal vein than it is to catheterize the right adrenal vein.

Microscopic Anatomy

Histologically, the adult cortex is composed of three zones: an outer zona glomerulosa, a zona fasciculata, and an inner zona reticularis (Figure 9–2). However, the inner two zones appear to function as a unit (see below). The **zona glomerulosa,** which produces aldosterone, is deficient in 17α-hydroxylase activity and thus cannot produce cortisol or androgens (see below and Chapter 10). The zona glomerulosa lacks a well-defined structure, and the small lipid-poor cells are scattered beneath the adrenal capsule. The **zona fasciculata** is the thickest layer of the adrenal cortex and produces cortisol and androgens. The cells of the zona fasciculata are larger and contain more lipid and thus are termed "clear cells." These cells extend in columns from the narrow zona reticularis to either the zona glomerulosa or to the capsule. The inner **zona reticularis** surrounds the medulla and also produces cortisol and androgens. The "compact" cells of this narrow zone lack significant lipid content but do contain lipofuscin granules. The zonae fasciculata and reticularis are regulated by ACTH; excess or deficiency of this hormone alters their structure and function. Thus, both zones atrophy when ACTH is deficient; when ACTH is present in excess, hyperplasia and hypertrophy of these zones occur. In addition, chronic stimulation with ACTH leads to a gradual depletion of the lipid from the clear cells of the zona fasciculata at the junction of the two zones; these cells thus attain the characteristic appearance of the compact reticularis cells. With chronic excessive stimulation, the compact reticularis

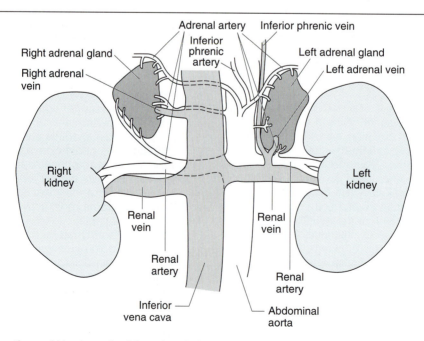

Figure 9–1. Location and blood supply of the adrenal glands (schematic). (Reproduced, with permission, from Baxter JD, Tyrrell JB: The adrenal cortex. In: *Endocrinology and Metabolism.* Felig P et al [editors]. 3rd ed. McGraw-Hill, 1995.)

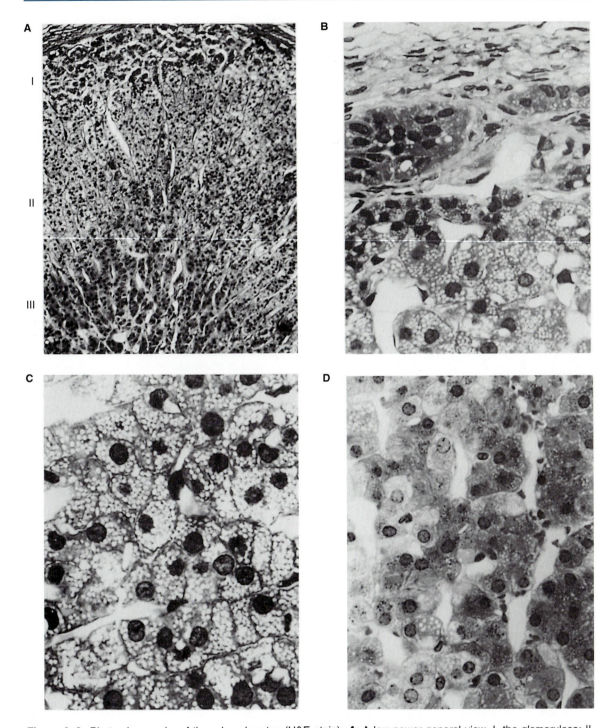

Figure 9–2. Photomicrographs of the adrenal cortex (H&E stain). **A:** A low-power general view. I, the glomerulosa; II, the fasciculata; III, the reticularis. × 80. **B:** The capsule and the zona glomerulosa. × 330. **C:** The zona fasciculata. × 330. **D:** The zona reticularis. × 330. (Reproduced, with permission, from Junqueira LC, Carneiro J: *Basic Histology,* 7th ed. Appleton & Lange, 1992.)

cells extend outward and may reach the outer capsule. It is postulated that the zona fasciculata cells can respond acutely to ACTH stimulation with increased cortisol production, whereas the reticularis cells maintain basal glucocorticoid secretion and that induced by prolonged ACTH stimulation.

BIOSYNTHESIS OF CORTISOL & ADRENAL ANDROGENS

Steroidogenesis

The major hormones secreted by the adrenal cortex are cortisol, the androgens, and aldosterone. The carbon atoms in the steroid molecule are numbered as shown in Figure 9–3, and the major biosynthetic pathways and hormonal intermediates are illustrated in Figures 9–4 and 9–5.

The scheme of adrenal steroidogenic synthesis has been clarified by analysis of the steroidogenic enzymes. Most of these enzymes belong to the family of cytochrome P450 oxygenases. In mitochondria, P450scc is responsible for side-chain cleavage of cholesterol. In humans, two separate but closely re-

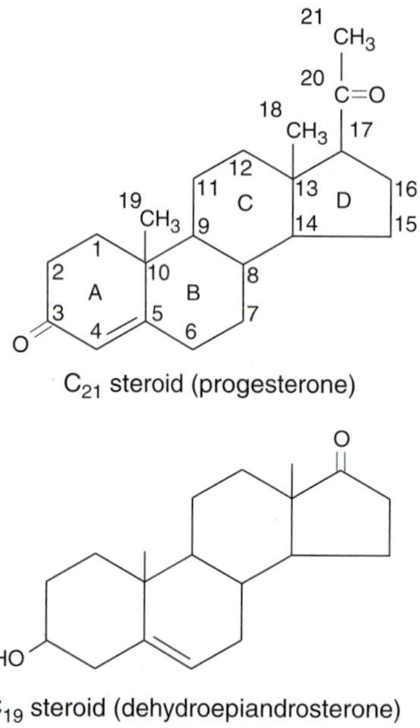

Figure 9–3. Structure of adrenocortical steroids. The letters in the formula for progesterone identify the A, B, C, and D rings; the numbers show the positions in the basic C-21 steroid structure. The angular methyl groups (positions 18 and 19) are usually indicated simply by straight lines, as in the lower formula. Dehydroepiandrosterone is a "17-ketosteroid" formed by cleavage of the side chain of the C-21 steroid 17-hydroxypregnenolone and its replacement by an O atom. (Reproduced, with permission, from Ganong WF: *Review of Medical Physiology,* 14th ed. Appleton & Lange, 1989.)

lated mitochondrial enzymes mediate 11β-hydroxylation, and the zona reticularis mediates conversion of 11-deoxycortisol to cortisol and 11-deoxycorticosterone to corticosterone. In the zona glomerulosa, P450aldo (also known as aldosterone synthase and P450cmo) mediates 11β-hydroxylation, 18-hydroxylation, and 18-oxidation to convert 11-deoxycorticosterone → corticosterone → 18-hydroxycorticosterone → aldosterone. In the endoplasmic reticulum, the single enzyme P450c17 mediates both 17α-hydroxylase activity and 17,20-lyase activity, while P450c21 mediates the 21-hydroxylation of both progesterone and 17-hydroxyprogesterone. The 3β-hydroxysteroid dehydrogenase:$\Delta^{5,4}$-isomerase activities are mediated by a single non-P450 microsomal enzyme.

A. Zones and Steroidogenesis: Because of enzymatic differences between the zona glomerulosa and the inner two zones, the adrenal cortex functions as two separate units, with differing regulation and secretory products. Thus, the zona glomerulosa, which produces aldosterone, lacks 17α-hydroxylase activity and cannot synthesize 17α-hydroxypregnenolone and 17α-hydroxyprogesterone, which are the precursors of cortisol and the adrenal androgens. The synthesis of aldosterone by this zone is primarily regulated by the renin-angiotensin system and by potassium, as discussed in Chapter 10.

The zona fasciculata and zona reticularis (Figure 12–4) produce cortisol, androgens, and small amounts of estrogens. These zones, primarily regulated by ACTH, do not contain the enzyme P450aldo (aldosterone synthase, P450cmo) and therefore cannot convert 11-deoxycorticosterone to aldosterone. (See Chapter 10.)

B. Cholesterol Uptake and Synthesis: Synthesis of cortisol and the androgens by the zonae fasciculata and reticularis begins with cholesterol, as does the synthesis of all steroid hormones. Plasma lipoproteins are the major source of adrenal cholesterol, though synthesis within the gland from acetate also occurs. A small pool of free cholesterol within the adrenal is available for rapid synthesis of steroids when the adrenal is stimulated. When stimulation occurs, there is also increased hydrolysis of stored cholesteryl esters to free cholesterol, increased uptake from plasma lipoproteins, and increased cholesterol synthesis within the gland.

C. Cholesterol Metabolism: The conversion of cholesterol to pregnenolone is the rate-limiting step in adrenal steroidogenesis and the major site of ACTH action on the adrenal. This step occurs in the mitochondria and involves two hydroxylations and then the side-chain cleavage of cholesterol. A single enzyme, P450scc, mediates this process; each step requires molecular oxygen and a pair of electrons. The latter are donated by NADPH to adrenodoxin reductase, a flavoprotein, and then to adrenodoxin, an iron-sulfur protein, and finally to P450scc. Both adrenodoxin reductase and adrenodoxin are also in-

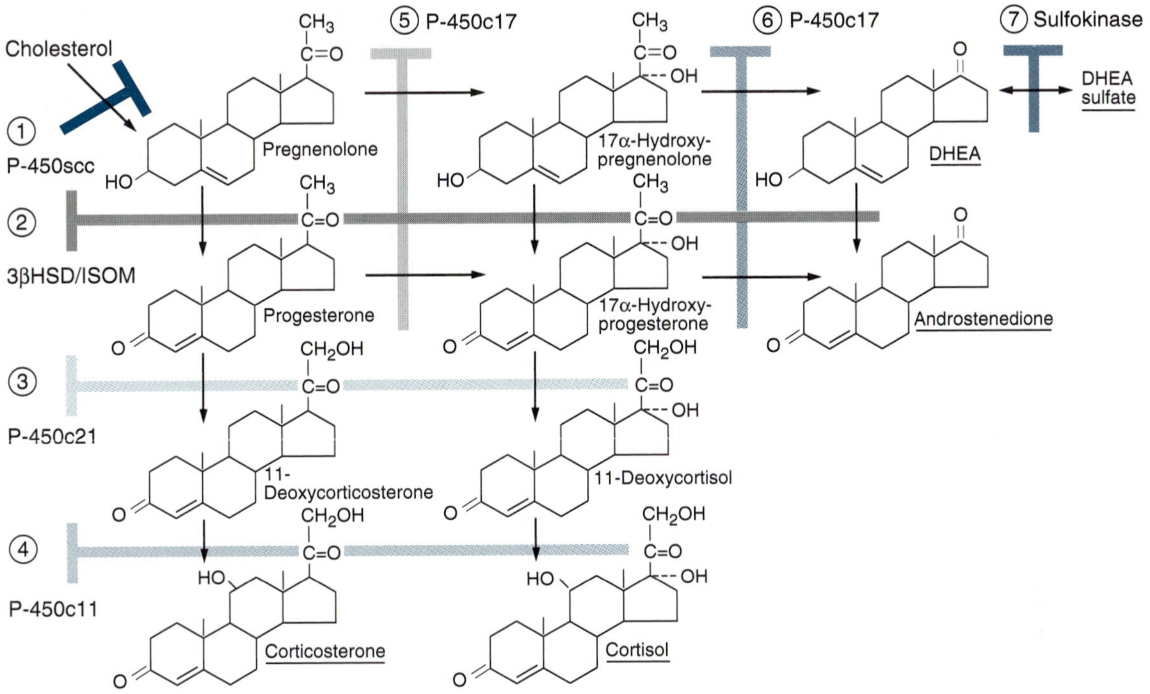

Figure 9–4. Steroid biosynthesis in the zona fasciculata and zona reticularis of the adrenal cortex. The major secretory products are underlined. The enzymes for the reactions are numbered on the left and at the top of the chart, with the steps catalyzed shown by the shaded bars. ① P450scc, cholesterol 20,22-hydroxylase:20,22 desmolase activity; ② 3βHSD/ISOM, 3-hydroxysteroid dehydrogenase:Δ^5-oxosteroid isomerase activity; ③ P450c21, 21α-hydroxylase activity; ④ P450c11 = 11β-hydroxylase activity; ⑤ P450c17, 17α-hydroxylase activity; ⑥ P450c17, 17,20-lyase/desmolase activity; ⑦ sulfokinase. (See also Figures 7–1, 9–2, 10–4, and 11–13.) (Modified and reproduced, with permission, from Ganong, WF: *Review of Medical Physiology,* 16th ed. Appleton & Lange, 1993.)

volved in the action of P450c11 (see above). Electron transport to microsomal cytochrome P450 involves P450 reductase, a flavoprotein distinct from adrenodoxin reductase. Pregnenolone is then transported outside the mitochondria before further steroid synthesis occurs.

D. Synthesis of Cortisol: Cortisol synthesis proceeds by P450c17 17α-hydroxylation of pregnenolone within the smooth endoplasmic reticulum to form 17α-hydroxypregnenolone. This steroid is then converted to 17α-hydroxyprogesterone after conversion of its 5,6 double bond to a 4,5 double bond by the 3β-hydroxysteroid dehydrogenase:$\Delta^{5,4}$-oxosteroid isomerase enzyme complex, which is also located within the smooth endoplasmic reticulum. An alternative but apparently less important pathway in the zonae fasciculata and reticularis is from pregnenolone → progesterone → 17α-hydroxyprogesterone (Figure 9–4).

The next step, which is again microsomal, involves the 21-hydroxylation by P450c21 of 17α-hydroxyprogesterone to form 11-deoxycortisol; this compound is further hydroxylated within mitochondria by 11β-hydroxylation (P450c11) to form cortisol. The zonae fasciculata and reticularis also pro-

duce 11-deoxycorticosterone (DOC), 18-hydroxydeoxycorticosterone, and corticosterone. However, as noted above, the absence of the mitochondrial enzyme P450aldo (aldosterone synthase, P450cmo) prevents production of aldosterone by these zones of the adrenal cortex (Figure 9–5).

E. Synthesis of Androgens: The production of adrenal androgens from pregnenolone and progesterone requires prior 17α-hydroxylation (P450c17) and thus does not occur in the zona glomerulosa. The major quantitative production of androgens is by conversion of 17α-hydroxypregnenolone to the 19-carbon compounds (C-19 steroids) DHEA and its sulfate conjugate DHEA sulfate. Thus, 17α-hydroxypregnenolone undergoes removal of its two-carbon side chain at the C_{17} position by microsomal 17,20-desmolase, yielding DHEA with a keto group at C_{17}. DHEA is then converted to DHEA sulfate by a reversible adrenal sulfokinase. The other major adrenal androgen, androstenedione, is produced from 17α-hydroxyprogesterone by 17,20-desmolase and to a lesser extent from DHEA. Androstenedione can be converted to testosterone, though adrenal secretion of this hormone is minimal. The adrenal androgens, DHEA, DHEA sulfate, and androstenedione, have

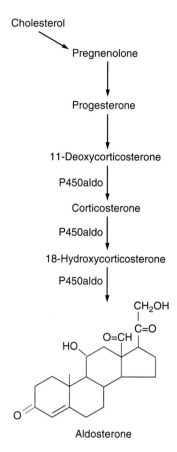

Cholesterol

↓

Pregnenolone

↓

Progesterone

↓

11-Deoxycorticosterone

P450aldo ↓

Corticosterone

P450aldo ↓

18-Hydroxycorticosterone

P450aldo ↓

Aldosterone

Figure 9–5. Steroid biosynthesis in the zona glomerulosa. The steps from cholesterol to 11-deoxycorticosterone are the same as in the zona fasciculata and zona reticularis. However, the zona glomerulosa lacks 17α-hydroxylase activity and thus cannot produce cortisol. Only the zona glomerulosa can convert corticosterone to 18-hydroxycorticosterone and aldosterone. The single enzyme P450aldo catalyses the conversion of 11-deoxycorticosterone → corticosterone → 18-hydroxycorticosterone → aldosterone. (See also Figures 7–1, 9–2, and 10–4.) (Modified and reproduced, with permission, from Ganong, WF: *Review of Medical Physiology,* 16th ed. Appleton & Lange, 1993.)

minimal intrinsic androgenic activity, and they contribute to androgenicity by their peripheral conversion to the more potent androgens testosterone and dihydrotestosterone. Although DHEA and DHEA sulfate are secreted in greater quantities, androstenedione is qualitatively more important, since it is more readily converted peripherally to testosterone (see Chapter 12).

Regulation of Secretion

A. Secretion of CRH and ACTH: ACTH is the trophic hormone of the zonae fasciculata and reticularis and the major regulator of cortisol and an-

drogen production by the adrenal cortex. ACTH in turn is regulated by the hypothalamus, vasopressin (AVP), and central nervous system via neurotransmitters and corticotropin-releasing hormone (CRH). The neuroendocrine control of CRH and ACTH secretion is discussed in Chapter 5 and involves three mechanisms to be discussed below.

B. ACTH Effects on the Adrenal Cortex: The delivery of ACTH to the adrenal cortex leads to the rapid synthesis and secretion of steroids; plasma levels of these hormones rise within minutes after ACTH administration. ACTH increases RNA, DNA, and protein synthesis. Chronic stimulation leads to adrenocortical hyperplasia and hypertrophy; conversely, ACTH deficiency results in decreased steroidogenesis and is accompanied by adrenocortical atrophy, decreased gland weight, and decreased protein and nucleic acid content.

C. ACTH and Steroidogenesis: ACTH binds to high-affinity plasma membrane receptors of adrenocortical cells, thereby activating adenylyl cyclase and increasing cAMP, which in turn activates intracellular phosphoprotein kinases (Figure 9–6). This process stimulates the rate-limiting step of cholesterol to Δ^5-pregnenolone conversion and initiates steroidogenesis. The exact mechanisms of ACTH stimulation of the side-chain cleavage enzyme (P450scc) are unknown, as is their relative impor-

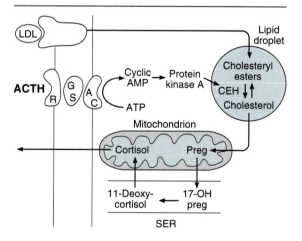

Figure 9–6. Mechanism of action of ACTH on cortisol-secreting cells in the inner two zones of the adrenal cortex. When ACTH binds to its receptor (R), adenylyl cyclase (AC) is activated via G_s. The resulting increase in cAMP activates protein kinase A, and the kinase phosphorylates cholesteryl ester hydrolase (CEH), increasing its activity. Consequently, more free cholesterol is formed and converted to pregnenolone in the mitochondria. Note that in the subsequent steps in steroid biosynthesis, products are shuttled between the mitochondria and the smooth endoplasmic reticulum (SER). (Reproduced, with permission, from Ganong WF: *Review of Medical Physiology,* 16th ed. Appleton & Lange, 1993.)

tance; however, ACTH has a number of effects, including increased free cholesterol formation as a consequence of increased cholesterol esterase activity and decreased cholesteryl ester synthetase, increased lipoprotein uptake by the adrenal cortex, increased content of certain phospholipids which may increase cholesterol side-chain cleavage, and increased binding of cholesterol to the cytochrome P450scc enzyme in mitochondria.

D. Neuroendocrine Control: Cortisol secretion is closely regulated by ACTH, and plasma cortisol levels parallel those of ACTH (Figure 9–7). There are three mechanisms of neuroendocrine control: (1) episodic secretion and the circadian rhythm of ACTH, (2) stress responsiveness of the hypothalamic-pituitary adrenal axis, and (3) feedback inhibition by cortisol of ACTH secretion.

1. Circadian rhythm–Circadian rhythm is superimposed on episodic secretion; it is the result of central nervous system events that regulate both the number and magnitude of CRH and ACTH secretory episodes. Cortisol secretion is low in the late evening and continues to decline in the first several hours of sleep, at which time plasma cortisol levels may be undetectable. During the third and fifth hours of sleep there is an increase in secretion, but the major secretory episodes begin in the sixth to eighth hours of sleep (Figure 9–7) and then begin to decline as wakefulness occurs. About half of the total daily cortisol output is secreted during this period. Cortisol secretion then gradually declines during the day, with fewer secretory episodes of decreased magnitude; however, there is increased cortisol secretion in response to eating and exercise.

Although this general pattern is consistent, there is considerable intra- and interindividual variability, and the circadian rhythm may be altered by changes in sleep pattern, light-dark exposure, and feeding times. The rhythm is also changed by (1) physical stresses such as major illness, surgery, trauma, or starvation; (2) psychologic stress, including severe anxiety, endogenous depression, and the manic phase of manic-depressive psychosis; (3) central nervous system and pituitary disorders; (4) Cushing's syndrome; (5) liver disease and other conditions that affect cortisol metabolism; (6) chronic renal failure; and (7) alcoholism. Cyproheptadine inhibits the circadian rhythm, possibly by its antiserotonergic effects, whereas other drugs usually have no effect.

2. Stress responsiveness–Plasma ACTH and cortisol secretion are also characteristically responsive to physical stress. Thus, plasma ACTH and cortisol are secreted within minutes following the onset of stresses such as surgery and hypoglycemia (Figure 9–8), and these responses abolish circadian periodicity if the stress is prolonged. Stress responses originate in the central nervous system and increase hypothalamic CRH and thus pituitary ACTH secretion. Stress responsiveness of plasma ACTH and cortisol is abolished by prior high-dose glucocorticoid administration and in spontaneous Cushing's syndrome; conversely, the responsiveness of ACTH secretion is enhanced following adrenalectomy. Regulation of the hypothalamic-pituitary-adrenal axis is linked to that of the immune system. For example, interleukin-1 (IL-1) stimulates ACTH secretion, and cortisol inhibits IL-2 synthesis.

3. Feedback inhibition–The third major regulator of ACTH and cortisol secretion is that of feedback inhibition by glucocorticoids of CRH, ACTH,

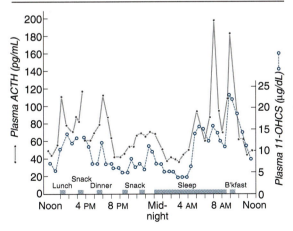

Figure 9–7. Fluctuations in plasma ACTH and glucocorticoids (11-OHCS) throughout the day. Note the greater ACTH and glucocorticoid rises in the morning before awakening. (Reproduced, with permission, from Krieger DT et al: Characterization of the normal temporal pattern of corticosteroid levels. J Clin Endocrinol Metab 1971;32:266.)

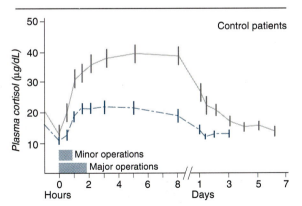

Figure 9–8. Plasma cortisol responses to major surgery (continuous line) and minor surgery (broken line) in normal subjects. Mean values and standard errors for 20 patients are shown in each case. (Reproduced, with permission, from Plumpton FS, Besser GM, Cole PV: Anaesthesia 1969;24:3.)

and cortisol secretion. Glucocorticoid feedback inhibition occurs at both the pituitary and hypothalamus and involves two distinct mechanisms—fast and delayed feedback inhibition (Figure 9–9).

Fast feedback inhibition of ACTH secretion is rate-dependent—ie, it depends on the rate of increase of the glucocorticoid but not the dose administered. This phase is rapid, and basal and stimulated ACTH secretion both diminish within minutes after the plasma glucocorticoid level increases. This fast feedback phase is transient and lasts less than 10 minutes, suggesting that this effect is not mediated via cytosolic glucocorticoid receptors but rather via actions on the cell membrane.

Delayed feedback inhibition after the initial rate-dependent effects of glucocorticoids further suppresses CRH and ACTH secretion by mechanisms that are both time- and dose-dependent. Thus, with continued glucocorticoid administration, ACTH levels continue to decrease and become unresponsive to stimulation. The ultimate effect of prolonged glucocorticoid administration is suppression of CRH and ACTH release and atrophy of the zonae fasciculata and reticularis as a consequence of ACTH deficiency. The suppressed hypothalamic-pituitary-adrenal axis fails to respond to stress and stimulation. Delayed feedback appears to act via the classic glucocorticoid receptor (see below), thus reducing synthesis of the messenger RNA for pro-opiomelanocortin, the precursor of ACTH.

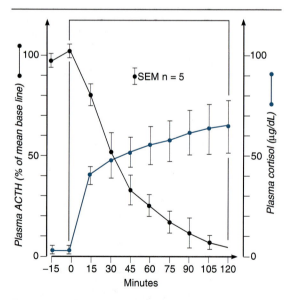

Figure 9–9. Feedback inhibition of plasma ACTH levels during intravenous cortisol infusion at a rate of 50 mg/h in patients with Addison's disease. ACTH values are expressed as percentages of mean basal levels. (Reproduced, with permission, from Fehm HL et al: J Clin Invest 1979;63:247.)

E. ACTH Effects on Regulation of Androgen Production: Adrenal androgen production in adults is also regulated by ACTH; both DHEA and androstenedione exhibit circadian periodicity in concert with ACTH and cortisol. In addition, plasma concentrations of DHEA and androstenedione increase rapidly with ACTH administration and are suppressed by glucocorticoid administration, confirming the role of endogenous ACTH in their secretion. DHEA sulfate, because of its slow metabolic clearance rate, does not exhibit a diurnal rhythm. Thus, adrenal androgen secretion is regulated by ACTH, and, in general, the secretion of these hormones parallels that of cortisol. The existence of a separate anterior pituitary hormone that regulates adrenal androgen secretion has been postulated but not yet proved. Several such factors have been identified in pituitary extracts.

CIRCULATION OF CORTISOL & ADRENAL ANDROGENS

Cortisol and the adrenal androgens circulate bound to plasma proteins. The plasma half-life of cortisol (70–90 minutes) is determined by the extent of plasma binding and by the rate of metabolic inactivation.

Plasma Binding Proteins

Cortisol and adrenal androgens are secreted in an unbound state; however, these hormones bind to plasma proteins upon entering the circulation. Cortisol binds mainly to corticosteroid-binding globulin (CBG, transcortin) and to a lesser extent to albumin, whereas the androgens bind chiefly to albumin. The precise physiologic role of plasma protein binding is unclear, since bound steroids are biologically inactive and the active fraction is that which circulates unbound. Furthermore, CBG is not required for cortisol transport to target tissues or for full biologic activity of the steroid. The plasma proteins may provide a pool of circulating cortisol by delaying metabolic clearance, thus preventing more marked fluctuations of plasma free cortisol levels during episodic secretion by the gland.

Free & Bound Cortisol

In basal conditions, about 10% of the circulating cortisol is free, about 75% is bound to CBG, and the remainder is bound to albumin. The plasma free cortisol level is approximately 1 µg/dL, and it is this biologically active cortisol which is regulated by ACTH.

A. Corticosteroid-Binding Globulin (CBG): CBG has a molecular weight of about 50,000, is produced by the liver, and binds cortisol with high affinity. The CBG in plasma has a cortisol-binding capacity of about 25 µg/dL. When total plasma cortisol concentrations rise above this level, the free concentration rapidly increases and exceeds its usual fraction of 10% of the total cortisol. Other endogenous steroids do not appreciably affect cortisol binding to CBG under usual circumstances; an exception is in late pregnancy, when progesterone may occupy about 25% of the binding sites on CBG. Synthetic steroids do not bind significantly to CBG—with the exception of prednisolone, which has a high affinity. CBG levels are increased in high-estrogen states (pregnancy; estrogen or oral contraceptive use), hyperthyroidism, diabetes, certain hematologic disorders, and on a genetic basis. CBG concentrations are decreased in familial CBG deficiency, hypothyroidism, and protein deficiency states such as severe liver disease or nephrotic syndrome.

B. Albumin: Albumin has a much greater capacity for cortisol binding but a lower affinity. It normally binds about 15% of the circulating cortisol, and this proportion increases when the total cortisol concentration exceeds the CBG binding capacity. Synthetic glucocorticoids are extensively bound to albumin; eg, 77% of dexamethasone in plasma is bound to albumin.

C. Androgen Binding: Androstenedione, DHEA, and DHEA sulfate circulate weakly bound to albumin. However, testosterone is bound extensively to a specific globulin, sex hormone-binding globulin (SHBG). (See Chapters 12 and 13.)

METABOLISM OF CORTISOL & ADRENAL ANDROGENS

The metabolism of the steroids renders them inactive and increases their water solubility, as does their subsequent conjugation with glucuronide or sulfate groups. These inactive conjugated metabolites are more readily excreted by the kidney. The liver is the major site of steroid catabolism and conjugation, and 90% of these metabolized steroids are excreted by the kidney.

Conversion & Excretion of Cortisol

Cortisol is modified extensively before excretion in urine; less than 1% of secreted cortisol appears in the urine unchanged.

A. Hepatic Conversion: Hepatic metabolism of cortisol involves a number of metabolic conversions of which the most important (quantitatively) is the irreversible inactivation of the steroid by Δ^4-reductases, which reduce the 4,5 double bond of the A ring. Dihydrocortisol, the product of this reaction, is then converted to tetrahydrocortisol by a 3-hydroxysteroid dehydrogenase. Cortisol is also converted extensively by 11-hydroxysteroid dehydrogenase to the biologically inactive cortisone, which is then metabolized by the enzymes described above to yield tetrahydrocortisone. Tetrahydrocortisol and tetrahydrocortisone can be further altered to form the cortoic acids. These conversions result in the excretion of approximately equal amounts of cortisol and cortisone metabolites. Cortisol and cortisone are also metabolized to the cortols and cortolones and to a lesser extent by other pathways. Cortisol is also converted to 6β-hydroxycortisol, which is water-soluble and excreted unchanged in the urine.

B. Hepatic Conjugation: Over 95% of cortisol and cortisone metabolites are conjugated by the liver and then reenter the circulation to be excreted in the urine. Conjugation is mainly with glucuronic acid at the 3α-hydroxyl position and to a lesser extent as the sulfate at the 21-hydroxyl group.

C. Variations in Clearance and Metabolism: The metabolism of cortisol is altered by a number of circumstances. It is decreased in infants and in the elderly. It is impaired in chronic liver disease, leading to decreased renal excretion of cortisol metabolites; however, the plasma cortisol level remains normal. Hypothyroidism decreases both metabolism and excretion; conversely, hyperthyroidism accelerates these processes. Cortisol clearance may be reduced in starvation and anorexia nervosa and is also decreased in pregnancy because of the elevated CBG levels. The metabolism of cortisol to 6β-hydroxycortisol is increased in the neonate, in pregnancy, with estrogen therapy, and in patients with liver disease or severe chronic illness. Cortisol metabolism by this pathway is also increased by drugs that induce hepatic microsomal enzymes, including barbiturates, phenytoin, mitotane, aminoglutethimide, and rifampin. These alterations generally are of minor physiologic importance, since secretion, plasma levels, and cortisol half-life are normal. However, they result in decreased excretion of the urinary metabolites of cortisol measured as 17-hydroxycorticosteroids. These conditions and drugs have a greater influence on the metabolism of synthetic glucocorticoids and may result in inadequate plasma levels of the administered glucocorticoid because of rapid clearance and metabolism.

D. Renal Conversion: Cortisol is also inactivated in the kidney by conversion to cortisone via the action of 11β-hydroxysteroid dehydrogenase. This inactivation is of major physiologic significance because it protects the mineralocorticoid receptor from occupancy by cortisol, and this prevents cortisol from causing a mineralocorticoid excess state. The quantitative role of this enzyme in total cortisol metabolism is unknown, but it has been demonstrated that plasma cortisone levels are reduced in patients with renal disease.

Conversion & Excretion of Adrenal Androgens

Adrenal androgen metabolism results either in degradation and inactivation or the peripheral conversion of these weak androgens to their more potent derivatives testosterone and dihydrotestosterone.

DHEA is readily converted within the adrenal to DHEA sulfate, the adrenal androgen secreted in greatest amount. DHEA secreted by the gland is also converted to DHEA sulfate by the liver and kidney, or it may be converted to Δ^4-androstenedione. DHEA sulfate may be excreted without further metabolism; however, both it and DHEA are also metabolized to 7α- and 16α-hydroxylated derivatives and by 17β-reduction to Δ^5-androstenediol and its sulfate. Androstenedione is converted either to testosterone or by reduction of its 4,5 double bond to etiocholanolone or androsterone, which may be further converted by 17α-reduction to etiocholanediol and androstanediol, respectively. Testosterone is converted to dihydrotestosterone in androgen-sensitive tissues by 5β-reduction, and it in turn is mainly metabolized by 3α-reduction to androstanediol. The metabolites of these androgens are conjugated either as glucuronides or sulfates and excreted in the urine. (See Figures 12–2 and 13–5.)

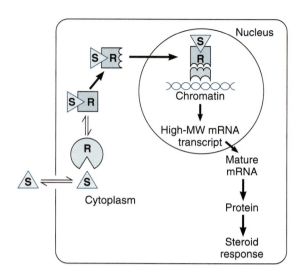

Figure 9–10. Steps in steroid hormone action. Activation of the intracellular receptors by steroid hormones is followed by nuclear binding of the complex and stimulation of mRNA synthesis. (R, receptor; S, steroid hormone.) (Reproduced, with permission, from Catt KJ, Dufau ML: Hormone action: Control of target-cell function by peptide, thyroid, and steroid hormones. In: *Endocrinology and Metabolism,* 3rd ed. Felig P, Baxter JD, Frohman LA [editors]. McGraw-Hill, 1995.)

BIOLOGIC EFFECTS

GLUCOCORTICOIDS

Although glucocorticoids were originally so called because of their influence on glucose metabolism, they are currently defined as steroids that exert their effects by binding to specific cytosolic receptors which mediate the actions of these hormones. These glucocorticoid receptors are present in virtually all tissues, and glucocorticoid-receptor interaction is responsible for most of the known effects of these steroids. Alterations in the structure of the glucocorticoids have led to the development of synthetic compounds with greater glucocorticoid activity. The increased activity of these compounds is due to increased affinity for the glucocorticoid receptors and delayed plasma clearance, which increases tissue exposure. In addition, many of these synthetic glucocorticoids have negligible mineralocorticoid effects and thus do not result in sodium retention, hypertension, and hypokalemia. This section describes the molecular mechanisms of glucocorticoid action and the effects on individual metabolic functions and tissues.

Molecular Mechanisms

A. Glucocorticoid Receptors: Glucocorticoid action is initiated by entry of the steroid into the cell and binding to the cytosolic glucocorticoid receptor proteins (Figure 9–10). These proteins probably originate in the nucleus but migrate into the cytosol in the presence of steroids. After binding, activated hormone-receptor complexes enter the nucleus and interact with nuclear chromatin acceptor sites. The 90-kDa heat shock protein hsp90 may be involved in hormone-induced glucocorticoid receptor activity. The DNA binding domain of the receptor is a cysteine-rich region which when it chelates zinc assumes a conformation called a "zinc finger." The receptor-glucocorticoid complex binds to specific sites in nuclear DNA, the glucocorticoid regulatory elements. This results in the expression of specific genes and the transcription of specific mRNAs. The resulting proteins affect the glucocorticoid response, which may be inhibitory or stimulatory depending on the specific tissue affected. Although glucocorticoid receptors are similar in many tissues, the proteins synthesized vary widely and are the result of expression of specific genes in different cell types. The mechanisms of this specific regulation are unknown. Analyses of cloned complementary DNAs for human glucocorticoid receptors have revealed marked structural and amino acid sequence homology between glucocorticoid receptors and receptors for other steroid hormones (eg, mineralocorticoids, estrogen, progesterone) as well as for thyroid hormone and the oncogene v-*erb* A. Although the steroid-binding domain of the glucocorticoid receptor confers specificity for glucocorticoid binding, glucocorticoids such as cortisol and corticosterone bind to the mineralocorticoid receptor with an affinity equal to that of aldosterone. Mineralocorticoid receptor specificity is maintained by the expression of 11β-hydroxysteroid dehydrogenase in classic mineralocorticoid-sensitive tissues. The expression in other tissues of this enzyme that inactivates these glucocorticoids may serve to protect these tissues from excessive glucocorticoid action.

B. Other Mechanisms: Although interaction of glucocorticoids with cytosolic receptors and their subsequent stimulation of gene expression are responsible for most glucocorticoid effects, other effects may occur through different mechanisms. The most significant example is that of glucocorticoid-induced fast feedback inhibition of ACTH secretion (see above). This effect occurs within minutes of glucocorticoid administration, and its rapidity suggests that it is not due to RNA and protein synthesis but rather to glucocorticoid-induced changes in secretory function or cell membranes.

Glucocorticoid Agonists & Antagonists

The study of glucocorticoid receptors has led to the definition of glucocorticoid agonists and antagonists. These studies have also identified a number of steroids with mixed effects termed partial agonists, partial antagonists, or partial agonist-partial antagonists.

A. Agonists: In humans, cortisol, synthetic glucocorticoids (eg, prednisolone, dexamethasone), corticosterone, and aldosterone are glucocorticoid agonists. The synthetic glucocorticoids have substantially higher affinity for the glucocorticoid receptor, and these have greater glucocorticoid activity than cortisol when present in equimolar concentrations. Corticosterone and aldosterone have substantial affinity for the glucocorticoid receptor; however, their plasma concentrations are normally much lower than that of cortisol, and thus these steroids do not have significant physiologic glucocorticoid effects.

B. Antagonists: Glucocorticoid antagonists bind to the glucocorticoid receptors but do not elicit the nuclear events required to cause a glucocorticoid response. These steroids compete with agonist steroids such as cortisol for the receptors and thus inhibit agonist responses. Other steroids have partial agonist activity when present alone;ie, they elicit a partial glucocorticoid response. However, in sufficient concentration, they compete with agonist steroids for the receptors and thus competitively inhibit agonist responses; ie, these partial agonists may function as partial antagonists in the presence of more active glucocorticoids. Steroids such as progesterone, 11-deoxycortisol, DOC, testosterone, and 17β-estradiol have antagonist or partial agonist-partial antagonist effects; however, the physiologic role of these hormones in glucocorticoid action is probably negligible, because they circulate in low concentrations. The antiprogestational agent RU 486

(mifepristone) has substantial glucocorticoid antagonist properties and has been used to block glucocorticoid action in patients with Cushing's syndrome.

Intermediary Metabolism

Glucocorticoids in general inhibit DNA synthesis. In addition, in most tissues they inhibit RNA and protein synthesis and accelerate protein catabolism. These actions provide substrate for intermediary metabolism; however, accelerated catabolism also accounts for the deleterious effects of glucocorticoids on muscle, bone, connective tissue, and lymphatic tissues. In contrast, RNA and protein synthesis in liver is stimulated.

A. Hepatic Glucose Metabolism: Glucocorticoids increase hepatic gluconeogenesis by stimulating the gluconeogenetic enzymes phosphoenolpyruvate carboxykinase and glucose 6-phosphatase. They also have a permissive effect in that they increase hepatic responsiveness to the gluconeogenetic hormones (glucagon, catecholamines), and they also increase the release of substrates from peripheral tissues, particularly muscle. This latter effect may be enhanced by the glucocorticoid-induced reduction in peripheral amino acid uptake and protein synthesis. Glucocorticoids also increase glycerol and free fatty acid release by lipolysis and increase muscle lactate release. These steroids also enhance hepatic glycogen synthesis and storage by stimulating glycogen synthetase activity and to a lesser extent by inhibiting glycogen breakdown. These effects are insulin-dependent.

B. Peripheral Glucose Metabolism: Glucocorticoids also alter carbohydrate metabolism by inhibiting peripheral glucose uptake in muscle and adipose tissue. This effect and the others described above may result in increased insulin secretion in states of chronic glucocorticoid excess.

C. Effects on Adipose Tissue: In adipose tissue, the predominant effect is increased lipolysis with release of glycerol and free fatty acids. This is partially due to direct stimulation of lipolysis by glucocorticoids, but it is also contributed to by decreased glucose uptake and enhancement by glucocorticoids of the effects of lipolytic hormones. Although glucocorticoids are lipolytic, increased fat deposition is a classic manifestation of glucocorticoid excess. This paradox may be explained by the increased appetite caused by high levels of these steroids and by the lipogenic effects of the hyperinsulinemia that occurs in this state. The reason for abnormal fat deposition and distribution in states of cortisol excess is unknown. In these instances, fat is classically deposited centrally in the face, cervical area, trunk, and abdomen; the extremities are usually spared.

D. Summary: The effects of the glucocorticoids on intermediary metabolism can be summarized as follows: (1) Effects are minimal in the fed state. However, during fasting, glucocorticoids contribute to the maintenance of plasma glucose levels by increasing gluconeogenesis, glycogen deposition, and the peripheral release of substrate. (2) Hepatic glucose production is enhanced, as is hepatic RNA and protein synthesis. (3) The effects on muscle are catabolic, ie, decreased glucose uptake and metabolism, decreased protein synthesis, and increased release of amino acids. (4) In adipose tissue, lipolysis is stimulated. (5) In glucocorticoid deficiency, hypoglycemia may result, whereas in states of glucocorticoid excess there may be hyperglycemia, hyperinsulinemia, muscle wasting, and weight gain with abnormal fat distribution.

Effects on Other Tissues & Functions

A. Connective Tissue: Glucocorticoids in excess inhibit fibroblasts, lead to loss of collagen and connective tissue, and thus result in thinning of the skin, easy bruising, stria formation, and poor wound healing.

B. Bone: The physiologic role of glucocorticoids in bone metabolism and calcium homeostasis is unknown; however, in excess, they have major deleterious effects. Glucocorticoids directly inhibit bone formation by decreasing cell proliferation and the synthesis of RNA, protein, collagen, and hyaluronate. Glucocorticoids also directly stimulate bone-resorbing cells, leading to osteolysis and increased urinary hydroxyproline excretion. In addition, they potentiate the actions of PTH and 1,25-dihydroxycholecalciferol ($1,25[OH]_2D_3$) on bone, and this may further contribute to net bone resorption.

C. Calcium Metabolism: Glucocorticoids also have other major effects on mineral homeostasis. They markedly reduce intestinal calcium absorption, which tends to lower serum calcium. This results in a secondary increase in PTH secretion, which maintains serum calcium within the normal range by stimulating bone resorption. In addition, glucocorticoids may directly stimulate PTH release. The mechanism of decreased intestinal calcium absorption is unknown, though it is not due to decreased synthesis or decreased serum levels of the active vitamin D metabolites; in fact, $1,25(OH)_2D_3$ levels are normal or even increased in the presence of glucocorticoid excess. Increased $1,25(OH)_2D_3$ synthesis in this setting may result from decreased serum phosphorus levels (see below), increased PTH levels, and direct stimulation by glucocorticoids of renal 1α-hydroxylase. Glucocorticoids also increase urinary calcium excretion, and hypercalciuria is a consistent feature of cortisol excess. They also reduce the tubular reabsorption of phosphate, leading to phosphaturia and decreased serum phosphorus concentrations.

Thus, glucocorticoids in excess result in negative calcium balance, with decreased absorption and increased urinary excretion. Serum calcium levels are maintained, but at the expense of net bone resorption. Decreased bone formation and increased resorption ultimately result in the disabling osteopenia that is often a major complication of spontaneous and iatrogenic glucocorticoid excess (see Chapter 8).

D. Growth and Development: Glucocorticoids accelerate the development of a number of systems and organs in fetal and differentiating tissues, although the mechanisms are unclear. As discussed above, glucocorticoids are generally inhibitory, and these stimulatory effects may be due to glucocorticoid interactions with other growth factors. Examples of these development-promoting effects are increased surfactant production in the fetal lung and the accelerated development of hepatic and gastrointestinal enzyme systems.

Glucocorticoids in excess inhibit growth in children, and this adverse effect is a major complication of therapy. This may be a direct effect on bone cells, although decreased growth hormone (GH) secretion and somatomedin generation also contribute (see Chapter 6).

E. Blood Cells and Immunologic Function:

1. Erythrocytes–Glucocorticoids have little effect on erythropoiesis and hemoglobin concentration. Although mild polycythemia and anemia may be seen in Cushing's syndrome and Addison's disease, respectively, these alterations are more likely to be secondary to altered androgen metabolism.

2. Leukocytes–Glucocorticoids influence both leukocyte movement and function. Thus, glucocorticoid administration increases the number of intravascular polymorphonuclear leukocytes by increasing PMN release from bone marrow, by increasing the circulating half-life of PMNs, and by decreasing PMN movement out of the vascular compartment. Glucocorticoid administration reduces the number of circulating lymphocytes, monocytes, and eosinophils, mainly by increasing their movement out of the circulation. The converse—ie, neutropenia, lymphocytosis, monocytosis, and eosinophilia—is seen in adrenal insufficiency. Glucocorticoids also decrease the migration of inflammatory cells (PMNs, monocytes, and lymphocytes) to sites of injury, and this is probably a major mechanism of the anti-inflammatory actions and increased susceptibility to infection that occur following chronic administration. Glucocorticoids also decrease lymphocyte production and the mediator and effector functions of these cells.

3. Immunologic effects–Glucocorticoids influence multiple aspects of immunologic and inflammatory responsiveness, including the mobilization and function of leukocytes, as discussed above. They inhibit phospholipase A_2, a key enzyme in the synthesis of prostaglandins. This inhibition is mediated by a class of peptides called lipocortins or annexins. They also impair release of effector substances such as the lymphokine interleukin-1, antigen processing, antibody production and clearance, and other specific bone marrow-derived and thymus-derived lymphocyte functions. The immune system, in turn, affects the hypothalamic-pituitary-adrenal axis; interleukin-I stimulates the secretion of CRH and ACTH.

F. Cardiovascular Function: Glucocorticoids may increase cardiac output, and they also increase peripheral vascular tone, possibly by augmenting the effects of other vasoconstrictors, eg, the catecholamines. Glucocorticoids also regulate expression of adrenergic receptors. Thus, refractory shock may occur when the glucocorticoid-deficient individual is subjected to stress. Glucocorticoids in excess may cause hypertension independently of their mineralocorticoid effects. Although the incidence and the precise cause of this problem are unclear, it is likely that the mechanism involves the renin-angiotensin system; glucocorticoids regulate renin substrate, the precursor of angiotensin I.

G. Renal Function: These steroids affect water and electrolyte balance by actions mediated either by mineralocorticoid receptors (sodium retention, hypokalemia, and hypertension) or via glucocorticoid receptors (increased glomerular filtration rate due to increased cardiac output or due to a direct renal effect and water retention). Thus, corticosteroids such as betamethasone or dexamethasone that have little mineralocorticoid activity increase sodium and water excretion. Glucocorticoid-deficient subjects have decreased glomerular filtration rates and are unable to excrete a water load. This may be contributed to by increased ADH secretion, which may occur in glucocorticoid deficiency.

H. Central Nervous System Function: Glucocorticoids readily enter the brain, and although their physiologic role in central nervous system function is unknown, their excess or deficiency may profoundly alter behavior and cognitive function.

1. Excessive glucocorticoids—In excess, the glucocorticoids initially cause euphoria; however, with prolonged exposure, a variety of psychologic abnormalities occur, including irritability, emotional lability, and depression. Hyperkinetic or manic behavior is less common; overt psychoses occur in a small number of patients. Many patients also note impairment in cognitive functions, most commonly memory and concentration. Other central effects include increased appetite, decreased libido, and insomnia, with decreased REM sleep and increased stage II sleep.

2. Decreased glucocorticoids—Patients with Addison's disease are apathetic and depressed and tend to be irritable, negativistic, and reclusive. They have decreased appetite but increased sensitivity of taste and smell mechanisms.

I. Effects on Other Hormones:

1. Thyroid function—Glucocorticoids in excess affect thyroid function. Although basal TSH levels are usually normal, TSH synthesis and release are inhibited by glucocorticoids, and TSH responsiveness to thyrotropin-releasing hormone (TRH) is frequently subnormal. Serum total thyroxine (T_4) concentrations are usually low normal because of a decrease in thyroxine-binding globulin, but free T_4 levels are normal. Total and free T_3 (triiodothyronine) concentrations may be low, since glucocorticoid excess decreases the conversion of T_4 to T_3 and increases conversion to reverse T_3. Despite these alterations, manifestations of hypothyroidism are not apparent.

2. Gonadal function—Glucocorticoids also affect gonadotropin and gonadal function. In males, they inhibit gonadotropin secretion, as evidenced by decreased responsiveness to administered gonadotropin-releasing hormone (GnRH) and subnormal plasma testosterone concentrations. In females, glucocorticoids also suppress LH responsiveness to GnRH, resulting in suppression of estrogens and progestins with inhibition of ovulation and amenorrhea.

J. Miscellaneous Effects:

1. Peptic ulcer—The role of steroid excess in the production or reactivation of peptic ulcer disease is controversial. Ulcers in spontaneous Cushing's syndrome and with modest exposure to glucocorticoid therapy are unusual, although current data suggest that steroid-treated patients with established ulcers and those on high-dose therapy may be at increased risk.

2. Ophthalmologic effects—Intraocular pressure varies with the level of circulating glucocorticoids and parallels the circadian variation of plasma cortisol levels. In addition, glucocorticoids in excess increase intraocular pressure in patients with open-angle glaucoma. Glucocorticoid therapy may also cause cataract formation. Central serous chorioretinopathy, an accumulation of subretinal detachment, may also complicate endogenous or exogenous glucocorticoid excess.

ADRENAL ANDROGENS

The direct biologic activity of the adrenal androgens (androstenedione, DHEA, and DHEA sulfate) is minimal, and they function primarily as precursors for peripheral conversion to the active androgenic hormones testosterone and dihydrotestosterone. Thus, DHEA sulfate secreted by the adrenal undergoes limited conversion to DHEA; this peripherally converted DHEA and that secreted by the adrenal cortex can be further converted in peripheral tissues to androstenedione, the immediate precursor of the active androgens.

The actions of testosterone and dihydrotestosterone are described in Chapter 12. This section will deal only with the adrenal contribution to androgenicity.

Effects in Males

In males with normal gonadal function, the conversion of adrenal androstenedione to testosterone accounts for less than 5% of the production rate of this hormone, and thus the physiologic effect is negligible. In adult males, excessive adrenal androgen secretion has no clinical consequences; however, in boys, it causes premature penile enlargement and early development of secondary sexual characteristics.

Effects in Females

In females, the adrenal substantially contributes to total androgen production by the peripheral conversion of androstenedione. In the follicular phase of the menstrual cycle, adrenal precursors account for two-thirds of testosterone production and one-half of dihydrotestosterone production. During midcycle, the ovarian contribution increases, and the adrenal precursors account for only 40% of testosterone production.

In females, abnormal adrenal function as seen in Cushing's syndrome, adrenal carcinoma, and congenital adrenal hyperplasia results in excessive secretion of adrenal androgens, and their peripheral conversion results in androgen excess, manifested by acne, hirsutism, and virilization.

LABORATORY EVALUATION

Cortisol and the adrenal androgens are measured by specific plasma assays. Certain urinary assays, particularly measurement of 24-hour urine free cortisol, are also useful. In addition, plasma concentrations of ACTH can be determined. The plasma steroid methods commonly used measure the total hormone concentration and are therefore influenced by alterations in plasma binding proteins. Furthermore, since ACTH and the plasma concentrations of the adrenal hormones fluctuate markedly (Figure 9–7), single plasma measurements are frequently unreliable. Thus, plasma levels must be interpreted cautiously, and more specific diagnostic information is usually obtained by performing appropriate stimulation and suppression tests.

Plasma ACTH

A. Methods of Measurement: Plasma ACTH measurements are extremely useful in the diagnosis of pituitary-adrenal dysfunction. The normal range for plasma ACTH, using a sensitive immunoradiometric assay, is 9–52 pg/mL (2.2–11.1 pmol/L).

B. Interpretation: Plasma ACTH levels are most useful in differentiating pituitary causes from adrenal causes of adrenal dysfunction: (1) In **adrenal insufficiency** due to primary adrenal disease, plasma ACTH levels are elevated. Conversely, in pituitary ACTH deficiency and secondary hypoadrenalism, plasma ACTH levels are less than 20 pg/mL. (2) In

Cushing's syndrome due to primary glucocorticoid-secreting adrenal tumors, plasma ACTH is suppressed, and a level less than 5 pg/mL (1.1 pmol/L) is diagnostic. In patients with Cushing's disease (pituitary ACTH hypersecretion), plasma ACTH levels are normal or elevated. Plasma ACTH levels are usually elevated in the ectopic ACTH syndrome, but there is a considerable amount of overlap with levels seen in Cushing's disease. In addition, values lower than expected may be observed occasionally in ectopic ACTH syndrome when the two-site immunoradiometric assay is used; this assay does not detect high-molecular-weight precursors of ACTH. (3) Plasma ACTH levels are also markedly elevated in patients with the common forms of **congenital adrenal hyperplasia** and are useful in the diagnosis and management of these disorders (see Chapters 10 and 14).

Plasma β-Lipotropin & β-Endorphin

β-Lipotropin (β-LPH) is secreted in equimolar amounts with ACTH and is measured by radioimmunoassay. Because of its greater stability and ease of measurement, it has some advantage over the measurement of ACTH. Alterations in β-LPH levels in disease states parallel those of ACTH as described above. Most assays of β-LPH also measure β-endorphin, and thus separation of these hormones is required for precise measurement of β-endorphin. This can be accomplished by chromatography; however, the clinical utility of β-endorphin measurements has not been established.

Plasma Cortisol

A. Methods of Measurement: The most comment method of measurement of plasma cortisol is radioimmunoassay. Other methods include high-performance liquid chromatography, competitive protein-binding assay, and fluorimetric assay. All these methods measure total cortisol (both bound and free) in plasma. Methods that measure plasma free cortisol—ie, that not bound to CBG—are also available. Since cortisol is present in saliva in its unbound or free state, salivary cortisol measurements provide a simple and accurate assessment of free cortisol concentration.

Radioimmunoassays of plasma cortisol depend on inhibition of binding of radiolabeled cortisol to an antibody by the cortisol present in a plasma sample. Current assays are very sensitive, so that small plasma volumes can be used. In addition, cross-reactivity of current antisera with other endogenous steroids is minimal, and radioimmunoassay thus gives a reliable measurement of total plasma cortisol levels. Cross-reactivity with some synthetic glucocorticoids, eg, prednisone, is variable. Other commonly used drugs and medications do not interfere with this assay.

B. Interpretation: The diagnostic utility of single plasma cortisol concentrations is limited by the episodic nature of cortisol secretion and its appropriate elevations during stress. As explained below, more information is obtained by dynamic testing of the hypothalamic-pituitary-adrenal axis.

1. Normal values–Normal plasma cortisol levels vary with the method used. With radioimmunoassay and the competitive protein-binding radioassay, levels at 8 AM range from 3 to 20 µg/dL (80–540 nmol/L) and average 10–12 µg/dL (275.9–331.1 nmol/L). Values obtained later in the day are lower and at 4 PM are approximately half of morning values. At 10 PM to 2 AM, the plasma cortisol concentrations by these methods are usually under 3 µg/dL (80 nmol/L). The normal salivary cortisol level at midnight is < 0.4 µg/dL (22 nmol/L).

2. Levels during stress–Cortisol secretion increases in patients who are acutely ill, during surgery, and following trauma. Plasma concentrations may reach 40–60 µg/dL (1100–1600 nmol/L).

3. High-estrogen states–The total plasma cortisol concentration is also elevated with increased CBG binding capacity, which occurs most commonly when circulating estrogen levels are high, eg, during pregnancy and when exogenous estrogens or oral contraceptives are being used. In these situations, plasma cortisol may reach levels two to three times normal.

4. Other conditions–CBG levels may be increased or decreased in other situations, as discussed above in the sections on circulation and metabolism. Total plasma cortisol concentrations may also be increased in severe anxiety, endogenous depression, starvation, anorexia nervosa, alcoholism, and chronic renal failure.

Urinary Corticosteroids

A. Free Cortisol:

1. Methods of measurement–The assay of unbound cortisol excreted in the urine is an excellent method for the diagnosis of Cushing's syndrome. Normally, less than 1% of the secreted cortisol is excreted unchanged in the urine. However, in states of excess secretion, the binding capacity of CBG is exceeded, and plasma free cortisol therefore increases, as does its urinary excretion. Urine free cortisol is measured in a 24-hour urine collection by radioimmunoassay or high-performance liquid chromatography (HPLC).

2. Normal values–The normal range for urine free cortisol is 20–90 µg/24 h (50-250 nmol/24 h) when radioimmunoassay techniques are used. Since HPLC provides a more specific measurement of cortisol, the normal range is < 50 µg/24 h (< 135 nmol/24 h) when this technique is used.

3. Diagnostic utility–This method is particularly useful in differentiating simple obesity from Cushing's syndrome, since levels are not elevated in obesity, as are the urinary 17-hydroxycorticosteroids (see below). The levels may be elevated in the same conditions that increase plasma cortisol (see above), including a slight elevation during pregnancy. This test is not useful in adrenal insufficiency, because of the lack of sensitivity of the method at low levels and because low cortisol excretion is often found in normal persons.

B. 17-Hydroxycorticosteroids:

These urinary steroids are less frequently measured at present, because of the greater utility of plasma cortisol and urine free cortisol measurements.

1. Methods of assay–Urine 17-hydroxycorticosteroids are assayed by the colorimetric Porter-Silber reaction, which detects cortisol and cortisone metabolites.

2. Normal values–Normal values are 3–15 mg/24 h (8.3–41.4 µmol/24 h) or 3–7 mg/g (0.9–2.2 mmol/mol) of urine creatinine.

3. Altered excretion–Total excretion is increased in obesity; however, these values are normal when corrected for creatinine excretion. 17-Hydroxycorticosteroids are increased in hyperthyroidism and decreased in hypothyroidism, starvation, liver disease, renal failure, and pregnancy. Drugs that induce hepatic microsomal enzymes increase cortisol conversion to 6β-hydroxycortisol, which is not measured by the 17-hydroxycorticosteroid method, and therefore reduce 17-hydroxycorticosteroid excretion (see section on metabolism).

d. Drug interference–Direct drug interference with the colorimetric reaction occurs with spironolactone, chlordiazepoxide, hydroxyzine, meprobamate, phenothiazines, and quinine.

Dexamethasone Suppression Tests

A. Low-Dose Tests: These procedures are used to establish the presence of Cushing's syndrome regardless of its cause. Dexamethasone, a potent glucocorticoid, normally suppresses pituitary ACTH release with a resulting fall in plasma and urine corticosteroids, thus assessing feedback inhibition of the hypothalamic-pituitary-adrenal axis. In Cushing's syndrome, this mechanism is abnormal, and steroid secretion fails to be suppressed in the normal way. Dexamethasone in the doses used does not interfere with the measurement of plasma and urinary corticosteroids.

1. Overnight 1-mg dexamethasone suppression test–This is a suitable screening test for Cushing's syndrome. Dexamethasone, 1 mg orally, is given as a single dose at 11 PM, and the following morning a plasma sample is obtained for cortisol determination. Cushing's syndrome is excluded if the plasma cortisol level is less than 3 µg/dL (80 nmol/L). If the level is greater than 10 µ/dL (279 nmol/L)—in the absence of conditions causing false-positive responses—Cushing's syndrome is the probable cause, and the diagnosis should be confirmed with other procedures.

Over 98% of patients with Cushing's syndrome have abnormal responses. Although false-negative results are rare, they may occur in patients in whom dexamethasone metabolism is abnormally slow, since plasma levels of dexamethasone in these patients are higher than normally achieved and result in apparently normal suppression of cortisol. Simultaneous measurement of plasma dexamethasone and cortisol levels will identify these patients; however, dexamethasone measurements may be available only in a research laboratory.

False-positive results occur in hospitalized and chronically ill patients. Acute illness, depression, anxiety, alcoholism, high-estrogen states, and uremia may also cause false-positive results. Patients taking phenytoin, barbiturates, and other inducers of hepatic microsomal enzymes may have accelerated metabolism of dexamethasone and thus fail to achieve adequate plasma levels to suppress ACTH.

2. Two-day low-dose test—This test is performed by administering dexamethasone, 0.5 mg every 6 hours for 2 days. Twenty-four-hour urine collections are obtained before and on the second day of dexamethasone administration. Although this test has been traditionally performed for the diagnosis of Cushing's syndrome, it is now recognized that many patients with mild hypercortisolism will suppress urine steroid levels to very low levels following low-dose dexamethasone administration. The sensitivity of this test in patients with mild Cushing's syndrome is only 55%, and it can never be used to exclude Cushing's syndrome. This test should be abandoned.

B. High-Dose Tests: High dose dexamethasone suppression testing has historically been used to differentiate Cushing's disease (pituitary ACTH hypersecretion) from ectopic ACTH and adrenal tumors. This rationale has been based on the fact that in some patients with Cushing's disease, the hypothalamic-pituitary-adrenal axis is suppressible with supraphysiologic doses of glucocorticoids, whereas cortisol secretion is autonomous in patients with adrenal tumors and in most patients with the ectopic ACTH syndrome. Unfortunately, exceptions to these rules are so common that high-dose dexamethasone suppression testing must be interpreted with extreme caution.

1. Overnight high-dose dexamethasone suppression test—This simple test is preferable to the 2-day high-dose dexamethasone suppression test described below. After a baseline morning cortisol specimen is obtained, a single dose of dexamethasone, 8 mg orally, is administered at 11:00 PM and plasma cortisol is measured at 8:00 AM the following morning. Generally, patients with Cushing's disease will suppress plasma cortisol level to less than 50% of baseline values—in contrast to patients with the

ectopic ACTH syndrome, who fail to suppress to this magnitude. Patients with cortisol-producing adrenal tumors will also fail to suppress: their cortisol secretion is autonomous, and ACTH secretion is already suppressed by the high endogenous levels of cortisol.

2. Two-day high-dose dexamethasone suppression test—This test is performed by administering dexamethasone, 2 mg orally every 6 hours for 2 days. Twenty-four-hour urine samples are collected before and on the second day of dexamethasone administration. Patients with Cushing's disease have a reduction of urine 17-hydroxycorticosteroid excretion to less than 50% of baseline values, whereas those with adrenal tumors or the ectopic ACTH syndrome usually have little or no reduction in urinary 17-hydroxycorticosteroids. However, some patients with an ectopic ACTH-secreting neoplasm suppress steroid secretion with high doses of dexamethasone, and some patients with pituitary ACTH-dependent Cushing's syndrome fail to suppress to these levels. The diagnostic sensitivity, specificity, and accuracy of high-dose dexamethasone suppression test are only about 80%. An analysis of the standard low- and high-dose dexamethasone suppression tests has shown better specificity and accuracy by utilizing new criteria. The decrease in urine free cortisol of more than 90% or in 17-hydroxycorticosteroid excretion of more than 64% had 100% diagnostic specificity for Cushing's disease and excluded ectopic ACTH syndrome in one series. However, several exceptions to these new criteria have been observed; and it has become increasingly clear that high-dose dexamethasone suppression testing, regardless of the criteria employed, cannot distinguish pituitary from nonpituitary ACTH hypersecretion with certainty.

Pituitary-Adrenal Reserve

Determinations of pituitary-adrenal reserve are used to evaluate the patient's adrenal and pituitary reserve and to assess the ability of the hypothalamic-pituitary-adrenal axis to respond to stress. ACTH administration directly stimulates adrenal secretion; metyrapone inhibits cortisol synthesis, thereby stimulating pituitary ACTH secretion; and insulin-induced hypoglycemia stimulates ACTH release by increasing CRH secretion. More recently, CRH has been utilized to directly stimulate pituitary corticotrophs to release ACTH. The relative utility of these procedures is discussed below in the section on adrenocortical insufficiency and also in Chapter 5.

A. ACTH Stimulation Testing:

1. Procedure and normal values—The rapid ACTH stimulation test measures the acute adrenal response to ACTH and is used to diagnose both primary and secondary adrenal insufficiency. A synthetic human α^{1-24}-ACTH called tetracosactrin or cosyntropin is used. Fasting is not required, and the test may be performed at any time of the day. A baseline cortisol sample is obtained; cosyntropin is administered in a dose of 0.25 mg intramuscularly or intravenously; and additional samples for plasma cortisol are obtained at 30 or 60 minutes following the injection. Because the peak concentration of ACTH with this test achieves a pharmacologic level exceeding 10,000 pg/mL, this study assesses maximal adrenocortical capacity. The peak cortisol response, 30–60 minutes later, should exceed 20 μg/dL (> 540 nmol/L). The 30-minute peak cortisol response to ACTH is constant and is unrelated to the basal cortisol level. In fact, there is no difference in the peak cortisol level at 30 minutes regardless of whether 250 μg, 5 μg, or even 1 μg of ACTH is administered. Use of a 1 μg dose of ACTH provides a more sensitive indication of adrenocortical function and has been better able to differentiate a subgroup of patients on long-term corticosteroid therapy who responded normally to the regular 250 μg test but who have a reduced response to 1 μg. The low-dose (1 μg) ACTH stimulation test is gaining greater acceptance and will probably emerge as the diagnostic procedure of choice in suspected adrenal insufficiency.

2. Subnormal responses–If the cortisol response to the rapid ACTH stimulation test is inadequate, adrenal insufficiency is present. In primary adrenal insufficiency, destruction of cortical cells reduces cortisol secretion and increases pituitary ACTH secretion. Therefore, the adrenal is already maximally stimulated, and there is no further increase in cortisol secretion when exogenous ACTH is given; ie, there is decreased adrenal reserve. In secondary adrenal insufficiency due to ACTH deficiency, there is atrophy of the zonae fasciculata and reticularis, and the adrenal thus is unresponsive to acute stimulation with exogenous ACTH. In either primary or secondary types, a subnormal response to the rapid ACTH stimulation test accurately predicts deficient responsiveness of the axis to insulin hypoglycemia, metyrapone, and surgical stress.

3. Normal responses–A normal response to the rapid ACTH stimulation test excludes both primary adrenal insufficiency (by directly assessing adrenal reserve) and overt secondary adrenal insufficiency with adrenal atrophy. However, a normal response does not rule out partial ACTH deficiency (decreased pituitary reserve) in patients whose basal ACTH secretion is sufficient to prevent adrenocortical atrophy. These patients may be unable to further increase ACTH secretion and thus may have subnormal pituitary ACTH responsiveness to stress or hypoglycemia. In such patients, further testing with metyrapone or hypoglycemia may be indicated. For further discussion, see the section on diagnosis of adrenocortical insufficiency.

4. Aldosterone secretion–The rapid ACTH stimulation test also increases aldosterone secretion and has been used to differentiate primary from secondary adrenocortical insufficiency. In the primary form with destruction of the cortex, both cortisol and aldosterone are unresponsive to exogenous ACTH. However, in secondary adrenal insufficiency, the zona glomerulosa, which is controlled by the renin-angiotensin system, is usually normal. Therefore, the aldosterone response to exogenous ACTH is normal. The normal peak plasma aldosterone response to ACTH on an unrestricted sodium diet is usually greater than 15 mg/dL (220 pg/L).

B. Metyrapone Testing: Metyrapone testing is used to diagnose adrenal insufficiency and to assess pituitary-adrenal reserve. The test procedures are detailed in Chapter 5. Metyrapone blocks cortisol synthesis by inhibiting the 11β-hydroxylase enzyme that converts 11-deoxycortisol to cortisol. This stimulates ACTH secretion, which in turn increases the secretion and plasma levels of 11-deoxycortisol. Urinary 17-hydroxycorticosteroid levels also increase because of increased excretion of the metabolites of 11-deoxycortisol that are measured by this method. The overnight metyrapone test is most commonly used and is best suited to patients with suspected pituitary ACTH deficiency; patients with suspected primary adrenal failure are usually evaluated with the rapid ACTH stimulation test as described above and discussed in the section on diagnosis of adrenocortical insufficiency. The normal response to the overnight metyrapone test is a plasma 11-deoxycortisol level greater than 7 μg/dL (190 nmol/L) and a plasma ACTH level greater than 100 pg/mL (22 pmol/L) and indicates both normal ACTH secretion and adrenal function. A subnormal response establishes adrenocortical insufficiency. A normal response to metyrapone accurately predicts normal stress responsiveness of the hypothalamic-pituitary axis and correlates well with responsiveness to insulin-induced hypoglycemia.

C. Insulin-Induced Hypoglycemia Testing: The details of this procedure are described in Chapter 5. Hypoglycemia induces a central nervous system stress response, increases CRH release, and in this way increases ACTH and cortisol secretion. It therefore measures the integrity of the axis and its ability to respond to stress. The normal plasma cortisol response is an increment greater than 8 μg/dL (220 nmol/L) and a peak level greater than 18–20 μg/dL (485–540 nmol/L). The plasma ACTH response to hypoglycemia is usually greater than 100 pg/mL (22 pmol/L). A normal plasma cortisol response to hypoglycemia excludes adrenal insufficiency and decreased pituitary reserve. Thus, patients with normal responses do not require cortisol therapy during illness or surgery.

D. CRH Testing: The procedure for CRH testing is described in Chapter 5. ACTH responses are exaggerated in patients with primary adrenal failure and absent in patients with hypopituitarism. Delayed responses may occur in patients with hypothalamic disorders.

Androgens

Androgen excess is usually evaluated by the measurement of basal levels of these hormones, since suppression and stimulation tests are not as useful as in disorders affecting the glucocorticoids.

A. Plasma Levels: Assays are available for total plasma levels of DHEA, DHEA sulfate, androstenedione, testosterone, and dihydrotestosterone; these tests are of greater diagnostic utility than the traditional measurement of urinary androgen metabolites measured as urinary 17-ketosteroids.

Because it is present in greater quantities, DHEA sulfate can be measured directly in unextracted plasma. However, because of their similar structures and lower plasma concentrations, the other androgens require extraction and purification steps prior to assay. This is accomplished by solvent extraction followed by chromatography, and the purified steroids are then measured by radioimmunoassay or competitive protein-binding radioassay. These methods allow measurement of multiple steroids in small volumes of plasma.

B. Free Testosterone: Plasma free testosterone (ie, testosterone not bound to SHBG) can be measured and is a more direct measure of circulating biologically active testosterone than the total plasma level. These methods require separation of the bound and free hormone prior to assay and are technically difficult. The plasma free testosterone concentration in normal women averages 5 pg/mL (17 pmol/L), representing approximately 1% of the total testosterone concentration. In hirsute women, average levels are 16 pg/mL (55 pmol/L), with a wide range (see Chapter 13).

C. SHBG Binding Capacity: The binding capacity of SHBG can be measured, although these methods are not in general use. SHBG binding capacity is higher in women; it is increased in pregnancy, in women receiving exogenous estrogens, in hepatic cirrhosis, and in hyperthyroidism and is decreased in hirsute women with increased androgens and in patients with acromegaly.

DISORDERS OF ADRENOCORTICAL INSUFFICIENCY

Deficient adrenal production of glucocorticoids or mineralocorticoids results in adrenocortical insufficiency, which is either the consequence of destruction or dysfunction of the cortex (primary adrenocortical insufficiency, Addison's disease) or secondary to deficient pituitary ACTH secretion (secondary adrenocortical insufficiency). Secondary adrenocortical insufficiency due to glucocorticoid therapy is the most common cause.

PRIMARY ADRENOCORTICAL INSUFFICIENCY (Addison's Disease)

Etiology & Pathology

The etiology of primary adrenocortical insufficiency has changed over time. Prior to 1920, tuberculosis was the major cause of adrenocortical insufficiency. Since 1950, autoimmune adrenalitis with adrenal atrophy has accounted for about 80% of cases. It is associated with a high incidence of other immunologic and autoimmune endocrine disorders (see below). Tuberculosis of the adrenal gland is now rare. Causes are listed in Table 9–1. Primary adrenocortical insufficiency, or Addison's disease, is rare, with a reported prevalence of 39 per million population in the United Kingdom and 60 per million in Denmark. It is more common in females, with a female:male ratio of 2.6:1. Addison's disease is usually diagnosed in the third to fifth decades. As the number of patients with acquired immunodeficiency syndrome (AIDS) increases, and as patients with malignant disease live longer, more cases of adrenal insufficiency will be seen.

A. Autoimmune Adrenocortical Insufficiency: Lymphocytic infiltration of the adrenal cortex is the characteristic histologic feature. The adrenals are small and atrophic, and the capsule is thickened. The adrenal medulla is preserved, though cortical cells are largely absent, show degenerative changes, and are surrounded by a fibrous stroma and lymphocytic infiltrates.

Autoimmune Addison's disease is frequently accompanied by other immune disorders. There are two different syndromes in which autoimmune adrenal insufficiency may occur. The best-characterized one is known as autoimmune polyendocrinopathy-candidiasis-ectodermal dystrophy syndrome (APECD), or autoimmune polyglandular disease type I. This is

Table 9–1. Causes of primary adrenocortical insufficiency.

Autoimmune
Metastatic malignancy or lymphoma
Adrenal hemorrhage
Infectious
   Tuberculosis, CMV, fungi (histoplasmosis,
     coccidioidomycosis)
Adrenoleukodystrophy
Infiltrative disorders
   Amyloidosis, hemochromatosis
Congenital adrenal hyperplasia
Familial glucocorticoid deficiency
Drugs
   Ketoconazole, metyrapone, aminoglutethimide, trilostane,
     mitotane, etomidate

an autosomal recessive disorder that usually presents in childhood and is accompanied by hypoparathyroidism, adrenal failure, and mucocutaneous candidiasis. These patients have a defect in T cell-mediated immunity, especially toward the *Candida* antigen. This disorder has no relationship to the HLA antigen and is often associated with hepatitis, dystrophy of dental enamel and nails, alopecia, vitiligo, and keratopathy and may be accompanied by hypofunction of the gonads, thyroid, pancreatic B cell, and gastric parietal cells. Autoantibodies against the cholesterol side-chain cleavage enzyme (P450ssc) have been described in patients with this disorder.

The more common presentation of autoimmune adrenocortical insufficiency is associated with HLA-related disorders including type I diabetes mellitus, autoimmune thyroid disease, alopecia areata, vitiligo, and celiac sprue. This disorder is often referred to as polyglandular autoimmune syndrome type II. The genetic susceptibility to this disorder is linked to HLA-DR3 or DR4 (or both). These patients have anti-adrenal cytoplasmic antibodies that may be important in the pathogenesis of this disorder, and autoantibodies directed against 21α-hydroxylase (P450c21) have recently been identified.

B. Adrenal Hemorrhage: Bilateral adrenal hemorrhage is now a relatively common cause of adrenal insufficiency in the United States. The diagnosis is usually made in critically ill patients in whom a CT scan of the abdomen is done. Bilateral adrenal enlargement is found, leading to an assessment of adrenocortical function. Anatomic factors predispose the adrenal glands to hemorrhage. The adrenal glands have a rich arterial blood supply, but they are drained by a single vein. Adrenal vein thrombosis may occur during periods of stasis or turbulence, thereby increasing adrenal vein pressure and resulting in a "vascular dam." This causes hemorrhage into the gland and is followed by adrenocortical insufficiency.

Most patients with adrenal hemorrhage have been taking anticoagulant therapy, have a underlying coagulopathy, or are predisposed to thrombosis. Heparin associated thrombosis thrombocytopenia syndrome may be accompanied by adrenal vein thrombosis and hemorrhage. The primary antiphospholipid syndrome (lupus anticoagulant) has emerged as one of the most common causes of adrenal hemorrhage.

C. Infectious: Although tuberculosis may represent a common cause of primary adrenal insufficiency in the rest of the world, it is a rare cause of this problem in the United States. Clinically significant adrenal insufficiency appears to occur in only about 5% of patients with disseminated tuberculosis. With the use of antituberculous chemotherapy, it may even be reversible if detected in early stages. It is important to recognized that rifampin may accelerate the metabolic clearance of cortisol, thereby increasing the replacement dose needed in these patients.

Fungal infections can also destroy the adrenal cortex. All commonly occurring fungi, except *Candida,* have been reported to cause adrenal insufficiency. Histoplasmosis is the most common fungal infection causing adrenal hypofunction in the United States. Another caveat regarding treatment is that the antifungal agent ketoconazole inhibits adrenal cytochrome P450 steroidogenic enzymes which are essential for cortisol biosynthesis. Thus, ketoconazole treatment in patients with marginal adrenocortical reserve due to fungal disease may precipitate adrenal crisis.

D. Adrenoleukodystrophy: X-linked adrenoleukodystrophy is an important cause of adrenal insufficiency in men. This disorder represents two distinct entities that may cause malfunction of the adrenal cortex and demyelination in the central nervous system. These disorders are characterized by abnormally high levels of very long chain fatty acids (VLCFAs) due to their defective beta oxidation within peroxisomes. The abnormal accumulation of VLCFAs in the brain, adrenal cortex, testes, and liver result in the clinical manifestations of this disorder.

Adrenoleukodystrophy has an incidence of approximately one in 25,000 and is an X-linked disorder with incomplete penetrance. The identification of restriction fragment length polymorphism in the region of the adrenoleukodystrophy gene permits use of DNA probes for genetic and diagnostic purposes, both in family screening and prenatal evaluation. Two clinical phenotypes have been described. Cerebral adrenoleukodystrophy usually presents in childhood, and its neurologic symptoms include cognitive dysfunction, behavioral problems, emotional lability, and visual and gate disturbances. It may progress to dementia. Because 30% of these patients develop adrenal insufficiency before the onset of neurologic symptoms, a young man with primary adrenal insufficiency should always be screened for adrenoleukodystrophy. A clinically milder phenotype, adrenomyeloneuropathy, usually presents in the second to fourth decades of life. Spinal cord and peripheral nerve demyelination occurs over years and may result in loss of ambulation, cognitive dysfunction, urinary retention, and impotence. Once again, adrenal insufficiency may occur before the onset of neurologic symptoms.

The diagnosis of adrenoleukodystrophy can be confirmed by demonstration of the defect in fatty acid metabolism with the abnormal accumulation of saturated VLCFAs, especially C26:0 fatty acid.

E. Metastatic Adrenal Disease: There is a common misconception that metastatic cancer to the adrenal glands rarely causes adrenal insufficiency. Prospective studies show that approximately 20% of patients with adrenal metastasis have a subnormal cortisol response to ACTH. The adrenal glands are common sites of metastasis for lung, gastrointestinal, breast, and renal neoplasia. In addition, non-Hodgkin's and Hodgkin's lymphoma may present primarily in the adrenal gland with primary adrenal insufficiency and bilateral adrenal enlargement.

F. AIDS: AIDS has been associated with pathologic involvement of the adrenal gland. Although adrenal necrosis is commonly seen in postmortem examination of patients with AIDS, primary adrenal insufficiency appears to complicate only approximately 5% of patients with this disorder. Primary adrenal insufficiency in AIDS is usually caused by opportunistic infections such as cytomegalovirus and tuberculosis. Adrenocortical insufficiency usually occurs as a late manifestation in AIDS patients with very low CD4 counts.

G. Familial Glucocorticoid Deficiency: Familial glucocorticoid deficiency is a rare disorder in which there is hereditary adrenocortical unresponsiveness to ACTH. This leads to adrenal insufficiency with subnormal glucocorticoid and adrenal androgen secretion as well as elevated plasma ACTH levels. As a rule, aldosterone secretion is preserved. At least two distinct types of this disorder have been described. One type is associated with mutations in the ACTH receptor on the cells of the adrenal cortex. Another type is often associated with achalasia and alacrima, but no mutations in the ACTH receptor have been seen in these patients.

H. Cortisol Resistance: Primary cortisol resistance is an unusual disorder representing target cell resistance to cortisol due to either qualitative or quantitative abnormalities of glucocorticoid receptor. This disorder is characterized by hypercortisolism without clinical manifestations of glucocorticoid excess. Pituitary resistance to cortisol results in hypersecretion of ACTH, which stimulates the adrenal gland to produce excessive amounts of cortisol, mineralocorticoids and adrenal androgens. The increased production of these nonglucocorticoid adrenal steroids may cause hypertension, hypokalemia, virilization, and sexual precocity. Because cortisol is essential for life, this disorder actually represents partial rather than complete resistance. Cortisol resistance has also been observed in patients with HIV infection.

Pathophysiology

Loss of more than 90% of both adrenal cortices results in the clinical manifestations of adrenocortical insufficiency. Gradual destruction such as occurs in the idiopathic and invasive forms of the disease leads to chronic adrenocortical insufficiency. However, more rapid destruction occurs in many cases; about 25% of patients are in crisis or impending crisis at the time of diagnosis. With gradual adrenocortical destruction, the initial phase is that of decreased adrenal reserve; ie, basal steroid secretion is normal, but secretion does not increase in response to stress. Thus, acute adrenal crisis can be precipitated by the stresses of surgery, trauma, or infection, which require increased corticosteroid secretion. With further

loss of cortical tissue, even basal secretion of mineralocorticoids and glucocorticoids becomes deficient, leading to the manifestations of chronic adrenocortical insufficiency. Destruction of the adrenals by hemorrhage results in sudden loss of both glucocorticoid and mineralocorticoid secretion, accompanied by acute adrenal crisis.

With decreasing cortisol secretion, plasma levels of ACTH are increased because of decreased negative feedback inhibition of their secretion. In fact, an elevation of plasma ACTH is the earliest and most sensitive indication of suboptimal adrenocortical reserve.

Clinical Features

A. Symptoms and Signs: Cortisol deficiency causes weakness, fatigue, anorexia, nausea and vomiting, hypotension, hyponatremia, and hypoglycemia. Mineralocorticoid deficiency produces renal sodium wasting and potassium retention and can lead to severe dehydration, hypotension, hyponatremia, hyperkalemia, and acidosis.

1. Chronic primary adrenocortical insufficiency—The chief symptoms (Table 9–2) are hyperpigmentation, weakness and fatigue, weight loss, anorexia, and gastrointestinal disturbances.

Hyperpigmentation is the classic physical finding, and its presence in association with the above manifestations should suggest primary adrenocortical insufficiency. Generalized hyperpigmentation of the skin and mucous membranes is one of the earliest manifestation of Addison's disease. It is increased in sun-exposed areas and accentuated over pressure areas such as the knuckles, toes, elbows, and knees. It is accompanied by increased numbers of black or dark-brown freckles. The classic hyperpigmentation of the buccal mucosa and gums is preceded by generalized hyperpigmentation of the skin; adrenal insufficiency should also be suspected when there is increased pigmentation of the palmar creases, nail beds, nipples, areolae, and perivaginal and perianal mucosa. Scars that have formed after the onset of ACTH excess become hyperpigmented, whereas older ones do not.

General weakness, fatigue and malaise, anorexia, and weight loss are invariable features of the disorder. Weight loss may reach 15 kg with progressive

Table 9–2. Clinical features of primary adrenocortical insufficiency.[1]

	Percent
Weakness, fatigue, anorexia, weight loss	100
Hyperpigmentation	92
Hypotension	88
Gastrointestinal disturbances	56
Salt craving	19
Postural symptoms	12

[1]Reproduced, with permission, from Baxter JD, Tyrrell JB, in: *Endocrinology and Metabolism.* Felig P, Baxter JD, Frohman LA (editors). 3rd Ed. McGraw-Hill, 1995.

adrenal failure. Gastrointestinal disturbances, especially nausea and vomiting, occur in most patients; diarrhea is less frequent. An increase in gastrointestinal symptoms during an acute adrenal crisis may confuse the diagnosis by suggesting a primary intra-abdominal process.

Hypotension is present in about 90% of patients and is accompanied by orthostatic symptoms and occasionally syncope. In more severe chronic cases and in acute crises, recumbent hypotension or shock is almost invariably present. Vitiligo occurs in 4–17% of patients with autoimmune Addison's disease but is rare in Addison's disease due to other causes. Salt craving occurs in about 20% of patients.

Severe hypoglycemia may occur in children. This finding is unusual in adults but may be provoked by fasting, fever, infection, or nausea and vomiting, especially in acute adrenal crisis.

Amenorrhea is common in Addison's disease. It may be due to weight loss and chronic illness or to primary ovarian failure. Loss of axillary and pubic hair may occur in women as a result of decreased secretion of adrenal androgens.

2. Acute adrenal crisis–Acute adrenal crisis represents a state of acute adrenocortical insufficiency and occurs in patients with Addison's disease who are exposed to the stress of infection, trauma, surgery, or dehydration due to salt deprivation, vomiting, or diarrhea.

The symptoms are listed in Table 9–3. Anorexia and nausea and vomiting increase and worsen the volume depletion and dehydration. Hypovolemic shock frequently occurs, and adrenal insufficiency should be considered in any patient with unexplained vascular collapse. Abdominal pain may occur and mimic an acute abdominal emergency. Weakness, apathy, and confusion are usual. Fever is usual and may be due to infection or to hypoadrenalism per se. Hyperpigmentation is present unless the onset of adrenal insufficiency is rapid and should suggest the diagnosis.

Additional findings that suggest the diagnosis are hyponatremia, hyperkalemia, lymphocytosis, eosinophilia, and hypoglycemia.

Shock and coma may rapidly lead to death in untreated patients.

3. Acute adrenal hemorrhage–(See Table 9–4.) Bilateral adrenal hemorrhage and acute adrenal destruction in an already compromised patient with major medical illness follow a progressively deterio-

Table 9–3. Clinical features of acute adrenal crisis.

Hypotension and shock
Fever
Dehydration, volume depletion
Nausea, vomiting, anorexia
Weakness, apathy, depressed mentation
Hypoglycemia

Table 9–4. Clinical features of adrenal hemorrhage.[1]

	Percent
General features	
Hypotension and shock	74
Fever	59
Nausea and vomiting	46
Confusion, disorientation	41
Tachycardia	28
Cyanosis or lividity	28
Local features	
Abdominal, flank, or back pain	77
Abdominal or flank tenderness	38
Abdominal distention	28
Abdominal rigidity	20
Chest pain	13
Rebound tenderness	5

[1]Reproduced, with permission, from Baxter JD, Tyrrell JB, In: *Endocrinology and Metabolism.* Felig P, Baxter JD, Frohman LA (editors). 3rd Ed. McGraw-Hill, 1995.

rating course. The usual manifestations are abdominal, flank, or back pain and abdominal tenderness. Abdominal distention, rigidity, and rebound tenderness are less frequent. Hypotension, shock, fever, nausea and vomiting, confusion, and disorientation are common; tachycardia and cyanosis are less frequent.

With progression, severe hypotension, volume depletion, dehydration, hyperpyrexia, cyanosis, coma, and death ensue.

The diagnosis of acute adrenal hemorrhage should be considered in the deteriorating patient with unexplained abdominal or flank pain, vascular collapse, hyperpyrexia, or hypoglycemia.

B. Laboratory and Electrocardiographic Findings and Imaging Studies:

1. Gradual adrenal destruction–Hyponatremia and hyperkalemia are classic manifestations of the mineralocorticoid deficiency of primary adrenal insufficiency and should suggest the diagnosis. Hematologic manifestations include normocytic, normochromic anemia, neutropenia, eosinophilia, and a relative lymphocytosis. Azotemia with increased concentrations of blood urea nitrogen and serum creatinine is due to volume depletion and dehydration. Mild acidosis is frequently present. Hypercalcemia of mild to moderate degree occurs in about 6% of patients.

Abdominal radiographs reveal adrenal calcification in half the patients with tuberculous Addison's disease and in some patients with other invasive or hemorrhagic causes of adrenal insufficiency. Computed tomography (CT scan) is a more sensitive detector of adrenal calcification and adrenal enlargement. Bilateral adrenal enlargement in association with adrenal insufficiency may be seen with tuberculosis, fungal infections, cytomegalovirus, malignant and nonmalignant infiltrative diseases, and adrenal hemorrhage.

Electrocardiographic features are low voltage, a vertical QRS axis, and nonspecific ST–T wave abnormalities secondary to abnormal electrolytes.

2. Acute adrenal hemorrhage–Hyponatremia and hyperkalemia occur in only a small number of cases, but azotemia is a usual finding. Increased circulating eosinophils may suggest the diagnosis. The diagnosis is frequently established only when imaging studies reveal bilateral adrenal enlargement.

SECONDARY ADRENOCORTICAL INSUFFICIENCY

Etiology

Secondary adrenocortical insufficiency due to ACTH deficiency is most commonly a result of exogenous glucocorticoid therapy. Pituitary or hypothalamic tumors are the most common causes of naturally occurring pituitary ACTH hyposecretion. These and other less common causes are reviewed in Chapter 5.

Pathophysiology

ACTH deficiency is the primary event and leads to decreased cortisol and adrenal androgen secretion. Aldosterone secretion remains normal except in a few cases. In the early stages, basal ACTH and cortisol levels may be normal; however, ACTH reserve is impaired, and ACTH and cortisol responses to stress are therefore subnormal. With further loss of basal ACTH secretion, there is atrophy of the zonae fasciculata and reticularis of the adrenal cortex; and, therefore, basal cortisol secretion is decreased. At this stage, the entire pituitary adrenal axis is impaired; ie, there is not only decreased ACTH responsiveness to stress but also decreased adrenal responsiveness to acute stimulation with exogenous ACTH.

The manifestations of glucocorticoid deficiency are similar to those described for primary adrenocortical insufficiency. However, since aldosterone secretion by the zona glomerulosa is usually preserved, the manifestations of mineralocorticoid deficiency are absent.

Clinical Features

A. Symptoms and Signs: Secondary adrenal insufficiency is usually chronic, and the manifestations may be nonspecific. However, acute crisis can occur in undiagnosed patients or in corticosteroid-treated patients who do not receive increased steroid dosage during periods of stress.

The clinical features of secondary adrenal insufficiency differ from those of primary adrenocortical insufficiency in that pituitary secretion of ACTH is deficient and hyperpigmentation is therefore not present. In addition, mineralocorticoid secretion is usually normal. Thus, the clinical features of ACTH and glucocorticoid deficiency are nonspecific.

Volume depletion, dehydration, and hyperkalemia are usually absent. Hypotension is usually not present except in acute presentations. Hyponatremia may occur as a result of water retention and inability to excrete a water load but is not accompanied by hyperkalemia. Prominent features are weakness, lethargy, easy fatigability, anorexia, nausea, and occasionally vomiting. Arthralgias and myalgias also occur. Hypoglycemia is occasionally the presenting feature. Acute decompensation with severe hypotension or shock unresponsive to vasopressors may occur.

B. Associated Features: Patients with secondary adrenal insufficiency commonly have additional features that suggest the diagnosis. A history of glucocorticoid therapy or, if this is not available, the presence of cushingoid features suggests prior glucocorticoid use. Hypothalamic or pituitary tumors leading to ACTH deficiency usually cause loss of other pituitary hormones (hypogonadism and hypothyroidism). Hypersecretion of GH or prolactin (PRL) from a pituitary adenoma may be present.

C. Laboratory Findings: Findings on routine laboratory examination consist of normochromic, normocytic anemia, neutropenia, lymphocytosis, and eosinophilia. Serum sodium, potassium, creatinine, and bicarbonate and blood urea nitrogen are usually normal; plasma glucose may be low, though severe hypoglycemia is unusual.

DIAGNOSIS OF ADRENOCORTICAL INSUFFICIENCY

Although the diagnosis of adrenal insufficiency should be confirmed by assessment of the pituitary adrenal axis, therapy should not be delayed nor should the patient be subjected to procedures that may increase volume loss and dehydration and further contribute to hypotension. If the patient is acutely ill, therapy should be instituted and the diagnosis established when the patient is stable.

Diagnostic Tests

Since basal levels of adrenocortical steroids in either urine or plasma may be normal in partial adrenal insufficiency, tests of adrenocortical reserve are necessary to establish the diagnosis (Figure 9–11). These tests are described in the section on laboratory evaluation and in Chapter 5.

Rapid ACTH Stimulation Test

The rapid ACTH stimulation test assesses adrenal reserve and is the initial procedure in the assessment of possible adrenal insufficiency, either primary or secondary. As previously discussed, the low-dose ACTH (1 μg cosyntropin) stimulation test has been shown to represent a more physiologic stimulus to the adrenal cortex and has emerged as a more sensitive indication of suboptimal adrenal function.

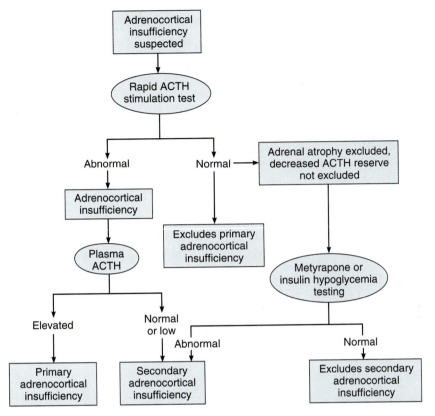

Figure 9–11. Evaluation of suspected primary or secondary adrenocortical insufficiency. Boxes enclose clinical decisions, and circles enclose diagnostic tests. (Redrawn and reproduced, with permission, from Baxter JD, Tyrrell JB: The adrenal cortex. In: *Endocrinology and Metabolism.* Felig P et al [editors]. McGraw-Hill, 1981.)

Subnormal responses to exogenous ACTH administration are an indication of decreased adrenal reserve and establish the diagnosis of adrenocortical insufficiency. Further diagnostic procedures are not required, since subnormal responses to the rapid ACTH stimulation test indicate lack of responsiveness to metyrapone, insulin-induced hypoglycemia, or stress. However, this test does not permit differentiation of primary and secondary causes. This is best accomplished by measurement of basal plasma ACTH levels, as discussed below.

A normal response to the rapid ACTH stimulation test excludes primary adrenal failure, since a normal cortisol response indicates normal cortical function. However, normal responsiveness does not exclude partial secondary adrenocortical insufficiency in those few patients with decreased pituitary reserve and decreased stress responsiveness of the hypothalamic-pituitary-adrenal axis who maintain sufficient basal ACTH secretion to prevent adrenocortical atrophy. If this situation is suspected clinically, pituitary ACTH responsiveness may be tested directly with metyrapone or insulin-induced hypoglycemia. (See section on laboratory evaluation and below.)

Plasma ACTH Levels

If adrenal insufficiency is present, plasma ACTH levels are used to differentiate primary and secondary forms. In patients with primary adrenal insufficiency, plasma ACTH levels exceed the upper limit of the normal range (> 52 pg/mL) and usually exceed 200 pg/mL (44 pmol/L). Plasma ACTH concentration is less than 30 pg/mL (7 pmol/L) in patients with secondary adrenal insufficiency (Figure 9–12). However, the basal ACTH level must always be interpreted in light of the clinical situation, especially because of the episodic nature of ACTH secretion and its short plasma half-life. For example, ACTH levels will frequently exceed the normal range during the recovery of the hypothalamic-pituitary-adrenal (HPA) axis from secondary adrenal insufficiency and may be confused with levels seen in primary adrenal insufficiency. Patients with primary adrenal insufficiency consistently have elevated ACTH levels. In fact, the ACTH concentration will be elevated early in the course of adrenal insufficiency even before a significant reduction in the basal cortisol level or its response to exogenous ACTH occurs. Therefore, plasma ACTH measurements serve as a

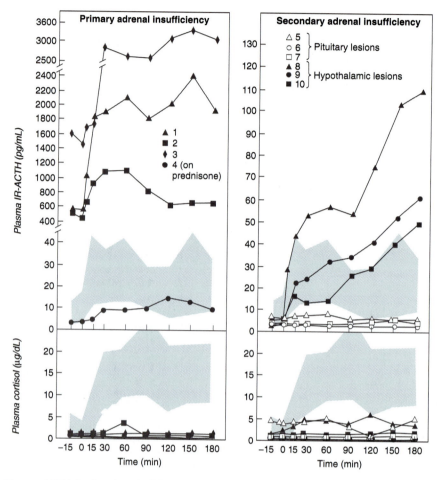

Figure 9–12. Plasma ACTH (top) and cortisol (bottom) responses to CRH in subjects with primary adrenal insufficiency (left) or secondary adrenal insufficiency (right). Patients with hypothalamic lesions had clearly distinct ACTH responses to CRH, different from those in three patients with pituitary adrenal insufficiency. *Shaded area:* Absolute range from 15 normal subjects. (Reproduced, with permission, from J. Clin Endocrinol Metab 1984;58:1066.)

valuable screening study for primary adrenal insufficiency.

Partial ACTH Deficiency

When partial ACTH deficiency and decreased pituitary reserve are suspected despite normal responsiveness to the rapid ACTH stimulation test, the following procedures may be used for more direct assessment of hypothalamic-pituitary function:

A. Methods of Testing: The overnight metyrapone test is used in patients with suspected hypothalamic or pituitary disorders when hypoglycemia is contraindicated and in those with prior glucocorticoid therapy. Insulin-induced hypoglycemia is used in patients with suspected hypothalamic or pituitary tumors, since both ACTH and GH responsiveness can be assessed (see Chapter 5).

B. Interpretation: A normal response to either metyrapone or hypoglycemia excludes secondary

adrenocortical insufficiency. (See section on laboratory evaluation.) Subnormal responses, in the presence of a normal response to ACTH administration, establish the diagnosis of secondary adrenal insufficiency.

TREATMENT OF ADRENOCORTICAL INSUFFICIENCY

The aim of treatment of adrenocortical insufficiency is to produce levels of glucocorticoids and mineralocorticoids equivalent to those achieved in an individual with normal hypothalamic-pituitary-adrenal function under similar circumstances.

Acute Addisonian Crisis (Table 9–5)

Treatment for acute addisonian crisis should be instituted as soon as the diagnosis is suspected. Ther-

Table 9–5. Treatment of acute adrenal crises.

Glucocorticoid replacement
(1) Administer cortisol (as hydrocortisone phosphate or hemisuccinate), 100 mg intravenously every 6 hours for 24 hours.
(2) When the patient is stable, reduce the dosage to 50 mg every 6 hours.
(3) Taper to maintenance therapy by day 4 or 5 and add mineralocorticoid therapy as required.
(4) Maintain or increase the dose to 200–400 mg/d if complications persist or occur.

General and supportive measures
(1) Correct volume depletion, dehydration, and hypoglycemia with intravenous saline and glucose.
(2) Evaluate and correct infection and other precipitating factors.

apy includes administration of glucocorticoids; correction of dehydration, hypovolemia, and electrolyte abnormalities; general supportive measures; and treatment of coexisting or precipitating disorders.

A. Cortisol (Hydrocortisone): Parenteral cortisol in soluble form (hydrocortisone hemisuccinate or phosphate) is the glucocorticoid preparation most commonly used. When administered in supraphysiologic doses, hydrocortisone has sufficient sodium-retaining potency so that additional mineralocorticoid therapy is not required in patients with primary adrenocortical insufficiency.

Cortisol in doses of 100 mg intravenously is given every 6 hours for the first 24 hours. The response to therapy is usually rapid, with improvement occurring within 12 hours or less. If improvement occurs and the patient is stable, 50 mg every 6 hours is given on the second day, and in most patients the dosage may then be gradually reduced to approximately 10 mg three times daily by the fourth or fifth day. (See section on maintenance therapy, below.)

1. In severely ill patients, especially in those with additional major complications (eg, sepsis), higher cortisol doses (100 mg intravenously every 6–8 hours) are maintained until the patient is stable.

2. In primary Addison's disease, mineralocorticoid replacement, in the form of fludrocortisone (see below), is added when the total cortisol dosage has been reduced to 50–60 mg/d.

3. In secondary adrenocortical insufficiency with acute crisis, the primary requirement is glucocorticoid replacement and is satisfactorily supplied by the administration of cortisol, as outlined above. If the possibility of excessive fluid and sodium retention in such patients is of concern, equivalent parenteral doses of synthetic steroids such as prednisolone or dexamethasone may be substituted.

4. Intramuscular cortisone acetate is contraindicated in acute adrenal failure for the following reasons: (1) absorption is slow; (2) it requires conversion to cortisol in the liver; (3) adequate plasma levels of cortisol are not obtained; and (4) there is in-

adequate suppression of plasma ACTH levels, indicating insufficient glucocorticoid activity.

B. Intravenous Fluids: Intravenous glucose and saline are administered to correct volume depletion, hypotension, and hypoglycemia. Volume deficits may be severe in Addison's disease, and hypotension and shock may not respond to vasopressors unless glucocorticoids are administered. Hyperkalemia and acidosis are usually corrected with cortisol and volume replacement; however, an occasional patient may require specific therapy for these abnormalities.

Maintenance Therapy (Table 9–6)

Patients with Addison's disease require life-long glucocorticoid and mineralocorticoid therapy. Cortisol (hydrocortisone) is the glucocorticoid preparation of first choice. The basal production rate of cortisol is approximately $8-12$ mg/m^2/d. The maintenance dose of hydrocortisone is usually 15–30 mg daily in adults. The oral dose is usually divided into 10–20 mg in the morning on arising and 5–10 mg later in the day. Other glucocorticoids such as oral cortisone acetate (37.5 mg/d), which is rapidly absorbed and converted to cortisol, or equivalent doses of synthetic steroids (eg, prednisone) may occasionally be used. Cortisol in twice-daily doses gives satisfactory responses in most patients; however, some patients may require only a single morning dose, and others may require three doses daily to maintain well-being and normal energy levels. Insomnia is a side effect of glucocorticoid administration and can usually be prevented by administering the last dose at 4:00–5:00 PM.

Fludrocortisone (9α-fluorocortisol) is used for mineralocorticoid therapy; the usual doses are 0.05–0.2 mg/d orally in the morning. Because of the long half-life of this agent, divided doses are not required. About 10–20% of addisonian patients can be managed with cortisol and adequate dietary sodium intake alone and do not require fludrocortisone.

Secondary adrenocortical insufficiency is treated with the cortisol dosages described above for the primary form. Fludrocortisone is rarely required. The recovery of normal function of the hypothalamic-pi-

Table 9–6. Regimen for maintenance therapy of primary adrenocortical insufficiency.[1]

(1) Cortisol, 15–20 mg in AM and 10 mg at 4–5 PM.
(2) Fludrocortisone, 0.05–0.1 mg orally in AM.
(3) Clinical follow-up: Maintenance of normal wieght, blood pressure, and electrolytes with regression of clinical features.
(4) Patient education plus identification card or bracelet.
(5) Increased cortisol dosage during "stress."

[1]Reproduced, with permission, from Baxter JD, Tyrrell JB, in: *Endocrinology and Metabolism.* Felig P, Baxter JD, Frohman LA (editors). 3rd Ed. McGraw-Hill, 1995.

tuitary-adrenal axis following suppression by exogenous glucocorticoids may take weeks to years, and its duration is not readily predictable. Consequently, prolonged replacement therapy may be required.

Response to Therapy

There are no currently available useful biochemical procedures for assessing the appropriateness of glucocorticoid replacement therapy in patients with primary or secondary adrenal insufficiency. The measurement of urine free cortisol or serum cortisol does not provide a reliable index for appropriate glucocorticoid replacement. Similarly, ACTH measurements are not a good indication of the adequacy of glucocorticoid replacement; marked elevations of plasma ACTH in patients with chronic adrenal insufficiency are often not suppressed into the normal range despite adequate hydrocortisone replacement.

General clinical signs, such as good appetite and sense of well-being, are the best guides to the adequacy of replacement. Obviously, signs of Cushing's syndrome indicate overtreatment. It is generally expected that the daily dose of hydrocortisone should be doubled during periods of minor stress, and the dose needs to be increased to as much as 200–300 mg/d during periods of major stress, such as a surgical procedure. Patients receiving excessive doses of glucocorticoids are also at risk for increased bone loss and clinically significant osteoporosis. Therefore, the replacement dose of glucocorticoid should be maintained at the lowest amount needed to provide the patient with a proper sense of well-being.

Adequate treatment results in the disappearance of weakness, malaise, and fatigue. Anorexia and other gastrointestinal symptoms resolve, and weight returns to normal. The hyperpigmentation invariably improves but may not entirely disappear. Inadequate cortisol administration leads to persistence of these symptoms of adrenal insufficiency, and excessive pigmentation will remain.

Adequate mineralocorticoid replacement may be determined by assessment of blood pressure and electrolyte composition. With adequate treatment, the blood pressure is normal without orthostatic change, and serum sodium and potassium remain within the normal range. Some endocrinologists monitor plasma renin activity (PRA) as an objective measure of fludrocortisone replacement. Upright PRA levels are usually < 5 ng/mL/h in adequately replaced patients. Hypertension and hypokalemia result if the fludrocortisone dose is excessive. Conversely, undertreatment may lead to fatigue and malaise, orthostatic symptoms, and subnormal supine or upright blood pressure, with hyperkalemia and hyponatremia.

Prevention of Adrenal Crisis

The development of acute adrenal insufficiency in previously diagnosed and treated patients is almost entirely preventable in cooperative individuals. The essential elements are patient education and increased glucocorticoid dosages during illness.

The patient should be informed about the necessity for lifelong therapy, the possible consequences of acute illness, and the necessity for increased therapy and medical assistance during acute illness. An identification card or bracelet should be carried or worn at all times.

The cortisol dose should be increased by the patient to 60–80 mg/d with the development of minor illnesses; the usual maintenance dosage may be resumed in 24–48 hours if improvement occurs. Increased mineralocorticoid therapy is not required.

If symptoms persist or become worse, the patient should continue increased cortisol doses and call the physician.

Vomiting may result in inability to ingest or absorb oral cortisol, and diarrhea in addisonian patients may precipitate a crisis because of rapid fluid and electrolyte losses. Patients must understand that if these symptoms occur, they should seek immediate medical assistance so that parenteral glucocorticoid therapy can be given.

Steroid Coverage for Surgery
(Table 9–7)

The normal physiologic response to surgical stress involves an increase in cortisol secretion. Thus, patients with primary or secondary adrenocortical insufficiency scheduled for elective surgery require increased glucocorticoid coverage. This problem is most frequently encountered in patients with pituitary-adrenal suppression due to exogenous glucocorticoid therapy. However, the increased glucocorticoid action may serve primarily to modulate the immunologic response to stress. The principles of management are outlined in Table 9–7. *Note:* Intramuscular cortisone acetate should not be used, for the reasons discussed above in the section on treatment of acute addisonian crisis.

Table 9–7. Steroid coverage for surgery.[1]

(1) Correct electrolytes, blood pressure, and hydration if necessary.
(2) Give cortisol (as hydrocortisone phosphate or hemisuccinate) 100 mg intramuscularly, on call to operating room.
(3) Give cortisol, 50 mg intramuscularly or intravenously, in the recovery room and every 6 hours for the first 24 hours.
(4) If progress is satisfactory, reduce dosage to 25 mg every 6 hours for 24 hours and then taper to maintenance dosage over 3–5 days. Resume previous fludrocortisone dose when the patient is taking oral medications.
(5) Maintain or increase cortisol dosage to 200–400 mg/d if fever, hypotension, or other complications occur.

[1]Modified and reproduced, with permission, from Baxter JD, Tyrrell JB, in *Endocrinology and Metabolism.* Felig P, Baxter JD, Frohman LA (editors), 3rd Ed. McGraw-Hill, 1995.

PROGNOSIS OF ADRENOCORTICAL INSUFFICIENCY

Before glucocorticoid and mineralocorticoid therapy became available, primary adrenocortical insufficiency was invariably fatal, with death usually occurring within 2 years after onset. Survival now depends upon the underlying cause of the adrenal insufficiency. In patients with autoimmune Addison's disease, survival approaches that of the normal population, and most patients lead normal lives. In general, death from adrenal insufficiency now occurs only in patients with rapid onset of disease who may die before the diagnosis is established and appropriate therapy started.

Secondary adrenal insufficiency has an excellent prognosis with glucocorticoid therapy.

Adrenal insufficiency due to bilateral adrenal hemorrhage is still often fatal, with most cases being recognized only at autopsy.

CUSHING'S SYNDROME

Chronic glucocorticoid excess, whatever its cause, leads to the constellation of symptoms and physical features known as Cushing's *syndrome*. It is most commonly iatrogenic, resulting from chronic glucocorticoid therapy. "Spontaneous" Cushing's syndrome is caused by abnormalities of the pituitary or adrenal or may occur as a consequence of ACTH secretion by nonpituitary tumors (**ectopic ACTH syndrome**). Cushing's *disease* is defined as the specific type of Cushing's syndrome due to excessive pituitary ACTH secretion from a pituitary tumor. This section will review the various types of spontaneous Cushing's syndrome and discuss their diagnosis and therapy. (See also Chapter 5.)

Classification & Incidence

Cushing's syndrome is conveniently classified as either ACTH-dependent or ACTH-independent (Table 9–8).

The ACTH-dependent types of Cushing's syndrome—ectopic ACTH syndrome and Cushing's disease—are characterized by chronic ACTH hypersecretion, which results in hyperplasia of the adrenal zonae fasciculata and reticularis and therefore increased adrenocortical secretion of cortisol, androgens, and DOC.

ACTH-independent Cushing's syndrome may be caused by a primary adrenal neoplasm (adenoma or carcinoma) or nodular adrenal hyperplasia. In these cases, the cortisol excess suppresses pituitary ACTH secretion.

Table 9–8. Cushing's syndrome: differential diagnosis.

ACTH-dependent
  Pituitary adenoma (Cushing's disease)
  Nonpituitary neoplasm (ectopic ACTH)
ACTH-independent
  Iatrogenic (glucocorticoid, megestrol acetate)
  Adrenal neoplasm (adenoma, carcinoma)
  Nodular adrenal hyperplasia
    Primary pigmented nodular adrenal disease
    Massive macronodular adrenonodular hyperplasia
    Food-dependent (GIP-mediated)
  Factitious

A. Cushing's Disease: This is the most frequent type of Cushing's syndrome and is responsible for about 70% of reported cases. Cushing's disease is much more common in women than in men (female:male ratio of about 8:1) and the age at diagnosis may range from childhood to 70 years.

B. Ectopic ACTH Hypersecretion: This disorder accounts for approximately 15–20% of patients with ACTH-dependent Cushing's syndrome. The production of ACTH from a tumor of nonpituitary origin may result in severe hypercortisolism, and many of these patients lack the classic features of glucocorticoid excess. This clinical presentation of ectopic ACTH secretion is most frequently seen in patients with small cell carcinoma of the lung; this tumor is responsible for about 50% of cases of this syndrome, though ectopic ACTH hypersecretion is estimated to occur in only 0.5–2% of patients with small cell carcinoma. The prognosis in these patients is very poor, with a mean survival of less than 1 month. The ectopic ACTH syndrome may also present in a fashion identical to classic Cushing's disease and pose a challenging diagnostic dilemma. The majority of these tumors are also located in the lung (bronchial carcinoids) and may be radiologically inapparent at the time of the presentation. The ectopic ACTH syndrome is more common in men, and the peak age incidence is 40–60 years.

C. Primary Adrenal Tumors: Primary adrenal tumors cause approximately 10% of cases of Cushing's syndrome. Most of these patients have benign adrenocortical adenomas. Adrenocortical carcinomas are uncommon, with an incidence of approximately 2 per million per year. Both adrenocortical adenomas and carcinomas are more common in women.

D. Childhood Cushing's Syndrome: Cushing's syndrome in childhood and adolescence is distinctly unusual; however, in contrast to the incidence in adults, adrenal carcinoma is the most frequent cause (51%), and adrenal adenomas are present in 14%. These tumors are more common in girls than in boys, and most occur between the ages of 1 and 8 years. Cushing's disease is more common in the adolescent population and accounts for 35% of cases; most of these patients are over 10 years of age at diagnosis, and the sex incidence is equal.

Pathology

A. Anterior Pituitary Gland:

1. Pituitary adenomas–Pituitary adenomas are present in over 90% of patients with Cushing's disease. These tumors are typically smaller than those secreting GH or PRL; 80–90% are less than 10 mm in diameter. A small group of patients have larger tumors (> 10 mm); these macroadenomas are frequently invasive, leading to extension outside the sella turcica. Malignant pituitary tumors occur rarely.

Microadenomas are located within the anterior pituitary; they are not encapsulated but surrounded by a rim of compressed normal anterior pituitary cells. With routine histologic stains, these tumors are composed of compact sheets of well-granulated basophilic cells in a sinusoidal arrangement. ACTH, β-LPH, and β-endorphin have been demonstrated in these tumor cells by immunocytochemical methods. Larger tumors may appear chromophobic on routine histologic study; however, they also contain ACTH and its related peptides. These ACTH-secreting adenomas typically show Crooke's changes (a zone of perinuclear hyalinization that is the result of chronic exposure of corticotroph cells to hypercortisolism). Electron microscopy demonstrates secretory granules that vary in size from 200 to 700 nm. The number of granules varies in individual cells; they may be dispersed throughout the cytoplasm or concentrated along the cell membrane. A typical feature of these adenomas is the presence of bundles of perinuclear microfilaments (average 7 nm in diameter) surrounding the nucleus; these are responsible for Crooke's hyaline changes visible on light microscopy.

2. Hyperplasia–Diffuse hyperplasia of corticotroph cells has been reported rarely in patients with Cushing's disease. These cases may be the consequence of excessive stimulation of the anterior pituitary by CRH.

3. Other conditions–In patients with adrenal tumors or ectopic ACTH syndrome, the pituitary corticotrophs show prominent Crooke hyaline changes and perinuclear microfilaments. The ACTH content of corticotroph cells is reduced consistent with their suppression by excessive cortisol secretion present in these conditions.

B. Adrenocortical Hyperplasia:
Bilateral hyperplasia of the adrenal cortex occurs with chronic ACTH hypersecretion. Three types have been described: simple, that associated with ectopic ACTH syndrome, and bilateral nodular hyperplasia.

1. Simple adrenocortical hyperplasia–This condition is usually due to Cushing's disease. Combined adrenal weight (normal, 8–10 g) is modestly increased, ranging from 12 to 24 g. On histologic study, there is equal hyperplasia of the compact cells of the zona reticularis and the clear cells of the zona fasciculata; consequently, the width of the cortex is increased. Electron microscopy reveals normal ultrastructural features.

2. Ectopic ACTH syndrome–In this disorder, the adrenals are frequently markedly enlarged; combined weights range from 24 g to more than 50 g. The characteristic microscopic feature is marked hyperplasia of the zona reticularis; columns of compact reticularis cells expand throughout the zona fasciculata and into the zona glomerulosa. The zona fasciculata clear cells are markedly reduced.

3. Bilateral nodular hyperplasia–Bilateral nodular hyperplasia with Cushing's syndrome has been identified as a morphologic consequence of several unique pathophysiologic disorders. Long-standing ACTH hypersecretion—either pituitary or nonpituitary—may result in nodular enlargement of the adrenal gland. These focal nodules may often be mistaken for an adrenal neoplasm and have led to unnecessary and unsuccessful unilateral adrenal surgery. These nodules may, over a period of time, even become autonomous or semiautonomous. Removal of the ACTH-secreting neoplasm will result in regression of the adrenal nodules as well as resolution of the hypercortisolism unless the nodules have already developed autonomy. A rare adrenal-dependent cause of Cushing's syndrome, primary pigmented nodular adrenocortical disease (PPNAD), presents in adolescence or young adulthood. It is a familial disorder with an autosomal dominant inheritance pattern and may be associated with unusual conditions such as myxomas (cardiac, cutaneous, and mammary), spotty skin pigmentation, endocrine overactivity (sexual precocity and acromegaly), and schwannomas. Interestingly, the adrenal glands in this disorder are often small or normal in size and have multiple black and brown nodules with intranodular cortical atrophy. The clinical manifestations of hypercortisolism usually become apparent in the second decade and can be mild, moderate, or severe. Primary pigmented nodular adrenocortical disease appears to be caused by adrenal stimulating immunoglobulins that bind to the ACTH receptor, provoking adrenal steroid biosynthesis. Another type of nodular adrenal hyperplasia has been termed massive macronodular adrenal hyperplasia. This ACTH-independent, adrenal-dependent cause of Cushing's syndrome is characterized by bilateral large nodules (3–6 cm in diameter). This disorder is rarely familial, and adrenal stimulating immunoglobulins have not been identified. The cause of this type of adrenal nodular hyperplasia is unknown; however, two patients with massive macronodular adrenal hyperplasia have been reported with food-dependent hypercortisolism. The adrenal cortex in these patients expressed abnormal receptors for gastrointestinal inhibitory polypeptide (GIP). Food consumption, therefore, stimulates GIP, which in turn binds to the receptors in the adrenal cortex, thereby stimulating adrenal growth and steroid biosynthesis. Because somatostatin inhibits GIP secretion, its long-acting analog, octreotide acetate, is used to attenuate GIP-dependent hypercortisolism.

C. Adrenal Tumors: Adrenal tumors causing Cushing's syndrome are independent of ACTH secretion and are either adenomas or carcinomas.

1. Glucocorticoid-secreting adrenal adenomas–These adenomas are encapsulated, weigh 10–70 g, and range in size from 1 cm to 6 cm. Microscopically, clear cells of the zona fasciculata type predominate, although cells typical of the zona reticularis are also seen.

2. Adrenal carcinomas–Adrenal carcinomas usually weigh over 100 g and may exceed several kilograms. Thus, they are commonly palpable as abdominal masses. Grossly, they are encapsulated and highly vascular; necrosis, hemorrhage, and cystic degeneration are common, and areas of calcification may be present. The histologic appearance of these carcinomas varies considerably; they may appear to be benign or may exhibit considerable pleomorphism. Vascular or capsular invasion is predictive of malignant behavior, as is local extension. These carcinomas invade local structures (kidney, liver, and retroperitoneum) and metastasize hematogenously to liver and lung.

3. Uninvolved adrenal cortex–The cortex contiguous to the tumor and that of the contralateral gland are atrophic in the presence of functioning adrenal adenomas and carcinomas. The cortex is markedly thinned, whereas the capsule is thickened. Histologically, the zona reticularis is virtually absent; the remaining cortex is composed of clear fasciculata cells. The architecture of the zona glomerulosa is normal.

Etiology & Pathogenesis

A. Cushing's Disease: The causes and natural history of Cushing's disease are reviewed in Chapter 5. Current evidence is consistent with the view that spontaneously arising corticotroph-cell pituitary adenomas are the primary cause and that the consequent ACTH hypersecretion and hypercortisolism lead to the characteristic endocrine abnormalities and hypothalamic dysfunction. This is supported by evidence showing that selective removal of these adenomas by pituitary microsurgery reverses the abnormalities and is followed by return of the hypothalamic-pituitary-adrenal axis to normal. In addition, molecular studies have shown that nearly all corticotroph adenomas are monoclonal.

Although these primary pituitary adenomas are responsible for the great majority of cases, a few patients have been described in whom pituitary disease has been limited to corticotroph-cell hyperplasia; these may be secondary to excessive CRH secretion by rare, benign hypothalamic gangliocytoma.

B. Ectopic ACTH Syndrome: This syndrome arises when nonpituitary tumors synthesize and hypersecrete biologically active ACTH. The related peptides β-LPH and β-endorphin are also synthesized and secreted, as are inactive ACTH fragments.

Production of CRH has also been demonstrated in ectopic tumors secreting ACTH, but whether CRH plays a role in pathogenesis is unclear. A few cases in which nonpituitary tumors produced only CRH have been reported.

Ectopic ACTH syndrome occurs predominantly in only a few tumor types (Table 9–9); small-cell carcinoma of the lung causes half of cases. Other tumors causing the syndrome are carcinoid tumors of lung, thymus, gut, pancreas, or ovary; pancreatic islet cell tumors; medullary thyroid carcinoma; and pheochromocytoma and related tumors. Other rare miscellaneous tumor types have also been reported (see Chapter 23).

C. Adrenal Tumors: Glucocorticoid-producing adrenal adenomas and carcinomas arise spontaneously. They are not under hypothalamic-pituitary control and autonomously secrete adrenocortical steroids. Rarely, adrenal carcinomas develop in the setting of chronic ACTH hypersecretion in patients with either Cushing's disease and nodular adrenal hyperplasia or congenital adrenal hyperplasia.

Pathophysiology

A. Cushing's Disease: In Cushing's disease, ACTH hypersecretion is random and episodic and causes cortisol hypersecretion with absence of the normal circadian rhythm. Feedback inhibition of ACTH (secreted from the pituitary adenoma) by physiologic levels of glucocorticoids is absent; thus, ACTH hypersecretion persists despite elevated cortisol secretion and results in chronic glucocorticoid excess. The episodic secretion of ACTH and cortisol results in variable plasma levels that may at times be within the normal range. However, measurement of the cortisol production rate, urine free cortisol, or sampling of multiple cortisol levels over 24 hours confirms cortisol hypersecretion (see sections on laboratory evaluation and diagnosis of Cushing's syndrome). In addition, because of the absence of diurnal variability, plasma ACTH and cortisol remain elevated throughout the day and night. This overall increase in glucocorticoid secretion causes the clinical manifestations of Cushing's syndrome; however, ACTH and β-LPH secretion are not usually elevated sufficiently to cause hyperpigmentation.

1. Abnormalities of ACTH secretion–Despite ACTH hypersecretion, stress responsiveness is ab-

Table 9–9. Tumors causing the ectopic ACTH syndrome.[1]

Small cell carcinoma of the lung (50% of cases)
Pancreatic islet cell tumors
Carcinoid tumors (lung, thymus, gut, pancreas, ovary)
Medullary carcinoma of the thyroid
Pheochromocytoma and related tumors

[1]Modified and reproduced, with permission, from Baxter JD, Tyrrell JB, in: *Endocrinology and Metabolism.* Felig P, Baxter JD, Frohman LA (editors). 3rd Ed. McGraw-Hill, 1995.

sent; stimuli such as hypoglycemia or surgery fail to further elevate ACTH and cortisol secretion. This is probably due to suppression of hypothalamic function and CRH secretion by hypercortisolism, resulting in loss of hypothalamic control of ACTH secretion (see Chapter 5).

2. Effect of cortisol excess–Cortisol excess not only inhibits normal pituitary and hypothalamic function, affecting ACTH, thyrotropin, GH, and gonadotropin release, but also results in all the systemic effects of glucocorticoid excess described in previous sections and in the section on clinical features below.

3. Androgen excess–Secretion of adrenal androgens is also increased in Cushing's disease, and the degree of androgen excess parallels that of ACTH and cortisol. Thus, plasma levels of DHEA, DHEA sulfate, and androstenedione may be moderately elevated in Cushing's disease; the peripheral conversion of these hormones to testosterone and dihydrotestosterone leads to androgen excess. In women, this causes hirsutism, acne, and amenorrhea. In men with Cushing's disease, cortisol suppression of LH secretion decreases testosterone secretion by the testis, resulting in decreased libido and impotence. The increased adrenal androgen secretion is insufficient to compensate for the decreased gonadal testosterone production.

B. Ectopic ACTH Syndrome: Hypersecretion of ACTH and cortisol is usually greater in patients with ectopic ACTH syndrome than in those with Cushing's disease. ACTH and cortisol hypersecretion is randomly episodic, and the levels are often greatly elevated. Usually, ACTH secretion by ectopic tumors is not subject to negative-feedback control; ie, secretion of ACTH and cortisol is nonsuppressible with pharmacologic doses of glucocorticoids (see section on diagnosis).

Plasma levels, secretion rates, and urinary excretion of cortisol, the adrenal androgens, and DOC are often markedly elevated; despite this, the typical features of Cushing's syndrome are usually absent, presumably because of rapid onset of hypercortisolism, anorexia, and other manifestations of the associated malignant disease. However, features of mineralocorticoid excess (hypertension and hypokalemia) are frequently due to DOC and the mineralocorticoid effects of cortisol.

C. Adrenal Tumors:

1. Autonomous secretion–Primary adrenal tumors, both adenomas and carcinomas, autonomously hypersecrete cortisol. Circulating plasma ACTH levels are suppressed, resulting in cortical atrophy of the uninvolved adrenal. Secretion is randomly episodic, and these tumors are typically unresponsive to manipulation of the hypothalamic-pituitary axis with pharmacologic agents such as dexamethasone and metyrapone.

2. Adrenal adenomas–Adrenal adenomas causing Cushing's syndrome typically present solely with clinical manifestations of glucocorticoid excess, since they usually secrete only cortisol. Thus, the presence of androgen or mineralocorticoid excess should suggest that the tumor is an adrenocortical carcinoma.

3. Adrenal carcinomas–Adrenal carcinomas frequently hypersecrete multiple adrenocortical steroids and their precursors. Cortisol and androgens are the steroids most frequently secreted in excess; 11-deoxycortisol is often elevated, and there may be increased secretion of DOC, aldosterone, or estrogens. Plasma cortisol, urine free cortisol, and urine 17-hydroxycorticosteroids are often markedly increased; androgen excess is usually even greater than that of cortisol. Thus, high levels of plasma DHEA and DHEA sulfate and of urinary 17-ketosteroids typically accompany the cortisol excess. Clinical manifestations of hypercortisolism are usually severe and rapidly progressive in these patients. In women, features of androgen excess are prominent; virilism may occasionally occur. Hypertension and hypokalemia are frequent and most commonly result from the mineralocorticoid effects of cortisol; less frequently, DOC and aldosterone hypersecretion also contribute.

Clinical Features
(Table 9–10)

A. Symptoms and Signs:

1. Obesity–Obesity is the most common manifestation, and weight gain is usually the initial symptom. It is classically central, affecting mainly the face, neck, trunk, and abdomen, with relative sparing of the extremities. Generalized obesity with central accentuation is equally common, particularly in children.

Accumulation of fat in the face leads to the typical "moon facies," which is present in 75% of cases and is accompanied by facial plethora in most patients. Fat accumulation around the neck is prominent in the supraclavicular and dorsocervical fat pads; the latter is responsible for the "buffalo hump."

Obesity is absent in a handful of patients who do not gain weight; however, they usually have central redistribution of fat and a typical facial appearance.

2. Skin changes–Skin changes are frequent, and their presence should arouse a suspicion of cortisol excess. Atrophy of the epidermis and its underlying connective tissue leads to thinning (a transparent appearance of the skin) and facial plethora. Easy bruisability following minimal trauma is present in about 40%. Striae occur in 50% but are very unusual in patients over 40 years of age; these are typically red to purple, depressed below the skin surface secondary to loss of underlying connective tissue, and wider (not infrequently 0.5–2 cm) than the pinkish white striae that may occur with pregnancy or rapid weight gain. These striae are most commonly abdominal but may also occur over the breasts, hips, buttocks, thighs, and axillae.

Table 9–10. Clinical features of Cushing's syndrome (% prevalence).

General
  Obesity 90%
  Hypertension 85%

Skin
  Plethora 70%
  Hirsutism 75%
  Striae 50%
  Acne 35%
  Bruising 35%

Musculoskeletal
  Osteopenia 80%
  Weakness 65%

Neuropsychiatric 85%
  Emotional lability
  Euphoria
  Depression
  Psychosis

Gonadal dysfunction
  Menstrual disorders 70%
  Impotence, decreased libido 85%

Metabolic
  Glucose intolerance 75%
  Diabetes 20%
  Hyperlipidemia 70%
  Polyuria 30%
  Kidney stones 15%

Acne may result from hyperandrogenism presenting as pustular lesions or as papular lesions from the glucocorticoid excess.

Minor wounds and abrasions may heal slowly, and surgical incisions sometimes undergo dehiscence.

Mucocutaneous fungal infections are frequent, including tinea versicolor, involvement of the nails (onychomycosis), and oral candidiasis.

Hyperpigmentation of the skin is rare in Cushing's disease or adrenal tumors but is common in ectopic ACTH syndrome.

3. Hirsutism–Hirsutism is present in about 80% of female patients owing to hypersecretion of adrenal androgens. Facial hirsutism is most common, but increased hair growth may also occur over the abdomen, breasts, chest, and upper thighs. Acne and seborrhea usually accompany hirsutism. Virilism is unusual except in cases of adrenal carcinoma, in which it occurs in about 20%.

4. Hypertension–Hypertension is a classic feature of spontaneous Cushing's syndrome; it is present in about 75% of cases, and the diastolic blood pressure is greater than 100 mm Hg in over 50%. Hypertension and its complications contribute greatly to the morbidity and mortality rates in spontaneous Cushing's syndrome.

5. Gonadal dysfunction–This is very common as a result of elevated androgens (in females) and cortisol (in males and to a lesser extent in females). Amenorrhea occurs in 75% of premenopausal women and is usually accompanied by infertility.

Decreased libido is frequent in males, and some have decreased body hair and soft testes.

6. Psychologic disturbances–Psychologic disturbances occur in the majority of patients. Mild symptoms consist of emotional lability and increased irritability. Anxiety, depression, poor concentration, and poor memory may also be present. Euphoria is frequent, and occasional patients manifest overtly manic behavior. Sleep disorders are present in most patients, with either insomnia or early morning awakening.

Severe psychologic disorders occur in a few patients and include severe depression, psychosis with delusions or hallucinations, and paranoia. Some patients have committed suicide.

7. Muscle weakness–This occurs in about 60% of cases; it is more often proximal and is usually most prominent in the lower extremities.

8. Osteoporosis–Owing to the profound effects of glucocorticoids on the skeleton, patients with Cushing's syndrome frequently have evidence of significant osteopenia. Patients may present with frequent unexplained fractures, typically of the feet, ribs, or vertebrae. Back pain may be the initial complaint. Compression fractures of the spine are demonstrated radiographically in 15–20% of patients. In fact, unexplained osteopenia in any young or middle-aged adult should always prompt an evaluation for Cushing's syndrome even in the absence of any other signs or symptoms of cortisol excess. Although avascular necrosis of bone has been associated with exogenous glucocorticoid administration, the problem is rarely observed in patients with endogenous hypercortisolism, suggesting a role for the underlying disorders in patients for whom glucocorticoids are prescribed.

9. Renal calculi–Calculi secondary to glucocorticoid-induced hypercalciuria occur in approximately 15% of patients, and renal colic may occasionally be a presenting complaint.

10. Thirst and polyuria–Polyuria is rarely due to overt hyperglycemia. Polyuria is usually due to glucocorticoid inhibition of vasopressin (antidiuretic hormone) secretion and the direct enhancement of renal free water clearance by cortisol.

B. Laboratory Findings: Routine laboratory examinations are described here. Specific diagnostic tests to establish the diagnosis of Cushing's syndrome are discussed in the section on diagnosis.

High normal hemoglobin, hematocrit, and red cell counts are usual; polycythemia is rare. The total white count is usually normal; however, both the percentage of lymphocytes and the total lymphocyte count may be subnormal. Eosinophils are also depressed, and a total eosinophil count less than $100/\mu L$ is present in most patients. Serum electrolytes, with rare exceptions, are normal in Cushing's disease; however, hypokalemic alkalosis occurs when there is marked steroid hypersecretion with the ectopic ACTH syndrome or adrenocortical carcinoma.

Fasting hyperglycemia or clinical diabetes occurs in only 10–15% of patients; postprandial hyperglycemia is more common. Glycosuria is present in patients with fasting or postprandial hyperglycemia. Most patients have secondary hyperinsulinemia and abnormal glucose tolerance tests.

Serum calcium is normal; serum phosphorus is low normal or slightly depressed. Hypercalciuria is present in 40% of cases.

C. Imaging Studies: Routine radiographs may reveal cardiomegaly due to hypertensive or atherosclerotic heart disease or mediastinal widening due to central fat accumulation. Vertebral compression fractures, rib fractures, and renal calculi may be present.

D. Electrocardiographic Findings: Hypertensive, ischemic, and electrolyte-induced changes may be present on the ECG.

Features Suggesting a Specific Cause

A. Cushing's Disease: Cushing's disease typifies the classic clinical picture: female predominance, onset generally between ages 20 and 40, and a slow progression over several years. Hyperpigmentation and hypokalemic alkalosis are rare; androgenic manifestations are limited to acne and hirsutism. Secretion of cortisol and adrenal androgens is only moderately increased.

B. Ectopic ACTH Syndrome (Carcinoma): In contrast, this syndrome occurs predominantly in males, with the highest incidence between ages 40 and 60. The clinical manifestations of hypercortisolism are frequently limited to weakness, hypertension, and glucose intolerance; the primary tumor is usually apparent. Hyperpigmentation, hypokalemia, and alkalosis are common, as are weight loss and anemia. The hypercortisolism is of rapid onset, and steroid hypersecretion is frequently severe, with equally elevated levels of glucocorticoids, androgens, and DOC.

C. Ectopic ACTH Syndrome (Benign Tumor): A minority of patients with ectopic ACTH syndrome due to more "benign" tumors, especially bronchial carcinoids, present a more slowly progressive course, with typical features of Cushing's syndrome. These patients may be clinically identical with those having pituitary-dependent Cushing's disease, and the responsible tumor may not be apparent. Hyperpigmentation, hypokalemic alkalosis, and anemia are variably present. Further confusion may arise, since a number of these patients with occult ectopic tumors may have ACTH and steroid dynamics typical of Cushing's disease (see below).

D. Adrenal Adenomas: The clinical picture in patients with adrenal adenomas is usually that of glucocorticoid excess alone, and androgenic effects such as hirsutism are usually absent. Onset is gradual, and

hypercortisolism is mild to moderate. Urinary 17-ketosteroids and plasma androgens are usually in the low normal or subnormal range.

E. Adrenal Carcinomas: In general, adrenal carcinomas have a rapid onset of the clinical features of excessive glucocorticoid, androgen, and mineralocorticoid secretion and are rapidly progressive. Marked elevations of both cortisol and androgens are usual; hypokalemia is common, as are abdominal pain, palpable masses, and hepatic and pulmonary metastases.

Diagnosis

The clinical suspicion of Cushing's syndrome must be confirmed with biochemical studies. Initially, a general assessment of the patient regarding the presence of other illnesses, drugs, alcohol, or psychiatric problems must be done since these factors may confound the evaluation. In the majority of cases, the biochemical differential diagnosis of Cushing's syndrome can be easily performed in the ambulatory setting (Figure 9–13).

A. Dexamethasone Suppression Test: The overnight 1 mg dexamethasone suppression test is the most valuable screening test in patients with suspected hypercortisolism. This study employs the administration of 1 mg of dexamethasone at bedtime (2300 hour), with determination of a plasma cortisol early the following the morning. Normal subjects should suppress plasma cortisol to less than 3 μg/dL (70 μg/L) following an overnight 1 mg test. Although a level of less than 5 μg/dL has been used in the past, several false negative studies have been discovered using this test criterion, presumably due to the exquisite sensitivity of glucocorticoid negative feedback in some patients with pituitary ACTH dependent Cushing's syndrome (Cushing's disease) as well the occasional intermittent nature of the hypercortisolism. This test should only be employed as a screening tool for the consideration of Cushing's syndrome and biochemical confirmation must rely on urine free cortisol excretion. False positive results of the overnight 1 mg dexamethasone suppression test may be caused by patients receiving drugs that accelerate dexamethasone metabolism (phenytoin, phenobarbital, rifampin). False-positive results also occur in patients with renal failure, in patients suffering from endogenous depression, or in any patients undergoing a stressful event or serious illness.

The low-dose dexamethasone suppression test in which 17-hydroxycorticosteroids excretion and free cortisol are measured during the administration of dexamethasone orally at a rate of 0.5 mg every 6 hours for two days has been used for many years. 17-Hydroxycorticosteroid excretion greater than 4 mg/24 h on the second day of dexamethasone administration is considered evidence for Cushing's syndrome. Critical analysis of this test has shown that it cannot be used reliably to exclude the diagnosis of

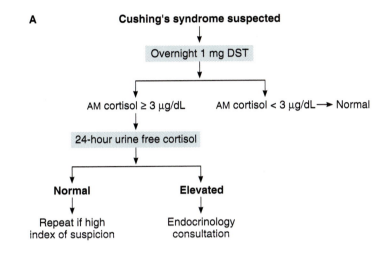

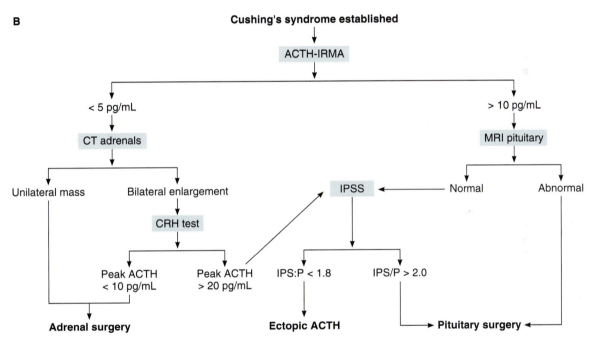

Figure 9–13. The diagnosis *(A)* and differential diagnosis *(B)* of Cushing's syndrome. (DST, dexamethasone suppression test; IRMA, immunoradiometric assay; IPSS, inferior petrosal sinus sampling; ISP:P, inferior petrosal sinus:peripheral ACTH ratio; CRH, corticotropin-releasing hormone.)

Cushing's syndrome. Many patients with mild hypercortisolism due to pituitary ACTH-dependent Cushing's syndrome may suppress urine steroid secretion to undetectable ranges even with low doses of dexamethasone. In addition, 15–25% of patients with a pseudo- Cushing's state (such as depression or alcoholism) may have false-positive tests. In patients with mild hypercortisolism, the test has an accuracy of only 70% and a sensitivity of only 55%. In light of the expense and cumbersome nature of consecutive urine collections and frequent dexamethasone administration, continued use of this 2-day low-dose

dexamethasone suppression test cannot be recommended.

B. Urine Free Cortisol: The most useful clinical study in the confirmation of Cushing's syndrome is the determination of cortisol secretion utilizing a 24-hour urine free cortisol determination. Most commercial laboratories use a solvent extraction of cortisol from urine and assay the extract by radioimmunoassay. The upper range of normal in this type of assay is usually 80–100 μg/24 h. More recently, methods involving HPLC have been introduced that provide more specific assessment of free cortisol.

Urinary free cortisol is usually less than 50 μg/24 h with HPLC. Urine free cortisol determinations usually provide clear discrimination between patients with hypercortisolism and obese non-Cushing patients, though exceptions occur. In obese patients, the cortisol production rate may be increased, and elevated levels of urinary 17-hydroxycorticosteroids may lead to an erroneous diagnosis of Cushing's syndrome. Less than 5% of obese subjects will have mild elevations of urine free cortisol, though as many as 10–15% will have elevations of 17-hydroxycorticosteroid excretion.

C. Diurnal Rhythm: The absence of diurnal rhythm has been considered the hallmark of the diagnosis of Cushing's syndrome. Normally, cortisol is secreted episodically with a diurnal rhythm paralleling the secretion of ACTH. Levels are usually highest early in the morning and decrease gradually throughout the day, reaching the nadir in the late evening. Because normal levels of plasma cortisol constitute a broad range, the levels found in Cushing's syndrome may often be normal. Documenting the presence or absence of diurnal rhythm is difficult, since single determinations obtained in the morning or evening are usually uninterpretable because of the pulsatility of pathologic and physiologic ACTH and cortisol secretion. Nonetheless, serum cortisol levels exceeding 7 μg/dL at midnight in nonstressed patients provide good specificity for the diagnosis of Cushing's syndrome. Since cortisol is secreted as free cortisol, the measurement of salivary cortisol may provide a simple and more convenient means of probing nighttime cortisol secretion in a practical fashion. Recent studies have shown that patients with Cushing's syndrome have midnight salivary cortisol levels that usually exceed 0.4 μg/dL (normal: 0.1–0.2 μg/dL).

Problems in Diagnosis

A major diagnostic problem is distinguishing patients with mild Cushing's syndrome from those with mild physiologic hypercortisolism due to conditions that are classified as "pseudo-Cushing's syndrome". These include the depressed phase of affective disorder, alcoholism, withdraw from alcohol intoxication, or eating disorders such as anorexia and bulimia nervosa. These conditions may have biochemical features of Cushing's syndrome, including elevations of urine free cortisol, disruptions in the normal diurnal pattern of cortisol secretion, and lack of suppression of cortisol after the overnight 1 mg dexamethasone suppression test. Although the history and physical examination may provide specific clues to the appropriate diagnosis, definitive biochemical confirmation may be difficult and may require repeated testing. The most definitive study available for distinguishing mild Cushing's syndrome from pseudo-Cushing conditions is the use of dexamethasone suppression followed by corticotropin-releasing hormone (CRH) stimulation. This new test takes advantage of the overt sensitivity of patients with Cushing's syndrome to both dexamethasone and CRH by combining these test in order to provide greater accuracy in the diagnosis. This study involves the administration of dexamethasone, 0.5 mg every 6 hours for eight doses, followed immediately by a CRH stimulation test, starting 2 hours after the completion of the low-dose dexamethasone suppression. A plasma cortisol concentration greater than 1.4 μg/dL measured 15 minutes after administration of CRH correctly identifies the majority of patients with Cushing's syndrome.

Differential Diagnosis

The differential diagnosis of Cushing's syndrome is usually very difficult and should always be performed with consultation by an endocrinologist. The introduction of several technologic advances over the past 10–15 years, including a specific and sensitive immunoradiometric assay for ACTH, CRH stimulation test, inferior petrosal sinus sampling (IPSS), and CT and MRI of the pituitary and adrenal glands have all provided means for an accurate differential diagnosis (Figure 9–13).

A. Plasma ACTH: Initially, the differential diagnosis for Cushing's syndrome must distinguish between ACTH-dependent Cushing's syndrome (pituitary or nonpituitary ACTH-secreting neoplasm) and ACTH-independent hypercortisolism. The best way to distinguish these forms of Cushing's syndrome is measurement of plasma ACTH by immunoradiometric assay. The development of this sensitive and specific test has made it possible to reliably identify patients with ACTH-independent Cushing's syndrome. The ACTH level is less than 5 pg/mL and exhibits a blunted response to CRH (peak response < 10 pg/mL) in patients with cortisol-producing adrenal neoplasms, autonomous bilateral adrenal cortical hyperplasia, and factitious Cushing's syndrome (Figure 9–14). Patients with ACTH-secreting neoplasms usually have plasma ACTH levels greater than 10 pg/mL and frequently greater than 52 pg/mL. The major challenge in the differential diagnosis of ACTH-dependent Cushing's syndrome is identifying the source of the ACTH-secreting tumor. The vast majority of these patients (90%) have a pituitary tumor, while the others harbor a nonpituitary neoplasm. Diagnostic studies needed to differentiate these two entities must yield nearly perfect sensitivity, specificity, and accuracy. Although plasma ACTH levels are usually higher in patients with ectopic ACTH than those with pituitary ACTH-dependent Cushing's syndrome, there is considerable overlap between these two entities. Many of the ectopic ACTH-secreting tumors are radiologically occult at the time of presentation and may not become clinically apparent for many years after the initial diagnosis. The introduction of pituitary microsurgery as the treatment of choice in patients with Cushing's disease mandates a precise diagnosis.

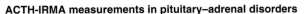

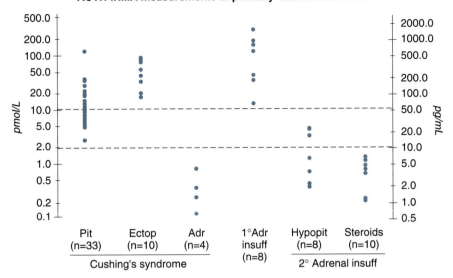

Figure 9–14. Plasma ACTH-IRMA (pmol/L or pg/mL) of patients with pituitary-adrenal disorders. Dashed horizontal lines indicate normal range. (Reproduced, with permission, from Findling JW: Clinical application of a new immunoradiometric assay for ACTH. The Endocrinologist 1992;2:360.)

B. Pituitary MRI: In the absence of ACTH-independent Cushing's syndrome, MRI of the pituitary gland with gadolinium enhancement should be performed and will identify an adenoma in 50–60% of the patients. If the patient has classic clinical laboratory findings of pituitary ACTH-dependent hypercortisolemia and an unequivocal pituitary lesion on MRI, the likelihood of Cushing's disease is 98–99%. However, it must be emphasized that approximately 10% of the population in the age group from 20 to 50 years will have incidental tumors of the pituitary demonstrable by MRI. Therefore, some patients with ectopic ACTH syndrome will have radiographic evidence of a pituitary lesion.

C. High-Dose Dexamethasone Suppression: Traditionally, high-dose dexamethasone suppression testing has been utilized in the differential diagnosis of Cushing's syndrome. The classic test employs the use of 2 mg of dexamethasone every 6 hours for 2 days, with collections of urine steroids. A greater than 50% decrease in urine steroid secretion on day 2 of the high-dose dexamethasone suppression test was considered to be indicative of pituitary disease, whereas an absence of suppression suggests a primary adrenal disease or ectopic ACTH. Unfortunately, these criteria cannot reliably distinguish ACTH-dependent from ACTH-independent Cushing's syndrome, much less pituitary from ectopic ACTH-secreting tumors. The diagnostic accuracy of this procedure is only 70–80% which is actually less than the pretest probability of Cushing's disease—on average about 90%. Recently, new criteria for this test have increased its sensitivity, speci-

ficity, and accuracy. The decrease in urine free cortisol of more than 90% and a decrease in 17-hydroxycorticosteroid secretion of more than 64% following the traditional high-dose dexamethasone suppression test has yielded 100% diagnostic specificity of Cushing's disease in one series. However, reports of false positives have been increasingly observed even with these new criteria.

An overnight 8 mg dexamethasone suppression test has also been used for distinguishing pituitary and nonpituitary ACTH-dependent Cushing's syndrome. This test used 8 mg of dexamethasone at bedtime (11 PM hours), with measurement of plasma cortisol the following morning. Suppression of plasma cortisol to less than 50% at baseline is most consistent with pituitary-dependent Cushing's syndrome. The test characteristics of this study provide approximately the same accuracy as the longer high-dose dexamethasone suppression test, and from the standpoints of cost and convenience it is preferred by most clinicians. Nonetheless, false-positive and false-negative results have been reported. Utilization of any dexamethasone suppression test in the differential diagnosis of Cushing's syndrome must be interpreted with caution as well as careful consideration of the patient's clinical presentation and other biochemical and radiographic studies.

D. Inferior Petrosal Sinus Sampling: The most definitive means of accurately distinguishing pituitary from nonpituitary ACTH-dependent Cushing's syndrome is the use of bilateral simultaneous IPSS with CRH stimulation. This study takes advantage of the means by which pituitary hormones reach the systemic circulation. Blood leaves the anterior lobe of the pituitary and drains into the cavernous sinuses, which then empty into the inferior petrosal sinuses and from there to the jugular bulb and vein. Simultaneous inferior petrosal sinus and peripheral ACTH measurement before and after CRH stimulation can reliably confirm the presence or absence of an ACTH-secreting pituitary tumor. An inferior petrosal sinus to peripheral (IPS:P) ratio greater than 2.0 is consistent with a pituitary ACTH-secreting tumor, and an IPS:P ratio less than 1.8 supports the diagnosis of ectopic ACTH. Since each petrosal sinus receives venous drainage from the ipsilateral side of the pituitary with little intracavernous sinus mixing, ACTH-secreting tumors with a lateral location should secrete ACTH mostly into the corresponding petrosal sinus. Interpetrosal sinus gradients have been utilized for preoperative localization of corticotroph adenomas, albeit with mixed results.

Bilateral IPSS with CRH stimulation does require a skilled invasive radiologist, but in experienced hands the procedure has yielded a diagnostic accuracy of 100% in the differential diagnosis of ACTH-dependent Cushing's syndrome.

E. Occult Ectopic ACTH: If the IPSS study is consistent with a nonpituitary ACTH-secreting tumor, a search for an occult ectopic ACTH-secreting tumor is needed. Since the majority of these lesions are in the thorax, high-resolution CT of the chest may be useful; MRI of the chest appears to have even better sensitivity in finding these lesions, which are usually small bronchial carcinoid tumors. Since some ectopic ACTH-secreting tumors express somatostatin receptors, utilization of a radiolabeled somatostatin analog scan (octreotide acetate scintigraphy) may also be employed to find these tumors.

F. Adrenal Localizing Procedures: CT scan (Figure 9–15), MRI, ultrasonography, and isotope scanning with iodocholesterol are used to define adrenal lesions. Their primary use is to localize adrenal tumors in patients with ACTH-independent Cushing's syndrome; most adenomas exceed 2 cm in diameter; carcinomas are usually much larger. False positive CT scans can be observed with nodular adrenal hyperplasia.

Treatment

A. Cushing's Disease: The aim of treatment of Cushing's syndrome is to remove or destroy the basic lesion and thus correct hypersecretion of adrenal hormones without inducing pituitary or adrenal damage, which requires permanent replacement therapy for hormone deficiencies.

Treatment of Cushing's disease is currently directed at the pituitary to control ACTH hypersecretion; available methods include microsurgery, various forms of radiation therapy, and pharmacologic inhibition of ACTH secretion. Treatment of hypercortisolism per se by surgical or medical adrenalec-

tomy is less commonly used. These methods are discussed in Chapter 5.

B. Ectopic ACTH Syndrome: Cure of ectopic ACTH syndrome is usually possible only in cases involving the more "benign" tumors such as bronchial or thymic carcinoids, or pheochromocytomas. Treatment is made difficult by the presence of metastatic malignant tumors and accompanying severe hypercortisolism. Therapy directed to the primary tumor is usually unsuccessful, and other means must be used to correct the steroid-excess state. Severe hypokalemia may require potassium replacement in large doses and spironolactone to block mineralocorticoid effects. Drugs that block steroid synthesis (ketoconazole, metyrapone, and aminoglutethimide) are useful, but they may produce hypoadrenalism, and steroid secretion must be monitored and replacement steroids given if necessary. The dosage of ketoconazole is 400–800 mg/d in divided doses and is usually well tolerated. Because of its slow onset of action and its side effects, mitotane is less useful, and several weeks of therapy may be required to control cortisol secretion (see below). Bilateral adrenalectomy is rarely required, but it may be necessary if hypercortisolism cannot otherwise be controlled.

C. Adrenal Tumors:

1. Adrenal adenomas–Patients with adrenal adenomas are successfully treated by unilateral adrenalectomy, and the outlook is excellent. Laparoscopic adrenal surgery has become widely used in patients with benign or small adrenal tumors and has significantly reduced the duration of the hospital stay. Since the hypothalamic-pituitary axis and the contralateral adrenal are suppressed by prolonged cortisol secretion, these patients have postoperative adrenal insufficiency and require glucocorticoid therapy both during and following surgery until the remaining adrenal recovers.

2. Adrenal carcinomas–Therapy in cases of adrenocortical carcinoma is less satisfactory, since the tumor has frequently already metastasized (usually to the retroperitoneum, liver, and lungs) by the time the diagnosis is made.

a. Operative treatment–Surgical cure is rare, but excision serves to reduce the tumor mass and the degree of steroid hypersecretion. Persisting nonsuppressible steroid secretion in the immediate postoperative period indicates residual or metastatic tumor.

b. Medical treatment–Mitotane is the drug of choice. The dosage is 6–12 g/d orally in three or four divided doses. The dose must often be reduced because of side effects in 80% of patients (diarrhea, nausea and vomiting, depression, somnolence). About 70% of patients achieve a reduction of steroid secretion, but only 35% achieve a reduction in tumor size. Since mitotane reduces urinary 17-hydroxycorticosteroid excretion by altering the hepatic metabolism of cortisol, these patients require follow-up by plasma cortisol or urine free cortisol assays.

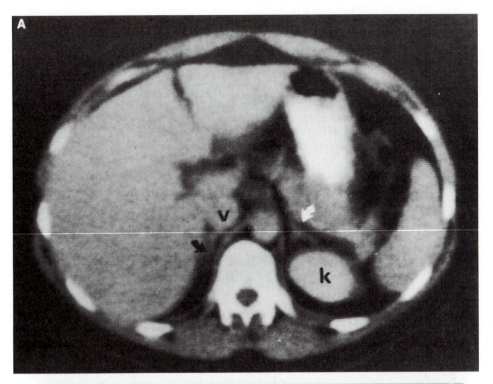

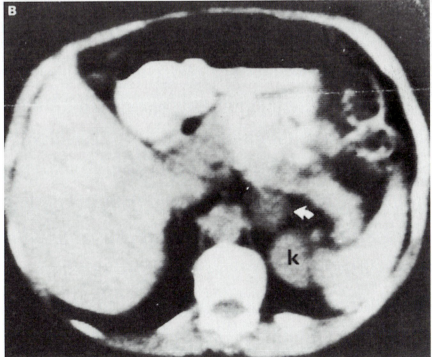

Figure 9–15. Adrenal CT scans in Cushing's syndrome. **A:** Patient with ACTH-dependent Cushing's syndrome. The adrenal glands are not detectably abnormal by this procedure. The curvilinear right adrenal (black arrow) is shown posterior to the inferior vena cava (V) between the right lobe of the liver and the right crus of the diaphragm. The left adrenal (white arrow) has an inverted Y appearance anteromedial to the left kidney (K). **B:** A 3-cm left adrenal adenoma (white arrow) is shown anteromedial to the left kidney (K). (Reproduced, with permission, from Korobkin MT et al: Computed tomography in the diagnosis of adrenal disease. Am J Roentgenol 1979;132:231.)

Ketoconazole, metyrapone, or aminoglutethimide (singly or in combination) are useful in controlling steroid hypersecretion in patients who do not respond to mitotane.

Radiotherapy and conventional chemotherapy have not been useful in this disease.

D. Nodular Adrenal Hyperplasia: When pituitary ACTH dependency can be demonstrated, macronodular hyperplasia may be treated like other cases of Cushing's disease. When ACTH dependency is not present, as in micronodular hyperplasia and in some cases of macronodular hyperplasia, bilateral adrenalectomy is appropriate.

Prognosis

A. Cushing's Syndrome: Untreated Cushing's syndrome is frequently fatal, and death may be due to the underlying tumor itself, as in the ectopic ACTH syndrome and adrenal carcinoma. However, in many cases, death is the consequence of sustained hypercortisolism and its complications, including hypertension, cardiovascular disease, stroke, thromboembolism, and susceptibility to infection. In older series, 50% of patients died within 5 years after onset.

B. Cushing's Disease: With current refinements in pituitary microsurgery and heavy particle irradiation, the great majority of patients with Cushing's disease can be treated successfully, and the operative mortality and morbidity rates that attended bilateral adrenalectomy are no longer a feature of the natural history of this disease. Survival in these patients is considerably longer than in older series. However, survival is still less than that of age-matched controls; the increased mortality rate is due to cardiovascular causes. Patients with Cushing's disease who have large pituitary tumors at the time of diagnosis have a much less satisfactory prognosis and may die as a consequence of tumor invasion or persisting hypercortisolism.

C. Adrenal Tumors: The prognosis in adrenal adenomas is excellent. In adrenal carcinoma, the prognosis is almost universally poor, and the median survival from the date of onset of symptoms is about 4 years.

D. Ectopic ACTH Syndrome: Prognosis is also poor in patients with ectopic ACTH syndrome due to malignant tumors, and in these patients with severe hypercortisolism, survival is frequently only days to weeks. Some patients respond to tumor resection or chemotherapy. The prognosis is better in patients with benign tumors producing the ectopic ACTH syndrome.

HIRSUTISM & VIRILISM

Excessive adrenal or ovarian secretion of androgens or excessive conversion of androgens in periph-eral tissues leads to hirsutism and virilism (see Chapter 13). As previously discussed, the adrenal secretory products DHEA, DHEA sulfate, and androstenedione are weak androgens; however, the peripheral conversion to testosterone and dihydrotestosterone can result in a state of androgen excess.

Excessive androgen production is seen in both adrenal and ovarian disorders. Adrenal causes include Cushing's syndrome, adrenal carcinoma, and congenital adrenal hyperplasia (see previous sections and Chapter 14). Mild adult-onset cases of congenital adrenal enzyme deficiencies have been described; these appear to be relatively uncommon. Biochemical diagnosis of late-onset 21-hydroxylase deficiency is best achieved by measurement of the 17-hydroxyprogesterone response to ACTH. Ovarian causes are discussed in Chapter 13.

In children, androgen excess is usually due to congenital adrenal hyperplasia or adrenal carcinoma. In women, hirsutism accompanied by amenorrhea, infertility, ovarian enlargement, and elevated plasma LH levels is typical of the polycystic ovary syndrome, whereas in Cushing's syndrome hirsutism is accompanied by features of cortisol excess. Late-onset 21-hydroxylase deficiency is accompanied by elevated levels of plasma 17-hydroxyprogesterone. Virilism and severe androgen excess in adults are usually due to androgen-secreting adrenal or ovarian tumors; virilism is unusual in the polycystic ovary syndrome and rare in Cushing's disease. In the absence of these syndromes, hirsutism in women is usually idiopathic or due to milder forms of polycystic ovary syndrome.

The diagnosis and therapy of hirsutism are discussed in Chapter 13.

INCIDENTAL ADRENAL MASS
(Figure 9–16)

The incidental adrenal mass has become a common diagnostic problem, since approximately 2% of patients undergoing CT studies of the abdomen are found to have focal enlargement of the adrenal gland. The major diagnostic concern is whether the lesion may represent a malignancy or a functioning adrenal neoplasm.

Adrenal masses in the adult may represent functional or nonfunctional cortical adenomas or carcinoma, pheochromocytomas, cysts, myelolipomas, or metastasis from other tumors. Congenital adrenal hyperplasia may also present as a focal enlargement of the adrenal gland, and adrenal hemorrhage will also cause enlargement, though usually bilateral.

The appropriate diagnostic approach to patients with an incidentally discovered adrenal mass is unresolved. The roentgenographic appearance taken in context with the clinical setting may provide some insight. The size of the lesion is important. Primary

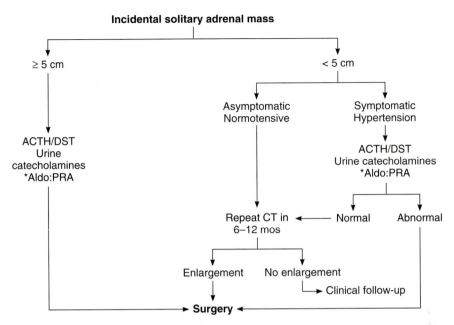

Figure 9–16. Incidental solitary adrenal mass. A proposed algorithm for the evaluation of an incidental solitary adrenal mass in a patient without a known malignancy. (ACTH, basal morning ACTH level by immunoradiometric assay [normal: 9–52 pg/mL]. DST, overnight 1 mg dexamethasone suppression test; Aldo:PRA, aldosterone [ng/dL]-to-plasma renin activity [ng/mL/h] ratio [Normal: < 25]; Enlgmt, enlargement > 0.5 cm. *If potassium < 3.7 mmol/L.) (Copyright © 1995 by the American College of Physicians. Reproduced with permission.)

adrenocortical carcinoma is exceedingly rare (1:10,000) in adrenal masses smaller than 5 cm; however, the presence of unilateral bilateral adrenal masses (> 3 cm) in a patient with a known malignancy (particularly lung, gastrointestinal, renal, or breast) probably represents metastatic disease. Adrenal lesions smaller than 3 cm in patients with a known malignancy actually represent metastases in only 20–30% of cases.

Other CT findings may be informative. The presence of fat within the adrenal mass may suggest a myelolipoma which is usually a benign lesion. Adrenocortical adenomas are usually round masses with smooth margins, and adrenal cysts can also be identified with either CT or ultrasound examination. Adrenal hemorrhage usually has irregular borders with some lack of homogeneity. Primary adrenocortical carcinoma usually presents as a lesion greater than 5 cm with irregular borders. MRI of the adrenal gland is usually not necessary but may be helpful in selected patients. Typically, malignancies and pheochromocytomas tend to have bright signal intensity with T2-weighted images, in contrast to benign lesions of the adrenal gland; however, exceptions to this rule have been seen, limiting the clinical utility of this technique.

Malignancy

Primary adrenocortical carcinoma usually presents with a large lesion, and most authorities recommend removing all adrenal masses greater than 5 cm. One series of 45 adrenal masses greater than 5 cm showed 30 benign lesions (16 pheochromocytomas, six adenomas, four adrenal cysts, two myelolipomas, one hematoma, one ganglioneuroma) and 15 malignancies (seven adrenocortical carcinomas, five adrenal metastases, and three adrenal lymphomas. Lesions less than 5 cm in diameter are of concern only in patients with a known malignancy or in those in whom there is a high index of suspicion based on other clinical information. In patients with primary malignancies of the lung, gastrointestinal tract, kidney, or breast, an ultrasound-or CT-guided needle biopsy may be helpful in establishing the presence or absence of metastatic disease. Metastatic disease can be identified with an accuracy of 75–85% in such patients; however, there are both false-negative and false-positive findings. Percutaneous adrenal biopsy really has no proved efficacy in patients with adrenal masses and no history of a malignancy. Percutaneous adrenal biopsy should be reserved for patients in whom the presence or absence of adrenal metastases may alter the therapy or prognosis of the patient.

Endocrine Evaluation

The appropriate biochemical evaluation with an incidental adrenal mass is also controversial. Certainly the endocrinopathies that constitute part of the differential diagnosis of the incidentally discovered adrenal mass are unusual. Statistical models based on epidemiologic data have concluded that no hormonal evaluation is necessary in the normotensive, symptomatic patient (Figure 9–6). Certainly, good clinical judgment is essential, and repeat CT imagining in 6–12 months is recommended to exclude neoplastic disease. Nonetheless, patients with hypertension, progressive hirsutism, hypokalemia, or obesity deserve biochemical evaluation.

Cortisol-Producing Adenoma

The most common functioning lesion in patients with an incidentally discovered adrenal mass appears to be the autonomous secretion of cortisol. Approximately 6–12% of patients with adrenal incidentalomas ranging from 2–5 cm in diameter have pathologic cortisol secretion. These benign adrenal adenomas secrete small amounts of cortisol that are often not sufficient to elevate urine cortisol excretion but are able to cause some suppression of the hypothalamic-pituitary axis. These patients can be easily identified by their failure to suppress cortisol to less than 3 μg/dL following an overnight 1 mg dexamethasone suppression test. In addition, the basal levels of ACTH in these patients are subnormal or frankly suppressed. The cortisol secretion by the tumor probably results in blunting of diurnal variation and eventually in lack of suppression by dexamethasone. The low plasma ACTH level exhibits a blunted response to CRH administration. Removal of these "silent" adrenocortical adenomas may be followed by clinically significant secondary adrenal insufficiency. Therefore, an overnight dexamethasone suppression test or measurement of plasma ACTH should be performed before surgical removal of any unknown adrenal neoplasm. These patients have been described as having "preclinical" Cushing's syndrome. The natural history of this autonomous cortisol secretion is unknown. Many of these patients described with this problem have hypertension, obesity, or diabetes, and improvements in these clinical problems have been reported following resection of these cortisol-producing adenomas. Consequently, adrenalectomy is recommended in young patients with preclinical Cushing's syndrome and in patients with clinical problems, potentially aggravated by glucocorticoid excess.

Pheochromocytoma

Pheochromocytoma is a potentially life-threatening tumor that may present as an incidental adrenal mass. Surprisingly, pheochromocytoma may account for as many as 2–3% of incidental adrenal lesions. Most of these patients will have hypertension and symptoms associated with catecholamine excess such as headache, diaphoresis, palpitations, or nervousness. A 24-hour urine measurement for catecholamines and metanephrines should be performed in patients with an incidental adrenal lesion. Supine resting plasma catecholamines may also be helpful as a screening test to exclude pheochromocytoma.

Aldosterone-Producing Adenoma

Although aldosterone-producing adenomas are more common than either pheochromocytomas or cortisol-producing adenomas, they actually represent a very unusual cause of an incidentally discovered adrenal mass. This appears to be due to the fact that aldosterone-producing adenomas are usually small and frequently missed with CT imaging of the adrenal gland. Because most of these patients have hypertension, this diagnosis needs to be considered only in patients with hypertension. The presence of hypokalemia should arouse suspicion of this diagnosis. It is virtually always present in patients with adrenal masses greater than 3 cm. It can be conclusively excluded by a single measurement of aldosterone and PRA. If the aldosterone (ng/dL):PRA (ng/mL/h) ratio is less than 25.0, an aldosterone-producing adenoma is excluded.

REFERENCES

General

Hadley ME: Adrenal steroid hormones. In: *Endocrinology,* 4th ed. Prentice Hall, 1996.

Loriaux DL: The adrenal glands. In: Becker KL (editor): *Principles and Practice of Endocrinology and Metabolism,* 2nd ed. Lippincott, 1995.

Miller, WL, Tyrrell JB: The adrenal cortex. In: *Endocrinology and Metabolism,* 3rd ed. Felig P, Baxter JD, Frohman LA (editors). McGraw-Hill, 1995.

Orth DN, Kovacs WJ, DeBold CR: The adrenal cortex. In: *Williams Textbook of Endocrinology,* 8th ed. Wilson JD, Foster DW (editors). Saunders, 1992.

Embryology, Anatomy, Biosynthesis, Circulation, and Metabolism of Cortisol and Adrenal Androgens

Brownie AC: The metabolism of adrenal cortical steroids. In: *The Adrenal Gland,* 2nd ed. James VHT (editor). Raven Press, 1992.

Chrousos GP: The hypothalamic-pituitary-adrenal axis and immune-mediated inflammation. N Engl J Med 1995;322:1351.

Demers LM: Biochemistry and laboratory measurement of androgens in women. In: *Androgenic Disorders.* Redmond JP (editor). Raven Press, 1995.

Fraser R: Biosynthesis of adrenocortical steroids. In:

The Adrenal Gland, 2nd ed. James VHT (editor). Raven Press, 1992.

McNicol AM: The human adrenal gland: Aspects of structure, function, and pathology. In: *The Adrenal Gland,* 2nd ed. James VHT (editor). Raven Press, 1992.

Reichlin S: Neuroendocrine-immune interactions. N Engl J Med 1993;329:1246.

Rosner W: Plasma steroid-binding proteins. Endocrinol Metab Clin North Am 1991;20:697.

Saeger W et al: Ultrastructural morphometry of normal adrenal cortex and of hyperplastic adrenals in Cushing's disease. Endocrinol Pathol 1991;2:40.

Biologic Effects and Glucocorticoid Therapy

Baxter JD: Minimizing the side effects of glucocorticoid therapy. Adv Intern Med 1990;35:173.

Christy NP: Corticosteroid withdrawal. In: *Current Therapy in Endocrinology and Metabolism.* Bardin WC (editor). Saunders, 1995.

Christy NP: Pituitary-adrenal function during corticosteroid therapy: Learning to live with uncertainty. N Engl J Med 1993;326:266.

Christy NP: Principles of systemic corticosteroid therapy in nonendocrine disease. In: *Current Therapy in Endocrinology and Metabolism.* Bardin WC (editor). Saunders, 1995.

Farese RV Jr et al: Licorice-induced hypermineralocorticoidism. N Engl J Med 1991;325:1223.

Frey FJ, Frey BM: Pharmacology of synthetic glucocorticoids: Alternate day glucocorticoid therapy—30 years later. In: *The Adrenal Gland,* 2nd ed. James VHT (editor). Raven Press, 1992.

Gomez MT et al: The pituitary corticotroph is not the rate limiting step in the postoperative recovery of the hypothalamic-pituitary-adrenal axis in patients with Cushing syndrome. J Clin Endocrinol Metab 1993; 77:173.

Hanania NA, Chapman KR, Kesten S: Adverse effects of inhaled corticosteroids. Am J Med 1995;98:196.

King RJB: Effects of steroid hormones and related compounds on gene transcription. Clin Endocrinol 1992; 36:1.

Lacomis D, Samuels MA: Adverse neurologic effects of glucocorticosteroids. J Gen Intern Med 1991;6:367.

LaRochelle GE Jr et al: Recovery of the hypothalamic-pituitary-adrenal (HPA) axis in patients with rheumatic disease receiving low-dose prednisone. Am J Med 1993;95:258.

Salem M et al: Perioperative glucocorticoid coverage. Ann Surg 1994;219:416.

Sawaya ME: Androgen action at the cellular level. In: *Androgenic Disorders.* Redmond JP (editor). Raven Press, 1995.

Schlaghecke R et al: The effect of long-term glucocorticoid therapy on pituitary-adrenal responses to exogenous corticotropin-releasing hormone. N Engl J Med 1992;326:226.

Spitz RM, Bardin CW: Mifepristone (RU 486): A modulator of progestin and glucocorticoid action. N Engl J Med 1993;329:404.

Ulick S et al: Cortisol inactivation overload: A mechanism of mineralocorticoid hypertension in the ectopic adrenocorticotropin syndrome. J Clin Endocrinol Metab 1992;74:963.

Walker BP, Edwards CRW: 11β-Hydroxysteroid dehydrogenase and enzyme-mediated receptor protection: Life after licorice? Clin Endocrinol 1991;35:281.

Walker BR, Williams BC: Corticosteroids and vascular tone: Mapping the messenger maze. Clin Sci 1992; 82:597.

Laboratory Evaluation

Baxter JD, Tyrrell JB: Evaluation of the hypothalamic-pituitary-adrenal axis: Importance in steroid therapy, AIDS, and other stress syndromes. Adv Intern Med 1994;39:667.

Broide J et al: Low-dose adrenocorticotropin test reveals impaired adrenal function in patients taking inhaled corticosteroids. J Clin Endocrinol Metab 1995;80: 1243.

Francis IR et al: Integrated imaging of adrenal disease. Radiology 1992;184:1.

Grinspoon SK, Biller BMK: Laboratory assessment of adrenal insufficiency. J Clin Endocrinol Metab 1994; 79:923.

Reznek RH, Armstrong P: Imaging in endocrinology: The adrenal gland. Clin Endocrinol 1994;40:561.

Snow K et al: Biochemical evaluation of adrenal dysfunction: The laboratory perspective. Mayo Clin Proc 1992;67:1055.

Tordjman K et al: The role of the low dose (1 μg) adrenocorticotropin test in the evaluation of patients with pituitary disease. J Clin Endocrinol Metab 1995;80:1301.

Adrenal Insufficiency

Ahonen P et al: Clinical evaluation of autoimmune polyendocrinopathy-candidiasis-ectodermal dystrophy (APCED) in a series of 68 patients. N Engl J Med 1990;322:1829.

Chodosh LA, Daniels GH: Addison's disease. The Endocrinologist 1993;3:166.

Chrousos GP, Detera-Wadleigh SD, Karl M: Syndromes of glucocorticoid resistance. Ann Intern Med 1993; 119:1113.

Findling J et al: Longitudinal evaluation of adrenocortical function in patients infected with the human immunodeficiency virus. J Clin Endocrinol Metab 1994; 79:1091.

Freda P et al: Primary adrenal insufficiency in patients with the acquired immunodeficiency syndrome: A report of five cases. J Clin Endocrinol Metab 1994;79: 1540.

Gamelin E et al: Non-Hodgkin's lymphoma presenting with primary adrenal insufficiency: A disease with an underestimated frequency? Cancer 1992;69:2333.

Grinspoon SK, Bilezikian JP: HIV disease and the endocrine system. N Engl J Med 1992;327:1360.

Javier EC, Reardon GE, Malchoff CD: Glucocorticoid resistance and its clinical presentations. The Endocrinologist 1991;1:141.

Kasperlik-Zaluska AA et al: Association of Addison's disease with autoimmune disorders: A long-term observation of 180 patients. Postgrad Med J 1991; 67:984.

Kong MF, Jeffcoate W: Eighty-six cases of Addison's disease. Clin Endocrinol 1994;41:757.

Leinung MC, Liporace R, Miller CH: Induction of

adrenal suppression by megestrol acetate in patients with AIDS. Ann Intern Med 1995;122:843.

Merry WH et al: Postoperative acute adrenal failure caused by transient corticotropin deficiency. Surgery 1994;116:1095.

Norbiato G et al: The syndrome of acquired glucocorticoid resistance in HIV infection. Ballieres Clin Endocrinol Metab 1994;8:777.

Opocherg G, Mantero F: Adrenal complications of HIV infection. Baillieres Clin Endocrinol Metab 1994; 8:769.

Provensale JM, Ortel TL, Nelson RC: Adrenal hemorrhage in patients with primary antiphospholipid syndrome: Imaging findings. AJR Am J Roentgenol 1995;165:361.

Riedel M et al: Quality of life in patients with Addison's disease: Effects of different cortisol replacement modes. Exp Clin Endocrinol 1993;101:106.

Rizzo WB: X-linked adrenoleukodystrophy: A cause of primary adrenal insufficiency in males. The Endocrinologist 1992;2:177.

Soni A et al: Adrenal insufficiency occurring during septic shock: Incidence, outcome, and relationship to peripheral cytokine levels. Am J Med 1995;98:266.

Werbel SS, Ober KP: Acute adrenal insufficiency. Endocrinol Metab Clin North Am 1993;22:303.

Cushing's Syndrome

Aron DC, Tyrrell JB (editors): Cushing's syndrome. Endocrinol Metab Clin North Am 1994;23:451, 925.

Atkinson AB: The treatment of Cushing's syndrome. Clin Endocrinol 1991;34:507.

Carney JA, Young WF Jr: Primary pigmented nodular adrenal hyperplasia and its associated conditions. The Endocrinologist 1992;2:6.

Danese RD, Aron DC: Principles of epidemiology and their application to the diagnosis of Cushing's syndrome: Rev. Bayes meets Dr. Cushing. The Endocrinologist 1994;5:339.

Extabe J, Vazquez JA: Morbidity and mortality in Cushing's disease: An epidemiological approach. Clin Endocrinol 1994;40:479.

Findling JW et al: Routine inferior petrosal sinus sampling in the differential diagnosis of adrenocorticotropin (ACTH)-dependent Cushing's syndrome: Early recognition of the occult ectopic ACTH syndrome. J Clin Endocrinol Metab 1991;73:408.

Flack MR et al: Urine free cortisol in the high-dose dexamethasone suppression test for the differential diagnosis of Cushing's syndrome. Ann Intern Med 1992;116:211.

Magiakow MA et al: Cushing's syndrome in children and adolescents. N Engl J Med 1994;331:752.

McCane DR et al: Assessment of endocrine function after transsphenoidal surgery for Cushing's disease. Clin Endocrinol 1993;38:79.

Miller J, Crapo L: The biochemical diagnosis of hypercortisolism. The Endocrinologist 1994;4:7.

Oldfield EH et al: Petrosal sinus sampling with and without corticotropin-releasing hormone for the differential diagnosis of Cushing's syndrome. N Engl J Med 1991;325:897.

Orth DN: Cushing's syndrome. N Engl J Med 1995;332:791.

Reznik Y et al: Food-dependent Cushing's syndrome mediated by aberrant adrenal sensitivity to gastric inhibitory polypeptide. N Engl J Med 1992;327:981.

Tsigos C, Chrousos GP: Clinical presentation, diagnosis, and treatment of Cushing's syndrome. Curr Opin Endocrinol Diabetes 1995;2:203.

Wajchenberg BL et al: Ectopic adrenocorticotropic hormone syndrome. Endocr Rev 1994;15:752.

Zeiger MA et al: Primary bilateral adrenocortical causes of Cushing's syndrome. Surgery 1991;110:1106.

Hirsutism and Virilization

Azziz R, Dewailly D, Owerbach D: Nonclassic adrenal hyperplasia: Current concepts. J Clin Endocrinol Metab 1994;78:810.

Ehrmann DA, Rosenfield RL: Hirsutism: Beyond the steroidogenic block. N Engl J Med 1990;323:909.

Miller WL: Genetics, diagnosis, and management of 21-hydroxylase deficiency. J Clin Endocrinol Metab 1994;78:241.

Redmond JP: Interpretation of androgen levels in women. In: *Androgenic Disorders.* Redmond JP (editor). Raven Press, 1995.

Vermeulen A, Rubens R: Adrenal virilism. In: *The Adrenal Gland,* 2nd ed. James VHT (editor). Raven Press, 1992.

New MI: 21-Hydroxylase deficiency congenital adrenal hyperplasia. Steroid Biochem Molec Biol 1994; 48:15.

Incidentally Discovered Adrenal Masses and Adrenal Cancer

Bukowski RM et al: Phase II trial of mitotane and cisplatin in patients with adrenal carcinoma: A Southwest Oncology Group Study. J Clin Oncol 1993;11:161.

Candel AG et al: Fine-needle aspiration biopsy of adrenal masses in patients with extraadrenal malignancy. Surgery 1993;114:1132.

Gross MD, Shapiro B: Clinically silent adrenal masses. J Clin Endocrinol Metab 1993;77:885.

Herrera MF et al: Incidentally discovered adrenal tumors: An institutional perspective. Surgery 1991;110:1014.

Jaresch S et al: Adrenal incidentaloma and patients with homozygous or heterozygous congenital adrenal hyperplasia. J Clin Endocrinol Metab 1992;74:685.

Jockenhovel F et al: Conservative and surgical management of incidentally discovered adrenal tumors (incidentalomas). J Endocrinol Invest 1992;15:331.

Pommier RF, Brennan MF: An eleven-year experience with adrenocortical carcinoma. Surgery 1992;112:963.

Reincke M et al: Preclinical Cushing's syndrome in adrenal "incidentalomas": Comparison with adrenal Cushing's syndrome. J Clin Endocrinol Metab 1992;75:826.

Ross NS, Aron DC: Hormonal evaluation of the patient with an incidentally discovered adrenal mass. N Engl J Med 1990;323:1401.

Turton DB, O'Brian JT, Shakir KMM: Incidental adrenal modules: Association with exaggerated 17-hydroxyprogesterone response to adrenocorticotropic hormone. J Endocrinol Invest 1992,15:789.

Endocrine Hypertension

10

Burl R. Don, MD, Edward G. Biglieri, MD, & Morris Schambelan, MD

Arterial hypertension is a prominent component of a number of endocrine disorders, most prominently those involving the adrenal glands (pheochromocytoma, primary aldosteronism) and the pituitary (ACTH-producing tumors). Although the kidney is not an endocrine organ per se, its role as both the origin of and target tissue for the hormones that comprise the renin-angiotensin-aldosterone system makes hypertensive disorders of renal origin an appropriate subject for a chapter on endocrine hypertension. Hypertension may also be a prominent feature of other endocrine disorders such as acromegaly, thyrotoxicosis, hypothyroidism, and hyperparathyroidism, but these topics are considered elsewhere in this volume and will not be discussed in any detail here.

ACRONYMS USED IN THIS CHAPTER	
ACE	Angiotensin-converting enzyme
ACTH	Adrenocorticotropic hormone
ANP	Atrial natriuretic peptide
BNP	Brain natriuretic peptide
CBG	Corticosteroid-binding globulin
CNP	C-type peptide
DHEA	Dehydroepiandrosterone
DHEAS	Dehydroepiandrosterone sulfate
DOC	Deoxycorticosterone
EDRF	Endothelium-derived relaxing factor
GFR	Glomerular filtration rate
MRI	Magnetic resonance imaging
THE	Tetrahydrocortisone
THF	Tetrahydrocortisol

HYPERTENSION OF ADRENAL ORIGIN

SYNTHESIS, METABOLISM, & ACTION OF MINERALOCORTICOID HORMONES

The biosynthetic pathways of the mineralocorticoid hormones are shown in Figure 10–1. The major adrenal secretory products with mineralocorticoid activity are aldosterone and 11-deoxycorticosterone (DOC). Cortisol also has high intrinsic mineralocorticoid activity, but, as discussed in a subsequent section, its actions in the kidney are blunted by local degradation. Aldosterone is produced exclusively in the zona glomerulosa and is primarily controlled by the renin-angiotensin system. Other regulators include Na^+ and K^+ levels, ACTH, and dopamine. With the exception of 18-hydroxycorticosterone, the precursors of aldosterone that originate in the zona glomerulosa are normally present in very low concentrations in the peripheral blood. In the zona fasciculata, the two major biosynthetic pathways are under the control of ACTH. The major product formed by the 17-hydroxy pathway is cortisol. The principal steroid product of the 17-deoxy pathway with significant mineralocorticoid activity is DOC. Corticosterone and 18-hydroxydeoxycorticosterone are also produced in substantial amounts, but these steroids have relative little mineralocorticoid activity in humans.

Aldosterone binds weakly to corticosteroid-binding globulin (CBG)—in contrast to steroids made in the zona fasciculata—and circulates mostly bound to albumin. Free aldosterone comprises 30–50% of its total plasma concentration, whereas the free fractions of the steroid products of the zona fasciculata comprise 5–10% of their total concentration. Consequently, aldosterone has a relatively short half-life, on the order of 15–20 minutes. Aldosterone is rapidly inactivated in the liver, with formation of tetrahydroaldosterone. Another metabolite, aldosterone-18-glucuronide, is formed by the kidney and usually represents 5–10% of the secreted aldosterone. A small amount of free aldosterone appears in the urine and can be easily quantitated. Aldosterone secretion rates

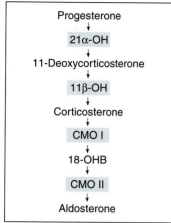
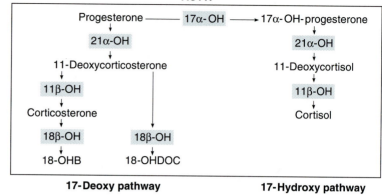

ACTH   = Adrenocorticotropic hormone
17α-OH = P450c17 (17α-hydroxylase) activity
21α-OH = P450c21 (21α-hydroxylase) activity
11β-OH = P450c11 (11β-hydroxylase) activity
18β-OH = P450c11 (18β-hydroxylase) activity

18-OHB   = 18-Hydroxycorticosterone
18-OHDOC = 18-Hydroxy-11-deoxycorticosterone
CMO I   = Corticosterone methyloxidase I
           (18β-hydroxylase) activity
CMO II   = Corticosterone methyloxidase II
           (18β-hydrogenase) activity
(CMO I and CMO II are also called aldosterone synthase)

Figure 10–1. Biosynthetic pathways of the mineralocorticoids. (See also Figures 2–6, 9–4, 9–5, and 14–13.)

vary from 50 to 250 mg/d on Na^+ intakes in the range of 100–150 mmol/d.

DOC is secreted at approximately the same rate as aldosterone. However, like cortisol, DOC is almost totally bound to CBG, with less than 5% appearing in the free form. It is metabolized in the liver to tetrahydrodeoxycorticosterone, conjugated with glucuronic acid, and excreted in the urine. There is virtually no free DOC detectable in the urine.

Mineralocorticoid activity reflects the availability of free hormone and the affinity of the hormone for the receptor. Aldosterone and DOC have approximately equal and high affinities for the mineralocorticoid receptors and circulate at roughly similar concentrations, but aldosterone is quantitatively the most important because much more of it is free. Cortisol has an affinity for the receptor similar to that of aldosterone and circulates at about 1000-fold higher concentrations. Because of this, cortisol is the major steroid that occupies the mineralocorticoid receptors in many tissues such as the pituitary and heart; however, at normal circulating levels, cortisol does not contribute much to mineralocorticoid action in typical target tissues (kidney, colon, salivary glands) because of local conversion (via 11β-hydroxysteroid dehydrogenase) to cortisone. Cortisol can lead to mineralocorticoid hypertension when this conversion is blunted by deficiency or inhibition of this enzyme (discussed subsequently).

Aldosterone and other mineralocorticoids influence certain cell types that have Na^+-K^+ ATPase ac-

tivity. The principal effects of the mineralocorticoids are on maintenance of normal Na^+ and K^+ concentrations and extracellular fluid volume. Mineralocorticoids cross the cell membrane and combine with a mineralocorticoid receptor in the cytosol (see Chapter 3 and Figure 3–12). The active steroid-receptor complex moves into the nucleus of the target cell, where it alters the rate of transcription of mineralocorticoid-responsive genes with subsequent changes in the levels of specific mRNAs and their protein products. The aldosterone-induced proteins include factors that regulate the luminal Na^+ channel, facilitating movement of Na^+ into cells, and components of the Na^+-K^+ ATPase pump. The metabolic effects of aldosterone in the collecting tubule and part of the distal renal tubule result from activation of the Na^+-K^+ ATPase in the serosal membrane to pump passively diffused Na^+ from the luminal side into the extracellular fluid. A subsidiary mechanism is activation of permease in the luminal membrane, favoring Na^+ transport into the tubular cell and subsequently to the extracellular fluid. The major effect of this action quantitatively is to increase the difference in potential across the renal tubule. The increased luminal negativity augments tubular secretion of K^+ by the principal cell and H^+ by the intercalated cell (Figure 10–2). Tubular Na^+, via the Na^+ pump, enters the extracellular fluid and helps maintain its normal composition and volume. All of these events occur in other secretory systems as well and can be measured in saliva, sweat, and feces.

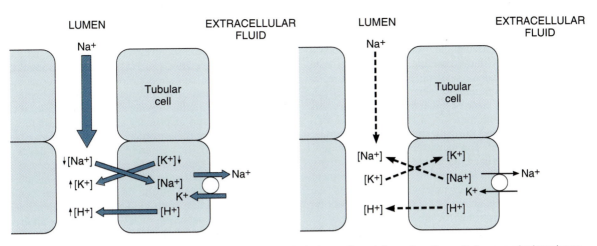

Figure 10–2. Mineralocorticoid action. On the left, rates of tubular sodium delivery together with increased mineralocorticoid action lead to K$^+$ and H$^+$ secretion and Na$^+$ movement into extracellular fluid. On the right, similar amounts of mineralocorticoid are ineffective when tubular sodium is reduced (eg, by dietary sodium restriction).

PATHOGENESIS OF MINERALOCORTICOID HYPERTENSION

Mineralocorticoid hormones produce hypertension by several mechanisms (Figure 10–3). The initiating events are the physiologic consequences of mineralo- corticoid-induced expansion of plasma and extracellular fluid volume. Insights into these early mechanisms come from studies in normal subjects given high doses of mineralocorticoids and from sequential observations made following discontinuation of spironolactone therapy in patients with aldosterone-secreting adenomas. Initially, Na$^+$ and fluid retention

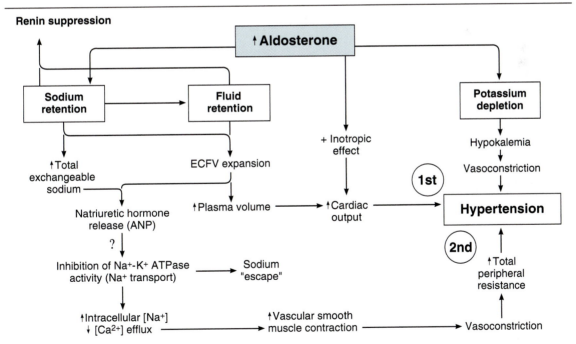

Figure 10–3. Mechanisms involved in mineralocorticoid hypertension. First, there is sodium retention, fluid retention, expansion of extracellular fluid volume and plasma volume, increased cardiac output, and hypertension. Second, there is vasoconstriction and increased total peripheral resistance and hypertension. (ANP, atrial natriuretic peptide; ECFV, extracellular fluid volume.) (See text for details.)

occur, with an increase in body weight, extracellular fluid volume, and cardiac output. After gaining 1–2 L of additional extracellular fluid, the phenomenon of Na⁺ "escape" follows, so that a new steady state is achieved. Renal K⁺ wasting persists and arterial blood pressure continues to increase, however. Typically, the chronic stage of mineralocorticoid excess is characterized by an increase in total peripheral vascular resistance and normalization of stroke volume and cardiac output. The increase in peripheral vascular resistance is related in part to increased sensitivity to catecholamines even without a distinct increment in plasma epinephrine or norepinephrine levels. An additional mechanism may be a direct central action of aldosterone: Intracerebroventricular infusion of aldosterone to rats produced hypertension that could not be reversed or prevented by infusion, at the same site, of a competitive aldosterone antagonist.

Primary mineralocorticoid excess is manifested by hypertension, hypokalemia, and suppression of the renin-angiotensin system. Primary aldosteronism is the prototypic disorder and will be described in the greatest detail. Clinically similar syndromes can result from increased adrenal production of other steroids with mineralocorticoid activity (eg, DOC), failure to inactivate cortisol (eg, syndrome of apparent mineralocorticoid excess), or as a consequence of mineralocorticoid-independent augmentation of renal Na⁺ reabsorption due to a constitutively activated epithelial Na⁺ channel (eg, Liddle's syndrome). The presence of these latter disorders is often suggested by clinical findings of primary mineralocorticoid excess in a patient with subnormal aldosterone levels.

PRIMARY ALDOSTERONISM

Increased production of aldosterone by abnormal zona glomerulosa tissue (adenoma or hyperplasia) initiates the series of events, described in the preceding sections, that result in the typical clinical manifestations of the syndrome of primary aldosteronism. A benign aldosterone-producing adenoma, as originally described by Conn, accounts for 75% of cases of primary aldosteronism. Idiopathic hyperaldosteronism, a disorder with many similar clinical features, accounts for most of the remaining cases. In idiopathic hyperaldosteronism the adrenals are either normal in appearance or, more commonly, reveal bilateral (or, rarely, unilateral) micro- or macronodular adrenal hyperplasia.

Increased renal Na⁺ retention results in expansion of the extracellular fluid volume and increased total body Na⁺ content. Although the effects on the kidney are greatest quantitatively, other mineralocorticoid target tissues are also affected. Fecal excretion of Na⁺, for example, can be decreased to almost nil, with a measurable effect on the rectal potential difference. Salivary electrolyte ratios can also reflect

the influence of hyperaldosteronism on that target tissue. The expanded extracellular fluid and plasma volumes are sensed by stretch receptors at the juxtaglomerular apparatus and Na⁺ flux at the macula densa, with resultant suppression of renin secretion, measured as suppressed plasma renin activity. Suppression of the renin-angiotensin system, while not of itself diagnostic of primary aldosteronism, is thus a major feature of this disorder.

In addition to Na⁺ retention, K⁺ depletion develops, decreasing the total body and plasma concentration of K⁺. The extrusion of K⁺ from its intracellular reservoir is followed by the intracellular movement of H⁺ and, together with aldosterone-dependent increases in renal secretion of H⁺, results in metabolic alkalosis. With moderate K⁺ depletion, decreased carbohydrate tolerance (as evidenced by an abnormal glucose tolerance test) and resistance to vasopressin (as evidenced by impaired urinary concentrating ability) occur. Severe K⁺ depletion blunts baroreceptor function, occasionally producing postural hypotension.

Primary aldosteronism is a disease of the zona glomerulosa. Other adrenal products formed in this zone such as DOC, corticosterone, and 18-hydroxycorticosterone may be present in increased amounts in the blood or urine of persons with an aldosterone-producing adenoma (Figure 10–1). Cells of this zone do not have the ability to make cortisol (owing to the absence of the P450c17, 17α-hydroxylase system). Thus, there are no abnormalities in either cortisol production or metabolism. Plasma and urine cortisol levels are normal.

Clinical Features

Patients typically come to medical attention because of symptoms of hypokalemia or detection of previously unsuspected hypertension during the course of a routine physical examination. The medical history reveals no characteristic symptoms other than nonspecific complaints of fatigue, loss of stamina, weakness, and lassitude—all of which are symptoms of K⁺ depletion. If K⁺ depletion is more severe, increased thirst, polyuria (especially nocturnal), and paresthesias may also be present. Headaches are frequent.

Excessive production of mineralocorticoids produces no characteristic physical findings. Blood pressure in patients with primary aldosteronism can range from borderline elevation to severely hypertensive levels. The mean blood pressure in the 136 patients reported by the Glasgow Hypertension Study unit was 205/123 mm Hg, with no significant difference between the groups with adenoma or hyperplasia. Accelerated or malignant hypertension is extremely rare. Retinopathy is mild, and hemorrhages are rarely present. Orthostatic decreases in blood pressure without reflex tachycardia are observed in the severely K⁺-depleted patient because of blunting of the baroreceptors. A positive Trousseau or Chvostek sign may be suggestive of alkalosis accompanying severe K^+ depletion. The heart is usually only mildly enlarged, and electrocardiographic changes reflect modest left ventricular hypertrophy and K^+ depletion. Clinical edema is uncommon.

Initial Diagnosis

A. Hypokalemia: Detection of spontaneous hypokalemia is often the initial clue that suggests a diagnosis of primary aldosteronism in a patient with hypertension. During the investigation, a high-K^+ diet or KCl supplements should be avoided, and all previous diuretic therapy must be discontinued for at least 3 weeks before a valid serum or plasma K^+ measurement can be obtained. The most common cause of hypokalemia in patients with hypertension is diuretic therapy.

In some series, up to 20% of patients with primary aldosteronism have had normal or low-normal serum K^+ concentrations. Serum K^+ concentration is closely related to and determined to a great extent by NaCl intake (Figure 10–2). A low Na^+ diet, by reducing delivery of Na^+ to aldosterone-sensitive sites in the distal nephron, can reduce renal K^+ secretion and thus correct hypokalemia. By the same token, increased distal delivery of Na^+ accompanying a high Na^+ diet can enhance K^+ loss, particularly when aldosterone is being secreted autonomously and is therefore not subject to normal suppression by the high Na^+ intake. These physiologic relationships serve to illustrate the importance of controlling the dietary Na^+ intake when evaluating patients suspected of having primary aldosteronism. In the presence of normal renal function and autonomous aldosterone production, salt loading will usually unmask hypokalemia. Normokalemic hyperaldosteronism under these conditions has been reported but is rare.

B. Salt Intake: In the USA, Japan, and many European countries, the average person consumes more than 120 mmol of Na^+ per day—enough to allow hypokalemia to become manifest. If a dietary history of high salt intake is obtained and K^+ concentrations are normal, a diagnosis of primary aldosteronism is unlikely. Patients who report a low Na^+ intake should be advised to take an unrestricted diet plus 1 g of NaCl with each meal for 4 days; blood samples for electrolyte determinations should be obtained in the fasting state on the following morning. This dietary regimen is also useful because it prepares the patient for optimal measurement of renin and aldosterone levels

C. Assessment of the Renin-Angiotensin-Aldosterone System: Assessment of the renin-angiotensin system can be accomplished by a random plasma renin activity measurement. If plasma renin activity is normal or high in a patient who has not been receiving diuretic therapy for at least 3 weeks, it is very unlikely that an aldosterone-producing ade-

noma is present. Some patients with idiopathic hyperaldosteronism may have low-normal levels of plasma renin activity, however. On the other hand, a subnormal plasma renin level is not alone sufficient to establish a diagnosis of primary aldosteronism, since a large subgroup of patients with essential hypertension have low plasma renin levels.

If hypokalemia and suppressed renin activity are detected, plasma and urinary aldosterone measurements should be obtained while the patient is taking an unrestricted salt diet with NaCl supplementation or if the dietary history reveals a high salt intake, as previously described. This is crucial, because with any significant diminution of salt intake, plasma aldosterone concentration and aldosterone production normally increase.

Assessment of aldosterone production can best be accomplished by measurement of urinary aldosterone excretion over a 24-hour period. Most laboratories measure excretion of the 18-glucuronide metabolite. The normal rates of urinary excretion of aldosterone-18-glucuronide range from 5 to 20 µg/24 h (14–56 nmol/24 h). In one large series, the mean values in patients with aldosterone-producing adenoma and idiopathic hyperaldosteronism were 45.2 ± 4 µg/24 h (125 ± 9 nmol/24 h) and 27.1 ± 2 µg/24 h (75 ± 5 nmol/24 h), respectively. Urinary measurements are superior to random measurements of plasma aldosterone for the detection of abnormal production of aldosterone but are not always able to discriminate between patients with adenoma and those with idiopathic hyperaldosteronism.

Samples for measurement of plasma aldosterone concentration should ideally be obtained at around 8:00 AM after at least 4 hours of recumbency and under the same dietary conditions as described above for measurement of urinary aldosterone. This measurement not only confirms the presence of hyperaldosteronism but also provides insight into the probable underlying pathology. When obtained under these conditions, a plasma aldosterone concentration greater than 25 ng/dL (695 pmol/L) usually indicates the presence of an aldosterone-producing adenoma (Figure 10–4).

The plasma aldosterone level should also be determined after 2–4 hours in the upright posture (which normally activates the renin system, with a resultant increase in the plasma aldosterone level). Ninety percent of patients with adenoma will show no significant change or a frank decrease in plasma aldosterone levels, whereas aldosterone levels almost always increase in those with idiopathic hyperaldosteronism (Figure 10–4). The difference is due to (1) the profound suppression of the renin system by excessive aldosterone production in patients with an adenoma; (2) the influence of ACTH, to which the adenoma is still responsive and which normally decreases between 8 AM and 12 noon; and (3) decreased responsiveness of adenomas to angiotensin

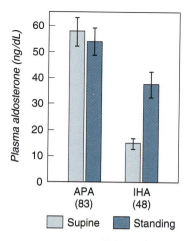

Figure 10–4. Response of plasma aldosterone to postural stimulation in primary aldosteronism. (APA, aldosterone-producing adenoma; IHA, idiopathic hyperaldosteronism.)

II. In contrast, in patients with idiopathic hyperaldosteronism, increased sensitivity of the gland to small increases in renin (and presumably of angiotensin II) levels that occur in the upright posture leads to an increased aldosterone level. Serum cortisol levels must be measured simultaneously. An increase in serum cortisol implies an ACTH discharge and invalidates the information obtained from the maneuver.

Measurement of other adrenal steroids may add to the precision of diagnosis. Plasma DOC, corticosterone, and, particularly, 18-hydroxycorticosterone levels are frequently increased in patients with adenoma, whereas they are rarely if ever increased in patients with idiopathic hyperaldosteronism. Increased urinary excretion of 18-hydroxycortisol and 18-oxocortisol, which is a characteristic finding in individuals with the dexamethasone-suppressible form of primary aldosteronism (described in a subsequent section), may also be present in some patients with aldosterone-producing adenomas.

The procedures just discussed can confirm a diagnosis of primary aldosteronism and differentiate adenoma from idiopathic hyperaldosteronism in most cases. Localization studies can also provide additional information. When uncertainty persists, the saline infusion test may also be useful.

D. Saline Infusion Test: Saline loading establishes aldosterone unresponsiveness to volume expansion and thereby identifies autonomy in patients with aldosterone-producing adenomas. Two liters of isotonic NaCl are administered over 2–4 hours. Blood samples for aldosterone and cortisol measurements are obtained before and after the infusion. Expansion of the extracellular fluid volume reduces plasma aldosterone concentration promptly in patients with "essential" hypertension but fails to suppress plasma aldosterone concentration into the normal range in patients with adenoma or hyperplasia. Moreover, the saline infusion test typically distinguishes patients with primary aldosteronism from those with low-renin essential hypertension. The ratio of aldosterone to cortisol is typically greater than 3.0 following administration of saline in patients with an aldosterone-producing adenoma, reflecting the limited effect of volume expansion in the setting of marked suppression of the renin-angiotensin system.

Rare Forms of Primary Aldosteronism

A. Dexamethasone (Glucocorticoid)-Remediable Aldosteronism: Dexamethasone-remediable aldosteronism is a rare form of genetic hypertension that has been recognized with increasing frequency since the molecular basis of this disorder was established. It is inherited in an autosomal dominant fashion. The primary defect is a gene duplication that results from an unequal crossing over event that fuses the regulatory region of the 11β-hydroxylase gene to the coding sequence of aldosterone synthase. With cortisol as a substrate, expression of this enzyme in the zona fasciculata results in the synthesis of 18-hydroxycortisol and 18-oxocortisol (phenotypic markers of this disorder). Aldosterone secretion also occurs in this zone and is ACTH-dependent, such that small doses of glucocorticoid (eg, 1–2 mg/d of dexamethasone) can ameliorate hypertension as well as the typical biochemical findings. However, the response to dexamethasone suppression may dissipate over the long term in many patients, and additional antihypertensive therapy may thus be necessary. The presence of glucocorticoid-remediable aldosteronism should be considered in any family in which more than one individual is found to have primary aldosteronism. The diagnosis can easily be established by measurement of the marker steroids (18-oxocortisol or 18-hydroxycortisol) or by detection of the abnormal gene in DNA samples obtained from peripheral blood leukocytes.

B. Aldosterone-Producing Adrenocortical Carcinoma: Malignant adrenocortical tumors producing aldosterone in the absence of hypercortisolism are rare, accounting for less than 3% of cases of primary aldosteronism. In general, the biochemical and hormonal features and the response to dynamic tests are similar to those typical in adenoma except that the magnitude of the abnormalities is usually greater. Hypercortisolism as well as hyperandrogenism or hyperestrogenism may occur during the progression of the disease.

Management of Aldosterone-Producing Adenomas

A. Location of Adenoma: Once the biochemical diagnosis is secure, procedures that identify the likely site of an adenoma can aid in establishing the appropriate surgical approach. A number of techniques have been developed including adrenal venography, adrenal scintigraphy, adrenal vein catheterization with sampling for aldosterone measurements, and CT or MRI imaging. The diagnostic information provided by CT scanning or MRI in locating adenomas has proved to be both accurate and practical and is the initial procedure of choice. Adrenal venography was associated with a number of problems, such as extravasation of dye, hemorrhage, and adrenal infarction and is no longer utilized. Scanning using intravenously administered ^{131}I-iodocholesterol can identify the site of an adenoma in about 80% of patients, although the success rate decreases markedly if tumors are less than 1 cm in diameter. The procedure takes several visits to accomplish, however. The use of ^{131}I-labeled 6β-iodomethyl-19-norcholesterol reduces the interval between injection and scintiscanning to about 3–7 days.

Adrenal vein catheterization to obtain samples for measurement and comparison of aldosterone levels in the venous effluent of both adrenal glands continues to be useful in lateralizing tumors after other techniques fail and biochemical evidence still supports the diagnosis of adenoma. The success of this procedure is highly dependent on the skill and experience of the interventional radiologist. Cortisol levels should always be measured simultaneously to confirm the source of the sample and the extent of contamination with nonadrenal venous blood. Prior treatment with ACTH is frequently employed to magnify the differences between affected and unaffected sides.

B. Treatment Options: Treatment depends for the most part on the accuracy of diagnosis. In patients with an aldosterone-producing adenoma and no contraindication to surgery, unilateral adrenalectomy is recommended. The degree of reduction of blood pressure and correction of hypokalemia achieved with prior spironolactone therapy provides a good indication of the likely response to surgery; in fact, greater reduction often occurs postoperatively, presumably because of a greater reduction of extracellular fluid volume. The surgical cure rate of hypertension associated with adenoma is excellent—more than 70% have benefited in several large series—with reduction of hypertension in the remainder.

Subtotal adrenalectomy will correct hypokalemia in patients with idiopathic aldosteronism, but hypertension is rarely cured. Therefore, other antihypertensive measures (including spironolactone) should be used to control hypertension, and such patients should not be routinely sent to surgery. A subset of patients with primary aldosteronism but no identifiable adenoma may benefit from surgical reduction of adrenal mass, ie, subtotal or total adrenalectomy. This group typically responds to stimulatory and suppressive maneuvers in a manner similar to patients with an aldosterone-producing adenoma. Pathologic examination of the adrenal tissue usually discloses micro- or macronodular hyperplasia. The autonomy of aldosterone production in this condition is difficult to explain, but the disease may be compared to the autonomy of cortisol production in nodular dysplasia associated with Cushing's syndrome.

C. Preoperative Preparation: Ideally, patients should be treated preoperatively with spironolactone until the blood pressure and serum K^+ are normal. This drug is particularly beneficial because of its unique mechanism of action in blocking the mineralocorticoid receptor. Spironolactone reduces the volume of the expanded extracellular fluid toward normal, promotes K^+ retention, and restores normal serum K^+ concentration. It often has the additional desirable effect of activating (after 1–2 months) the suppressed renin-angiotensin system and, consequently, of aldosterone secretion by the contralateral adrenal gland. Postoperative hypoaldosteronism with hyperkalemia is unlikely with this treatment. Preoperative treatment will also permit reversal to some extent of some of the changes in target organs that were produced by the hypertensive and hypokalemic states. Spironolactone is usually well tolerated; the side effects of rashes, gynecomastia, impotence, and epigastric discomfort are rare over a short time interval. Once blood pressure and serum K^+ levels are normal on an initial dose of 200–300 mg/d, the dose can be tapered to a maintenance dose of approximately 100 mg/d until the time of surgery. In patients who develop one or more of these side effects, the K^+-sparing diuretic amiloride, in doses of 20–40 mg/d, can be used as an alternative. Other antihypertensive drugs may also be required and should be used to obtain optimal blood pressure control. Calcium channel blockers appear to be effective in this setting.

D. Surgical and Postoperative Medical Treatment: When the diagnosis and lateralization are certain, surgical removal of the adenoma is advised. Current preoperative lateralization techniques easily identify the site of tumor, and a unilateral posterior approach should be used. Some centers have begun to remove these tumors via a laparoscope with success. Postoperative morbidity is usually not significant with either of these procedures.

Over 70% of patients with primary aldosteronism who have undergone surgery have had unilateral adenoma. Bilateral tumors are rare. The characteristic adenoma is readily identified by its golden-yellow color. In addition, small satellite adenomas are often found, and distinction from micro- or macronodular hyperplasia is occasionally difficult. In patients with adenoma, the contiguous adrenal gland can show hyperplasia throughout the gland. Hyperplasia is also present in the contralateral adrenal gland but is not associated with aldosterone abnormalities after removal of the primary adenoma.

If the tumor is identified at surgery in a patient who had a unilateral lesion detected preoperatively, exploration of the contralateral adrenal is not indicated. If surgery is contraindicated or refused, prolonged treatment with spironolactone can be effective. The initial dose of 200–400 mg of spironolactone per day must be continued for 4–6 weeks before the full effect on blood pressure is realized. With prolonged treatment, aldosterone production does not increase even though K^+ replenishment and activation of the renin-angiotensin system occur. In addition, spironolactone directly inhibits aldosterone synthesis by adenomas. A chronic dose of 75–100 mg is usually sufficient to maintain a normal blood pressure.

Patients who have had unilateral adrenalectomy for removal of an aldosterone-producing tumor occasionally have a transient period of relative hypomineralocorticoidism with negative Na^+ balance, K^+ retention, and mild acidosis. Full recovery of the chronically unstimulated, contralateral zona glomerulosa usually takes place in 4–6 months following surgery but may take longer. Restitution of the suppressed renin-angiotensin system to normal is required for a completely normal adrenocortical response similar to the need for recovery of pituitary function after removal of a cortisol-producing adenoma (Cushing's syndrome). No specific treatment is usually necessary other than adequate Na^+ intake. A small percentage of patients (1%) do not have normal recovery of their renin-angiotensin-aldosterone system and require mineralocorticoid replacement (fludrocortisone) therapy for life. Preexisting renal disease that impairs renin secretion is usually evident in such individuals.

SYNDROMES DUE TO EXCESS DEOXYCORTICOSTERONE PRODUCTION

Deoxycorticosterone is the second most important naturally occurring mineralocorticoid hormone. Accordingly, excess DOC production should be suspected in any hypertensive patient with hypokalemia and suppression of renin and aldosterone production.

17α-Hydroxylase Deficiency

17α-Hydroxylase deficiency syndrome is usually recognized at the time of puberty in young adults by the presence of hypertension, hypokalemia, and primary amenorrhea (with sexual infantilism) in the female or pseudohermaphroditism in the male (Chapter 14). In contrast to the clinical manifestations in 21- and 11β-hydroxylation deficiencies, there is no virilization or restricted growth. Patients often present with eunuchoid proportions and appearance. The virtual absence of 17α-hydroxyprogesterone, pregnanetriol, and 17-ketosteroids is diagnostic of this type of hydroxylase deficiency.

The key location of the 17α-hydroxylating system (cytochrome P450c17α) in the steroid biosynthetic pathway prevents normal production of androgens and estrogens (Figure 9–4). There has been no instance in which the adrenal defect has appeared without a concomitant gonadal defect. The defect occurs in a single gene (in chromosome 10), which codes for the enzyme or the expression of the enzyme. The diminution of cortisol production induces increased production of ACTH. Initially, activity of the entire biosynthetic pathway of non-17-hydroxylated steroids is increased—namely, progesterone, DOC, corticosterone, 18-OH DOC, and aldosterone. Subsequently, expansion of extracellular fluid and blood volumes, hypertension, and profound suppression of the renin-angiotensin system results, in most cases, in reduced aldosterone levels. Thus, the principal steroids present in excess are DOC, corticosterone, 18-hydroxycorticosterone, and 18-OH DOC.

11β-Hydroxylase Deficiency

Congenital adrenal hyperplasia due to 11β-hydroxylase deficiency is usually recognized in newborns and infants because of virilization and the presence of both hypertension and hypokalemia. Plasma androgens, 11-deoxycortisol, 17α-hydroxyprogesterone, urinary 17-ketosteroids, and 17-hydroxycorticosteroids are increased. (See Chapter 14 and Figure 14–13.)

The defect (in the gene mapped to chromosome 8) is usually partial, so that some cortisol is produced, but it does not increase with further stimulation by ACTH. Blood levels and production rates of cortisol are usually within normal limits. A partial defect of 11β-hydroxylation results in increased production and blood levels of DOC, 11-deoxycortisol (Figure 10–1), and androgens. Hypertension results from excessive production of DOC by mechanisms similar to those previously described for aldosterone.

The blood levels and production rates of aldosterone are low-normal or reduced. Two mechanisms are proposed. Originally, a partial deficiency of the 11β-hydroxylation activity in the zona glomerulosa was postulated, with a block in aldosterone synthesis. This concept was supported by the observation that after normalization of DOC production and correction of the hypertension (by ACTH suppression), aldosterone production remained normal or reduced and a Na^+-losing state could be provoked. Currently, it is felt that there is no zona glomerulosa defect but that suppression of renin by the increased production of DOC reduces the production of aldosterone in the zona glomerulosa. Thus, after chronic salt restriction and ACTH suppression, both renin and aldosterone dynamics return to normal, implying an intact zona glomerulosa.

Treatment of 17α- and 11β-Hydroxylase Deficiency

Treatment of both of these disorders is similar to that of all non-Na$^+$-losing forms of congenital adrenal hyperplasia. Treatment with physiologic replacement doses of glucocorticoid, such as hydrocortisone or dexamethasone, restores blood pressure to normal levels, corrects K$^+$ depletion, reduces excessive DOC and corticosterone production in 17α-hydroxylase deficiency, and reduces DOC and 11-deoxycortisol production in 11β-hydroxylase deficiency. In 17α-hydroxylase deficiency syndrome, restoration of normal levels of DOC results in a return of plasma renin activity and aldosterone to normal values. A delay in return of the suppressed renin-aldosterone system toward normal can result in hypovolemic crises with the initial natriuresis and diuresis. It may take several years before the aldosterone and renin systems become normal. The amount of glucocorticoid administered must be carefully determined because of apparently exquisite tissue sensitivity to glucocorticoid hormones. Addition of estrogen-progestogen combined cyclic therapy may be necessary in the adult patient with 17α-hydroxylase deficiency (see Chapter 14).

Androgen- & Estrogen-Producing Adrenal Tumors

Most of the C-19 steroids produced by the adult adrenocortical zona reticularis have weak androgen activity, especially dehydroepiandrosterone (DHEA) and its sulfate (DHEAS) as well as androstenedione. Disturbances in both internal zona reticularis regulatory mechanisms (ie, enzyme activity) and its extra-adrenal regulators (ACTH and an androgen-stimulating peptide of possible hypothalamic-pituitary origin) may lead to excessive adrenal sex steroid production, resulting in syndromes of hirsutism and virilization in the female or feminization in men.

Although the zona reticularis has no intrinsic capacity to synthesize any effective glucocorticoid or mineralocorticoid, it has the potential, under conditions of chronic stimulation by ACTH, to transform some cellular function into the fasciculata cell type (by the induction of specific enzyme complexes) and produce cortisol and presumably other typical zona fasciculata steroids.

Some patients with malignancies originating in the zona reticularis (androgen- or estrogen-producing tumors, or both types) may have clinical features of mineralocorticoid excess, with hypertension, hypokalemia, and renin suppression. Aldosterone levels are generally not elevated and are often reduced. Urinary or plasma steroid profiling in some of these patients suggests that there may be inhibition of 11β-hydroxylase activity in association with the increased production of androgens or estrogens. Administration of methylandrostanediol to experimental animals and

testosterone to humans suggests that exogenous androgen excess can block the conversion of 11-deoxycortisol and DOC to cortisol and corticosterone, respectively. Excessive secretion of DOC could then lead to a state of mineralocorticoid excess. Increased urinary excretion of DOC metabolites or plasma DOC concentrations have been found in several patients with androgen- or estrogen-producing adrenocortical carcinomas who have hypertension and hypokalemia.

The inhibition of 11β-hydroxylase in these carcinomas may be due to inactivation of the enzyme cytochrome P450c11 by the high intra-adrenal concentration of androgens (androstenedione) that act as a pseudosubstrate for the reaction. This mechanism is similar to that occurring in Cushing's syndrome, in which cortisol appears to serve as the enzymatic inhibitor.

Syndrome of Primary Cortisol Resistance

Peripheral resistance to cortisol action is a very rare condition—reported only in a few families—in which severe hypertension, hypokalemia, and renin suppression are associated with elevated plasma and urinary levels of cortisol without causing clinical manifestations of Cushing's syndrome. The basic defect is at the glucocorticoid receptor level; both the number of receptors and the affinity of the receptors for cortisol are reduced in the target tissues. In this condition, plasma levels of ACTH are elevated as a result of block of cortisol feedback at the corticotroph. Cortisol production is thus increased, but it does not result in the typical clinical stigmas of hypercortisolism. However, chronic stimulation by excess ACTH of the 17-deoxy pathway of the zona fasciculata results in abnormal production of DOC and corticosterone, causing hypertension, hypokalemia, and suppression of renin and aldosterone production. The clinical and biochemical abnormalities are partially relieved by treatment with high doses of dexamethasone.

CUSHING'S SYNDROME

Hypertension is a common finding of endogenous hypercortisolism (present in more than 80% of cases; see Chapter 9) but occurs in only 10–20% of patients receiving therapy with synthetic glucocorticoids. ACTH-dependent hypercortisolism (Cushing's disease and ectopic ACTH production) is frequently accompanied by increased levels of other ACTH-dependent steroids, especially DOC and corticosterone. Elevated DOC (Figure 10–5) and cortisol levels probably contribute to the mineralocorticoid excess state. Plasma renin activity varies but is typically normal as a consequence of concomitant increase in the production of angiotensinogen. Serum K$^+$ levels are also normal in most patients, implying the ab-

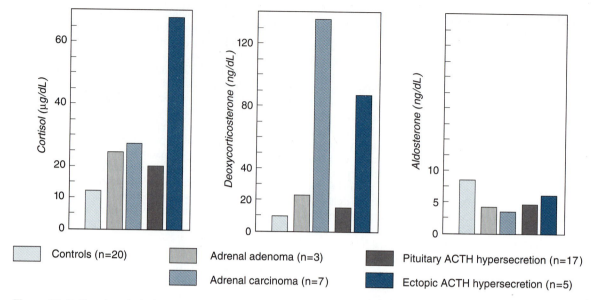

Figure 10–5. Basal cortisol, deoxycorticosterone, and aldosterone levels in patients with Cushing's syndrome according to their etiology.

sence of a mineralocorticoid excess state. However, a small subset of patients have hypokalemia and suppressed plasma renin levels. Most of these patients have ectopic ACTH hypersecretion or adrenal tumors. Even when there is evidence for mineralocorticoid excess (suppressed plasma renin and hypokalemia), levels of aldosterone and 18-hydroxycorticosterone are consistently within or below the low normal range.

Hypertension in Cushing's syndrome is usually more frequent in patients with adrenocortical hyperplasia (due to ACTH excess) than in patients with cortical adenomas, which implies that, in addition to cortisol, other ACTH-dependent steroids (eg, DOC, corticosterone, or 18-hydroxyDOC) may contribute to the development or maintenance of hypertension. In addition, urinary excretion of the potent naturally occurring mineralocorticoid 19-nor-DOC, produced in the kidney by the conversion of an oxygenated form of DOC, is elevated in both the primary (adrenal) and secondary (pituitary) forms of Cushing's syndrome.

Since most patients with Cushing's syndrome do not have findings consistent with hypermineralocorticoidism (eg, hypokalemia and hyporeninemia), glucocorticoids appear to cause hypertension by mineralocorticoid-independent mechanisms (Figure 10–6). These include increased production of angiotensin II due to glucocorticoid-induced increases in the hepatic synthesis of angiotensinogen; enhanced glucocorticoid-mediated vascular reactivity to vasoconstrictors; inhibition of extraneuronal uptake and degradation of catecholamines; inhibition of vasodilatory systems such as kinins and prostaglandins;

shift in Na^+ from the intracellular to the extracellular compartment, resulting in increased plasma volume; and an increase in cardiac output from the increased production of epinephrine due to enhanced phenylethanolamine-N-methyl transferase activity in the adrenal medulla.

PSEUDOHYPERALDOSTERONISM

The term pseudohyperaldosteronism comprises a heterogeneous group of disorders in which endogenous mineralocorticoid secretion is abnormally low owing to suppressed renin production. Renin secretion is suppressed by increased Na^+ retention and volume expansion, resulting either from the presence of endogenous or exogenous mineralocorticoids or mineralocorticoid-like substances or from a renal tubular defect. Hypertension, hypokalemia, and metabolic alkalosis are the usual manifestations. In addition to the syndromes that result from excess production of DOC as described above, continuous use of fluorinated steroids with powerful mineralocorticoid-like activity contained in some topical preparations such as nasal sprays and dermatologic creams can be associated with hypertension, hypokalemia, and renin and aldosterone suppression. Withdrawal of these medications or adjustment of the dosage easily controls undesirable side effects. Pseudohyperaldosteronism can also occur as a prominent feature of several rare syndromes, the pathophysiologic features of which have only recently been established. These are described in the following sections.

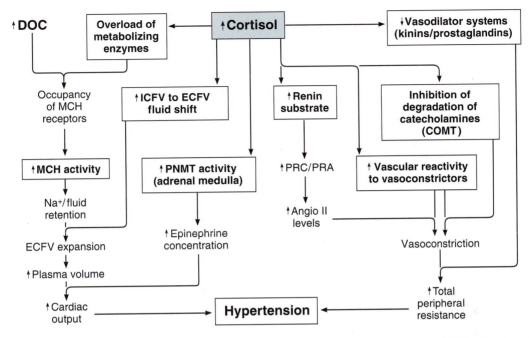

Figure 10–6. Mechanisms involved in glucocorticoid hypertension. (DOC, deoxycorticosterone; MCH, mineralocorticoid hormone; ECFV, extracellular fluid volume; ICFV, intracellular fluid volume; PRC, plasma renin concentration; PRA, plasma renin activity; COMT, catechol-O-methyltransferase; PNMT, phenylethanolamine-*N*-methyltransferase.)

Syndrome of Apparent Mineralocorticoid Excess (11β-Hydroxysteroid Dehydrogenase Deficiency)

A rare disorder, initially designated as the syndrome of apparent mineralocorticoid excess, is characterized by findings suggestive of a hypermineralocorticoid state (hypertension, hypokalemia, suppressed renin levels, and amelioration by spironolactone) despite low levels of aldosterone and DOC. Most of the reported cases have been in children who have severe—often lethal—hypertension. Although the pathogenesis remained elusive for more than a decade, it is now evident that the primary abnormality in this disorder is reduced peripheral metabolism of cortisol due to one or more mutations in the gene encoding 11β-hydroxysteroid dehydrogenase type 2, the isoenzyme that is present in greatest abundance in the renal tubule. Impaired conversion of cortisol to cortisone (Figure 10–7) in the cells of the renal tubule results in an accumulation of cortisol and subsequent occupancy of mineralocorticoid receptors. Despite normal plasma cortisol levels, urinary cortisol is increased, reflecting impairment of the kidney's ability to convert cortisol to cortisone. The increased urinary excretion of tetrahydrocortisol (THF) and reduced excretion of tetrahydrocortisone (THE) leads to a marked increase in the THF/THE ratio (Figure 10–8), a finding considered diagnostic of this disorder. Treatment consists of the administration of small doses of dexamethasone (0.75–1 mg/d) to suppress ACTH and to limit thereby the production of cortisol and its accumulation in mineralocorticoid target tissues in the kidney.

Chronic Ingestion of Licorice

Chronic ingestion of large amounts of substances containing "mineralocorticoid-like activity"—eg, certain candies, infusions, and some chewing tobaccos containing licorice—results in a syndrome of hypertension, hypokalemia, renal Na+ retention, volume expansion, suppressed plasma renin activity, and metabolic alkalosis. Aldosterone secretion and excretion are low or undetectable, however, as are other mineralocorticoid precursors in the aldosterone pathway. The responsible agent for this syndrome is the active principle of licorice, glycyrrhizic acid, and its metabolite glycyrrhetinic acid, that are present in certain commercially available products. Both of these alkaloids inhibit 11β-hydroxysteroid dehydrogenase in the kidney, which increases free cortisol locally to act as the mineralocorticoid in a manner similar to the syndrome of apparent mineralocorticoid excess. Pseudohyperaldosteronism can be induced by licorice and its derivatives such as carbenoxolone (an anti-gastric ulcer drug), the Na+ hemisuccinate of 18β-glycyrrhetinic acid. Electrolyte abnormalities and hypertension disappear within a few weeks upon discontinuation of licorice ingestion or withdrawal of carbenoxolone treatment.

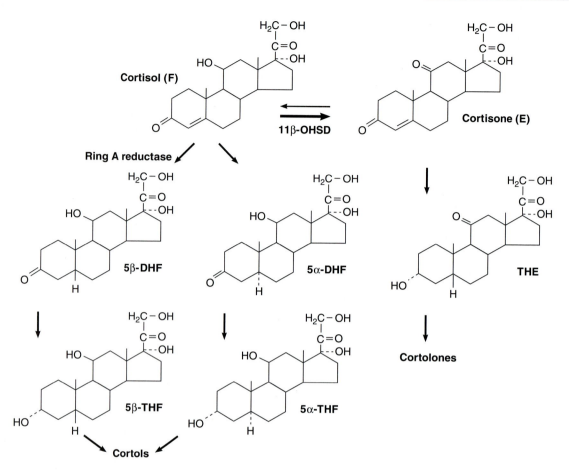

Figure 10–7. Principal pathways of cortisol metabolism. (11β-OHSD, 11β-hydroxysteroid dehydrogenase; DHF, dihydrocortisol; THF, tetrahydrocortisol; THE, tetrahydrocortisone.)

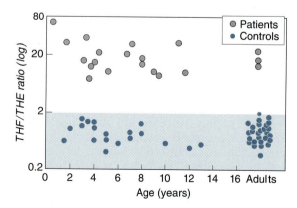

Figure 10–8. Ratio of the urinary metabolites of cortisol (THF, tetrahydrocortisol; 5α-THF, allotetrahydrocortisol) to cortisone (THE, tetrahydrocortisone) in the syndrome of apparent mineralocorticoid excess. (Modified from Shackleton CHL, Stewart PM: The hypertension of apparent mineralocorticoid excess syndrome. In: *Endocrine Hypertension.* Biglieri EG [editor]. Raven Press, 1990.)

Liddle's Syndrome

In 1963, Liddle and his colleagues reported the results of studies in a large family in which the affected members had clinical manifestations resembling those of classic primary aldosteronism: hypertension, hypokalemia with renal K^+ wasting, metabolic alkalosis, and suppressed plasma renin activity. Aldosterone production, however, was negligible. The inheritance pattern in this large family was that of an autosomal dominant disorder, and the phenotype was soon identified in several additional families as well as in sporadic cases.

Although these findings suggested the possibility of excessive production of another mineralocorticoid to explain the clinical manifestations, in contrast to patients with excess DOC production or those with the syndrome of apparent mineralocorticoid excess, administration of the mineralocorticoid antagonist spironolactone did not correct either the hypertension or the hypokalemia. Furthermore, the adrenocortical synthesis-blocking agent metyrapone, which inhibits

11β- and 18-hydroxylation of aldosterone precursors, also had no effect. In contrast, administration of triamterene, a diuretic agent with K^+-sparing activity independent of mineralocorticoid antagonism, was effective in correcting the abnormalities. The investigators proposed that a primary abnormality in the renal tubule that enhanced Na^+ reabsorption was responsible.

Recent studies in the original kindred of Liddle as well as in individuals from several other kindreds similarly affected proved this hypothesis to be remarkably prescient. Using linkage analysis as well as electrophysiologic techniques, it has been established that patients with Liddle's syndrome have a defect in the cytoplasmic domain of either the β or γ subunit of the epithelial Na^+ channel that results in constitutive activation of the channel. Since amiloride as well as triamterene are relatively specific inhibitors of this channel, treatment with these agents will correct the electrolyte abnormalities and ameliorate the hypertension as well.

TYPE II PSEUDOHYPOALDOSTERONISM (Arnold-Healy-Gordon Syndrome)

The term type II pseudohypoaldosteronism has been used to describe a rare clinical syndrome in which hypertension is present in association with hyperkalemia, impairment of renal K^+ excretion, hyperchloremic metabolic acidosis, and hyporeninemic hypoaldosteronism. The glomerular filtration rate (GFR) is usually normal. Mineralocorticoid resistance is apparent by persistence of hyperkalemia and a subnormal kaliuretic response to large doses of exogenously administered mineralocorticoid hormone. However, in contrast to patients with the classic form of mineralocorticoid resistance (type I pseudohypoaldosteronism), salt wasting is not present and both the antinatriuretic and antichloruretic responses to mineralocorticoid are intact.

An impairment in renal K^+ secretion was initially proposed as the primary defect. However, whereas fractional renal K^+ excretion was subnormal and increased only minimally when Na^+ was delivered to distal nephron segments as NaCl, distal renal K^+ secretion increased greatly when Na^+ was delivered distally in the presence of non-Cl^- anions (sulfate and bicarbonate). These findings indicate that the renal K^+ secretory mechanism is intact and suggested an alternative hypothesis in which the primary defect was proposed to increase the reabsorptive avidity of the distal nephron for Cl^-. This, in turn, would (1) limit the Na^+ and mineralocorticoid-dependent driving force for K^+ and H^+ secretion, resulting in hyperkalemia and acidosis; and (2) augment distal NaCl reabsorption, resulting in hyperchloremia, volume expansion, and hypertension. Consistent with the presence of such a "chloride shunt," restriction of dietary NaCl or administration of a chloruretic diuretic (furosemide, thiazides) ameliorates hyperkalemia and acidosis in such patients.

HYPERTENSION OF RENAL ORIGIN

THE RENIN-ANGIOTENSIN SYSTEM

The term "renin" was first suggested by Tigerstedt and Bergman in 1898 to denote the pressor material in saline extracts of rabbit kidneys. Pioneer studies by Page and Helmer and Braun-Menendez in the 1930s demonstrated that renin enzymatically cleaves an α_2 globulin substrate (angiotensinogen) to form a decapeptide (angiotensin I) that is subsequently cleaved by angiotensin-converting enzyme (ACE) to form an octapeptide with potent vasoconstrictor effects (angiotensin II). During this same period, Goldblatt noted that reducing the flow of blood to the kidney in experimental animals was followed by an increase in blood pressure. Subsequently, these two landmark observations were found to be related; reducing blood flow to the kidney stimulates the renin-angiotensin system, resulting in an increase in blood pressure. The integration of these concepts is a key paradigm in understanding blood pressure regulation and has served as one of the important models in evaluating mechanisms of hypertension.

Renin

As the afferent arteriole enters the glomerulus (Figure 10–9), the smooth muscle cells become modified to perform a secretory function. These juxtaglomerular cells produce and secrete renin, a proteolytic enzyme with a molecular weight of approximately 40,000. In close proximity to the juxtaglomerular cells are specialized tubular cells of the cortical thick ascending limb of the loop of Henle known as the macula densa. The juxtaglomerular cells of the afferent arteriole and the macula densa are referred to collectively as the juxtaglomerular apparatus and the interplay of these specialized cells has an important role in the secretion of renin.

The synthesis of renin involves a series of steps beginning with the translation of renin mRNA into preprorenin. The 23-amino-acid amino terminal sequence of preprorenin directs trafficking of the protein into the endoplasmic reticulum, where it is subsequently cleaved, resulting in the formation of prorenin. Prorenin is glycosylated in the Golgi apparatus and is either secreted directly into the circulation by a nonregulated constitutive pathway or is processed in secretory granules to form active renin.

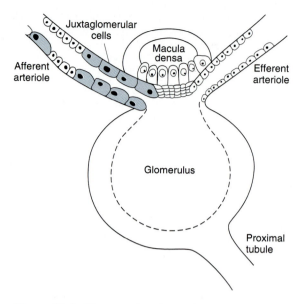

Figure 10–9. Diagram of a glomerulus, showing juxta-glomerular apparatus and macula densa.

cholamines and increased direct neural stimulation of juxtaglomerular cells via β_1-adrenergic receptors; and (3) cells of the macula densa that appear to be stimulated by a reduction in Na^+ or Cl^- ion concentrations in the tubular fluid delivered to this site. The chloride ion may be the primary mediator of this effect.

Once secreted, renin initiates a series of steps beginning with the enzymatic cleavage of a decapeptide, angiotensin I from the amino terminal of angiotensinogen. Angiotensin I is then converted to the octapeptide angiotensin II (Figure 10–10) by ACE. The concentration of ACE is greatest in the lung but is also localized to the luminal membrane of endothelial cells, the glomerulus, the brain, and other organs. The half-life of angiotensin II in plasma is less than 1 minute as a result of the action of multiple angiotensinases located in most tissues of the body.

Angiotensinogen

Angiotensinogen (renin substrate) is an α_2-globulin secreted by the liver. It has a molecular weight of approximately 60,000 and is usually present in human plasma at a concentration of 1 mmol/L. Although the rate of production of angiotensin II is normally determined by changes in plasma renin concentration, the concentration of angiotensinogen is below the V_{max} for the reaction. Thus, if angiotensinogen concentration increases, the amount of angiotensin produced at the same plasma renin concentration will increase. As will be discussed later, increased levels of angiotensinogen have been noted in patients with essential hypertension, and there appears to be linkage between a variant allele for the angiotensinogen gene and the presence of essential hypertension. Hepatic production of angiotensinogen is increased by glucocorticoids and by estrogens. Stimulation of angiotensinogen production by estrogen-containing contraceptive pills may contribute to some of the hypertension encountered as a side effect of this treatment.

In situations such as Na^+ depletion, where there is a sustained high circulating level of renin, the rate of

Although prorenin constitutes 50–90% of the total circulating renin, it has no clear physiologic role. Prorenin can be converted into renin in vitro by a number of methods, but it is unlikely that significant extrarenal conversion of prorenin occurs. Plasma prorenin levels tend to be elevated in patients with type I diabetes mellitus in association with microvascular complications.

The release of renin from secretory granules into the circulation is controlled by three major effectors: (1) baroreceptors in the wall of the afferent arteriole that are stimulated by decreases in renal arteriolar perfusion pressure, perhaps mediated by local production of prostaglandins; (2) cardiac and systemic arterial receptors that activate the sympathetic nervous system, resulting in increased circulating cate-

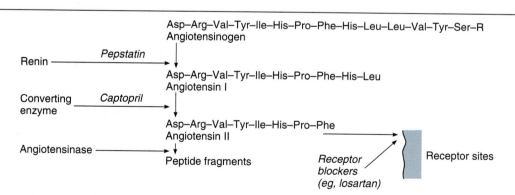

Figure 10–10. Sequence of formation of angiotensin II. Drugs that can be used to block various steps are shown in italics.

breakdown of angiotensinogen is greatly increased. Because the plasma concentration of angiotensinogen remains constant in these situations, hepatic production must increase to match the increased rate of breakdown. The mechanism of this increase is not clear, though angiotensin II itself is a stimulus to substrate production.

Angiotensin Converting Enzyme

Angiotensin converting enzyme is a dipeptidyl carboxypeptidase, a glycoprotein of MW 130,000–160,000, that cleaves dipeptides from a number of substrates. In addition to angiotensin I, these include bradykinin, enkephalins, and substance P. Inhibitors of ACE are widely used to prevent the formation of angiotensin II in the circulation and thus block its biologic effects (Figure 10–10). Since ACE acts on a number of substrates, blockade of the enzyme may not always exert its effects solely via the renin-angiotensin system.

Angiotensin II

Similar to other peptide hormones, angiotensin II binds to receptors on the plasma membrane of target cells. Two major classes of angiotensin II receptors (AT1 and AT2) have been characterized and their respective mRNAs isolated and cloned. AT1 appears to mediate virtually all the known cardiovascular, renal, and adrenal-stimulatory effects of angiotensin II; AT2 may be involved in cell differentiation and growth. Both receptors have a seven-transmembrane-spanning motif. AT1 is linked to a G protein that activates phospholipase C, resulting in the hydrolysis of phosphoinositide to form inositol triphosphate and diacylglycerol. Generation of these second messengers results in a cascade of intracellular events including increases in calcium concentration, activation of protein kinases, and possible decreases in intracellular cAMP. The precise signaling mechanism associated with the AT2 receptor is still unknown.

Angiotensin II is a potent pressor agent, exerting its effects on peripheral arterioles to cause vasoconstriction and thus increasing total peripheral resistance. Vasoconstriction occurs in all tissue beds, including the kidney, and has been implicated in the phenomenon of renal autoregulation. Angiotensin may also increase the rate and strength of cardiac contraction. The possible role of increased circulating levels of angiotensin II in the pathogenesis of hypertension is discussed below.

Angiotensin II also acts directly on the adrenal cortex to stimulate aldosterone secretion and in most situations is the most important regulator of aldosterone secretion. Aldosterone thus plays a central role in regulating Na^+ balance. For example, during dietary Na^+ depletion, extracellular fluid volume is reduced. Subsequent stimulation of the renin-angiotensin system is important in two ways: Its vaso-constrictor actions help to maintain blood pressure in the face of reduced extracellular fluid volume, whereas its actions to stimulate aldosterone secretion and thus Na^+ retention allow volume to be conserved.

During chronic intravascular volume depletion, such as occurs during a low Na^+ intake, the persistent increases in angiotensin II levels results in AT1 receptor down-regulation in the vasculature. In this setting, there is less vasoconstriction for a given plasma level of angiotensin II. In contrast, intravascular volume depletion increases the number of AT1 receptors in the adrenal glomerulosa, resulting in augmented aldosterone secretion. It has been suggested that these opposite and apparently contradictory effects of chronic intravascular volume depletion on responsiveness of the vasculature and the adrenal glomerulosa to angiotensin II may be physiologically appropriate; in the setting of a low-Na^+ diet, the greater increase in aldosterone secretion allows Na^+ reabsorption to occur without a major rise in blood pressure. As will be discussed later, this so-called "Na^+ modulation" of adrenal and vascular responsiveness to angiotensin II may be modified in some patients with essential hypertension.

Angiotensin II modulates activity at sympathetic nerve endings in peripheral blood vessels and in the heart. It increases sympathetic activity partly by facilitating adrenergic transmitter release and partly by increasing the responsiveness of smooth muscle to norepinephrine. Angiotensin II also stimulates the release of catecholamines from the adrenal medulla.

Blockade of the formation or peripheral effects of angiotensin II is useful therapeutically. For example, in low-output congestive cardiac failure, plasma levels of angiotensin II are high. These high circulating levels promote salt and water retention and, by constricting arterioles, raise peripheral vascular resistance, thus increasing cardiac afterload. Treatment with ACE inhibitors such as captopril results in peripheral vasodilation, thereby improving tissue perfusion and cardiac performance as well as aiding renal elimination of salt and water. The use of ACE inhibitors as well as of AT1 receptor antagonists (losartan) in the treatment of hypertension is discussed in a subsequent section.

Effects of Angiotensin II in the Brain

Angiotensin II is a polar peptide that does not cross the blood-brain barrier. Circulating angiotensin II, however, may affect the brain by acting through one or more of the circumventricular organs. These specialized regions within the brain lack a blood-brain barrier, so that receptive cells in these areas are sensitive to plasma composition. Of particular significance to the actions of angiotensin are the subfornical organ, the organum vasculosum of the lamina terminalis, and the area postrema.

Angiotensin II is a potent dipsogen when injected directly into the brain or administered systemically. The major receptors for the dipsogenic action of circulating angiotensin II are located in the subfornical organ. Angiotensin II also stimulates vasopressin secretion, particularly in association with raised plasma osmolality. As such, the renin-angiotensin system may have an important part to play in the control of water balance, particularly during hypovolemia.

Production of angiotensin II in the brain has been implicated in several models of hypertension. Angiotensin also acts on the brain to increase blood pressure, though its effects at this site seem to be less potent than those exerted directly in the systemic circulation. In most animals, the receptors are located in the area postrema. Other central actions of angiotensin II include stimulation of ACTH secretion, suppression of plasma renin activity, and stimulation of Na^+ appetite, particularly in association with raised mineralocorticoid levels. The full implications of these (and other) central actions of angiotensin remain to be elucidated.

Local Renin-Angiotensin Systems

In addition to the circulating renin-angiotensin system, there is an increasing appreciation that all of the components of the renin-angiotensin system may be present in various tissues and function thereby to promote local production of angiotensin II. Such tissues include the kidney, brain, heart, ovary, adrenal, testis, and peripheral blood vessels. In the kidney, for example, local generation of angiotensin II directly stimulates Na^+ reabsorption in the early proximal tubule, in part by activation of the Na^+-H^+ antiporter in the luminal membrane. Angiotensin II of either local or systemic origin is also of critical importance in the maintenance of GFR during hypovolemia and reduced renal arterial flow. Angiotensin II appears to induce a relatively greater increase in efferent arteriole vasoconstriction, resulting in an increase in hydraulic pressure in the glomerular capillary. This increased pressure protects against a fall in GFR during a reduction in renal perfusion.

THE RENIN-ANGIOTENSIN SYSTEM & HYPERTENSION

Essential Hypertension

Blood pressure is the product of cardiac output and peripheral vascular resistance. The hemodynamic abnormality that appears to underlie essential hypertension is an elevation in peripheral vascular resistance. The determinants of peripheral vascular resistance include a complex array of systemic and locally produced hormones and growth factors as well as neurogenic factors. However, the specific factor or factors that underlie the pathogenesis of essential hypertension remain to be determined. Since the origi-

nal observation that impaired renal perfusion leads to secretion of renin and an increase in blood pressure, the renin-angiotensin system has been implicated in the etiology of essential hypertension.

In the early 1970s, Laragh and his colleagues suggested that plasma renin activity could be used to categorize the relative contributions of vasoconstriction and intravascular volume expansion in patients with essential hypertension. This so-called "renin profiling" divided patients with essential hypertensive into two subgroups: those with high renin levels, who were said to have a vasoconstrictor mechanism; and those with low renin levels, who were said to have a volume-expanded mechanism. While this bipolar model of hypertension is intellectually attractive, it has not generally been supported by hemodynamic measurements, and for that reason renin profiling of patients with essential hypertension is not generally advocated as part of routine practice.

As noted earlier, dietary Na^+ restriction enhances the adrenal but reduces the vascular response to angiotensin II; Na^+ loading produces the opposite effect. Thus, for normal subjects ingesting a high-Na^+ diet, the Na^+-induced modulation of adrenal and vascular activities increases renal blood flow while attenuating renal reabsorption of Na^+; both events facilitate excretion of the Na^+ load. It has been observed that about one-half of patients with essential hypertension with normal or high plasma renin levels may not modulate their adrenal and vascular responsiveness to a Na^+ load. These so-called "nonmodulators" do not increase their renal blood flow in response to a high-salt diet or increase aldosterone secretion in response to a low-salt diet. Thus, according to this model, these patients have an impaired ability to excrete a Na^+ load, leading to elevations in blood pressure. The proponents of this hypothesis suggest that there is an abnormality related either to local angiotensin II production or the angiotensin receptor such that target tissue responsiveness is not modified when Na^+ intake is altered. Adrenal and vascular responsiveness can be restored in these patients by reducing angiotensin II levels using ACE inhibitors.

Approximately 25% of patients with essential hypertension have low plasma renin levels. There is an increased frequency in blacks and the elderly, and it has been suggested that the increases in blood pressure in this population are more likely to be salt-sensitive and that the greatest antihypertensive response may be achieved with a diuretic or calcium channel blocker. Although it was initially suggested that ACE inhibitors would not be effective in this low-renin hypertensive population, recent studies suggest that plasma renin levels are not predictive of efficacy of this class of drugs. Conceivably, ACE inhibitors may be effective in this population by increasing levels of bradykinin or by reducing local angiotensin II generation in the kidney, brain, and vasculature. This notion is supported by recent experimental studies in transgenic rats harboring a mouse renin gene. These rats experience a severe and lethal form of hypertension that can be ameliorated by treatment with an ACE inhibitor or angiotensin II receptor antagonist. Although plasma renin activity, plasma angiotensin II levels and renal vein renin content are subnormal, adrenal renin content and plasma prorenin levels are increased in this model, and adrenalectomy attenuates the hypertension. This lends further support to the concept that measurements of systemic renin activity may not reflect the relative importance of local renin-angiotensin systems and their potential role in the pathogenesis of hypertension.

Recent studies using techniques of molecular genetics have further implicated the renin-angiotensin system in the pathogenesis of essential hypertension. A genetic linkage has been described between an allele of the angiotensinogen gene and essential hypertension in affected siblings. It is interesting to note that there is a correlation between plasma concentration of angiotensinogen and blood pressure and that increased levels of angiotensinogen are observed in patients with essential hypertension. Furthermore, normotensive offspring of hypertensive patients tend to have higher levels of angiotensinogen compared with normal control subjects.

Renovascular Hypertension

The most common cause of renin-dependent hypertension is renovascular hypertension. Various studies have reported it to be present in 1–4% of patients with hypertension, and it is the most common correctable cause of secondary hypertension. Both renovascular disease, defined as the presence of lesions in the renal artery, and renovascular hypertension, defined as renovascular disease that is causal of hypertension, are less common in African-Americans. Renovascular hypertension is usually due either to atherosclerosis or to fibromuscular hyperplasia of the renal arteries. These lesions result in decreased perfusion in the renal segment distal to the obstructed vessel, resulting in increased renin release and angiotensin II production. Blood pressure increase and high angiotensin II levels suppress renin release from the contralateral kidney. Consequently, total plasma renin activity may be only slightly elevated or even normal. Other anatomic lesions may cause hypertension as well: renal infarction, solitary cysts, hydronephrosis, and other parenchymal lesions.

Because of the relatively low incidence of the disorder, screening all hypertensives for renovascular hypertension is generally not recommended. Instead, most physicians look for indications that the hypertension is inappropriate before deciding to evaluate the patient for renovascular hypertension. The following clinical conditions are settings in which renovascular hypertension should be suspected: (1) severe hypertension (diastolic blood pressure greater than 120 mm Hg with either progressive renal insufficiency or refractoriness to aggressive medical therapy; (2) accelerated or malignant hypertension with grade III or grade IV retinopathy; (3) moderate to severe hypertension in a patient with diffuse atherosclerosis or an incidentally detected asymmetry of kidney size; (4) an acute elevation in plasma creatinine concentration in a hypertensive patient that is either unexplained or follows therapy with an ACE inhibitor; (5) an acute rise in blood pressure over a previously stable baseline; (6) a systolic-diastolic abdominal bruit; (7) onset of hypertension below age 20 or above age 50; (8) moderate to severe hypertension in patients with recurrent acute pulmonary edema; (9) hypokalemia with normal or elevated plasma renin levels in the absence of diuretic therapy; and (10) a negative family history of hypertension. An acute deterioration in renal function following therapy with an ACE inhibitor should suggest the possibility of bilateral renal artery stenosis. In that situation, both kidneys are dependent on angiotensin II to maintain intraglomerular pressure by its vasoconstrictor effect on the efferent arteriole; loss of this angiotensin II-mediated vasocontriction will result in a decrease in intraglomerular pressure and GFR.

The standard test for diagnosing renal vascular disease is renal arteriography. Because of risks such as contrast-induced acute tubular necrosis, attempts have made to use newer noninvasive imaging tests and pharmacologic probes as screening tests for renovascular disease. Current noninvasive screening tests for renovascular disease include (1) captopril stimulation with measurement of plasma renin activity; (2) captopril renography; (3) Doppler ultrasound; (4) magnetic resonance imaging; and (5) spiral CT scan.

Basal plasma renin levels by themselves do not serve to diagnose renovascular hypertension inasmuch as levels are increased in only 50–80% of affected patients. The administration of the ACE inhibitor captopril normally induces a reactive hyperreninemia by preventing the negative feedback exerted by angiotensin II. This response is exaggerated in patients with renal artery stenosis such that renin levels measured 1 hour after the oral administration of captopril are much greater than those observed in patients with essential hypertension. The sensitivity and specificity of this test has been reported to range from 93% to 100% and 80% to 95%, respectively. The test has less sensitivity in blacks, in the young, and in patients with reduced renal function as well as in the presence of concomitant antihypertensive therapy.

Normally, stenosis of a renal artery stimulates the renin-angiotensin system of the ipsilateral kidney such that angiotensin II-mediated vasoconstriction of the efferent arteriole helps maintain intraglomerular pressure and filtration. Administration of an ACE inhibitor (eg, captopril) will result in a reduction in angiotensin II production and thus lower intraglomerular pressure and GFR. Performance of a renal isotope scan prior to and after the administration of captopril scan can optimize detection of unilateral renal ischemia. Both the sensitivity and the specificity of this test have been reported to be in the 90% range.

The combination of direct ultrasound imaging of the renal arteries (B-mode imaging) and measurement of renal arterial flow by Doppler technique has recently been become a popular screening test for renal artery stenosis. Studies suggest that the positive and negative predictive values for these procedures are in the upper 90% range. Having an experienced operator is important to achieve this level of performance. Visualization of the renal arteries can be impaired by the presence of a large amount of bowel gas, obesity, recent surgery, or the presence of an accessory renal artery.

Magnetic resonance imaging (MRI) has recently been advocated as a good screening test for renal artery stenosis. Initial sensitivities have been reported in the 92–97% range. A recent study suggests that spiral CT scan may be the most sensitive noninvasive imaging test to evaluate for renal artery stenosis, with sensitivity and specificity of 98% and 94%, respectively. These results are promising, and more studies are needed to clarify the utility of these imaging tests for renal vascular disease.

Given that there is no noninvasive imaging test that is sensitive enough to totally exclude renal artery stenosis, clinicians are frequently confronted with the dilemma of when and how a patient with hypertension should be evaluated for renovascular hypertension. Based on the index of clinical suspicion (Table 10–1), Mann and Pickering have developed a practical algorithm for the evaluation of renovascular hypertension and for the selection of patients for renal arteriography (Figure 10–11).

Anatomic correction is the preferred therapy for renovascular hypertension when it is possible and the patient is considered able to tolerate the procedure. Recent advances in transluminal angioplasty have made this the procedure of choice except for lesions at the orifice. In special situations, other surgical approaches such as endarterectomy are used. Prior to correction of a stenotic renal artery, it had been suggested that measurements of renal vein renins be performed to determine whether the stenosis is hemodynamically significant. In selective venous sampling, blood samples are obtained from the venous effluent of the affected portion of the kidney and from the contralateral kidney. The renin level is ordinarily significantly higher in the sample from the affected kidney than in that from the contralateral kidney. When the value for the affected kidney sample is divided by the value for the unaffected sample, a ratio greater than 1.5 generally indicates a functional abnormality, though a lower ratio does not exclude the diagnosis. Giving an ACE inhibitor prior to the renal vein sam-

Table 10–1. Testing for renovascular hypertension: Clinical index of suspicion as a guide to workup.[1]

Low index (should not be tested)
   Borderline, mild, or moderate hypertension in the absence of clinical clues

Moderate (noninvasive tests recommended)
   Severe hypertension (diastolic blood pressure > 120 mm Hg)
   Hypertension refractory to standard therapy
   Abrupt onset of sustained moderate to severe hypertension at age < 20 or > 50 years
   Hypertension with a suggestive abdominal bruit (long, high-pitched, and localized to the region of the renal artery)
   Moderate hypertension (diastolic blood pressure exceeding 105 mm Hg) in a smoker, a patient with evidence of occlusive vascular disease (cerebrovascular, coronary, peripheral vascular), or a patient with unexplained but stable elevation of serum creatinine
   Normalization of blood pressure by an angiotensin-converting enzyme inhibitor in a patient with moderate or severe hypertension (particularly in a smoker or A patient with recent onset of hypertension)

High index (may consider proceeding directly to arteriography)
   Severe hypertension (diastolic blood pressure > 190 mm Hg) with either progressive renal insufficiency or refractoriness to aggressive treatment (particularly in a patient who has been a smoker or has other evidence of occlusive arterial disease)
   Accelerated or malignant hypertension (grade III or grade IV retinopathy)
   Hypertension with recent elevation of serum creatinine, either unexplained or reversibly induced by an angiotensin-converting enzyme inhibitor.
   Moderate to severe hypertension with incidentally detected asymmetry of renal size

[1]Reprinted, with permission, from Mann SJ, Pickering TG: Detection of renovascular hypertension. State of the art: 1992. Ann Intern Med 1992;117:845.

pling may increase the sensitivity of this test. Over 90% of patients with renal artery stenosis and lateralizing renal vein renins will have an improvement in blood pressure control. However, since many patients with renal vein renin ratios less than 1.5 (nonlateralizing) will have an amelioration of their hypertension after angioplasty or surgery, it is no longer routine to perform such studies in patients with a high-grade renal artery stenosis. Measurement of renal vein renin levels may be helpful in evaluating hypertensive patients with bilateral or segmental renal artery stenosis in order to determine which kidney or region of a kidney is the source of the augmented renin release.

Renovascular hypertension can also be treated medically; this treatment is used when the patient is considered unable to tolerate a surgical procedure or the diagnosis is uncertain. The ACE inhibitors and selective AT1 antagonists are particularly effective, although they can lower intrarenal efferent arteriolar resistance and so decrease renal function in patients with bilateral renal artery stenosis. Renovascular hy-

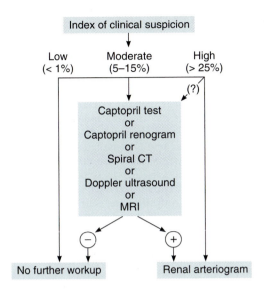

Index of clinical suspicion

Low (< 1%)   Moderate (5–15%)   High (> 25%)

(?)

Captopril test
or
Captopril renogram
or
Spiral CT
or
Doppler ultrasound
or
MRI

(−)   (+)

No further workup   Renal arteriogram

Figure 10–11. Suggested workup for renovascular hypertension. (Reproduced, with permission, from Mann SJ, Pickering TG: Detection of renovascular hypertension. State of the art: 1992. Ann Intern Med 1992;117:845.

pertension may also respond to beta-adrenergic and calcium channel blockers.

Renin-Secreting Tumors

Renin-secreting tumors are extremely rare. The tumors are usually hemangiopericytomas containing elements of the juxtaglomerular cells. They can be located by CT scan and the presence confirmed by measurement of renin in the venous effluent. Other renin-secreting neoplasms (eg, Wilms' tumor) have been reported, including a pulmonary tumor that secreted excessive amounts of renin, producing hypertension and hypokalemia with secondary aldosteronism.

Accelerated Hypertension

Accelerated hypertension is characterized by marked elevations of diastolic blood pressure that can be abrupt in onset. This disorder is associated with progressive arteriosclerosis. The plasma levels of renin and aldosterone may be extremely high. It is believed that the intense vasospastic events that occur and the excessive renal cortical nephrosclerosis lead to hyperreninemia and accelerate the hypertensive process. Vigorous antihypertensive therapy usually will result in a reduction in the vasospastic process and an amelioration of hyperreninemia with time.

Estrogen Therapy

Aldosterone levels may be increased during treatment with replacement estrogen therapy or oral contraceptives. This is due to an increase in angiotensinogen production and presumed increase in angiotensin II levels. Aldosterone levels increase secondarily, but hypokalemia rarely occurs during estrogen administration.

OTHER HORMONE SYSTEMS & HYPERTENSION

INSULIN

Hyperinsulinemia and insulin resistance have been implicated as potential factors in the generation of hypertension, particularly in obese patients. It has been argued that insulin resistance is present in most obese patients with hypertension and in some nonobese hypertensive patients. In the setting of obesity, there is impaired insulin-mediated glucose uptake resulting in both type II diabetes mellitus and increased insulin secretion by the pancreas (hyperinsulinemia). The distribution of body fat may also be a key factor, inasmuch as hypertension and insulin resistance are seen more commonly in patients with abdominal obesity (upper body, male-type subcutaneous fat distribution). The association of hypertension, diabetes mellitus, abdominal obesity, and hyperlipidemia has been referred to as "syndrome X" or the syndrome of insulin resistance.

The hypertension observed in this clinical syndrome may be due in part to the hyperinsulinemia. Insulin accentuates the activity of the sympathetic nervous system, leading to greater vasoconstriction. In addition, insulin increases Na^+ reabsorption by the kidney, resulting in increased intravascular volume and blood pressure. Although insulin usually induces vasodilation to counterbalance these pressor forces, in the setting of obesity this action is attenuated. Thus, in these insulin-resistant states, it is postulated that the stimulation of both the sympathetic nervous system and renal Na^+ reabsorption by hyperinsulinemia combined with impaired vasodilation results in increases in blood pressure. It is noteworthy that weight loss lowers both blood pressure, insulin levels, and insulin resistance in these patients.

Increased insulin levels alone are probably not sufficient to cause hypertension given the observations that experimental animals receiving high doses of insulin and patients with insulinomas do not develop hypertension. In addition, there are a substantial number of patients with obesity, insulin resistance, and type II diabetes mellitus who do not have hypertension (eg, Pima Indians). Thus, there is probably a critical interplay of genetic and hormonal factors in the pathogenesis of hypertension in patients with insulin resistance. (See Chapter 18.)

ATRIAL NATRIURETIC PEPTIDE

Extracts of atrial but not ventricular tissue cause marked natriuresis when injected into rats. The material is contained in densely staining granules in the atria of most mammalian species. Atrial natriuretic peptide (ANP) is a 28-amino-acid peptide derived from cleavage of the carboxyl terminal of a 126-amino-acid precursor located primarily in the storage vesicles in the atrial cells. At least three other natriuretic peptides have subsequently been identified: a brain natriuretic peptide (BNP; 32-amino acids), C-type peptide (CNP; 22-amino acids), and a renal natriuretic peptide (urodilatin; 32-amino acids). Although originally described in the brain, the major source of BNP is the cardiac ventricle, and its action is similar to that of ANP. CNP is mainly produced in the brain, where it serves as a neurotransmitter. Urodilatin is produced in the kidney, where it acts locally to affect Na^+ transport.

These natriuretic peptides bind to membrane receptors linked to guanylyl cyclase, resulting in production of the second messenger, cGMP. The major effects seen following the administration of ANP are vasodilation, hyperfiltration, and natriuresis. Although the peptide can cause relaxation of smooth muscle, the fall in blood pressure is due to reduction of venous return and depression of cardiac output in intact animals. In the kidney, ANP increases GFR probably by inducing a relative afferent arteriolar dilation and efferent arteriolar vasoconstriction and an increase in glomerular permeability. The natriuresis is due both to the increase in GFR and to the direct inhibition by ANP of Na^+ and water reabsorption by inner medullary and cortical collecting duct cells. ANP inhibits secretion of renin, aldosterone, vasopressin, and ACTH as well as the stimulation of heart rate mediated by the baroreceptors.

Maneuvers that expand plasma volume and increase atrial pressure are associated with increased levels of ANP in plasma. Thus, when blood volume increases, the associated increase in atrial pressure and atrial stretch may trigger secretion of the peptide and lead to natriuresis and blood pressure reduction. However, the precise role ANP plays in the control of Na^+ balance, blood volume, and blood pressure regulation under normal physiologic conditions is not clear, and there are no known roles for impaired ANP secretion in the pathogenesis or maintenance of essential hypertension. Because of the pharmacologic effects of the natriuretic peptides to induce vasodilation, hyperfiltration, and natriuresis, studies are under way to determine if these peptides may have a therapeutic role in the treatment of hypertension, heart failure, and renal failure. Whether ANP will be a useful therapy for congestive heart failure is uncertain inasmuch as patients with chronically increased atrial pressures already have increased plasma levels of the peptide.

ENDOTHELIUM-DERIVED RELAXING FACTOR

The vascular endothelium produces a labile substance, endothelium-derived relaxing factor (EDRF), that mediates the vasorelaxant actions of various endogenous hormones including acetylcholine. EDRF has been identified as the free radical, nitric oxide, which is synthesized from the guanidine nitrogen atom of the amino acid L-arginine by the enzyme nitric oxide synthase. Nitric oxide diffuses within the cell or to adjacent cells such as smooth muscle cells, where it stimulates soluble guanylyl cyclase. The resultant increase in cyclic guanosine monophosphate leads to a relaxation of vascular smooth muscle cells and therefore vasodilation. A number of recent studies in laboratory animals and human subjects have shown that nitric oxide synthesized by the vascular endothelium is an important determinant of resting peripheral vascular resistance and blood pressure. In anesthetized rabbits, inhibition of the activity of nitric oxide synthase activity using substituted arginine analogs (L-monomethyl arginine) acutely increased blood pressure. This hypertensive effect can be reversed by the infusion of arginine. In normal subjects, infusion of L-arginine decreases peripheral vascular resistance, causing hypotension and a reflex tachycardia. Because of this apparently important role of nitric oxide in maintaining basal blood pressure, it has been proposed that the nitric oxide pathway may be abnormal in patients with hypertension. This view has been supported by recent studies in humans. For example, patients with essential hypertension have a diminished vasoconstrictor response to an infusion of arginine analogs and a reduced arterial vasodilatory response to acetylcholine, suggesting that both the basal and stimulated release of nitric oxide is reduced in this disease. In contrast, the response to the endothelium-independent vasodilator nitroprusside was normal in patients with essential hypertension, suggesting that abnormality is a result of reduced nitric oxide production by the endothelium rather than impaired response by vascular smooth muscle. The mechanisms for this endothelial dysfunction are not known.

ENDOTHELIN

In addition to the production of the potent vasodilator, nitric oxide, the vascular endothelium produces a potent vasoconstrictor peptide, endothelin. At least three endothelin peptides have been identified: endothelin-1, endothelin-2, and endothelin-3. The predominant vascular vasoconstrictor, endothelin-1, is formed from proendothelin-1 by the action of a metalloprotease, endothelin-converting enzyme. Endothelin-1 binds to receptors in vascular smooth muscle which are linked to phospholipase C, resulting in the hydrolysis of phosphoinositide to inositol triphosphate.

Increased endothelin activity has been observed in disorders associated with vasoconstriction such as in malignant hypertension, heart failure, pulmonary hypertension, contrast-induced acute tubular necrosis, and myocardial infarction. A rare tumor, hemangioendothelioma, can cause hypertension by the secretion of large quantities of endothelin. In addition, the hypertension associated with the use of cyclosporine may be due to increased endothelin production. However, a conclusive role for endothelin in the pathogenesis of essential hypertension has not been demonstrated.

KALLIKREIN-KININ SYSTEM

Kinins are potent vasodilators formed in blood vessels and cleaved from kininogen by the enzymatic action of kallikrein. Kallikrein activity has been noted to be reduced in patients with essential hypertension, suggesting lower vasodilatory kinin production. Given that ACE inactivates bradykinin, it has been argued that the hypotensive effect of ACE inhibitors may be due, in part, to increased bradykinin level. Moreover, the improved insulin sensitivity and glucose utilization observed in diabetic patients treated with ACE inhibitors may be the result of increased kinin levels rather than reduced angiotensin II production.

OTHER HORMONES & AUTACOIDS

Prostaglandins, vasopressin, calcitonin gene-related peptide, parathyroid hormone, and parathyroid hormone-related peptide are vasoactive hormones or autacoids that have been implicated in the regulation of blood pressure. Although vasopressin is both a potent vasoconstrictor and a prime factor in water reabsorption by the kidney, it does not appear to be a factor in the pathogenesis of essential hypertension. Calcitonin gene-related peptide is a potent vasodilator produced in the central nervous system and nerves innervating blood vessels. It has been suggested that calcitonin gene-related peptide may mediate the hypotensive effect of calcium supplements given to hypertensive patients. Both infusions of parathyroid hormone and parathyroid hormone-related peptide can produce hypotension. Thus, the hypertension commonly seen in primary hyperparathyroidism is probably due to other factors.

SYMPATHETIC NERVOUS SYSTEM

Increased activity of the sympathetic nervous system has been implicated as a contributing factor in the pathogenesis of essential hypertension. This may be due to both genetic and environmental factors. Some patients with hypertension, particularly during the early stages, as well as normotensive offspring of hypertensive patients have enhanced sympathetic nervous system activity. It has been postulated that impaired baroreceptor function may prevent the normal inhibitory check on increases in sympathetic activity. In addition, the role of stress in the generation and maintenance of hypertension probably is mediated, in part, by activation of the sympathetic nervous system. The mechanisms by which increased sympathetic nervous system activity and catecholamines increase blood pressure is multifactorial, including augmented vasoconstriction, increased cardiac output, increased activity of the renin-angiotensin system, and enhanced Na^+ reabsorption by the kidney. Disorders of catecholamine metabolism are discussed in further detail in Chapter 11.

REFERENCES

Anderson GH Jr et al: The effect of age on prevalence of secondary forms of hypertension in 4429 consecutively referred patients. J Hypertens 1994;12:609.

Baxter JD et al: The endocrinology of hypertension. In: *Endocrinology and Metabolism,* 3rd ed. Felig P, Baxter JD, Frohman LA (editors). McGraw-Hill, 1995.

Biglieri EG, Kater CE: 17α-Hydroxylation deficiency. Endocrinol Metab Clin North Am 1991;20:257.

Davidson RA, Wilcox CS: Newer tests for the diagnosis of renovascular disease. JAMA 1992;268:3353.

Derkx FHM, Schalekamp MADH: Renal artery stenosis and hypertension. Lancet 1994;344:237.

Duh Q-Y et al: Adrenals. In: Current Surgical Diagnosis & Treatment, 10th ed. Way LW (editor). Appleton & Lange, 1994.

Funder JW et al: Mineralocorticoid action: Target tissue specificity is enzyme, not receptor, mediated. Science 1988;242:583.

Genest J, Cantin M: The atrial natriuretic factor: Its physiology and biochemistry. Rev Physiol Biochem Pharmacol 1988;110:1.

Gordon RD: Mineralocorticoid hypertension. Lancet 1994;344:240.

Irony I et al: Correctable subsets of primary aldosteronism: Primary adrenal hyperplasia and renin responsive adenoma. Am J Hypertens 1990;3:576.

Kater CE et al: Stimulation and suppression of the mineralocorticoid hormones in normal subjects and adrenocortical disorders. Endocr Rev 1989;11:149.

Krieger JE, Dzau VJ: Molecular biology of hypertension. Hypertension 1991;18(Suppl):13.

Lifton RP: Genetic determinants of human hypertension. Proc Soc Natl Acad Sci U S A 1995;92:11495.

Lifton RP et al: A chimaeric 11β-hydroxylase/aldosterone synthase gene causes glucocorticoid-remediable aldosteronism and human hypertension. Nature 1992;355:262.

Lowenstein CJ et al: Nitric oxide: A physiologic messenger. Ann Intern Med 1994;120:227.

Mann SJ, Pickering TG: Detection of renovascular hypertension. State of the art: 1992. Ann Intern Med 1992;117:845.

Reaven GM: Pathophysiology of insulin resistance in human disease. Physiol Rev 1995;75:473.

Rodriguez-Portales JA: 11β-Hydroxylation deficiency. In: *Endocrine Hypertension.* Biglieri EG (editor). Raven Press, 1990.

Schambelan M: Liquorice ingestion and blood pressure regulating hormones. Steroids 1994;59:127.

Shiffrin EL: Endothelin: Potential role in hypertension and vascular hypertrophy. Hypertension 1995;25:1135.

Shimkets RA et al: Liddle's syndrome: Heritable human hypertension caused by mutations in the β subunit of the epithelial sodium channel. Cell 1994;79:407.

Ulick S: Two uncommon causes of mineralocorticoid excess: Syndrome of apparent mineralocorticoid excess and glucocorticoid-remediable aldosteronism. Endocrinol Metab Clin North Am 1991;20:269.

Williams GH: Guardian of the gate: Receptors, enzymes, and mineralocorticoid function. (Editorial.) J Clin Endocrinol Metab 1991;74:961.

Wilson RC et al: Several homozygous mutations in the gene for 11β-hydroxysteroid dehydrogenase type 2 in patients with apparent mineralocorticoid excess. J Clin Endocrinol Metab 1995;80:3145.

White PC: Disorders of aldosterone biosynthesis and action. N Engl J Med 1994;331:250.

Adrenal Medulla

11

Alan Goldfien, MD

The adrenal medulla was first distinguished from the adrenal cortex at the beginning of the 19th century. Its major secretory product, **epinephrine,** was isolated, purified, and synthesized a century later. **Norepinephrine** was synthesized in 1904, but not until 1946 was it recognized as a secretory product of the adrenal medulla and as the major neurotransmitter of the postganglionic sympathetic nerves. The adrenal medulla, a highly specialized part of the sympathetic nervous system, functions under stress or whenever marked deviations from normal homeostasis occur—in contrast to the rest of the sympathetic nervous system, which is involved in the minute-to-minute fine regulation of most physiologic processes.

ANATOMY

Embryology
(Figure 11–1)

The sympathetic nervous system arises in the fetus from the primitive cells of the neural crest (sympathogonia). At about the fifth week of gestation, these cells migrate from the primitive spinal ganglia in the thoracic region to form the sympathetic chain posterior to the dorsal aorta. They then begin to migrate anteriorly to form the remaining ganglia.

At 6 weeks, groups of these primitive cells migrate along the central vein and enter the fetal adrenal cortex to form the adrenal medulla, which is detectable by the eighth week. The adrenal medulla at this time is composed of sympathogonia and pheochromoblasts, which then mature into pheochromocytes. The cells appear in rosette-like structures, with the more primitive cells occupying a central position. Storage granules can be found in these cells by electron microscopy at 12 weeks. Pheochromoblasts and pheochromocytes also collect on both sides of the aorta to form the paraganglia. The principal collection of these cells is found at the level of the inferior mesenteric artery. They fuse anteriorly to form the organ of Zuckerkandl, which is quite prominent in fetal life. This organ is thought to be a major source of catecholamines during the first year of life, after

---

ACRONYMS USED IN THIS CHAPTER

ACTH	Adrenocorticotropic hormone
ATP	Adenosine triphosphate
cAMP	Cyclic adenosine monophosphate
COMT	Catechol-O-methyltransferase
DHMA	Dihydroxymandelic acid
DHPG	Dihydroxyphenylglycol
IP$_3$	Inositol triphosphate
MAO	Monoamine oxidase
MEN	Multiple endocrine neoplasia
MIBG	[131]Metaiodobenzylguanidine
PGE	Prostaglandin E
PNMT	Phenylethanolamine-N-methyl-transferase
VIP	Vasoactive intestinal polypeptide
VMA	Vanillylmandelic acid (3-methoxy-4-hydroxymandelic acid)

---

which it begins to atrophy. Pheochromocytes (chromaffin cells) also are found scattered throughout the abdominal sympathetic plexuses as well as in other parts of the sympathetic nervous system.

Gross Structure

The anatomic relationships between the adrenal medulla and the adrenal cortex are different in different species. These organs are completely separate structures in the shark. They remain separate but in close contact in amphibians, and there is some intermingling in birds. In mammals, the medulla is surrounded by the adrenal cortex. In humans, the adrenal medulla occupies a central position in the widest part of the gland, with only small portions extending into the narrower parts. It constitutes approximately one-tenth of the weight of the gland, although the proportions vary from individual to individual. There is no clear demarcation between cortex and medulla. The central vein is usually surrounded by a cuff of adrenal cortical cells, and there may be islands of cortex elsewhere in the medulla.

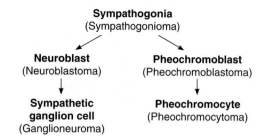

Sympathogonia
(Sympathogonioma)

Neuroblast
(Neuroblastoma)

Pheochromoblast
(Pheochromoblastoma)

**Sympathetic
ganglion cell**
(Ganglioneuroma)

Pheochromocyte
(Pheochromocytoma)

Figure 11–1. The embryonic development of adrenergic cells and tumors that develop from them. Sympathogonia are primitive cells derived from the neural crest. Neuroblasts are also called sympathoblasts; ganglion cells are the same as sympathocytes; and pheochromocytes are mature chromaffin cells.

Microscopic Structure

The **chromaffin cells,** or **pheochromocytes,** of the adrenal medulla are large ovoid columnar cells arranged in clumps or cords around blood vessels. They derive their name from the observation that their granules turn brown (*pheo-*) when stained with chromic acid. The color is due to the oxidation of epinephrine and norepinephrine to melanin. These cells have large nuclei and a well-developed Golgi apparatus. They contain large numbers of vesicles or granules containing catecholamines. Vesicles containing norepinephrine are darker than those containing epinephrine.

The pheochromocytes may be arranged in nests, alveoli, or cords and are surrounded by a rich network of capillaries and sinusoids. The adrenal medulla also contains some sympathetic ganglion cells, singly or in groups. Ganglion cells are also found in association with the viscera, the carotid body, the glomus jugulare, and the cervical and thoracic ganglia.

Nerve Supply

The cells of the adrenal medulla are innervated by preganglionic fibers of the sympathetic nervous system, which release acetylcholine and enkephalins at the synapses. Most of these fibers arise from a plexus in the capsule of the posterior surface of the gland and enter the adrenal glands in bundles of 30–50 fibers without synapsing. They follow the course of the blood vessels into the medulla without branching into the adrenal cortex. Some reach the wall of the central vein, where they synapse with small autonomic ganglia. However, most fibers end in relationship to the pheochromocytes.

Blood Supply

The human adrenal gland derives blood from the superior, middle, and inferior adrenal branches of the inferior phrenic artery, directly from the aorta and from the renal arteries. Upon reaching the adrenal gland, these arteries branch to form a plexus under the capsule supplying the adrenal cortex. A few of these vessels, however, penetrate the cortex, passing directly to the medulla. The medulla is also nourished by branches of the arteries supplying the central vein and cuff of cortical tissue around the central vein. Capillary loops passing from the subcapsular plexus of the cortex also supply blood as they drain into the central vein. It would appear, then, that most of the blood supply to the medullary cells is via a portal vascular system arising from the capillaries in the cortex. There is also a capillary network of lymphatics that drain into a plexus around the central vein.

In mammals, the enzyme that catalyzes the conversion of norepinephrine to epinephrine (phenylethanolamine-*N*-methyltransferase, PNMT) is induced by cortisol. The chromaffin cells containing epinephrine therefore receive most of their blood supply from the capillaries draining the cortical cells, whereas cells containing predominantly norepinephrine are supplied by the arteries that directly supply the medulla. (See Biosynthesis, below.)

On the right side, the central vein is short and drains directly into the vena cava, although some branches go to the surface of the gland and reach the azygos system. On the left, the vein is somewhat longer and drains into the renal vein.

HORMONES OF THE ADRENAL MEDULLA

CATECHOLAMINES

Biosynthesis
(Figure 11–2)

Catecholamines are widely distributed in plants and animals. In mammals, **epinephrine** is synthesized mainly in the adrenal medulla, whereas **norepinephrine** is found not only in the adrenal medulla but also in the central nervous system and in the peripheral sympathetic nerves. **Dopamine,** the precursor of norepinephrine, is found in the adrenal medulla and in noradrenergic neurons. It is present in high concentrations in the brain, in specialized interneurons in the sympathetic ganglia, and in the carotid body, where it serves as a neurotransmitter. Dopamine is also found in specialized mast cells and in enterochromaffin cells.

The proportions of epinephrine and norepinephrine found in the adrenal medulla vary with the species (Table 11–1). In humans, the adrenal contains 15–20% norepinephrine.

A. Conversion of Tyrosine to Dopa: The catecholamines are synthesized from **tyrosine,** which

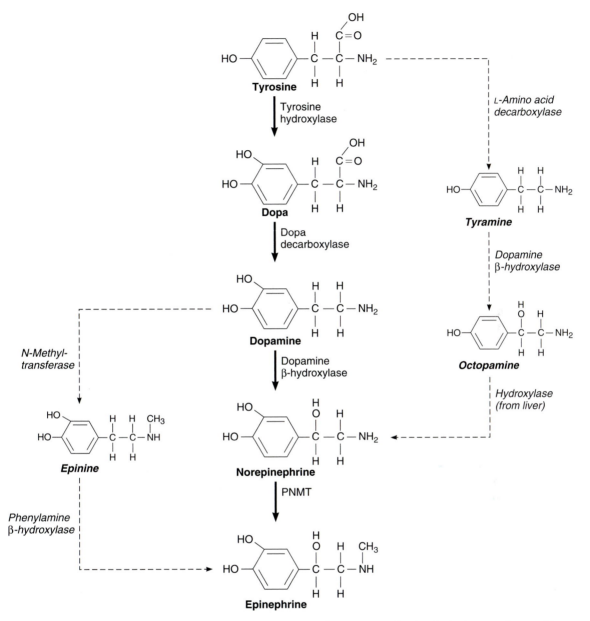

Figure 11–2. Biosynthesis of catecholamines. The alternative pathways shown by the dashed arrows have not been found to be of physiologic significance in humans. (PNMT, phenylethanolamine-*N*-methyltransferase.)

may be derived from ingested food or synthesized from phenylalanine in the liver. Tyrosine circulates at a concentration of 1–1.5 mg/dL of blood. It enters neurons and chromaffin cells by an active transport mechanism and is converted to **dihydroxyphenylalanine (dopa).** The reaction is catalyzed by **tyrosine hydroxylase,** which is transported via axonal flow to the nerve terminal. Tyrosine hydroxylase activity may be inhibited by a variety of compounds. Alpha-methylmetatyrosine is effective and is sometimes used in the therapy of malignant pheochromo-

cytomas (see below). Substances that chelate iron or compete for the pteridine cofactor also inhibit the enzyme but are not useful clinically. Activity of tyrosine hydroxylase is a reliable marker of intact sympathetic nerve tissue and neurotransmitter synthesis.

B. Conversion of Dopa to Dopamine: Dopa is converted to dopamine by the enzyme aromatic L-amino acid decarboxylase (dopa decarboxylase). This enzyme is found in all tissues, with the highest concentrations in liver, kidney, brain, and vas deferens. The various enzymes have different substrate

Table 11–1. Approximate percentages of total adrenal medullary catecholamines present as norepinephrine in various species.

Whale	70	Horse	25
Chicken	70	Squirrel	25
Lion	55	Cow	25
Frog	50	Human	20
Pig	45	Guinea pig	15
Cat	40	Rat	15
Gazelle	35	Zebra	13
Sheep	35	Rabbit	5
Goat	35	Baboon	0
Dog	30		

specificities depending upon the tissue source. Competitive inhibitors of dopa decarboxylase such as methyldopa are converted to substances (an example is α-methylnorepinephrine) that are then stored in granules in the nerve cell and released in place of norepinephrine. These products (false transmitters) were thought to mediate the antihypertensive action of drugs at peripheral sympathetic synapses but are now believed to stimulate the alpha receptors of the inhibitory corticobulbar system, reducing sympathetic discharge peripherally.

C. Conversion of Dopamine to Norepinephrine: The conversion of dopamine to norepinephrine is catalyzed by dopamine β-hydroxylase, a mixed-function oxidase requiring oxygen and an external electron donor. The enzyme does not occur in tissues outside the neuron. Part of the biologic specificity of dopamine β-hydroxylase may result from its compartmentalization. Newly synthesized dopamine β-hydroxylase is incorporated directly into storage vesicles that take up, synthesize, and store the catecholamines. The membranes of these vesicles contain dopamine β-hydroxylase, ATPase, cytochrome P561, and cytochrome P561:NADH reductase. Dopamine β-hydroxylase is also found within the granule and is released with norepinephrine during secretion. Inhibitors of the enzyme, such as disulfuramic and picolinic acid, have no clinical importance.

D. Conversion of Norepinephrine to Epinephrine: Phenylethanolamine-N-methyltransferase is a cytosolic enzyme that catalyzes the N-methylation of norepinephrine to epinephrine, using S-adenosylmethionine as a methyl donor. It is found in the adrenal medulla and in a few neurons in the central nervous system. Norepinephrine leaves the granule and after methylation reenters different granules. This enzyme is induced by the high levels of glucocorticoids (100 times the systemic concentration) found in the adrenal medulla. PNMT indistinguishable from adrenal PNMT occurs in pancreas, kidney, and lung, and the kidney enzyme may contribute as much as half of the urinary epinephrine. A nonspecific NMT that can be distinguished from PNMT is widely distributed and correlates with tissue epinephrine levels. The conversion of dopamine to epinephrine is also catalyzed by nonspecific N-methyltransferase.

Catecholamine biosynthesis is coupled to secretion, so that the stores of norepinephrine at the nerve endings remain relatively unchanged even in the presence of marked nerve activity. In the adrenal medulla, it is possible to deplete stores with prolonged hypoglycemia. Biosynthesis appears to be increased during nerve stimulation by activation of tyrosine hydroxylase. Prolonged stimulation leads to the induction of increased amounts of this enzyme.

Storage

The catecholamines are found in the adrenal medulla and various sympathetically innervated organs, and their concentration reflects the density of sympathetic neurons. The adrenal medulla contains about 0.5 mg/g; the spleen, vas deferens, brain, spinal cord, and heart contain 1–5 μg/g; liver, gut, and skeletal muscle contain 0.1–0.5 μg/g. The catecholamines are stored in electron-dense granules approximately 1 μm in diameter that contain catecholamines and ATP in a 4:1 molar ratio, several neuropeptides, calcium, magnesium, and water-soluble proteins called **chromogranins.** The ratio of catecholamines to ATP is much higher in granules isolated from pheochromocytomas. The interior surface of the membrane contains dopamine β-hydroxylase and ATPase. The Mg^{2+}-dependent ATPase facilitates the uptake and inhibits the release of catecholamines by the granules. This activity is inhibited by reserpine. Adrenal medullary granules appear to contain and release a number of active peptides including adrenomedullin, ACTH, vasoactive intestinal polypeptide (VIP), chromogranins, and enkephalins. The peptides derived from the chromogranins are physiologically active and may modulate catecholamine release.

Secretion

Adrenal medullary catecholamine secretion is increased by exercise, angina pectoris, myocardial infarction, hemorrhage, ether anesthesia, surgery, hypoglycemia, anoxia and asphyxia, and many other stressful stimuli. The rate of secretion of epinephrine increases more than that of norepinephrine in the presence of hypoglycemia and most other stimuli (Figure 11–3). However, anoxia and asphyxia produce a greater increase in adrenal medullary release of norepinephrine than is observed with other stimuli (Figure 11–4).

Secretion of the adrenal medullary hormones is mediated by the release of acetylcholine from the terminals of preganglionic fibers. The resulting depolarization of the axonal membrane triggers an influx of calcium ion. The contents of the storage vesicles, including the chromogranins and soluble dopamine β-hydroxylase, are released by exocytosis by the calcium ion increase. Membrane-bound dopamine β-hy-

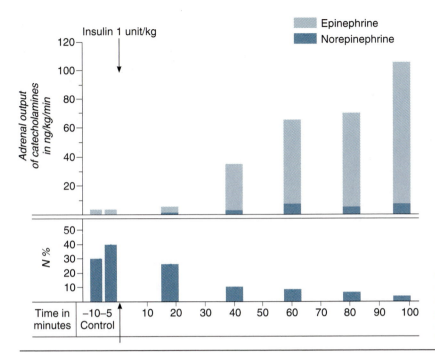

Figure 11–3. Rate of secretion of amines from one adrenal following injection of insulin. The percentage of the total released as norepinephrine is shown below.

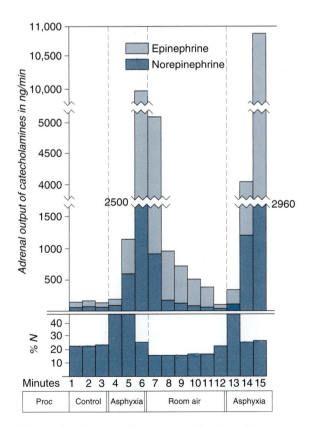

Figure 11–4. Rate of secretion of amines from one adrenal during asphyxia. The percentage of the total released as norepinephrine is shown below.

droxylase is not released. **Tyramine,** however, releases norepinephrine primarily from the free store in the cytosol. Cocaine and monoamine oxidase inhibitors inhibit the effect of tyramine but do not affect the release of catecholamines by nervous stimulation. The rate of release in response to nerve stimulation is increased or decreased by a wide variety of neurotransmitters acting at specific receptors on the presynaptic neuron. Norepinephrine has an important role in modulating its own release by activating the alpha receptors on the presynaptic membrane. Alpha$_2$ receptor antagonists inhibit this reaction. Conversely, presynaptic beta receptors enhance norepinephrine release, whereas beta receptor blockers increase it. The effect of such substances are shown in Table 11–2. The accumulation of excess

Table 11–2. Substances altering the release of norepinephrine at nerve endings by binding to specific presynaptic membrane receptors.

Increase	Decrease
Norepinephrine (beta receptor)	Norepinephrine (alpha receptor)[1]
Angiotensin	Serotonin
Epinephrine	Dopamine
	PGE$_2$
	Purines
	Metenkephalin
	Substance P
	Acetylcholine

[1]The alpha receptor-mediated inhibition of norepinephrine release is the dominant effect.

catecholamines that are not in the storage granules is prevented by the presence of intraneuronal monoamine oxidase.

Transport

When released into the circulation, the amines are bound to albumin or a closely associated protein with low affinity and high capacity (K_d 10^{-7}).

Metabolism & Inactivation

The actions of catecholamines are terminated rapidly. Compared to hormones with a more prolonged action they have a relatively low affinity for their receptor and rapidly dissociate from it. The free hormone is removed by several mechanisms. These include reuptake by the sympathetic nerve ending, metabolism by the enzymes catechol-*O*-methyltransferase (COMT) and monoamine oxidase (Figure 11–5), conjugation with sulfate ion, and direct excretion by the kidney. Estimates of the metabolic clearance rates for epinephrine and norepinephrine are 4000–5000 L/d.

Uptake

A. Neuronal (Uptake 1): A large proportion (85–90%) of the amines released at the synapse are taken up locally by the nerve endings from which they are released (uptake 1). Circulating amines can also be taken up by this mechanism. However, this mechanism plays a less important role in the inactivation of circulating catecholamines. The axonal membrane uptake process is energy-requiring, saturable, stereoselective, and sodium-dependent. It is blocked by cocaine, other sympathomimetic amines such as metaraminol and amphetamine, and agents such as tricyclic antidepressants and phenothiazines. Neither calcium nor magnesium ion has any effect on uptake 1. There is also an uptake process for dopamine in neurons of the central nervous system, but this process is not inhibited by tricyclic antidepressants. After being taken up by the neuron, the amines are reutilized or deaminated by monoamine oxidase and the metabolites are released (Figure 11–6). The intraneuronal monoamine oxidase is a flavoprotein and is localized to the outer mitochondrial membrane. Its substrate specificity favors norepinephrine, which it oxidizes to dihydroxyphenylglycol (DHPG) or dihydroxymandelic acid (DHMA). The major functions of monoamine oxidase are (1) to regulate dopamine and norepinephrine content of the neurons; (2) to destroy ingested amines; and (3) to metabolize the circulating catecholamines and their O-methyl metabolites. Progesterone increases the level of monoamine oxidase in women, whereas estrogens inhibit the enzyme.

B. Extraneuronal (Uptake 2): Extraneuronal tissues also take up catecholamines. This process,

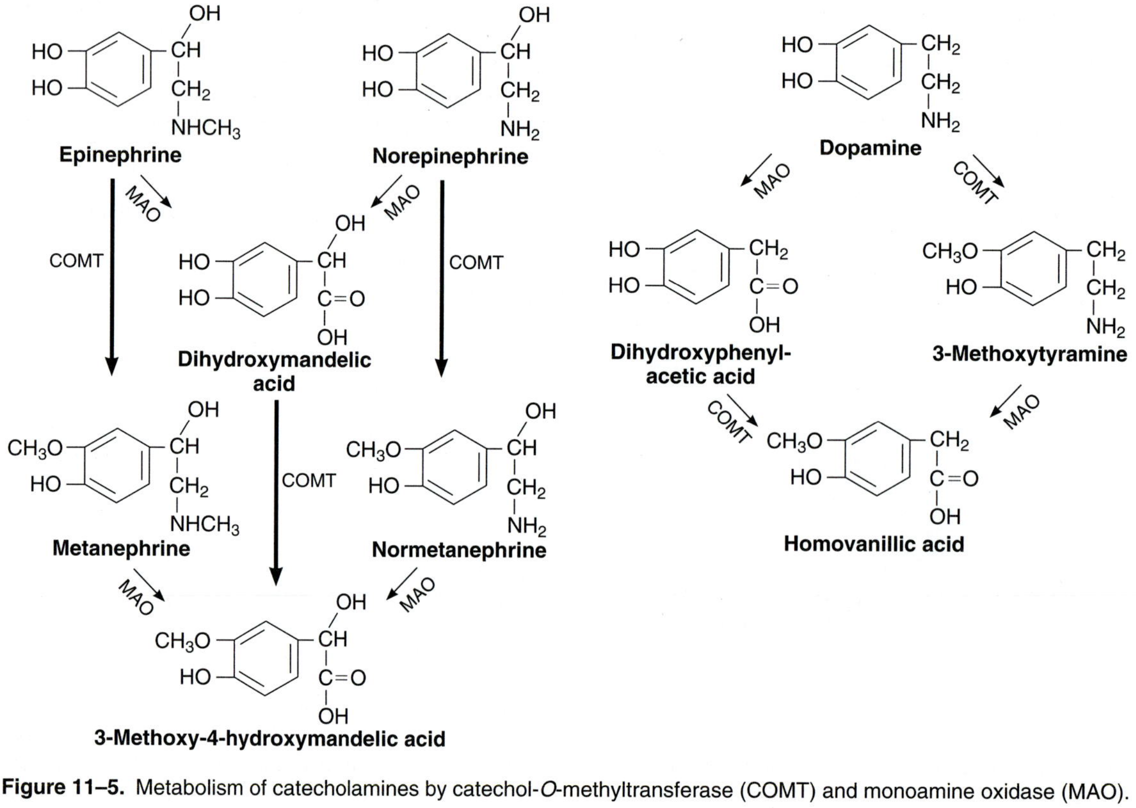

Figure 11–5. Metabolism of catecholamines by catechol-*O*-methyltransferase (COMT) and monoamine oxidase (MAO).

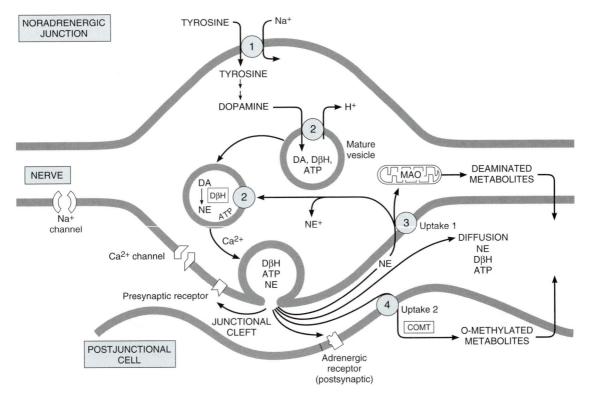

Figure 11–6. Schematic diagram of the neuroeffector junction of the peripheral sympathetic nervous system. The nerves terminate in complex networks with varicosities or enlargements that form synaptic junctions with effector cells. The neurotransmitter at these junctions is norepinephrine, which is synthesized from tyrosine. Tyrosine uptake ① is linked to sodium uptake and transport into the varicosity where the secretory vesicles form. Tyrosine is hydroxylated by tyrosine hydroxylase to dopa, which is then decarboxylated by dopa decarboxylate to dopamine in the cytoplasm. Dopamine (DA) is transported into the vesicle by a carrier mechanism ② that can be blocked by reserpine. The same carrier transports norepinephrine (NE) and several other amines into these granules. Dopamine is converted to norepinephrine through the catalytic action of dopamine β-hydroxylase (DβH). ATP is also present in high concentration in the vesicle. Release of transmitter occurs when an action potential is conducted to the varicosity by the action of voltage-sensitive sodium channels. Depolarization of the varicosity membrane opens voltage-sensitive calcium channels and results in an increase in intracellular calcium. The elevated calcium facilitates exocytotic fusion of vesicles with the surface membrane and expulsion of norepinephrine, ATP, and some of the dopamine β-hydroxylase. Release is blocked by drugs such as guanethidine and bretylium. Norepinephrine reaching either pre- or postsynaptic receptors modifies the function of the corresponding cells. Norepinephrine also diffuses out of the cleft, or it may be transported into the cytoplasm of the varicosity (uptake 1, blocked by cocaine, tricyclic antidepressants) ③ or into the postjunctional cell (uptake 2) ④. (Reproduced, with permission, from Katzung BG [editor]: Basic & Clinical Pharmacology, 5th ed. Appleton & Lange, 1992.)

uptake 2, is saturable, is not specific for catecholamines, and is inhibited by various steroids, phenoxybenzamine, and normetanephrine but not by cocaine and other drugs that inhibit neuronal uptake.

At uptake 2, the catecholamines are metabolized to their O-methyl derivatives by COMT (Figure 11–6). This enzyme is found mainly in the soluble fraction of tissue homogenates, with the highest levels in the liver and kidney. S-Adenosylmethionine is the methyl donor, and divalent ions are required for the reaction. It is predominantly an extraneuronal enzyme and acts on circulating catecholamines as well as on the locally released norepinephrine. It is the most important enzyme in the metabolism of circulating amines.

Approximately 70% of circulating epinephrine in humans is methoxylated, and about 24% is also deaminated. These enzymes also metabolize dopamine to homovanillic acid. Although normetanephrine is fairly active at the alpha receptor of the nictitating membrane, the metabolites of the catecholamines are generally devoid of biologic or physiologic activity.

Conjugation

The phenolic hydroxyl group of the catecholamines and their metabolites may be conjugated with sulfate or glucuronide. Liver and gut appear to be important sites of this reaction, and circulating red blood cells are also a significant site of sulfation in humans.

Connective tissue binds catecholamines by a process that is inhibited by oxytetracycline. The significance of this binding is unknown.

Mechanism of Action

The catecholamines exert their physiologic effects by activating signaling pathways in their target cells. Early studies of sympathetic activation suggested that there were two classes of responses designated as inhibitory or excitatory. Cannon and his colleagues in the 1930s postulated that this difference was produced by the release of different neurotransmitters: sympathin I and sympathin E. The discovery by von Euler and others that norepinephrine was the neurotransmitter released by peripheral sympathetic nerve endings and was responsible for both types of responses led to the proposal by Ahlquist in 1948 that there were two types of receptors that he designated alpha and beta, based on the relative potencies of a series of adrenergic agonists. The subsequent development of relatively specific antagonists confirmed this hypothesis and allowed the development of binding assays for the alpha, beta, and dopaminergic receptors. Subsequent pharmacologic and biochemical studies indicate that alpha, beta, and dopaminergic receptors can be further divided into subtypes. Although these receptors were first classi-

fied by the relative potencies of a series of adrenergic agonists and antagonists, each of the subtypes is now known to be coded for by one or more separate genes (Table 11–3). The characteristic interactions of these receptors with various agonists and antagonists are shown in Table 11–4. The physiologic effects mediated by them are summarized in Table 11–5.

The adrenergic receptors are transmembrane proteins with an extracellular amino terminus and an intracellular carboxyl terminus. Each of their seven hydrophobic regions spans the cell membrane. Although these regions of the adrenergic receptor subtypes exhibit significant amino acid homology, differences in the fifth and sixth segments determine the specificity of agonist binding. Differences in the fifth and seventh segments determine which of the guanylyl nucleotide binding proteins (G proteins) is coupled to the receptor. The G proteins consist of α, β, and γ subunits. There are many G proteins that have different α subunits while the β and γ subunits are similar. When hormone binds to the receptor, the β and γ subunits dissociate from the α subunits, allowing GDP to be replaced by GTP on the α subunits and causing the β and γ subunits to dissociate from it. The GTP-bound α subunits activate the postreceptor pathways. (See also Chapter 3 and Figure 3–3.)

Table 11–3. Adrenoceptor types and subtypes.[1]

Receptor	Agonist	Antagonist	Effects	Gene on Chromosome
Alpha₁ type	Phenylephrine, methoxamine, cirazoline	Prazosin, corynanthine	↑ IP_3, DAG common to all	
Alpha₁A		WB4101, prazosin	↑ IP_3, DAG; ↑Ca^{2+} influx	
Alpha₁B		CEC (irreversible)	↑ IP_3, DAG	C5
Alpha₁C		WB4101, CEC	↑ IP_3, DAG	C8
Alpha₁D		WB4101	?↑ Ca^{2+} influx	C20
Alpha₂ type	Clonidine, BHT920	Rauwolscine, yohimbine	↓ cAMP common to all	
Alpha₂A	Oxymetazoline		↓ cAMP; ↑ K⁺ channels; ↓ Ca^{2+} channels	C10
Alpha₂B		Prazosin	↓ cAMP; ↓ Ca^{2+} channels	C2
Alpha₂C		Prazosin	↓ cAMP	C4
Beta type	Isoproterenol	Propranolol	↑ cAMP common to all	
Beta₁	Dobutamine	Betaxolol	↑ cAMP	
Beta₂	Procaterol, terbutaline	Butoxamine	↑ cAMP	
Beta₃	BRL37344		↑ cAMP	
Dopamine type	Dopamine			
D₁	Fenoldopam		↑ cAMP	C5
D₂	Bromocriptine		↓ cAMP; ↑ K⁺ channels; ↓ Ca^{2+} channels	C11
D₄		Clozapine	↓ cAMP	
D₅			↑ cAMP	C4

[1]Reproduced, with permission, from Katzung BG (editor): *Basic & Clinical Pharmacology,* 6th ed. Appleton & Lange, 1995.
Key:

BRL37344	= Sodium-4-(2-[2-hydroxy-{3-chlorophenyl}ethylamino]propyl)phenoxyacetate
BHT920	= 6-Allyl-2-amino-5,6,7,8-tetrahydro-4*H*-thiazolo-[4,5-*d*]-azepine
CEC	= Chloroethylclonidine
DAG	= Diacylglycerol
IP_3	= Inositol trisphosphate
WB4101	= *N*-[2-(2,6-dimethoxyphenoxy)ethyl]-2,3-dihydro-1,4-benzodioxan-2-methanamine

Table 11–4. Characteristic interactions of agonists and antagonists at the adrenergic receptors.

Receptor	Agonist Potency[1]	Antagonist Potency	Agonist Effect on Adenylyl Cyclase Activity
Alpha$_1$	Same for α_1 and α_2.	Prazosin > phentolamine > yohimbine.	None
Alpha$_2$	Epinephrine slightly > norepinephrine >> isoproterenol.	Phentolamine slightly > yohimbine >> prazosin.	Decrease
Beta$_1$	Isoproterenol > epinephrine $\cong$ norepinephrine.	Metoprolol > butoxamine.	Increase
Beta$_2$	Isoproterenol > epinephrine >> norepinephrine.	Butoxamine > metoprolol.	Increase

[1]These potencies are defined by studies of binding competition and pharmacologic response.

Table 11–5. Adrenergic responses of selected tissues.

Organ or Tissue	Receptor	Effect
Heart (myocardium)	β_1	Increased force of contraction Increased rate of contraction
Blood vessels	α	Vasoconstriction
	β_2	Vasodilation
Kidney	β	Increased renin release
Gut	α, β	Decreased motility and increased sphincter tone
Pancreas	α	Decreased insulin release Decreased glucagon release
	β	Increased insulin release Increased glucagon release
Liver	α, β	Increased glycogenolysis
Adipose tissue	β	Increased lipolysis
Most tissues	β	Increased calorigenesis
Skin (apocrine glands on hands, axillae, etc)	α	Increased sweating
Bronchioles	β_2	Dilation
Uterus	α	Contraction
	β_2	Relaxation

A. Alpha-Adrenergic Receptors: The α_1 subtypes are postsynaptic receptors that typically mediate vascular and other smooth muscle contraction. When agonist binds to this receptor, the alpha subunit of the guanylyl nucleotide binding protein G_q is released and activates phospholipase C. This enzyme catalyzes the conversion of phosphatidylinositol phosphate to 1,4,5-inositol trisphosphate (IP_3) and diacylglycerol. IP_3 releases calcium ion from intracellular stores to stimulate physiologic responses. Diacylglycerol activates kinase C, which in turn phosphorylates a series of other proteins that initiate or sustain effects stimulated by the release of IP_3 and calcium ion (Figure 3–5). Epinephrine and norepinephrine are potent agonists for this receptor, while isoproterenol is weakly active.

Alpha$_2$ receptors were first identified at the presynaptic sympathetic nerve ending and, when activated, served to inhibit the release of norepinephrine. However, these receptors have been found in platelets and postsynaptically in the nervous system, adipose tissue, and smooth muscle.

Agonist binding to the α_2 receptor releases G_i alpha, which inhibits the enzyme adenylyl cyclase and reduces the formation of cAMP. Prazosin is a selective antagonist at the α_1 receptor and yohimbine is selective for the α_2, whereas phentolamine and phenoxybenzamine act at both (Table 11–3).

B. Beta-Adrenergic Receptors: Agonist binding to the beta-adrenergic receptors activates adenylyl cyclase via the G_s alpha subunit to increase the production of cAMP, which in turn converts protein kinase A to its active form. Kinase A then phosphorylates a variety of proteins, including enzymes, ion

channels, and receptors (see Figure 3–4). There are three major beta-receptor subtypes. The β_1 receptor, which mediates the direct cardiac effects, is more responsive to isoproterenol than to epinephrine or norepinephrine, whose potencies are similar. The β_2 receptor mediates vascular, bronchial, and uterine smooth muscle relaxation, probably by phosphorylating myosin light chain kinase. Isoproterenol is also the most potent agonist at this receptor, but epinephrine is much more potent than norepinephrine. The β_3 receptors are found in adipose tissue, and mutations of the gene are associated with earlier onset of NIDDM in Pima Indians.

C. Dopamine Receptors: Dopaminergic receptors are found in the central nervous system, presynaptic adrenergic nerve terminals, pituitary, heart, renal and mesenteric vascular beds, and other sites. Two subtypes of the dopaminergic receptor, D_1 and D_2, have been identified. The binding affinity of the D_1 receptor is greater for dopamine than for haloperidol; the reverse is true for the D_2 receptor. The effects of the D_1 receptor are mediated by stimulation of the adenylyl cyclase system and are found postsynaptically in the brain. Those in the pituitary are D_2 receptors that inhibit the formation of cAMP, open potassium channels, and decrease calcium influx.

Regulation of Activity

The major physiologic control of sympathoadrenal activity is exerted by alterations in the rate of secretion of the catecholamines. However, the receptors and postreceptor events serve as sites of fine regulation.

As noted above, presynaptically, norepinephrine released during nerve stimulation binds to alpha receptors and reduces the amount of norepinephrine released. Nerve endings have also been found to have receptors for many other agents presynaptically (Table 11–2).

The number of receptors on the effector cell surface can be reduced by binding of agonist to receptor (antagonists do not have the same effect). This reduction is called "down-regulation." Thyroid hormone, however, has been shown to increase the number of beta receptors in the myocardium. Estrogen, which increases the number of alpha receptors in the myometrium, increases the affinity of some vascular alpha receptors for norepinephrine.

The mechanisms involved in some of these changes are known. For example phosphorylation of the beta-adrenergic receptor by beta-adrenergic receptor kinase results in their sequestration into membrane vesicles, internalization, and degradation. The phosphorylated receptor also has a greater affinity for β-arrestin, another regulatory protein, which prevents its interaction with G_{sa}.

The finding that most cells in the body have adrenergic receptors has led to an appreciation of the important regulatory role of the peripheral sympathetic nervous system. In contrast, the effects of the adrenal medulla are mediated via the circulating amines and, therefore, are much more generalized in nature. Furthermore, adrenal medullary secretion increases significantly only in the presence of stress or marked deviation from homeostatic or resting conditions. For example, a minor reduction in the available glucose leads to sympathetic activation of fat mobilization from adipose tissue, whereas the adrenal medulla may not release large amounts of epinephrine until the blood sugar falls to 40–50 mg/dL (3 mmol/L) in normal individuals. A summary of physiologic effects of the catecholamines in various tissues is presented in Table 11–5.

Physiologic Effects

A. Cardiovascular Effects: Catecholamines increase the rate and frequency of contraction and increase the irritability of the myocardium by activating myocardial β_1 receptors. The contractile effects of the catecholamines on vascular smooth muscle are mediated via alpha receptors. Although beta receptors are present and cause dilatation, other mechanisms of vascular dilatation are probably more important. The release or injection of catecholamines can therefore be expected to increase heart rate and cardiac output and cause peripheral vasoconstriction—all leading to an increase in blood pressure. These events are mod-

ulated by reflex mechanisms, so that, as the blood pressure increases, reflex stimulation may slow the heart rate and tend to reduce cardiac output. Although norepinephrine in the usual doses will have these effects, the effect of epinephrine may vary depending on the smooth muscle tone of the vascular system at the time. For example, in an individual with increased vascular tone, the net effect of small amounts of epinephrine may be to reduce the mean blood pressure while increasing the heart rate and cardiac output. In an individual with a reduction in vascular tone, the mean blood pressure would be expected to increase. In addition to the reflex mechanisms, vascular output is integrated by the central nervous system, so that, under appropriate circumstances, one vascular bed may be dilated while others remain unchanged. The central organization of the sympathetic nervous system is such that its ordinary regulatory effects are quite discrete—in contrast to periods of stress, when stimulation may be rather generalized and accompanied by release of catecholamines into the circulation. The infusion of catecholamines leads to a rapid reduction in plasma volume, presumably to accommodate to the reduced volume of the arterial and venous beds (Figure 11–7).

B. Effects on Extravascular Smooth Muscle: The catecholamines also regulate the activity of smooth muscle in tissues other than blood vessels.

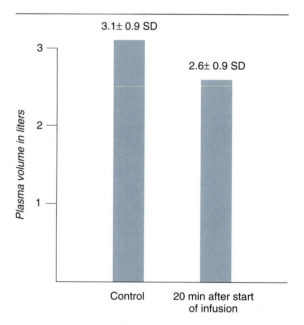

Figure 11–7. Changes in plasma volume produced by infusion of norepinephrine for 20 minutes in a dose sufficient to increase mean arterial pressure from 96 ± 10 mm Hg to 150 ± 16 mm Hg. (Data from Finnerty FA Jr, Buchholz JH, Guillaudeu RL: Blood volumes and plasma protein during arterenol-induced hypertension. J Clin Invest 1958;37:425.)

These effects include relaxation and contraction of uterine myometrium, relaxation of intestinal and bladder smooth muscle, contraction of the smooth muscle in the bladder and intestinal sphincters, and relaxation of tracheal smooth muscle and pupillary dilatation.

C. Metabolic Effects: The catecholamines increase oxygen consumption and heat production. Although the effects appear to be mediated by the beta receptor, the mechanism is unknown. The catecholamines also regulate glucose and fat mobilization from storage depots. Glycogenolysis in heart muscle and in liver leads to an increase in available carbohydrate for utilization. Stimulation of adipose tissue leads to lipolysis and the release of free fatty acids and glycerol into the circulation for utilization at other sites. In humans, these effects are mediated by the beta receptor.

The plasma levels of catecholamines required to produce some cardiovascular and metabolic effects in humans are shown in Table 11–6.

The catecholamines have effects on water, sodium, potassium, calcium, and phosphate excretion in the kidney. However, the mechanisms and the significance of these changes are not clear.

The Regulatory Role of Catecholamines in Hormone Secretion

The sympathetic nervous system plays an important role in the regulation and integration of hormone secretion at two levels. Centrally, norepinephrine and dopamine play important roles in the regulation of secretion of the anterior pituitary hormones. Dopamine, for example, has been identified as the prolactin-inhibiting hormone, and the hypothalamic releasing hormones appear to be under sympathetic nervous system control. Peripherally, the secretion of renin by the juxtaglomerular cells of the kidney is regulated by the sympathetic nervous system via the renal nerves and circulating catecholamines. The catecholamines release renin via a beta receptor mechanism. The B cell of the pancreatic islets is stimulated by activation of the beta receptors in the presence of alpha-adrenergic blockade. However, the dominant effect of nor-

epinephrine or epinephrine is inhibition of insulin secretion, which is mediated by the alpha receptor. Similar effects have been observed in the secretion of glucagon by pancreatic A cells. The catecholamines have also been found to increase the release of thyroxine, calcitonin, parathyroid hormone, and gastrin by a beta receptor-mediated mechanism.

OTHER HORMONES

In addition to the catecholamines, the chromaffin cells of the adrenal medulla and peripheral sympathetic neurons synthesize and secrete opiate-like peptides, including met- and leu-enkephalin (see Chapter 5). They are stored in the large, dense-cored vesicles with the catecholamines in the adrenal medulla and at sympathetic nerve endings. These peptides are also found in the terminals of the splanchnic fibers that innervate the adrenal medulla. The observation that naloxone increases plasma catecholamine levels suggests that these peptides may inhibit sympathetic activity.

Adrenomedullin, a peptide originally isolated from pheochromocytoma tissue, is produced in the adrenal medulla. It consists of 52 amino acids, has slight homology with calcitonin gene-related peptide, and exerts its effects by elevation of cAMP levels. It exhibits potent depressor and vasorelaxant activity. It has also been found in the heart, lung, kidney, and brain as well as vascular endothelium. Adrenomedullin circulates in blood, and plasma levels in patients with hypertension have been reported to be higher than those of normotensive controls. It is thought to play a role in blood pressure regulation. The amino terminal 20-amino-acid peptide of proadrenomedullin from which adrenomedullin is derived is also found in the same tissues. This peptide also exhibits hypotensive effects, but it appears to do so by inhibiting neural transmission at sympathetic nerve endings rather than directly relaxing vascular smooth muscle like adrenomedullin.

Extracts of normal adrenals have also been found to contain corticotropin-releasing factor, growth hor-

Table 11–6. Approximate circulating plasma levels of epinephrine and norepinephrine required to produce hemodynamic and metabolic changes duirng infusions of epinephrine and norepinephrine.[1]

	Norepinephrine	Epinephrine
Systolic blood pressure	↑ at 2500 pg/mL (15 nmol/L)	↑ at 500 pg/mL (3 nmol/L)
Diastolic blood pressure	↑ at 2500 pg/mL (15 nmol/L)	↓ at 500 pg/mL (3 nmol/L)
Pulse	↓ at 2500 pg/mL (15 nmol/dL)	↑ at 250 pg/mL (1.5 nmol/L)
Plasma glucose	↑ at 2500 pg/moL (15 nmol/L)	↑ at 250–500 pg/mL (1.5–3 nmol/L)

[1]Data from Silverberg AB et al: Am J Physiol 1978:234:E252; and from Clutter WE et al: J Clin Invest 1980:66:94.

mone-releasing hormone, somatostatin, and peptide histidine methionine. Although these and other active peptides are secreted by tumors of the adrenal medulla and contribute to the symptomatology, little is known of their function in the normal gland.

DISORDERS OF ADRENAL MEDULLARY FUNCTION

HYPOFUNCTION

Hypofunction of the adrenal medulla alone probably occurs only in individuals receiving adrenocortical steroid replacement therapy following adrenalectomy. Such individuals with otherwise intact sympathetic nervous systems suffer no clinically significant disability. Patients with autonomic insufficiency, which includes deficiency of adrenal medullary epinephrine secretion, can be demonstrated to have minor defects in recovery from insulin-induced hypoglycemia (Figure 11–8). It should be

noted, however, that in patients with diabetes mellitus in whom the glucagon response is also deficient, the additional loss of adrenal medullary response leaves them more susceptible to severe bouts of hypoglycemia. This is the result of a decrease in the warning symptoms as well as an impaired response. (See Chapter 19.) Patients with generalized autonomic insufficiency usually have orthostatic hypotension. The causes of disorders associated with autonomic insufficiency are listed in Table 11–7.

When a normal individual stands, a series of physiologic adjustments occur that maintain blood pressure and ensure adequate circulation to the brain. The initial lowering of the blood pressure stimulates the baroreceptors, which then activate central reflex mechanisms that cause arterial and venous constriction, increase cardiac output, and activate the release of renin and vasopressin. Interruption of afferent, central, or efferent components of this autonomic reflex results in autonomic insufficiency.

The treatment of symptomatic orthostatic hypotension is dependent upon maintenance of an adequate blood volume. If physical measures such as raising the head of the bed at night and using support garments do not alleviate the condition, pharmacologic measures may be used. Although agents producing

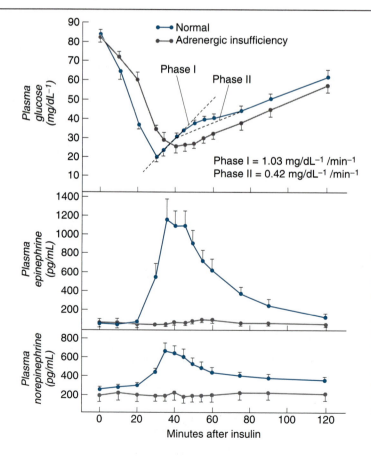

Figure 11–8. Plasma glucose, epinephrine, and norepinephrine levels after insulin administration in 14 normal subjects (•—•) and seven patients with idiopathic orthostatic hypotension (•—•) with low or absent epinephrine responses. Results are expressed as mean ± SEM. (Reproduced, with permission, from Polinsky RJ et al: The adrenal medullary response to hypoglycemia in patients with orthostatic hypotension. J Clin Endocrinol Metab 1980;51:1404.)

Table 11–7. Disorders associated with autonomic insufficiency.

Familial dysautonomia
Shy-Drager syndrome
Parkinson's disease
Tabes dorsalis
Syringomyelia
Cerebrovascular disease
Peripheral neuropathy due to diabetes
Idiopathic orthostatic hypotension
Sympathectomy
Drugs: antihypertensives, antidepressants

constriction of the vascular bed, including ephedrine, phenylephrine, metaraminol, monoamine oxidase inhibitors, levodopa, propranolol, and indomethacin, have been used, volume expansion with fludrocortisone is the most effective treatment.

HYPERFUNCTION

The adrenal medulla is not known to play a significant role in essential hypertension. However, the role of the sympathetic nervous system in the regulation of blood flow and blood pressure has led to extensive investigations of its role in various types of hypertension. Some of the abnormalities observed, such as a resetting of baroreceptor activity, are thought to be secondary to the change in blood pressure. Others, such as the increased cardiac output found in early essential hypertension, have been thought by some investigators to play a primary role.

Catecholamines can increase blood pressure by increasing cardiac output, by increasing peripheral resistance through their vasoconstrictive action on the arteriole, and by increasing renin release from the kidney, leading to increased circulating levels of angiotensin II. Although many studies show an increase in circulating free catecholamine levels, evidence of increased sympathetic activity has not been a uniform finding in patients with essential hypertension.

PHEOCHROMOCYTOMA

Pheochromocytomas are tumors arising from chromaffin cells in the sympathetic nervous system. They release epinephrine or norepinephrine (or both)—and in some cases dopamine—into the circulation, causing hypertension and other signs and symptoms.

In addition to the catecholamines, pheochromocytomas have been reported to produce a wide variety of active peptides. These include somatostatin, substance P, corticotropin-releasing hormone, adrenocorticotropin, β endorphin, lipotropin, vasoactive intestinal polypeptide, interleukin-6, parathyroid hormone-related protein, neuropeptide Y, calcitonin, calcitonin gene-related peptide, met-enkephalin, serotonin, gastrin, neurotensin, pancreastatin, galanin, insulin-like growth factor II, and others. Secretion of large amounts of these substances may result in atypical clinical presentations.

It is estimated that 0.1% of patients with diastolic hypertension have pheochromocytomas. These tumors are found at all ages and in both sexes and are most commonly diagnosed in the fourth or fifth decades. An analysis of data from the National Cancer Registry in Sweden indicates an incidence of about two per million in that population.

Although uncommon, this disorder is important to diagnose, because undiagnosed it may be fatal in pregnant women during delivery or in patients undergoing surgery for other disorders. However, with early diagnosis and proper management, almost all patients with benign tumors recover completely.

Clinical Features

A. Symptoms and Signs: Although most patients with functioning tumors have symptoms most of the time, these vary in intensity and are perceived to be mainly episodic or paroxysmal by about half of the patients. Most patients with persistent hypertension also have superimposed paroxysms. A few patients are entirely free of symptoms and hypertension between attacks and give no evidence of excessive catecholamine release during these intervals. In some instances, these tumors occur with minimal clinical manifestations and are only found incidentally on CT or MRI scan. Commonly reported symptoms and signs are listed in Table 11–8.

B. Description of an Attack: In patients with paroxysmal release of catecholamines, the symptoms resemble those produced by injections of epinephrine or norepinephrine, and the symptom complex is far more consistent than is suggested by the variability

Table 11–8. Common symptoms in patients with hypertension due to pheochromocytoma.

Symptoms during or following paroxysms
Headache
Sweating
Forceful heartbeat with or without tachycardia
Anxiety or fear of impending death
Tremor
Fatigue or exhaustion
Nausea and vomiting
Abdominal or chest pain
Visual disturbances
Symptoms between paroxysms
Increased sweating
Cold hands and feet
Weight loss
Constipation

of patients' complaints. An episode usually begins with a sensation of something happening deep inside the chest, and a stimulus to deeper breathing is noted. The patient then becomes aware of a pounding or forceful heartbeat, caused by the β_1 receptor-mediated increase in cardiac output. This throbbing spreads to the rest of the trunk and head, causing headache or a pounding sensation in the head. The intense alpha receptor-mediated peripheral vasoconstriction causes cool, moist hands and feet and facial pallor. The combination of increased cardiac output and vasoconstriction causes marked elevation of the blood pressure when large amounts of catecholamines are released. The decreased heat loss and increased metabolism may cause a rise in temperature or flushing and lead to reflex sweating, which may be profuse and usually follows the cardiovascular effects that begin in the first few seconds after onset of an attack. The increased glycolysis and alpha receptor-mediated inhibition of insulin release cause an increase in blood sugar levels. Patients experience marked anxiety during all but the mildest attacks, and when episodes are prolonged or severe, there may be nausea, vomiting, visual disturbances, chest or abdominal pain, paresthesias, or seizures. A feeling of fatigue or exhaustion usually follows these episodes unless they are very mild or of short duration.

C. Frequency of Attacks: In patients with paroxysmal symptoms, attacks usually occur several times a week or oftener and last for 15 minutes or less though they may occur at intervals of months or as often as 25 times daily and may last from minutes to days. As time passes, the attacks usually increase in frequency but do not change much in character. They are frequently precipitated by activities that compress the tumor (eg, changes in position, exercise, lifting, defecation, or eating) and by emotional distress or anxiety.

D. Variability of Manifestations: Although the pattern of the manifestations described above can be elicited in almost all patients capable of clear communication, the variability of presenting complaints may be confusing and is sometimes misleading. Women whose episodes are first noted around the time of menopause may be thought to be experiencing "hot flushes." The diagnosis may only be made when hormonal therapy has failed to alleviate the "hot flush" or the episode is observed and the blood pressure taken during an attack. When a pheochromocytoma causes hypertension late in pregnancy, it may be confused with preeclampsia. As noted above, when tumors secrete other peptides in significant amounts, they may produce atypical manifestations such as fever with leukotrienes, hypercalcemia with parathyroid hormone-related protein, and Cushing's syndrome with secretion of ACTH or CRH. Other causes of increased sympathetic activity must be distinguished from pheochromocytomas (see below) (Table 11–9).

Table 11–9. Disorders presenting with features of sympathetic discharge or hypermetabolism.

Apnea due to coronary vasospasm
Severe anxiety and panic states
Hypertension
Hypertensive crises associated with–
Surgery
Cerebrovascular accidents
Acute pulmonary edema
Paraplegia
Tabes dorsalis
Lead poisoning
Acute porphyria
Menopausal hot flushes
Autonomic epilepsy
Thyrotoxicosis
Migraine and cluster headache
Hyperdynamic beta-adrenergic states
Sympathomimetic drug ingestion

E. Chronic Symptoms: Patients with persistently secreting tumors and chronic symptoms usually experience the symptom complex described above in response to transient increases in the release of catecholamines. In addition, in these patients the increased metabolic rate usually causes heat intolerance, increased sweating, and weight loss or (in children) lack of weight gain. The effects on glycogenolysis and insulin release can produce hyperglycemia and glucose intolerance, and patients may present with diabetes mellitus. Hypertension is usually present. Wide fluctuations of blood pressure are characteristic, and marked increases may be followed by hypotension and syncope. When pressure is elevated, postural hypotension is present. Typically, the hypertension does not respond to commonly used antihypertensive regimens, and such drugs as guanethidine and ganglionic blockers can induce paradoxic pressor responses. On examination, these patients, usually thin, have a forceful heartbeat that is often visible and easily palpable. They feel warm, may have pallor of the face and chest, perspire, have cool and moist hands and feet, and prefer a cool room. A mass may be palpable in the abdomen or neck, and deep palpation of the abdomen may produce a typical paroxysm. Chronic constriction of the arterial and venous beds leads to a reduction in plasma volume in most of these patients. The inability to further constrict these vessels upon arising contributes to the postural hypotension that is characteristically observed.

Familial Syndromes & Other Tumors

Pheochromocytoma may also occur as a heritable disorder, either alone or more commonly in association with other endocrine tumors. In one syndrome, multiple endocrine neoplasia (MEN) type IIa (Sipple's syndrome), the patient may also have a calcitonin-producing carcinoma of the thyroid (medullary carcinoma) and a parathyroid hormone-producing adenoma of the parathyroid. In the other group (MEN type

IIb), pheochromocytomas occur in association with medullary carcinoma and mucosal neuromas, which are numerous and small and are found around the mouth and in the bowel. Transmission of these disorders follows the pattern of an autosomal dominant gene with incomplete penetrance. (See Chapter 24.)

Pheochromocytomas occurring as part of the familial syndromes appear to be the expression of a stimulus to tumor formation in patients with genetic abnormalities that predispose them to respond with neoplasia. *RET* proto-oncogene germline mutations in exons 10 and 11 on chromosome 10 are responsible for inherited multiple endocrine neoplasia type II (MEN type II) syndromes. The *RET* proto-oncogene encodes a receptor type tyrosine kinase. Recently, codon mutations of *RET* have been described in multiple endocrine neoplasia types IIa and IIb. The expression of *RET* has been observed in human tumors of neural crest origin, and recent studies demonstrate that the *RET* protooncogene plays important roles in the development of the tissues derived from the neural crest, including pheochromocytomas. The *RET* proto-oncogene is normally expressed in the adrenal medulla and cerebellum. *RET* transcripts have been detected in sporadic and familial pheochromocytomas. The levels of *RET* mRNA were higher in pheochromocytomas than in the normal adrenal medulla, suggesting that *RET* may be overexpressed in many sporadic pheochromocytomas. In MEN type IIa, bilateral pheochromocytomas are common and may develop from hyperplasia of the adrenal medulla. Medullary carcinoma of the thyroid in these patients is commonly bilateral and is preceded by parafollicular or "C" cell hyperplasia. Multiple tumors of the parathyroid gland are also quite typical and are found predominantly in patients with MEN type IIa and rarely in those with MEN type IIb. The thyroid tumors have been reported to secrete ACTH, serotonin, prostaglandins, and kallikreins, which may contribute to the clinical manifestations in these patients. Usually, the thyroid tumor (medullary carcinoma) is diagnosed by finding an elevated serum calcitonin level under basal conditions or after provocative testing with stimuli such as calcium or pentagastrin (see Chapters 7 and 8). Ganglioneuromas (which are usually small, well-differentiated tumors arising from ganglion cells) and neuroblastomas (which are highly malignant tumors arising from more primitive sympathoblastic cells) can produce catecholamines and present a similar clinical picture. Dopamine is usually the major active catecholamine produced, and its production leads to elevated concentrations of dopamine in plasma and of homovanillic acid in urine.

Pathology

A. Location of Tumor: Pheochromocytomas occur wherever chromaffin tissue is found (Figure 11–9). The adrenal medulla contains the largest col-

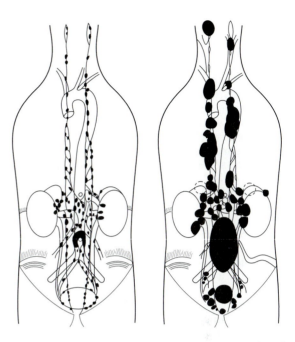

Figure 11–9. Left: Anatomic distribution of extra-adrenal chromaffin tissue in the newborn. **Right:** Locations of extra-adrenal pheochromocytomas reported before 1965. (Reproduced, with permission, from Coupland R: *The Natural History of the Chromaffin Cell.* Longmans, Green, 1965.)

lection of chromaffin cells. They are also found in the organ of Zuckerkandl, which is very large in the fetus but is gradually replaced by fibrous tissue after delivery and is small in the adult. Chromaffin cells are also found in association with sympathetic ganglia, nerve plexuses, and nerves.

Over 95% of pheochromocytomas are found in the abdomen, and 85% of these are in the adrenal. Common extra-adrenal sites are near the kidney and in the organ of Zuckerkandl. Those found in the chest are in the heart or the posterior mediastinal area. The intracranial lesions reported are thought to be metastatic in origin. The tumors may be multicentric in origin, particularly when they are familial or part of the syndromes of multiple endocrine neoplasia and when they are seen in children. Although fewer than 10% of adults have multiple tumors, they are found in about one-third of affected children.

B. Size of Tumor: Pheochromocytomas vary in size from less than 1 g to several kilograms. However, they are usually small, most weighing under 100 g. They are vascular tumors and commonly contain cystic or hemorrhagic areas. The cells tend to be large and contain typical catecholamine storage granules similar to those in the adrenal medulla. Multinucleated cells, pleomorphic nuclei, mitoses, and extension into the capsule and vessels are sometimes seen but do not indicate that the tumor is malignant. The incidence of malignant tumors in reported studies varies from less than 5% to more than 10%. These can be recognized during surgery when there is significant local infiltration or when metastases are identified. About 5–10% of patients thought to have been cured will recur later. Using cell sorting and DNA staining methods, it has been found that patients with tumors whose cells contain increased amounts of nuclear DNA and patients with extra-adrenal tumors are at higher risk of recurrence and should be screened at regular intervals following surgery.

C. Adrenal Medullary Hyperplasia: This has also been described as the cause of an indistinguishable clinical picture and is found in the syndrome of multiple endocrine neoplasia (see Chapter 24).

Complications

Patients with persistent symptoms and hypertension may develop hypertensive retinopathy or nephropathy. Postmortem studies indicate that there are a significant number of patients with pheochromocytomas who have myocarditis characterized by focal degeneration and necrosis of myocardial fibers with infiltration of histiocytes, plasma cells, and other signs of inflammation. Platelet aggregates and fibrin deposition are found in pulmonary arterioles. These changes may be associated with abnormal findings on the ECG but may not become apparent until the patient is exposed to marked cardiovascular stress and heart failure results. In patients harboring pheochromocytomas for long periods, the serious sequelae of hypertension are observed. Cerebrovascular accidents, congestive heart failure, and myocardial infarction have been observed. Some of the causes of death in unoperated patients are shown in Table 11–10.

Differential Diagnosis

The diagnosis of pheochromocytoma should be considered in all patients with paroxysmal symptoms; in children with hypertension; in adults with severe hypertension not responding to therapy; in hypertensive patients with diabetes or hypermetabolism; in patients with hypertension in whom symptoms resemble those described above or can be

Table 11–10. Causes of death in patients with unsuspected pheochromocytomas.

Myocardial infarction
Cerebrovascular accident
Arrhythmias
Irreversible shock
Renal failure
Dissecting aortic aneurysm

evoked by exercise, position change, emotional distress, or antihypertensive drugs such as guanethidine and ganglionic blockers; and in patients who become severely hypertensive or go into shock during anesthesia, surgery, or obstetric delivery. Patients who have disorders sometimes associated with pheochromocytomas (neurofibromatosis, mucosal adenomas, von Hippel's disease, medullary carcinoma of the thyroid) and those with first-degree relatives who have pheochromocytoma or other manifestations of MEN should be investigated. Other disorders associated with marked sympathetic stimulation may cause confusion and are listed in Table 11–9. Levels may also be elevated in patients undergoing severe mental or physical stress or other severe illness. Plasma catecholamine levels at rest and with exercise and various disorders are shown in Table 11–11.

In these and other disorders in which elevated plasma catecholamine levels are under sympathetic nervous system control, it may be possible to reduce catecholamine release by autonomic blockade or sympathetic suppression. Pentolinium and clonidine have been used for this purpose. The reliability and safety of such procedures have not been established. Patients with migraine and cluster headaches, menopausal symptoms, anxiety disorders, autonomic hyperreflexia, and perioperative hypertension may have symptoms suggestive of a pheochromocytoma but have normal catecholamine levels that do not increase during attacks.

As noted below, the use of CT and MRI to localize these tumors is indicated only after the diagnosis has been confirmed. However, since these procedures are frequently employed diagnostic tools, masses in the region of the adrenal are diagnosed as **incidental findings** in approximately 2% of such scans. These

Table 11–11. Range of plasma catecholamine levels observed in healthy subjects and patients.

	Norepinephrine	Epinephrine
Healthy subjects		
Basal	150–400 pg/mL (0.9–2.4 nmol/L)	25–100 pg/mL (0.1–0.6 nmol/L)
Ambulatory	200–800 pg/mL (1.2–4.8 nmol/L)	30–100 pg/mL (0.1–1 nmol/L)
Exercise	800–4000 pg/mL (4.8–24 nmol/L)	100–1000 pg/mL (0.5–5 nmol/L)
Symptomatic hypoglycemia	200–1000 pg/mL (1.2–6 nmol/L)	1000–5000 pg/mL (5–25 nmol/L)
Patients		
Hypertension	200–500 pg/mL (1.2–3 nmol/L)	20–100 pg/mL (0.1–0.6 nmol/L)
Surgery	500–2000 pg/mL (3–12 nmol/L)	199–500 pg/mL (0.5–3 nmol/L)
Myocardial infarction	1000–2000 pg/mL (6–12 nmol/L)	800–5000 pg/mL (4–25 nmol/L)

images can represent cysts, lipomas, nonfunctioning adenomas, infections, hemorrhage, or metastases as well as pheochromocytomas. These patients should be screened for pheochromocytomas clinically and chemically. The workup of these patients is discussed in more detail in Chapter 9.

Diagnostic Tests & Procedures

Assay of catecholamines and their metabolites has markedly simplified the diagnosis of this disorder. Operative exploration for pheochromocytoma should not be done in the absence of chemical confirmation of the diagnosis. With currently available methods, it is possible to avoid unnecessary surgery and to successfully locate a tumor in almost all patients.

A. Hormone Assay: In patients with continuous hypertension or symptoms, levels of plasma or urine catecholamines and their metabolites are usually clearly increased. Therefore, in the selection of a particular assay, it is more important that the test be performed well by the laboratory than that a particular substance be measured. A reliable assay of the catecholamines, metanephrines, or vanillylmandelic acid (VMA) is usually sufficient to confirm the diagnosis. Patients with large tumors may excrete disproportionately greater amounts of catecholamine metabolites, because the amines can be metabolized by enzymes in the tumor cells prior to their release. Malignant tumors may release large amounts of dopamine, leading to increased plasma dopamine and to the excretion of large amounts of homovanillic acid in the urine. It is important that the appropriate assay procedure be chosen to avoid misleading results and that drugs and foods that interfere with these assays be eliminated (Table 11–12).

In patients having brief and infrequent paroxysms with symptom-free intervals, confirmation of the diagnosis may be more difficult. Although large amounts of catecholamines are produced during the brief episode, the total amount excreted during the 24-hour urine collection period may not be clearly abnormal—in contrast to patients whose tumors secrete continuously. The latter group will accumulate larger amounts of catecholamines and metabolites in the urine even though secretion rates are lower and symptoms are less severe. Therefore, sampling of blood or timed urine collections during a carefully observed episode may be necessary to confirm the diagnosis.

B. Glucagon Test: In patients with infrequent episodes, glucagon can be used to induce a paroxysm. This is rarely necessary and should not be done in patients who have angina, visual changes, or other severe symptoms during spontaneous attacks. Phentolamine should be available to terminate the induced episode. Injection of 1 mg of glucagon intravenously will induce an attack in more than 90% of patients with pheochromocytoma. A typical response in such a patient is shown in Figure 11–10. In those instances in which glucagon has failed to evoke a paroxysm and the clinical suspicion is very strong, histamine given intravenously in doses of 25–50 µg may also be tried. However, histamine injection is associated with flushing and a brief but severe episode of headache. In general, the provoked episodes are no more severe than those occurring spontaneously. Provocative tests should be reserved for patients in whom it is necessary to rule out the presence of pheochromocytoma when they are seen (eg, prior to surgery or obstetric delivery). At all other times, a timed urine collection during an episode can provide more accurate information.

C. Clonidine Suppression Test: In patients whose catecholamine levels are elevated because of neurogenic stimulation rather than release of catecholamine from a tumor, the administration of 0.3 mg of clonidine 2–3 hours before sampling of blood may be useful in reducing plasma norepinephrine levels. This procedure can be used during an office visit or whenever it is not possible to obtain blood under resting conditions.

D. Trial of Phenoxybenzamine or Other α_2 Receptor Blockers: In the occasional patient in whom the chemical tests are inconclusive, it may be useful or convenient to institute therapy with phenoxybenzamine over a period of 1–2 months to

Table 11–12. Maximal normal concentrations of the catecholamines and their metabolism in urine.[1] Substances interfering with their measurement are listed.

Compound	Excreted	Interfering Substances
Epinephrine Norepinephrine Dopamine	0.02 mg/24 h (0.1 nmol/24 h) 0.08 mg/24 h (0.5 nmol/24 h) 0.4 mg/24 h (2.5 nmol/24 h)	May be increased by highly fluorescent compounds such as tetracyclines and quinidine; by foods[2] and drugs containing catecholamines; and by levodopa, methyldopa, and ethanol.
Metanephrine Normetanephrine	0.4 mg/24 h (2.5 nmol/24 h) 0.9 mg/24 h (5 nmol/24 h)	Increased by catecholamines, monoamine oxidase inhibitors, and others, depending on the method.
Vanillylmandelic acid Homovanillic acid	8 mg/24 h (7 nmol/24 h) 7 mg/24 h (45 nmol/24 h)	Increased by catecholamines, by foods containing vanillin, or by levodopa. Decreased by clofibrate, disulfiram, and monoamine oxidase inhibitors.

[1]Values may be higher under unusual stress, illness, or strenuous activity.
[2]For example, bananas contain significant amounts of norepinephrine.

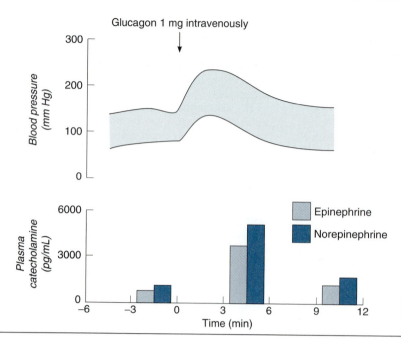

Figure 11–10. Blood pressure and plasma catecholamine levels following glucagon injection in a patient with a paroxysmally secreting pheochromocytoma. The blood sugar at 12 minutes was 180 mg/dL.

observe effects both on the nature and frequency of attacks and on the blood pressure. A salutary effect will sometimes be observed for a few weeks but seldom longer than that in the absence of pheochromocytoma. A good response indicates the need for reappraisal of the patient.

Screening for Pheochromocytoma

In addition to screening patients with typical clinical manifestations, assays for catecholamines and their metabolites can be used to screen other patients at high risk. The indications for screening are listed in Table 11–13. When the presence of an undetected pheochromocytoma is particularly dangerous, as in pregnancy or prior to surgery, screening should be considered even when clinical manifestations are less typical. In families with suspected MEN type IIa, DNA analysis for the *RET* proto-oncogene mutations provides unambiguous identification of individuals at risk.

Localization of Tumors

When the diagnosis has been established, the tumor must be located in order to facilitate its surgical removal. CT and MRI are of great value in localizing these tumors (Figure 11–11). MRI is somewhat more successful in locating extra-adrenal tumors and has the advantage of producing brighter images of pheochromocytomas with T2 weighting in contrast to most other adrenal tumors. Only the smallest tumors or those shielded by clips and other metal objects from previous surgery have been elusive.

Although not as widely available, scintigrams following the injection of ^{131}I labeled metaiodobenzyl-

guanidine (MIBG) are quite specific for identifying masses producing catecholamines, including neuroblastomas and pheochromocytomas. Administration of MIBG in these patients results in detectable images in 48–72 hours. It is particularly useful in identifying extra-adrenal tumors and metastases. Very small tumors can be safely and conveniently located by this method. Although not all pheochromocytomas will produce detectable images, the specificity of the method seems high, and it has been possible to locate tumors not found by other methods.

Table 11–13. Patients to be screened for pheochromocytoma.

Young hypertensives
Hypertensive patients with–
  Symptoms listed in Table 11–8
  Weight loss
  Seizures
  Orthostatic hypotension
  Unexplained shock
  Family history of pheochromocytoma or medullary
    carcinoma of thyroid
  Neurofibromatosis and other neurocutaneous syndromes
  Mucosal neuromas
  Hyperglycemia
  Cardiomyopathy
Marked lability of blood pressure
Family history of pheochromocytoma
Shock or severe pressor responses with–
  Induction of anesthesia
  Parturition
  Surgery
  Invasive procedures
  Antihypertensive drugs
Radiologic evidence of adrenal mass

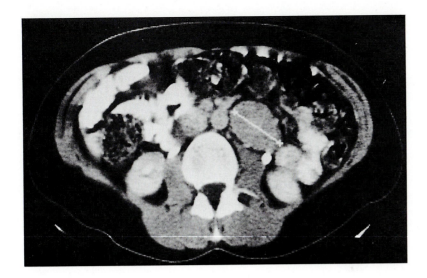

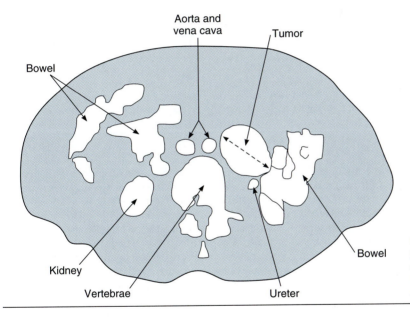

Figure 11–11. Left infrarenal pheochromocytoma shown by CT scanning. The lower diagram identifies many of the visible structures.

Analysis of blood samples obtained via percutaneous venous catheterization can be of great value in locating small tumors in unusual locations. An example of the use of this technique is shown in Figure 11–12. Because of a small risk of complications and the discomfort and cost of this procedure, it should be used only after simpler methods fail.

Management

Optimal management of patients with pheochromocytomas requires an understanding of the pathophysiology produced by excessive catecholamines and an acquaintance with the action of adrenergic antagonists and other drugs used in the treatment of these patients.

A. Treatment With Adrenergic Antagonists: As soon as the diagnosis has been confirmed, therapy with adrenergic antagonists should be instituted. Treatment is directed toward reduction of symptoms, lowering of blood pressure, and amelioration of paroxysms occurring spontaneously or induced by studies undertaken to localize the tumors. Such treatment will allow expansion of the vascular bed and plasma volume and will reduce the amount of transfused blood required for maintenance of blood pressure during surgery.

Although only a few days of therapy are required for preoperative study and preparation of most patients for surgery, prolonged medical therapy is advantageous in patients who have had recent myocardial infarctions, those with electrocardiographic or clinical evidence of catecholamine cardiomyopathy, or those in the last trimester of pregnancy. They can

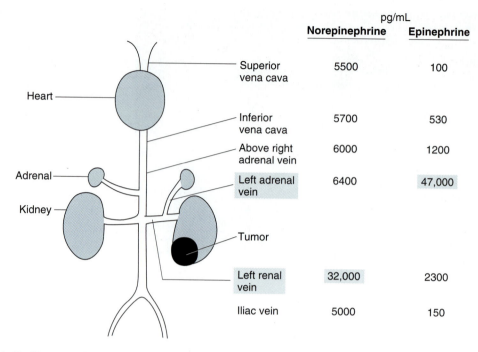

	pg/mL	
	Norepinephrine	**Epinephrine**
Superior vena cava	5500	100
Inferior vena cava	5700	530
Above right adrenal vein	6000	1200
Left adrenal vein	6400	47,000
Tumor		
Left renal vein	32,000	2300
Iliac vein	5000	150

Figure 11–12. Plasma norepinephrine and epinephrine levels in samples of blood obtained from the vena cava. Note that the level of epinephrine is very high in the left adrenal vein sample, distinguishing it from the drainage of the tumor, which secretes mainly norepinephrine. Note the relatively normal peripheral levels of epinephrine (as seen in the iliac vein or the superior vena cava)

be maintained on this regimen until the infant is delivered or the complication resolved, at which time the tumor can be removed.

Agents commonly used in therapy include phentolamine, prazosin, and phenoxybenzamine. Propranolol is occasionally helpful to control marked tachycardia and arrhythmias, but it should not be given until alpha receptor blockade is established.

In patients with persistent hypertension or frequent paroxysms, **phenoxybenzamine** (Dibenzyline), a noncompetitive alpha-adrenergic antagonist with a prolonged effect, is indicated. Treatment is begun with doses of 20–40 mg/d orally and can be increased by 10–20 mg every 1–2 days until the desired effect is achieved. Postural hypotension may be marked at the beginning of therapy, and care should be taken to prevent syncope. However, postural hypotension usually disappears when adequate blockade is achieved. Completely normal blood pressures (< 140/90 mm Hg) may not be achieved and are not required. A dose of 60–80 mg daily is usually adequate, but two to three times that amount may be necessary. When marked tachycardia or arrhythmias occur prior to or during surgery, small doses of **propranolol** may be required. Patients with infrequent paroxysms and an absence of interval manifestations can be treated in a similar manner.

Rapid titration of the dose may be difficult using

phenoxybenzamine, because of its long half-life (36 hours). However, **prazosin,** an alpha antagonist with a shorter duration of activity, has been found to be useful. Prazosin is predominantly an α_1 antagonist and has not been found to be effective in all patients.

B. Preparation for Surgery: Preparation of the patient as described above minimizes the hazards of anesthesia and surgery. The patient's blood pressure and electrocardiographic patterns should be continuously monitored, and phentolamine and particularly sodium nitroprusside are useful to reduce blood pressure if necessary. Suspected intra-abdominal tumors are usually approached through a transabdominal incision, since this allows exploration of the adrenals, sympathetic ganglia, bladder, and other pelvic structures. However, posterior and flank incisions are preferred by some surgeons for removal of larger tumors. In skilled hands, these tumors have been successfully removed via laparoscopic surgery. This approach can significantly reduce postoperative morbidity. When bilateral adrenal tumors are found and the adrenals removed, adrenocortical steroid replacement is required (see Chapter 9).

C. Postoperative Care: When the tumor is removed, the blood pressure usually falls to about 90/60 mm Hg. Persistence of low blood pressures or poor peripheral perfusion may require blood volume expansion with whole blood, plasma, or other fluids as indicated. Pressor therapy is not usually required and should not be substituted for volume expansion.

Lack of a fall in pressure at the time of tumor removal (even in the presence of adrenergic blockade) indicates the presence of additional tumor tissue.

In patients with tumors producing persistent hypertension, the initial fall in blood pressure may be followed by an elevation of blood pressure in the postoperative period. However, the accompanying symptoms of sympathetic stimulation are gone, and the pressure returns to normal over the next few weeks. If the blood pressure remains elevated but the patient is otherwise asymptomatic, another cause for the elevated blood pressure should be considered. Essential hypertension and renal vascular hypertension have been reported in patients harboring pheochromocytomas. In patients whose tumors secrete little or no excess of catecholamines and who are free of signs and symptoms other than fixed hypertension, tumor removal will not usually eliminate the elevated blood pressure.

D. Long Term Follow-Up: As noted above, the incidence of malignant tumors in reported studies varies from less than 5% to more than 10%. These can be recognized during surgery only when there is significant local infiltration or when metastases are identified. Since 5–10% of patients thought to have been cured later have recurrences, patients should be followed carefully. Patients with extra-adrenal tumors and those whose tumor cells contain increased amounts of nuclear DNA are at higher risk of recurrence and should be screened at regular intervals for many years.

E. Treatment of Malignant Tumors: Patients with nonresectable malignant tumors or metastases or those who for other reasons are not amenable to successful surgical treatment can be managed medically for prolonged periods. Phenoxybenzamine and

Table 11–14. Distribution of metastases in 41 cases of malignant pheochromocytoma.[1]

	Autopsy Cases (n = 26)	Nonautopsy Cases (n = 15)	Percentage
Skeleton	12	6	44
Liver	12	3	37
Lymph node	11	4	37
Lungs	9	2	27
Central nervous system	4	0	10
Pleura	4	0	10
Kidneys	2	0	5
Pancreas	1	0	2
Omentum	1	0	2

[1]Reproduced, with permission, from Schönebeck J: Scand J Urol Nephrol 1969;3:66.

perhaps prazosin can be used chronically as described above. Patients with malignant tumors have also benefited symptomatically from treatment with α-methylmetatyrosine, an inhibitor of tyrosine hydroxylase, the rate-limiting enzyme in the biosynthetic process. Although some patients with malignant pheochromocytomas die early because of disseminated disease, there are long-term survivors. Sites of metastases are shown in Table 11–14. The most common site of metastases is the skeleton, and bone lesions tend to respond well to radiation therapy. The use of combinations of chemotherapeutic agents such as cyclophosphamide, vincristine, and dacarbazine is effective in controlling soft tissue lesions in some patients.

[131]I-labeled metaiodobenzylguanidine has been used in the treatment of malignant pheochromocytomas. Preliminary reports indicate that half of the patients treated have partial remissions and that the side effects of this therapy are acceptable.

REFERENCES

General

Coupland RE: *The Natural History of the Chromaffin Cell.* Longmans, Green, 1965.

Cryer PE: Physiology and pathophysiology of the human sympathoadrenal neuroendocrine system. N Engl J Med 1980;303:436.

Gross MD, Shapiro B: Clinically silent masses. J Clin Endocrinol Metab 1993;77:885.

Liggett S: Functional properties of human β_2-adrenergic receptor polymorphisms. News Physiol Sci 1995; 10:265.

Hormones of the Adrenal Medulla

Ahlquist RP: A study of the adrenotropic receptors. Am J Physiol 1948;153:586.

Axelrod J: The metabolism, storage and release of catecholamines. Recent Prog Horm Res 1965;21:597.

Brown MR, Fisher LA: Brain peptide regulation of adrenal epinephrine secretion. Am J Physiol 1984; 247:E41.

Clutter WE et al: Epinephrine plasma metabolic clearance rates and physiologic thresholds for metabolic and hemodynamic actions in man. J Clin Invest 1980;66:94.

Ganong WF, Reid IA: Role of the sympathetic nervous system and central alpha- and beta-adrenergic receptors in regulation of renin activity. Am J Physiol 1976;230:1733.

Goldfien A: Effects of glucose deprivation on the sympathetic outflow to the adrenal medulla and adipose tissue. Pharmacol Rev 1966;18:303.

Goldstein DS, Eisenhofer G: Plasma catechols: What do they mean? News Physiol Sci 1988;3:139.Handbook of Psychopharmacology. Section 1, Vol. 3. Plenum Press, 1975.

Kennedy B, Bigby TD, Ziegler MB: Nonadrenal epinephrine-forming enzymes in humans: Characteristics, distribution, regulation, and relationship to epinephrine levels. J Clin Invest 1995;95:2896.

Mannelli M et al: Endogenous dopamine (DA) and DA2 receptors: A mechanism limiting excessive sympathetic-adrenal discharge in humans. J Clin Endocrinol Metab 1988;66:626.

Murray E et al: Determination of norepinephrine apparent release rate and clearance in humans. Life Sci 1979;25:1461.

Robertson D et al: Use of alpha$_2$ adrenoceptor agonists and antagonists in the functional assessment of the sympathetic nervous system. J Clin Invest 1986;78:576.

Satoh F et al: Adrenomedullin in human brain, adrenal glands, and tumor tissues of pheochromocytoma, ganglioneuroblastoma, and neuroblastoma. J Clin Endocrinol Metab 1995;80:1750.

Shimosawa T et al: Proadrenomedullin NH$_2$-terminal 20 peptide, a new product of the adrenomedullin gene, inhibits norepinephrine overflow from nerve endings. J Clin Invest 1995;96:1672.

Simon JP, Bader MF, Aunis D: Secretion from chromaffin cells is controlled by chromogranin A-derived peptides. Proc Natl Acad Sci USA 1988;85:1712.

Trendelenburg U, Weiner N (editors): Catecholamines. Vol 90 of Handbook of Experimental Pharmacology. Springer-Verlag, 1988. Annu Rev Pharmacol 1970;10:273.

Woods SC, Porte D Jr: Neural control of the endocrine pancreas. Physiol Rev 1974;54:596.

Disorders of Adrenal Medullary Function; Pheochromocytoma

Auerbach SD et al: Malignant pheochromocytoma: Effective treatment with a combination of cyclophosphamide, vincristine, and dacarbazine. Ann Intern Med 1988;109:267.

Beldjord C et al: The RET protooncogene in sporadic pheochromocytomas: Frequent MEN 2-like mutations and new molecular defects. J Clin Endocrinol Metab 1995;80:2063.

Cornelis JM et al: Clinical screening as compared with DNA analysis in families with multiple endocrine neoplasia type 2A. N Engl J Med 1994;331:828.

Engelman K, Sjoerdsma A: Chronic medical therapy for pheochromocytoma. Ann Intern Med 1964;61:229.

Freier DT, Thompson NW: Pheochromocytoma and pregnancy: The epitome of high risk. Surgery 1993;114:1148.

Gagel RF et al: The clinical outcome of prospective screening for multiple endocrine neoplasia type 2a: An 18-year experience. N Engl J Med 1988;318:478.

Goldfien A: Pheochromocytoma: Diagnosis and anesthetic and surgical management. Anesthesiology 1963;24:462.

Goldstein DS: Plasma norepinephrine in essential hypertension. Hypertension 1981;3:48.

Griffing GT: A-I-D-S: The new endocrine epidemic. J Clin Endocrinol Metab 1994;79:1530.

Hosaka Y et al: Pheochromocytoma: Nuclear DNA patterns studied by flow cytometry. Surgery 1986;100:1003.

Krempf M et al: Use of m-[^{131}I]iodobenzylguanidine in the treatment of malignant pheochromocytoma. J Clin Endocrinol Metab 1991;72:455.

Landsberg L: Catecholamines and hyperthyroidism. Clin Endocrinol Metab 1977;6:697.

Ledger GA et al: Genetic testing in the diagnosis and management of multiple endocrine neoplasia type II. Ann Intern Med 1995;122:218.

Lindor NM et al: Mutations in the RET protooncogene in sporadic pheochromocytomas. J Clin Endocrinol Metab 1995;80:627.

Manger WM, Gifford RW: Pheochromocytoma. Springer, 1977.

Modlin IM et al: Pheochromocytomas in 72 patients: Clinical and diagnostic features, treatment and long-term results. Br J Surg 1979;66:456.

Ponder BA, Jackson CE (editors): The second international workshop on multiple endocrine neoplasia type 2 syndromes. Henry Ford Hosp Med J 1987;35:1. [Entire 2 issues.]

Proye C et al: Dopamine-secreting pheochromocytoma: An unrecognized entity. Classification of pheochromocytomas according to their type of secretion. Surgery 1986;100:1154.

Ross NS, Aron DC: Hormonal evaluation of the patient with an incidentally discovered adrenal mass. N Engl J Med 1990;323:1401.

Schenker JG, Chowers U: Pheochromocytoma and pregnancy: Review of 89 cases. Obstet Gynecol Surv 1971;26:739.

Shapiro B et al: Iodine-131 metaiodobenzylguanidine for the locating of suspected pheochromocytoma: Experience in 400 cases. J Nucl Med 1985;26:576.

Sheps SG et al: Recent development in the diagnosis and treatment of pheochromocytoma. Mayo Clin Proc 1990;65:88.

Sisson JC, Wieland DM: Radiolabeled metaiodobenzylguanidine: Pharmacology and clinical studies. Am J Physiol Imaging 1986;1:96.

Sjoerdsma A: Chronic medical therapy for pheochromocytoma. Ann Intern Med 1964;61:229.

Stenström G, Svärdsudd K: Pheochromocytoma in Sweden 1958-1981: An analysis of the National Cancer Registry data. Acta Med Scand 1986;220:225.

Sutton MGSJ, Sheps SG, Lie JT: Prevalence of clinically unsuspected pheochromocytoma: Review of a 50-year autopsy series. Mayo Clin Proc 1981;56:354.

Troncone L et al: The diagnostic and therapeutic utility of radioiodinated metaiodobenzylguanidine (MIBG). Eur J Nucl Med 1990;16:325.

Tsai MS et al: Identification of MEN type 2 gene carriers using linkage analysis and analysis of the RET oncogene. J Clin Endocrinol Metab 1994;78:1261.

Visser J, Axt R: Bilateral adrenal medullary hyperplasia: A clinicopathological entity. J Clin Pathol 1975;28:298.

Yanese T et al: Studies on adrenorphin in pheochromocytoma. J Clin Endocrinol Metab 1987;64:692.

Adrenal Medullary Hypofunction

Robertson D et al: Autonomic insufficiency Isolated failure of autonomic noradrenergic neurotransmission: Evidence for impaired β-hydroxylation of dopamine. N Engl J Med 1986;314:1494.

Schatz IJ: Orthostatic hypotension. Arch Intern Med 1984;144:733.

Testes

12

Glenn D. Braunstein, MD

The testes contain two major components which are structurally separate and serve different functions. The **Leydig cells,** or **interstitial cells,** comprise the major endocrine component. The primary secretory product of these cells, testosterone, is responsible either directly or indirectly for embryonic differentiation along male lines of the external and internal genitalia, male secondary sexual development at puberty, and maintenance of libido and potency in the adult male. The **seminiferous tubules** comprise the bulk of the testes and are responsible for the production of approximately 30 million spermatozoa per day during male reproductive life (puberty to death).

Both of these testicular components are interrelated, and both require an intact hypothalamic-pituitary axis for initiation and maintenance of their function. In addition, several accessory genital structures are required for the functional maturation and transport of spermatozoa. Thus, disorders of the testes, hypothalamus, pituitary, or accessory structures may result in abnormalities of androgen or gamete production, infertility, or a combination of these problems.

ACRONYMS USED IN THIS CHAPTER	
ACTH	Adrenocorticotropic hormone
cAMP	Cyclic adenosine monophosphate
DHEA	Dehydroepiandrosterone
FSH	Follicle-stimulating hormone
GnRH	Gonadotropin-releasing hormone
hCG	Human chorionic gonadotropin
LH	Luteinizing hormone
mRNA	Messenger ribonucleic acid
PRL	Prolactin
SHBG	Sex hormone-binding globulin

ANATOMY & STRUCTURE-FUNCTION RELATIONSHIPS (Figure 12–1)

TESTES

The adult testis is a prolate spheroid with a mean volume of 18.6 ± 4.8 mL. The average length is 4.6 cm (range, 3.6–5.5 cm), and the average width is 2.6 cm (range, 2.1–3.2 cm). The testes are located within the scrotum, which not only serves as a protective envelope but also helps to maintain the testicular temperature approximately 2 °C (3.6 °F) below abdominal temperature. Three layers of membranes— visceral tunica vaginalis, tunica albuginea, and tunica vasculosa—comprise the testicular capsule. Extensions of the tunica albuginea into the testicle as fibrous septa result in the formation of approximately 250 pyramidal lobules each of which contains coiled seminiferous tubules. Within each testis there are almost 200 m of seminiferous tubules, and these structures account for 80–90% of the testicular mass. The approximately 350 million androgen-producing Leydig cells, as well as the blood and lymphatic vessels, nerves, and fibroblasts, are interspersed between the seminiferous tubules.

The blood supply to the testes is derived chiefly from the testicular arteries, which are branches of the internal spermatic arteries. After traversing a complicated capillary network, blood enters multiple testicular veins that form an anastomotic network, the pampiniform plexus. The pampiniform plexuses coalesce to form the internal spermatic veins. The right spermatic vein drains directly into the vena cava; the left enters the renal vein.

The seminiferous tubules in the adult average 165 μm in diameter and are composed of Sertoli cells and germinal cells. The Sertoli cells line the basement membrane and form tight junctions with other Sertoli cells. These tight junctions prevent the passage of

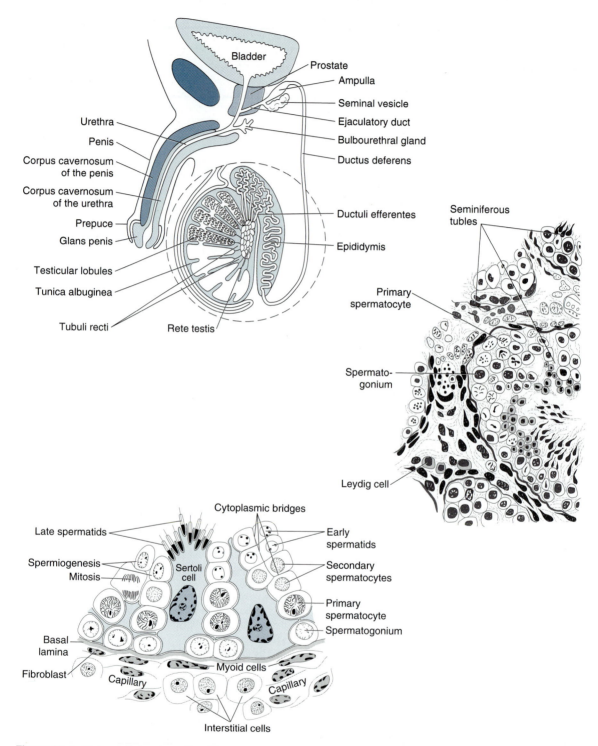

Figure 12–1. Male genital system. **Top:** The testis and the epididymis are in different scales from the other parts of the reproductive system. Observe the communication between the testicular lobules. **Bottom:** Structural organization of the human seminiferous tubule and interstitial tissue. This figure does not show the lymphatic vessels frequently found in the connective tissue. (Both illustrations reproduced, with permission, from Junqueira LC, Carneiro J, Kelley RO: *Basic Histology,* 7th ed. Appleton & Lange, 1992.) At right: Section of human testis. (Reproduced, with permission, from Ganong WF: *Review of Medical Physiology,* 15th ed. Appleton & Lange, 1991.)

proteins from the interstitial space into the lumen of the seminiferous tubules, thus establishing a "blood-testis barrier." Through extension of cytoplasmic processes, the Sertoli cells surround developing germ cells and provide an environment essential for germ cell differentiation. In addition, these cells have been shown to be responsible for the movement of germ cells from the base of the tubule toward the lumen and for the release of mature sperm into the lumen. These cells also actively phagocytose damaged germ cells and residual bodies, which are portions of the germ cell cytoplasm not used in the formation of spermatozoa. Finally, in response to follicle-stimulating hormone (FSH) or testosterone, the Sertoli cells secrete androgen-binding protein, a molecule with high affinity for androgens. This substance, which enters the tubular lumen, provides a high concentration of testosterone to the developing germinal cells during the process of spermatogenesis.

More than a dozen different types of germ cells have been described in males. Broadly, they can be classified as spermatogonia, primary spermatocytes, secondary spermatocytes, spermatids, and spermatozoa. Spermatogenesis occurs in an orderly fashion, with the spermatocytes being derived from the spermatogonia via mitotic division. Through meiotic (or reduction) division, the spermatids are formed; they contain a haploid number of chromosomes (23). The interval from the beginning of spermatogenesis to release of mature spermatozoa into the tubular lumen is approximately 74 days. Although there is little variation in the duration of the spermatogenic cycle, a cross section of a seminiferous tubule will demonstrate several stages of germ cell development.

ACCESSORY STRUCTURES

The seminiferous tubules empty into a highly convoluted anastomotic network of ducts called the rete testis. Spermatozoa are then transported through efferent ductules and into a single duct, the epididymis, by testicular fluid pressure, ciliary motion, and contraction of the efferent ductules. During the approximately 12 days required for transit through the epididymis, spermatozoa undergo morphologic and functional changes essential to confer upon the gametes the capacity for fertilizing an ovum. The epididymis also serves as a reservoir for sperm. Spermatozoa stored in the epididymis enter the vas deferens, a muscular duct 35–50 cm long that propels its contents by peristaltic motion into the ejaculatory duct.

In addition to the spermatozoa and the secretory products of the testes, retia testis, and epididymides, the ejaculatory ducts receive fluid from the seminal vesicles. These paired structures, 10–20 cm long, are composed of alveolar glands, connective tissue, and muscle. They are the source of seminal plasma fructose, which provides nourishment to the spermatozoa. In addition, the seminal vesicles secrete phosphorylcholine, ergothioneine, ascorbic acid, flavins, and prostaglandins. About 60% of the total volume of seminal fluid is derived from the seminal vesicles.

The ejaculatory ducts terminate in the prostatic urethra. There additional fluid (approximately 20% of total volume) is added by the prostate, a tubuloalveolar gland with a fibromuscular stroma that weighs about 20 g and measures 4 × 2 × 3 cm. The constituents of the prostate fluid include spermine, citric acid, cholesterol, phospholipids, fibrinolysin, fibrinogenase, zinc, acid phosphatase, and prostate-specific antigen, a 34-kDa kallikrein-like serine protease. Fluid is also added to the seminal plasma by the bulbourethral (Cowper) glands and urethral (Littre) glands during its transit through the penile urethra.

PHYSIOLOGY OF THE MALE REPRODUCTIVE SYSTEM

GONADAL STEROIDS (Figure 12–2)

The three steroids of primary importance in male reproductive function are testosterone, dihydrotestosterone, and estradiol. From a quantitative standpoint, the most important androgen is testosterone. Over 95% of the testosterone is secreted by the testicular Leydig cells; the remainder is derived from the adrenals. In addition to testosterone, the testes secrete small amounts of the potent androgen dihydrotestosterone and the weak androgens dehydroepiandrosterone (DHEA) and androstenedione. The Leydig cells also secrete small quantities of estradiol, estrone, pregnenolone, progesterone, 17α-hydroxypregnenolone, and 17α-hydroxyprogesterone. The steps in testicular androgen biosynthesis are illustrated in Figure 12–2.

Dihydrotestosterone and estradiol are derived not only by direct secretion from the testes but also by conversion in peripheral tissues of androgen and estrogen precursors secreted by both the testes and the adrenals. Thus, about 80% of the circulating concentrations of these two steroids is derived from such peripheral conversion. Table 12–1 summarizes the approximate contributions of the testes, adrenals, and peripheral tissues to the circulating levels of several sex steroid hormones in men.

In the blood, androgens and estrogens exist in either a free (unbound) state or bound to serum proteins. Although about 38% of testosterone is bound to albumin, the major binding protein is sex hor-

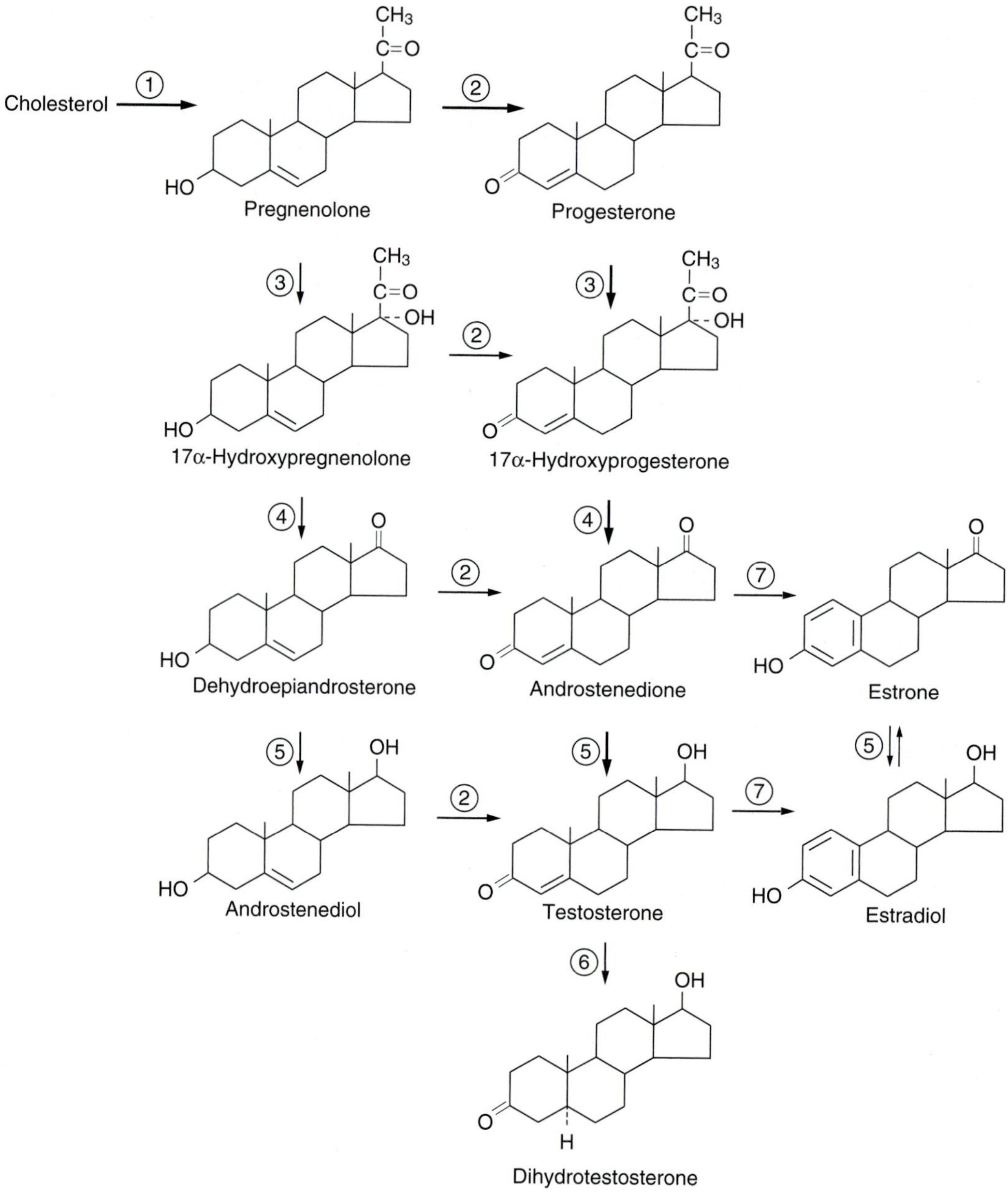

Figure 12–2. Pathways for testicular androgen and estrogen biosynthesis. Heavy arrows indicate major pathways. Circled numbers represent enzymes as follows: ①, 20,22-desmolase (P-450scc); ②, 3β-hydroxysteroid dehydrogenase and Δ^5,Δ^4-isomerase; ③, 17-hydroxylase (P-450c17); ④, 17,20-desmolase (P-450c17); ⑤, 17-ketoreductase; ⑥, 5α-reductase; ⑦, aromatase. (See also Figures 9–4, 13–4, and 14–13.)

mone-binding globulin (SHBG), which binds 60% of the testosterone. This glycosylated dimeric protein is homologous to, yet distinct from, the androgen-binding protein secreted by the Sertoli cells. SHBG is synthesized in the liver, with the gene located on the short arm of chromosome 17. The serum concentra-

tions of this protein are increased by estrogen, tamoxifen, phenytoin, or thyroid hormone administration and by hyperthyroidism and cirrhosis and are decreased by exogenous androgens, glucocorticoids, or growth hormone and by hypothyroidism, acromegaly, and obesity. About 2% of the circulating testosterone

Table 12–1. Relative contributions (approximate percentages) of the testes, adrenals, and peripheral tissues to circulating levels of sex steroids in men.

	Testicular Secretion	Adrenal Secretion	Peripheral Conversion of Precursors
Testosterone	95	< 1	< 5
Dihydrotestosterone	20	< 1	80
Estradiol	20	< 1	80
Estrone	2	< 1	98
DHEA sulfate	< 10	90	...

is not bound to serum proteins and is able to enter cells and exert its metabolic effects. In addition, some of the protein-bound testosterone may dissociate from the protein and enter target tissues; thus, the amount of bioavailable testosterone may be greater than just the amount of non-protein-bound testosterone.

As noted below, testosterone may be converted to dihydrotestosterone within specific androgen target tissues. Most circulating testosterone is converted primarily by the liver into various metabolites such as androsterone and etiocholanolone, which, after conjugation with glucuronic or sulfuric acid, are excreted in the urine as 17-ketosteroids. However, it should be noted that only 20–30% of the urinary 17-ketosteroids are derived from testosterone metabolism. The majority of the 17-ketosteroids are formed from the metabolism of adrenal steroids. Therefore, 17-ketosteroid determinations do not reliably reflect testicular steroid secretion.

Testosterone leaves the circulation and rapidly traverses the cell membrane (Figure 12–3). In most androgen target cells, testosterone is enzymatically converted to the more potent androgen dihydrotestosterone by the microsomal isoenzyme 5α-reductase-2, which has a pH optimum of 5.5. Another isoenzyme, 5α-reductase-1, has a pH optimum near 8.0 and may involve androgen action in the skin, but it is not active in the urogenital tract. Dihydrotestosterone as well as testosterone then binds to the same specific intracellular receptor protein (R_c in Figure 12–3) that is distinct from both androgen-binding protein and SHBG. The genes that encode for this protein are located on the X chromosome. The androgen receptor, a phosphoprotein of about 110 kDa, is a member of the steroid-thyroid hormone nuclear superfamily. It is synthesized in the cytoplasm and is associated with several heat shock proteins. When testosterone or dihydrotestosterone binds to the carboxyl terminal androgen-binding portion of the receptor, the heat shock proteins dissociate and conformational changes in the receptor take place that allow it to be translocated into the nucleus (R_n in Figure 12–3). Some studies suggest that androgen binding to the receptor takes place only in the nucleus and not in the

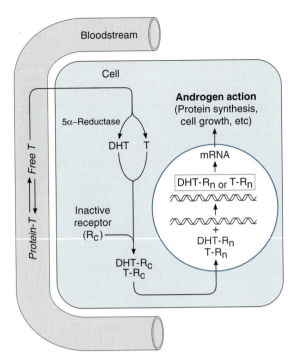

Figure 12–3. Mechanisms of androgen action. (T, testosterone; DHT, dihydrotestosterone; R_n, activated nuclear receptor; mRNA, messenger RNA; R_c, inactive receptor.)

cytoplasm. In the nucleus, the androgen-androgen receptor complex binds to DNA through the DNA-binding domain of the receptor, which allows the polymorphic transactivating amino terminal portion of the receptor to initiate transcriptional activity. This results in the synthesis of messenger RNA (mRNA), which is eventually transported to the cytoplasm, where it directs new protein synthesis and other changes that together constitute androgen action.

A variety of biologic effects of androgens have been defined in males. As discussed in Chapter 14, they are essential for appropriate differentiation of the internal and external male genital system during fetal development. During puberty, androgen-mediated growth of the scrotum, epididymis, vas deferens, seminal vesicles, prostate, and penis occurs. The functional integrity of these organs requires androgens. Androgens stimulate skeletal muscle growth and growth of the larynx, which results in deepening of the voice; and of the epiphysial cartilaginous plates, which results in the pubertal growth spurt. Both ambisexual (pubic and axillary) hair growth and sexual (beard, mustache, chest, abdomen, and back) hair growth are stimulated, as is sebaceous gland activity. Other effects include stimulation of erythropoiesis and social behavioral changes.

CONTROL OF TESTICULAR FUNCTION

Hypothalamic-Pituitary-Leydig Cell Axis (Figure 12–4)

The hypothalamus synthesizes a decapeptide, gonadotropin-releasing hormone (GnRH), and secretes it in pulses every 90–120 minutes into the hypothalamohypophysial portal blood. After reaching the anterior pituitary, GnRH binds to the gonadotrophs and stimulates the release of both luteinizing hormone (LH) and, to a lesser extent, FSH into the general circulation. LH is taken up by the Leydig cells, where it binds to specific membrane receptors. The LH receptor is a G protein-coupled receptor containing seven transmembrane domains with a serine and threonine-rich cytoplasmic region containing a phosphorylation site and a 350- to 400-amino-acid extracellular hormone-binding domain. The binding of LH to the receptor leads to activation of adenylyl cyclase and generation of cAMP and other messengers that ultimately result in the secretion of androgens. In turn, the elevation of androgens inhibits the secretion of LH from the anterior pituitary through a direct action on the pituitary and an inhibitory effect at the hypothalamic level. Both the hypothalamus and the pituitary have androgen and estrogen receptors. Experimentally, pure androgens such as dihydrotestosterone (DHT) reduce LH pulse frequency, while estradiol reduces LH pulse amplitude. However, the major inhibitory effect of androgen on the hypothalamus appears to be mediated principally by estradiol, which may be derived locally through the aromatization of testosterone. Leydig cells also secrete small quantities of oxytocin, renin, insulin-like growth factor I, transforming growth factors α and β, interleukin-1, lipotropin, β-endorphin, dynorphin, angiotensin, and prostaglandins, which may be important for paracrine regulation of testicular function.

Hypothalamic-Pituitary-Seminiferous Tubular Axis (Figure 12–4)

After stimulation by GnRH, the gonadotrophs secrete FSH into the systemic circulation. This glycoprotein hormone binds to specific receptors in the Sertoli cells and stimulates the production of androgen-binding protein. FSH is necessary for the initiation of spermatogenesis. However, full maturation of the spermatozoa appears to require not only an FSH effect but also testosterone. Indeed, the major action of FSH on spermatogenesis may be via the stimulation of androgen-binding protein production, which allows a high intratubular concentration of testosterone to be maintained.

In addition to androgen-binding protein, the Sertoli cell secretes several other substances including GnRH-like peptide, transferrin, plasminogen activator, ceruloplasmin, müllerian duct inhibitory factor, H-Y antigen, and inhibin. At least three genes have been found to direct inhibin synthesis. Two forms of inhibin have been identified, inhibin A and inhibin B. Both are 32-kDa proteins composed of the same alpha subunit cross-linked with different beta subunits, and each can selectively inhibit FSH release from the pituitary without affecting LH release. FSH directly stimulates the Sertoli cells to secrete inhibin, and therefore inhibin is probably a physiologic regulator of pituitary FSH secretion, possibly together with the gonadal steroids. Inhibin levels decline with advancing age.

Two additional inhibin-related proteins that have been identified in porcine follicular fluid may also be present in the testes. These factors, designated follicle regulatory protein and activin, are composed of

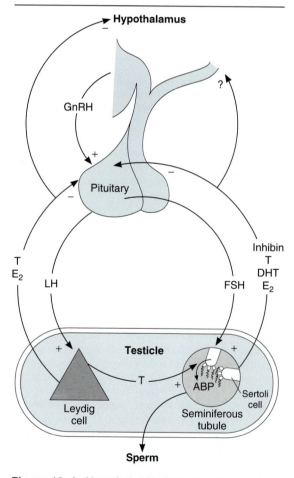

Figure 12–4. Hypothalamic-pituitary-testicular axis. (GnRH, gonadotropin-releasing hormone; LH, luteinizing hormone; FSH, follicle-stimulating hormone; T, testosterone; DHT, dihydrotestosterone; ABP, androgen-binding protein; E_2, estradiol; +, positive influence; –, negative influence.)

inhibin beta subunit dimers and can selectively stimulate pituitary FSH secretion in vitro. They are structurally similar to transforming growth factor-β (TGFβ), which can also stimulate pituitary FSH release. The physiologic role, if any, that follicle regulatory protein, activin, and TGFβ have in the regulation of FSH secretion is unknown.

EVALUATION OF MALE GONADAL FUNCTION

CLINICAL EVALUATION

Clinical Presentation

The clinical presentation of patients with deficient testosterone production or action depends upon the age at onset of hypogonadism. Androgen deficiency during the second to third months of fetal development results in varying degrees of ambiguity of the genitalia and male pseudohermaphroditism. If the deficiency develops during the third trimester, defects in testicular descent leading to cryptorchidism as well as micropenis may occur. These topics are covered in Chapters 14 and 15.

Prepubertal androgen deficiency leads to poor secondary sexual development and eunuchoid skeletal proportions. The penis fails to enlarge, the testes remain small, and the scrotum does not develop the marked rugae characteristic of puberty. The voice remains high-pitched and the muscle mass does not develop fully, resulting in less than normal strength and endurance. The lack of appropriate stimulation of sexual hair growth results in sparse axillary and pubic hair (which receive some stimulation from adrenal androgens) and absent or very sparse facial, chest, upper abdominal, and back hair. Although the androgen-mediated pubertal growth spurt will fail to take place, the epiphysial plates of the long bones will continue to grow under the influence of insulin-like growth factor-I and other growth factors. Thus, the long bones of the upper and lower extremities will grow out of proportion to the axial skeleton. Healthy white men have an average upper segment (crown to pubis) to lower segment (pubis to floor) ratio of >1, whereas prepubertal hypogonadism results in a ratio of <1. Similarly, the ratio of total arm span to total height averages 0.96 in white men. Because of the relatively greater growth in the upper extremities, the arm span of eunuchoid individuals exceeds height by 5 cm or more.

If testosterone deficiency develops after puberty, the patient may complain of decreased libido, impotence, and low energy. Patients with mild androgen deficiency or androgen deficiency of recent onset may not note a decrease in facial or body hair growth; it appears that although adult androgen levels must be achieved to *stimulate* male sexual hair growth, relatively low levels of androgens are required to *maintain* sexual hair growth. With longstanding hypogonadism, the growth of facial hair will diminish, and the frequency of shaving may also decrease (Figure 12–5). In addition, fine wrinkles may appear in the corners of the mouth and eyes and, together with the sparse beard growth, result in the classic hypogonadal facies.

Genital Examination

Adequate assessment of the genitalia is essential in the evaluation of male hypogonadism. The examination should be performed in a warm room in order to relax the dartos muscle of the scrotum. The penis should be examined for the presence of hypospadias, epispadias, and chordee (abnormal angulation of the penis due to a fibrotic plaque), which may interfere with fertility. The fully stretched dorsal penile length should be measured in the flaccid state from the pubopenile skin junction to the tip of the glans. The normal range in adults is 11–16 cm (10th and 90th percentiles, respectively).

Assessment of testicular volume is also vital to the evaluation of hypogonadism. Careful measurement of the longitudinal and transverse axes of the testes may be made and testicular volume (V) calculated from the formula for a prolate spheroid: $V = 0.52 \times \text{length} \times \text{width}^2$. The mean volume for an adult testis is 18.6 ± 4.8 mL. Alternatively, volume may be estimated with the Prader orchidometer, which consists of a series of plastic ellipsoids ranging in volume from 1 mL to 25 mL (Figure 12–6). Each testis is compared with the appropriate ellipsoid. Adults normally have volumes greater than 15 mL by this method.

Since 80–90% of testicular volume is composed of seminiferous tubules, decrease in volume indicates lack of tubular development or regression of tubular size. The consistency of the testicle should be noted. Small, firm testes are characteristic of hyalinization or fibrosis, as may occur in Klinefelter's syndrome. Small, rubbery testes are normally found in prepubertal males; in an adult, they are indicative of deficient gonadotropin stimulation. Testes with a mushy or soft consistency are characteristically found in individuals with postpubertal testicular atrophy.

The epididymis and vas deferens should also be examined. One of the most important parts of the examination is evaluation of the presence of varicocele resulting from incompetence of the internal spermatic vein. As will be discussed later, this is an important and potentially correctable cause of male infertility. The patient should be examined in the upright position while performing the Valsalva maneuver. The examiner should carefully palpate the spermatic cords above the testes. A varicocele can be felt

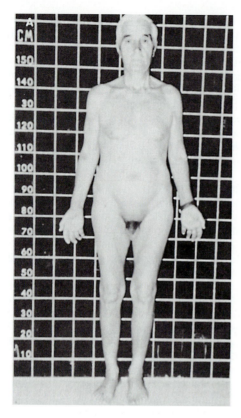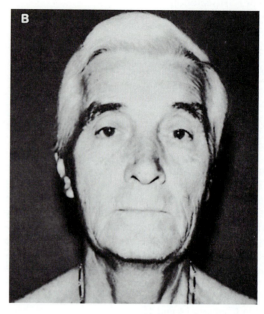

Figure 12–5. *A:* Hypogonadal habitus. Note absence of body and facial hair as well as feminine body distribution. ***B:*** Hypogonadal facies. Note absence of facial hair and fine wrinkles around the corners of the eyes and lips.

as an impulse along the posterior portion of the cord. About 85% of varicoceles are located on the left side, and 15% are bilateral.

LABORATORY TESTS OF TESTICULAR FUNCTION

Semen Analysis

With some exceptions, a normal semen analysis excludes gonadal dysfunction. However, a single abnormal semen analysis is not a sufficient basis for a diagnosis of disturbance of testicular function, since marked variations in several of the parameters may be seen in normal individuals: At least three semen samples must be examined over a 2- to 3-month interval in order to evaluate this facet of male gonadal function. As noted above, approximately 3 months are required for completion of the spermatogenic cycle and movement of the mature spermatozoa through the ductal system. Therefore, when an abnormal semen sample is produced, one must question the patient about prior fever, trauma, drug exposure, and other factors that may temporarily damage spermatogenesis.

The semen should be collected by masturbation after 1–3 days of sexual abstinence. If the patient will not masturbate, a specially designed plastic condom (Mylex Corporation, Chicago) can be used during intercourse. Ordinary condoms cannot be used for this purpose, since they contain spermicidal chemicals. If neither of these methods is satisfactory, coitus interruptus may be used as long as the complete ejaculate is collected. It should be stressed to the patient that the highest concentration of spermatozoa is in the first portion of the ejaculate and that this is the portion most often lost as a result of coitus interruptus.

The specimen should be examined within 2 hours after collection. Normal semen has a volume of 2–5 mL, with 20×10^6 or more sperm per milliliter. Over half of the spermatozoa should exhibit progressive motility, and 30% or more should have normal morphology.

Steroid Measurements

Each of the gonadal steroids may be measured by radioimmunoassay. Although single determinations may distinguish between normal individuals and patients with severe hypogonadism, mild defects in an-

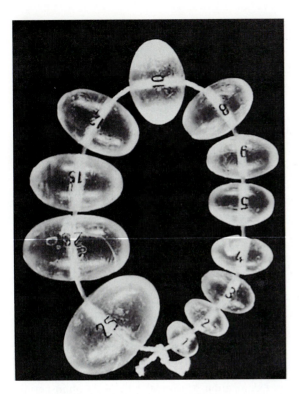

Figure 12–6. Prader orchidometer.

Table 12–2. Normal ranges for gonadal steroids, pituitary gonadotropins, and prolactin in men.

	Ranges
Testosterone, total	300–1100 ng/dL (10.4–38.2 nmol/L)
Testosterone, free	50–210 pg/mL (173–729 pmol/L)
Dihydrotestosterone	27–75 ng/dL (0.9–2.6 nmol/L)
Androstenedione	50–200 ng/dL (1.7–6.9 nmol/L)
Estradiol	15–40 pg/mL (55–150 pmol/L)
Estrone	15–65 pg/mL (55.5–240 pmol/L)
FSH	2–15 mIU/mL (2–15 IU/L)
LH	2–15 mIU/mL (2–15 IU/L)
PRL	4–18 ng/mL (4–18 µg/L)

drogen production may be missed. In normal individuals, there are frequent, rapid pulsatile changes in serum testosterone concentration as well as a slight nocturnal elevation. Therefore, at least three separate blood samples should be collected at 20- to 40-minute intervals during the morning for testosterone measurement. The testosterone may be measured in each of the serum samples, or equal aliquots of each of the three serum samples may be combined, mixed, and subjected to testosterone analysis. The latter procedure provides a savings in cost as well as a mean serum testosterone concentration that takes into account the pulsatile release of testosterone.

Androgen and estrogen radioimmunoassays measure total serum steroid concentrations. This is the sum of the free, biologically active hormone and the protein-bound moiety. Although in most circumstances it is not necessary to determine the actual quantity of free steroid hormones, in some situations alterations in the binding protein concentration may occur. Lowered concentrations of SHBG are seen in patients with hypothyroidism, obesity, and acromegaly. In these circumstances, the free testosterone concentration should be directly measured, since it may be normal when the total serum testosterone level is decreased. The normal male serum concentrations of gonadal steroids collected in the basal state are given in Table 12–2.

Gonadotropin & Prolactin Measurements

LH and, to a lesser extent, FSH are released in pulsatile fashion throughout the day. Therefore, as with testosterone, at least three blood samples should be obtained at 20- to 40-minute intervals during the day. FSH and LH may be measured in each of the samples or in a single pooled specimen. Although many laboratories give a numerical value for the lower limits of normal for gonadotropins, some normal males have concentrations of FSH and LH undetectable by presently available radioimmunoassay techniques. Furthermore, the concentrations of gonadotropins measured in one laboratory may not be directly comparable to those measured in another because of differences in the reference preparations used. The primary use of basal FSH and LH concentrations is to distinguish between hypergonadotropic hypogonadism, in which either or both of the gonadotropins are elevated, and hypogonadotropic hypogonadism, in which the gonadotropins are low or inappropriately normal in the presence of decreased androgen production.

Elevations of serum prolactin (PRL) inhibit the normal release of pituitary gonadotropins (shown by a reduced LH pulse frequency), probably through an effect on the hypothalamus. Thus, serum PRL measurements should be performed in any patient with hypogonadotropic hypogonadism. Serum PRL concentrations are generally stable throughout the day; therefore, measurement of this hormone in a single sample is usually sufficient. However, the patient should abstain from eating for 3 hours before the blood sample is obtained, since a protein meal may acutely stimulate the release of PRL from the pituitary. The normal ranges for serum PRL and gonadotropins are shown in Table 12–2.

Dynamic Tests

A. Chorionic Gonadotropin Stimulation Test: Human chorionic gonadotropin (hCG) is a glycoprotein hormone with biologic actions similar to those of LH. Following an injection of chorionic gonadotropin, this hormone binds to the LH receptors on the Leydig cells and stimulates the synthesis and secretion of testicular steroids. Therefore, the Leydig cells may be directly assessed by the intramuscular injection of 4000 IU of chorionic gonadotropin daily for 4 days. A normal response is a doubling of the testosterone level following the last injection. Alternatively, a single intramuscular dose of chorionic gonadotropin (5000 IU/1.7 m^2 in adults or 100 IU/kg in children) may be given, with blood samples taken for testosterone measurements 72 and 96 hours later. Patients with primary gonadal disease will have a diminished response following administration of chorionic gonadotropin, while patients with Leydig cell failure secondary to pituitary or hypothalamic disease will have a qualitatively normal response.

B. Clomiphene Citrate Stimulation Test: Clomiphene citrate is a nonsteroid compound with weak estrogenic activity. It binds to estrogen receptors in various tissues, including the hypothalamus. By preventing the more potent estrogen estradiol from occupying these receptors, the hypothalamus in effect "sees" less estradiol. As noted above, most if not all of the hypothalamic-pituitary feedback control by testicular androgens is mediated by estradiol, which is derived from the peripheral conversion of androgens. The apparent estradiol deficiency leads to an increase of GnRH release the net result of which is stimulation of the gonadotrophs to secrete increased quantities of LH and FSH.

The test is performed by giving clomiphene citrate, 100 mg orally twice daily for 10 days. Three blood samples are collected at 20-minute intervals (see comments above, under Steroid Measurements) 1 day before the drug is administered and again on days 9 and 10 of drug administration. LH, FSH, and testosterone should be measured in pooled aliquots from each of these samples. Healthy men have a 50–250% increase in LH, a 30–200% increase in FSH, and a 30–220% increase in testosterone on day 10 of the test. Patients with pituitary or hypothalamic disease do not show a normal increment in LH or FSH.

C. Gonadotropin-Releasing Hormone Test: The decapeptide GnRH (gonadorelin; Factrel) directly stimulates the gonadotrophs of the anterior pituitary to secrete LH and FSH. It was expected that measurement of LH and FSH following the administration of GnRH would be useful in distinguishing between hypothalamic and pituitary lesions, but this has not proved to be the case. Patients with destructive lesions of the pituitary and those with longstanding hypogonadism due to hypothalamic disorders may not show a response to a GnRH test. However, if the releasing factor is administered by repeated injections every 60–120 minutes or by a programmable pulsatile infusion pump for 7–14 days, patients with hypothalamic lesions may have their pituitary responsiveness to GnRH restored, whereas patients with pituitary insufficiency do not. Conversely, a normal LH and FSH response to GnRH in a hypogonadal male does not eliminate hypopituitarism as the cause of the gonadal failure, since patients with mild hypogonadotropic hypogonadism may demonstrate a normal response.

The test is performed by administering 100 µg of gonadorelin by rapid intravenous bolus. Blood is drawn at −15, 0, 15, 30, 45, 60, 90, 120, and 180 minutes for LH and FSH measurements. Normal adult males have a two- to fivefold increase in LH over baseline concentrations and an approximately twofold rise of FSH. However, some normal males fail to have an increase in FSH following GnRH. Patients with primary testicular disease may respond with exaggerated increases in LH and FSH. If seminiferous tubule damage alone is present, abnormal FSH rise and normal LH response may be seen.

Testicular Biopsy

Testicular biopsy in hypogonadal men is primarily indicated in patients with normal-sized testes and azoospermia in order to distinguish spermatogenic failure and ductal obstruction. Although germinal aplasia, hypoplasia, maturation arrest, and other abnormalities of spermatogenesis may be diagnosed by examination of testicular tissue in oligospermic males, knowledge of the type of defect does not alter therapy. Therefore, testicular biopsy is not usually indicted for evaluation of mild to moderate oligospermia.

Evaluation for Male Hypogonadism

Figure 12–7 outlines an approach to the diagnosis of male gonadal disorders. Semen analysis and determination of the basal concentrations of testosterone, FSH, and LH allow the clinician to distinguish patients with primary gonadal failure who have poor semen characteristics, low or normal testosterone, and elevated FSH or LH from those with secondary gonadal failure and abnormal semen analysis, decreased testosterone, and low or inappropriately normal gonadotropins.

In patients with elevations of gonadotropins resulting from primary testicular disease, chromosomal analysis will help to differentiate between genetic abnormalities and acquired testicular defects. Since no therapy exists that will restore spermatogenesis in an individual with severe testicular damage, androgen replacement is the treatment of choice. Patients with isolated seminiferous tubule failure may have normal or elevated FSH concentrations in association with normal LH and testosterone levels and usually severe oligospermia. Patients with azoospermia require evaluation for the possible presence of ductal obstruction, since this defect may be surgically correctable. Fructose is added to seminal plasma by the seminal vesicles, and an absence of fructose indicates

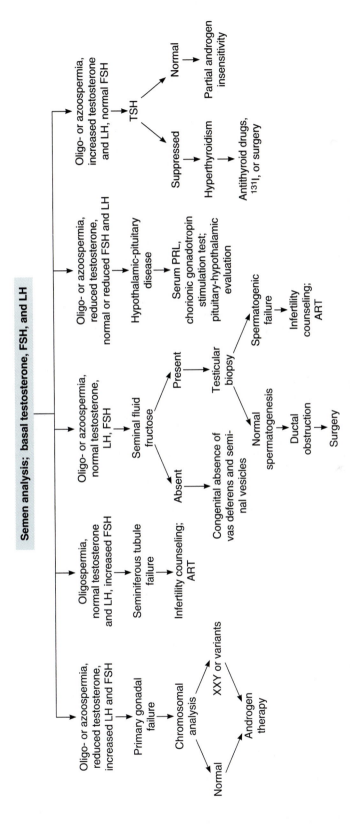

Figure 12–7. Scheme for evaluation of clinical hypogonadism. (ART, assisted reproductive technologies such as in vitro fertilization and sperm injection into ova.)

that the seminal vesicles are absent or bilaterally obstructed. The combination of a poor semen analysis with low testosterone, FSH, and LH is indicative of a hypothalamic or pituitary defect. Such patients need further evaluation of anterior and posterior pituitary gland function with appropriate pituitary function tests, as well as neuroradiologic and neuro-ophthalmologic studies (Chapter 5).

PHARMACOLOGY OF DRUGS USED TO TREAT MALE GONADAL DISORDERS

ANDROGENS

A variety of drugs are available for the treatment of androgen deficiency. Preparations for sublingual or oral administration such as methyltestosterone, oxymetholone, and fluoxymesterone have the advantage of ease of administration but the disadvantage of erratic absorption, potential for cholestatic jaundice, and decreased effectiveness when compared to the intramuscular preparations. Testosterone propionate is a short-acting androgen. Its main use is in initiating therapy in older men, whose prostate glands may be exquisitely sensitive to testosterone. A dose of 50 mg two or three times per week is adequate. Obstructive symptoms due to benign prostatic hypertrophy following therapy with this androgen usually resolve rapidly because of its short duration of action.

Androgen deficiency is usually treated with testosterone enanthate or cyclopentylpropionate (cypionate) given intramuscularly. The duration of action of these preparations is usually 2 weeks, although some patients note an effect for up to 4 weeks. Unlike the oral androgen preparations, both of these agents are capable of completely virilizing the patients. Therapy may be initiated with 200 mg intramuscularly every 1–2 weeks for 1–2 years. After adequate virilization has been achieved, the androgen effect may be maintained by doses of 100–200 mg every 2–3 weeks (average wholesale price about $100 per year). Testosterone pellets may be implanted subcutaneously for a longer duration of effect. However, this therapy has not enjoyed much popularity. Transdermal delivery via membranes impregnated with testosterone is a new method of replacement therapy. One variety (Testoderm, Alza Pharmaceuticals) is placed on the scrotum. The patches, which are replaced daily, provide physiologic levels of testosterone that closely mimic the normal diurnal testosterone fluctuation. Elevated serum concentrations of dihydrotestosterone—a finding of unknown clinical significance—have been noted in patients using these patches. Another type of transdermal delivery system (Androderm, Smith-Kline Beecham Pharmaceuticals) can be placed on the skin of the back, shoulder, or abdomen and provides normal androgen concentrations without elevation in dihydrotestosterone.

Androgens, both oral and intramuscular, have been used (illegally) by some athletes to increase muscle mass and strength. Although this may achieve the anticipated result in some individuals, adverse effects include oligospermia and testicular atrophy—in addition to some of the complications noted below.

Androgen therapy is contraindicated in patients with prostatic carcinoma. About 1–2% of patients receiving oral methyltestosterone or fluoxymesterone develop intrahepatic cholestatic jaundice that resolves when the drug is discontinued. Rarely, these methylated or halogenated androgens have been associated with benign and malignant hepatocellular tumors.

Androgen therapy may also cause premature fusion of the epiphyses in an adolescent, and this may result in some loss of potential height. Therefore, androgen therapy is usually withheld until a hypogonadal male reaches 13 years of age. Water retention may be associated with hypertension or congestive heart failure in susceptible individuals. Since androgens stimulate erythropoietin production, erythrocytosis may occur during therapy. This is not usually clinically significant. Inhibition of spermatogenesis is mediated through suppression of gonadotropins by the androgens. Gynecomastia may develop during initiation of androgen therapy but usually resolves with continued administration of the drug. Sleep apnea may be precipitated. Priapism, acne, and aggressive behavior are dose-related adverse effects and generally disappear after reduction of dosage. Androgens decrease the production of thyroxine-binding globulin and corticosteroid-binding globulin by the liver. Therefore, total serum thyroxine and cortisone concentrations may be decreased though the free hormone concentrations remain normal. High-density lipoprotein concentrations may also be reduced.

GONADOTROPINS

In patients with hypogonadism due to inadequate gonadotropin secretion, spermatogenesis and virilization may be induced by exogenous gonadotropin injections. Since the gonadotropins are proteins with short half-lives, they must be administered parenterally two or three times a week.

The expense and inconvenience of this type of therapy preclude its routine use for the treatment of androgen deficiency. The two major indications for exogenous gonadotropins are treatment of cryptorchidism (see below) and induction of spermatogenesis in hypogonadal males who wish to father children.

To induce spermatogenesis, 2000 IU of chorionic gonadotropin may be given intramuscularly three times a week for 12–18 months (average wholesale price about $800 per year). In some individuals with partial gonadotropin deficiencies, this may induce adequate spermatogenesis. In patients with more severe deficiencies, menotropins (Pergonal), available in bottles containing 75 IU each of FSH and LH, is added to chorionic gonadotropin therapy after 12–18 months and is administered in a dosage of one vial intramuscularly three times a week (average wholesale price about $200 per week).

Adverse reactions with such therapy are minimal. Acne, gynecomastia, or prostatic enlargement may be noted due to excessive Leydig cell stimulation. Reduction of the chorionic gonadotropin dosage or a decrease in the frequency of chorionic gonadotropin injections generally result in resolution of the problem.

GONADOTROPIN-RELEASING HORMONE

GnRH (gonadorelin acetate), administered in pulses every 60–120 minutes by portable infusion pumps, effectively stimulates the endogenous release of LH and FSH in hypogonadotropic hypogonadal patients. This therapy does not currently appear to offer any major advantage over the use of exogenous gonadotropins for induction of spermatogenesis or the use of testosterone enanthate or cypionate for virilization. A long-acting analog of GnRH, leuprolide acetate, is available for the treatment of prostatic carcinoma. Daily subcutaneous administration of 1 mg or monthly intramuscular injections of 7.5 mg of a depot preparation (average wholesale price about $5700 per year) results in desensitization of the pituitary GnRH receptors, which reduces LH and FSH levels and so ultimately testosterone concentrations. Similar results are produced with a 3.6-mg subcutaneous injection of the depot form of the GnRH analog goserelin (average wholesale price about $4300 per year). With these therapies, initial remission rates for prostatic carcinoma are similar to those found with orchiectomy or treatment with diethylstilbestrol (about 70%). In patients with benign prostatic hypertrophy, prostate size has been reduced with this therapy. Another potent intranasally administered GnRH analog, nafarelin acetate, is available for the treatment of endometriosis and central precocious puberty. Central precocious puberty also may be treated with leuprolide acetate and a new analog, histrelin acetate. Long-acting GnRH agonists combined with testosterone have been studied as a possible male contraceptive, but they do not uniformly induce azoospermia.

CLINICAL MALE GONADAL DISORDERS

Hypogonadism may be subdivided into three general categories (Table 12–3). A thorough discussion of the hypothalamic-pituitary disorders that cause hypogonadism is presented in Chapters 5 and 15. The defects in androgen biosynthesis and androgen action are described in Chapter 14. The following section emphasizes the primary gonadal abnormalities.

KLINEFELTER'S SYNDROME (XXY Seminiferous Tubule Dysgenesis)

Klinefelter's syndrome is the most common cause of male hypogonadism. An extra X chromosome is present in about 0.2% of male conceptions and 0.1% of live-born males. Sex chromosome surveys of mentally retarded males have revealed an extra X chromosome in 0.45–2.5% of such individuals. Patients with an XXY genotype have classic Klinefelter's syndrome; those with an XXXY, XXXXY, or XXYY genotype or with XXY/chromosomal mosaicism are considered to have variant forms of the syndrome.

Table 12–3. Classification of male hypogonadism.

Hypothalamic-pituitary disorders
Panhypopituitarism
Isolated LH deficiency (fertile eunuch)
LH and FSH deficiency
  a. With normal sense of smell
  b. With hyposmia or anosmia (Kallmann's syndrome)
Prader-Willi syndrome
Laurence-Moon-Biedl syndrome
Cerebellar ataxia
Biologically inactive LH

Gonadal abnormalities
Klinefelter's syndrome
Other chromosomal defects (XX male, XY/XXY, XX/XXY, XXXY, XXXXY, XXYY, XYY)
Bilateral anorchia (vanishing testes syndrome)
Leydig cell aplasia
Cryptorchidism
Noonan's syndrome
Myotonic dystrophy
Adult seminiferous tubule failure
Adult Leydig cell failure
Defects in androgen biosynthesis

Defects in androgen action
Complete androgen insensitivity (testicular feminization)
Incomplete androgen insensitivity
  a. Type I
  b. Type II (5α-reductase deficiency)

Etiology & Pathophysiology

The XXY genotype is usually due to maternal meiotic nondisjunction, which results in an egg with two X chromosomes. Meiotic nondisjunction during spermatogenesis has also been documented. Both observations correlate positively with the epidemiologic findings that both the mother and the father tend to be older than average at the time of the patient's birth.

At birth there are generally no physical stigmas of Klinefelter's syndrome, and during childhood there are no specific signs or symptoms. The chromosomal defect is expressed chiefly during puberty. As the gonadotropins increase, the seminiferous tubules do not enlarge but rather undergo fibrosis and hyalinization, which results in small, firm testes. Obliteration of the seminiferous tubules results in azoospermia.

In addition to dysgenesis of the seminiferous tubules, the Leydig cells are also abnormal. They are present in clumps and appear to be hyperplastic upon initial examination of a testicular biopsy. However, the Leydig cell mass is not increased, and the apparent hyperplasia is actually due to the marked reduction in tubular volume. Despite the normal mass of tissue, the Leydig cells are functionally abnormal. The testosterone production rate is reduced, and there is a compensatory elevation in serum LH. Stimulation of the Leydig cells with exogenous chorionic gonadotropin results in a subnormal rise in testosterone. The clinical manifestations of androgen deficiency vary considerably from patient to patient. Thus, some individuals have virtually no secondary sexual developmental changes, whereas other are indistinguishable from healthy individuals.

The elevated LH concentrations also stimulate the Leydig cells to secrete increased quantities of estradiol and estradiol precursors. The relatively high estradiol:testosterone ratio is responsible for the variable degrees of feminization and gynecomastia seen in these patients. The elevated estradiol also stimulates the liver to produce SHBG. This may result in total serum testosterone concentrations that are within the low normal range for adult males. However, the free testosterone level may be lower than normal.

The pathogenesis of the eunuchoid proportions, personality, and intellectual deficits and associated medical disorders is presently unclear.

Testicular Pathology

Most of the seminiferous tubules are fibrotic and hyalinized, although occasional Sertoli cells and spermatogonia may be present in some sections. Absence of elastic fibers in the tunica propria is indicative of the dysgenetic nature of the tubules. The Leydig cells are arranged in clumps and appear hyperplastic, although the total mass is normal.

Clinical Features
(Figure 12–8)

A. Symptoms and Signs: There are usually no symptoms before puberty other than poor school performance in some affected individuals. Puberty may be delayed, but not usually by more than 1–2 years. During puberty, the penis and scrotum undergo varying degrees of development, with some individuals appearing normal. Most patients (80%) have diminished facial and torso hair growth. The major complaint is often persistent gynecomastia, which is clinically present in over half of patients. The testes are uniformly small (< 2 cm in longest axis) and firm as a result of fibrosis and hyalinization. Other complaints include infertility or insufficient libido and potency. The patient may have difficulty putting into words his embarrassment in situations where he must disrobe in the presence of other men, and the subnormal development of the external genitalia along with gynecomastia may lead to feelings of inadequacy that may be partly responsible

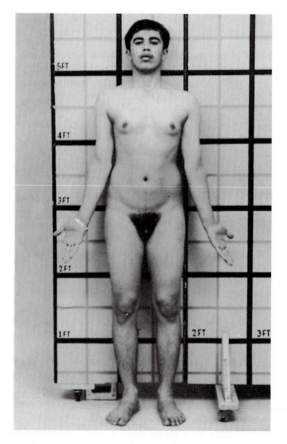

Figure 12–8. Klinefelter's syndrome in a 20-year-old man. Note relatively increased lower/upper body segment ratio, gynecomastia, small penis, and sparse body hair with a female pubic hair pattern.

for the dyssocial behavior some patients exhibit. Osteopenia may be severe in patients with long-standing androgen deficiencies.

Patients with Klinefelter's syndrome have abnormal skeletal proportions that are not truly eunuchoid. Growth of the lower extremities is relatively greater than that of the trunk and upper extremities; therefore, pubis-to-floor height is greater than crown-to-pubis height, and span is less than total height. Thus, the abnormal skeletal proportions are not the result of androgen deficiency per se (which results in span greater than height).

Intellectual impairment is noted in many patients with Klinefelter's syndrome, but the true proportion of affected individuals with subnormal intelligence is not known. Dyssocial behavior is common (see above). Patients generally show want of ambition, difficulties in maintaining permanent employment, and a tendency to ramble in conversations.

Several clinical and genotypic variants of Klinefelter's syndrome have been described. In addition to small testes with seminiferous tubular hyalinization, azoospermia, deficient secondary sexual development, and elevated gonadotropins, patients with three or more X chromosomes uniformly have severe mental retardation. The presence of more than one Y chromosome tends to be associated with aggressive antisocial behavior and macronodular acne. Skeletal deformities such as radioulnar synostosis, flexion deformities of the elbows, and clinodactyly are more commonly seen in Klinefelter variants. Patients with sex chromosome mosaicism (XX/XXY) may have only a few of the Klinefelter stigmas. These patients may have normal testicular size and may be fertile if their testes contain the XY genotype.

Medical disorders found to be associated with Klinefelter's syndrome with greater than chance frequency include chronic pulmonary disease (emphysema, chronic bronchitis), varicose veins, cerebrovascular disease, glucose intolerance, primary hypothyroidism, and a 20-fold increased risk of breast cancer.

B. Laboratory Findings: Serum testosterone is low or normal; FSH and LH concentrations are elevated. Azoospermia is present. The buccal smear is chromatin-positive (>20% of cells having a Barr body), and chromosomal analysis reveals a 47,XXY karyotype.

Differential Diagnosis

Klinefelter's syndrome should be distinguished from other causes of hypogonadism. Small, firm testes should suggest Klinefelter's syndrome. Hypothalamic-pituitary hypogonadism may be associated with small, rubbery testes if puberty has not occurred or atrophic testes if normal puberty has occurred. The consistency of the testes in Klinefelter's syndrome is also different from that noted in acquired forms of

adult seminiferous tubular damage. The elevated gonadotropins place the site of the lesion at the testicular level, and chromosomal analysis confirms the diagnosis. Chromosomal analysis is also required to differentiate classic Klinefelter's syndrome from the variant forms.

Treatment

A. Medical: Androgen deficiency should be treated with testosterone replacement. Patients with personality defects should be virilized gradually to decrease the risk of aggressive behavior. Testosterone enanthate or cypionate, 100 mg intramuscularly, may be given every 2–4 weeks initially and increased to 200 mg every 2 weeks if well tolerated. Patients with low normal androgen levels may not require androgen replacement therapy.

B. Surgical: If gynecomastia presents a cosmetic problem, mastectomy may be performed.

Course & Prognosis

Patients generally feel better after androgen replacement therapy has begun. However, the personality defects do not improve, and these patients often require long-term psychiatric counseling. Life expectancy is not affected.

BILATERAL ANORCHIA
(Vanishing Testes Syndrome)

Approximately 3% of phenotypic boys undergoing surgery to correct unilateral or bilateral cryptorchidism are found to have absence of one testis, and in about 1% of cryptorchid males both testes are absent. Thus, bilateral anorchia is found in approximately one out of every 20,000 males.

Etiology & Pathophysiology

Functional testicular tissue must be present during the first 14–16 weeks of embryonic development in order for wolffian duct growth and müllerian duct regression to occur and for the external genitalia to differentiate along male lines. Absence of testicular function before this time will result in varying degrees of male pseudohermaphroditism with ambiguous genitalia. Prenatal testicular injury occurring after 16 weeks of gestation as a result of trauma, vascular insufficiency, infection, or other mechanisms may result in loss of testicular tissue in an otherwise normal phenotypic male; hence the term "vanishing testes syndrome."

Testicular Pathology

In most instances, no recognizable testicular tissue has been identified despite extensive dissections. Wolffian duct structures are generally normal, and the vas deferens and testicular vessels may terminate blindly or in a mass of connective tissues in the inguinal canal or scrotum.

Clinical Features

A. Symptoms and Signs: At birth, patients appear to be normal phenotypic males with bilateral cryptorchidism. Growth and development are normal until secondary sexual development fails to occur at puberty. The penis remains small; pubic and axillary hair does not fully develop despite the presence of adrenal androgens; and the scrotum remains empty. If the patient does not receive androgens, eunuchoid proportions develop. Gynecomastia does not occur.

An occasional patient will undergo partial spontaneous virilization at puberty. Although anatomically no testicular tissue has been identified in such patients, catheterization studies have demonstrated higher testosterone concentrations in venous blood obtained from the spermatic veins than in the peripheral venous circulation. This suggests that functional Leydig cells are present in some patients, although they are not associated with testicular germinal epithelium or stroma.

B. Laboratory Findings: Serum testosterone concentrations are generally quite low, and both LH and FSH are markedly elevated. Serum testosterone concentrations do not rise following a chorionic gonadotropin stimulation test. Chromosomal analysis discloses a 46,XY karyotype.

C. Imaging Studies: Testicular artery arteriograms and spermatic venograms show vessels that taper and end in the inguinal canal or scrotum without an associated gonad.

D. Special Examinations: Thorough inguinal and abdominal laparoscopic examination or retroperitoneal examination at laparotomy may locate the testes. If testicular vessels and the vas deferens are identified and found to terminate blindly together, it may be assumed that the testis is absent.

Differential Diagnosis

Bilateral cryptorchidism must be differentiated from congenital bilateral anorchia. A normal serum testosterone concentration that rises following stimulation with chorionic gonadotropin is indicative of functional Leydig cells and probable bilateral cryptorchidism. Elevated serum LH and FSH and a low testosterone that fails to rise after administration of exogenous chorionic gonadotropin indicate bilateral absence of functional testicular tissue.

Treatment

Androgen replacement therapy is discussed in the section of pharmacology (see Androgens, above).

Implantation of testicular prostheses for cosmetic purposes may be beneficial after the scrotum has enlarged in response to androgen therapy.

LEYDIG CELL APLASIA

Defective development of testicular Leydig cells is a rare cause of male pseudohermaphroditism with ambiguous genitalia.

Etiology & Pathophysiology

Testes are present in the inguinal canal and contain prepubertal-appearing tubules with Sertoli cells and spermatogonia without germinal cell maturation. The interstitial tissue has a loose myxoid appearance with an absence of Leydig cells. The binding of hCG or LH to testicular extracts from these patients is absent. It is not known whether this represents a primary defect in Leydig cell development due to an abnormality in the Leydig cell precursor cells or is the result of a deficiency of Leydig cell receptors for gonadotropins that may be responsible for inducing Leydig cell differentiation. The presence of a vas deferens and epididymis in these patients indicates that the local concentration of testosterone was high enough during embryogenesis to result in differentiation of the wolffian duct structures. However, the ambiguity of the genitalia indicates that the androgen concentration in these patients was insufficient to bring about full virilization of the external genitalia. The absence of müllerian duct structures is compatible with normal fetal secretion of müllerian duct inhibitory factor from the Sertoli cells.

Clinical Features

A. Symptoms and Signs: These patients may present in infancy with variable degrees of genital ambiguity, including a bifid scrotum, clitoral phallus, urogenital sinus, and blind vaginal pouch. Alternatively, they may appear as normal phenotypic females and escape detection until adolescence, when they present with primary amenorrhea, with or without normal breast development. The gonads are generally located in the inguinal canal. Axillary and pubic hair, although present, may be sparse.

B. Laboratory Findings: Serum gonadotropins are elevated, and testosterone levels are below normal limits for a male and within the low normal range for females. There is no increase in testosterone following chorionic gonadotropin administration.

Differential Diagnosis

Leydig cell aplasia should be differentiated from the vanishing testes syndrome, from testosterone biosynthetic defects, from disorders of androgen action, and from 5α-reductase deficiency. The differential diagnostic features of these disorders are discussed in Chapter 14.

Treatment

Patients with Leydig cell aplasia respond well to the exogenous administration of testosterone, and it would be anticipated that they would be fully virilized and even develop some degree of spermatogenesis with exogenous testosterone administration. However, since the few patients that have been reported have been discovered either late in childhood or as adolescents and have been raised as females, it would be inappropriate to attempt a gender reversal at such a late period. Removal of the cryptorchid testes and feminization with exogenous estrogens would appear to be the most prudent course of therapy.

CRYPTORCHIDISM

Cryptorchidism is unilateral or bilateral absence of the testes from the scrotum because of failure of normal testicular descent from the genital ridge through the external inguinal ring. About 5% of full-term male infants have cryptorchidism. In most cases of cryptorchidism noted at birth, spontaneous testicular descent occurs during the first year of life, reducing the incidence to 0.2–0.8% by 1 year of age. Approximately 0.75% of adult males are cryptorchid. Unilateral cryptorchidism is five to ten times more common than bilateral cryptorchidism.

Almost 50% of cryptorchid testes are located at the external inguinal ring or in a high scrotal position; 19% lie within the inguinal canal between the internal and external inguinal rings (canalicular); 9% are intra-abdominal; and 23% are ectopic, ie, located away from the normal pathway of descent from the abdominal cavity to the scrotum. Most ectopic testes are found in a superficial inguinal pouch above the external inguinal ring.

Etiology & Pathophysiology

Testicular descent usually occurs between the twelfth week of fetal development and birth. Both mechanical and hormonal factors appear to be important for this process: Cryptorchidism is common in patients with congenital defects in androgen synthesis or action and in patients with congenital gonadotropin deficiency, and experimental studies have demonstrated that dihydrotestosterone is required for normal testicular descent. These observations suggest that prenatal androgen deficiency may be of etiologic importance in the development of cryptorchidism.

It is not known whether pathologic changes in the testes are due to the effects of cryptorchidism or to intrinsic abnormalities in the gonad. Experimental studies in animals have shown that an increase in the temperature of the testes by 1.5–2 °C (2.7–3.6 °F) (the temperature differential between the abdomen and scrotum) results in depression of spermatogenesis. Serial testicular biopsies in cryptorchid patients have demonstrated partial reversal of the histologic abnormalities following surgical correction, suggesting that the extrascrotal environment is partly responsible for the observed pathologic abnormalities.

An intrinsic abnormality in the testes in patients with unilateral cryptorchidism is suggested by the observation that such patients are at increased risk for development of germ cell neoplasms in the scrotal testis. Similarly, the observation that adults with unilateral cryptorchidism surgically corrected before puberty had low sperm counts, high basal serum LH and FSH concentrations, and an exaggerated FSH response to GnRH suggests either that both testes are intrinsically abnormal or that the cryptorchid gonad somehow suppresses the function of the scrotal testis.

Pathology

Histologic studies on cryptorchid testes have demonstrated a decrease in the size of the seminiferous tubules and number of spermatogonia and an increase in peritubular tissue. The Leydig cells usually appear normal. It is unclear at what age these changes first appear. Abnormalities have been detected as early as 18 months to 2 years. It is well established that the longer a testis remains cryptorchid, the more likely it is to show pathologic changes. More severe changes are generally found in intra-abdominal testes than in canalicular testes.

Clinical Features

A. Symptoms and Signs: There are usually no symptoms unless a complication such as testicular torsion, trauma, or malignant degeneration occurs. School-age children may have gender identity problems. Adults may complain of infertility, especially if they have a history of bilateral cryptorchidism.

Absence of one or both testes is the cardinal clinical finding. This may be associated with a small scrotum (bilateral cryptorchidism) or hemiscrotum (unilateral cryptorchidism). Signs of androgen deficiency are not present.

B. Laboratory Findings: Basal or stimulated serum FSH, LH, and testosterone concentrations are not helpful in evaluating prepubertal unilaterally cryptorchid males. However, serum FSH and LH concentrations and the testosterone response to exogenous chorionic gonadotropin are useful in differentiating cryptorchid patients from those with congenital anorchia. The latter have high basal gonadotropins, low serum testosterone, and absent or diminished testosterone rise following chorionic gonadotropin stimulation.

Postpubertal adults may have oligospermia, elevated basal serum FSH and LH concentrations, and an exaggerated FSH increase following GnRH stimulation. Such abnormalities are more prevalent in patients with a history of bilateral cryptorchidism than with unilateral cryptorchidism.

C. Imaging Studies: Intravenous urography will disclose an associated abnormality of the upper urinary tract in 10% of cases—horseshoe kidney, renal hypoplasia, ureteral duplication, hydroureter, and hydronephrosis.

Differential Diagnosis

Retractile testis (pseudocryptorchidism) is due to a hyperactive cremasteric reflex, which draws the testicle into the inguinal canal. Cold temperature, fear, and genital manipulation commonly activate the reflex, which is most prominent between the ages of 5 and 6 years. The child should be examined with warm hands in a warm room. The testis can usually be "milked" into the scrotum with gentle pressure over the lower abdomen in the direction of the inguinal canal.

Bilateral anorchia is associated with elevated gonadotropins, decreased testosterone, and an absent or subnormal response to stimulation with chorionic gonadotropin.

The virilizing forms of congenital adrenal hyperplasia may result in prenatal fusion of the labial-scrotal folds and clitoral hypertrophy (Chapter 14). Severely affected females have the appearance of phenotypic males with bilateral cryptorchidism. Because of the potentially disastrous consequences (acute adrenal insufficiency) if this diagnosis is missed, a buccal smear should be performed on bilaterally cryptorchid phenotypic male infants.

Complications & Sequelae

A. Hernia: Approximately 90% of cryptorchid males have associated ipsilateral inguinal hernia resulting from failure of the processus vaginalis to close. This is rarely symptomatic.

B. Torsion: Because of the abnormal connection between the cryptorchid testis and its supporting tissues, torsion may occur. This should be suspected in any patient with abdominal or pelvic pain and an ipsilateral empty scrotum.

C. Trauma: Testes that lie above the pubic tubercle are particularly susceptible to traumatic injury.

D. Neoplasms: A cryptorchid testis is 20–30 times more likely to undergo malignant degeneration than are normal testes. The incidence of such tumors is greater in patients with intra-abdominal testes than in patients with canalicular testes. Seminomas are the neoplasms most commonly associated with maldescended testes. Because of the increased risk of neoplasia, many urologists recommend orchiectomy for a unilaterally undescended testicle in a patient first seen during or after puberty. Patients who present with bilateral cryptorchidism after puberty should have bilateral orchiopexy and testicular biopsies to preserve testicular endocrine function and to make palpation for detection of neoplasia easier.

E. Infertility: Over 90% of untreated bilaterally cryptorchid males are infertile. About 30–50% of bilaterally cryptorchid patients who undergo prepubertal orchiopexy have been found to be fertile. About half of patients with untreated unilateral cryptorchidism are infertile, whereas infertility is found in less than one-fourth of such patients whose cryptorchidism is surgically repaired before puberty.

Prevention

Although cryptorchidism cannot be prevented, the complications can. It is clear that the adverse changes that take place in the testes are related in part to the location of the maldescended testis and the duration of the cryptorchidism. Most testes that are undescended at birth enter the scrotum during the first year of life. However, it is rare for a cryptorchid testis to descend spontaneously after the age of 1 year. Since adverse histologic changes have been noted around the age of 2 years, hormonal or surgical correction should be undertaken at or before that time.

Treatment

A. Medical:

1. Intramuscular chorionic gonadotropin therapy–Because growth of the vas deferens and testicular descent are at least partially dependent upon androgens, stimulation of endogenous testosterone secretion by chorionic gonadotropin may correct the cryptorchidism. Cryptorchidism is corrected in less than 25% of patients treated with a course of chorionic gonadotropin, and recent studies suggest that patients with conditions that respond to hormonal therapy may actually have retractile testes rather than true cryptorchidism. Nevertheless, this therapy should be tried prior to orchiopexy, since it is innocuous and may avoid the need for surgery. For bilateral cryptorchidism, give a short course of chorionic gonadotropin consisting of 3300 units intramuscularly every other day over a 5-day period (three injections). For unilateral cryptorchidism, give 500 units intramuscularly three times a week for 6½ weeks (20 injections).

2. Intranasal GnRH therapy–GnRH given three times a day for 28 days by nasal spray has been shown to be as effective as chorionic gonadotropin injections in correcting cryptorchidism in some patients. This preparation of GnRH has not yet been released for clinical use in the USA.

B. Surgical: Several procedures have been devised to place the maldescended testis into the scrotum (orchiopexy). The operation may be performed in one or two stages. Inguinal hernia should be repaired if present.

NOONAN'S SYNDROME
(Male Turner's Syndrome)

Phenotypic and genotypic males with many of the physical stigmas of classic Turner's syndrome have been described under a variety of names, including Noonan's syndrome and male Turner's syndrome. The incidence and cause of this syndrome are unknown. It may occur sporadically or may be familial, inherited in an autosomal dominant fashion with variable penetrance. A number of pathologic features have been noted, including reduced seminiferous tubular size with or without sclerosis, diminished or absent germ cells, and Leydig cell hyperplasia.

Clinical Features

A. Symptoms and Signs: The most common clinical features are short stature, webbed neck, and cubitus valgus. Other somatic defects are variably observed in these patients. Congenital cardiac anomalies are common and involve primarily the right side of the heart—in contrast to patients with XO gonadal dysgenesis.

Cryptorchidism is frequently present. Although some affected individuals are fertile, with normal testes, most have small testes and mild to moderate hypogonadism.

B. Laboratory Findings: Serum testosterone concentrations are usually low or low normal, and serum gonadotropins are high. The karyotype is 46,XY.

Differential Diagnosis

The clinical features of Noonan's syndrome are sufficiently distinct so that confusion with other causes of hypogonadism is usually not a problem. However, a rare individual with XY/XO mosaicism may have similar somatic anomalies requiring chromosomal analysis for differentiation.

Treatment

If the patient is hypogonadal, androgen replacement therapy is indicated.

MYOTONIC DYSTROPHY

Myotonic dystrophy is one of the familial forms of muscular dystrophy. About 80% of affected males have some degree of primary testicular failure.

The disorder is transmitted in an autosomal dominant fashion, with marked variability in expression. The underlying lesion is an expansion repeat of a hypervariable region of the *DM* gene located on chromosome 19.

Testicular histology varies from moderate derangement of spermatogenesis with germinal cell arrest to regional hyalinization and fibrosis of the seminiferous tubules. The Leydig cells are usually preserved and may appear in clumps.

The testes are normal in affected prepubertal individuals, and puberty generally proceeds normally. Testosterone secretion is normal, and secondary sexual characteristics develop. After puberty, seminiferous tubular atrophy results in a decrease in testicular size and change of consistency from firm to soft or mushy. Infertility is a consequence of disrupted spermatogenesis. If testicular hyalinization and fibrosis are extensive, Leydig cell function may also be impaired.

Clinical Features

A. Symptoms and Signs: The disease usually becomes apparent in adulthood. Progressive weakness and atrophy of the facial, neck, hand, and lower extremity muscles is commonly observed. Severe atrophy of the temporalis muscles, ptosis due to weakness of the levator muscles of the eye with compensatory wrinkling of the forehead muscles, and frontal baldness comprise the myopathic facies characteristic of the disorder. Myotonia is present in several muscle groups and is characterized by inability to relax the muscle normally after a strong contraction.

Testicular atrophy is not noted until adulthood, and most patients develop and maintain normal facial and body hair growth and libido. Gynecomastia is usually not present.

Associated features include mental retardation, cataracts, cranial hyperostosis, diabetes mellitus, and primary hypothyroidism.

B. Laboratory Findings: Serum testosterone is normal to slightly decreased. FSH is uniformly elevated in patients with atrophic testes. LH is also frequently elevated, even in patients with normal serum testosterone levels. Leydig cell reserve is generally diminished, with subnormal increases in serum testosterone following stimulation with chorionic gonadotropin. An excessive rise in FSH and, to a lesser extent, LH is found following GnRH stimulation.

Differential Diagnosis

Myotonic dystrophy should be distinguished from forms of muscular dystrophy not associated with hypogonadism.

Treatment

There is no therapy that will prevent progressive muscular atrophy in this disorder. Testosterone replacement therapy is not indicated unless the serum testosterone levels are subnormal.

ADULT SEMINIFEROUS TUBULE FAILURE

Adult seminiferous tubule failure encompasses a spectrum of pathologic alterations of the seminiferous tubules that results in hypospermatogenesis, germinal cell arrest, germinal cell aplasia, and tubular hyalinization. Almost half of infertile males exhibit some degree of isolated seminiferous tubule failure.

Etiology, Pathology, & Pathophysiology

Etiologic factors in seminiferous tubule failure include mumps or gonococcal orchitis, leprosy, cryptorchidism, irradiation, uremia, alcoholism, paraplegia, lead poisoning, and therapy with antineoplastic agents such as cyclophosphamide, chlorambucil, vincristine, methotrexate, and procarbazine. Vascular insufficiency resulting from spermatic artery damage during herniorrhaphy, testicular torsion, or sickle cell anemia may also selectively damage the tubules. Similar pathologic changes may be found in oligospermic patients with varicoceles. In many patients, no etiologic factors can be identified, and the condition is referred to as "idiopathic."

The rapidly dividing germinal epithelium is more susceptible to injury than are the Sertoli or Leydig cells. Thus, pressure necrosis (eg, mumps or gonococcal orchitis), increased testicular temperature (eg, cryptorchidism and perhaps varicocele and paraplegia), and the direct cytotoxic effects of irradiation, alcohol, lead, and chemotherapeutic agents primarily injure the germ cells. Although the Sertoli and Leydig cells appear to be morphologically normal, severe testicular injury may result in functional alterations in these cells.

Several different lesions may be found in testicular biopsy specimens. The pathologic process may involve the entire testes or may appear in patches. The least severe lesion is hypospermatogenesis, in which all stages of spermatogenesis are present but there is a decrease in the number of germinal epithelial cells. Some degree of peritubular fibrosis may be present. Cessation of development at the primary spermatocyte or spermatogonial stage of the spermatogenic cycle is classified as germinal cell arrest. More severely affected testes may demonstrate a complete absence of germ cells with maintenance or morphologically normal Sertoli cells (Sertoli cell only syndrome). The most severe lesion is fibrosis or hyalinization of the tubules. This latter pattern may be indistinguishable from that seen in Klinefelter's syndrome.

Irrespective of the etiologic factors involved in damage to the germinal epithelium, the alterations in spermatogenesis result in oligospermia. If the damage is severe, as in the Sertoli cell only syndrome or tubular hyalinization, azoospermia may be present. Since testicular volume consists chiefly of tubules, some degree of testicular atrophy is often present in these patients. Some patients have elevations in basal serum FSH concentrations and demonstrate a hyperresponsive FSH rise following GnRH, suggesting that the Sertoli cells are functionally abnormal despite their normal histologic appearance.

Clinical Features

A. Symptoms and Signs: Infertility is usually the only complaint. Mild to moderate testicular atrophy may be present. Careful examination should be made for the presence of varicocele by palpating the spermatic cord during Valsalva's maneuver with the patient in the upright position. The patients are fully virilized, and gynecomastia is not present.

B. Laboratory Findings: Semen analysis shows oligospermia or azoospermia, and serum testosterone and LH concentrations are normal. Basal serum FSH levels may be normal or high, and an excessive FSH rise following GnRH may be present.

Differential Diagnosis

Patients with hypothalamic or pituitary disorders may have oligospermia or azoospermia and testicular atrophy. The serum FSH and LH concentrations are often in the low normal range, and the testosterone level is usually (not always) diminished. The presence of neurologic and ophthalmologic abnormalities, diabetes insipidus, anterior pituitary trophic hormone deficiencies, or an elevated serum PRL concentration distinguishes these patients from those with primary seminiferous tubule failure. Other causes of primary testicular failure are associated either with clinical signs and symptoms of androgen deficiency or with enough somatic abnormalities to allow differentiation from isolated seminiferous tubule failure.

Prevention

In many instances, damage to the seminiferous tubules cannot be prevented. Early correction of cryptorchidism, adequate shielding of the testes during diagnostic radiologic procedures or radiotherapy, and limitation of the total dose of chemotherapeutic agents may prevent or ameliorate the adverse effects.

Treatment

A. Medical: Attempts to treat oligospermia and infertility medically have included testosterone rebound therapy, low-dose testosterone, exogenous gonadotropins, thyroid hormone therapy, vitamins, and clomiphene citrate. None of these agents have been found to be uniformly beneficial, and several may actually lead to a decrease in the sperm count.

B. Surgical: Some of the pathologic changes in the testes have been reversed by early orchiopexy in cryptorchid individuals. If a varicocele is found in an oligospermic, infertile male, it should be ligated.

Course & Prognosis

Patients who have received up to 300 cGy of testicular irradiation may show partial or full recovery of spermatogenesis months to years following exposure. The prognosis for recovery is better for individuals who receive the irradiation over a short interval than for those who are exposed over several weeks.

Recovery of spermatogenesis may also occur months to years following administration of chemotherapeutic agents. The most important factor determining prognosis is the total dose of chemotherapy administered.

Improvement in the quality of the semen is found in 60–80% of patients following successful repair of varicocele. Restoration of fertility has been reported in about half of such patients.

The prognosis for spontaneous improvement of idiopathic oligospermia due to infection or infarction is poor.

ADULT LEYDIG CELL FAILURE
(Andropause)

In contrast to the menopause in women, men do not experience an abrupt decline or cessation of gonadal function. However, a gradual diminution of testicular function does occur in many men as part of the aging process (Chapter 25). It is not known how many men develop symptoms directly attributable to this phenomenon.

Etiology, Pathology, & Pathophysiology

There have been many studies of the relationships between age and testicular function, often with conflicting results. Several investigators have found that after age 50, there is a gradual decrease in the total serum testosterone concentration, although the actual values remain within the normal range. The levels of free testosterone decrease to a greater extent because of an increase in SHBG. The testosterone production rate declines, and Leydig cell responsiveness to hCG also decreases. A gradual compensatory increase in serum LH levels has also been noted.

Histologic studies of the aging testes have shown patchy degenerative changes in the seminiferous tubules with a reduction in number and volume of Leydig cells. The pathologic changes are first noted in the regions most remote from the arterial blood supply. Thus, microvascular insufficiency may be the etiologic basis for the histologic tubular changes and the decrease in Leydig cell function noted with aging. In addition, virtually all of the conditions that cause adult seminiferous tubule failure may lead to Leydig cell dysfunction if testicular injury is severe enough.

Clinical Features

A. Symptoms and Signs: A great many symptoms have been attributed to the male climacteric (andropause), including decreased libido and potency, emotional instability, fatigue, decreased strength, decreased concentrating ability, vasomotor instability (palpitations, hot flushes, diaphoresis), and a variety of diffuse aches and pains. There are usually no associated signs unless the testicular injury is severe. In such patients, a decrease in testicular volume and consistency may be present as well as gynecomastia.

B. Laboratory Findings: Serum testosterone may be low or low normal; serum LH concentration is usually high normal or slightly high. Oligospermia is usually present. Bone mineral density may be decreased.

C. Special Examinations: Because many men with complaints compatible with Leydig cell failure have testosterone and LH concentrations within the normal adult range, a diagnostic trial of testosterone therapy may be attempted. The test is best performed double-blind over an 8-week period. During the first or last 4 weeks, the patient receives testosterone enanthate, 200 mg intramuscularly per week; during the other 4-week period, placebo injections are administered. The patient is interviewed by the physician 2 weeks after the last course of injections. After the interview, the code is broken; if the patient notes amelioration of symptoms during the period of androgen administration but not during the placebo period, the diagnosis of adult Leydig cell failure is substantiated. If the patient experiences no subjective improvement following testosterone, of if improvement is noted following both placebo and testosterone injections, Leydig cell failure is effectively ruled out.

Differential Diagnosis

Impotence from vascular, neurologic, or psychologic causes must be distinguished from Leydig cell failure. A therapeutic trial of androgen therapy will not help impotence that is not due to androgen deficiency.

Treatment

Androgen replacement therapy is the treatment of choice for both symptomatic and asymptomatic Leydig cell failure. This results in increases in lean body mass, hemoglobin, libido, strength, and sense of well being and decreases in total and HDL cholesterol and urine hydroxyproline.

IMPOTENCE
(Erectile Dysfunction)

Impotence implies erectile dysfunction with or without associated disturbances of libido or ejaculatory ability. The overall prevalence of impotence in the general population is unknown, though it is probable that most men experience occasional episodes of impotence at some time during their lives.

Etiology & Pathophysiology

Penile erection occurs when blood flow to the penile erectile tissue (corpora cavernosa and spongiosum) increases as a result of dilation of the urethral artery, the artery of the bulb of the penis, the deep artery of the penis, and the dorsal artery of the penis following psychogenic or sensory stimuli transmitted to the limbic system and then to the thoracolumbar and sacral autonomic nervous system. The relaxation of the cavernosal arterial and cavernosal trabecular sinusoidal smooth muscles occurs following stimulation of the sacral parasympathetic (S_{2-4}) nerves, which results in the release of acetylcholine, vasoactive intestinal peptide, and an endothelial cell-derived relaxing factor which is most likely nitrous oxide. As the sinusoids become engorged, the subtunical venous plexus is compressed against the tunica albuginea, preventing egress of blood from the penis. Contraction of the bulbocavernosus muscle through stimulation of the somatic portion of the S_{2-4} pudendal nerves further increases the intracavernosal pressure. These processes result in the distention, engorgement, and rigidity of the penis that constitute erection.

Broadly speaking, erectile dysfunction may be divided into psychogenic and organic causes. Table 12–4 lists various pathologic conditions and drugs that may be associated with impotence.

Most organic causes of impotence result from disturbances in the neurologic pathways essential for the initiation and maintenance of erection or in the blood supply to the penis. Many of the endocrine disorders, systemic illnesses, and drugs associated with impotence affect libido, the autonomic pathways essential for erection, or the blood flow to the penis. Venous incompetence because of anatomic defects in the corpora cavernosa or subtunical venous plexus is being recognized with increasing frequency. Local urogenital disorders such as Peyronie's disease (idiopathic fibrosis of the covering sheath of the corpus cavernosum) may mechanically interfere with erection. In some patients, the cause of impotence is multifactorial. For example, some degree of erectile dysfunction is reported by over 50% of men with diabetes mellitus. The basis of the impotence is usually autonomic neuropathy. However, vascular insufficiency, antihypertensive medication, uremia, and depression may also cause or contribute to the problem in diabetics.

Clinical Features

A. Symptoms and Signs: Patients may complain of constant or episodic inability to initiate or maintain an erection, decreased penile turgidity, decreased libido, or a combination of these difficulties. Besides the specific sexual dysfunction symptoms, symptoms and signs of a more pervasive emotional or psychiatric problem may be elicited. If an underlying neurologic, vascular, or systemic disorder is the cause of impotence, additional symptoms and signs referable to the anatomic or metabolic disturbances may be present. A history of claudication of the buttocks or lower extremities should direct attention toward arterial insufficiency.

The differentiation between psychogenic and organic impotence can usually be made on the basis of the history. Even though the patient may be selectively unable to obtain or maintain a satisfactory erection to complete sexual intercourse, a history of repeated normal erections at other times is indicative of psychogenic impotence. Thus, a history of erections that occur nocturnally, during masturbation, or

Table 12–4. Organic causes of impotence.

Neurologic
Anterior temporal lobe lesions
Spinal cord lesions
Autoimmune neuropathy

Vascular
Leriche's syndrome
Pelvic vascular insufficiency
Sickle cell disease
Venous leaks
?Aging

Endocrine
Diabetes mellitus
Hypogonadism
Hyperprolactinemia
Adrenal insufficiency
Feminizing tumors
Hypothyroidism
Hyperthyroidism

Urogenital
Trauma
Castration
Priapism
Peyronie's disease

Systemic illness
Cardiac insufficiency
Cirrhosis
Uremia
Respiratory insufficiency
Lead poisoning

Postoperative
Aortoiliac or aortofemoral reconstruction
Lumbar sympathectomy
Perineal prostatectomy
Retroperitoneal dissection

Drugs
Endocrinologic
Antiandrogens
Estrogens
5α-Reductase inhibitors
GnRH agonists
Antihypertensives
Diuretics
Psychotropic agents
Tranquilizers
Monoamine oxidase inhibitors
Tricyclic antidepressants
Other
Tobacco
Alcohol
Opioids
H_2-receptor antagonists
Gemfibrozil
Amphetamines
Cocaine

during foreplay or with other sexual partners eliminates significant neurologic, vascular, or endocrine causes of impotence. Patients with psychogenic impotence often note a sudden onset of sexual dysfunction concurrently with a significant event in their lives such as loss of a friend or relative, an extramarital affair, or the loss of a job.

Patients with organic impotence generally note a more gradual and global loss of potency. Initially, such individuals may be able to achieve erections with strong sexual stimuli, but ultimately they may be unable to achieve a fully turgid erection under any circumstances. In contrast to patients with psychogenic impotence, patients with organic impotence generally maintain a normal libido. However, patients with systemic illness may have a concurrent diminution of libido and potency. Hypogonadism should be suspected in a patient who has never had an erection (primary impotence).

B. Laboratory Findings and Special Examinations: The integrity of the neurologic pathways and the ability of the blood vessels to deliver a sufficient amount of blood to the penis for erection to occur may be objectively examined by placement of a strain gauge behind the glans penis and at the base of the penis at the time the patient retires for sleep. The occurrence of nocturnal penile tumescence can thus be recorded. Healthy men and those with psychogenic impotence have three to five erections a night associated with rapid eye movement (REM) sleep. Absence or reduced frequency of nocturnal tumescence indicates an organic lesion. Penile rigidity as well as tumescence can be evaluated with an ambulatory monitor called RigiScan (Dacomed Corporation, Minneapolis, MN 55420).

Rather than perform nocturnal penile tumescence monitoring, many clinicians elect to initially try an intracavernous injection of a vasoactive drug with evaluation of the quality of the erection. A full erection indicates adequate penile arterial and venous systems. The presence of a partial or no erection is usually further evaluated as to the cause, though after ruling out an endocrine causes (see below), a cost-effective approach is to proceed directly to therapy.

The vascular integrity of the penis may be examined by Doppler ultrasonography with spectral analysis following intracorporal injection of a vasoactive drug. This method allows detection of venous leaks with a sensitivity of 55–100% and specificity of 69–88%. Arterial problems are also detected with a sensitivity of 82–100% and specificity of 64–96%.

Neural innervation of the penis may be assessed by measurement of the bulbocavernosus reflex response latency period or cystometrography. These tests are rarely needed, since patients with autonomic neuropathy due to a generalized disease process like diabetes mellitus or the Shy-Drager syndrome will exhibit other features of autonomic dysfunction such as vasomotor instability and incontinence.

Serum testosterone measurements may uncover a mild and otherwise asymptomatic androgen deficiency. If the testosterone level is low, serum PRL should be measured, since hyperprolactinemia, whether drug-induced or due to a pituitary or hypothalamic lesion, may inhibit androgen production. Because diabetes mellitus is a relatively common cause of impotence and impotence may be the presenting symptom of diabetes, fasting and 2-hour postprandial blood glucose measurements should be ordered. The choice of other laboratory tests such as cavernosometry, cavernosography, or arteriography depends upon associated organic symptoms or signs.

Treatment

A. Psychogenic Impotence: Simple reassurance and explanation, formal psychotherapy, and various forms of behavioral therapy have a reported 40–70% success rate. Androgen therapy should not be used in patients with psychogenic impotence, since androgens exert no more than a placebo effect and may focus the patient's attention on a nonexistent organic problem.

B. Organic Impotence: Discontinuation of an offending drug usually results in a return of potency. Similarly, effective therapy of an underlying systemic or endocrine disorder may cure the erectile dysfunction. Patients with permanent impotence due to organic lesions that cannot be corrected should be counseled in noncoital sensate focus techniques.

Vasoactive drugs including prostaglandin E_1, papaverine hydrochloride, and phentolamine mesylate, either alone or in combination, may induce an erection following an intracavernous injection. Of these, the only FDA-approved agent is prostaglandin E_1 (alprostadil), which needs to be individualized within the dose range of 2.5–60 μg per injection (average wholesale price about $18 for 20 μg). In clinical studies, up to 80% of men with impotence developed erections. Side effects include penile pain (33% of patients), hematoma (3%), penile fibrosis (3%), and priapism (0.4%). Trials are currently under way to evaluate the intraurethral instillation of prostaglandin E_2, which appears to have an approximately 60% success rate.

Devices have been developed that use suction to induce penile engorgement and constrictive bands to maintain the ensuing erection. Erections are achieved in 90% of patients with approximately a 70% couple satisfaction rate. Alternatively, a penile prosthesis may be surgically implanted. Three major types of such prostheses have been developed. These include semirigid silicone rubber rods that are implanted in the corpora, malleable rods, or inflatable penile prostheses that allow the penis to remain flaccid until erection is desired. Prostheses have given satisfactory results in 85–90% of cases.

There has been a variable success rate in repairing venous leaks and in microsurgical revascularization of arterial lesions.

MALE INFERTILITY

About 15% of married couples are unable to produce offspring. Male factors are responsible in about 40% of cases, female factors in about 40%, and couple factors in 20%.

Etiology & Pathophysiology

In order for conception to occur, spermatogenesis must be normal, the sperm must complete its maturation during transport through patent ducts, adequate amounts of seminal plasma must be added to provide volume and nutritional elements, and the male must be able to deposit the semen near the female's cervix. Any defect in this pathway can result in infertility due to a male factor problem. The spermatozoa must also be able to penetrate the cervical mucus and reach the uterine tubes, where conception takes place. These latter events may fail to occur if there are female reproductive tract disorders or abnormalities of sperm motility or fertilizing capacity.

Table 12–5 lists the identified causes of male infertility. Disturbances in the function of the hypothalamus, pituitary, adrenals, or thyroid are found in approximately 4% of males evaluated for infertility. Sex chromosome abnormalities, cryptorchidism, adult seminiferous tubule failure, and other forms of primary testicular failure are found in 15% of infertile males. Congenital or acquired ductal problems are found in approximately 6% of such patients, and poor coital technique, sexual dysfunction, ejaculatory disturbances, and anatomic abnormalities such as hypospadias are causative factors in 4–5% of patients evaluated for infertility. Idiopathic infertility, in which no cause can be identified with certainty, accounts for approximately 35% of patients. Autoimmune disturbances that lead to sperm agglutination and immobilization causes infertility in only a small fraction of patients. Varicoceles are found in 25–40% of patients classified as having idiopathic infertility. The significance of this finding is uncertain, since 8–20% of males in the general population have varicoceles.

Clinical Features

A. Symptoms and Signs: The clinical features of the hypothalamic-pituitary, thyroid, adrenal, testicular, and sexual dysfunctional disorders have been discussed in preceding sections of this chapter. Evaluation for the presence of varicocele has also been described.

Patients with immotile cilia syndrome have associated mucociliary transport defects in the lower airways that result in chronic pulmonary obstructive disease. Some patients with this disorder also have Kartagener's syndrome, with sinusitis, bronchiectasis, and situs inversus. Infections of the epididymis or vas deferens may be asymptomatic or associated with scrotal pain that may radiate to the flank, fever, epididymal swelling and tenderness, and urethral discharge. The presence of thickened, enlarged epididymis and vas is indicative of chronic epididymitis. Chronic prostatitis is usually asymptomatic, although a perineal aching sensation or low back pain may be described. A boggy or indurated prostate may be found on rectal palpation. A careful examination for the presence of penile anatomic abnormalities such as chordee, hypospadias, or epispadias should be made, since these defects may prevent the deposit of sperm in the vagina.

B. Laboratory Findings: A carefully collected and performed semen analysis is mandatory. A normal report indicates normal endocrine function and spermatogenesis and an intact transport system. Semen analysis should be followed by a postcoital test, which consists of examining a cervical mucus sample obtained within 2 hours after intercourse. The presence of large numbers of motile spermatozoa in mucus obtained from the internal os of the cervix rules out the male factor as a cause of infertility. If a postcoital test reveals necrospermia (dead sperm), asthenospermia (slow-moving sperm), or agglutination of sperm, examination of the female partner for the presence of sperm-immobilizing antibodies or cervical mucus abnormalities should be carried out.

If semen analysis shows abnormalities, at least two more specimens should be obtained at monthly intervals. Persistent oligospermia or azoospermia should be evaluated by studies outlined in Figure 12–7.

The female partner should be thoroughly examined to verify patency of the uterus and uterine tubes, normal ovulation, and normal cervical mucus. This examination must be done even in the presence of a male factor abnormality, since infertility is due to a combination of male and female factors in about 20% of cases.

Table 12–5. Causes of male infertility.

Endocrine
Hypothalamic-pituitary disorders
Testicular disorders
Defects of androgen action
Hyperthyroidism
Hypothyroidism
Adrenal insufficiency
Congenital adrenal hyperplasia

Systemic illness

Defects in spermatogenesis
Immotile cilia syndrome
Drug-induced
Adult seminiferous tubule failure

Ductal obstruction
Congenital
Acquired

Seminal vesicle disease

Prostatic disease

Varicocele

Retrograde ejaculation

Antibodies to sperm or seminal plasma

Anatomic defects of the penis

Poor coital technique

Sexual dysfunction

Idiopathic

Treatment

A. Endocrine Disorders: Correction of hyperthyroidism, hypothyroidism, adrenal insufficiency, and congenital adrenal hyperplasia generally restores fertility. Patients with hypogonadotropic hypogonadism may have spermatogenesis initiated with gonadotropin therapy. Chorionic gonadotropin (2000 units given intramuscularly three times per week) with menotropins (75 units given intramuscularly three times per week) added after 12–18 months if sperm do not appear in the ejaculate, will restore spermatogenesis in most hypogonadotropic men. The sperm count following such therapy usually does not exceed 10 million/mL but may still allow impregnation. Patients with isolated deficiency of LH may respond to chorionic gonadotropin alone. There is no effective therapy for adult seminiferous tubule failure not associated with varicocele or cryptorchidism. However, if the oligospermia is mild (10–20 million/mL), cup insemination of the female partner with concentrates of semen may be tried. In vitro fertilization and other assisted reproductive techniques, including direct injection of a spermatozoon into an egg, are increasingly being utilized as a method for achieving pregnancy in couples in which the male is oligospermic.

B. Defects of Spermatogenesis: There is no treatment for immotile cilia syndrome or for chromosomal abnormalities associated with defective spermatogenesis. Drugs that interfere with spermatogenesis should be discontinued. These include the antimetabolites, phenytoin, marijuana, alcohol, monoamine oxidase inhibitors, and nitrofurantoin. Discontinuing use of these agents may be accompanied by restoration of normal sperm density.

C. Ductal Obstruction: Localized obstruction of the vas deferens may be treated by vasovasotomy. Sperm are detected in the ejaculate of 60–80% of patients following this procedure. However, the subsequent fertility rate is only 30–35%; the presence of antisperm antibodies that agglutinate or immobilize sperm probably accounts for the high failure rate.

Epididymovasostomy may be performed for epididymal obstruction. Sperm in the postoperative ejaculate have been found in approximately half of patients treated with this procedure, but subsequent fertility has been demonstrated in only 20% of cases.

D. Genital Tract Infections: Acute prostatitis may be treated with daily sitz baths, prostatic massage, and antibiotics. A combination of trimethoprim (400 mg) and sulfamethoxazole (2000 mg), twice a day for 10 days followed by the same dosage once a day for another 20 days, has been used with some success. Acute epididymitis may respond to injections of local anesthetic into the spermatic cord just above the testicle. Appropriate antibiotic therapy should also be given. The prognosis for fertility following severe bilateral chronic epididymitis or extensive scarring from acute epididymitis is poor.

E. Varicocele: The presence of varicocele in an infertile male with oligospermia is an indication for surgical ligation of the incompetent spermatic veins. Improvement in the semen is noted in 60–80% of treated patients, and about half are subsequently fertile.

F. Retrograde Ejaculation: Ejaculation of semen into the urinary bladder may occur following disruption of the internal bladder sphincter or with neuropathic disorders such as diabetic autonomic neuropathy. Normal ejaculation has been restored in a few patients with the latter problem following administration of phenylpropanolamine, 15 mg orally twice daily in timed-release capsules. Sperm can also be recovered from the bladder following masturbation for the purpose of direct insemination of the female partner.

G. Antibodies to Sperm or Seminal Plasma: Antibodies in the female genital tract that agglutinate or immobilize sperm may be difficult to treat. Older methods such as condom therapy or administration of glucocorticoids have not been uniformly successful. Currently, intrauterine insemination with washed spermatozoa, in vitro fertilization, and gamete intrafallopian transfer are considered the most effective treatments.

H. Anatomic Defects of the Penis: Patients with hypospadias, epispadias, or severe chordee may collect semen by masturbation for use in insemination.

I. Poor Coital Technique: Couples should be counseled not to use vaginal lubricants or postcoital douches. In order to maximize the sperm count in cases of borderline oligospermia, intercourse should not be more frequent than every other day. Exposure of the cervix to the seminal plasma is increased by having the woman lie supine with her knees bent up for 20 minutes after intercourse.

Course & Prognosis

The prognosis for fertility depends upon the underlying cause. It is good for patients with nontesticular endocrine abnormalities, varicoceles, retrograde ejaculation, and anatomic defects of the penis. If fertility cannot be restored, the couple should be counseled regarding artificial donor insemination, in vitro fertilization, or adoption.

GYNECOMASTIA

Gynecomastia is common during the neonatal period and is present in about 70% of pubertal males (Chapter 15). Clinically apparent gynecomastia has been noted at autopsy in almost 1% of adult males, and 40% of autopsied males have histologic evidence of gynecomastia.

Etiology & Pathophysiology

The causes of gynecomastia are listed in Table 12–6. Several mechanisms have been proposed to account for this disorder. All involve a relative imbalance between estrogen and androgen concentrations

Table 12–6. Causes of gynecomastia.

Physiologic
  Neonatal
  Pubertal
  Involutional
Drug-induced
  Hormones
    Androgens and anabolic steroids
    Chorionic gonadotropin
    Estrogens and estrogen agonists
    Growth hormone
  Antiandrogens or inhibitors of androgen synthesis
    Cyproterone
    Flutamide
    Finasteride
  Antibiotics
    Isoniazid
    Ketoconazole
    Metronidazole
  Antiulcer medications
    Cimetidine
    Omeprazole
    Ranitidine
  Cancer chemotherapeutic agents (especially alkylating agents)
  Cardiovascular drugs
    Amiodarone
    Captopril
    Digitoxin
    Enalapril
    Methyldopa
    Nifedipine
    Reserpine
    Spironolactone
    Verapamil
  Psychoactive agents
    Diazepam
    Haloperidol
    Phenothiazines
    Tricyclic antidepressants
  Drugs of abuse
    Alcohol
    Amphetamines
    Heroin
    Marijuana
  Other
    Phenytoin
    Penicillamine
Endocrine
  Primary hypogonadism with Leydig cell damage
  Hyperprolactinemia
  Hyperthyroidism
  Androgen receptor disorders
Systemic diseases
  Hepatic cirrhosis
  Uremia
  Recovery from malnourishment
Neoplasms
  Testicular germ cell or Leydig cell tumors
  Feminizing adrenocortical adenoma or carcinoma
  hCG-secreting nontrophoblastic neoplasms
Idiopathic

or action at the mammary gland level. Decrease in free testosterone may be due to primary gonadal disease or an increase in SHBG as is found in hyperthyroidism and some forms of liver disease (eg, alcoholic cirrhosis). Decreased androgen action in patients with the androgen insensitivity syndromes results in unopposed estrogen action on the breast glandular tissue. Acute or chronic excessive stimulation of the Leydig cells by pituitary gonadotropins alters the steroidogenic pathways and favors excessive estrogen and estrogen precursor secretion relative to testosterone production. This mechanism may be responsible for the gynecomastia found with hypergonadotropic states such as Klinefelter's syndrome and adult Leydig cell failure. The rise of gonadotropins during puberty may lead to an estrogen-androgen imbalance by similar mechanisms. Patients who are malnourished or have systemic illness may develop gynecomastia during refeeding or treatment of the underlying disorder. Malnourishment and chronic illness are accompanied by a reduction in gonadotropin secretion, and during recovery the gonadotropins rise and may stimulate excessive Leydig cell production of estrogens relative to testosterone.

Excessive stimulation of Leydig cells may also occur in patients with hCG-producing trophoblastic or nontrophoblastic tumors. In addition, some of these tumors are able to convert estrogen precursors into estradiol. Feminizing adrenocortical and Leydig cell neoplasms may directly secrete excessive quantities of estrogens. The mechanisms by which PRL-secreting pituitary tumors and hyperprolactinemia produce gynecomastia are unclear. Elevated serum PRL levels may lower testosterone production and diminish the peripheral actions of testosterone, which may result in an excessive estrogen effect on the breast that is not counteracted by androgens.

Drugs such as phenothiazines, methyldopa, and reserpine may induce gynecomastia through elevations of PRL. Other drugs may reduce androgen production (eg, spironolactone), peripherally antagonize androgen action (spironolactone, cimetidine), or interact with breast estrogen receptors (spironolactone, digitoxin, phytoestrogens in marijuana).

Finally, it has been proposed that patients with idiopathic and familial gynecomastia have breast glandular tissue that is inordinately sensitive to normal circulating levels of estrogen or excessively converts estrogen precursors to estrogens.

Pathology

Three histologic patterns of gynecomastia have been recognized. The florid pattern consists of an increase in the number of budding ducts, proliferation of the ductal epithelium, periductal edema, and a cellular fibroblastic stroma. The fibrous type has dilated ducts, minimal duct epithelial proliferation, no periductal edema, and a virtually acellular fibrous stroma. An intermediate pattern contains features of both types.

Although it has been proposed that different causes of gynecomastia are associated with either the florid or the fibrous pattern, it appears that the duration of gynecomastia is the most important factor in determining the pathologic picture. Approximately 75% of patients with gynecomastia of 4 months' duration or less exhibit the florid pattern, while 90% of patients with gynecomastia lasting a year or more have the fibrous type. Between 4 months and 1 year, 60% of patients have the intermediate pattern.

Clinical Features

A. Symptoms and Signs: The principal complaint is unilateral or bilateral concentric enlargement of breast glandular tissue. Nipple or breast pain is present in one-fourth of patients and objective tenderness in about 40%. A complaint of nipple discharge can be elicited in 4% of cases. Histologic examination has demonstrated that gynecomastia is almost always bilateral, although grossly it may be detected only on one side. The patient will often complain of discomfort in one breast despite obvious bilateral gynecomastia. Breast or nipple discomfort generally lasts less than 1 year. Chronic gynecomastia is usually asymptomatic, with the major complaint being the cosmetic one.

Symptoms and signs of underlying disorders may be present. Gynecomastia may be the earliest manifestation of an hCG-secreting testicular tumor; therefore, it is mandatory that careful examination of the testes be performed in any patient with gynecomastia. Enlargement, asymmetry, and induration of a testis may be noted in such patients.

B. Laboratory Findings: Once pubertal and drug-induced gynecomastia have been excluded, a biochemical screen for liver and renal abnormalities should be performed. If those are normal, then serum hCG, LH, testosterone, and estradiol levels should be measured. The interpretation of the results is outlined in Figure 12–9.

Differential Diagnosis

Gynecomastia should be differentiated from lipomas, neurofibromas, carcinoma of the breast, and obesity. Breast lipomas, neurofibromas, and carcinoma are usually unilateral, painless, and eccentric, whereas gynecomastia characteristically begins in the subareolar areas and enlarges concentrically. The differentiation between gynecomastia and enlarged breasts due to obesity may be difficult. The patient should be supine. Examination is performed by spreading the thumb and index fingers and gently palpating the breasts during slow apposition of the fingers toward the nipple. In this manner, a concentric ridge of tissue can be felt in patients with gynecomastia but not in obese patients without glandular tissue enlargement. The examination may be facilitated by applying soap and water to the breasts.

Complications & Sequelae

There are no complications other than possible psychologic damage from the cosmetic defect. Patients with gynecomastia may have a slightly increased risk of development of breast carcinoma.

Treatment

A. Medical: The underlying disease should be corrected if possible, and offending drugs should be discontinued. Antiestrogens such as tamoxifen and clomiphene citrate have been found useful for relieving pain and reversing gynecomastia in a few patients. Whether this therapy will be useful in most patients with gynecomastia remains to be seen.

B. Surgical: Reduction mammoplasty should be considered for cosmetic reasons in any patient with long-standing gynecomastia that is in the fibrotic stage.

C. Radiologic: Patients with prostatic carcinoma may receive low-dose radiation therapy (900 cGy or less) to the breasts before initiation of estrogen therapy. This may prevent or diminish the gynecomastia that usually results from such therapy. Radiotherapy should not be given to other patients with gynecomastia.

Course & Prognosis

Pubertal gynecomastia usually regresses spontaneously over 1–2 years. Patients who develop drug-induced gynecomastia generally have complete or near-complete regression of the breast changes if the drug is discontinued during the early florid stage. Once gynecomastia from any cause has reached the fibrotic stage, little or no spontaneous regression occurs.

TESTICULAR TUMORS

Testicular neoplasms account for 1–2% of all male-related malignant neoplasms and 4–10% of all genitourinary neoplasms. They are the second most frequent type of cancer in men between 20 and 34 years of age. The incidence is 2–3 per 100,000 men in the USA and 4–6 per 100,000 men in Denmark. The incidence is lower in nonwhite than in white populations. Ninety-five percent of testicular tumors are of germ cell origin; 5% are composed of stromal or Leydig cell neoplasms.

Etiology & Pathophysiology

The cause of testicular tumors is not known. Predisposing factors include testicular maldescent and dysgenesis. About 4–12% of testicular tumors are found in association with cryptorchidism, and such a testicle has a 20- to 30-fold greater risk of developing a neoplasm than does a normally descended one. Almost 20% of testicular tumors associated with cryptorchidism arise in the contralateral scrotal testis, suggesting that testicular dysgenesis may be of etio-

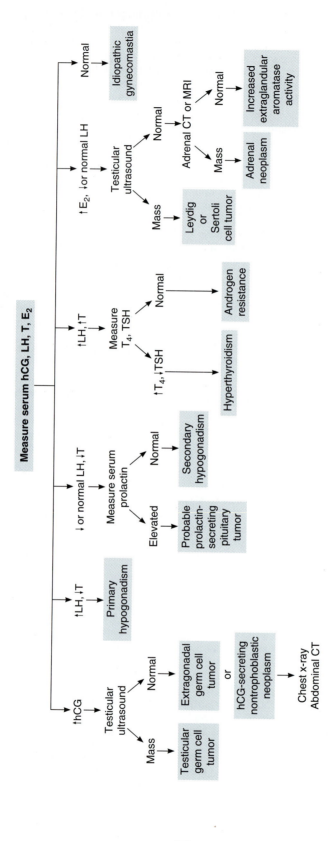

Figure 12–9. Diagnostic evaluation for endocrine causes of gynecomastia. (hCG, human chorionic gonadotropin; LH, luteinizing hormone; T, testosterone; E₂, estradiol; T₄, thyroxine; TSH, thyrotropic hormone.) (Reproduced, with permission, from Braunstein GD: Gynecomastia. N Engl J Med 1993;328:490.)

logic importance in the development of germ cell neoplasms. Although trauma is frequently cited as an etiologic factor in testicular tumors, no causal relationship has been established. What is more likely is that testicular trauma serves to call the patient's attention to the presence of a testicular mass.

Bilateral gynecomastia is uncommon in patients who present with testicular cancer. It is generally associated with production of hCG by the trophoblastic elements in the tumor. The hCG stimulates the Leydig cells to produce excessive estrogens relative to androgen production, resulting in estrogen-androgen imbalance and gynecomastia. In addition, the trophoblastic tissue in some of the tumors may convert estrogen precursors to estrogens.

Pathology

A. Germ Cell Tumors: Seminomas account for 33–50% of all germ cell tumors. They are composed of round cells with abundant cytoplasm, prominent nuclei, and large nucleoli. The cells are arranged in cords and nests and have a thin delicate network of stromal connective tissue. Embryonal cell neoplasms comprise 20–33% of germ cell tumors. These tumors have multiple histologic patterns composed of cuboidal pleomorphic cells. One distinct pattern of cellular arrangement is the endodermal sinus tumor (yolk sac tumor), the most frequent germ cell neoplasm found in infants. Immunohistochemical techniques have localized alpha-fetoprotein to the embryonal cells. About 10% of germ cell tumors are teratomas, which are composed of well-differentiated cells derived from all three germ layers. When one or more of the teratoid elements are malignant or are mixed with embryonal carcinoma cells, the term teratocarcinoma is applied. These tumors account for one-tenth to one-third of germ cell neoplasms. Choriocarcinoma is the rarest form of germ cell tumor (2%) and is composed of masses of large, polymorphic, multinucleated syncytiotrophoblastic cells. Although pure choriocarcinoma is rare, many testicular tumors contain an occasional trophoblastic giant cell. Immunohistochemical techniques have shown that these cells are the source of hCG in such tumors.

B. Leydig Cell Tumors: Leydig cell (interstitial cell) tumors are rare. Most are benign and are composed of sheets of oval to polygonal cells arranged in lobules separated from one another by thin strands of connective tissue. Malignant Leydig cell tumor disseminates by both lymphatic and venous channels, with initial metastatic deposits being found in the regional lymph nodes, followed by metastases to liver, lung, and bone.

Clinical Features

A. Symptoms and Signs:

1. Germ cell tumors–Testicular tumors usually present as painless enlargement of a testicle with an associated feeling of fullness or heaviness in the scrotum. Thus, about 80% of patients note a testicular swelling or mass, whereas only 25% complain of testicular pain or tenderness. About 6–25% of patients give a history of testicular trauma that brought the testicular mass to their attention. Gynecomastia may be present initially in 2–4% of patients and develops subsequently in another 10%. About 5–10% of patients present with symptoms of distant metastatic disease, including backache, skeletal pains, gastrointestinal and abdominal pains, inguinal adenopathy, and neurologic dysfunction.

A testicular mass or generalized enlargement of the testis is often present on examination. In 5–10% of patients, a coexisting hydrocele may be present. In the presence of metastatic disease, supraclavicular and retroperitoneal lymph node enlargement may be present.

2. Leydig cell tumors–In children, Leydig cell tumors of the testes may produce sexual precocity, with rapid skeletal growth and development of secondary sexual characteristics. Adults with such tumors usually present with a testicular mass and occasionally gynecomastia. Decreased libido may also be present in such patients.

B. Laboratory Findings:

1. Germ cell tumors–The tumor markers hCG and alpha-fetoprotein should be measured in every male presenting with a testicular mass. hCG is found in the sera of 5–10% of males with seminoma, over half of patients with teratocarcinoma or embryonal cell carcinoma, and all patients with choriocarcinoma. hCG should be measured by the beta subunit or other hCG-specific radioimmunoassay method. Elevated serum immunoreactive alpha-fetoprotein concentrations are found in almost 70% of patients with nonseminomatous forms of germ cell neoplasms. Both markers are elevated in over 50% of patients with nonseminomatous germ cell tumors, and at least one of the markers is elevated in 85% of such patients. These markers can also be used to monitor the results of therapy.

2. Leydig cell tumors–Urinary 17-ketosteroids and serum DHEA sulfate concentrations are increased. Both urinary and serum estrogen levels may also be increased. Serum testosterone concentrations tend to be low or within the normal adult range.

C. Imaging Studies: Staging of testicular tumors requires several radiologic procedures, including chest tomograms, intravenous urograms, liver scans, gallium scans, and bipedal lymphangiography. CT scans of the abdomen and retroperitoneum have replaced lymphangiograms in many institutions.

Differential Diagnosis

Testicular tumors are sometimes misdiagnosed as epididymitis or epididymo-orchitis. An inflammatory reaction of the epididymis often involves the vas deferens. Therefore, both the vas and the epididymis will be thickened and tender on examination during the acute disease. Pyuria and fever also help to differentiate between epididymitis and testicular tumor. Because hydrocele may coexist with testicular tumor, the testes should be carefully examined following aspiration of the hydrocele.

Other conditions that can cause confusion with testicular tumors include inguinal hernia, hematocele, hematoma, torsion, spermatocele, varicocele, and (rarely) sarcoidosis, tuberculosis, and syphilitic gumma. Ultrasonic examination of the scrotum may help distinguish between testicular tumors and extratesticular disease such as acute or chronic epididymitis, spermatocele, or hydrocele.

Benign Leydig cell tumors of the testes must be differentiated from adrenal rest tumors in patients with congenital adrenal hyperplasia. Since the testes and the adrenals are derived from the same embryologic source, ectopic adrenal tissue may be found to migrate with the testes. This tissue can enlarge under the influence of ACTH in patients with congenital adrenal hyperplasia or Cushing's disease. Adrenal rest tumors tend to be bilateral, whereas patients with Leydig cell tumors generally have unilateral disease. Both may be associated with elevated urine 17-ketosteroids and elevated serum DHEA sulfate concentrations. Elevated serum and urinary estrogen concentrations are found with both disorders. However, patients with congenital adrenal hyperplasia or Cushing's disease will have a decrease in 17-ketosteroids, DHEA sulfate, and estrogen concentrations, as well as a decrease in tumor size, following administration of dexamethasone.

Treatment

A. Germ Cell Tumors: Seminomas are quite radiosensitive, and disease localized to the testes is usually treated with orchiectomy and 2000–4000 cGy of conventional radiotherapy delivered to the ipsilateral inguinal-iliac and bilateral para-aortic lymph nodes to the level of the diaphragm. For disease that has spread to the lymph nodes below the diaphragm, additional whole abdominal radiotherapy and prophylactic mediastinal and supraclavicular lymph node irradiation are usually given. Widely disseminated disease is generally treated with a combination of radiotherapy and chemotherapy, especially with alkylating agents.

Nonseminomatous tumors are treated with orchiectomy, retroperitoneal lymph node dissection, and, if necessary, radiotherapy or chemotherapy (or both). Although many chemotherapeutic agents have been used, combinations of etoposide (VP-16), bleomycin, and cisplatin currently appear to produce the best overall results. Patients with nonseminomatous tumors treated by these means should be monitored with serial measurements of serum hCG and alpha-fetoprotein.

B. Leydig Cell Tumors: Benign Leydig cell tumors of the testes are treated by unilateral orchiectomy. Objective remissions of malignant Leydig cell tumors have been noted following treatment with mitotane.

Course & Prognosis

A. Germ Cell Tumors: In patients with seminoma confined to the testicle, the 5-year survival rates after orchiectomy and radiotherapy are 98–100%. Disease in the lymph nodes below the diaphragm also has an excellent prognosis, with 5-year survival rates of 80–85%. Disease above the diaphragm and disseminated disease have 5-year survival rates as low as 18%.

In patients with nonseminomatous germ cell tumors, aggressive surgery and combination chemotherapy have raised the 5-year survival rates from less than 20% to 60–90%.

B. Leydig Cell Tumors: Removal of a benign Leydig cell tumor is accompanied by regression of precocious puberty in children or feminization in adults. The prognosis for malignant Leydig cell tumor is poor, with most patients surviving less than 2 years from the time of diagnosis.

REFERENCES

Physiology

Burger HG: Clinical utility of inhibin measurements. J Clin Endocrinol Metab 1993;76:1391.

Quigley CA et al: Androgen receptor defects: Historical, clinical, and molecular perspectives. Endocr Rev 1995;16:271.

Saez JM: Leydig cells: Endocrine, paracrine, and autocrine regulation. Endocr Rev 1994;15:574.

Saez JM et al: Cell-cell communication in the testis. Horm Res 1991;36:104.

Shenker A: G protein-coupled receptor structure and function: the impact of disease-causing mutations. Clin Endocrinol Metab 1995;9:427.

Williams GR, Franklyn JA: Physiology of the steroid-thyroid hormone nuclear receptor superfamily. Clin Endocrinol Metab 1994;8:241.

Wu FCW: Testicular steroidogenesis and androgen use and abuse. Clin Endocrinol Metab 1992;6:373.

Androgen Therapy

Bardin CW, Swerdloff RS, Santen RJ: Androgens: Risks and benefits. J Clin Endocrinol Metab 1991;73:4.

Bhasin S: Androgen treatment of hypogonadal men. J Clin Endocrinol Metab 1992;74:1221.

Lukas SE: Current perspectives on anabolic-androgenic steroid abuse. Trends Pharm Sci 1993;14:61.

Morley JE et al: Effects of testosterone replacement therapy in old hypogonadal males: A preliminary study. J Am Geriatr Soc 1993;41:149.

Rudman D, Shetty KR: Unanswered questions concerning the treatment of hyposomatotropism and hypogonadism in elderly men. J Am Geriatr Soc 1994;42:522.

Tenover JS: Effects of testosterone supplementation in the aging male. J Clin Endocrinol Metab 1992;75:1092.

Hypogonadism

Castro-Magaña M, Bronsther B, Angulo MA: Genetic forms of male hypogonadism. Urology 1990;35:195.

Giwercman A et al: Evidence for increasing incidence of abnormalities of the human testis: A review. Environ Health Perspect 1993;101(Suppl 2):65.

Hudson RW, Edwards AL: Testicular function in hyperthyroidism. J Androl 1992;13:117.

Martinez-Mora J et al: Male pseudohermaphroditism due to Leydig cell agenesia and absence of testicular LH receptors. Clin Endocrinol 1991;34:485.

Palmer JM: The undescended testicle. Endocrinol Metab Clin North Am 1991;20:231.

Schwartz ID, Root AW: The Klinefelter syndrome of testicular dysgenesis. Endocrinol Metab Clin North Am 1991;20:153.

Smith NM, Byard RW, Bourne AJ: Testicular regression syndrome: A pathological study of 77 cases. Histopathology 1991;19:269.

Swerdloff RS, Wang C: Androgen deficiency and aging in men. West J Med 1993;159:579.

Vazquez JA: Hypothalamic-pituitary-testicular function in 70 patients with myotonic dystrophy. J Endocrinol Invest 1990;13:375.

Vermeulen A: The male climacterium. Ann Med 1993;25:531.

Whitcomb RW, Crowley WF Jr.: Male hypogonadotropic hypogonadism. Endocrinol Metab Clin North Am 1993;22:125.

Infertility

Gangi GR, Nagler HM: Clinical evaluation of the subfertile male. Infertil Reprod Med Clin North Am 1992;3:299.

Howards SS: Varicocele. Infertil Reprod Med Clin North Am 1992;3:429.

Overstreet JW, Davis RO, Katz DF: Semen evaluation. Infertil Reprod Med Clin North Am 1992;3:329.

Impotence

Brock GB, Lue TF: Drug-induced male sexual dysfunction: An update. Drug Safety 1993;8:414.

Korenman SG: Advances in the understanding and management of erectile dysfunction. J Clin Endocrinol Metab 1995;80:1985.

Lerner SE, Melman A, Christ GJ: A review of erectile dysfunction: New insights and more questions. J Urol 1993;149:1246.

NIH Consensus Statement: Impotence. 1992;10:1.

von Heyden B et al: Intracavernous pharmacotherapy for impotence: Selection of appropriate agent and dose. J Urol 1993;149:1288.

Wespes E, Schulman C: Venous impotence: Pathophysiology, diagnosis and treatment. J Urol 1993;149:1238.

Gynecomastia

Braunstein GD: Gynecomastia. N Engl J Med 1993;328:490.

Testicular Cancer

Roth BJ, Nichols CR (editors): Testicular cancer. Semin Oncol 1992;19:117.

13

Ovaries

Alan Goldfien, MD, & Scott E. Monroe, MD

ANATOMY OF THE OVARIES

The mature ovaries are paired nodular structures 2.5–5 × 2 × 1 cm, weighing from 4 to 8 g, the weight varying during the menstrual cycle. They are situated behind the peritoneum attached to the posterior surface of the broad ligament by a fold of the peritoneum called the mesovarium, which contains the blood vessels and nerves leading to the hilum. The ovaries are attached to the uterus by the ovarian ligament and lie in close association with the uterine tubes (oviducts, fallopian tubes) (Figure 13–1).

The ovaries develop from the genital ridges situated between the base of the dorsal mesentery and the mesonephros on either side of the celomic cavity. The primordial germ cells that originate in the endoderm of the yolk sac at the third week begin to migrate through the hindgut to invade the genital ridges at about the sixth week. These primary oocytes are surrounded by a layer of epithelium and mesenchymal cells that give rise to the primordial follicles. About 1700 germ cells are present before migration to the genital ridge begins; however, these multiply during the process of migration and within the genital ridge, reaching a peak of 7 million oocytes at mid gestation. The primordial germ cells increase in size early in their development and become oogonia. At mid gestation they begin the first meiotic division, becoming primary oocytes. This prophase lasts until just before ovulation, which may occur 12–40 or more years later. In this state, they are no longer capable of multiplication and in fact steadily decline in number (Figure 13–2). About 400 ova are lost through the process of ovulation during a woman's lifetime. The remainder undergo degeneration so that, by the time of the menopause, few are present.

Blood Supply

The arterial vessels supplying the ovary are derived from branches of the ovarian and uterine arteries that enter through the mesovarium and divide into branches leading into the stroma of the medulla and then to the cortex. The small arteries of the ovary are characteristically spiral. The capillary blood gathers in veins that form a large, thin-walled plexus of vessels called the pampiniform plexus, leaving the ovary by way of the ovarian vein at the hilum. Lymphatics arise in the outer or cortical portion of the ovary and anastomose centrally, leaving through the hilum. Although the lymphatic channels are numerous in the

---

ACRONYMS USED IN THIS CHAPTER

ACTH	Adrenocorticotropic hormone
ALT	Alanine aminotransferase
BSP	Bromsulphalein
CBG	Corticosteroid-binding globulin
DHEA	Dehydroepiandrosterone
DHT	Dihydrotestosterone
EI	Eosinophilic index
FSH	Follicle-stimulating hormone
GH	Growth hormone
GnRH	Gondotropin-releasing hormone
hCG	Human chorionic gonadotropin
HDL	High-density lipoprotein(s)
KPI	Karyopyknotic index
LDL	Low-density lipoprotein(s)
LH	Luteinizing hormone
LHRH	Luteinizing hormone-releasing hormone
LRH	Luteotropin-releasing hormone
MCR	Metabolic clearance rate
MI	Maturation index
PMN	Polymorphonuclear neutrophil
PMS	Premenstrual syndrome
PRL	Prolactin
PTH	Parathyroid hormone
RNA	Ribonucleic acid
SHBG	Sex hormone-binding globulin
TBG	Thyroid hormone-binding globulin
VLDL	Very low density lipoprotein(s)

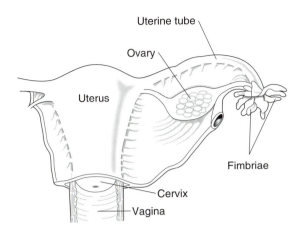

Figure 13–1. Internal organs of the female reproductive system: ovary, fimbriae of infundibulum, uterine tube, uterus, cervix, and vagina. (Reproduced, with permission, from Junqueira LC, Carneiro J, Kelley RO: *Basic Histology,* 6th ed. Appleton & Lange, 1989.)

theca externa, corpora lutea, and corpora albicantia, they are not seen in the theca interna, granulosa, or tunica albuginea.

Nerve Supply

The ovary has a rich autonomic innervation arising from the intermesenteric nerves and renal plexus; from the superior hypogastric plexus or presacral nerve and the hypogastric nerve; and from the inferior hypogastric plexus or pelvic plexus. The nerves appear to be mainly sympathetic in origin.

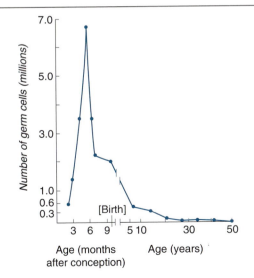

Figure 13–2. Total number of germ cells in the human ovary at different ages. (Reproduced, with permission, from Baker TG: *Reproduction in Mammals.* Austin CR, Short RV [editors]. Cambridge Univ Press, 1972.)

Microscopic Anatomy

As shown in Figure 13–3, the ovary consists of many different structures. The mature ovary is covered by a layer of columnar cells that constitute the **germinal epithelium.** The dense layer of connective tissue under the epithelium is called the tunica albuginea. The remainder of the organ is divided into outer cortical and inner medullary portions, of which the cortex is the larger. The cortex contains follicular structures in all stages of development, surrounded by the connective tissue elements of the stroma and the hilar cells, a group of steroid-secreting cells that histologically resemble the Leydig, or interstitial, cells of the testes. The medulla consists of a connective tissue stroma containing elastic fibers, blood vessels, nerves, lymphatics, and smooth muscle fibers.

The follicular complex contains the ova as well as the cells responsible for production of the ovarian hormones and their precursors. Structural changes and hormonal activity that occur throughout the menstrual cycle are discussed below.

HORMONES OF THE OVARY

The mature ovary actively synthesizes and secretes a variety of hormones. Among these are the sex steroids, which include estrogens, progesterone, androgens, and their precursors. In addition, the ovary produces relaxin, inhibin, activins, and locally active agents such as follistatin and prostaglandins.

STEROID HORMONES

The ovary is normally the major source of estrogens, although the conversion of androgen precursors in other tissues is clinically important after the menopause and in some women with disorders of ovarian function. The ovary also produces and secretes large amounts of progesterone during the luteal phase of the cycle. It is also the source of small amounts of testosterone and other androgens that serve not only as precursors to estrogen synthesis but also are released into the circulation to act on peripheral tissues.

Biosynthesis of Steroid Hormones

The biochemical pathways, including the major enzymes and their intracellular localizations, are similar in the ovary, testis, and adrenal. The process in the ovary is outlined in Figure 13–4. The steroid hormones are synthesized from cholesterol, which is present in the gland both free and esterified to fatty

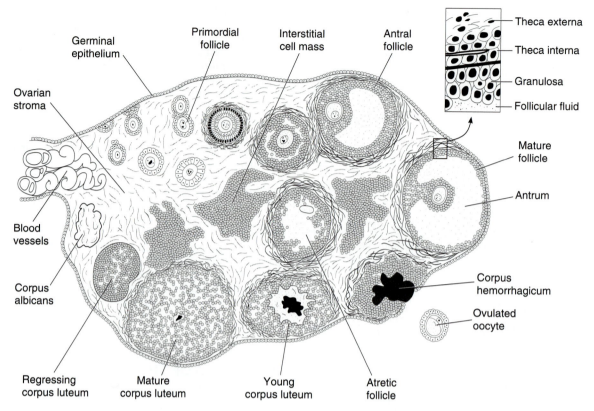

Figure 13–3. Diagram of a mammalian ovary, showing the sequential development of a follicle, formation of a corpus luteum, and, in the center, follicular atresia. A section of the wall of a mature follicle is enlarged at the upper right. The interstitial cell mass is not prominent in primates. (After Patten and Eakin. Reproduced, with permission, from Katzung BG [editor]: *Basic and Clinical Pharmacology,* 3rd ed. Appleton & Lange, 1987.)

acids (cholesteryl esters). Cholesterol derived either from circulating lipoproteins (LDL) or from cholesteryl esters in the gland is converted to pregnenolone by the enzyme P450scc which removes a six-carbon fragment, isocaproic acid. This reaction or group of reactions is the rate-limiting step in the biosynthetic process and is controlled by luteinizing hormone (LH) from the anterior pituitary.

Pregnenolone formed by this reaction may be converted either to progesterone or to 17α-hydroxypregnenolone. The conversion to progesterone requires the action of 3β-hydroxysteroid dehydrogenase and $\Delta^{5,4}$-ketosteroid isomerase, which shifts the double bond from the Δ^5 to the Δ^4 position. Progesterone is secreted by the corpus luteum in large amounts following ovulation (see below). However, it also serves as a precursor for androgen and estrogen, since it is a substrate for P450c17 (17α-hydroxylase), which converts it to 17α-hydroxyprogesterone in the endoplasmic reticulum. Following 17α-hydroxylation, the two-carbon (20–21) side chain may be cleaved by the P450c17α (17,20-lyase) enzyme to form androgens (see Figure 13–4).

17α-Hydroxypregnenolone is converted by the P450c17α (lyase) enzyme to dehydroepiandrosterone (DHEA). This compound can then be converted to androstenedione. The relative importance of these pathways to androgen production is not clear. Androstenedione is the major androgen secreted by the ovary, but small amounts of DHEA and testosterone are also released.

Estradiol, the most active estrogen produced by the ovary, is synthesized from androgens by the enzyme P45O aromatase. The process involves three steps: hydroxylation of the methyl group at carbon 19, oxidation of this group, and hydroxylation at the 3α position. These steps are thought to occur in the microsomal fraction (see Chapter 9).

During the menstrual cycle, regulation of biosynthesis and release is controlled by the gonadotropins as well as by local factors.

Secretion of Steroid Hormones

The secretory activity of the steroid-producing granulosa and theca cells is closely coupled to their biosynthetic activity, since little hormone is stored in

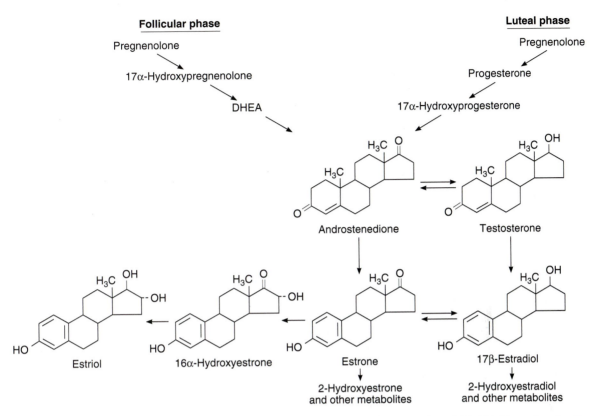

Figure 13–4. Biosynthesis and metabolism of estrogens. (See also Figures 9–4, 12–2, and 14–13.) (Reproduced, with permission, from Katzung BG [editor]: *Basic and Clinical Pharmacology,* 4th ed. Appleton & Lange, 1989.)

the cells. Direct measures of secretion rates in humans require an accurate measure of the concentration of the hormone in the effluent blood from the gland and a measure of blood flow through the gland. Such samples and measurements are difficult to obtain without interfering with blood flow and normal gland activity. Therefore, indirect measures have been widely used. Some of the most useful information has been obtained by measuring the metabolic clearance rate (MCR) with an in vivo isotope dilution technique. Multiplying MCR by the concentration of the hormone in blood provides a total production rate for the hormone. However, the production rate also includes production of the hormone at other sites from circulating precursors, and it may therefore be greater than the amount secreted by the gland. The production rates, plasma levels, and MCRs of various ovarian steroids are shown in Table 13–1.

During pregnancy, the fetal-placental unit produces a large amount of steroid hormone. The placenta produces progesterone, which is released into the maternal circulation, and large amounts of pregnenolone, which is released into the fetal circulation. Enzymatic conversion of pregnenolone by the fetal adrenal and liver produces steroids, including 16-hy-droxydehydroepiandrosterone sulfate, which are subsequently converted to estriol and other estrogens in the placenta and released into the maternal circulation (see Chapter 16).

Transport of Steroid Hormones

When released into the circulation, the gonadal steroids bind to plasma proteins. Estradiol binds avidly to a transport globulin called sex hormone-binding globulin (SHBG) and binds with less affinity to albumin. Progesterone binds strongly to corticosteroid-binding globulin (CBG) and weakly to albumin. The percentages of various steroids that bind to these carrier proteins are listed in Table 13–2. The concentration of these binding proteins is increased by estrogen and thyroxine and decreased by androgens and progestins. SHBG is synthesized in the liver, and because its synthesis is stimulated by estrogens and inhibited by androgen, levels are twice as high in women as in men. The proportions of free and bound estradiol do not vary significantly during the menstrual cycle. However, differences in binding may assume clinical importance after the menopause or in women with abnormal ovarian function associated with excess androgens.

Table 13–1. Approximate concentrations, metabolic clearance rates (MCR), production rates, and ovarian secretion rates of steroids in blood.[1]

	MCR (L/d)	Phase of Menstrual Cycle	Plasma Concentration		Production Rate		Secretion Rate (Both Ovaries)	
			(μg/dL)	(nmol/L)	(mg/d)	(μmol/d)	(mg/d)	(μmol/d)
Estradiol	1350	Early follicular	0.006	(0.22)	0.081	(0.3)	0.07	(0.26)
		Late follicular	0.033–0.07	(1.21–2.57)	0.445–0.945	(1.63–3.47)	0.4–0.8	(1.63–2.93)
		Midluteal	0.02	(0.73)	0.27	(1)	0.25	(0.92)
Estrone	2210	Early follicular	0.005	(0.18)	0.11	(0.41)	0.08	(0.3)
		Late follicular	0.015–0.03	(0.55–1.11)	0.331–0.662	(0.86–2.45)	0.25–0.5	(0.92–1.85)
		Midluteal	0.011	(0.41)	0.243	(0.9)	0.16	(0.59)
Progesterone	2200	Late follicular	0.095	(3.02)	2.1	(6.68)	1.5	(4.77)
		Luteal	1.13	(35.9)	25	(79.5)	24	(76.3)
Androstenedione	2010	...	0.159	(5.1)	3.2	(11.1)	0.8–1.6	(2.77–5.55)
Testosterone	690	...	0.038	(1.32)	0.26	(0.9)	...	...
Dehydroepiandrosterone	1640	...	0.49	(16.8)	8	(27.5)	0.3–3	(1.03–10.3)
Dihydrotestosterone	400	...	0.02	(0.69)	0.05	(0.17)	0.01–0.02	(0.03–0.06)

[1]Modified from Lipsett, MB: Steroid hormones. Page 84 in: *Reproductive Endocrinology.* Yen SSC, Jaffe RB (editors). Saunders, 1978.

Metabolism of Steroid Hormones

A. Estrogens: Circulating estradiol is rapidly converted in the liver to estrone by 17β-hydroxysteroid dehydrogenase (Figure 13–5). Some of the estrone reenters the circulation; however, most of it is further metabolized to 16α-hydroxyestrone (which is then converted to estriol) or to 2- or 4-hydroxyestrone (catechol estrogen). The catechol estrogens that have biologic activity are converted to the 2- and 4-methoxy compounds by catechol-*O*-methyltransferase. Much of the remaining estrone is conjugated to form estrone sulfate. Estriol is converted largely to estriol 3-sulfate-16-glucuronide before excretion by the kidney.

B. Progesterone: Progesterone is rapidly cleared from the circulation, having an initial half-life of about 5 minutes. As indicated by its high clearance rate (Table 13–1), it is rapidly converted to pregnanediol and conjugated to glucuronic acid in the liver. Pregnanediol glucuronide is excreted in the urine and may be used as an index of progesterone production. In addition, small amounts of 20α-hydroxyprogesterone are formed (Figure 13–5). This compound has one-fifth the activity of progesterone.

Physiologic Effects of Steroid Hormones

The biologic effects of the ovarian steroids are mediated by specific hormone receptors. Plasma estradiol is thought to enter its target cell by diffusion and is transported to the nucleus, where it binds to the estrogen receptors. The estrogen receptors are found in the nucleus bound to a number of different heat shock proteins. Binding of the hormone to its receptor leads to dissociation of the receptor from the heat shock protein complex and alterations in the receptor structure. The ligand-receptor complex forms a homodimer that binds to the estrogen response element on the gene and in association with other transcription factors leads to the formation of specific messenger RNA (see Figure 3–12).

There are estimated to be between 5000 and 20,000 estrogen receptor molecules per cell. These

Table 13–2. Total plasma concentration and percentage of steroid hormone that is free or bound to plasma transport proteins in healthy women in the early follicular phase. During the luteal phase, the total concentrations of estradiol (0.72 nmol/L) and progesterone (38 nmol/L) are higher, but the distrubution is the same.[1]

	Total Plasma Concentration (nmol/L)	Percentage Distribution of Steroid			
		Free	SHBG	CBG	Albumin
Estradiol	0.29	1.8	37.3	0.1	60.8
Estrone	0.23	3.6	16.3	0.1	80.1
Progesterone	0.65	2.4	0.6	17.7	79.3
Testosterone	1.3	1.4	66	2.3	30.4
Dihydrotestosterone	0.65	0.5	78.4	0.1	21
Androstenedione	5.4	7.5	6.6	1.4	84.5
Cortisol	400	3.8	0.2	89.7	6.3

[1]Data from Dunn JF, Nisula BC, Rodbard D: *J Clin Endocrinol Metab* 1981;**53:**58.

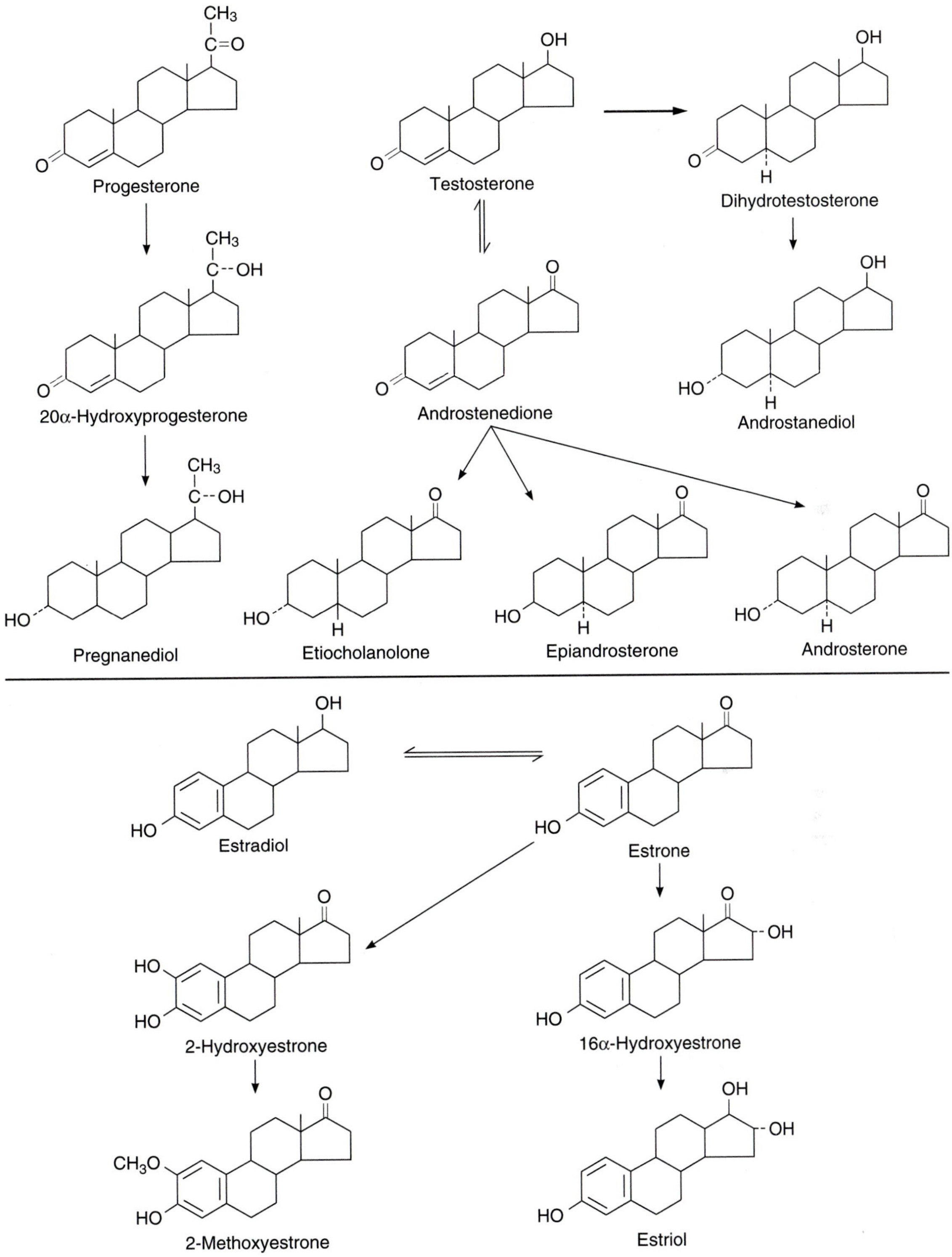

Figure 13–5. Metabolism of ovarian steroid hormones. (See also Figures 12–2 and 14–14.)

receptors also serve as sites for regulation of hormonal activity. For example, estrogens induce development of increased numbers of estrogen receptors in some tissues and also stimulate the synthesis of progesterone receptors. By contrast, progesterone may cause a reduction in the number of estrogen and progesterone receptors.

Progesterone also enters the cell by diffusion and binds to progesterone receptors, which are distributed between the nucleus and the cytoplasmic domains. The ligand-receptor complex binds to a response element to activate gene transcription. The response element for progesterone appears to be similar to the corticoid response element, and the specificity of the response is determined by which receptor is present in the cell as well as by other cell-specific transcription factors. The progesterone receptor also forms a dimer before binding to DNA. However, in contrast to the estrogen receptor, it can form heterodimers. Although it is clear that these intracellular receptors mediate many of the important effects of steroid hormones, some effects, such as the anesthetic effect of progesterone and the stimulatory effect of estrogens on uterine blood flow, the acrosome reaction in sperm, the meiotic maturation of frog oocytes, and granulosa cell Ca^{2+} uptake, suggest that these steroids also act at the cell membrane.

A. Estrogens: Estrogens are required for the normal maturation of the female. They stimulate the maturation of the vagina, uterus, and uterine tubes at puberty as well as the secondary sex characteristics. They stimulate stromal development and ductal growth in the breast and are responsible for the accelerated growth phase and the closing of the epiphyses of the long bones that occurs at puberty. They alter the distribution of body fat so as to produce typical female body contours, including some accumulation of body fat around the hips and breasts. Larger quantities also stimulate development of pigmentation in the skin, most prominently in the region of the nipples and areolae and in the genital region.

In addition to its effects on growth of uterine muscle, estrogen also plays an important role in development of the endometrial lining. Continuous exposure to estrogens for prolonged periods leads to an abnormal hyperplasia of the endometrium that is usually associated with abnormal bleeding patterns. When estrogen production is properly coordinated with the production of progesterone during the normal human menstrual cycle, regular periodic bleeding and shedding of the endometrial lining occur.

Estrogens have a number of important metabolic effects. They seem to be partially responsible for maintenance of the normal structure of the skin and blood vessels in women. Estrogens decrease the rate of resorption of bone by antagonizing the effect of parathyroid hormone (PTH) on bone; they do not stimulate bone formation. Estrogens may have important effects on intestinal absorption, because they

reduce the motility of bowel. In addition to stimulating the synthesis of enzymes leading to uterine growth, they alter the production and activity of many other enzymes in the body. In the liver, there is an increase in the synthesis of binding or transport proteins, including those for estrogen, testosterone, and thyroxine.

Estrogens enhance the coagulability of blood. Many changes in factors influencing coagulation have been reported, including increased circulating levels of factors II, VII, IX, and X and decreased levels of antithrombin III. Increased plasminogen levels and decreased platelet adhesiveness have been reported.

Estrogens decrease adipose tissue lipid oxidation to ketones and increase synthesis of triglycerides. Alterations in the composition of the plasma lipids include an increase in high-density lipoproteins (HDL), a slight reduction in low-density lipoproteins (LDL), and a reduction in plasma cholesterol levels. Plasma triglyceride levels are increased, as is fat deposition as well.

Estrogens have many other effects. They are responsible for estrous behavior in animals and influence libido in humans. They facilitate the loss of intravascular fluid into the extracellular space, producing edema. The resulting decrease in plasma volume causes a compensatory retention of sodium and water by the kidney. Estrogens also modulate sympathetic nervous system control of smooth muscle function.

B. Progesterone: The effects of progesterone on reproductive organs include the glandular development of the breasts and the cyclic glandular development of the endometrium described below (see Menstrual Cycle) and are critical for successful reproduction. However, progesterone exhibits important metabolic effects in other organs and tissues, producing changes in carbohydrate, protein, and lipid metabolism.

A dose of 50 mg of progesterone intramuscularly daily can lead to increased insulin levels and decreased response of blood glucose levels to insulin as observed in normal pregnancy.

Progesterone can compete with aldosterone at the renal tubule, causing a decrease in Na^+ reabsorption. This leads to an increased secretion of aldosterone by the adrenal cortex—eg, in pregnancy. Progesterone increases the body temperature in humans. The mechanism of this effect is not known, but an alteration of the temperature-regulating centers in the hypothalamus has been suggested. Progesterone also alters the function of the respiratory centers. The ventilatory response to CO_2 is increased, leading to a measurable reduction in arterial and alveolar P_{CO_2} during pregnancy and in the luteal phase of the menstrual cycle. Synthetic progestins with an ethinyl group do not have these respiratory effects. Progesterone and related steroids also have hypnotic effects on the brain.

C. Androgens: The normal ovary produces potent androgens, including testosterone and dihydrotestosterone, as well as androstenedione, Δ^5-androstenediol, and DHEA. Only testosterone and dihydrotestosterone have significant androgenic activity, although androstenedione is converted to testosterone in peripheral tissues. The healthy woman produces less than 300 μg of testosterone in 24 hours, and about one-fourth of this is probably formed in the ovary directly. The physiologic significance of these small amounts of androgens is not established, but they may be partly responsible for normal hair growth at puberty and may have other important metabolic effects. Androgen production by the ovary may be markedly increased in some abnormal states (usually in association with amenorrhea), and less active precursors (eg, androstenedione) may be converted to more active hormones in target tissues such as the hair follicle and sebaceous glands.

Dehydroepiandrosterone (DHEA) and dehydroepiandrosterone sulfate (DHEAS) in large amounts and androstenedione and testosterone in smaller amounts are also secreted by the adrenal cortex. Although they are thought to contribute to the normal maturation process (adrenarche), they do not stimulate or support other androgen-dependent pubertal changes in the human. Some studies suggest that DHEA and DHEAS may have other important metabolic effects which inhibit atherosclerosis and prolong life in rabbits and perhaps in humans. The therapeutic uses of this hormone are currently being explored.

RELAXIN

Relaxin is a polypeptide that has been extracted from the ovary. In certain animal species, it appears to play an important role at the time of parturition, causing relaxation of the pelvic ligaments and softening of the uterine cervix. The three-dimensional structure of relaxin is similar to that of insulin and related growth-promoting polypeptides, although the amino acid sequences are different. It consists of two chains linked by disulfide bonds, cleaved from a prohormone. It is found in the ovary, placenta, and uterus and in the blood. Relaxin synthesis has been demonstrated in luteinized granulosa cells of the corpus luteum. In addition to changing the mechanical properties of tissues such as the cervix and pubic ligaments, it increases glycogen synthesis and water uptake by the myometrium and decreases its contractility. It may also have mammotropic effects.

In women, relaxin has been measured by immunoassay. During the menstrual cycle, levels were highest immediately after the LH surge and during menstruation. Circulating levels of relaxin are reported to be 25% higher by the end of the first trimester than during the second and third trimesters of pregnancy.

OTHER OVARIAN HORMONES & REGULATORY SUBSTANCES

Several nonsteroidal substances that may be important in the regulation of both intra- and extraovarian processes have been found in follicular fluid. These substances include factors that can decrease (eg, inhibin) or increase (eg, activin) FSH secretion, modulate steroid secretion from granulosa cells, and delay the maturation of the oocyte in the developing preovulatory follicle (follistatin, a binding protein for activin and inhibin). See below for additional information concerning nonsteroidal ovarian regulatory factors.

THE MENSTRUAL CYCLE

The female reproductive system undergoes a series of regular cyclic changes termed the menstrual cycle. The most obvious of these changes is periodic vaginal bleeding, resulting from shedding of the endometrial lining of the uterus. Normal menstrual function results from the interaction of the hypothalamus, pituitary, and ovaries and associated changes in the target tissues of the reproductive tract. Although each component is essential for normal reproductive function, the ovary plays a central role in this process, since it appears to be responsible for regulating both the cyclic changes and the length of the menstrual cycle. In most women in the middle reproductive years, menstrual bleeding recurs every 25–35 days, with a median cycle length of 28 days (Figure 13–6). In women with ovulatory cycles, the interval from the onset of menses to ovulation—the follicular (proliferative) phase—is variable in duration and accounts for the range of cycle lengths observed in ovulating women. The interval from ovulation to the onset of menstrual bleeding—the luteal (secretory) phase—is relatively constant and averages 14 ± 2 days in most women. The greatest variability in cycle length is found in the first few years after menarche and the years immediately preceding the menopause. There is a high incidence of anovulatory vaginal bleeding at these times.

HORMONAL PROFILES DURING THE MENSTRUAL CYCLE

Pituitary Gonadotropins

Luteinizing hormone (LH) and follicle-stimulating hormone (FSH) are glycoproteins with molecular weights of about 28,000 and 33,000, respectively. Each hormone is composed of an alpha subunit and a

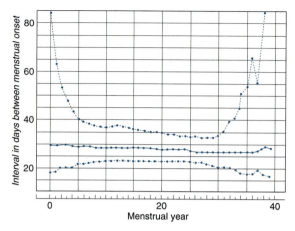

Figure 13–6. Median lengths of menstrual cycles (solid line) throughout reproductive life in women from menarche (year 0) to menopause (year 40). Ninety percent of all cycles fall within the upper and lower dotted lines. (After Treolar AE et al. Reproduced, with permission, from Yen SSC, Jaffe RB [editors]: *Reproductive Endocrinology.* Saunders, 1978.)

beta subunit. The alpha subunits have essentially the same amino acid sequences. The beta subunits, however, are unique and are responsible for the characteristic biologic activities of each hormone. The initial plasma half-life of LH is approximately 30 minutes, whereas the half-life of FSH is 3 hours. The profiles of LH and FSH throughout the menstrual cycle are illustrated in Figure 13–7. Because of the diversity of standards used to quantitate gonadotropins, the LH and FSH values for the same serum sample reported by different laboratories may vary 2- or 3-fold. The clinician must therefore be aware of the laboratory's upper and lower limits of normal. Serum FSH levels persistently greater than 40 mIU/mL (mIU of the Second International Reference Preparation of Human Menopausal Gonadotropin; mIU-2nd IRP-HMG) usually indicate declining or absent ovarian follicular activity.

In the normal menstrual cycle, serum concentrations of both LH and FSH begin to increase a few days prior to menses. FSH concentrations initially increase more rapidly than those of LH and attain maximum levels during the first half of the follicular phase. FSH levels gradually decline in the latter half of the follicular phase and, with the exception of a brief peak at midcycle, continue to fall until the lowest concentrations in the cycle are reached during the second half of the luteal phase. The preovulatory decline in serum concentrations of FSH is a consequence of the rising concentration of estradiol in this period. LH levels increase gradually throughout the follicular phase. At midcycle, there is a large peak in serum concentration of LH (midcycle LH surge) last-

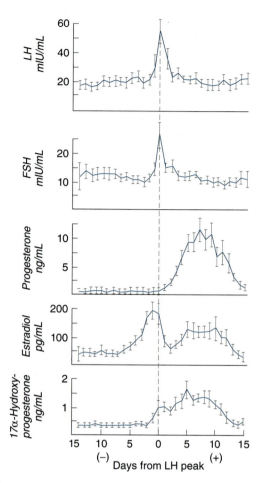

Figure 13–7. Mean values of LH, FSH, progesterone, estradiol, and 17α-hydroxyprogesterone in daily serum samples from 9 women during ovulatory menstrual cycles. Data from different cycles have been combined using the day of the midcycle LH peak as the reference day (day 0). The vertical bars represent one standard error of the mean. (Reproduced, with permission, from Thorneycroft IH et al: Am J Obstet Gynecol 1971;111:947).

ing 1–3 days. Subsequently, LH levels gradually decline, also reaching their lowest concentrations late in the luteal phase (Figure 13–7). Frequent measurements of serum gonadotropin levels in individual women indicate that gonadotropin secretion—particularly LH—is pulsatile. These pulses of gonadotropins are dependent upon the pulsatile secretion of gonadotropin-releasing hormone (GnRH) from the hypothalamus. During the follicular phase, pulses of LH occur approximately every hour. During the luteal phase, these pulses gradually decrease in frequency, occurring as infrequently as once every 4-8 hours. The decrease in frequency is secondary to rising levels of progesterone, which slow down the hypothalamic GnRH pulse generator.

Prolactin (PRL)

In contrast to LH and FSH profiles, there are no consistent cyclic changes in individual PRL profiles during the normal menstrual cycle. In studies of large numbers of women, however, mean PRL levels in the preovulatory and luteal phases of the menstrual cycle may be slightly higher than in the follicular phase. There is also a significant diurnal variation in plasma concentrations of PRL, with peak levels during the night and early morning hours. Laboratories vary in their reporting of PRL levels (as they do also in reporting gonadotropin levels) because of the use of standards with different biologic and immunologic potencies. The upper limit of normal may thus vary from 15 ng/mL to 30 ng/mL (0.68–1.4 nmol/L), depending upon the laboratory.

Ovarian Steroids

The ovary secretes progestins, androgens, and estrogens. Many of these steroids are also secreted by the adrenal gland or can be formed by peripheral conversion of other steroid precursors; consequently, plasma concentrations of these hormones may not directly reflect ovarian steroidogenic activity. Table 13–1 summarizes the plasma concentrations, metabolic clearance rates, and production rates of the major steroids secreted by the ovary in normal women.

A. Estrogens: Estradiol (E_2) is perhaps the most important secretory product of the ovary, because of its biologic potency and diverse physiologic effects on peripheral target tissues. Plasma concentrations of estradiol during the first half of the follicular phase are low, generally less than 50 pg/mL (0.18 nmol/L) (Figure 13–7). About 1 week prior to the midcycle gonadotropin surge, estradiol concentrations begin to increase rapidly, and peak levels of approximately 200–300 pg/mL (0.73–1.1 nmol/L) are attained on the day preceding—or, less commonly, the day of—the LH surge. The rise in plasma estradiol levels correlates closely with the increase in size of the preovulatory follicle. After the LH surge, serum estradiol levels fall rapidly for several days. There is a secondary increase in plasma estradiol levels that reaches a peak in the midportion of the luteal phase, reflecting estrogen secretion by the corpus luteum. Plasma patterns of estrone during the menstrual cycle are similar to those of estradiol, but the changes in concentrations are less than those of estradiol; thus, the ratio of estrone to estradiol varies throughout the cycle. The ratio is highest at the time of menses, when estradiol secretion is minimal, and lowest in the preovulatory period, when estradiol secretion is maximal. While most of the estradiol in the peripheral circulation results from direct ovarian secretion, a significant fraction of the circulating estrone arises from estradiol and the peripheral conversion of androstenedione. Catheterization studies have shown that increased plasma concentrations of estradiol in the preovulatory and midluteal phases of the cycle principally reflect secretion from the ovary containing the dominant or preovulatory follicle, which later becomes the corpus luteum.

B. Progesterone: Throughout the follicular phase, serum concentrations of progesterone are low—less than 1 ng/mL (3.18 nmol/L). At the time of the LH surge, there is a small increase in plasma concentrations of progesterone, followed by a rise over the next 4–5 days (Figure 13–7). Progesterone levels reach a plateau at concentrations between 10 and 20 ng/mL (32–64 nmol/L) during the midportion of the luteal phase. Thereafter, progesterone levels decline rapidly, reaching concentrations of about 1 ng/mL (3.18 nmol/L) by the first day of menses. Although catheterization studies have shown that progesterone is secreted by both ovaries during the first half of the follicular phase, most of the circulating progesterone at this time appears to be derived from the extraglandular conversion of the adrenal steroids, pregnenolone and pregnenolone sulfate, and from the direct secretion of small amounts of progesterone by the adrenal glands.

During the luteal phase of the cycle, virtually all of the circulating progesterone arises by direct secretion from the corpus luteum. Measurement of plasma concentrations of progesterone is widely used to monitor ovulation. Concentrations greater than 4–5 ng/mL (12.7–15.9 nmol/L) suggest that ovulation has occurred.

C. Androgens: In healthy women, circulating androgens can be derived from secretion by the ovaries and the adrenal glands and also by peripheral conversion of steroid precursors of ovarian and adrenal origin. In healthy women, testosterone is secreted in small quantities by the ovaries and adrenal glands. About 50–70% of the circulating testosterone, however, arises primarily from the peripheral conversion of androstenedione. Mean plasma concentrations of testosterone range from 0.2 ng/mL to 0.4 ng/mL (0.69–1.39 nmol/L) during most of the follicular and luteal phases and increase slightly in the preovulatory phase. Androstenedione arises primarily from direct secretion by the ovaries and adrenal glands. Only a small percentage (about 10%) is formed by peripheral conversion. Secretion of androstenedione by the adrenal does not vary significantly during different phases of the menstrual cycle, although there is a diurnal variation in adrenal secretion of androstenedione similar to that of cortisol. Ovarian secretion of androstenedione, however, fluctuates throughout the menstrual cycle, and the pattern of secretion resembles that of estradiol. Serum concentrations of androstenedione increase in the late follicular phase of the cycle and are maximal at the time of the midcycle gonadotropin surge. There is a small secondary peak of androstenedione during the midluteal phase. Plasma concentrations of both DHEA and DHEA sulfate vary independently of the phase of the menstrual cycle. Both hormones are secreted primarily by the adrenal gland.

THE OVARIAN CYCLE

Ovarian Structure

Throughout adult reproductive years, the structural composition and hormonal activity of the ovary are continually changing (Figures 13–3 and 13–8). These changes in composition and activity are responsible for many of the physiologic events in the normal menstrual cycle. The two major functions of the adult ovary—the synthesis and secretion of sex steroids and the release of a mature ovum every 28–30 days—normally progress in concert with one another and are closely interrelated. The basic reproductive unit of the ovary is the small **primordial follicle,** consisting of (1) a small oocyte (< 25 μm in diameter) arrested in the diplotene stage of meiotic prophase; (2) a few, or a complete ring of, poorly differentiated granulosa cells; and (3) a basement membrane that surrounds the granulosa cells, separating them from the adjacent ovarian stroma. Primordial follicles are found principally in the outer cortex just beneath the fibrous capsule of the ovary.

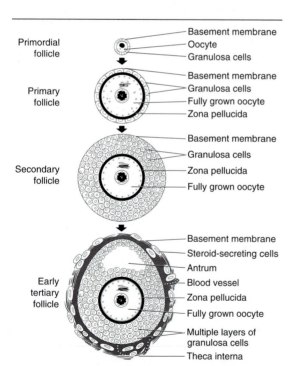

Figure 13–8. Morphologic changes that occur in ovarian follicles during growth and development. (Reproduced, with permission, from Erickson GF: Follicular growth and development. In: *Gynecology and Obstetrics.* Vol 5. Sciarra JJ [editor]. Harper & Row, 1981.)

These primordial follicles constitute an inactive or resting pool from which all ovulatory follicles will eventually develop. During late fetal life and throughout the prepubertal years, a small percentage of these small, inactive follicles are continually resuming growth. At an early stage of development and prior to antrum formation, however, growth is arrested and the follicles undergo atresia. Although ovulation does not occur, the continual process of limited growth and atresia in the prepubertal ovary depletes a large portion of the small primordial follicles, so that only about 400,000 primordial follicles remain at puberty (Figure 13–2). Of these follicles, only about 400 will reach full development and release an oocyte during ovulation in the adult.

The earliest morphologic change indicating that the primordial follicle has left the pool of resting follicles and resumed the process of growth is an increase in size of the oocyte. As the oocyte enlarges, the zona pellucida, a membrane that will eventually surround the oocyte, begins to form. The flat, poorly differentiated granulosa cells, which form a single layer, assume a cuboidal shape as the oocyte approaches its maximum size of 80–100 μm. At this stage of development, the follicular unit is known as a **primary follicle.** Subsequently, the granulosa cells rapidly proliferate, forming a multilayered covering around the oocyte. Small patches of fluid form between the granulosa cells. Blood vessels, however, do not penetrate the basement membrane surrounding the granulosa cells, and the granulosa layer remains avascular until after ovulation has occurred. As the follicle continues to enlarge, cells that are indistinguishable from mesenchymal fibroblasts align themselves concentrically outside the basement membrane. These cells form the thecal layer and complete the formation of the **secondary follicle (preantral follicle).** As the granulosa cells continue to multiply, there is further production and accumulation of fluid within the granulosa cell layer, leading to the formation of a follicular cavity, or **antrum.** The oocyte and a portion of the surrounding granulosa cells (cumulus cells) are gradually displaced to one side of the follicular cavity, and a **tertiary follicle (antral follicle)** is formed. There is both a rapid accumulation of follicular fluid and additional growth of granulosa cells, causing further enlargement of the **preovulatory (graafian) follicle.** The follicle reaches a diameter of 2–2.5 cm shortly before ovulation. Following ovulation, the antrum fills with blood and lymph fluid (Figure 13–3). The wall of the follicle collapses and becomes convoluted, and vessels from the thecal layer invade the granulosa layer. The appearance of the granulosa cells changes markedly after ovulation, and they become luteinized. In conjunction with the contiguous thecal layer or adjacent stromal cells, the luteinized granulosa layer forms the **corpus luteum.** If pregnancy does not follow ovulation, the corpus luteum lasts about 14 days and is gradually replaced by fibrous tissue, forming a **corpus albicans.** The mechanisms responsible for regression (luteolysis) of the corpus luteum after 14 days in humans are incompletely understood. In nonprimates, prostaglandins appear to play an important role in luteolysis.

Control of Growth
& Steroidogenesis
in Ovarian Follicles

The factors that stimulate resting primordial follicles to resume growth and development are unknown. Pituitary gonadotropins, however, are not involved in initiating these events. Cohorts of primordial follicles in prepubertal girls—in whom LH and FSH levels are undetectable—and in hypophysectomized laboratory animals are continually leaving the large pool of inactive primordial follicles and resuming growth. Development beyond the preantral or early antral stage, however, depends upon the interaction of pituitary gonadotropins, ovarian steroids, and other local factors within the follicle.

Receptors for FSH have been found only in granulosa cells. Each cell is estimated to contain about 1000 receptors. The binding of FSH to its receptor stimulates the synthesis of enzymes which have aromatase activity and which convert androgen precursors to estrogens. Estradiol, in turn, plays a critical role in follicular growth and development both by a local effect on granulosa cells and via positive and negative feedback regulation of FSH and LH secretion (see below). In small follicles, estradiol induces the proliferation of granulosa cells. In the absence of FSH, estradiol per se can stimulate follicular growth to the preantral stage, but further development is dependent upon gonadotropin stimulation. FSH and estradiol, working in concert, also induce the formation of LH receptors in granulosa cells. In contrast to FSH receptors, which are restricted to granulosa cells, LH receptors also have been found in theca, interstitial, and luteal cells.

The cellular origin of estradiol in large ovarian follicles in primates remains controversial. In the rat, granulosa cells lack the enzyme P450c17 (17α-hydroxylase and 17,20-lyase) and thus are unable to directly synthesize androgens or estrogens from C21 precursors—eg, progesterone or pregnenolone. Therefore, estradiol production by granulosa cells is dependent upon the availability of C19 androgenic precursors (testosterone and androstenedione), which can be aromatized to estrogens. These observations have led to the formation of the "two-cell theory" to explain estradiol formation within the follicular complex (Figure 13–9). According to this hypothesis, LH stimulates the synthesis of androgenic precursors, primarily androstenedione and to a lesser extent testosterone, by the theca cells. The androgens diffuse across the basement membrane that separates the theca and granulosa cells. Some of the androstenedione and testosterone enters the antral fluid, while the remainder is converted to estradiol by the

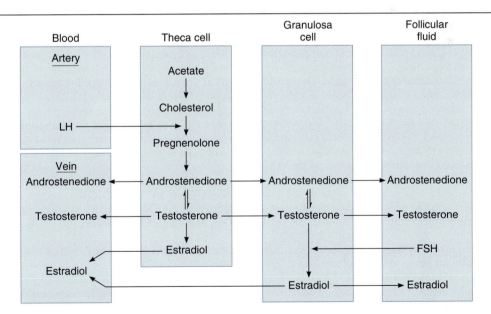

Figure 13–9. Pathways involved in the synthesis and secretion of androgens and estradiol by the preovulatory follicle. In primates, it is not known if the theca cells or granulosa cells are the major source for estradiol in plasma. (Reproduced, with permission, from Peters H, McNatty KP: *The Ovary: A Correlation of Structure and Function in Mammals.* Granada Publishing, 1980.)

granulosa cells. Studies in primates, however, have shown that both the thecal layer and the granulosa cells of antral follicles are able to synthesize estradiol; consequently, it is unclear whether it is the theca cells or the granulosa cells that are the principal site of estradiol synthesis in the mid and late follicular phases of the menstrual cycle. A study in the rhesus monkey suggested that most of the estradiol production in the preovulatory period was of theca cell—not granulosa cell—origin. It is possible that most of the estradiol produced by the granulosa cells remains within the follicular fluid, while estradiol in the serum arises primarily from the thecal layer.

In the normal ovary, androgens produced by the thecal layer—particularly androstenedione—serve, in part, as precursors of estrogen synthesis by granulosa cells. Androgens utilized in this fashion thus indirectly facilitate follicular growth via estradiol stimulation. However, high concentrations of testosterone or dihydrotestosterone—or increased ratios of androgen to estrogen—have been found in follicles undergoing atresia, and this suggests an inhibitory action of androgens on follicular development. This could explain, in part, the lack of normal follicular development in polycystic ovary syndrome and other disorders associated with increased androgen levels.. In polycystic ovary syndrome, high levels of LH may promote excessive androgen production by the thecal layer. Since FSH levels are low, granulosa cells may have a reduced capacity to convert these androgens to estrogens.

All of the developing follicles within the ovary are initially exposed to similar concentrations of FSH and LH. Since fewer than 1% of these follicles will eventually reach full maturity and ovulate, local factors must play a critical role in selection of the dominant preovulatory follicle. There are significant differences in the concentrations of protein and steroid hormones in the antral fluid of follicles of differing sizes and at differing stages of the menstrual cycle. The presence of this fluid-filled cavity provides a mechanism by which the granulosa cells and oocyte of one developing follicle can be exposed to a unique microenvironment that differs from that of the other developing follicles within the ovary. Studies have shown that it is the concentrations of pituitary gonadotropins and ovarian steroids within the follicular fluid rather than the serum concentrations of these hormones that correlate most closely with both the mitotic and synthetic activity of the granulosa cells as well as with the future viability of the oocyte. The highest concentrations of FSH and LH in antral fluid are found in the largest follicles during the late follicular phase of the menstrual cycle. Prolactin (PRL) levels, in contrast, are highest in small follicles and lower in large follicles in the late follicular phase. The concentrations of LH and FSH in follicular fluid are generally lower than corresponding serum levels,

but the concentrations of ovarian steroids—androstenedione, testosterone, dihydrotestosterone, and estradiol—may be 10-40,000 times greater than their serum levels. Although androgen concentrations do not differ greatly in follicular fluid from either small or large follicles, mean estradiol concentrations in antral fluid increase markedly, reaching levels in excess of 1500 ng/mL (5507 nmol/L) in large follicles in the late follicular phase of the menstrual cycle. It is not known at present whether these increases in the absolute concentration of estradiol and the ratio of estradiol to androgen in antral fluid are a consequence of follicular growth and development or play an important role in the process that leads to selection of a single preovulatory follicle.

Nonsteroidal Ovarian Regulatory Factors

Several proteins that can alter the secretion of FSH and/or modify estradiol secretion by granulosa cells have been identified in ovarian follicular fluid. The best characterized of these are the inhibins A and B, which are glycoprotein heterodimers with two subunits. Both inhibins have a common alpha subunit but somewhat different beta subunits, called β_a and β_b. Inhibin preferentially inhibits the secretion of FSH; it is thought to be produced by ovarian granulosa cells. If the beta subunits of inhibin are combined, forming a dimer without the usual alpha subunit, the resultant proteins, known as activins, can stimulate the secretion of FSH. The exact physiologic roles of inhibins and activins during the menstrual cycle remain to be elucidated; however, studies in primates indicate that inhibin has no direct effect on ovarian steroidogenesis but that activin modulates the response to LH and FSH. For example; cotreatment with activin and human FSH enhances FSH stimulation of progesterone synthesis and aromatase activity in granulosa cells. Activin, when combined with LH, suppresses the LH-induced progesterone response by 50% while markedly stimulating basal and LH-stimulated aromatase activity. Activin may also act as a growth factor in other tissues.

HORMONE INTERACTION & REGULATION DURING THE MENSTRUAL CYCLE

Gonadotropin-Releasing Hormone (GnRH)

GnRH (also referred to as luteinizing hormone-releasing hormone [LHRH]; luteotropin-releasing hormone [LRH]; and luteotropin-releasing factor [LRF]) is a decapeptide synthesized by neurosecretory cells located primarily within the hypothalamus. It regulates the secretion of LH and FSH and is essential for their synthesis and release. LH and FSH cannot be detected in serum from peripheral blood of women with congenital absence of hypothalamic GnRH. Ovarian sex steroids are not essential for the synthesis of LH and FSH, but they modulate release of these hormones by altering either gonadotroph response to GnRH or secretion of hypothalamic GnRH. Concentrations of GnRH in serum from peripheral blood are very low, and the pattern of GnRH secretion throughout the menstrual cycle in humans has not been well characterized. However, studies in humans suggest that GnRH secretion may be increased in the preovulatory period. GnRH has been measured in the pituitary portal blood of rhesus monkeys. In these nonhuman primates, GnRH is secreted in pulses every 1–3 hours. Concentrations of GnRH in the portal blood of nonhuman primates during the follicular phase of the menstrual cycle range from less than 10 pg/mL (which is undetectable) to 200 pg/mL. Studies in sheep have shown that each episode of LH release is triggered by a pulse of GnRH from the hypothalamus. Continuous infusions of GnRH initially increase the secretion of LH and FSH. After several hours or days of continuous infusion, desensitization and receptor "down-regulation" occur, and the pituitary gonadotrophs become refractory to further stimulation by GnRH.

Regulation of GnRH Secretion

In both rhesus monkeys and humans, intermittent pulses of GnRH every 60–90 minutes stimulate indefinitely the release of LH and FSH. In rhesus monkeys, changes in the frequency of the GnRH pulses can selectively increase or decrease the serum concentration of either LH or FSH. This observation suggests a mechanism by which a single releasing hormone, GnRH, can alter the ratio of LH to FSH in serum and further supports the concept that GnRH is the only hypothalamic hormone required for the regulation of both LH and FSH secretion.

Effects of Ovarian Steroids & Peptides on Gonadotropin Secretion

A. Negative Feedback: Under most conditions, ovarian steroids limit or reduce the secretion of pituitary gonadotropins. Serum concentrations of both FSH and LH increase markedly following ovariectomy or menopause, whereas the administration of estrogen (or estrogen and progesterone) lowers serum gonadotropin levels. Throughout most of the normal menstrual cycle, the negative feedback effects of ovarian steroids predominate and plasma gonadotropin concentrations remain below 25 mIU/mL. The physiologic importance of inhibin and other inhibitory peptides of ovarian origin during the normal menstrual cycle has not yet been determined.

B. Positive Feedback: Estradiol and progesterone, under certain conditions, can induce the release of LH and FSH. During the menstrual cycle, rising concentrations of estradiol in the latter part of the follicular phase initiate the preovulatory surge of LH via this mechanism. This increase in LH secretion in turn stimulates a small but significant increase in the secretion of progesterone that further augments the LH surge and, coupled with estradiol, initiates the midcycle surge of FSH. Although the negative feedback action of ovarian steroids may become apparent within a few hours, positive feedback develops more slowly, and 48–72 hours of sustained estrogen stimulation is generally required before an increase in LH secretion is observed. It is probable that the negative and positive feedback actions of ovarian sex steroids result from both (1) a direct effect of the steroids on the pituitary gonadotrophs that alters their sensitivity to GnRH and (2) modulation of the frequency and magnitude of the pulses of hypothalamic GnRH.

Neural Regulation of the Menstrual Cycle

In nonhuman primates—and perhaps in humans as well—the neural components that control both the tonic and surge secretion of gonadotropins are located within the medial basal hypothalamus. When the medial basal hypothalamus, which includes the median eminence, the arcuate nucleus, and portions of the ventromedial nucleus, was surgically isolated from the remainder of the brain without disrupting the hypothalamic-pituitary-portal vasculature, gonadotropin secretion in rhesus monkeys was not significantly altered. Both the negative and positive feedback actions of estradiol remained intact, and many monkeys continued to have spontaneous ovulatory menstrual cycles. It is probable, however, that other neural areas outside the hypothalamus (eg, limbic structures) normally modify gonadotropin secretion.

GnRH plays a permissive, though still essential, role in the regulation of LH and FSH secretion throughout the menstrual cycle. Pulsatile administration of exogenous GnRH every 60–90 minutes induced ovulatory menstrual cycles in monkeys with hypothalamic lesions or in humans with congenital absence of hypothalamic GnRH. In these cycles, the serum profiles of pituitary gonadotropins and ovarian steroids were within normal limits. These observations suggest that the cyclic nature of the menstrual cycle in primates is regulated by the ovary and not by the brain. The length of the menstrual cycle thus is determined by both the time required for development of a mature follicle and by the functional life span of the corpus luteum. Following luteolysis, follicular development resumes, and a new menstrual cycle begins. The major hypothalamic-pituitary-gonadal interactions that regulate the menstrual cycle are summarized in Figure 13–10.

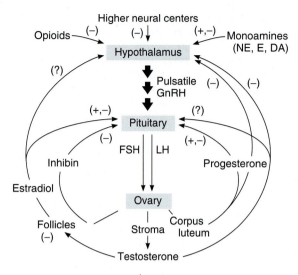

Figure 13–10. The major hypothalamic-pituitary-gonadal interactions thought to regulate the menstrual cycle. Ovarian sex steroids and neural monoamines may exert stimulatory (+) or inhibitory (–) (or both) effects on the secretion of GnRH or pituitary gonadotropins (or both).

CYCLIC CHANGES IN THE FEMALE REPRODUCTIVE TRACT

As a consequence of the changing rates of secretion of estrogen and progesterone throughout the menstrual cycle, the female reproductive tract undergoes a series of regular and cyclic changes. These changes can be recognized by histologic study of the endometrium, the composition and appearance of the cervical mucus, and the cytologic features of the vaginal epithelium. The end of each cycle is marked by uterine bleeding that continues for 3–7 days.

HISTOLOGY OF THE ENDOMETRIUM THROUGHOUT THE MENSTRUAL CYCLE

The endometrium consists of two distinct layers or zones differing in both histologic appearance and functional responsiveness to hormonal stimulation: a **basal layer** and a **functional layer.** The basal layer is in direct contact with the myometrium, undergoes little change throughout the menstrual cycle, and is not sloughed during menses. The functional layer arises from the basal layer and eventually surrounds the entire lumen of the uterine cavity. The functional layer can be subdivided further into two components:

a thin superficial **compact layer** and a deeper **spongiosa layer,** of which most of the secretory or fully developed endometrium is composed. The blood supply of the endometrium consists of a highly specialized network of arterial and venous channels. The **spiral arteries** arise within the myometrium from branches of the uterine artery, pass through the basal endometrial layer, and extend into the functional zone. The proximal portion of the spiral artery, the **straight artery,** distributes blood to tissues of the basal layer and is not influenced by changes in estrogen and progesterone secretion. The spiral arteries, however, undergo cyclic regeneration and degeneration during each menstrual cycle in response to hormonal changes.

The endometrial cycle can be subdivided into three major phases: proliferative, secretory, and menstrual. The morphologic changes of the endometrium that occur during the normal menstrual cycle have been described in great detail and are summarized in Figure 13–11. For convenience, the changes described in this figure and the following discussion are based on a hypothetical menstrual cycle of 28 days, in which the follicular and luteal phases are each approximately 14 days in length.

Proliferative Phase

When menstrual flow ceases, a thin layer of basal endometrial tissue remains. This tissue, consisting of the remnants of glands and stroma, grows rapidly. Epithelial cells from the glands proliferate and cover the raw stromal surfaces with a layer of simple columnar epithelium. In the early proliferative phase, most of the glands are straight, short, and narrow. The glandular epithelium exhibits increasing mitotic activity. Throughout the proliferative phase, there is continued and rapid growth of both the epithelial and stromal components of the endometrium. By the late proliferative phase of the menstrual cycle, the surface of the endometrium is somewhat undulant. The glands are becoming tortuous and are lined by tall columnar cells with basal nuclei. Pseudostratification of nuclei is prominent. The stroma at this time is moderately dense, with many mitotic figures.

Secretory Phase

During the secretory phase, histologic changes occur very rapidly. During the first half of this phase, the appearance of the glandular epithelium is most useful in precise dating of the endometrium, whereas in the second half, accurate dating depends largely on the characteristics of the stroma. On the 16th day of the cycle (second postovulatory day), subnuclear glycogen-rich vacuoles become prominent in the glandular epithelium. The vacuoles push the epithelial cell nuclei into a central position within the cells. By the 19th day (fifth postovulatory day), few vacuoles remain within the cells. Acidophilic intraluminal glandular secretory material is most apparent on

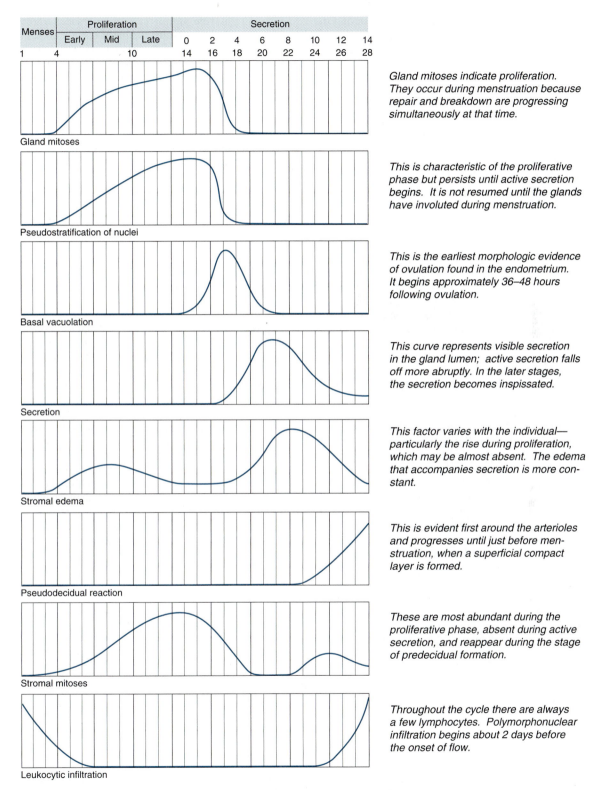

Menses	Proliferation			Secretion							
	Early	Mid	Late	0	2	4	6	8	10	12	14
1	4		10	14	16	18	20	22	24	26	28

Gland mitoses

Gland mitoses indicate proliferation. They occur during menstruation because repair and breakdown are progressing simultaneously at that time.

Pseudostratification of nuclei

This is characteristic of the proliferative phase but persists until active secretion begins. It is not resumed until the glands have involuted during menstruation.

Basal vacuolation

This is the earliest morphologic evidence of ovulation found in the endometrium. It begins approximately 36–48 hours following ovulation.

Secretion

This curve represents visible secretion in the gland lumen; active secretion falls off more abruptly. In the later stages, the secretion becomes inspissated.

Stromal edema

This factor varies with the individual—particularly the rise during proliferation, which may be almost absent. The edema that accompanies secretion is more constant.

Pseudodecidual reaction

This is evident first around the arterioles and progresses until just before menstruation, when a superficial compact layer is formed.

Stromal mitoses

These are most abundant during the proliferative phase, absent during active secretion, and reappear during the stage of predecidual formation.

Leukocytic infiltration

Throughout the cycle there are always a few lymphocytes. Polymorphonuclear infiltration begins about 2 days before the onset of flow.

Figure 13–11. Morphologic changes in the endometrium that are useful in determining the stage of the menstrual cycle. (After Noyes, Hertig, and Rock. Reproduced, with permission, from Benson RC [editor]: *Current Obstetric and Gynecologic Diagnosis and Treatment,* 5th ed. Lange, 1984.)

day 21. Stromal edema, which is variable during the proliferative phase, also becomes prominent at this time and peaks on day 22. By day 24, pseudodecidual or predecidual changes begin to appear within the stroma. These changes are initially most apparent near the spiral arteries and eventually encompass large areas of the stroma. Lymphocytic infiltration of the stroma increases markedly in conjunction with the appearance of pseudodecidual changes, and by day 26, PMN invasion also is apparent.

If the blastocyst implants successfully, serum concentrations of hCG and, secondarily, progesterone begin to increase 7–10 days after ovulation (ie, days 21–24 of the menstrual cycle). The rising levels of progesterone produce a type of endometrial change known as decidualization. The decidua of pregnancy consists primarily of plump, eosinophilic stromal cells that have a pavement-like appearance. In the early stages of pregnancy, the cells of the glandular epithelium become distended with clear cytoplasm and possibly with enlarged and hyperchromatic nuclei, a feature called the Arias-Stella phenomenon. With advancing pregnancy, the endometrial glands gradually atrophy.

Menstrual Phase

In the absence of pregnancy, changes in the endometrium secondary to declining hormone production by the corpus luteum can be observed by day 24. The functional layer of the stroma begins to shrink, and the endometrial glands become more tortuous and saw-toothed in appearance. Intermittent constriction of the spiral arteries leads to stasis within the capillaries of the functional layer, tissue ischemia, and extravasation of blood into the stroma with formation of small hematomas. Eventually, desquamation and sloughing of the entire functional layer of the endometrium occurs.

Endometrial biopsy has been used extensively in the past to assess progesterone secretion in women with menstrual dysfunction and infertility. With the widespread availability of reliable radioimmunoassays to measure serum concentrations of progesterone, the need for endometrial biopsy is limited; it should be used primarily to assess the response of the endometrium to hormonal stimulation. Endometrial biopsy is most informative when performed a few days before the anticipated menstrual period. Although biopsy late in the luteal phase may potentially interrupt a pregnancy if conception has occurred, the risk is minimal.

CERVICAL MUCUS

Cervical mucus is a complex secretion produced by the glands of the endocervix. It is composed of 92–98% water and approximately 1% inorganic salts, of which NaCl is the main constituent. The mucus also contains free simple sugars, polysaccharides, proteins, and glycoproteins. Its pH is usually alkaline and ranges from 6.5 to 9.0. Several physical characteristics of cervical mucus can be evaluated readily by the clinician. Since these characteristics are influenced by serum estrogen and progesterone levels, it is often possible to gain an approximate assessment of the hormonal status of a patient by examination of cervical mucus. Estrogen stimulates the production of copious amounts (up to 700 mg/d) of clear, watery mucus through which sperm can penetrate most readily. Progesterone, however, even in the presence of high plasma levels of estrogen, reduces the secretion of mucus. Both during the luteal phase of the menstrual cycle and during pregnancy, the mucus is scant, viscous, and cellular. During most of the menstrual cycle, 20–60 mg of mucus is produced each day.

Figure 13–12 summarizes those characteristics of cervical mucus that the clinician can readily determine and correlates them with the day of the menstrual cycle.

Spinnbarkeit is the property that allows cervical mucus to be stretched or drawn into a thread. Spinnbarkeit can be estimated by stretching a sample of mucus between 2 glass slides and measuring the maximum length of the thread before it breaks. At midcycle, spinnbarkeit usually exceeds 10 cm. **Ferning,** or **arborization,** refers to the characteristic microscopic pattern cervical mucus forms when dried on a slide (Figure 13–13). Ferning results from the crystallization of inorganic salts around small and optimal amounts of organic material present in cervical mucus. As serum concentrations of estradiol increase, the composition of cervical mucus changes, so that dried mucus begins to demonstrate ferning in the latter part of the follicular phase. In the periovulatory interval, when estradiol levels are maximal and prior to significant progesterone secretion, ferning is most prominent and the mucus is thin, watery, and contains few cells. As serum progesterone concentrations increase following ovulation, the quality of the mucus changes and ferning disappears. The absence of ferning can reflect either inadequate stimulation of endocervical glands by estrogen or inhibition by increased secretion of progesterone. Persistent ferning throughout the menstrual cycle suggests anovulatory cycles or insufficient progesterone secretion.

VAGINAL EPITHELIUM

The vaginal mucosa is composed of a stratified squamous epithelium and does not contain glands. Cells in the outer layer during the reproductive years are flattened and may contain keratohyaline granules, but true cornification does not normally occur. The epithelial cells of the vagina, like other tissues of the

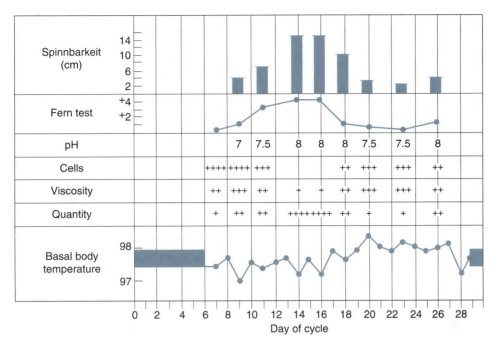

Figure 13–12. Changes in the composition and properties of cervical mucus throughout the menstrual cycle. (Modified and reproduced, with permission, from Moghissi KS: Composition and function of cervical secretion. In: *Handbook of Physiology,* Section 7: Endocrinology, Vol 2, Part 2. Greep RO [editor]. American Physiological Society, 1973.)

female reproductive tract, respond to changing levels of ovarian sex steroids. Estrogen stimulates the proliferation and maturation of the epithelial cells, resulting in a thickening of the vaginal mucosa and increased glycogen content of the epithelial cells. This glycogen is fermented to lactic acid by the normal bacterial flora of the vagina, thus accounting for the mildly acid pH of vaginal fluid. The histologic and cytologic changes of the vaginal epithelium of women during the normal menstrual cycle are less marked than those occurring in the estrous cycle of rodents.

Cytologists describe three types of exfoliated vaginal epithelial cells—superficial, intermediate, and basal-parabasal—which do not refer to the locations of the cells within the epithelium but to their degree of cellular maturity or differentiation. Exfoliated cells, obtained by light scrapings from the midportion of the lateral vaginal wall, are most useful for cytohormonal assessment.

Superficial cells are mature, flat, usually polygonal, squamous epithelial cells with pyknotic, hyperchromatic nuclei. These cells develop in response to high levels of unopposed estrogen stimulation.

Intermediate cells are relatively mature squamous epithelial cells with eosinophilic or cyanophilic cytoplasm and a vesicular, nonpyknotic nucleus. The appearance of the nucleus is the critical factor in differentiating intermediate cells from superficial cells. Intermediate cells predominate in endocrinologic

states in which progesterone levels are high, such as in pregnancy or in the midluteal phase of the menstrual cycle.

Basal-parabasal cells are thick, small, oval or round, immature cells with large vesicular nuclei and cyanophilic cytoplasm. Parabasal cells usually indicate estrogen deficiency and are the predominant cell type in the prepubertal and postmenopausal periods.

Among the various indices that describe the ratio or percentage of superficial, intermediate, and basal-parabasal cells are (1) the karyopyknotic index (KPI), the ratio of superficial cells to intermediate cells; (2) the eosinophilic index (EI), the ratio of mature eosinophilic cells to mature cyanophilic cells; and (3) the maturation index (MI), the percentage of parabasal, intermediate, and superficial cells present, in that order. Since only MI includes as a factor the presence of all three cell types, it may provide more information than the other two indices.

In general, only two diagnostic patterns of vaginal epithelial cells are clinically useful. When the vaginal epithelium has been stimulated by estrogen, MI may range from (0/40/60) at mid cycle, when estradiol concentrations are highest, to (0/70/30) late in the luteal phase, when progesterone effects are most prominent. A finding of parabasal cells with a few intermediate cells and no superficial cells indicates that the vaginal epithelium has received little or no estrogen stimulation. The MI in this instance may be

Normal cycle, 14th day

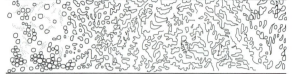

Midluteal phase, normal cycle

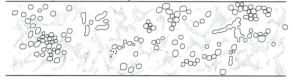

Anovulatory cycle with estrogen present

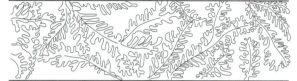

Figure 13–13. Patterns formed when cervical mucus is smeared on a slide, permitted to dry, and examined under the microscope. Progesterone makes the mucus thick and cellular. In the smear from a patient who failed to ovulate (bottom), there is no progesterone to inhibit the estrogen-induced fern pattern. (Reproduced, with permission, from Ganong WF: *Review of Medical Physiology,* 14th ed. Appleton & Lange, 1989.)

(100/0/0) or (80/20/0). The vaginal smear can be used to provide a qualitative assessment of estrogen production in women with amenorrhea.

EXTRAGENITAL SYMPTOMS ASSOCIATED WITH NORMAL MENSTRUAL FUNCTION

PREMENSTRUAL SYNDROME

Premenstrual syndrome (PMS) is a complex of symptoms occurring in the luteal phase of the cycle in ovulating women. Behavioral symptoms include fatigue, irritability, anxiety, depression, emotional lability, insomnia, increased appetite, and difficulty in working effectively. Physical symptoms may include bloating, breast tenderness, ankle edema, and headaches.

Recent epidemiologic studies indicate that in the populations studied, about 5–10% of women in the reproductive age group have moderate to severe symptoms temporally related to the menstrual cycle, and most of these women seek medical care. Another 20–40% of women feel less well during the late luteal and early menstrual phase of the cycle and for a day or so in mid cycle. PMS appears to be limited to women with ovulatory cycles. In patients with more severe symptoms, interrelationships at home and at work can be disrupted. Among the serious consequences commonly reported are marital discord, parenting problems, poor work or school performance, and social isolation.

Although many theories of causation have been proposed, none account for the entire symptom complex, and the syndrome is probably the result of hormonal as well as environmental and psychologic factors. Women with moderate to severe PMS experience more stressful events than other women. However, it is not clear whether these events are etiologically related nor whether they exacerbate the syndrome or result from it. Studies in twins indicate that genetic factors may also be involved.

Diagnosis

The physician must take a careful history, including detailed inquiry into the stresses associated with the patient's work and family life, and perform a complete physical examination to properly assess the nature and severity of the complaints. It may also be helpful to interview the patient's spouse or housemate. It is important to rule out other causes of the complaints, particularly the somatic complaints, since they may be amenable to therapy..

When symptoms are severe and maneuvers such as ovulation suppression or anxiolytic and antidepressant drugs are contemplated, it is best to document the cyclic nature and severity of the symptoms and behaviors to be treated. Several instruments are available for this purpose; however, it is sufficient to have the patient select the symptoms she finds most bothersome and rate them daily on a calendar through two or more cycles using the following scale:

0   No symptoms.
1+ Changes are noticed by the patient and family, but normal activities are not affected.
2+ Family or occupational relationships and activities are disturbed but functioning.
3+ Family or occupational relationships are seriously disturbed, and normal activities cannot continue.

Treatment

The objective of therapy is to make the patient more comfortable and enable her to function more normally. Simple life-style changes, a diet exercise program, and stress management strategies are a useful way to begin treatment. Reductions in alcohol and caffeine intake can reduce irritability and anxiety, respectively. Salt restriction may reduce swelling and bloating. Empiric treatment of physical manifestations is helpful. Spironolactone, a potassium-sparing agent, given in doses of 50–100 mg from day 12 to menses, reduces swelling, breast tenderness, and bloating and can be useful when salt restriction and exercise are ineffective in relieving swelling. Naproxen, 550 mg twice daily, or ibuprofen, 600 mg three times daily, taken from onset of symptoms until bleeding commences, is effective for headaches, cramping, and back and muscle aches, and in some patients these agents reduce irritability and depression. Danazol, tamoxifen, and bromocriptine are useful for breast pain. Preliminary studies suggest that danazol in doses of 200 mg/d taken from the onset of symptoms to the start of menses provides modest but significant overall improvement without side effects or ovulation suppression.

When anxiety and irritability are the dominant symptoms, alprazolam in doses of 0.125–0.25 mg three times daily from day 20 to the second day of menses, followed by the same dose twice daily on day 3 and one dose on day 4, is effective and unassociated with withdrawal symptoms. Buspirone is also effective and free of sedative effects in a dose of 25 mg/d from the onset of symptoms until menses. Fluoxetine, 20–60 mg daily, or fenfluramine, 20 mg three times daily, has been found to be helpful when depression is a prominent symptom. Psychiatric referral is advisable when there is a risk of suicide, violence toward others, or exacerbation of psychiatric illness or when the physician requires assistance with the use of psychotropic drugs.

In many studies, women treated with placebos have shown as much as 50% or more improvement for short periods of time. Pyridoxine, vitamin E, evening primrose oil (a rich source of γ-linoleic acid—a precursor of prostenoids), or vitamin and mineral supplements as well as progesterone are commonly used but have not been shown to be more effective than placebo.

When symptoms last more than a week or are unduly severe, ovulation suppression can be tried. Patients responding to ovulation suppression with danazol, gonadotropin-releasing hormone, medroxyprogesterone, depot medroxyprogesterone acetate, or estrogen implants or patches may have relief which continues after a period (1 year) of treatment. If symptoms return and persist, ovariectomy can be discussed with appropriate patients. In a patient with a well-documented symptom complex that responds to induction of anovulation with GnRH analogs, danazol, or estrogen and in whom the syndrome causes a major disruption of the patient's life, ovariectomy is a rational therapeutic option if the desire for further childbearing is not a factor and the patient can anticipate many more years of ovulatory function.

DYSMENORRHEA

Dysmenorrhea unrelated to any identifiable disorder almost always begins before age 20 but seldom within the first year or so after menarche. It is one of the most important causes of lost working hours and failure to attend school. The pain is colicky in nature and thought to be related to uterine contractions caused by prostaglandins released at the time of endometrial breakdown. When severe, the pain may radiate from the pelvic region to the back and thighs and is frequently accompanied by nausea and in some women vomiting and diarrhea. Treatment with aspirin before the onset of pain is effective in milder cases; however, the nonsteroidal anti-inflammatory compounds that are active inhibitors of prostaglandin synthesis are more effective when the pain is severe. Naproxen, 250 mg twice daily, and ibuprofen, 400 mg three times daily, are useful for this purpose, as is indomethacin, 25 mg three or four times daily, or mefenamic acid, 250 mg four times daily. These compounds are often more effective if started before the pain begins. Since dysmenorrhea rarely accompanies bleeding in the absence of ovulation, suppression of ovulation with oral contraceptives is also effective treatment.

DISORDERS OF OVARIAN & MENSTRUAL FUNCTION

Abnormal ovarian endocrine function is manifested by (1) evidence of inappropriate estrogen secretion (eg, precocious puberty); (2) deficient estrogen secretion (eg, delayed puberty); (3) disturbances or alterations of the menstrual cycle in mature women; or (4) evidence of excessive androgen production. In this chapter, emphasis will be placed on disorders occurring in postpubertal adults, since these comprise the vast majority of disorders encountered and because disorders of development and differentiation are described in Chapters 14 and 15 and pituitary disorders in Chapter 5.

The pattern of menstrual bleeding with regard to the frequency, duration, and amount of flow tends to be fairly consistent in most healthy women. Periodic, regular menstrual cycles are usually ovulatory. However, there are a wide variety of organic and functional disturbances of menstrual flow. In general, when the basic pattern of bleeding is undisturbed and there are superimposed episodes of spotting or bleeding, the cause is likely to be a local organic lesion or hematologic disorder. When the basic pattern of bleeding is changed, it is more often due to lack of ovulation and disturbances in the pattern of hormone secretion. Table 13–3 sets forth the terms frequently used to describe abnormalities of menses, their definitions, and some common causes.

The great majority of disorders of ovarian function causing amenorrhea occur without known or identifiable structural changes in the components of the complex system required for normal ovulatory cycles. They can result from abnormalities in function of the central mechanism that regulates the pulsatile secretion of GnRH; from abnormalities in feedback; or from changes in intraovarian regulatory mechanisms. Environmental changes, physical and emotional stress, extreme weight loss, and drugs seem to be able to interfere with the functioning of the hypothalamic centers and their control of GnRH secretion. In such cases, a variety of hormonal abnormalities may be identified. In some patients, follicle stimulation by FSH is insufficient to produce adequate growth and maturation of ovarian follicles, with a resulting decrease in ovarian estradiol secretion. Failure of the preovulatory LH surge to occur even though follicles have developed and produced estrogen will also disrupt normal ovarian and menstrual function. However, the continuous secretion of increased amounts of LH in the absence of normally developing follicles may result in overproduction of androgens and lead to amenorrhea and hirsutism. The role of estrogens, androgens, and other local hormones in the ovary is not presently well delineated, but these hormones may be responsible for abnormalities in ovarian function in some patients. Abnormalities of gonadotropin secretion leading to anovulation are sometimes associated with the release of increased amounts of PRL in the absence of any demonstrable lesion of the pituitary. In such patients, amenorrhea may be associated with galactorrhea.

Treatment of these disorders depends to some extent on their causes and manifestations. However, the desired outcome is the critical consideration. It would be fruitless, for example, to treat hirsutism secondary to excess production of ovarian androgens by suppressing the ovary with oral contraceptives in a patient whose main objective was to achieve a pregnancy.

In considering the possible causes of amenorrhea in a given patient, it is useful to review the requirements for normal cyclic ovarian function: (1) a normal outflow tract, (2) normal ovaries, (3) a normal pituitary gland, and (4) a normal central nervous system. Each of these systems can be examined by means of the history, direct observation, and appropriate laboratory tests or procedures. The problem may be more complex in young women with primary amenorrhea and no evidence of sexual maturation. In women with secondary amenorrhea, however, the process may require very few laboratory tests. By the time one has begun to speak to the patient, one has already observed her approximate age, appearance, stature, and extent of sexual development; this information provides some direction for taking her history and doing the physical examination.

Table 13–3. Types of abnormal vaginal bleeding.

	Definition	Causes
Hypermenorrhea (menorrhagia)	Cyclic bleeding in excessive amount.	Uterine myomas and endometrial polyps, hyperplasia, adenomyosis, endometritis, von Willebrand's disease
Hypomenorrhea	Cyclic bleeding in abnormally small amount	Cervical obstruction, synechia of endometrium, tuberculosis of endometrium.
Polymenorrhea	Frequent periods (cycle length of < 21 days).	Shortening of follicular phase, luteal insufficiency, frequent anovulatory bleeding.
Oligomenorrhea	Infrequent periods (cycle length of > 35 days).	Anovulation, systemic disturbances.
Amenorrhea	More than 6 months since last menstrual period	Anovulation or outflow tract disorder
Metrorrhagia	Bleeding between normal cycles.	Except for ovulatory bleeding or spotting, this symptom usually indicates disease of the vagina, cervix, or uterus.

AMENORRHEA IN THE ABSENCE OF SEXUAL MATURATION

The diagnostic considerations for a young, immature woman are quite different from those for a mature woman with secondary amenorrhea. In the otherwise healthy but sexually immature patient over 16 years of age, the first question to resolve is whether normal puberty is merely delayed. This question can sometimes be answered by finding a normal level of gonadotropins and a history of late puberty in the family. No conclusion can be drawn if the levels of gonadotropins are low. In these patients, LH and FSH responses to testing with GnRH or a GnRH agonist analog may help to differentiate delayed puberty from a more serious disorder (see Chapter 15).

Elevated concentrations of FSH and LH indicate unresponsiveness or absence of functioning ovarian tissue. If the patient is short in stature and has obvious stigmas of Turner's syndrome (gonadal dysgenesis), gonadotropins will be elevated. Chromosomal analysis will confirm the diagnosis, determine the genotype, and indicate the need for gonadectomy if a Y chromosome mosaicism is found. If the patient is of normal height or has relatively longer arms and legs compared with the length of the trunk (eunuchoid proportions), gonadal absence or agenesis must be differentiated from selective hypogonadotropism. FSH will be elevated in the former and low in the latter. If height and stature are normal and gonadotropins are low, one must also consider a central nervous system defect such as Kallmann's syndrome. These patients also have anosmia, which can be determined by the history or by testing the ability to smell.

Patients with amenorrhea and hypogonadism in whom the levels of gonadotropins are normal or lower than normal may be experiencing a delay in onset of puberty. However, after age 16, this is sufficiently unusual to warrant further investigation. When the cause is craniopharyngioma or pituitary tumor, there is commonly an interference with growth secondary to deficient GH secretion. Clinical or laboratory evidence of thyroid or adrenal insufficiency or decreased reserve also may be present. These and other pituitary disorders causing amenorrhea and conditions of abnormal pubertal development are discussed in Chapters 5 and 15.

Primary Ovarian Disorders

A. Gonadal Agenesis: Hypogonadism may result from absent or incomplete development of the ovary. This abnormality could result from environmentally induced abnormalities in development early in pregnancy (see Chapter 14).

B. Turner's Syndrome (Gonadal Dysgenesis): Turner's syndrome and related variants of gonadal dysgenesis are the most common cause of congenital hypogonadism. The karyotype in affected patients is most frequently 45,X, showing an absence of the second X chromosome. Clinical features, in addition to the lack of sexual maturation, include short stature, webbed neck, shield chest, and valgus deformity of the elbow. This syndrome and its variants are described in detail in Chapter 14. Gonadal dysgenesis may also occur in the presence of multiple cell lines with varying chromosomal composition. This is called "mosaicism." Many patients with mosaicism have typical phenotypic characteristics of Turner's syndrome, and the diagnosis may be made before puberty. A karyotype should be performed on all of these patients to determine whether or not a Y chromosome is present. Patients having Y chromosomes require laparotomy and excision of the gonadal area to prevent development of gonadoblastomas. It should also be noted that patients having an XX constituent to their mosaicism may have functional ovarian tissue. In some of these, normal puberty (including menses) occurs, and they are able to reproduce. These individuals frequently experience premature menopause.

C. P450c17α (17α-Hydroxylase) Deficiency: Hypogonadism and elevated levels of gonadotropin can be found in patients with 17α-hydroxylase deficiency, a rare form of congenital adrenal hyperplasia in which there is impaired conversion of pregnenolone and progesterone to cortisol and to androgens and estrogens. The impairment leads to increased production of deoxycorticosterone and corticosterone, resulting in hypokalemia and hypertension (see Chapters 10 and 14).

Disorders Due to Central Nervous System Disease

A. Hypogonadotropism and Anosmia: This syndrome, similar to Kallmann's syndrome in the male, is a rare cause of amenorrhea. Patients fail to mature at the expected time for puberty and are found to have low gonadotropins, normal stature, anosmia, and a female karyotype. The disorder is believed to involve failure of development of the olfactory lobe and a deficiency of GnRH. Ovulation can be induced by injection of menopausal gonadotropins and by pulsatile injection of GnRH.

B. Prepubertal Pituitary and Central Nervous System Tumors: Pituitary and central nervous system disorders which interfere with ovarian function, or tumors such as craniopharyngiomas and pituitary adenomas are discussed in Chapters 5 and 15.

AMENORRHEA IN PATIENTS WITH NORMAL SECONDARY SEX CHARACTERISTICS

The evaluation of women with amenorrhea but otherwise normal sexual development begins with the history and physical examination plus a few laboratory tests (Figure 13–14). This initial evaluation will localize the underlying cause of the amenorrhea to dysfunction of either the outflow tract, the ovary, or the hypothalamic-pituitary complex. In most cases, further diagnostic procedures will not be required. The medical history should include a complete description of prior menstrual patterns, the presence or absence of breast discharge, and any changes that might suggest increased androgen secretion. The possibility of pregnancy should always be considered.

The initial evaluation consists of a qualitative assessment of the patient's endogenous estrogen level and determination of the serum PRL concentration. The presence of endogenous estrogens can be established by measuring estradiol levels or attempting to induce withdrawal uterine bleeding by administering progesterone. An oral progestin with no estrogenic activity—eg, medroxyprogesterone, 10 mg daily for 5–7 days—or a single intramuscular injection of 200 mg of progesterone in oil may be used. The presence of vaginal bleeding within 7 days after conclusion of the progesterone treatment indicates that the outflow tract is intact and that the patient is producing suffi-

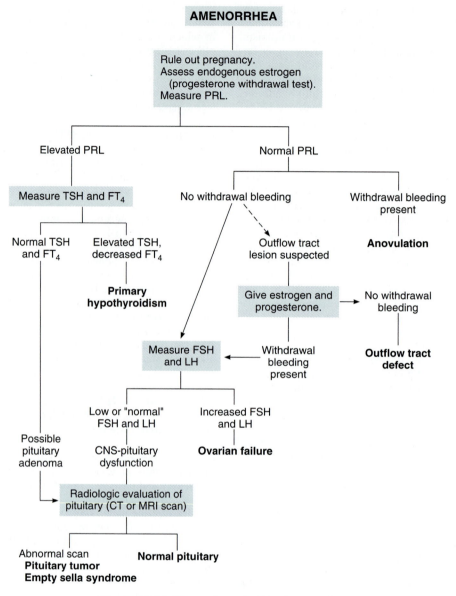

Figure 13–14. Diagnostic evaluation of amenorrhea.

cient estrogen to stimulate endometrial growth. If the serum PRL concentration is also within normal limits, a pituitary tumor is very unlikely. These patients can be considered to be anovulatory, and in most cases no further evaluation is required. The choice of treatment, if any, will depend upon the objectives of the patient.

Failure to induce menstrual bleeding by exogenous progestin indicates either a defect of the outflow tract with normal estrogen production (an infrequent cause of secondary amenorrhea) or insufficient estrogen production secondary to hypothalamic-pituitary-ovarian dysfunction. To differentiate between these possibilities in women with normal PRL levels, gonadotropin levels are obtained to differentiate between ovarian failure and hypothalamic-pituitary dysfunction. If an abnormality of the outflow tract is suspected, its integrity can be assessed by administering oral estrogen (1.25–2.5 mg of conjugated estrogens or 50 μg of ethinyl estradiol per day) for 21 days. A progestin should be added during the last 5 days of treatment. Lack of withdrawal bleeding following treatment usually indicates an abnormality of the outflow tract. In most instances, however, bleeding will occur and the outflow tract is found to be normal.

To differentiate between ovarian failure and hypothalamic-pituitary dysfunction, gonadotropin levels are obtained. If ovarian failure is the primary cause of amenorrhea, serum FSH and LH levels will be elevated because of the loss of negative feedback by ovarian sex steroids. If serum concentrations of FSH and LH are low or low normal or if prolactin levels are elevated, radiologic or magnetic resonance examination of the pituitary gland is indicated to rule out a pituitary tumor. Therapy for these disorders is discussed below.

Abnormalities of the Outflow Tract

Patients with amenorrhea in whom gonadal tissue is presumed to be present because they have undergone normal sexual maturation may have abnormalities of the outflow tract. Patients who cannot be induced to bleed by treatment with a progestational agent and who fail to bleed following administration of estrogens in conjunction with a progestational agent after several attempts can be presumed to have an abnormality of the outflow tract. In these patients, the presence or absence of ovulation can be determined by following the basal body temperature over a month or more or by measuring serum progesterone levels once a week for several weeks.

A. Müllerian Defects: In women with no history of vaginal bleeding, developmental abnormalities of the müllerian tube must be considered. These abnormalities range from the presence of an imperforate hymen to the total absence of müllerian structures. In the presence of a uterus lined with endometrium, interruption of the outflow tract by an abnormal cervix, interruptions of the vaginal canal, or imperforate hymen may be accompanied by collection of the menstruum proximal to the point of obstruction. This leads to pain and distention of the proximal structures or accumulation of blood in the peritoneal cavity. **Absence of the vagina,** with varying degrees of uterine development associated with normal ovarian function, is one of the more common abnormalities of müllerian development (Mayer-Rokitansky-Küster-Hauser syndrome). Affected patients commonly have developmental abnormalities of the urinary and skeletal systems. Surgical creation of an artificial vagina is indicated when there is evidence that a functioning uterus exists and that fertility might be restored. Otherwise, progressive dilation by the use of vaginal dilators can be used to form a functional vagina.

B. Asherman's Syndrome (Uterine Synechia): In women in whom menses have once been established, destruction of the endometrial cavity by chronic infections such as tuberculosis or destruction of the endometrium by curettage can lead to amenorrhea. Such scarring (Asherman's syndrome) is uncommon and can be treated by careful dilation under hysteroscopic view, followed by insertion of a small Foley catheter or other device to prevent adhesions from recurring. Treatment should include the use of broad-spectrum antibiotics for 10 days following the procedure and cyclic stimulation of endometrial development with large doses of estrogen plus a progestin.

Primary Gonadal Disorders

In patients with amenorrhea and a normal outflow tract, abnormal ovarian function may result from disorders of the ovary itself or disorders of the controlling mechanisms. A plasma FSH of more than 40 mIU/mL accompanied by high levels of LH is evidence of failure of ovarian hormone production. This is a very serious diagnosis, not only because of the hormone deficiency, which is correctable, but also—and more importantly from the patient's point of view—because lack of a functioning follicular apparatus results in sterility. For this reason, it is worth repeating the test to be sure there is no error. In women near menopause, elevated gonadotropin levels are sometimes found in the presence of ovulatory cycles. However, a misdiagnosis in this group of patients is rarely clinically important unless the patient is pregnant.

A. Premature Ovarian Failure: Ovarian failure occasionally occurs in women under the age of 35 following spontaneous sexual maturation. In some patients, ovarian failure is associated with ovarian autoantibodies and is probably due to autoimmune destruction of the ovary. It is frequently associated with autoantibodies to other glands such as the thyroid and adrenal (Schmidt's syndrome) (see Chapters 7, 9, and 24). In other patients, the ovaries show a few primordial follicles, and in some they resemble menopausal ovaries. Chromosomal abnormalities are sometimes found in these patients.

B. Testicular Feminization: This disorder in its classic form is characterized by primary amenorrhea, an absent uterus, and the absence of pubic and axillary hair. Affected patients are male pseudohermaphrodites with testes and an XY karyotype. Incomplete forms of this disorder have also been described. They are discussed in detail in Chapter 14.

C. Resistant Ovary Syndrome: Rarely, women exhibit amenorrhea and elevated gonadotropin levels in the presence of potentially functional ovarian follicles. It may be possible to induce follicular growth and estrogen secretion in these patients by administration of large amounts of exogenous gonadotropins. However, it is usually difficult or impossible to induce ovulation and subsequent pregnancy in these patients. Although this disorder can only be diagnosed with certainty by ovarian biopsy, the infrequency of the disorder and the poor prognosis dictate that ovarian biopsy be performed only rarely in patients with high gonadotropins and normal karyotype.

D. Functioning Ovarian Tumors: Hormone-producing tumors of the ovary presenting clinically as endocrine disorders are uncommon. Classification of these tumors is made difficult by the uncertainty of embryonic origin in some and the lack of correlation between the functional and morphologic characteristics. However, it is convenient to divide them into broad morphologic categories, keeping in mind that the diagnostic approach will be based on the clinical presentation. Detection of androgen-producing tumors is considered in the section on amenorrhea with excess androgen production (see below). The estrogen-producing tumors cause amenorrhea or anovulatory bleeding in premenopausal women, irregular bleeding after the menopause, and precocious puberty in children. A classification of these tumors is presented in Table 13–4.

1. Germ cell tumors–

a. Germinomas (dysgerminoma, seminoma, gonocytoma, embryonal carcinoma)–These tumors of the ovary are usually found on routine examination in young women. They are generally small and asymptomatic unless associated with teratomatous elements that produce hCG. When hCG is produced, the patient will develop amenorrhea and other signs and symptoms of early pregnancy.

b. Teratomas–Teratomas arising in gonadal tissue are common. Although rarely active hormonally, they may contain hormone-secreting elements. Tumors containing thyroid tissue (struma ovarii) can release thyroxine. Carcinoid tumors producing serotonin have also been reported.

Choriocarcinoma of the ovary is usually secondary to uterine choriocarcinoma and very rarely arises within the ovary. It is composed of trophoblastic tissue, usually with extensive hemorrhage and necrosis. These tumors produce large amounts of hCG. The elevated plasma levels of this hormone are useful in diagnosing the tumor and in monitoring treatment. Treatment is similar to that of tumors of trophoblastic origin in the uterus. However, the prognosis is less favorable.

c. Gonadoblastomas–These rare tumors arise in dysgenetic gonads. They are typically seen in phenotypic females with a Y chromosome. They are

morphologically similar to germinomas but also have cells of mesenchymal or sex cord origin. The latter may differentiate into Leydig or granulosa cells and secrete androgens or estrogens. Prophylactic removal of the dysgenetic gonads is recommended in patients with a Y chromosome (see Chapter 14).

2. Sex cord-mesenchymal tumors–

a. Granulosa-theca cell tumors–These tumors constitute 5–10% of ovarian neoplasms. They are usually associated with some clinical or pathologic evidence of estrogen secretion. Androgen-producing tumors of this type have been reported but are rare. Granulosa cell tumors are unilateral in 90% of patients. They are usually solid and vary in appearance from mature granulosa cells arranged in circumferential rows around spaces ("Call-Exner bodies") to immature cells with a sarcomatous appearance. The cells may take on the polyhedral appearance of the luteinized granulosa cells of the corpus luteum. Although the prognosis following removal of these tumors is better than for ovarian carcinomas, about 20% recur in 5 years and about 40% in 10 years. The recurrences may be circumscribed and can be quite sensitive to radiation.

b. Sertoli-Leydig cell tumors (arrhenoblastoma, androblastoma)–This group of tumors, as noted above, may cause feminization. They more commonly produce virilization and under these circumstances are commonly called arrhenoblastomas or androblastomas. They are not common, accounting for fewer than 5% of ovarian tumors. They vary in size and, although usually small, may become large. The histologic pattern varies from that of well-differentiated testicular tubules (Pick's adenoma) to an undifferentiated sarcomatous appearance and mixtures of both.

Typically, the first manifestation of an androgen-producing tumor is amenorrhea, followed rapidly by hirsutism, acne, and breast atrophy; clitoral hypertrophy, balding, and deepening of the voice occur later. Plasma androgen levels are usually in the normal male range (testosterone $\geq$ 3 ng/mL) and usually cannot be suppressed by administration of estrogens or

Table 13–4. Classification and clinical features of functioning ovarian tumors.

	Hormones[1]	Usual Age at Onset	Percent Palpable	Percent Bilateral	Percent Malignant
Germ cell tumors					
Germinomas-teratomas					
Struma ovarii	Thyroxine	10–40	90	10	Rare
Carcinoid tumors	Serotonin	10–40	90	10	Rare
Choriocarcinomas	Chorionic gonadotropin	6–15	100	Rare	100
Gonadoblastomas	Androgens, estrogens	10–30		40	50
Sex cord–mesenchymal tumors					
Granulosa–theca cell tumors	Estrogens, androgens, progestins	30–70	90	10	20
Sertoli–Leydig cell tumors (arrhenoblastomas)	Androgens, estrogens	20–50	80	Rare	20
Hilar cell tumors	Androgens, estrogens	45–75	50	Rare	Rare

[1]Steroid-producing tumors may produce estrogens or androgens. The usual hormone released is listed first.

estrogen-containing oral contraceptives. Removal of the tumor is followed by a return of menses and partial or complete loss of abnormal hair. The tumors are seldom bilateral and usually benign.

3. Hilar cell (lipoid cell) tumors–These androgen-producing tumors usually occur in older patients and cause severe masculinization, including hirsutism, balding, clitoral enlargement, and deepening of the voice. They are usually small and less likely to be palpated than other ovarian tumors. Histologically, they are typical steroid-producing cells and contain Reinke crystalloids, which are characteristically found in the interstitial cells of the testis. They are almost always benign and are treated by extirpation, which reverses the hirsutism, baldness, and metabolic changes, though clitoral enlargement and voice changes persist.

Disorders of the Pituitary

The anterior pituitary gland plays a key role in normal ovarian function. In adults, the loss of pituitary gonadotropic activity is usually noted before the loss of other pituitary trophic functions when the organ is damaged by vascular, inflammatory, or neoplastic processes.

A. Pituitary Tumors: Most patients with amenorrhea and low gonadotropin levels have decreased or altered secretion of GnRH secondary to altered hypothalamic or central nervous system activity. However, the presence of a pituitary tumor must be considered and excluded. Amenorrhea may be the only clue to a nonfunctioning tumor. Most apparently nonsecreting tumors of the pituitary arise from gonadotrops and can be recognized by an increase in the β chain of LH in response to TRH injection. Most commonly, however, pituitary tumors in young women with amenorrhea cause hyperprolactinemia, and galactorrhea is found in more than 50% of patients with PRL-secreting adenomas (see Chapter 5). In contrast, GH-secreting tumors are associated with clinical signs of acromegaly. Although this is an unusual cause of amenorrhea, it is important to consider the diagnosis in appropriate clinical circumstances, since early diagnosis and treatment can prevent the permanently disfiguring effects of excessive GH. Amenorrhea may also be the presenting symptom in patients with Cushing's syndrome due to a pituitary tumor (Cushing's disease).

B. Empty Sella Syndrome: Amenorrhea and galactorrhea may occur in the presence of the empty sella syndrome (see Chapter 5). In this condition, there appears to be an extension of the subarachnoid space into the pituitary fossa, which leads to flattening of pituitary tissue against the wall of the sella and may lead to its enlargement. The disorder is found in 5% of patients at autopsy. It is benign and requires no treatment unless associated abnormalities of pituitary function are present. This condition can be differentiated from tumor by CT or MRI scanning.

Disorders Due to Central Nervous System Abnormalities of Regulation of Gonadotropin Secretion

A. Hypothalamic Amenorrhea: This term is used to described amenorrhea due to functional abnormalities in the neural mechanisms that regulate the pulsatile secretion of GnRH. Young women commonly fail to ovulate at times of increased stress such as may be occasioned by academic or career pressures, disruption of personal life-styles, change in residences, or illness. These events may mark the onset of periods of amenorrhea.

In most instances, the period of amenorrhea is self-limited and ovulatory menstrual function returns spontaneously. If this does not occur, treatment is dependent upon the expectations of the patient. If she wishes to become pregnant, induction of ovulation by clomiphene would be the initial treatment. If this does not induce ovulation, treatment with clomiphene plus chorionic gonadotropin, with menotropins (Pergonal), or with pulsatile administration of GnRH will be required. If the patient does not want to become pregnant, her estrogenic status will help to determine treatment. Most of these women will have a positive progesterone challenge test (withdrawal bleeding) and either normal or only moderately reduced levels of estrogen. Cyclic treatment with a progestational agent will prevent endometrial hyperplasia in these women. Rarely, these women will have a negative progesterone challenge test (no withdrawal bleeding) and may have significant loss of calcium with the eventual development of osteoporosis secondary to low levels of estrogen. In these patients, preventative treatment with estrogen and a cyclic progestin should be considered.

B. Amenorrhea in Athletes: Menstrual abnormalities are sufficiently common in female athletes to suggest a causal relationship between vigorous physical effort and amenorrhea. About one-third of long-distance runners experience amenorrhea or oligomenorrhea. The incidence appears to vary with the degree of stress and effort in other activities. The incidence of amenorrhea correlates directly with the amount of weight lost and inversely with the percentage of body weight as fat. It is less frequent in multiparous women. No consistent changes in plasma estradiol, testosterone, or gonadotropin levels have been reported. In general, these menstrual abnormalities disappear with a reduction of physical activity and a return to the individual's natural weight and proportion of body weight as fat. Some of these women with prolonged amenorrhea show excessive bone loss in spite of their intense physical activity, and appropriate hormone replacement therapy should be instituted. Amenorrhea in swimmers differs from other exercise amenorrheas in that these women have a normal body mass index and increased androsterone, DHEAS, and LH levels.

C. Anorexia: Anorexia nervosa in its classic form is a serious but uncommon disorder characterized by extreme malnutrition and hypogonadotropism. It is considered to be a severe behavioral disorder, with endocrine changes secondary to both psychologic and nutritional disturbances. Amenorrhea may precede weight loss. Psychiatric treatment is required, and hospitalization may be necessary to prevent death from starvation, suicide, or intercurrent illnesses. Women who resort to induced vomiting (bulimia), laxative use, or other drastic methods of weight loss or control may also present with amenorrhea. These patients may respond to psychotherapy and antidepressant drug therapy.

D. Post-Pill Amenorrhea: Although it has not been possible to clearly demonstrate an increase in prolactinomas or a reduction in the fertility rate of women following the use of oral contraceptives, some studies show a moderate increase in the incidence of amenorrhea with galactorrhea in women treated with oral contraceptives. However, most women who develop amenorrhea following the use of contraceptive pills would probably have developed amenorrhea without them, and the disorder must be investigated as in other women.

Amenorrhea With Galactorrhea

Galactorrhea may be induced by a wide variety of stimuli ranging from local irritation or stimulation of the chest wall to ingestion of drugs that interfere with the hypothalamic release of dopamine or its binding to the pituitary lactotrophs (see Chapter 8). The secretion may be present in only one breast at any given time.

Whether or not galactorrhea is present, however, prolactin levels should be measured in patients with persistent amenorrhea (Figure 13–14). When a detectable tumor is present, prolactin levels are usually elevated. In the presence of nonsecreting tumors impinging on the pituitary stalk but not secreting prolactin, prolactin levels may be only minimally elevated. It is advisable to obtain CT or MRI studies of the pituitary in most patients with galactorrhea or elevated prolactin levels. Studies of pituitary function, including the gonadotropin response to GnRH and the effect of levodopa and other drugs on prolactin secretion, do not reliably identify patients with pituitary tumors. However, these and other tests of pituitary function are useful in assessing residual pituitary function. CT scanning will detect microadenomas as small as 3–5 mm in size. Bulging and demineralization of the sella turcica usually occur when the tumor exceeds 1 cm in diameter, and larger tumors are usually found in patients presenting with visual field defects. About 10–20% of women examined at autopsy show small pituitary adenomas. The natural history of the disorder is not well understood.

Although clomiphene or gonadotropins may induce ovulation in these patients, bromocriptine is more effective. Bromocriptine mesylate is an ergot alkaloid that acts by binding to the dopaminergic receptors in the pituitary, resulting in inhibition of PRL secretion. In 90% or more of these patients, treatment leads to the onset of menses in 3–5 weeks. The usual dose is 2.5 mg two or three times a day. Since there are side effects of nausea and mild dizziness, it is useful to start with a small dose, such as 2.5 mg daily—or half that amount given at bedtime in sensitive patients—and increase to 2.5 mg twice daily. PRL levels should be depressed to normal if treatment is adequate. Pergolide taken once daily is as effective as bromocriptine.

The long-term use of bromocriptine induces some regression of pituitary tumors in most patients. Even incomplete regression may be useful in patients whose tumors are too large to favor the transsphenoidal approach to the removal of the tumor. Transsphenoidal tumor removal will restore normal gonadal function and normal PRL levels in the large majority of these patients. However, patients must be followed carefully with PRL levels and radiologic reevaluation of the sella every 1–2 years, since recurrences are common. Larger tumors and those invading other structures such as the cavernous sinus that cannot be completely removed may require radiotherapy as well. (See Chapter 5.)

DISORDERS OF ANDROGEN METABOLISM

Production & Metabolism of Androgens in Women

The major circulating androgens in women are testosterone, dihydrotestosterone, androstenedione, dehydroepiandrosterone (DHEA), and DHEA sulfate. The relative androgenic activity, serum concentrations, and sources of these androgens are summarized in Table 13–5. Testosterone is the principal circulating androgen in normal women. Both the ovaries and the adrenals normally secrete testosterone. Approximately 50% of the testosterone in serum, however, is derived from the peripheral conversion of steroid precursors, principally androstenedione and to a lesser extent DHEA. In many androgen-sensitive tissues, such as hair follicles, the enzyme 5α-reductase converts testosterone to dihydrotestosterone. It is believed that dihydrotestosterone per se (and not testosterone) is mainly responsible for stimulating hair growth in many areas of the body. Virtually all of the dihydrotestosterone in the circulation is formed in androgen-dependent peripheral tissues by 5α-reductase conversion of testosterone and androstenedione. Most of the dihydrotestosterone formed in these target tissues is metabolized further to androstanediols. Circulating androstenedione, in contrast to testosterone and dihydrotestosterone, is derived primarily from direct secretion by the ovaries and adrenals. Although an-

Table 13–5. Circulating androgens and their relative androgenic activity, serum concentration, and site of formation in women.

Hormone	Relative Androgenic Activity[1]	Serum Concentration[2]		Source of Circulating Hormone (Percentage of Total)		
		(ng/mL)	(nmol/L)	Adrenal	Ovary	Peripheral Conversion
Testosterone	100	0.2–0.7	(0.69–2.43)	5–25	5–25	50–70
Dihydrotestosterone	250	0.05–0.3	(0.17–1.03)	. . .	. . .	100
Androstenedione	10–20	0.5–2.5	(1.72–8.6)	30–45	45–60	10
DHEA	5	1.3–9.8	(4.5–34)	80	20	. . .
DHEA sulfate	Minimal	400–3200	(790–6318)	>95	<5	. . .

[1]Testosterone has been assigned a potency of 100. Values are approximate and may vary depending upon the biologic system in which the hormones are evaluated.
[2]Normal ranges will vary in different laboratories.

drostenedione is a relatively weak androgen, possessing only 10–20% of the biologic activity of testosterone, it can be converted to testosterone and dihydrotestosterone in androgen-sensitive target tissues. Increased production and secretion of androstenedione thus may play a role in promoting the development of hirsutism in many women. DHEA is a very weak androgen with little biologic activity. DHEA sulfate has little or no androgenic activity. Most of the DHEA sulfate in the serum is derived from the adrenal glands. Measurement of serum DHEA sulfate is useful in assessing adrenal androgen production.

Androgen metabolism in skin and hair follicles is an important factor in the etiology of hirsutism. Alterations in the activity of 5α-reductase can influence the androgenic activity of testosterone. In vitro studies utilizing skin biopsies from hair-bearing regions have demonstrated increased 5α-reductase activity in hirsute women; thus, many women presently thought to have idiopathic hirsutism may actually have increased formation of dihydrotestosterone in hair follicles. This mechanism also is suggested by the relatively high percentage of women with hirsutism and normal levels of testosterone who have been found to have increased serum levels of androstanediol glucuronide, a major metabolite of dihydrotestosterone. The factors responsible for the development of androgen-dependent hirsutism are summarized in Figure 13–15.

Amenorrhea With Androgen Excess

The presence of excessive amounts of circulating androgen is usually associated with oligomenorrhea or amenorrhea. Causes of androgen excess are shown in Table 13–6.

A. Functional Ovarian Hyperandrogenism (Polycystic Ovary Syndrome): This is a complex of varying symptoms ranging from amenorrhea to anovulatory bleeding often associated with obesity and hirsutism. The latter term has been used to describe such a variety of symptom complexes (Table 13–7) that it is almost a barrier to communication. In this discussion, we are referring to patients who are anovulatory with continuous stimulation of the ovary by normal or disproportionately high levels of LH. The chronic stimulation leads to increased ovarian androgen secretion and characteristic morphologic changes in the ovaries. The ovaries are commonly enlarged and may reach several times their normal size; one ovary may be significantly larger than the other. The ovaries typically appear glistening white because of a thickened capsule and show many small follicles in various stages of development and atresia at the surface. They also may appear normal. The theca cells are often hyperplastic and luteinized.

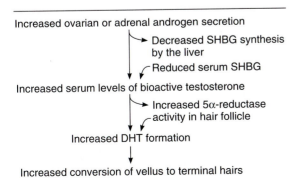

Figure 13–15. Development factors of androgen-dependent hirsutism.

Table 13–6. Causes of increased androgen production, hirsutism, or both.

Ovarian causes
  Polycystic ovary syndrome (LH-dependent androgen excess, hyperandrogenic chronic anovulation)
  Hyperthecosis
  Androgen-producing ovarian tumors
  Virilization of pregnancy (luteoma)

Adrenal causes
  Congenital or adult-onset adrenal hyperplasia
  Androgen-producing adrenal tumors
  Cushing's syndrome

Other
  Idiopathic or familial hirsutism
  Incomplete testicular feminization
  Postmenopausal state
  Iatrogenic (androgens, cyclosporine, danazol, diazoxide, minoxidil, phenytoin)

Table 13–7. Incidence of various clinical findings in women with functional ovarian hyperandrogenism polycystic ovary syndrome. Data are derived from 187 references comprising a total of 1079 cases.[1]

	Incidence (%)	
	Mean	Range
Infertility	74	35–94
Hirsutism	69	17–83
Amenorrhea	51	15–77
Obesity	41	16–49
Functional bleeding	29	6–65
Dysmenorrhea	23	
Corpus luteum at surgery	22	0–71
Virilization	21	0–28
Biphasic basal body temperature	15	12–40
Cyclic menses	12	7–28

[1]Reproduced, with permission, from Goldzieher JW: Polycystic ovarian disease. In: *Progress in Infertility*, 2nd ed. Behrman SH, Kistner RW (editors). Little, Brown, 1975.

These findings are not specific and are seen with androgen excess from any source. Estrogen production in these patients is usually a result of the peripheral conversion of androgens to estrogens, predominantly androstenedione to estrone, and may be increased. This can produce endometrial hyperplasia and eventually lead to adenocarcinoma of the endometrium, since the estrogen action is unopposed by progesterone. As a group, patients with this disorder often have elevated fasting levels of insulin with insulin resistance, an increased incidence of diabetes and hypertension, and a late menopause.

1. Etiology–The cause of this syndrome is unknown, and it is possible that there are several causes. Each of the functional changes that occur tends to maintain the cycle of functional abnormalities as shown in Figure 13–16. It has been suggested that in some patients this disorder may be initiated by

excessive adrenal androgen production at the time of puberty or by a stress-induced increase in adrenal androgen secretion. The peripheral conversion of androgen to estrogen could facilitate the secretion of increased amounts of LH, leading to increased ovarian androgen production and impaired follicular maturation. In the ovary, aromatase is inhibited, reducing androgen conversion to estradiol. The lack of estrogen locally reduces IGF-1, which normally sensitizes the follicle to FSH. In some patients, there is a strong family history, and the pattern of inheritance suggests that the trait is dominant and may be linked to the X chromosome. A group of patients have also been found in whom amenorrhea and androgen excess are associated with acanthosis nigricans and insulin resistance.

Although androgen production is quite variable, it seldom reaches the levels seen in the presence of androgen-producing ovarian tumors. As a result, the vast majority of women show hirsutism and increased activity of the sebaceous glands often associated with acne. Signs of more severe virilization, such as male pattern (bitemporal) balding, clitoral hypertrophy, and voice changes, are rare. In patients with amenorrhea, there is a good correlation between levels of free testosterone and clinical evidence of androgen excess.

2. Management–The major manifestations of functional ovarian hyperandrogenism (polycystic ovary syndrome) are hirsutism secondary to increased circulating levels of androgens or increased 5α-reductase activity (or both) in the hair follicles and failure of ovulation causing amenorrhea and infertility. The goals of therapy in the individual patient are of prime importance in determining the appropriate therapeutic program.

Induction of ovulation is required for anovulatory patients who wish to conceive. Most women ovulate

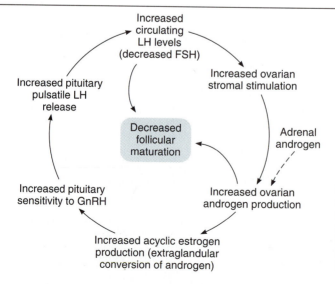

Figure 13–16. Pathophysiology of chronic anovulation in women with polycystic ovary syndrome. (Reproduced, with permission, from Yen SSC, Jaffe RB [editors]: *Reproductive Endocrinology.* Saunders, 1978.)

in response to clomiphene citrate (see Ovulation Induction, below). In women whose ovaries fail to respond, combined therapy consisting of adrenal suppression and clomiphene may be more successful. The use of pulsatile GnRH to induce ovulation has generally not been effective. Wedge resection of the ovaries is rarely employed today.

In patients who have amenorrhea but do not wish to become pregnant, treatment may not be required. Some obese patients have been reported to resume ovulation and reduce androgen secretion on a program of weight reduction alone. In patients producing moderate to large amounts of estrogen continuously, endometrial hyperplasia with consequent bleeding and even endometrial carcinoma may develop. In such patients, the cyclic administration of a progestational agent may be required (see Anovulatory Bleeding, below). Hirsutism can be treated by suppression of ovarian androgen production or by antiandrogen therapy, as discussed in the Treatment of Hirsutism section, below.

B. Adult-onset Congenital Adrenal Hyperplasia: An infrequent cause of amenorrhea and hirsutism is adult-onset congenital adrenal hyperplasia. The incidence is 1–5% (about 5% in Hispanics, Ashkenazi Jews, and Yugoslavs, and highest in Alaskan Eskimos). These women most often have a reduction in P450c21 (21-hydroxylase) activity (see Chapter 14). This defect in cortisol synthesis leads to an increase in ACTH and 17-hydroxyprogesterone production. The latter is the basis for making the diagnosis (Figure 13–17). Levels of 17-hydroxyprogesterone below 300 ng/dL are normal, and levels of more than 800 ng/dL are considered to be diagnostic. When levels fall between these values, ACTH stimulation is required to make the diagnosis.

C. Other Causes of Androgen Excess: Excessive production of androgens is more commonly of ovarian than adrenal origin. The exact cause needs to be established to rule out androgen-producing adrenal and ovarian tumors, and Cushing's syndrome. Other causes of androgen excess are shown in Table 13–6. The general clinical approach to the evaluation of patients with excess androgen production is discussed above and summarized in Figure 13–17.

HIRSUTISM

Hair can be classified as either vellus or terminal. Vellus hairs are fine, soft, and nonpigmented. They are found over most of the body and predominate prior to puberty. They are often so fine that they are barely visible. Terminal hairs are coarse and pigmented. Before puberty, terminal hairs normally are found only on the scalp and eyebrows. Under the influence of increasing levels of androgen at puberty, vellus hairs are transformed into terminal hairs. In women, this conversion to terminal hairs involves principally the axillary and pubic regions and to a lesser extent the extremities. Under conditions of excessive androgen production or increased 5α-reductase activity (which increases conversion of testosterone to dihydrotestosterone), there is increased conversion of vellus to terminal hairs. Terminal hairs may thus develop in body regions where such hair growth is normally considered to be a male secondary sex characteristic. The presence of increasing numbers of terminal hairs on the face, chest, back, lower abdomen, and inner thighs is referred to as hirsutism. In many women, hirsutism in combination with increased circulating levels of androgen is accompanied by menstrual dysfunction (usually oligomenorrhea but sometimes amenorrhea). Rarely, abnormal androgen production increases to levels normally found only in men. In such instances, the high circulating levels of androgen also produce somatic changes referred to as virilization. These changes include frontal balding, deepening of the voice, breast atrophy, clitoral enlargement, increased muscle mass, and loss of normal female body contours.

Pathophysiology of Hirsutism

A. Increased Androgen Production: Studies in which women with mild to moderate hirsutism have been evaluated with sensitive and specific laboratory techniques have shown that most women with excessive hair growth have increased serum androgen levels (ie, increased concentrations of free testosterone) or increased 5α-reductase activity. Thus, fewer women are currently classified as having "idiopathic" hirsutism. The source (adrenal, ovarian, or both) of the increased production of androgens in women with mild to moderate hirsutism is sometimes difficult to establish. Some published reports support a combined adrenal-ovarian source for the increased serum levels of androgens, with the ovary as the major contributor in most instances. Approximately 1–5% of women with mild hirsutism and menstrual abnormalities have elevated serum levels of 17-hydroxyprogesterone and are thought to have increased androgen production secondary to adult-onset congenital adrenal hyperplasia.

B. Serum Binding Proteins and the Serum Transport of Androgens: As reviewed earlier (Table 13–2), circulating steroid hormones are bound, to varying degrees, to plasma proteins, eg, albumin and specific transport proteins. In normal women, approximately 65% of the circulating testosterone is tightly bound to SHBG, while most of the remaining hormone is loosely bound to albumin. Only 1–2% of the total testosterone is free (not bound to protein). It is generally thought that testosterone bound to SHBG is not readily available to intracellular androgen receptors at target tissues and therefore has little biologic activity. Factors that can

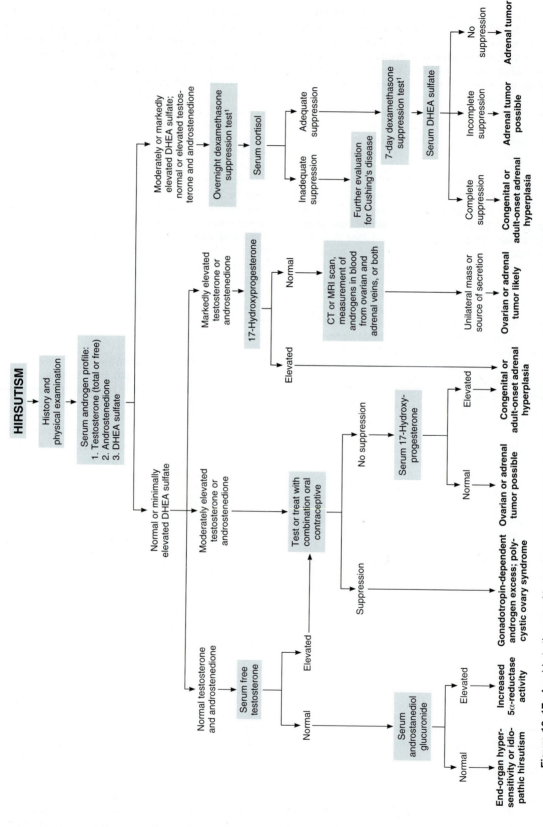

Figure 13–17. A guide to the use of hormone measurements in the evaluation of hirsutism. [1]See text for discussion of dexamethasone suppression tests.

alter the serum concentration of SHBG are shown in Table 13–8. Hirsute women often have reduced serum concentrations of SHBG. Thus, a small increase in total testosterone, accompanied by a decrease in the concentration of SHBG, may result in a significant increase in biologically active hormone. The measurement of free, or non-SHBG bound, testosterone levels in serum is a more sensitive indicator of androgen activity. A greater proportion of women with mild to moderate hirsutism have elevated concentrations of free—as compared to total—plasma testosterone.

Evaluation of Women With Hirsutism

The common causes of increased androgen production and hirsutism are listed in Table 13–6. The initial assessment of hirsute women should include a thorough history and physical examination. Hirsutism is usually secondary to a mild increase in androgen activity. The increase in body hair occurs gradually and may be accompanied by other symptoms of mild androgen excess such as acne, oily skin, and oligomenorrhea or amenorrhea. The sudden appearance of rapid hair growth and amenorrhea associated with virilization, however, suggests an ovarian or adrenal androgen-producing tumor (see Chapter 9 and Table 13–4). The physical examination should detect signs of associated endocrine dysfunction, such as Cushing's syndrome or virilization. The degree and extent of growth of terminal hairs should be carefully recorded. This will help the physician decide if further endocrine investigation is warranted and help assess the effects of any future therapy. A pelvic examination also should be included in the initial evaluation of the patient, especially if she has oligomenorrhea or amenorrhea.

The laboratory evaluation of women with hirsutism is important for ruling out a serious underlying disease process such as an ovarian or adrenal androgen-producing tumor, steroid enzymatic defect (eg, partial 21-hydroxylase deficiency), or Cushing's syndrome. Once therapy has been initiated, measurement of serum androgen levels also can be used to determine if androgen secretion has been reduced.

Table 13–8. Conditions affecting SHBG synthesis and therefore the percentage of plasma testosterone that is free.

	SHBG Synthesis
Hypothyroidism Androgen therapy Corticosteroid therapy Obesity Acromegaly	Decreased
Hyperthyroidism Pregnancy Estrogen therapy Cirrhosis	Increased

Suppression of androgen production or action at the hair follicle will, in most women, reduce but not eliminate the extent of excessive hair growth.

A general approach to the hormonal evaluation of women with hirsutism is shown in Figure 13–17. The rate of ovarian and adrenal androgen secretion can be estimated initially by measuring the serum concentrations of testosterone (total or free), androstenedione, and DHEA sulfate. In many women with hirsutism, serum testosterone or androstenedione will be somewhat elevated. Patients with raised levels of these hormones and normal or minimally increased levels of DHEA sulfate can be evaluated further by administering a combination oral contraceptive to suppress pituitary LH and FSH secretion. If the excess production of androgen is gonadotropin-dependent and of ovarian origin (eg, as in polycystic ovary syndrome), serum androgen levels (especially free testosterone levels) also will be suppressed after a 1-month trial of oral contraceptives. Treatment may be continued in those women with LH-dependent androgen secretion. Failure of serum androgens to suppress indicates that the excessive production is either of adrenal origin (eg, a tumor or enzyme defect) or secondary to an ovarian neoplasm. Women with adult-onset adrenal hyperplasia secondary to a 21-hydroxylase deficiency will have elevated serum levels of 17-hydroxyprogesterone, which are readily suppressed by dexamethasone.

Women with initially normal serum levels of total testosterone and androstenedione can be evaluated further by measuring free testosterone. If free testosterone levels also are within normal limits, 5α-reductase activity in the hair follicles can be estimated by measuring serum levels of androstenediol glucuronide (measurement of serum androstenediol glucuronide is rarely justified for clinical management). Only a small percentage of hirsute women eventually will be found to have both normal androgen production and 5α-reductase activity. These women can be diagnosed as having idiopathic hirsutism.

Women with signs or symptoms of virilization generally will have greatly elevated testosterone levels (> 3 ng/mL [10.4 nmol/L]), androstenedione levels above 5 ng/mL (17.3 nmol/L), or both. These women are most likely to have an androgen-producing >*ovarian* tumor if DHEA sulfate levels are normal or an androgen-producing *adrenal* tumor if DHEA sulfate levels are elevated. Rarely, an androgen-secreting adrenal tumor can be found in the presence of normal serum DHEA sulfate levels. Women with 21-hydroxylase deficiencies may also have normal or minimally elevated levels of DHEA sulfate. Further evaluation of women with virilization should include suppression tests (dexamethasone for adrenal suppression and an oral contraceptive for ovarian suppression) as well as CT or MRI scans of the adrenals and ovaries. If the androgens are not suppressible, surgical exploration is required. A few patients have been found to have tumors with LH-dependent androgen secretion.

Moderately to markedly elevated serum levels of DHEA sulfate indicate increased adrenal androgen secretion resulting from excessive stimulation (eg, Cushing's disease) or indicate adrenal hyperplasia secondary to an enzyme defect, stress, or a tumor. In these cases, serum testosterone and androstenedione levels may vary from minimally to markedly elevated. Initially, women in this group should be evaluated by an overnight dexamethasone suppression test (1 mg of dexamethasone given at bedtime, and serum cortisol levels measured in the morning) to rule out Cushing's syndrome. Suppression of serum cortisol levels to less than 5 μg/dL (138 nmol/L) excludes this disorder. If suppression to this level is not achieved, further assessment of adrenal function, as described in Chapter 9, is required. An overnight dexamethasone suppression test, however, is inadequate to assess adrenal androgen production as reflected by levels of DHEA sulfate, since this hormone has a long plasma half-life. In women who have elevated levels of DHEA sulfate but in whom Cushing's syndrome has been excluded, dexamethasone (2 mg/d) given for 4–7 days will differentiate an adrenal tumor (no suppression) from other causes of increased adrenal androgen production.

Treatment of Hirsutism

Medical therapies directed at reducing the production of ovarian or adrenal androgens are effective primarily in reducing or preventing the formation of new hair growth. For the most part, such treatment has limited effect on terminal hairs previously formed, since the cycle of hair growth ordinarily occurs only every 6 months to 2 years. Consequently, an effective approach to the management of hirsutism usually consists of both medical and cosmetic treatment.

A. Suppression of Androgen Production: The reduction of serum levels of androgens by trials with combination oral contraceptives, progestins, or glucocorticoids should provide a rational basis for choosing one or another of these various forms of therapy. However, most women with hirsutism have only slightly increased androgen production, and its precise source or sources cannot be identified readily. In these patients, estrogen-containing oral contraceptives are generally more effective and are most often the initial form of treatment.

1. Oral contraceptives or progestins–Oral contraceptives containing both an estrogen and a progestin suppress the secretion of LH and FSH and reduce LH-dependent ovarian androgen production. The progestin component also increases the metabolic clearance rate of testosterone, while the estrogen component stimulates the production of SHBG. Although treatment with a progestin alone (ie, oral or injectable medroxyprogesterone acetate) suppresses

the secretion of LH and increases the metabolic clearance rate of androgens, there is no concomitant increase in SHBG levels. Progestins are therefore generally less effective than combination oral contraceptives. They may be useful when estrogens are contraindicated.

The available combination oral contraceptives are listed in Table 13–9. In selecting a particular contraceptive for the treatment of hirsutism, the physician should avoid compounds containing the more androgenic progestins. Contraceptives containing a minimum of 35–50 μg of ethinyl estradiol may increase serum concentrations of SHBG and reduce the levels of both total and free testosterone in most patients. If significant clinical improvement—eg, a decrease in acne, skin oiliness, and rate of hair growth—is not apparent after 3 months of treatment, serum androgen levels should be reevaluated to make certain that adequate suppression of ovarian function has occurred. Treatment with oral contraceptives is discussed in a subsequent section of this chapter.

2. Glucocorticoids–If increased androgen production is predominantly or entirely of adrenal origin—such as occurs in adult-onset adrenal hyperplasia—treatment with glucocorticoids is indicated. In these cases, dexamethasone, 0.5–0.75 mg/d, or prednisone, 5–7.5 mg/d, has been used to reduce the production of adrenal androgens. In most women with hirsutism, however, excess androgen secretion is generally of ovarian origin, and glucocorticoids are not effective.

3. Gonadotropin-releasing hormone analogs–GnRH analogs are effective in the management of hirsutism due to excessive ovarian androgens. They inhibit pituitary FSH and LH secretion and thus decrease ovarian androgen production. Since ovarian estradiol production will also be reduced, treatment with GnRH analogs will produce symptoms and other changes of estrogen deficiency. These can be prevented by concurrent low-dose estrogen replacement. A progestin with low androgenicity should also be administered. Progestins without androgenic activity include desogestrel, gestodine, and norgestimate. Although not available in the USA or Canada, an oral contraceptive containing cyproterone, a progestin with antiandrogenic properties, is available in Europe. The combination of oral contraceptives or spironolactone with GnRH gives a more rapid response and may be slightly more effective.

B. Antiandrogens: Cyproterone acetate was the first antiandrogen to be employed extensively for the treatment of hirsutism. Clinical studies with this drug in Europe have resulted in a high rate of improvement. Cyproterone acetate is a derivative of the progestin chlormadinone acetate and possesses both progestational and antiandrogenic activity. It suppresses the secretion of LH, with a subsequent decrease in ovarian androgen production, and blocks

Table 13–9. Some oral and implantable contraceptive agents in use. The estrogen-containing compounds are arranged in order of increasing content of estrogen (ethinyl estradiol and mestranol have similar potencies).[1]

	Estrogen (mg)		Progestin (mg)[2]	
Monophasic combination tablets				
Loestrin 1/20	Ethinyl estradiol	0.02	Norethindrone acetate	1.0
Loestrin 1.5/30	Ethinyl estradiol	0.03	Norethindrone acetate	1.5
Desogen	Ethinyl estradiol	0.03	Desogestrel	0.15
Orthosept 13–9	Ethinyl estradiol	0.03	Desagestryl	0.15
Lo/Ovral	Ethinyl estradiol	0.03	DL-Norgestrel	0.3
Nordette	Ethinyl estradiol	0.03	L-Norgestrel	0.15
Brevicon, Modicon	Ethinyl estradiol	0.035	Norethindrone	0.5
Demulen 1/35	Ethinyl estradiol	0.035	Ethynodiol diacetate	1.0
Genora 1/35, Nelova 1/35 E, Norinyl 1/35, Ortho-Novum 1/35	Ethinyl estradiol	0.035	Norethindrone	1.0
Ortho-Cyclen	Ethinyl estradiol	0.035	Norgestimate	0.25
Ovcon 35	Ethinyl estradiol	0.035	Norethindrone	0.4
Demulen 1/50	Ethinyl estradiol	0.05	Ethynodiol diacetate	1.0
Norlestrin 1/50	Ethinyl estradiol	0.05	Norethindrone acetate	1.0
Norlestrin 2.5/50	Ethinyl estradiol	0.05	Norethindrone acetate	2.5
Ovcon 50	Ethinyl estradiol	0.05	Norethindrone	1.0
Ovral	Ethinyl estradiol	0.05	DL-Norgestrel	0.5
Genora 1/50, Norinyl 1/50, Ortho-Novum 1/50	Mestranol	0.05	Norethindrone	1.0
Enovid 5	Mestranol	0.075	Norethynodrel	5.0
Norinyl 1/80, Ortho-Novum 1/80	Mestranol	0.08	Norethindrone	1.0
Enovid E	Mestranol	0.1	Norethynodrel	2.5
Norinyl-2, Ortho-Novum-2	Mestranol	0.1	Norethindrone	2.0
Ovulen	Mestranol	0.1	Ethynodiol diacetate	1.0
Biphasic combination tablets				
Ortho-Novum 10/11 Days 1–10	Ethinyl estradiol	0.035	Norethindrone	0.5
Days 11–21	Ethinyl estradiol	0.035	Norethindrone	1.0
Triphasic combination tablets				
Triphasil Days 1–6	Ethinyl estradiol	0.03	L-Norgestrel	0.05
Days 7–11	Ethinyl estradiol	0.04	L-Norgestrel	0.075
Days 12–21	Ethinyl estradiol	0.03	L-Norgestrel	0.125
Ortho-Novum 7/7/7 Days 1–7	Ethinyl estradiol	0.035	Norethindrone	0.5
Days 8–14	Ethinyl estradiol	0.035	Norethindrone	0.75
Days 15–21	Ethinyl estradiol	0.035	Norethindrone	1.0
Tri-Norinyl Days 1–7	Ethinyl estradiol	0.035	Norethindrone	0.5
Days 8–16	Ethinyl estradiol	0.035	Norethindrone	1.0
Days 17–21	Ethinyl estradiol	0.035	Norethindrone	0.5

(*continued*)

Table 13–9. Some oral and implantable contraceptive agents in use. The estrogen-containing compounds are arranged in order of increasing content of estrogen (ethinyl estradiol and mestranol have similar potencies).[1] (continued)

	Estrogen (mg)		Progestin (mg)[2]	
Triphasic combination tablets (cont.) Ortho-Tri-Cyclen				
Days 1–7	Ethinyl estradiol	0.035	Norgestimate	0.18
Days 8–14	Ethinyl estradiol	0.035	Norgestimate	0.215
Days 15–21	Ethinyl estradiol	0.035	Norgestimate	0.25
Daily progestin tablets Micronor	. . .		Norethindrone	0.35
Nor-QD	. . .		Norethindrone	0.35
Ovrette	. . .		D,L-Norgestrel	0.075
Implantable progestin preparation Norplant	. . .		l-Norgestrel (6 tubes of 36 mg each)	

[1]Modified and reproduced, with permission, from Katzung BG (editor): *Basic & Clinical Pharmacology,* 7th ed. Appleton & Lange, 1997.
[2]Progestational potency.

the binding of androgens to receptors in the hair follicles. Estrogen is usually administered concurrently, since endogenous estrogen production also is reduced during treatment. Although few serious side effects have been reported, cyproterone acetate is not available in the USA. A commonly used dosage is 2 mg of cyproterone acetate plus 50 μg of ethinyl estradiol daily on days 5–20 of each menstrual cycle. In preliminary studies, treatment with flutamide or finasteride, a 5α-reductase inhibitor, produces effects comparable to those achieved with cyproterone.

Spironolactone, a competitive inhibitor of aldosterone, has been shown to possess antiandrogenic properties and competes with dihydrotestosterone for androgenic receptors in target tissues. It also decreases 17α-hydroxylase activity and thus reduces serum levels of testosterone and androstenedione. Doses ranging from 50 to 200 mg/d have been used to treat hirsutism. Spironolactone is especially useful for therapy in women in whom oral contraceptives are contraindicated or ineffective. Irregular uterine bleeding is a common side effect of treatment with spironolactone. Combined therapy consisting of spironolactone and an oral contraceptive may be employed when neither alone has been effective in reducing hair growth.

C. Cosmetic Therapy: The initial response to medical treatment is generally slow, and 3–6 months of therapy may be required before there is noticeable improvement in hirsutism. During the initial period of treatment, the patient can either continue with or start a simple and inexpensive method for the temporary removal of hair, eg, shaving or use of a depilatory or hot wax. After several

months of medical treatment, the rate of formation of new terminal hairs will be reduced markedly, and permanent hair removal by electrolysis can be initiated, if desired. If permanent hair removal is tried prior to adequate medical treatment, the results will be transient, since new terminal hairs will continue to be formed.

ANOVULATORY BLEEDING

In the absence of ovulatory cycles, the pattern of bleeding (Table 13–3) is dependent upon the amount and timing of estrogen secretion, since the bleeding is due to estrogen stimulation of the endometrium. When estrogen secretion is low, there is usually no bleeding. However, the heaviest bleeding is observed in association with continuous secretion of substantial amounts of estrogen. In these instances, the estrogen produces proliferation of the endometrium, leading to hyperplasia or adenomatous hyperplasia. In some of these women, endometrial carcinoma will develop over long periods.

When the level of estrogen fluctuates, bleeding will occur during periods of reduced secretion. However, when the secretion is continuous and maturation is not synchronized by progesterone, the tissue is subject to spontaneous breakdown and bleeding of differing portions of the endometrium at different times. Furthermore, local factors such as the coiling and contraction of the spiral vessels do not contribute to the hemostasis, and bleeding may be severe. Such bleeding is more common in postpubertal teenagers and in the premenopausal period in older women. It is also seen in some patients in association with polycystic ovary syndrome and in women receiving estrogen therapy.

OVULATION INDUCTION

CLOMIPHENE CITRATE

Clomiphene citrate is a partial agonist of estrogen that effectively inhibits the action of stronger estrogens and stimulates the secretion of gonadotropins; it is used for the treatment of anovulatory patients in whom ovulation is desired. In general, a single ovulation is induced by a single course of therapy, and the patient must be treated repeatedly until pregnancy is achieved. The compound is of no use in the treatment of ovarian or pituitary failure.

The recommended initial dose of clomiphene citrate is 50 mg/d for 5 days. If ovulation occurs, this same course may be repeated until pregnancy is achieved. If ovulation does not occur, the dose is doubled to 100 mg/d for 5 days. If ovulation and menses occur, the next course can be started on the fifth day of the cycle. About 80% of patients with anovulatory disorders or amenorrhea can be expected to respond to this treatment by having ovulatory cycles. Approximately half of these patients will become pregnant. In patients in whom pregnancy is achieved, the incidence of early abortion seems to be slightly increased, as is the occurrence of multiple pregnancy (10%). Although a variety of congenital defects have been described in the offspring of these pregnancies, the incidence does not appear to be greater than that of the general population. Ovulation can be induced in some of the patients not responding to 50 or 100 mg of clomiphene daily for 5 days by using larger doses (up to 200 mg/d) for longer periods or by injecting 5000 units of chorionic gonadotropin at the time of expected ovulation. The combination of clomiphene and bromocriptine has also been reported to be successful in some patients with normal PRL levels. Clomiphene has also been used in combination with menotropins to reduce the amount of the latter required to induce ovulation.

The effective use of clomiphene is associated with some stimulation of the ovaries and usually with ovarian enlargement. The degree of enlargement tends to be greater and its incidence higher in patients who have enlarged ovaries at the beginning of therapy.

The most common side effects in patients treated with this drug are hot flushes, which resemble those experienced by menopausal patients. These tend to be mild and disappear when the drug is discontinued.

There have been occasional reports of visual disturbances consisting of intensification and prolongation of afterimages. These are generally of short duration. Headache, constipation, allergic skin reactions, and reversible hair loss have been reported occasionally. Treatment with clomiphene for more than a year may be associated with an increased risk for low-grade ovarian cancer.

HUMAN MENOPAUSAL GONADOTROPINS (Menotropins)

Human menopausal gonadotropins, or menotropins, in conjunction with chorionic gonadotropin, are used to stimulate ovulation in anovulatory patients who have potentially functional ovarian tissue. Patients with ovarian failure should not be considered for therapy. Menotropins are generally used only after less complicated therapies, such as clomiphene citrate or bromocriptine, have been unsuccessful. Since therapy is difficult and expensive, it is also important to exclude other factors that might preclude pregnancy (eg, obstruction of the uterine tubes or abnormalities in sperm production by the husband) prior to initiating treatment. The possibility of multiple births must be acceptable to the patient. This treatment has induced ovulation in patients with hypopituitarism and other defects of gonadotropin secretion and in patients with amenorrhea or anovulatory cycles in whom ovulatory disturbances are associated with galactorrhea or hirsutism. In patients undergoing in vitro fertilization, menotropins are used to stimulate the development of multiple large follicles to increase the number of available ova.

Contraindications & Cautions

The most common problem encountered is excessive ovarian stimulation. Ovarian enlargement is common. When marked, as in the ovarian hyperstimulation syndrome, it may be accompanied by pain, ascites, and pleural effusion. A few patients experience fever and swelling along with discomfort at the injection site. Undesirable results of therapy include a high incidence of multiple pregnancy and abortion. The frequency of birth defects has not been increased in the offspring of patients who have succeeded in carrying their pregnancies to term.

The typical outcome of therapy in properly selected patients treated by experienced physicians is shown in Table 13–10. Menotropins are potentially dangerous and should be administered by physicians with experience in endocrine disturbances and problems of reproductive function. This mode of therapy is complicated, time-consuming, and expensive and should not be undertaken unless simpler therapeutic measures have failed.

Table 13–10. Results of treatment with menotropins.

Pregnancy achieved: 25–40%
Multiple births
Twins, 10–20%
Triplets, etc, 5–10%
Abortions, 20%
Hyperstimulation syndrome: 0.5–1.5%

Dosages

Human menopausal gonadotropins (menotropins, Pergonal) are supplied in lyophilized form in ampules containing 75 units each of FSH and LH and 10 mg of lactose. The usual dosage is one or more ampules intramuscularly daily until estrogen production is optimal—ie, plasma levels of 600–1000 pg/mL (2.2–3.7 nmol/L). Growth of ovarian follicles should also be monitored by ultrasonography to assist in determining the optimal dosage and duration of treatment. Chorionic gonadotropin (see Chapter 16) in doses of 5000–10,000 units intramuscularly is then administered once to induce ovulation from the mature follicle and then several times after ovulation to support corpus luteum function. If estrogen production becomes excessive during the preovulatory treatment phase, chorionic gonadotropin should be withheld to avoid the ovarian hyperstimulation syndrome. Patients must be examined frequently (daily or on alternate days) for 2 weeks following the last injection to detect signs of overstimulation and should be advised to have intercourse at least every other day near the time of expected ovulation.

GONADOTROPIN-RELEASING HORMONE

The pulsatile administration of GnRH in doses of 1–10 μg per pulse at 60- to 120-minute intervals will induce ovulation in most patients with amenorrhea due to hypothalamic dysfunction associated with decreased secretion of endogenous GnRH. GnRH can be given intravenously or subcutaneously using a peristaltic pump. Although the method is somewhat cumbersome, less frequent monitoring of the patient is required and ovarian hyperstimulation is less likely to occur.

BROMOCRIPTINE

Although bromocriptine is occasionally effective in treating patients with amenorrhea in the absence of elevated serum levels of PRL, its use is generally reserved for patients with hyperprolactinemia or galactorrhea. Its use in such patients is described elsewhere in this chapter.

THERAPEUTIC USE OF OVARIAN HORMONES & THEIR SYNTHETIC ANALOGS

Estrogens are used in combination with progestins by more than 40 million women for contraception and are widely used after the menopause. Estrogens are also used to limit the height of tall girls and to replace absent or deficient endogenous hormone in patients with hypogonadism or after gonadectomy. It is therefore important to understand the effects of these agents and problems engendered by their use.

TREATMENT OF PRIMARY HYPOGONADISM

Treatment of primary hypogonadism is usually begun at 11–13 years of age in order to stimulate the development of secondary sex characteristics and menses and to promote optimal growth. Treatment consists mainly of the administration of estrogens and progestins. Androgens and anabolic agents have also been used in these patients to stimulate growth, but no further increase in final height was achieved. Furthermore, acne, hirsutism, clitoromegaly, and premature closure of the epiphyses have occurred as unwanted effects of androgens and anabolic agents. Progestins are advisable in conjunction with estrogens, because long-term replacement therapy, even when used cyclically in modest doses, has been associated with an increase in the incidence of endometrial hyperplasia and endometrial carcinoma. Oral contraceptives have also been used for replacement therapy.

OVARIAN SUPPRESSION

Estrogen-progestin combinations (oral contraceptives) are used to suppress ovarian function in patients with LH-dependent excess androgen production or endometriosis and are discussed elsewhere in this chapter.

Progestational hormones alone are used to produce long-term ovarian suppression when estrogens are contraindicated. When used parenterally in large doses—eg, medroxyprogesterone acetate, 150 mg intramuscularly every 90 days—prolonged anovulation and amenorrhea are produced. This procedure has been employed in the treatment of dysmenorrhea, endometriosis, hirsutism, and bleeding disorders. The major problem encountered with this regimen is the prolonged time required for ovulatory function to return after cessation of therapy in some patients. Irregular spotting also occurs. This treatment should not be used for patients planning a pregnancy in the near future.

THREATENED ABORTION

Progestins do not appear to have any place in the therapy of threatened or habitual abortion. Early reports of the usefulness of these agents were based on the unwarranted assumption that after several abortions the likelihood of repeated abortions was over 90%. When progestational agents were administered to patients with previous abortions, a salvage rate of 80% was achieved. It is now recognized that similar patients abort only 20% of the time even when untreated.

In some patients with "threatened" abortion, progesterone production is decreased. It is likely that the decrease in progesterone reflects damage to the placenta or fetus and is a result of events leading to abortion rather than a cause of the abortion. Administration of progesterone in these circumstances, especially in the presence of declining serum levels of hCG, does not appear to be useful and may allow retention of the dead fetus, thus delaying recognition of an abortion that has occurred. Prolonged postpartum bleeding has also been reported in some patients treated with repository medroxyprogesterone or hydroxyprogesterone caproate.

INADEQUATE LUTEAL PHASE

Progesterone and medroxyprogesterone have been used in the treatment of women who have difficulty in conceiving and who demonstrate a slow rise in basal body temperature. Some investigators believe that these patients suffer from a relative luteal insufficiency, and progesterone or related compounds are given to replace the deficiency. There is no convincing evidence that this treatment is effective. In the absence of satisfactory controls, the successes reported are impossible to distinguish from placebo effects.

DIAGNOSTIC USES

Progesterone is also used as a test of estrogen secretion. A single intramuscular injection of 200 mg of progesterone in oil or a course of medroxyprogesterone, 10 mg/d for 5–7 days, is followed by withdrawal bleeding in amenorrheic patients only when the endometrium has been stimulated by estrogens. In the absence of withdrawal bleeding, a combination of estrogen and progestin can be given to test the responsiveness of the endometrium in patients with amenorrhea.

INHIBITORS OF OVARIAN FUNCTION

GONADOTROPIN-RELEASING HORMONE ANALOGS & ANTAGONISTS

As noted above, GnRH administered in a pulsatile manner will induce ovulation in patients with amenorrhea. However, when large amounts are administered continuously, inhibition of gonadotropin release occurs. This property has been exploited by the development of highly potent agonist analogs, such as leuprolide, buserelin, and nafarelin. These analogs can be administered subcutaneously or intranasally. In sufficient doses, they can inhibit ovarian function, both reducing the secretion of sex steroids and inhibiting ovulation. GnRH analogs have been used to treat patients with sex hormone-dependent disorders such as precocious puberty, endometriosis, uterine fibroids, and hirsutism secondary to excess ovarian androgen production.

ANTIESTROGENS

Antagonists acting at the estrogen receptor are divided into four classes determined by the configuration of the receptor to which they bind. Tamoxifen, a partial estrogen agonist, is a type II nonsteroidal competitive inhibitor of estradiol at its receptor. It can be given orally and is being used in the palliative treatment of advanced breast cancer in postmenopausal women (see Chapter 22). Peak plasma levels are reached in a few hours. It has an initial half-life of 7–14 hours in the circulation and is predominantly excreted by the liver. It is dispensed as the citrate in the form of tablets containing the equivalent of 10 mg of tamoxifen. It is used in doses of 10–20 mg twice daily. Hot flushes and nausea and vomiting occur in 25% of patients, and many other adverse effects have been reported.

Studies of patients given tamoxifen as adjuvant therapy for early breast cancer have shown a 35% decrease in contralateral breast cancer. Prevention of the expected loss of lumbar spine bone density and plasma lipid changes consistent with a reduction in the risk for atherosclerosis have also been reported in these patients following spontaneous or surgical menopause.

CI-164,384, a type II pure antagonist, inhibits dimerization of the occupied estrogen receptor and interferes with its binding to DNA. It has been used in breast cancer patients who have become resistant to tamoxifen.

DANAZOL

Danazol, an isoxazole derivative of ethisterone (17α-ethinyl testosterone) with weak progestational and androgenic activities, is used to suppress ovarian function. It inhibits the midcycle surge of LH and FSH and can prevent the compensatory increase in LH and FSH following castration in animals, but it does not significantly lower or suppress basal LH or FSH levels in healthy humans. Danazol binds to androgen, progesterone, and glucocorticoid receptors and can initiate androgen-specific RNA synthesis. It does not bind to intracellular estrogen receptors, but it does compete with steroids for binding to sex hormone-binding globulin (SHBG) and corticosteroid-binding globulins (CBG). It inhibits P450scc (the cholesterol side chain-cleaving enzyme), 3β-HSD (3β-hydroxysteroid dehydrogenase), P450c17 (17,20-lyase; 17α-hydroxylase), P450c11 (11β-hydroxylase), and P450c21 (21-hydroxylase), but it does not inhibit aromatase. It increases the mean clearance rate of progesterone, probably by competing with the hormone for binding proteins, and may have similar effects on other active steroid hormones. Ethisterone, a major metabolite, has both progestational and mild androgenic effects.

Danazol has been employed as an inhibitor of gonadal function and has found its major use in the treatment of endometriosis. For this purpose, it can be given in a dose of 600 mg/d. The dose is reduced to 400 mg/d after 1 month and to 200 mg/d in 2 months. About 85% of patients show marked improvement in 3–12 months.

The major side effects are weight gain, edema, decreased breast size, acne and oily skin, mild hirsutism, deepening of the voice, headache, hot flushes, changes in libido, and muscle cramps. Although these side effects do not present any health risks, many women discontinue treatment because of them.

Danazol should be used with great caution in patients with hepatic dysfunction, since it has been reported to produce mild to moderate hepatocellular damage in some patients, as evidenced by enzyme changes. Danazol treatment also markedly decreases the HDL:LDL ratio in most women. It is contraindicated during pregnancy and breast-feeding, as it can produce urogenital abnormalities in the offspring.

Several aromatase inhibitors are undergoing clinical trials in patients with breast cancer. Formestane (4-hydroxyandrostenedione) in doses of 250–500 mg daily, reduced estradiol levels by 40% when given to women with breast cancer. Related compounds being tested appear to be more effective. Letrozole (CGS 20267), a triazole derivative, is a new, once-daily oral nonsteroidal inhibitor of aromatase. IC 182780 is a pure antiestrogen that has been somewhat more effective than those with agonist effects and is effective in some patients who have become resistant to tamoxifen. 4-Hydroxyandrostenedione is also an effective estrogen antagonist.

ANTIPROGESTINS

Mifepristone (17β-hydroxy-11β[4-dimethylaminophenyl]-17α[1-propynyl]estra-4,9-dien-3-one; RU 486), a 19 norsteroid, binds strongly to the progesterone receptor (in addition to binding to the glucocorticoid receptor) and inhibits the binding and activity of progesterone. Preliminary studies indicate that it has luteolytic properties in many women when given in the midluteal period and may be useful as a contraceptive. The mechanism of this effect is unknown. These luteolytic properties could make mifepristone useful as a contraceptive. However, its long half-life and large dose requirement may prolong the follicular phase of the subsequent cycle and make it difficult to use for this purpose. This drug has been used for the termination of early pregnancy. The combination of a single oral dose of 600 mg of mifepristone and a vaginal pessary containing 1 mg of prostaglandin E_1 or oral misoprostol has been found to effectively terminate pregnancy in 95% of patients when administered during the first 7 weeks after conception. The side effects of the medications included vomiting, diarrhea, and abdominal pain. However, the major side effect was prolonged bleeding that did not require treatment. As many as 5% of patients have vaginal bleeding requiring intervention with dilation and curettage.

ZK 98,734 is another potent progesterone inhibitor and abortifacient in doses of 25 mg twice daily. It also appears to have antiglucocorticoid activity.

Preliminary studies have found that epostane, a 3β-hydroxysteroid dehydrogenase inhibitor, decreases the synthesis of progesterone and can terminate early pregnancy.

ANTIANDROGENS

The possibility of using antiandrogens to treat hirsutism and other disorders due to excessive amounts of testosterone has led to a search for effective drugs. **Cyproterone** and **cyproterone acetate** are effective antiandrogens that inhibit the action of the androgens at the target organ. The acetate form has a marked progestational effect that suppresses LH and FSH, thus leading to a more effective antiandrogen effect. These compounds have been used to decrease excessive sexual drive in disturbed individuals and are being studied in other conditions in which reduction of androgenic effects would be useful. In Europe, they are used in the treatment of hirsutism (see above). They are not available in the USA. **Flutamide** and **casodex** are nonsteroid competitive inhibitors at the androgen receptor. They have been widely used in the treatment of prostatic cancer, and limited experience indicates that they may be useful in the treatment of hirsutism. Drospirenome, a progestational agent, has some antiandrogenic and antimineralocorticoid activity. It has no estrogenic or glucocorticoid effects.

Ketoconazole, an imidazole derivative used for the treatment of fungal disease, is a potent inhibitor of adrenal and gonadal steroid synthesis. This compound inhibits P450scc (cholesterol side chain cleavage enzyme), P450c17 (17α-hydroxylase and 17,20-lyase), 3β-hydroxysteroid dehydrogenase, and P450c11 (11β-hydroxylase) enzymes. The sensitivity of the P450 enzymes to this compound in mammalian tissues is much lower than that of the fungal enzymes, so that the inhibitory effects are seen only at high doses. Ketoconazole also has other endocrine effects. It displaces estradiol and dihydrotestosterone from SHBG in vitro and increases the estradiol-testosterone ratio in plasma in vivo by a different mechanism. The latter effect may be responsible for the gynecomastia that occurs in men with ketoconazole therapy. This compound has been used with some success for the treatment of Cushing's syndrome. However, it does not appear to be clinically useful in women with increased androgens because of the toxicity associated with prolonged use of the 400–800 mg/d required.

MENOPAUSE

Menopause begins with the last episode of menstrual bleeding induced by the cyclic endogenous secretion of ovarian hormones. It normally occurs between the ages of 42 and 60 years. It occurs prematurely as a result of surgical removal, irradiation, or abnormalities of the ovaries.

HORMONAL CHANGES

The changes in endocrine function are not abrupt in women undergoing spontaneous menopause. The circulating levels of gonadotropins begin to increase several years before ovulation ceases. Production of estrogen and progesterone decreases, and irregular cycles and anovulatory bleeding are not uncommon (Table 13–11). The increase in FSH is greater than that of LH and reflects the lack of feedback inhibition by estrogen or inhibin, or both. The stromal cells of the ovary respond to increased LH stimulation by producing more androstenedione but only tiny amounts of estrogen.

The average production rate of estradiol falls to 12 μg/24 h (44 nmol/24 h), and the clearance rate is reduced. Since very little estradiol is found in ovarian or adrenal veins, most of the circulating estradiol is derived from estrone, which in itself is produced by the peripheral conversion of androstenedione. The average production rate for estrone is 55 μg/24 h (202 nmol/24 h), and there is a 20% reduction in its clearance.

Progesterone levels are approximately 30% of the concentration seen in young women during the follicular phase. The source of this progesterone is the adrenal.

Androgen levels are also reduced postmenopausally. Androstenedione falls to about half of the concentration found in young women, and most of that apparently comes from the adrenal, as suggested by its peak concentrations at 8 AM and nadir concentrations at 3–4 PM. The clearance rate does not change. The average production rate is about 1.5 mg/24 h (5200 nmol/24 h). About 20% of it is thought to come from the ovary. Testosterone production rates are approximately 150 μg/24 h (520 nmol/24 h), as compared to about 200 μg/24 h (693 nmol/24 h) in younger women. This fall is less than that seen after ovariectomy, indicating that testosterone is produced by conversion of androstenedione as well as being secreted by the adrenal and ovary. It is of interest that DHEA and DHEA sulfate also fall

Table 13–11. Serum concentrations (mean ± SEM) of steroids in premenopausal and postmenopausal women.[1]

Steroid	Premenopausal[2]		Postmenopausal	
	(ng/mL)	(nmol/L)	(ng/mL)	(nmol/L)
Progesterone	0.47 ± 0.03	(1.49 ± 0.1)	0.17 ± 0.02	(0.54 ± 0.06)
DHEA	4.2 ± 0.5	(14.5 ± 1.7)	1.8 ± 0.2	(6.2 ± 0.69)
DHEA sulfate	1600 ± 350	(3159 ± 691)	300 ± 70	(592 ± 138)
Androstenedione	1.5 ± 0.1	(5.2 ± 0.35)	0.6 ± 0.01	(2.08 ± 0.03)
Testosterone	0.32 ± 0.02	(1.11 ± 0.07)	0.25 ± 0.03	(0.87 ± 0.1)
Estrone	0.08 ± 0.01	(0.29 ± 0.04)	0.029 ± 0.002	(0.11 ± 0.01)
Estradiol	0.05 ± 0.005	(0.18 ± 0.02)	0.013 ± 0.001	(0.05 ± 0.004)

[1]Reproduced, with permission, from Pernoll ML, Benson RC (editor): *Current Obstetric & Gynecologic Diagnosis & Treatment,* 6th ed. Appleton & Lange, 1987.
[2]Follicular phase concentrations.

with age, although almost all of these steroids come from the adrenal gland.

CLINICAL MANIFESTATIONS OF MENOPAUSE

1. EARLY MANIFESTATIONS

Menstrual Changes

The interval prior to the menopause is usually characterized sequentially by cycles with a shortening of the follicular phase, an interval of very irregular cycles, and an interval of anovulatory bleeding. Fertility is usually very low during this time. Although menses may cease abruptly, usually there is a gradual diminution in the amount of menstrual flow as well as its duration. However, if secretion of estrogen is prolonged in the absence of ovulation, endometrial hyperplasia may occur and cause heavy bleeding. It is sometimes difficult to clinically distinguish this type of bleeding from that produced by organic diseases, including endometrial carcinoma. Any bleeding that occurs more than a year after the last previous period is likely to be an indication of organic disease.

Vasomotor Symptoms

The most common menopausal complaint is hot flushes, which occur in 75% of women at the menopause. They are due to declining estrogen levels. Women with estrogen deficiency from childhood do not develop hot flushes unless they have been treated with exogenous estrogens and treatment is interrupted. Episodes of flushing are associated with periodic increases in core temperature, causing reflex peripheral vasodilation, a small increase in pulse rate, and sweating. They are synchronous with the pulsatile release of LH but are not caused by increased secretion of gonadotropins. Rather, they appear to be linked to the central mechanism controlling the release of GnRH. These symptoms occur most frequently in a warm environment and are common at night, contributing to insomnia.

The hot flush often starts with a sensation of pressure in the head, followed by a feeling of warmth in the head and neck and upper thorax. It may be associated with palpitations and gradually spreading waves of heat over the entire body. The feeling of warmth and flushing is quickly followed by sweating. The sweating and vasodilation lead to heat loss and a decrease in core temperature of approximately 0.2 °C. These episodes last 10–20 minutes.

In 20% of patients, hot flushes are a transient phenomenon lasting for less than 1 year, but 25–50% of women experience them for more than 5 years. Estrogen therapy is remarkably effective in controlling hot flushes in over 90% of patients.

Atrophic Changes in the Genitourinary System

The decline in estrogen production results in reduction in mucus secretion and gradual atrophy of the vaginal and urethral epithelium. The rugae progressively disappear with thinning of the epithelium. The surface may appear vascular at first but then becomes pale. These changes lead to itching, dyspareunia, and burning. Similar changes in the urinary tract may give rise to atrophic cystitis, with symptoms of urgency, incontinence, and frequency. The cervix decreases in size, and the mucus secretion diminishes. The endometrium and myometrium also undergo atrophy. Myomas become smaller and endometriosis less symptomatic. The adverse symptoms can be treated by administration of estrogens locally as well as systemically (see below).

Skin & Hair Changes

At the time of the menopause, changes in the skin due to aging are noticeable. There is some thinning and wrinkling. Although estrogen creams are widely used cosmetically, it is not clear that they have any effects other than enhancement of the dermal water content. Changes in hair include loss of some underarm and pubic hair and occasionally replacement of vellus hair on the chin and upper lip by terminal hairs.

Emotional Changes

Anxiety, depression, and irritability are commonly reported around the time of the menopause. There is no good evidence that these symptoms are directly related to estrogen deficiency. However, sleep disturbances caused by hot flushes may contribute to the irritability. The majority of women treated with estrogens report some improvement in their sense of well-being and relief of insomnia and other symptoms produced by estrogen deficiency.

2. LATER MANIFESTATIONS

In addition to the signs and symptoms that follow closely upon the cessation of normal ovarian function, there are changes which over many years influence the health and well-being of postmenopausal women. These include an acceleration of bone loss, which in susceptible women may lead to vertebral, hip, and wrist fractures, and lipid changes that may contribute to the acceleration of cardiovascular disease noted in postmenopausal women. The effects of estrogens on bone have been extensively studied, and the effects of hormone withdrawal and replacement are well characterized. However, the roles of estrogen and progestins in the cause and prevention of cardiovascular disease, which is responsible for 350,000 deaths per year, and breast cancer, which causes 35,000 deaths per year, are less well understood.

Osteoporosis

Osteoporosis results from a combination of increased bone resorption and decreased bone formation. In its early stages, it is predominantly a disease of trabecular bone. Affected patients show increased calcium loss from bone. The problem is enhanced in winter months because of decreased activity and decreased exposure to sunlight and by the difficulty of maintaining calcium balance at normal levels of intake (see Chapters 8 and 25).

During the first few years following menopause, women lose an average of about 1% of their metacarpal cortical bone mass per year (Figure 13–18). The initial rapid bone loss is inhibited by estrogen. Loss of bone mass leads to reduced skeletal strength and susceptibility to fractures. There is, for example, a tenfold increase in the incidence of Colles' fractures in women between the ages of 35 and 55, although a similar increase is not seen in men (Figure 13–19). Hip fractures, which are ultimately fatal in about one-third of patients and disable others for life, also occur more frequently.

Studies indicate that bone density decreases in women as the years advance. However, the loss is accelerated at menopause. Other studies indicate that estrogen therapy started at that time can prevent the loss (Figure 13–18). If estrogens are administered subsequently, the process can be arrested. However, when treatment is delayed for 5–6 years, less effect is noted. Treatment with estrogen decreases plasma Ca^{2+} and increases plasma PTH and $1,25(OH)_2D_3$, which, in turn, increases calcium absorption. The risk for osteoporosis is highest in smokers who are thin, Caucasian, inactive, and have a low calcium intake and a strong family history of osteoporosis. (See Chapters 8 and 25.)

Cardiovascular Disease

When normal ovulatory function ceases and the estrogen levels fall after the menopause or oophorectomy, there is an accelerated rise in cholesterol, and

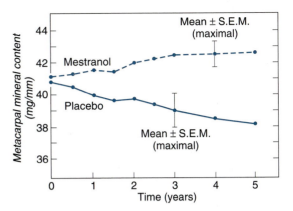

Figure 13–18. Metacarpal mineral content in postmenopausal women treated with mestranol or placebo for 5 years. Note loss of bone density in placebo but not mestranol treatment group. (Reproduced, with permission, from Lindsay R et al: Long-term prevention of postmenopausal osteoporosis by oestrogen. Lancet 1976; 1:1038.)

LDL and LDL receptors decline. HDL is not much affected, and levels remain higher than in men. VLDL and triglyceride levels are not much different. Since cardiovascular disorders account for most deaths in this age group, the risk for these disorders constitutes a major consideration in deciding whether or not hormonal therapy is indicated and influences the selection of hormones to be administered. The effects of estrogen replacement therapy on circulating lipids and lipoproteins is shown in Figure 13–20. These changes are associated with a reduction in myocardial infarction by about 50% and fatal strokes by as much as 40%. Some progestins antagonize the effects on LDL and HDL to a variable extent.

Patients at higher risk for cardiovascular disease should be encouraged to stop smoking, to exercise, and make appropriate dietary adjustments, and their plasma lipids should be checked. Diabetes and hyper-

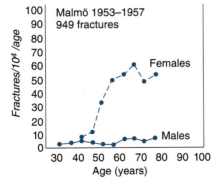
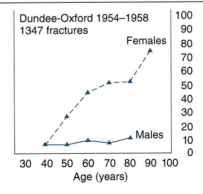

Figure 13–19. Indices of Colles' fracture in relation to age in Malmö and Dundee-Oxford. (Reproduced, with permission, from Cope E: Physical changes associated with post-menopausal years. Page 4 in: Management of the Menopause and Post-Menopause Years. Campbell S [editor]. MTP Press Ltd, 1976.)

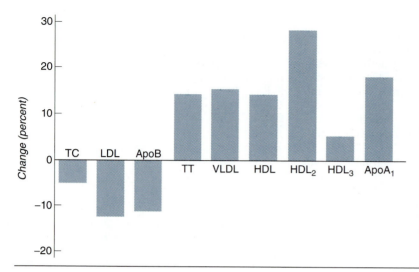

Figure 13–20. Percentage changes in lipids and lipoproteins with the use of oral estrogen (equivalent to 0.625 mg for at least 3 months). (TC, total cholesterol; TT, total triglycerides.) (Redrawn and reproduced, with permission, from Lobo RA: Effects of hormonal replacement on lipids and lipoproteins in postmenopausal women. J Clin Endocrinol Metab 1991;79:925.)

tension should be brought under control when present. Antioxidant vitamins, small amounts of alcohol, and aspirin may also be useful (see Chapter 20).

MANAGEMENT OF MENOPAUSE

Optimal management requires careful assessment of the patient's symptoms as well as consideration of her age; the risk for cardiovascular disease, osteoporosis, and breast and endometrial cancer; and knowledge of the effects of the gonadal hormones on each of these disorders. The goals of therapy can then be defined and the risks of therapy assessed and discussed with the patient.

Hormonal Therapy

If the main indication for therapy is hot flushes, therapy with the lowest dose of estrogen required for symptomatic relief is recommended. Treatment may only be required for a limited period of time and the possible increased risk for breast cancer thus avoided. In women who have had hysterectomies, estrogens alone can be given 5 days a week or every day, since progestins are not required to reduce the risk for endometrial hyperplasia and cancer. In women who have not undergone hysterectomy, estrogen therapy should be given for the first 25 days of each month and a progestational agent administered during the last 10–14 days of estrogen administration. The recommended daily dosage of estrogen is 0.3–1.25 mg of conjugated estrogens or 0.01–0.02 mg of ethinyl estradiol. Doses in the middle of these ranges have been shown to be maximally effective in preventing the decrease in bone density occurring at the menopause. In order to prevent osteoporosis, it is important to begin therapy as soon as possible after the menopause. Studies indicate that addition of 10 mg medroxyprogesterone

acetate orally daily for the last 10–14 days of estrogen therapy markedly reduces the risk of endometrial carcinoma.

On this regimen, some women will experience a return of symptoms during the period off estrogen therapy. In these patients, the estrogen can be given every day. If the progestin produces sedation or other undesirable effects, the dose can be reduced to 2.5–5 mg for the last 10 days of the cycle, with only a slight increase in the risk for endometrial hyperplasia. These regimens are usually accompanied by bleeding at the end of each cycle.

Women who object to the cyclic bleeding associated with sequential therapy can consider uninterrupted therapy. Therapy with 0.625 mg of conjugated estrogens and 2.5–5 mg of medroxyprogesterone will eliminate cyclic bleeding, control vasomotor symptoms, prevent genital atrophy, maintain bone density, and show a favorable lipid profile with a small decrease in LDL and an increase in HDL. Short-term studies indicate that these women have endometrial atrophy on biopsy. About half of them experience breakthrough bleeding during the first few months of therapy. After the first 4 months, 70–80% become amenorrheic, and most remain so. The main disadvantage of uninterrupted therapy is the need for uterine biopsy when bleeding occurs after the first few months.

The above combination of hormones can also be given 5 days a week, withholding medication on the weekends. This regimen controls bleeding about as well as daily therapy and results in an increase in HDL with little change in LDL.

Patients at low risk for development of osteoporosis with only mild atrophic vaginitis can be treated with local vaginal preparations. This route of application is also useful in treatment of urinary tract symptoms. It is important to realize, however, that locally administered estrogens are almost completely absorbed into the circulation and should be used intermittently or with a progestin.

Although the estrogens share most, if not all, of their hormonal effects, their relative potencies vary depending on the agent and the route of administration. As noted above, estradiol is the most active endogenous estrogen and has the highest affinity for the estrogen receptor. However, its metabolites estrone and estriol have weak uterotropic effects. 2-Hydroxyestrone, another important metabolite, possesses neurotransmitter activity in the brain. It also competes with catecholamines for catechol-O-methyltransferase and inhibits tyrosine hydroxylase. For a given level of gonadotropin suppression, oral compounds have a greater effect on the circulating levels of corticosteroid and sex hormone-binding proteins. This effect, which is thought to be due to larger concentrations of hormone reaching the liver by this route, has led to the development of transdermal preparations. When administered transdermally, 50–100 µg of estradiol had effects similar to those of 0.625–1.25 mg conjugated oral estrogens on gonadotropin levels, endometrium, and vaginal epithelium. However, only the oral estrogen increased levels of renin substrate, CBG, and TBG and had favorable effects on high- and low-density lipoprotein levels.

In patients in whom estrogen replacement therapy is contraindicated (eg, those with estrogen-sensitive tumors), relief of vasomotor symptoms may be obtained by the use of progestational agents. Medroxyprogesterone acetate, 150 mg intramuscularly once a month, norgestrel, 250 µg orally daily, or medroxyprogesterone, 10 mg orally daily, can be useful. Mild tranquilizers and clonidine are also effective in some patients, as are atropine-barbiturate mixtures. Calcium carbonate supplements (eg, Os-Cal) are useful in bringing the total daily calcium intake up to 1500 mg. Vitamin D therapy may be useful when calcium intake is less than optimal. Preliminary studies show that fluoride in adequate amounts can increase bone density but that it may not reduce the rate of fracture. Bisphosphonate therapy may be useful in the management of osteoporosis (see Chapters 8 and 25).

Adverse Effects of Therapy

Nausea and breast tenderness are common and can be minimized by using the smallest effective dose. These symptoms may be more marked at the beginning of therapy. The presence of cystic mastitis or fibroids that increase in size during treatment may also interfere with the use of estrogen. Hyperpigmentation also occurs. Estrogen therapy is associated with an increase in frequency of hypertension and gallbladder disease. Some women experience migraine headaches during the last few days of the cycle. The use of a continuous estrogen regimen will often prevent their occurrence.

The relationship of hormonal therapy to cancer in postmenopausal women continues to be the subject of active investigation. The risk of endometrial carcinoma is increased in patients taking estrogens without adjunct progestins and varies with the dose and duration of treatment. It increases 15 times in patients taking large doses of estrogen for 5 or more years but only two to four times in patients receiving lower doses for 2 years. The concomitant use of a progestin not only prevents this increased risk but actually reduces the incidence of endometrial cancer below that in the general population.

Although short-term estrogen therapy has not been shown to increase the incidence of breast cancer, a small increase in the incidence of this tumor may occur with prolonged therapy. Although the increased risk factor is small (1.25), the impact is great since this tumor occurs in 10% of women. The effect of progesterone has not been determined as yet. As noted above, studies indicate that following unilateral excision of breast cancer, women receiving tamoxifen show a 35% decrease in contralateral breast cancer compared with controls. These studies also demonstrate that tamoxifen is well tolerated by most patients, produce estrogen-like alterations in plasma lipid levels, and stabilize bone mineral loss. Studies bearing on the possible use of tamoxifen in postmenopausal women at high risk for breast cancer are under way.

HORMONAL CONTRACEPTION (Oral Contraceptives)

A large number of oral contraceptives containing estrogens or progestins (or both) are now available for clinical use (Table 13–9). These preparations vary in chemical composition and, as might be expected, have many properties in common, but there are also differences. Two types of preparations are used for oral contraception: (1) monophasic, biphasic, and triphasic combinations of estrogens and progestins; and (2) progestins without concomitant administration of estrogens.

PHARMACOLOGIC EFFECTS OF ESTROGENS & SYNTHETIC PROGESTINS

Mechanisms of Contraceptive Action

Estrogens and progestin combinations inhibit gonadotropin secretion, which prevents ovulation. They also change the cervical mucus, the endometrium, and tubal motility and secretion, all of which decrease the likelihood of conception and implantation. Continuous use of progestins alone does not inhibit ovulation, and the other effects play a major role in prevention of pregnancy when these agents are used.

Genital Effects of Oral Contraceptives

Chronic use of estrogen-progestin combinations depresses ovarian function. The ovary shows minimal follicular development and an absence of corpora lutea and other morphologic features normally seen in ovulating women. Estrogen production is decreased, and progesterone secretion is minimal. The ovaries usually become smaller even when previously enlarged.

Cytologic findings on vaginal smears vary depending on the preparation used. However, with almost all of the combined drugs, a midzone maturation index is found because of the presence of progestational agents.

Effects on the uterus include hypertrophy of the cervix and polyp formation after prolonged use. The cervical mucus becomes thick and less copious and contains much cellular debris. Stromal deciduation occurs toward the end of the cycle. The agents containing 19-nortestosterone derivatives combined with smaller amounts of estrogen tend to produce more glandular atrophy and less bleeding than agents containing progestins that stimulate glandular development.

Stimulation of the breasts occurs in most patients receiving estrogen-containing agents. Some enlargement is generally noted. These agents tend to suppress lactation, but when the doses are small, the effects on breast feeding are not appreciable. Preliminary studies of transport of oral contraceptives into the breast milk suggest that only small amounts of these compounds are found and they have not been considered to be of importance.

Extragenital Effects of Oral Contraceptives

It is important to understand the extragenital effects of oral contraceptives, because of the large and growing number of normal individuals using them.

A. Central Nervous System Effects: The effects of the oral contraceptives on the central nervous system have not been well studied in humans. In animals, estrogens tend to lower the threshold of excitability in the brain, whereas progesterone tends to increase it. In addition, the increased respiration and thermogenic actions of progesterone and some of the synthetic progestins are thought to be due to effects on the central nervous system. The suppression of ovarian function results in part from inhibition of GnRH secretion by the hypothalamus.

It is very difficult to evaluate any behavioral or emotional effects of these compounds. Although there is a low incidence of pronounced changes in mood, affect, and behavior in most studies, milder changes are common.

B. Endocrinologic Effects: The combined agents inhibit the secretion of pituitary gonadotropins, as mentioned above. Estrogens increase the plasma concentration of CBG. This increases plasma cortisol concentrations but does not lead to chronic alteration in the rate of cortisol secretion. It has also been observed that the ACTH response to the administration of metyrapone is attenuated by estrogens and the oral contraceptives.

These preparations alter the angiotensin-aldosterone system, increasing plasma renin activity and therefore aldosterone secretion. The relationship between these alterations and the hypertension that occurs in some patients taking oral contraceptives is not clear.

TBG is increased, resulting in higher circulating thyroxine levels. However, the free thyroxine level in these patients is normal.

C. Hematologic Effects: Serious thromboembolic phenomena occurring in women taking oral contraceptives have stimulated a great many studies of their effects on blood coagulation. In general, the changes observed are similar to those reported in pregnancy and include an increase in factors VII, VIII, IX, and X. Increased amounts of coumarin derivatives are required to prolong prothrombin time in patients taking oral contraceptives. The platelet aggregation response to catecholamines is also increased.

Oral contraceptives inhibit the conversion of polyglutamic folate found in food to the monoglutamic folate that is absorbed in the gastrointestinal tract, thereby causing folic acid deficiency anemias, which can be reversed by folic acid supplementation or by discontinuing oral contraceptives.

D. Hepatic Effects: The liver plays an important role in the metabolism of the estrogens and progestins used in oral contraceptives. These hormones also affect liver function. (See Adverse Effects of Oral Contraceptives, below.)

Estrogens increase the synthesis of the various transport globulins and fibrinogen and decrease the synthesis of serum haptoglobins.

Important alterations in drug excretion and metabolism also occur in the liver. Estrogens in the amounts present during pregnancy or ingested in oral contraceptive agents delay the clearance of sulfobromophthalein (BSP) and reduce bile flow.

Oral contraceptives increase the saturation of cholesterol in bile, and the ratio of cholic acid to chenodeoxycholic acid is increased. These changes may cause the observed increase in cholelithiasis associated with use of these agents.

E. Effects on Lipid Metabolism: Estrogens increase plasma high-density lipoproteins (HDL) and very low density lipoproteins (VLDL) while lowering low-density lipoproteins (LDL). In young women with normal lipids, this results in higher circulating triglyceride and free and esterified cholesterol levels. In older women with higher cholesterol levels, a reduction is usually observed because of the reduction of LDL. Phospholipid levels are increased. Although the effects are marked with doses of 100 µg of mestranol or ethinyl estradiol, doses of 50 µg or less have minimal effects. The progestins—particularly the 19-nortestosterone derivatives—tend to antagonize the effects of estrogen. Preparations containing small amounts of estrogen and a progestin may slightly decrease triglycerides and high-density lipoproteins.

F. Effects on Carbohydrate Metabolism: The administration of oral contraceptives produces alterations in carbohydrate metabolism similar to those observed in pregnancy (see Chapter 16). There is a reduction in the rate of absorption of carbohydrates from the gastrointestinal tract. These agents antagonize the effects of insulin, causing decreases in glucose tolerance or increased secretion of insulin following administration of glucose. Studies in experimental animals indicate that estrogens enhance islet cell function, whereas progesterone interferes with insulin action. The changes in glucose tolerance are reversible on discontinuing medication.

G. Cardiovascular Effects: These agents cause small increases in cardiac output associated with slightly higher systolic and diastolic blood pressure and heart rate. Pathologic increases in blood pressure occur in a small number of patients, in whom the pressure slowly returns to normal when treatment is terminated. It is important that blood pressure be followed in each patient.

H. Dermatologic Effects: Oral contraceptives have been noted to increase pigmentation of the skin (chloasma). This effect seems to be enhanced in women with dark complexions and by exposure to ultraviolet light. Agents with larger amounts of androgenic progestins may increase the production of sebum and cause acne. However, estrogen-dominant oral contraceptive preparations usually decrease sebum production by suppressing the ovarian production of androgens.

CLINICAL USES OF ORAL CONTRACEPTIVES

The most important use of estrogen and progestin compounds is for prevention of pregnancy. Many preparations are available, and they are packaged to provide for ease of administration. When these agents are taken according to directions, the risk of conception is estimated to be about 0.5–1 per 100 woman years.

These compounds are also used in the treatment of endometriosis. When severe dysmenorrhea is the major symptom of this disorder, suppression of ovulation with estrogen may be followed by painless periods. In some patients, long-term continuous administration of large doses of progestins or estrogen-progestin combinations to prevent cyclic breakdown of the endometrial tissue leads to endometrial fibrosis and prevents the reactivation of implants for prolonged periods.

As is true with most hormonal preparations, many of the adverse effects are physiologic or pharmacologic effects of the drug that are objectionable only because they are not pertinent to the situation for which they are being used. Therefore, the product containing the smallest amounts of hormones should be selected for use.

The differences between preparations can be used to advantage for individualized treatment. These preparations differ in amounts and types of estrogen and progestin (Table 13–9). Preparations containing larger amounts of estrogen tend to produce more withdrawal bleeding, nausea, and mastalgia. Preparations containing 19-nortestosterone derivatives tend to reduce the amount of withdrawal bleeding and have more anabolic or androgenic effects.

ADVERSE EFFECTS OF ORAL CONTRACEPTIVES

The incidence of serious adverse effects associated with the use of these drugs is low. Minor adverse effects are frequent but transient and may respond to simple changes in pill formulation. Although it is not often necessary to discontinue taking the pills because of these adverse effects, one-third of patients started on oral contraception discontinue therapy for reasons other than a desire to become pregnant.

Mild Adverse Effects

Breakthrough bleeding is the most common problem in the use of progestational agents alone for contraception, occurring in as many as 25% of patients. It also occurs in patients taking combined agents and is more common with preparations containing less than 50 µg of ethinyl estradiol (or equivalent). The newer biphasic and triphasic formulations containing 35 µg of ethinyl estradiol and varying doses of progestin (Table 13–11) reduce breakthrough bleeding without increasing the total amount of hormone administered during a cycle.

Nausea, mastalgia, excessive withdrawal bleeding, and edema are more common with larger amounts of estrogen and can often be alleviated by a shift to a preparation containing smaller amounts of estrogen or more potent progestational compounds.

Psychologic changes are often transient and are not predictable with any of the preparations. In general, most patients "feel better" because they are relieved of anxiety about becoming pregnant. Some patients experience symptoms of irritability and depression throughout the cycle. Depression and fatigue may respond to a reduction in progestin content.

Withdrawal bleeding sometimes fails to occur and may cause confusion with regard to pregnancy. If this is disturbing to the patient, a preparation with higher estrogenic or lower progestational potency may be tried or another method of contraception used. Increased estrogen potency can also reduce early and midcycle spotting.

Moderately Severe Adverse Effects

Any of the following may require discontinuation of oral contraceptives:

Mild and transient headaches may occur. Migraine is often made worse and is associated with an increased frequency of cerebrovascular accidents. Therefore, when migraine becomes more severe or has its onset during therapy with these agents, treatment should be discontinued.

Weight gain is more common with the combination agents containing more potent progestins. It can usually be controlled by shifting to preparations with less progestin effect or by dieting.

Increased skin pigmentation occurs in 5% of women at the end of the first year and about 40% after 8 years. It is thought to be exacerbated by vitamin B deficiency. The condition improves upon discontinuance of medication, but pigmentation may disappear very slowly.

Acne may be exacerbated by agents containing androgenic progestins, whereas agents containing larger amounts of estrogen frequently cause marked improvement in acne in women with androgen excess.

Hirsutism may be aggravated by the 19-nortestosterone derivatives. This effect is seldom seen, because the suppression of ovarian androgens usually causes a net reduction in androgen effect.

Ureteral dilation similar to that observed in pregnancy has been reported, and bacteriuria is more frequent.

Vaginal infections are more common and more difficult to treat in patients who are receiving oral contraceptives.

When therapy is terminated, the great majority of patients return to normal menstrual patterns. About 75% will ovulate in the first posttreatment cycle and 97% by the third posttreatment cycle. Patients with a history of irregular cycles more commonly develop amenorrhea following cessation of therapy.

About 2% of patients remain amenorrheic for up to several years after stopping the pills, and the prevalence of amenorrhea, often with galactorrhea, is higher in women who have used this form of contraception.

Severe Adverse Effects

A. Vascular Disorders: Thromboembolism was one of the earliest of the serious unanticipated effects to be reported and has been the most thoroughly studied. It should be kept in mind that almost all of these studies have been conducted in Great Britain, the USA, and Scandinavia and that effects in other populations might be somewhat different. During the past 15 years, the amounts of estrogen used in these preparations have been reduced, and this decline has been associated with a reduction in frequency of many of these effects. The most important adverse effect of the oral contraceptives is the increased risk of cardiovascular disease, including venous thromboembolism, myocardial infarction, and stroke.

1. Venous thromboembolic disease–Epidemiologic studies indicate that about one woman per 1000 woman years not using oral contraceptives will develop superficial or deep thromboembolic disease. The overall incidence of these disorders in patients taking oral contraceptives is about 3 per 1000 woman years. Data obtained by studying changes in plasma fibrinogen or by ^{125}I fibrinogen uptake studies suggest that subclinical thrombosis occurs much more frequently than overt disease. The risk for this disorder is increased during the first month of contraceptive use and remains constant for several years or more. The risk returns to normal within a month when treatment is discontinued. The risk of venous thrombosis or pulmonary embolism among women with predisposing conditions may be higher than that in healthy women.

The incidence of this complication is related to the estrogen content of oral contraceptives. A reduction from 100–150 µg to 50–80 µg reduced the incidence of pulmonary embolism by 50% or more. The most recent studies employing contraceptives containing 30 µg of estrogen indicate that the risk of death from pulmonary embolism is even lower. There is no clear relationship between progestin content and the incidence of this complication. The risk of superficial or deep thromboembolic disease in patients treated with oral contraceptives is not related to age, parity, mild obesity, or cigarette smoking. However, the risk of idiopathic deep venous thromboembolic disease in women with blood types A, B, or AB is twice as great as in those with blood type O who are not taking contraceptives and three times as great in type O women using these compounds. These studies indicate a genetic susceptibility to this disorder and suggest that oral contraceptives magnify the effect. Decreased venous blood flow, endothelial proliferation in veins and arteries, and increased coagulability of blood due to changes in platelet coagulation and fibrinolytic systems contribute to the increased incidence of thrombosis. In general, these changes are similar to those seen in pregnancy. It has been proposed that the main factor responsible is a decrease in the ability to halt the progression of intravenous coagulation and inhibition of fibrin clot dissolution. The major plasma inhibitor of thrombin is antithrombin 3, which is substantially decreased during oral contraceptive use. This change occurs in the first month of treatment and lasts as long as treatment persists.

2. Myocardial infarction–Myocardial infarction occurs more frequently in oral contraceptive users but is unrelated to the duration of use. The attributable risk of myocardial infarction is about 5–7 per 100,000 current user years at age 30–39, rising to approximately 60 at age 40–44. The risk is related to the dose of estrogen and is significantly lower in women using low-dose estrogen compounds. There are also data indicating that the risk is increased in women using oral contraceptives containing 3–4 mg, as compared to 1 or 2 mg, of the progestin norethindrone acetate.

The use of oral contraceptives is associated with a higher risk of myocardial infarction in women who smoke 15 or more cigarettes a day, who have a history of preeclampsia or hypertension, or who have type II hyperlipoproteinemia or diabetes. The risk attributable to oral contraceptives in women 30–39 years of age who do not smoke is about 4 cases per 100,000 users per year, as compared to 185 cases per 100,000 among women 40–44 who smoke heavily. The pathogenesis of myocardial infarction is thought to be related to acceleration of atherogenesis, decreased levels of HDL, and increased platelet aggregation. However, the facilitation of coronary arterial spasm may play a role in some of these patients. The progestational component of oral contraceptives decreases HDL cholesterol, whereas the estrogenic component increases it. The net difference, therefore, will depend entirely on the specific composition of the pill used and the patient's susceptibility to the particular effects. Preparations containing norgestrel, 0.5 mg, or norethindrone acetate, 2.5 mg, have been reported to have strong antiestrogenic effects and to decrease HDL cholesterol, while some of the others have no effect.

3. Cerebrovascular disease–The risk of stroke is concentrated in women over 35. It is increased in current users but not in past users. However, the incidence of subarachnoid hemorrhage is increased among both current and past users and may increase with time. The risk of thrombotic or hemorrhagic stroke attributable to oral contraceptives is about 37 cases per 100,000 users per year. Ten percent of these strokes are fatal, and most of them are due to subarachnoid hemorrhage. Insufficient data are available on which to base an assessment of the effects of smoking and other risk factors.

Elevations in blood pressure may also increase the risk, since there is a three- to sixfold increase in the incidence of overt hypertension in women taking oral contraceptives.

In summary, the information available indicates that oral contraceptives increase the risk of various cardiovascular disorders at all ages and among both smokers and nonsmokers. *However, this risk appears to be concentrated in women 35 years of age or older who are heavy smokers. The presence of these risk factors must be considered in each individual patient for whom oral contraceptives are considered.*

B. Gastrointestinal Disorders: Many cases of cholestatic jaundice have been reported in patients taking progestin-containing drugs. The differences in incidence of these disorders from one population to another suggest that genetic factors are involved. The jaundice caused by these agents is similar to that produced by other 17-alkyl-substituted steroids. It is most often observed in the first 3 cycles and is particularly common in women with a history of cholestatic jaundice during pregnancy. Liver biopsies from such women show bile thrombi in the canaliculi and occasional areas of focal necrosis. Serum alkaline phosphatase and ALT are increased. The BSP retention and serum enzyme changes observed in some patients may indicate liver damage. Jaundice and pruritus disappear 1-8 weeks after the drug is discontinued.

These agents have also been found to increase the incidence of symptomatic gallbladder disease, including cholecystitis and cholangitis. This is probably the result of alterations in bile secretion and content.

It also appears that the incidence of hepatic adenomas is increased in women taking oral contraceptives. Ischemic bowel disease secondary to thrombosis of celiac and superior and inferior mesenteric arteries and veins has also been reported in women using these drugs.

An increase in abnormal cervical smears has been reported involving glandular cells. The neoplastic changes were usually mild. The increase may have also reflected the increased frequency of examination in these women.

C. Depression: Depression severe enough to require stopping the pills occurs in about 6% of patients taking some preparations.

NONCONTRACEPTIVE ADVANTAGES OF HORMONAL CONTRACEPTION

The advent of oral contraceptives with low hormone content has significantly reduced the incidence of serious adverse effects. Furthermore, it has become apparent that their use is associated with important health benefits such as less risk of developing ovarian and endometrial cancer, iron deficiency anemia, benign breast disease, functional ovarian cysts, premenstrual syndrome, and dysmenorrhea.

These and other benefits make hormonal contraception with low-dose, low-potency combination pills an excellent contraceptive method for younger women who do not smoke.

CONTRAINDICATIONS & CAUTIONS

Oral contraceptives are contraindicated in patients with thrombophlebitis, thromboembolic phenomena, and cerebrovascular disorders or a past history of these conditions. They should not be used to treat vaginal bleeding when the cause is unknown. They should be avoided in patients known or suspected to have a tumor of the breast or other estrogen-dependent neoplasm. They are contraindicated in adolescents in whom epiphysial closure has not yet been completed, because they may prevent attainment of normal adult height.

Since these preparations have caused aggravation of preexisting disorders, they should be avoided or used with caution in patients with liver disease, hypertriglyceridemia, asthma, eczema, migraine, diabetes, hypertension, congestive heart failure, optic neuritis, retrobulbar neuritis, or convulsive disorders.

Estrogens may increase the rate of growth of fibroids. Therefore, for women with these tumors, agents with the smallest amounts of estrogen and the most potent progestins should be selected. The use of progestational agents alone for contraception might be especially useful in such patients (see below).

CONTRACEPTION WITH PROGESTINS

Small doses of progestins administered orally can be used for contraception (Table 13–9). They are particularly suited for patients who should not take estrogens. They are about as effective as intrauterine devices or combination pills containing 20–30 μg of ethinyl estradiol. There is a high incidence of spotting or irregular bleeding.

Effective contraception can also be achieved by injecting 150 mg of depot medroxyprogesterone every 3 months. During the first year, random vaginal bleeding is common, but more than 50% become amenorrheic thereafter. No increase in the risk of breast, cervical, ovarian, or endometrial cancer has been noted. Several women have developed benign intracranial hypertension. This agent is also used in the therapy of endometriosis, dysmenorrhea, and hemoglobinopathy. A slight reversible loss of bone density occurs.

Subcutaneous implants of capsules containing levonorgestrel are extremely effective for 5–6 years. These capsules release one-fifth to one-third the amount of progestin required by oral administration. The low circulating levels of hormone have little effect on blood pressure or carbohydrate and lipid metabolism. The disadvantages of this method include the need for surgical insertion and removal of the capsules and some irregular bleeding.

Table 13–12. Schedules for use of postcoital contraceptives.

Conjugated estrogens: 10 mg 3 times daily for 5 days
Ethinyl estradiol: 2.5 mg twice daily for 5 days
Diethylstilbestrol: 50 mg daily for 5 days
Norgestrel, 0.5 mg, with ethinyl estradiol, 0.05 mg: 2 tablets and 2 in 12 hours

Contraception with progestins is useful in patients with hepatic disease, hypertension, psychosis or mental retardation, and prior thromboembolism. The side effects include headache, dizziness, bloating, and weight gain of 1–2 kg. Reduction of glucose tolerance and lipid changes have been reported.

POSTCOITAL CONTRACEPTIVES

Pregnancy can be prevented following coitus by the administration of estrogens alone or in combination with progestins. Insertion of an intrauterine device within 5 days has also been effective.

A variety of schedules have been tested and found effective, and these are shown in Table 13–12. When treatment is begun within 72 hours, the failure rate is less than 1%. Since 40% of patients treated experience nausea or vomiting, antiemetics are recommended. Headache, dizziness, breast tenderness, and abdominal and leg cramps have also been reported as adverse effects. Because these compounds have serious teratogenic effects early in pregnancy and because vaginal adenosis and cancer, cervical abnormalities, and impairment of reproductive function have been found in the offspring of women treated with diethylstilbestrol during gestation, voluntary termination of pregnancy is advised when conception occurs in these patients.

Mifepristone (see above), an antiprogestin, when given in the midluteal phase or at intervals during the menstrual cycle, can also prevent pregnancy. Its use for this purpose is under study.

INFERTILITY

Infertility is usually defined as failure of conception by a couple who have been having regular intercourse for 1 year or more without contraception. The intensity of the patients' concern varies, and a physician may be consulted after only a few months or many years of trying to become pregnant. Some of the more common problems encountered are listed in Table 13–13.

Table 13–13. Causes of infertility.

Male (40–50%)	Female (50–60%)
Abnormalities of sperm	Tubal disease (20%)
Infection (mumps)	Anovulation (15%)
Failure to liquefy	Cervical factors (5%)
Agglutination	Unknown (10–20%)
Chronic infection (epididymitis,	Immunologic abnor-
prostatitis)	malities[1]
High scrotal temperature	
Varicocele	
Baths	
Jockey shorts	
Prolonged sitting	
Radiation exposure	
Drugs (cimetidine, sulfasalazine,	
nitrofurantoin, etc)	
Retrograde ejaculation	
Severe allergic reactions (rare)	
Endocrine disorders	
Immunologic abnormalities[1]	

[1]Failure of conception correlates best with agglutinating antibodies to sperm in the male and with agglutinating and immobilizing antibodies in the female.

SEMEN ABNORMALITIES

Semen analysis is usually performed early in the investigation of infertile couples, because male factors are responsible for 40% of cases of infertility and because the test is relatively simple and inexpensive; furthermore, sperm abnormalities may compound the problem in women who fail to ovulate or have other problems reducing fertility. The characteristics of normal semen and sperm are discussed in Chapter 12. Male infertility is commonly attributed to varicocele of the left internal spermatic vein. Although this hypothesis is controversial, surgical correction of this disorder usually results in marked improvement in sperm motility, and even when lower than normal sperm counts remain, pregnancy is achieved about half the time. The quality and concentration of sperm can also be improved in some men by the use of split ejaculates. In about 90% of men, the first few drops of semen contain a higher concentration of sperm with better motility than the remainder of the ejaculate. The combination of this technique with artificial insemination increases the chances of pregnancy in some couples.

OVULATORY DISORDERS

Absent or infrequent ovulation accounts for about 15% of infertility problems. Whether ovulation is completely absent or occurs infrequently, the opportunity for conception is diminished, and the patient should be treated by ovulation induction (see above).

Women who have menstrual bleeding at regular intervals preceded by recognizable symptoms or who have dysmenorrhea almost always ovulate regularly. The occurrence of ovulation can be confirmed by the finding of a progesterone level greater than 4 ng/mL. However, it is useful to obtain daily basal body temperatures in order to determine the length of the luteal phase and to find out whether coitus has occurred at the time of ovulation. The timing of coitus is important, since the egg is fertilizable for only 12–24 hours, and sperm retain their ability to fertilize for 24–48 hours. Ideally, coitus should occur every other day for the 3 days preceding and following ovulation.

INFERTILITY IN THE PRESENCE OF OVULATION

When conception has not occurred in spite of a normal sperm analysis in the man and regular ovulation in the woman, a postcoital test of cervical mucus should be done near the time of expected ovulation as indicated by basal body temperature charts, length of cycle, or the patient's observation of increased amounts of clear mucus at an appropriate time of the cycle. The cervical mucus at this time is under the influence of high estrogen levels and is clear and abundant. It can be stretched between a slide and cover slip as much as 10 cm at this time ("spinnbarkeit"). When the mucus is dried on the slide, the interaction of the electrolytes and protein results in a crystalline pattern called "ferning" (Figure 13–13). This mucus contains chains of glycoproteins that form channels through which the sperm can migrate. In order to perform the test, mucus is obtained from the cervix following intercourse, preferably within 8 hours. If the mucus is thick and cloudy, the specimen may have been obtained too late in the cycle, and the test should be repeated. Absence of spermatozoa in the specimen indicates the need for a more careful study of the semen specimen, as does the presence of dead sperm cells without motility. The presence of 20 or more motile sperm per high dry field is associated with a higher fertility rate than when few sperm are found. However, pregnancies occur even when no motile sperm cells are found in this test. The finding of dead cells suggests the use of spermicidal lubricants or may indicate the need for sperm antibody testing.

Tests of Tubal Patency

When there is a history of pelvic infection or pelvic surgery, tubal patency should be examined by hysterosalpingography or at the time of diagnostic laparoscopy. Such examinations are also indicated in patients in whom other factors have not been identified that might explain the infertility. Hysterosalpingography is best performed a few days following cessation of menstrual flow, thus avoiding the disruption of an early pregnancy. It is contraindicated in the presence of active pelvic inflammatory disease, as indicated by the presence of pelvic masses, tenderness, or an elevated sedimentation rate. Radiation should be minimized by the use of image intensification fluoroscopy and by taking the minimum number of films. An increased number of conceptions has been reported following this procedure when oil-based dye is used. The increase has been attributed to various mechanical and chemical effects of lavage with an iodine-containing and possibly bacteriostatic substance.

When semen analysis and the above tests are found to be normal in the infertile couple, the possibility of endometriosis should be considered even in the absence of typical signs and symptoms such as severe dysmenorrhea, dyspareunia, thickening of the broad ligament, nodularity and tenderness, or fixation of the uterus on pelvic examination. In these instances, laparoscopy may detect the presence and indicate the extent of any intrapelvic disease. Surgical treatment of minimal endometriosis established in this manner is followed by conception in half of women so treated. Hormonal treatment (eg, danazol or GnRH analogs) also may be effective in some patients.

IN VITRO FERTILIZATION

In vitro fertilization and transfer of the fertilized ovum into the uterus is now a therapeutic option to achieve pregnancy. After thorough fertility evaluation and study of the patient's menstrual cycles, the patient is given clomiphene citrate, menotropins, or both to increase the number of large mature follicles. Just before ovulation, several ova are obtained by laparoscopy or percutaneously under ultrasound guidance. The ova are incubated for several hours, and washed sperm are added to the culture medium. After 2–3 days of incubation, several four- to six-cell conceptuses are transferred to the uterus via the cervix.

Seventy to 80 percent of mature ova obtained can be fertilized. Early abortion is frequent, and the overall success rate is less than 30% but is increasing with experience. The process is very expensive and time-consuming. It is estimated to cost between $40,000 and $200,000 per successful pregnancy. However, the risks of fetal abnormalities and maternal complications are low and it copes with the problem of tubal obstruction.

GAMETE INTRA-FOLLICULAR TRANSFER (GIFT)

In this process, the fertilized gamete is transferred into the uterine tube. The preparation of the patient and fertilization technique are similar to that for in vitro fertilization. However, the transfer of the gamete takes place shortly after fertilization. The injection of single sperm directly into the oocyte can also be done.

Enormous amounts of money are spent and millions of visits to physicians occur every year for the complaint of infertility. Recent focus on advanced technologies has overshadowed what can be accomplished with less sophisticated management. It is also important to recognize that there is a significant spontaneous cure rate in almost every category of infertility, including failed in-vitro fertilization and GIFT. In one study of infertile couples, pregnancy occurred in 41% of treated couples and 35% of untreated couples.

REFERENCES

General

Adashi EY: Intraovarian peptides: Stimulators and inhibitors of follicular growth and differentiation. Endocrinol Metab Clin North Am 1992;21:1.

Carr BR, Blackwell RE (editors): *Textbook of Reproductive Endocrinology.* Appleton & Lange, 1993.

Chen CL: Inhibin and activin as paracrine/autocrine factors. Endocrinology 1993;132:4.

Griffing GT: Editorial: Dinosaurs and steroids J Clin Endocrinol Metab 1993;77:1450.

Hodgen GD: The dominant ovarian follicle. Fertil Steril 1982;38:281.

Speroff L, Glass RH, Kase NG: *Clinical Gynecologic Endocrinology and Infertility,* 4th ed. Williams & Wilkins, 1989.

Taylor AE et al: Midcycle levels of sex steroids are sufficient to recreate the follicle-stimulating hormone but not the luteinizing hormone midcycle surge: Evidence for the contribution of other ovarian factors to the surge in normal women. J Clin Endocrinol Metab 1995;80:1541.

Disorders of Ovarian Function

Conn MP, Crowley WF: Gonadotropin releasing hormone and its analogs. N Engl J Med 1001;324:93.

Constantini MW, Warren MP: Menstrual function in swimmers: A distinct entity. J Clin Endocrinol Metab 1995;80:2740.

Conte FA et al: A syndrome of female pseudohermaphroditism, hypergonadotropic hypogonadism, and multicystic ovaries associated with missense mutations in the gene encoding aromatase (P450arom). J Clin Endocrinol Metab 1994;78:1287.

Kirschner MA, Samojlik E, Szmal E: Clinical usefulness of plasma androstanediol glucuronide measurements in women with idiopathic hirsutism. J Clin Endocrinol Metab 1987;65:597.

Malkasian GD Jr et al: Functioning tumors of the ovary in women under 40. Obstet Gynecol 1965;26:669.

Prior JC et al: Spinal bone loss and ovulatory disturbances. N Engl J Med 1990;323:1221.

Schlechte J et al: The natural history of untreated hyperprolactinemia: A prospective analysis. J Clin Endocrinol Metab 1989;68:412.

Smith. BR: Adrenal and gonadal autoimmune diseases. J Clin Endocrinol Metab 1995;80:1502.

Hirsutism

Apter D et al: Metabolic features of polycystic ovary syndrome are found in adolescent girls with hyperandrogenism. J Clin Endocrinol Metab 1995;80:2966.

Azziz R: Leuprolide and estrogen versus oral contraceptive pills for the treatment of hirsutism: a prospective randomized study. J Clin Endocrinol Metab 1995; 80:3406.

Burkman RT Jr: The role of oral contraceptives in the treatment of hyperandrogenic disorders. Am J Med 1995;98:130S.

Cummings DC et al: Treatment of hirsutism with spironolactone. JAMA 1982;247:1295.

Ehrmann DA, Barnes RB, Rosenfield RL: Polycystic ovary syndrome as a form of functional ovarian hyperandrogenism due to dysregulation of androgen secretion. Endocr Rev 1995;16:322.

Ferriman D, Gallwey JD: Clinical assessment of body hair growth in women. J Clin Endocrinol Metab 1961;21:1440.

Franks S: Polycystic ovary syndrome. N Engl J Med 1995;333:1995.

Fruzzetti F et al: Effects of finasteride, a Sa-reductase inhibitor, on circulating androgen and gonadotropin secretion in hirsute women. J Clin Endocrinol Metab 1994;79:811.

Leemay A: Attenuation of mild hyperandrogenic activity in postpubertal acne by a triphasic oral contraceptive containing low doses of ethynyl estradiol and d,l-norgestrel. J Clin Endocrinol Metab 1990;71:8.

Mooradian AD, Morley JD, Korenman SG: Biological action of androgens. Endocr Rev 1987;8:1.

Mortola JF, Yen SSC: The effects of oral dehydroepiandrosterone on endocrine-metabolic parameters in postmenopausal women. J Clin Endocrinol Metab 1990;71:696.

Pittaway DE, Maxson WS, Wentz AC: Spironolactone in combination drug therapy for unresponsive hirsutism. Fertil Steril 1985;43:878.

Tropiano G et al: Insulin, C-peptide, androgens and β-endorphin response to oral glucose in patients with polycystic ovary syndrome. J Clin Endocrinol Metab 1994;78:305.

Venturoli S et al: Ketoconazole therapy for women with acne and/or hirsutism. J Clin Endocrinol Metab 1990; 71:335.

Therapeutic Use of Ovarian & Hypothalamic Hormones & Inhibitors

Chetkowski RJ et al: Biologic effects of transdermal estradiol. N Engl J Med 1986;314:1615.

Christiansen C, Riis BJ: 17β-estradiol and continuous norethisterone: A unique treatment for established osteoporosis in elderly women. J Clin Endocrinol Metab 1990;71:836.

Conn MP, Crowley WF Jr: Gonadotropin-releasing hormone and its analogues. N Engl J Med 1991;324:93.

Crooij MJ et al: Termination of early pregnancy by the 3β-hydroxysteroid dehydrogenase inhibitor epostane. N Engl J Med 1988;319:813.

D'Amato G et al: Serum and bile lipid levels in a postmenopausal woman after percutaneous and oral natural estrogens. Am J Obstet Gynecol 1989;169:600.

Davidson NE: Tamoxifen: Panacea or Pandora's box? N Engl J Med 1992;326:885.

Hill NCW, Furguson J, MacKenzie IZ: The efficacy of oral mifepristone (RU 38,486) with a prostaglandin E_1 analog vaginal pessary for the termination of early pregnancy: Complications and patient acceptability. Am J Obstet Gynecol 1990;162:414.

Love RR et al: Effects of tamoxifen on bone mineral density in postmenopausal women with breast cancer. N Engl J Med 1992;326:852.

Mishell DR (editor): Interdisciplinary review of estrogen replacement therapy. Am J Obstet Gynecol 1989;161 (Suppl Part 2):1825.

Riggs BL: Overview of osteoporosis. West J Med 1991; 154:63.

Rittmaster RS: Medical treatment of androgen-dependent hirsutism. J Clin Endocrinol Metab 1995;80: 2559.

Rossing AM et al: Ovarian tumors in a cohort of infertile women. N Engl J Med 1994;331:731.

Sherwin BB: The impact of different doses of estrogen and progestin on mood and sexual behavior in postmenopausal women. J Clin Endocrinol Metab 1991; 72:336.

Spitz IM, Bardin WC: Mifepristone (RU-486): A modulator of progestin and glucocorticoid action. N Engl J Med 1993;329:404.

Stampfer MJ et al: A prospective study of past use of oral contraceptive agents and risk of cardiovascular diseases. N Engl J Med 1988;319:1313.

Steiner M et al: Fluoxetine in the treatment of premenstrual dysphoria. N Engl J Med 1995;332:1529.

Taylor AE et al: Midcycle levels of sex steroids are sufficient to recreate the follicle-stimulating hormone but not the luteinizing hormone midcycle surge: Evidence for the contribution of other ovarian factors to the surge in normal women. J Clin Endocrinol Metab 1995;80:1541.

Wong IL et al: A prospective randomized trial comparing finasteride to spironolactone in the treatment of hirsute women. J Clin Endocrinol Metab 1995;80: 233.

Menopause

Civitelli R et al: Bone turnover in postmenopausal osteoporosis: Effect of calcitonin treatment, J Clin Invest 1988;82:1268.

Colditz GA et al: The use of estrogens and progestins and the risk of breast cancer in postmenopausal women. N Engl J Med 1995;332:1589.

Godsland IF et al: The effects of different formulations of oral contraceptive agents on lipid and carbohydrate metabolism. N Engl J Med 1990;323:1375.

Grey AX et al: The effect of the anti-estrogen tamoxifen on cardiovascular risk factors in normal postmenopausal women. J Clin Endocrinol Metab 1995; 80:8192.

Liberman UA et al: Effect of oral alendronate on bone mineral density and the incidence of fractures in menopausal osteoporosis. N Engl J Med 1995;333: 1437.

Lindsay R et al: Bone response to termination of oestrogen treatment. Lancet 1978;1:1325.

Mishell DR et al: Postmenopausal replacement with a combination estrogen-progestin regimen for five days per week. J Reprod Med 1991;36:351.

Prough SG et al: Continuous estrogen/progestin therapy in menopause. Am J Obstet Gynecol 1987;157:1449.

Rockwell JC et al: Weight training decreases vertebral bone density in premenopausal women: A prospective study. J Clin Endocrinol Metab 1990;71:988.

Sherman BM, West JH, Korenman SG: The menopausal transition: Analysis of LH, FSH, estradiol, and progesterone concentrations during menstrual cycles of older women. J Clin Endocrinol Metab 1976;42:629.

Weinstein L, Bewtra C, Gallagher JC: Evaluation of a continuous combined low-dose regimen of estrogen-progestin for treatment of the menopausal patient. Am J Obstet Gynecol 1990;162:1534.

Williams SR et al: A study of combined continuous ethynyl estradiol and norethindrone acetate for postmenopausal hormone replacement. Am J Obstet Gynecol 1990;162:438.

Wolfe BM, Huff MW: The effects of combined estrogen and progestin administration on plasma lipoprotein metabolism in postmenopausal women. J Clin Invest 1989;83:40.

Hormonal Contraception

Grimes DA, Mishell DR, Speroff L (editors): Contraceptive choices for women with medical problems. Am J Obstet Gynecol 1993;168:No. 6 (part II), 1993.

Kuhl H, Goethe JW (editors): Pharmacokinetics of oral contraceptive steroids and drug interaction. Am J Obstet Gynecol 1990;163(Suppl Part 2):2113.

Herbst AL, Berek JS: Impact of contraception on gynecologic cancers. Am J Obstet Gynecol 1993;168:1980.

Ortmeier BG et al: A cost-benefit analysis of four hormonal contraceptive methods. Clin Therap 1994;16: 707.

Polaneczky M et al: The use of levonorgestrel implants (Norplant) for contraception in adolescent mothers. N Engl J Med 1994;331:1201.

Rich-Edwards,JW: et al: The primary prevention of coronary heart disease in women. N Engl J Med 1995; 332:1758.

Sivin I. Contraception with Norplant implants. Human Reproduction 9: 1818, 1993

Infertility

Collins JA et al: Treatment-independent pregnancy among infertile couples. N Engl J Med 1983;309:1201.

Penzias, AS and DeCherney, AH: Advances in clinical in vitro fertilization. J Clin Endocrinol Metab 1994; 78:503.

Speroff L, Glass RH, Kase NG: *Clinical Gynecologic Endocrinology and Infertility,* 4th ed. Williams & Wilkins, 1989.

Abnormalities of Sexual Determination & Differentiation

14

Felix A. Conte, MD, & Melvin M. Grumbach, MD

Advances in molecular genetics, experimental embryology, steroid biochemistry, and methods of evaluation of the interaction between the hypothalamus, pituitary, and gonads have helped to clarify problems of sexual determination and differentiation. Anomalies may occur at any stage of intrauterine maturation and lead to gross ambisexual development or to subtle abnormalities that do not become manifest until sexual maturity is achieved.

NORMAL SEX DIFFERENTIATION

Chromosomal Sex

The normal human diploid cell contains 22 autosomal pairs of chromosomes and two sex chromosomes (two X or one X and one Y). When arranged serially and numbered according to size and centromeric position, they are known as a karyotype. Advances in the techniques of staining chromosomes (Figure 14–1) permit positive identification of each chromosome by its unique "banding" pattern. Bands can be produced in the region of the centromere (C bands), with the fluorescent dye quinacrine (Q bands), and with Giemsa stain (G bands). Fluorescent banding (Figure 14–2) is particularly useful because the Y chromosome stains so brightly that it can be identified easily in both interphase and metaphase cells. A new technique called fluorescent in situ hybridization (FISH) has been developed. This technique has been found to be particularly useful in identifying "marker" chromosomes, especially deleted sex chromosomes that are not readily identifiable by standard banding techniques. The standard nomenclature for describing the human karyotype is shown in Table 14–1. Recently, a complete clone map of the euchromatic region of the Y chromosome was described. This is the first map of this type for a human chromosome, and it spans about 35 million base pairs.

Studies in animals as well as humans with abnormalities of sexual differentiation indicate that the sex chromosomes (the X and Y chromosomes) and the autosomes carry genes that influence sexual differentiation by causing the bipotential gonad to develop

<table>
<tr><th colspan="2">ACRONYMS USED IN THIS CHAPTER</th></tr>
<tr><td>AMH</td><td>Anti-müllerian hormone</td></tr>
<tr><td>AS</td><td>Aldosterone synthetase</td></tr>
<tr><td>CAH</td><td>Congenital adrenal hyperplasia</td></tr>
<tr><td>DAX-1</td><td>DSS-AHC-critical region on the X gene</td></tr>
<tr><td>DAZ</td><td>Deleted in azoospermia</td></tr>
<tr><td>DHEA</td><td>Dehydroepiandrosterone</td></tr>
<tr><td>DHT</td><td>Dihydrotestosterone</td></tr>
<tr><td>DMD</td><td>Duchenne muscular dystrophy</td></tr>
<tr><td>DSS</td><td>Dosage-sensitive sex reversal</td></tr>
<tr><td>FISH</td><td>Fluorescent in situ hybridization</td></tr>
<tr><td>FSH</td><td>Follicle-stimulating hormone</td></tr>
<tr><td>GK</td><td>Glycerol kinase</td></tr>
<tr><td>GM-CSF</td><td>Granulocyte-macrophage colony-stimulating factor</td></tr>
<tr><td>GnRH</td><td>Gonadotropin-releasing hormone</td></tr>
<tr><td>hCG</td><td>Human chorionic gonadotropin</td></tr>
<tr><td>HH</td><td>Hypogonadotropic hypogonadism</td></tr>
<tr><td>HMG</td><td>High mobility group</td></tr>
<tr><td>LH</td><td>Leutinizing hormone</td></tr>
<tr><td>PAR</td><td>Pseudoautosomal region</td></tr>
<tr><td>POLA</td><td>RNA polymerase</td></tr>
<tr><td>SF-1</td><td>Steroidogenic factor-1</td></tr>
<tr><td>SHBG</td><td>Sex hormone-binding globulin</td></tr>
<tr><td>SOX 9</td><td>SRY-like HMG box-9</td></tr>
<tr><td>SRY</td><td>Sex-determining region Y</td></tr>
<tr><td>StAR</td><td>Steroidogenic acute regulatory protein</td></tr>
<tr><td>T</td><td>Testosterone</td></tr>
<tr><td>TDF</td><td>Testis-determining factor</td></tr>
<tr><td>WAGR</td><td>Wilms tumor-aniridia-genital anomalies-mental retardation syndrome</td></tr>
<tr><td>WT-1</td><td>Wilms tumor repressor gene</td></tr>
<tr><td>XIST</td><td>X-inactive specific transcripts</td></tr>
<tr><td>XIC</td><td>X inactivation center</td></tr>
<tr><td>Xm</td><td>X-linked serum macroglobulin</td></tr>
<tr><td>ZFY</td><td>Zinc finger Y</td></tr>
<tr><td>ZFX</td><td>Zinc finger X</td></tr>
</table>

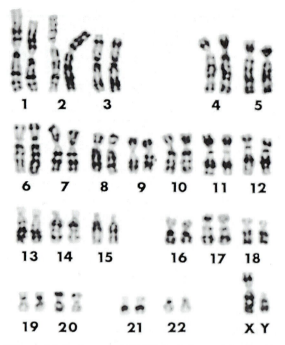

Figure 14–1. A normal 46,XY karyotype stained with Giemsa's stain to produce G bands. Note that each chromosome has a specific banding pattern.

either as a testis or as an ovary. Two intact and normally functioning X chromosomes, in the absence of a Y chromosome (and the genes for testicular organogenesis), lead to the formation of an ovary, whereas a Y chromosome or the presence of the male-determining region of the short arm of the Y chromosome—the "testis determining factor" (TDF)—will lead to testicular organogenesis.

In humans, there is a marked discrepancy in size between the X and Y chromosomes. Gene dosage compensation is achieved in all persons with two or more X chromosomes in their genetic constitution by partial inactivation of all X chromosomes except one. This phenomenon is thought to be a random process that occurs in each cell in the late blastocyst stage of embryonic development in which either the maternally or the paternally derived X chromosome undergoes heterochromatinization. The result of this process is formation of an X chromatin body (Barr body) in the interphase cells of persons having two or more X chromosomes (Figure 14–3). A gene termed *XIST* (X inactive, specific transcripts) has been found in the region of the putative X inactivation center (XIC) at Xq13.2 on the paracentromeric region of the long arm of the X chromosome. *XIST* is expressed only by the inactive X chromosome.

The distal portion of the short arm of the X chromosmome escapes inactivation and has a short (2.5 megabase) segment homologous to a segment on the distal portion of the short arm of the Y chromosome. This segment is called the "pseudoautosomal" region (PAR); it is these two limited regions of the X and Y that pair during meiosis, undergo obligatory chiasm formation, and allow for exchange of DNA between these specific regions of the X and Y chromosomes. At least seven genes have been localized to the PAR on the short arm of the X and Y chromosomes. Among these are *MIC2,* a gene coding for a cell surface antigen recognized by the monoclonal antibody, 12E7; the gene for the granulocyte-macrophage colony-stimulating factor receptor (GM-CSF); the human interleukin-3 receptor; and a gene for short stature. A pseudoautosomal region has also been described for the distal ends of the long arms of the X and Y chromosomes. Only one gene has been localized to this region (Figures 14–4 and 14–5).

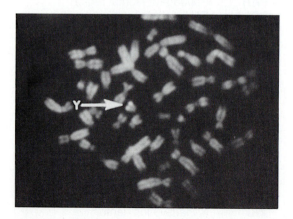

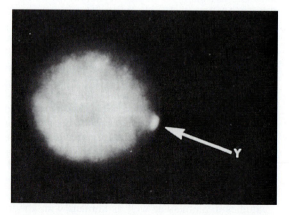

Figure 14–2. Metaphase chromosomes stained with quinacrine and examined through a fluorescence microscope. Note the bright fluorescence of the distal arms of the Y chromosome, which can also be seen in interphase cells ("Y body" at right).

Table 14–1. Nomenclature for describing the human karyotype pertinent to designating sex chromosome abnormalities.

ISCN 1995	Description	Former Nomenclature
46,XX	Normal female karyotype	XX
46,XY	Normal male karyotype	XY
47,XXY	Karyotype with 47 chromosomes including an extra Y chromosome	XXY
45,X	Monosomy X	XO
45,X/46,XY	Mosaic karyotype composed of 45,X and 46,XY cell lines	XO/XY
p	Short arm	p
q	Long arm	q
46,X,del (X) (p21)	Deletion of the short arm of the X distal to band Xp21	XXp–
46,X,del (X) (q21)	Deletion of the long arm of the X distal to band Xq21	XXq–
46,X,i(Xq10)	Isochromosome of the long arm of X. q10 = centromeric band	XXqi
46,Xr(X)(p22q25)	Ring X chromosome with breaks at p22 and q25	XXr
46,XY,der(7)t(Y;7)(q11; q13)	Translocation of the distal fluorescent portion of the Y chromosome to the long arm of chromosome 7	46,XYt (Yq–7q+)

In buccal mucosal smears of 46,XX females, a sex chromatin body is evident in 20–30% of the interphase nuclei examined, whereas in normal 46,XY males, a comparable sex chromatin body is absent. In patients with more than two X chromosomes, the maximum number of sex chromatin bodies in any diploid nucleus is one less than the total number of X chromosomes. Using sex chromatin and Y fluorescent staining, one can determine indirectly the sex chromosome complement of an individual (Table 14–2).

Sex Determination (SRY = Testis-Determining Factor)

Over the past 20 years, interest has focused on several proteins as candidates for the "testis-determining factor" produced by a gene on the Y chromosome. Experimental and clinical data do not support the candidacy of H-Y antigen or zinc finger Y (ZFY) as the testis-determining factor. In studies of 46,XX males with very small Y-to-X translocations, a gene was localized to the region just proximal to the pseudoautosomal boundary of the Y chromosome (Figure 14–5). This gene has been cloned, expressed, and named sex-determining region Y (SRY). Sry (the murine analog of the human SRY gene) is expressed in the embryonic genital ridge of the mouse between days 10.5 and 12.5, just prior to and during the time at which testis differentiation first occurs. Furthermore, deletions or mutations of the human SRY gene occur in about 15–20% of 46,XY females with "complete XY gonadal dysgenesis." However, the most compelling evidence to indicate that SRY is the testis-determining factor is that transfection of the SRY gene into 46,XX mouse embryos results in transgenic 46,XX mice with testes and male sex differentiation.

The SRY gene encodes for a DNA-binding protein that has an 80-amino-acid domain similar to that found in "high mobility group" (HMG) proteins. This domain binds to DNA in a sequence-specific manner (A/TAACAAT). It bends the DNA and is thus thought to facilitate interaction between DNA-bound proteins to affect the transcription of "downstream genes." Almost all the mutations thus far described in 46,XY females with gonadal dysgenesis have occurred in the nucleotides of the SRY gene encoding the DNA binding region (the HMG box) of the SRY protein.

An unknown number of genes are involved in the testis-determining cascade (Figures 14–6A and 14–6B). Heterozygous mutations and deletions of the Wilms tumor repressor gene (WT-1) located on 11p13 result in urogenital malformations as well as Wilms' tumors. "Knockout" of the WT-1 gene in mice results in apoptosis of the metanephric blastema with the resultant absence of the kidneys and gonads. Thus, WT-1, a transcriptional regulator, appears to act on metanephric blastema early in urogenital development.

SF-1 (steroidogenic factor-1) is an orphan nuclear receptor involved in transcriptional regulation. It is

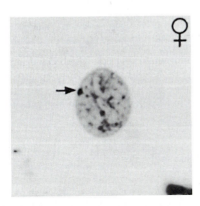

Figure 14–3. X chromatin (Barr) body in the nucleus of a buccal mucosal cell from a normal 46,XX female.

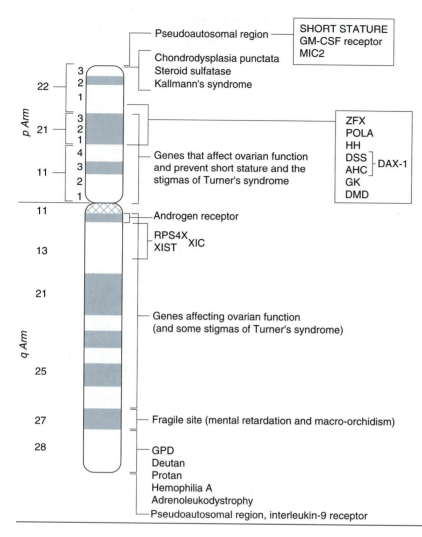

Figure 14–4. Diagrammatic representation of G-banded X chromosome. Selected X-linked genes are shown. (GM-CSF, granulocyte-macrophage colony-stimulating factor; MIC2, a cell surface antigen recognized by monoclonal antibody 12E7; ZFX, zinc finger X; POLA, RNA polymerase; HH, hypogonadotropic hypogonadism; AHC, congenital adrenal hypoplasia; DSS, dosage-sensitive sex reversal; DAX-1, DSS-AHC-critical region on the X_1 gene 1; GPD, glucose-6-phosphate dehydrogenase; deutan and protan, color blindness genes; Xm, X-linked serum macroglobulin; GK, glycerol kinase; DMD, Duchenne muscular dystrophy; RPS4X, ribosomal protein S4; XIST, Xi-specific transcripts; XIC, X inactivation center.) (Reproduced, with permission, from Grumbach MM, Conte FA: Disorders of sex differentiation. In: *Williams Textbook of Endocrinology,* 8th ed. Wilson JD, Foster DW [editors]. Saunders, 1992.)

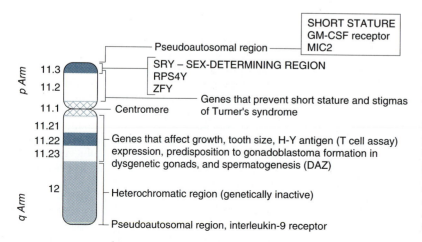

Figure 14–5. Diagrammatic representation of a G-banded Y chromosome. Y-linked genes are shown. (ZFY, zinc finger Y; SRY, sex-determining region Y; GM-CSF, granulocyte-macrophage colony-stimulating factor; MIC2, gene for a cell surface antigen recognized by monoclonal antibody 12E7; RPS4Y, ribosomal protein S4; DAZ, deleted in azoospermia.) (Reproduced, with permission, from Grumbach MM, Conte FA: Disorders of sex differentiation. In: *Williams Textbook of Endocrinology,* 8th ed. Wilson JD, Foster DW [editors]. Saunders, 1992.)

Table 14–2. Sex chromosome complement correlated with X chromatin and Y bodies in somatic interphase nuclei.[1]

Sex Chromosomes	Maximum Number in Diploid Somatic Nuclei	
	X Bodies	Y Bodies
45,X	0	0
46,XX	1	0
46,XY	0	1
47,XXX	2	0
47,XXY	1	1
47,XYY	0	2
48,XXXX	3	0
48,XXXY	2	1
48,XXYY	1	2
49,XXXXX	4	0
49,XXXXY	3	1
49,XXXYY	2	2

[1]The maximum number of X chromatin bodies in diploid somatic nuclei is one less than the number of Xs, whereas the maximum number of Y fluorescent bodies is equivalent to the number of Ys in the chromosome constitution.

expressed in both the female and male urogenital ridges as well as in steroidogenic tissues, where it is required for the synthesis of testosterone, and in Sertoli cells, where it regulates the anti-müllerian hormone gene. SF-1 is encoded by the mammalian homolog of the *Drosophila* gene *FTZ-F1*. "Knockout" of the *SF-1* gene in mice results in apoptosis of the cells of the genital ridge that give rise to the adrenals and gonads and thus lack of gonadal and adrenal gland morphogenesis in both males and females. This gene thus appears to play a critical role in the formation of all steroid-secreting glands, ie, the adrenals, testes, and ovaries.

XY gonadal dysgenesis with resulting female differentiation in 46,XY patients with intact *SRY* function has been reported in individuals with duplications of Xp21. A locus at this site has been called DSS (dosage-sensitive sex reversal). A gene, *DAX-1,* whose mutation results in X-linked congenital adrenal hypoplasia and hypogonadotropic hypogonadism maps within the DSS critical region. Deletion of the DSS locus in 46,XY individuals has not resulted in an abnormality of either testicular differentiation or function. Similarly, duplication of the DSS locus appears not to affect ovarian morphogenesis and function in 46,XX females. It has been hypothesized that the DSS locus may contain an ovarian differentiation gene which is normally repressed in 46,XY individuals by *SRY*. However, duplication of DSS and, hence, the putative ovarian differentiation gene, may prevent repression and result in gonadal dysgenesis and sex reversal in 46,XY individuals (Figure 14–6B).

Campomelic dysplasia is a skeletal dysplasia associated with sex reversal due to gonadal dysgenesis in 46,XY individuals. The gene for campomelic dysplasia *(CMPD1)* has been localized to 17q24.3–q25.1.

Mutations in one allele of the *SOX 9* gene, a gene related to *SRY* (called a *SOX* gene because it has an *SRY* HMG b*ox* which is more than 60% homologous to that of SRY), can result in both *CMPD1* and XY gonadal dysgenesis with sex reversal. XY individuals with 9p– or 10q– deletions exhibit gonadal dysgenesis and male pseudohermaphroditism, which suggests that autosomal genes at these loci are important in the gonadal differentiation cascade (Figure 14–6B).

TESTICULAR & OVARIAN DIFFERENTIATION

Until the 12-mm stage (approximately 42 days of gestation), the embryonic gonads of males and females are indistinguishable. By 42 days, 300–1300 primordial germ cells have seeded the undifferentiated gonad from their extragonadal origin in the yolk sac dorsal endoderm. These large cells are the progenitors of oogonia and spermatogonia; lack of these cells is incompatible with further ovarian differentiation but not testicular differentiation. Under the influence of *SRY* and other genes that encode for male sex determination (Figure 14–6B), the gonad will begin to differentiate as a testis at 43–50 days of gestation. Leydig cells are apparent by about 60 days, and differentiation of male external genitalia occurs by 65–77 days of gestation.

In the gonad destined to be an ovary, the lack of differentiation persists. At 77–84 days—long after differentiation of the testis in the male fetus—a significant number of germ cells enter meiotic prophase to characterize the transition of oogonia into oocytes, which marks the onset of ovarian differentiation from the undifferentiated gonads. Primordial follicles (small oocytes surrounded by a single layer of flat granulosa cells and a basement membrane) are evident after 90 days. Preantral follicles are seen after 6 months, and fully developed oocytes with fluid-filled cavities and multiple layers of granulosa cells are present at birth. As opposed to the testes, there is little evidence of hormone production by the fetal ovaries (Figure 14–7).

Differentiation of Genital Ducts (Figure 14–8)

By the seventh week of intrauterine life, the fetus is equipped with the primordia of both male and female genital ducts. The müllerian ducts, if allowed to persist, form the uterine (fallopian) tubes, the corpus and cervix of the uterus, and the upper third of the vagina. The wolffian ducts, on the other hand, have the potential for differentiating into the epididymis, vas deferens, seminal vesicles, and ejaculatory ducts of the male. In the presence of a functional testis, the müllerian ducts involute under the influence of "anti-müllerian hormone" (AMH), a dimeric glycoprotein secreted by fetal Sertoli cells. This hormone acts "lo-

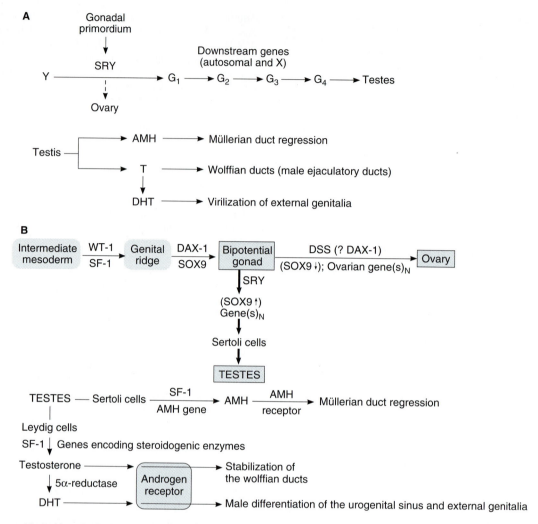

Figure 14–6. Hypothetical diagrammatic representation of the cascade of genes involved in testes determination and hormones involved in male sex differentiation. WT-1, Wilms tumor suppressor; SF-1, steroidogenic factor-1; DSS, dosage-sensitive sex reversal; SRY, sex-determining region Y; SOX 9, SRY-like HMG box gene 9; AMH, Antimüllerian hormone; DAX-1, OSS-AHC critical region on the X gene; DHT, dihydrotestosterone. (Reproduced, with permission, from Grumbach MM, Conte FA: Abnormalities of sex differentiation. In: *Williams Textbook of Endocrinology,* 9th ed. Wilson JD, Foster DW [editors]. Saunders, 1996.)

cally" to cause müllerian duct repression ipsilaterally. The differentiation of the wolffian duct is stimulated by testosterone secretion from the testis. In the presence of an ovary or in the absence of a functional fetal testis, müllerian duct differentiation occurs, and the wolffian ducts involute. Data indicate that *SF-1* regulates steroidogenesis by the Leydig cell by binding to the promoter of the genes encoding P450scc and P450c17.

The gene for AMH encodes a 560-amino-acid protein whose carboxyl terminal domain shows marked homology with TGFβ and the B chain of inhibin and activin. The gene has been localized on the short arm of chromosome 19. AMH is secreted by human fetal and postnatal Sertoli cells until 8–10 years of age and

can be used as a marker for the presence of these cells. *SF-1,* an orphan nuclear receptor, has been shown to regulate AMH gene expression. The human AMH receptor gene has been cloned and mapped to the q13 band of chromosome 12. The receptor has been identified as being similar to other type II receptors of the TGF-β family.

Differentiation of External Genitalia (Figure 14–9)

Up to the eighth week of fetal life, the external genitalia of both sexes are identical and have the capacity to differentiate into the genitalia of either sex. Female sex differentiation will occur in the presence of an ovary or streak gonads or if no gonad is present

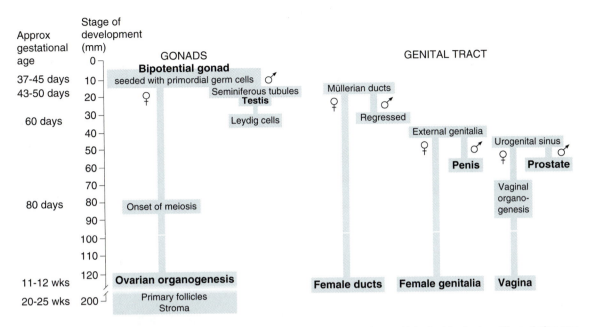

Figure 14–7. Schematic sequence of sexual differentiation in the human fetus. Note that testicular differentiation precedes all other forms of differentiation. (Reproduced, with permission, from Grumbach MM, Conte FA: Disorders of sex differentiation. In: *Williams Textbook of Endocrinology,* 8th ed. Wilson JD, Foster DW [editors]. Saunders, 1992.)

(Figure 14–10). Differentiation of the external genitalia along male lines depends on the action of testosterone and particularly dihydrotestosterone, the 5α-reduced metabolite of testosterone. In the male fetus, testosterone is secreted by the Leydig cells, perhaps autonomously at first and thereafter under the influence of hCG, and then by stimulation from fetal pituitary LH. Masculinization of the external genitalia and urogenital sinus of the fetus results from the action of dihydrotestosterone, which is converted from testosterone in the target cells by the enzyme 5α-reductase. Dihydrotestosterone (as well as testosterone) is bound to a specific protein receptor in the nucleus of the target cell. The transformed steroid-receptor complex dimerizes and binds with high affinity to specific DNA domains, initiating DNA-directed, RNA-mediated transcription. This results in androgen-induced proteins that lead to differentiation and growth of the cell. The gene that encodes the intracellular androgen-binding protein has been localized to the paracentromeric portion of the long arm of the X chromosome (Figure 14–4). Thus, an X-linked gene controls the androgen response of all somatic cell types by specifying the androgen receptor protein.

As in the case of the genital ducts, there is an inherent tendency for the external genitalia and urogenital sinus to develop along female lines. Differentiation of the external genitalia along male lines requires androgenic stimulation early in fetal life. The testosterone metabolite dihydrotestosterone and its specific nuclear receptor must be present to effect masculinization of the external genitalia of the fetus. Dihydrotestosterone stimulates growth of the genital tubercle, fusion of the urethral folds, and descent of the labioscrotal swellings to form the penis and scrotum. Androgens also inhibit descent and growth of the vesicovaginal septum and differentiation of the vagina. There is a critical period for action of the androgen. After about the 12th week of gestation, fusion of the labioscrotal folds will not occur even under intense androgen stimulation, although phallic growth can be induced. Incomplete masculinization of the male fetus results from (1) impairment in the synthesis or secretion of fetal testosterone or in its conversion to dihydrotestosterone, (2) deficient or defective androgen receptor activity, or (3) defective production and local action of anti-müllerian hormone. Exposure of the female fetus to abnormal amounts of androgens from either endogenous or exogenous sources, especially before the 12th week of gestation, can result in virilization of the external genitalia.

PSYCHOSEXUAL DIFFERENTIATION

Psychosexual differentiation may be classified into four broad categories: (1) gender identity, defined as the identification of self as either male or female; (2) gender role, ie, those aspects of behavior in which males and females differ from one another in our culture at this time; (3) gender orientation, the choice of sexual partner; and (4) cognitive differences.

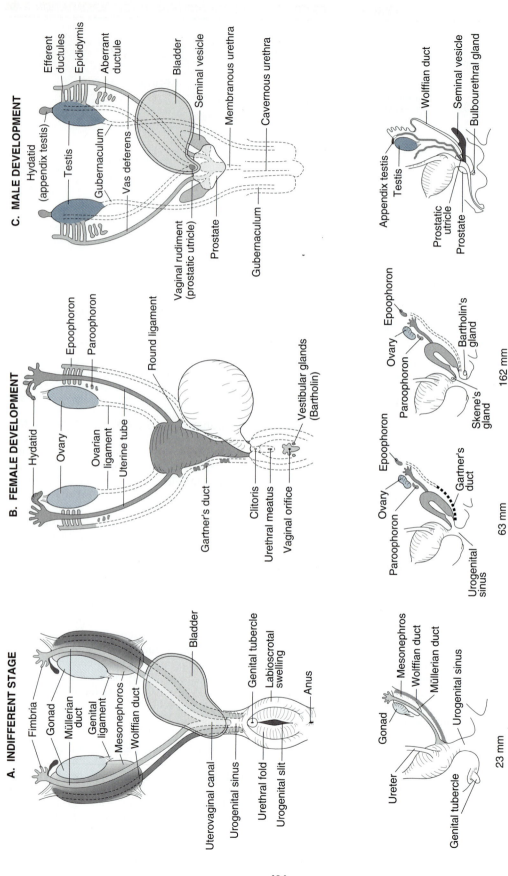

Figure 14–8. Embryonic differentiation of male and female genital ducts from wolffian and müllerian primordia. *A:* Indifferent stage showing large mesonephric body. *B:* Female ducts. Remnants of the mesonephros and wolffian ducts are now termed the epoophoron, paroophoron, and Gartner's duct. *C:* Male ducts before descent into the scrotum. The only müllerian remnant is the testicular appendix. The prostatic utricle (vagina masculina) is derived from the urogenital sinus. (Redrawn from Corning and Wilkins.)

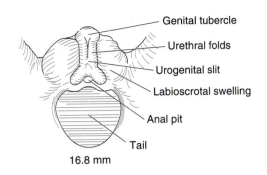

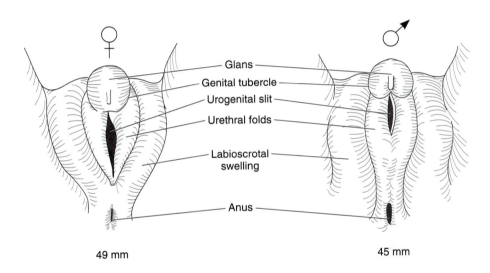

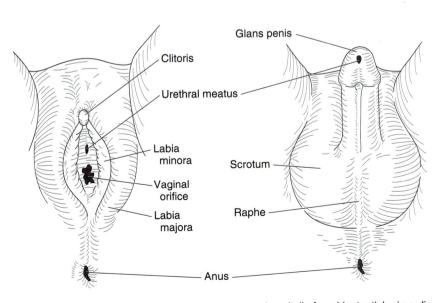

Figure 14–9. Differentiation of male and female external genitalia from bipotential primordia.

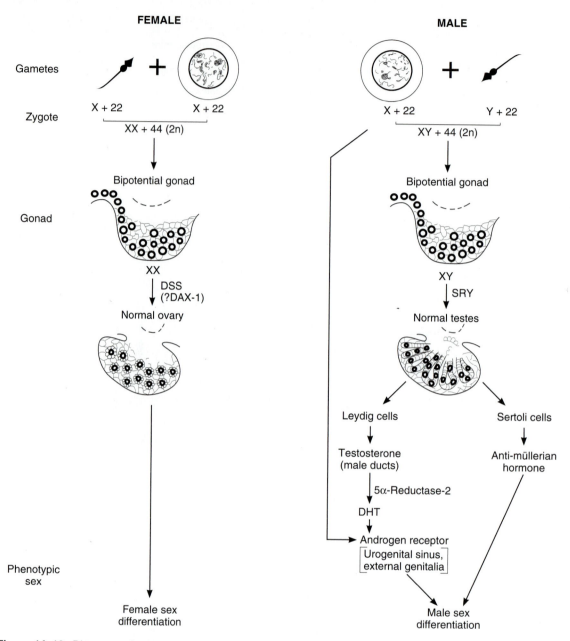

Figure 14–10. Diagrammatic summation of human sexual differentiation. (DHT, dihydrotestosterone.) (Reproduced, with permission, from Grumbach MM, Conte FA: Disorders of sex differentiation. In: *Williams Textbook of Endocrinology*, 8th ed. Wilson JD, Foster DW [editors]. Saunders, 1992.)

Studies in individuals who have been reared in a sex opposite to their chromosomal or gonadal sex, as well as prenatally androgenized females with virilizing adrenal hyperplasia, provide strong evidence that gender identity is not determined primarily by sex chromosomes or prenatal sex steroid exposure. Rather, it is imprinted postnatally by words, attitudes, and comparisons of one's body with that of others. Generally, gender identity agrees with the sex of assignment in the intersex patient, provided the child is reared *unambiguously* as a person of that gender and provided also that appropriate surgical and hormonal therapy is instituted so that the child has an unambiguous male or female phenotype. Under these circumstances, gender identity is usually established by 18–30 months of age. If, at puberty, discordant secondary sexual characteristics are allowed to develop and persist, some intersex individuals may develop doubts about their gender identity and request a change of sex. This phenomenon has been observed primarily in patients with 5α-reductase deficiency, 17β-oxidoreductase deficiency, or 45,X/46,XY mosaicism in whom androgen secretion from the retained gonad has caused virilization at puberty.

Gender identity may be more plastic than previously thought. At puberty, sex steroids as well as socialization play a role in the function and maintenance of gender identity. However, the weight of evidence still supports environmental factors as the principal determinant of gender identity in our culture.

ABNORMAL SEX DIFFERENTIATION

Classification of Errors in Sex Differentiation (Table 14–3)

Disorders of sexual differentiation are the result of abnormalities in complex processes that originate in genetic information on the X and Y chromosomes as well as on the autosomes. A true hermaphrodite is defined as a person who possesses both ovarian and testicular tissue. A male pseudohermaphrodite is one whose gonads are exclusively testes but whose genital ducts or external genitalia (or both) exhibit incomplete masculinization. A female pseudohermaphrodite is a person whose gonadal tissue is exclusively ovarian but whose genital development exhibits ambiguous or male appearance.

SEMINIFEROUS TUBULE DYSGENESIS: CHROMATIN-POSITIVE KLINEFELTER'S SYNDROME & ITS VARIANTS

Klinefelter's syndrome is one of the most common forms of primary hypogonadism and infertility in males. The invariable clinical features in adults are a male phenotype, firm testes less than 3 cm in length, and azoospermia. Gynecomastia is common. Affected patients usually have a 47,XXY sex chromosome constitution and an X chromatin-positive buccal smear, though subjects with a variety of sex chromosome constitutions, including mosaicism, have been described. Virtually all of these variants have in common the presence of at least two X chromosomes and a Y chromosome, except for the rare group in which only an XX sex chromosome complement is found.

Surveys of the prevalence of 47,XXY fetuses by karyotype analysis of unselected newborn infants indicate an incidence of about 1:1000 newborn males. Prepubertally, the disorder is characterized by small testes, disproportionately long legs, personality and behavioral disorders, and a lower mean verbal IQ score when compared with that of controls but no significant difference in full-scale IQ. Severe mental

---

Table 14–3. Classification of anomalous sexual development.

I. Disorders of gonadal differentiation
  A. Seminiferous tubule dysgenesis (Klinefelter's syndrome)
  B. Syndrome of gonadal dysgenesis and its variants (Turner's syndrome)
  C. Complete and incomplete forms of XX and XY gonadal dysgenesis
  D. True hermaphroditism

II. Female pseudohermaphroditism
  A. Congenital virilizing adrenal hyperplasia
  B. P450 aromatase (placental) deficiency
  C. Androgens and synthetic progestins transferred from maternal circulation
  D. Associated with malformations of intestine and urinary tract (non-androgen-induced female pseudohermaphroditism)
  E. Other teratologic factors

III. Male pseudohermaphroditism
  A. Testicular unresponsiveness to hCG and LH (Leydig cell agenesis or hypoplasia due to hcG/LH receptor defect)
  B. Inborn errors of testosterone biosynthesis
    1. Enzyme defects affecting synthesis of both corticosteroids and testosterone (variants of congenital adrenal hyperplasia)
      a. StAR deficiency (congenital lipoid adrenal hyperplasia)
      b. 3β-Hydroxysteroid dehydrogenase deficiency
      c. P450c17 (17α-hydroxylase) deficiency
    2. Enzyme defects primarily affecting testosterone biosynthesis by the testes
      a. P450c17 (17,20-1yase) deficiency
      b. 17β-Hydroxysteroid oxidoreductase deficiency
  C. Defects in androgen-dependent target tissues
    1. End-organ resistance to androgenic hormones (androgen receptor and postreceptor defects)
      a. Syndrome of complete androgen resistance and its variants (testicular feminization and its variant forms)
      b. Syndrome of partial androgen resistance and its variants (Reifenstein's syndrome)
      c. Androgen resistance in infertile men
      d. Androgen resistance in fertile men
    2. Defects in testosterone metabolism by peripheral tissues
      a. 5α-Reductase deficiency (pseudovaginal perineoscrotal hypospadias)
  D. Dysgenetic male pseudohermaphroditism
    1. XY gonadal dysgenesis (incomplete)
    2. XO/XY mosaicism, structurally abnormal Y chromosome, Xp+, 9p–, 10q–
    3. Denys-Drash (*WT-1* mutation)
    4. WAGR (*WT-1* deletion)
    5. Campomelic dysplasia (SOX 9 mutation)
    6. ?SF-1 mutation
    7. Testicular regression syndrome
  E. Defects in synthesis, secretion, or response to AMH
    1. Female genital ducts in otherwise normal men—"herniae uteri inguinale"; persistent müllerian duct syndrome
  F. ?Environmental chemicals

IV. Unclassified forms of abnormal sexual development
  A. In males
    1. Hypospadias
    2. Ambiguous external genitalia in 46,XY males with multiple congenital anomalies
  B. In females
    1. Absence or anomalous development of the vagina, uterus, and uterine tubes (Rokitansky-Küster syndrome)

Modified from Grumbach MM, Conte FA, Abnormalities of sex differentiation. In: *Williams Textbook of Endocrinology*, 8th ed. Wilson JD, Foster D (editors). Saunders, 1992.

retardation requiring special schooling is uncommon. Gynecomastia and other signs of androgen deficiency such as diminished facial and body hair, a small phallus, poor muscular development, and a eunuchoid body habitus occur postpubertally in affected patients. Adult males with a 47,XXY karyotype tend to be taller than average, with adult height close to the 75th percentile, mainly because of the disproportionate length of their legs. Untreated adult males are at increased risk for the development of osteoporosis. They also have an increased incidence of mild diabetes mellitus, varicose veins, stasis dermatitis, cerebrovascular disease, chronic pulmonary disease, and carcinoma of the breast; the incidence of breast carcinoma in patients with Klinefelter's syndrome is 20 times higher than that in normal men. Patients with Klinefelter's syndrome often have a delay in the onset of adolescence. There is an increased risk for developing malignant extragonadal germ cell tumors, including central nervous system germinomas and mediastinal tumors, which may be hCG-secreting and cause sexual precocity in the prepubertal patient.

The testicular lesion is progressive and gonadotropin-dependent. It is characterized in the adult by extensive seminiferous tubular hyalinization and fibrosis, absent or severely deficient spermatogenesis, and pseudoadenomatous clumping of the Leydig cells. Although hyalinization of the tubules is usually extensive, it varies considerably from patient to patient and even between testes in the same patient. Azoospermia is the rule, and patients who have been reported to be fertile invariably have been 46,XY/47,XXY mosaics.

Nondisjunction during the first or second meiotic division of gametogenesis plays an important role in the genesis of a 47,XXY karyotype. Fifty-three percent of cases appear to result from paternal nondisjunction at the first meiotic division, 34% from meiotic nondisjunction during the first maternal meiotic division, and 9% from nondisjunction at the second meiotic division. Only 3% of patients appear to have arisen from postzygotic meiotic nondisjunction.

The diagnosis of Klinefelter's syndrome is suggested by the classic phenotype and hormonal changes. It is confirmed by the finding of an X chromatin-positive buccal smear and demonstration of a 47,XXY karyotype in blood, skin, or gonads. After puberty, levels of serum and urinary gonadotropins (especially FSH) are raised. The testosterone production rate, the total and free levels of testosterone, and the metabolic clearance rates of testosterone and estradiol tend to be low, while plasma estradiol levels are normal or high. Testicular biopsy reveals the classic findings of hyalinization of the seminiferous tubules, severe deficiency of spermatogonia, and pseudoadenomatous clumping of Leydig cells.

Treatment of patients with Klinefelter's syndrome is directed toward androgen replacement, especially in patients in whom puberty is delayed or fails to progress or in those who have subnormal testosterone levels for age and developmental stage. Testosterone therapy may help to enhance secondary sexual characteristics and sexual performance, prevent osteoporosis, prevent or cause regression of gynecomastia, and improve general well-being in most patients. If testosterone deficiency is present, testosterone therapy early in adolescence should commence with 50 mg of testosterone enanthate in oil intramuscularly every 4 weeks, gradually increasing to the adult replacement dose of 200 mg every 2 weeks. A marked decrease in gynecomastia may result from testosterone therapy; however, once advanced, gynecomastia may not be amenable to hormone therapy but can be surgically corrected if it is severe or psychologically disturbing to the patient. Early diagnosis, support, and appropriate counseling may improve the overall prognosis. (See also Chapter 12.)

Variants of Chromatin-Positive Seminiferous Tubule Dysgenesis

A. Variants of Klinefelter's Syndrome: Variants of Klinefelter's syndrome include 46,XY/47,XXY mosaics as well as patients with multiple X and Y chromosomes. With increasing numbers of X chromosomes in the genome, both mental retardation and other developmental anomalies such as radioulnar synostosis become prevalent.

B. 46,XX Males: Phenotypic males with a 46,XX karyotype have been described since 1964; the incidence of 46,XX males is approximately 1:20,000 births. In general, these individuals have a male phenotype, male psychosocial gender identity, and testes with histologic features similar to those observed in patients with a 47,XXY karyotype. At least 10% of patients have hypospadias or ambiguous external genitalia. XX males have normal body proportions and a mean final height that is shorter than that of patients with an XXY sex chromosome constitution or normal males but taller than that of normal females. As in XXY patients, testosterone levels are low or low normal, gonadotropins are elevated, and spermatogenesis is impaired postpubertally. Gynecomastia is present in approximately one-third of cases.

The presence of testes and male sexual differentiation in 46,XX individuals has been a perplexing problem. However, the paradox has been clarified by the use of recombinant DNA studies. Males with a 46,XX karyotype have been shown by genetic linkage studies and X chromosome restriction fragment length polymorphisms (RFLPs) to possess one X chromosome from each of their parents. Approximately 80% of XX males have a Y chromosome-specific DNA segment from the distal portion of the Y short arm translocated to the distal portion of the short arm of the paternal X chromosome. This translocated segment is heterologous in length but always includes the *SRY* gene, which codes for TDF as well as the pseudoautosomal region of the Y chromosome. Thus, in 80% of XX males, an abnormal X-Y terminal exchange during paternal meiosis, has resulted in two products: an X chromosome with an *SRY* gene and a Y chromosome deficient in this gene (the latter would result in a female with XY gonadal dysgenesis). Fewer than 20% of XX males tested have been shown to lack Y chromosome-specific DNA sequences, including the *SRY* gene and the pseudoautosomal region of the Y chromosome. These XX, Y, DNA-negative males tend to have hypospadias and may have relatives with true hermaphroditism.

The finding of XX males who lack any evidence of Y chromosome-specific genes suggests that testicular determination—and, thus, male differentiation—can occur in the absence of a gene or genes from the Y chromosome. This could be a result of (1) mutation of a "downstream" autosomal gene involved in male sex determination; or (2) mutation, deletion, or aberrant inactivation of a gene sequence on the X chromosome, critical to testis determination and differentiation; or (3) circumscribed Y chromosome mosaicism (eg, occurring only in the gonads). Further studies will be necessary to elucidate the pathogenesis of male sex determination and differentiation in those 46,XX males who lack ascertainable Y-to-X chromosome translocations.

SYNDROME OF GONADAL DYSGENESIS: TURNER'S SYNDROME & ITS VARIANTS

Turner's Syndrome: 45,X Gonadal Dysgenesis

One in 5000 newborn females has a 45,X or XO sex chromosome constitution. It has been estimated that 99% of 45,X fetuses do not survive beyond 28 weeks of gestation, and 15% of all first-trimester abortuses have a 45,X karyotype. In about 70–80% of instances, the origin of the normal X chromosome is maternal. Patients with a 45,X karyotype represent approximately 50% of all patients with X chromosome abnormalities. The cardinal features of 45,X gonadal dysgenesis are a variety of somatic anomalies, sexual infantilism at puberty secondary to gonadal dysgenesis, and short stature. Patients with a 45,X karyotype can be recognized in infancy, usually because of lymphedema of the extremities and loose skin folds over the nape of the neck. In later life, the typical patient is often recognizable by her distinctive facies in which micrognathia, epicanthal folds, prominent low-set ears, a fish-like mouth, and ptosis are present to varying degrees. The chest is shield-like and the neck short, broad, and webbed (40% of patients). Additional anomalies associated with Turner's syndrome include coarctation of the aorta (10%), hypertension, renal abnormalities (50%), pigmented nevi, cubitus valgus, a tendency to keloid formation,

puffiness of the dorsum of the hands and feet, short fourth metacarpals and metatarsals, Madelung deformity of the wrist, scoliosis, and recurrent otitis media, which may lead to conductive hearing loss. Routine intravenous urography or renal sonography is indicated for all patients to rule out a surgically correctable renal abnormality. The internal ducts as well as the external genitalia of these patients are invariably female except in rare patients with a 45,X karyotype, in whom a Y-to-autosome or Y-to-X chromosome translocation has been found.

Short stature is an invariable feature of the syndrome of gonadal dysgenesis. Mean final height in 45,X patients is 143 cm, with a range of 133–153 cm. Current data suggest that the short stature found in patients with the syndrome of gonadal dysgenesis is not due to a deficiency of growth hormone, somatomedin, sex steroids, or thyroid hormone. However, administration of high-dose biosynthetic human growth hormone results in an apparent increase in final height (see Chapter 6).

Gonadal dysgenesis is another feature of patients with a 45,X chromosome constitution. The gonads are typically streak-like and usually contain only fibrous stroma arranged in whorls. Longitudinal studies of both basal and GnRH-evoked gonadotropin secretion in patients with gonadal dysgenesis indicate a lack of feedback inhibition of the hypothalamic-pituitary axis by the dysgenetic gonads in affected infants and children (Figure 14–11). Thus, plasma and urinary gonadotropin levels, particularly FSH levels, are high during early infancy and after 9–10 years of age. Since ovarian function is impaired, puberty does not usually ensue spontaneously; hence, sexual infantilism is a hallmark of this syndrome. Rarely, patients with a 45,X karyotype may undergo spontaneous pubertal maturation, menarche, and pregnancy.

A variety of disorders are associated with this syndrome, including obesity, osteoporosis, diabetes mellitus, Hashimoto's thyroiditis, rheumatoid arthritis, inflammatory bowel disease, intestinal telangiectasia with bleeding, and anorexia nervosa. Because an increased prevalence of bicuspid aortic valve and aortic dilation with aneurysm formation and rupture has been reported in patients with Turner's syndrome, echocardiography is indicated in all patients with a 45,X cell line.

Phenotypic females with the following features should have a karyotype analysis: (1) short stature (> 2.5 SD below the mean value for age); (2) somatic anomalies associated with the syndrome of gonadal dysgenesis; and (3) delayed adolescence with an increased level of plasma FSH.

Therapy should be directed toward maximizing final height and inducing secondary sexual characteristics and menarche at an age commensurate with that of normal peers. The results of recent clinical trials suggest that patients treated with recombinant growth hormone (0.375 mg/kg/wk divided into seven once-

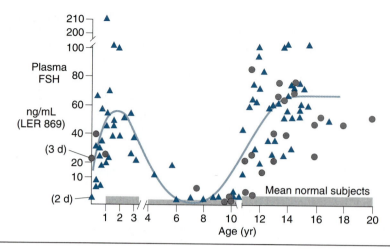

Figure 14–11. Diphasic variation in basal levels of plasma FSH (ng/mL-LER 869) in patients with a 45,X karyotype (solid triangles) and patients with structural abnormalities of the X chromosome and mosaics (solid circles). Note that mean basal levels of plasma FSH in patients with gonadal dysgenesis are in the castrate range before 4 years and after 10 years of age. (Reproduced, with permission, from Conte FA, Grumbach MM, Kaplan SL: A diphasic pattern of gonadotropin secretion in patients with the syndrome of gonadal dysgenesis. J Clin Endocrinol Metab 1975;40:670.)

daily doses), with or without oxandrolone (0.0625 mg/kg/d by mouth), had an increase in growth rate that was sustained and resulted in a mean 8–10 cm increase in height after 3–7 years of therapy. Before initiation of growth hormone therapy, a thorough analysis of the costs, benefits, and possible side effects must be discussed with the parents and the child. Long-term studies with low-dose estrogen therapy have not demonstrated a significant positive effect on final height in girls with Turner's syndrome. No synergistic effect of combined estrogen and growth hormone therapy on final height has been found. In patients who have been treated with growth hormone and have achieved an acceptable height and in those who have refused growth hormone therapy, estrogen replacement therapy is usually initiated at 12–13 years of age. Conjugated estrogens (0.3 mg or less) or ethinyl estradiol (5 μg) are given orally for the first 21 days of the calendar month. Thereafter, the dose of estrogen is gradually increased over the next several years to 0.6–1.25 mg of conjugated estrogens or 10 μg of ethinyl estradiol daily for the first 21 days of the month. The minimum dose of estrogen necessary to maintain secondary sexual characteris-

tics and menses and prevent osteoporosis should be administered. After the first year of estrogen therapy, medroxyprogesterone acetate, 5 mg daily, or a comparable progestin is given on the 10th–21st days of the menstrual cycle to ensure physiologic menses and to reduce the risk of endometrial carcinoma, which is associated with unopposed estrogen stimulation. (See also Chapter 13.)

X Chromatin-Positive Variants of the Syndrome of Gonadal Dysgenesis

Patients with structural abnormalities of the X chromosome (deletions and additions) and sex chromosome mosaicism with a 45,X cell line may manifest the somatic as well as the gonadal features of the syndrome of gonadal dysgenesis (Table 14–4). Evidence suggests that genes on both the long and short arms of the X chromosome control gonadal differentiation, whereas genes primarily on the short arms of the X prevent the short stature and somatic anomalies that are seen in 45,X patients (Figure 14–4). In general, 45,X/46,XX mosaicism will modify the 45,X phenotype toward normal and can even result in nor-

Table 14–4. Relationship of structural abnormalities of the X and Y to clinical manifestations of the syndrome of gonadal dysgenesis.

Type of Sex Chromosome Abnormality	Karyotype	Phenotype	Sexual Infantilism	Short Stature	Somatic Anomalies of Turner's Syndrome
Loss of an X or Y	45,X	Female	+	+	+
Deletion of short arm of an X[1]	46,XXqi	Female	+ (occ. ±)	+	+
	46,XXp–	Female	+, ±, or –	+ (–)	+ (–)
Deletion of long arm of an X[1]	46,XXq–	Female	+	– (+)	– (±)
Deletion of ends of both arms of an X[2]	46,XXr	Female	– or +	+	+ or (±)
Deletion of short arm of Y	46,XYp–	Female	+	+	+

[1]In Xp and Xq–, the extent and site of the deleted segment are variable.
Xqi = Isochromosome for long arm of an X; Xp– = deletion of short arm of an X; Xq– = deletion of long arm of an X; Xr = ring chromosome derived from an X.
[2]Patients with small ring X chromosomes can have mental retardation and somatic abnormalities not usually associated with the Turner phenotype due to noninactivation of genes on the small ring X chromosome.

mal gonadal function. Some patients with mosaicism and a 45,X/46,Xr(X) karyotype may manifest mental retardation and congenital anomalies not usually associated with Turner's syndrome. Recent data indicate that these abnormalities are related to lack of inactivation of small ring X chromosomes and, hence, functional disomy for genes on the ring X chromosome and the normal X chromosome.

X Chromatin-Negative Variants of the Syndrome of Gonadal Dysgenesis

These patients usually have mosaicism with a 45,X and a Y-bearing cell line—45,X/46,XY; 45,X/47,XXY; 45,X/46,XY/47,XYY—or perhaps a structurally abnormal Y chromosome. They range from phenotypic females with the features of Turner's syndrome through patients with ambiguous genitalia to completely virilized males with few stigmas of Turner's syndrome. The variations in gonadal differentiation range from bilateral streaks to bilateral dysgenetic testes to apparently "normal" testes, and there may be asymmetric development, ie, a streak on one side and a dysgenetic testicle or, rarely, a normal testis on the other side—sometimes called "mixed gonadal dysgenesis." The development of the external genitalia and of the internal ducts correlates with the degree of testicular differentiation and, presumably, the capacity of the fetal testes to secrete anti-müllerian hormone and testosterone.

The risk of development of gonadal tumors is greatly increased in patients with 45,X/46,XY mosaicism and streak or dysgenetic gonads; hence, prophylactic removal of streak gonads or dysgenetic undescended testes in this syndrome is indicated. Breast development at or after the age of puberty in these patients is commonly associated with a gonadal neoplasm, usually a gonadoblastoma. Pelvic sonography, CT scanning, or MRI may be useful in screening for neoplasms in these patients. Gonadoblastomas are calcified and so may be visible even on a plain film of the abdomen.

The diagnosis of 45,X/46,XY mosaicism can be established by the demonstration of both 45,X and 46,XY cells in blood, skin, or gonadal tissue. In some mosaics, a "marker" chromosome is found that is cytogenetically indistinguishable as X or Y. In these cases, either FISH or molecular analyses with X- and Y-specific probes is indicated to definitively determine the origin of the marker chromosome, since gonadoblastomas have been reported in patients with deleted Y chromosomes—even those with deletions of the *SRY* gene. The decision regarding the sex of rearing should be based on the age at diagnosis and the potential for normal function of the external genitalia. Most patients with 45,X/46,XY mosaicism ascertained by amniocentesis have normal male genitalia and normal testicular histology. Thus, the ambiguity of the genitalia invariably described in

patients with 45,X/46,XY mosaicism is due to ascertainment bias. We have observed a short, 30-year-old male with documented 45,X/46,XY mosaicism who has normal male genitalia and is fertile.

In patients assigned a female gender role, the gonads should be removed and the external genitalia repaired as soon as possible. Estrogen therapy should be initiated at the age of puberty, as in patients with a 45,X karyotype (see above). In affected infants who are assigned a male gender role, all gonadal tissue except that which appears histologically normal and is in the scrotum should be removed. Removal of the müllerian structures and repair of hypospadias are also indicated. At puberty, depending on the functional integrity of the retained gonads, androgen replacement therapy may be indicated in doses similar to those for patients with the incomplete form of XY gonadal dysgenesis. In patients with retained scrotal testes, a repeat gonadal biopsy is indicated postpubertally to rule out the possibility of carcinoma in situ, a premalignant lesion (see below).

In infants and children with 45,X/46,XY mosaicism who have normal genitalia, and normal testicular integrity as assessed by gonadotropin levels and pelvic MRI, gonadal biopsy may be deferred until adolescence. The risk of gonadal malignancies in males with 45,X/46,XY mosaicism who have normal male genitalia and histologically and functionally normal testes in the scrotum is still to be ascertained.

46,XX & 46,XY GONADAL DYSGENESIS

The terms XX and XY gonadal dysgenesis have been applied to 46,XX or 46,XY patients who have bilateral streak gonads, a female phenotype, and no somatic stigmas of Turner's syndrome. After the age of puberty, these patients exhibit sexual infantilism, castrate levels of plasma and urinary gonadotropins, normal or tall stature, and eunuchoid proportions.

46,XX Gonadal Dysgenesis

Familial and sporadic cases of XX gonadal dysgenesis have been reported with an incidence as high as 1:8300 females in Finland. Pedigree analysis of familial cases is consistent with autosomal recessive inheritance.

Analysis of familial cases in Finland revealed that a locus on chromosome 2p was linked to XX gonadal dysgenesis in females. The gene for the follicle-stimulating hormone receptor has been localized to chromosome 2p. Analysis of this gene revealed a mutation in exon 7 of the FSH receptor which segregated with XX gonadal dysgenesis. This mutation affected the extracellular ligand-binding domain of the FSH receptor and reduced the binding capacity of the receptor and consequently signal transduction, resulting in "streak ovaries" and hypergonadotropic hypogonadism in XX females at puberty. Preliminary data suggests that males homozygous for this mutation are phenotypically normal, with spermatogenesis varying from normal to absent.

Studies of familial cohorts have revealed apparent marked heterogeneity in pathogenesis. Siblings, one with a 46,XX karyotype and the other with a 46,XY karyotype, both with gonadal "agenesis," have been reported, supporting the involvement of an autosomal gene in this family. However, in view of the normal phenotype in XY males observed with a mutation in the FSH receptor, it seems unlikely that these patients have an FSH receptor defect. Rather, they may have a mutation in an autosomal recessive gene involved in gonadal determination. In one family, four affected women had an inherited interstitial deletion of the long arm of the X chromosome involving the q21–q27 region. This region seems to contain a gene or genes "critical" to ovarian development and function. In three families, XX gonadal dysgenesis was associated with deafness of the sensorineural type. In several affected groups of siblings, a spectrum of clinical findings occurred, eg, varying degrees of ovarian function, including breast development and menses followed by secondary amenorrhea. In contrast to Turner's syndrome, stature is normal. The diagnosis of 46,XX gonadal dysgenesis should be suspected in phenotypic females with sexual infantilism and normal müllerian structures who lack the somatic stigmas of the syndrome of gonadal dysgenesis (Turner's syndrome). Karyotype analysis reveals only 46,XX cells. As in Turner's syndrome, gonadotropin levels are high, estrogen levels are low, and treatment consists of cyclic estrogen and progesterone replacement.

Sporadic cases of XX gonadal dysgenesis, similar to familial cases, may represent a heterogeneous group of patients from a pathogenetic point of view. XX gonadal dysgenesis should be distinguished from ovarian failure due to infections such as mumps, antibodies to gonadotropin receptors, biologically inactive FSH, gonadotropin-insensitive ovaries, and galactosemia as well as errors in steroid (estrogen) biosynthesis. In the latter group, ultrasound or MRI should reveal polycystic ovaries.

46,XY Gonadal Dysgenesis

46,XY gonadal dysgenesis occurs both sporadically and in familial aggregates. Patients with the complete form of this syndrome have female external genitalia, normal or tall stature, bilateral streak gonads, müllerian duct development, sexual infantilism, eunuchoid habitus and a 46,XY karyotype. Clitoromegaly is quite common, and, in familial cases, a continuum of involvement ranging from the complete syndrome to ambiguity of the external genitalia has been described. The phenotypic difference between the complete and incomplete forms of XY gonadal dysgenesis is due to the degree of differentiation of testicular tissue and the functional capacity of the fetal testis to produce testosterone and anti-müllerian hormone. Early in infancy and after the age of puberty, plasma and urinary gonadotropin levels are markedly elevated.

Analysis of familial and sporadic cases of 46,XY gonadal dysgenesis indicates that about 15–20% of patients have a mutation in the HMG box of the SRY gene that affects DNA binding and/or bending by the SRY protein. So far, all patients in whom mutations have been detected have had "complete" gonadal dysgenesis. Patients with large deletions of the short arm of the Y chromosome may have, in addition to gonadal dysgenesis, stigmas of Turner's syndrome. Mutations outside the HMG box region of the SRY gene as well as in X-linked or autosomal genes may be responsible for those patients in whom no molecular abnormality has as yet been found. A mutation in the HMG box of the SRY gene has been described in three normal 46,XY fathers and their "daughters" with 46,XY gonadal dysgenesis. These three familial cohorts suggest that these mutations may affect either the level or the timing of SRY expression and in this manner result in either normal or abnormal testicular differentiation.

Approximately 20 patients with 46,XY gonadal dysgenesis have been reported with a duplication of the Xp21.2 → p22.11 region of the X chromosome. This region contains two overlapping loci: a locus for X-linked congenital hypoplasia with a gene called DAX-1 and another locus called DSS (dosage-sensitive sex reversal). Deletion of the DSS locus in 46,XY males with adrenal hypoplasia and hypogonadotrophic hypogonadism, and normal sex differentiation suggests that it is not required for testicular differentiation; duplicating the locus, however, impairs testes differentiation. Thus, it appears that one or more genes in the DSS locus function in the gonadal differentiation pathway; they have been postulated to be ovarian differentiation genes which, when duplicated in a 46,XY individual, result in gonadal dysgenesis and consequent sex reversal.

XY gonadal dysgenesis associated with campomelic dysplasia is due to a mutation of one allelle of an SRY-related gene, SOX 9 on chromosome 17. In addition, XY gonadal dysgenesis has been associated with 9p– and 10q– deletions, which suggests the presence of other autosomal genes that affect testicular morphogenesis.

Therapy for patients with 46,XY gonadal dysgenesis who have female external genitalia involves prophylactic gonadectomy at diagnosis and estrogen substitution at puberty. In the incomplete form of XY gonadal dysgenesis, assignment of a male gender role may be possible. It depends upon the degree of ambiguity of the genitalia and the potential for normal sexual function. Prophylactic gonadectomy must be considered, since fertility is unlikely and there is an increased risk of malignant transformation of the dysgenetic gonads in these patients. Biopsy of all retained gonads should be done pre- and postpubertally in order to detect early malignant changes (carcinoma in situ). In affected individuals raised as males, prosthetic testes should be implanted at the time of gonadectomy, and androgen substitution therapy is instituted at the age of puberty. Testosterone enanthate in oil (or another long-acting testosterone ester) is used, beginning with 50 mg intramuscularly every 4 weeks and gradually increasing over 3–4 years to a full replacement dose of 200 mg intramuscularly every 2 weeks.

TRUE HERMAPHRODITISM

In true hermaphroditism, both ovarian and testicular tissue are present in one or both gonads. Differentiation of the internal and external genitalia is highly variable. The external genitalia may simulate those of a male or female, but most often they are ambiguous. Cryptorchidism and hypospadias are common. A testis or ovotestis, if present, is located in the labioscrotal folds in one-third of patients, in the inguinal canal in one-third, and in the abdomen in the remainder. A uterus is usually present, though it may be hypoplastic or unicornuate. The differentiation of the genital ducts usually follows that of the ipsilateral gonad. The ovotestis is the most common gonad found in true hermaphrodites (60%), followed by the ovary and, least commonly, by the testis. At puberty, breast development is usual in untreated patients, and menses occur in over 50% of cases. Whereas the ovary or the ovarian portion of an ovotestis may function normally, the testis or testicular portion of an ovotestis is almost always dysgenetic.

Sixty percent of true hermaphrodites have been reported to have a 46,XX karyotype, 20% 46,XY, and about 20% mosaicism or 46,XX/46,XY chimerism. 46,XX true hermaphroditism appears to be a genetically heterogeneous entity. A small proportion of 46,XX true hermaphrodites, including some in family cohorts with 46,XX males, have been reported to be SRY-positive. Hence, Y-to-X and Y-to-autosome translocations, hidden sex chromosome mosaicism, or chimerism can explain the pathogenesis in these patients. The majority of 46,XX true hermaphrodites, however, are SRY-negative. A number of families have been reported which had both SRY-negative 46,XX males and 46,XX true hermaphrodites. This latter observation suggests a common genetic pathogenesis in these patients. Possible genetic mechanisms to explain SRY-negative true hermaphroditism include (1) mutation of a downstream autosomal gene or genes involved in testicular determination; (2) mutation, deletion, duplication, or anomalous inactivation of an X-linked locus involved in testes determination; or (3) circumscribed chimerism or mosaicism that occurred only in the gonads.

The diagnosis of true hermaphroditism should be considered in all patients with ambiguous genitalia. The finding of a 46,XX/46,XY karyotype or a bilobate gonad compatible with an ovotestis in the inguinal region or labioscrotal folds suggests the diagnosis. Basal plasma testosterone levels are elevated above 40 ng/dL in affected patients under 6 months of age, and testosterone levels increase after hCG stimulation. If all other forms of male and female pseudohermaphroditism have been excluded, laparotomy and histologic confirmation of both ovarian and testicular tissue establish the diagnosis. The management of true hermaphroditism is contingent upon the age at diagnosis and a careful assessment of the functional capacity of the gonads, genital ducts, and external genitalia. In general, true hermaphrodites should be raised as females, with the possible exception of the well-virilized patient in whom no uterus is found.

Gonadal Neoplasms in Dysgenetic Gonads

While gonadal tumors are rare in patients with 47,XXY Klinefelter's syndrome and 45,X gonadal dysgenesis, the prevalence of gonadal neoplasms is greatly increased in patients with certain types of dysgenetic gonads. The frequency is increased in 45,X/46,XY mosaicism, especially in those with female or ambiguous genitalia; in patients with a structurally abnormal Y chromosome; and in those with XY gonadal dysgenesis, either with a female phenotype or with ambiguous genitalia. Gonadoblastomas, germinomas, seminomas, and teratomas are found most frequently. Prophylactic gonadectomy is advised in these patients as well as in those with gonadal dysgenesis who manifest signs of virilization, regardless of karyotype. Gonadoblastomas have been reported in patients with "marker" chromosomes of Y origin lacking the SRY gene. The testis should be preserved in patients who are to be raised as males only if it is histologically normal and is or can be situated in the scrotum. The fact that a testis is palpable in the scrotum does not preclude malignant degeneration and tumor dissemination, as seminomas tend to metastasize at an early stage before a mass is obvious. If a testis is preserved in the scrotum in a patient with 45,X/46XY mosaicism or in rare cases of true hermaphroditism, it is prudent to follow the patient closely with sonography or pelvic MRI and a biopsy postpubertally in order to monitor for the development of a premalignant or malignant lesion.

FEMALE PSEUDOHERMAPHRODITISM

Affected individuals have normal ovaries and müllerian derivatives associated with ambiguous external genitalia. In the absence of testes, a female fetus will be masculinized if subjected to increased circulating levels of androgens derived from a fetal or maternal source. The degree of masculinization depends upon

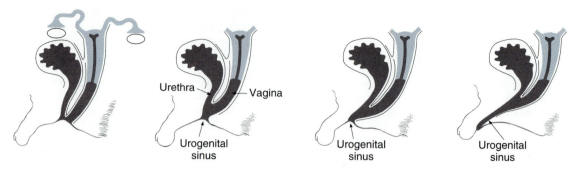

Figure 14–12. Female pseudohermaphroditism induced by prenatal exposure to androgens. Exposure after the 12th fetal week leads only to clitoral hypertrophy (diagram at left). Exposure at progressively earlier stages of differentiation (depicted from left to right in drawings) leads to retention of the urogenital sinus and labioscrotal fusion. If exposure occurs sufficiently early, the labia will fuse to form a penile urethra. (Reproduced, with permission, from Grumbach MM, Ducharme J: The effects of androgens on fetal sexual development: Androgen-induced female pseudohermaphroditism. Fertil Steril 1960;11:757.)

the stage of differentiation at the time of exposure (Figure 14–12). After 12 weeks of gestation, androgens will produce only clitoral hypertrophy. Rarely, ambiguous genitalia that superficially resemble those produced by androgens are the result of other teratogenic factors.

Congenital Adrenal Hyperplasia (Figure 14–13)

There are six major types of congenital adrenal hyperplasia (CAH), all transmitted as autosomal recessive disorders. The common denominator of all six types is a defect in the synthesis of cortisol that results in an increase in ACTH and consequently in adrenal hyperplasia. Both males and females can be affected, but males are rarely diagnosed at birth unless they have ambiguous genitalia, are salt losers and manifest adrenal crises, are identified during newborn screening, or are at known risk because they have an affected sibling. Defects of types I–III are confined to the adrenal gland and produce virilization. Defects of types IV–VI have in common blocks in cortisol and sex steroid synthesis in both the adrenals and the gonads. The latter three types produce chiefly incomplete masculinization in the male and little or no virilization in the female (Table 14–5). Consequently, these will be discussed primarily as forms of male pseudohermaphroditism. (See also Chapters 9, 12, and 13.)

P450c21 Hydroxylase Deficiency

21-Hydroxylase activity in mediated by P450c21, a microsomal cytochrome P450 enzyme. A deficiency of this enzyme results in the most common type of adrenal hyperplasia, with an overall prevalence of 1:14,000 live births in Caucasians. Over 95% of patients with CAH have 21-hydroxylase deficiency. The locus for the gene that encodes for 21-hydroxylation is on the short arm of chromosome 6, close to the locus for C4 (complement) between HLA-B and HLA-D. DNA analysis has detected two genes, designated *P450c21A* and *P450c21B*, in this region in tandem with the two genes for complement, *C4A* and *C4B*. *P450c21A* is a nonfunctional "pseudogene," ie, it is missing critical sequences and does not code for a functional 21-hydroxylase. Patients with P450c21B (21α-hydroxylase) deficiency have either a point mutation, a deletion, or a "gene conversion" (the transfer of nonfunctioning sequences from the *21-OHA* gene to the *21-OHB* gene) in the *P450c21B* gene. Seventy-five percent of patients with "classic" P450c21 deficiency have point mutations which change a small portion of the *P450c21B* to a sequence similar to that in the nonfunctional *P450c21A* gene—hence a "microgene conversion." The remainder have gene deletions and macrogene conversions. Recent work has demonstrated that classic salt-wasting 21-hydroxylase deficiency is associated with a mutation, deletion, or gene conversion that abolishes or severely reduces 21-hydroxylase activity. Most patients with 21-hydroxylase deficiency are compound heterozygotes, ie, they have a different genetic lesion in each of their *P450c21B* allelic genes. The phenotypic spectrum observed—salt loss, simple virilization, or late onset of virilization—is a consequence of the degree of enzymatic deficiency. The latter is determined by the functionally less severely mutated *P450c21B* allele. The gene for P450c21 (21-hydroxylase) deficiency is not only closely linked to the HLA supergene complex, but certain specific HLA subtypes are found to be statistically increased in patients with 21-hydroxylase deficiency. These include Bw51 in the simple virilizing form, Bw47 in the salt-losing form, and B14 in the nonclassic form.

A. Type I—P450c21 Hydroxylase Deficiency With Virilization: This defect in P450c21 (21-hydroxylase) activity results in impaired cortisol synthesis, increased ACTH levels, and increased adrenal androgen precursor and androgen secretion. Prior to

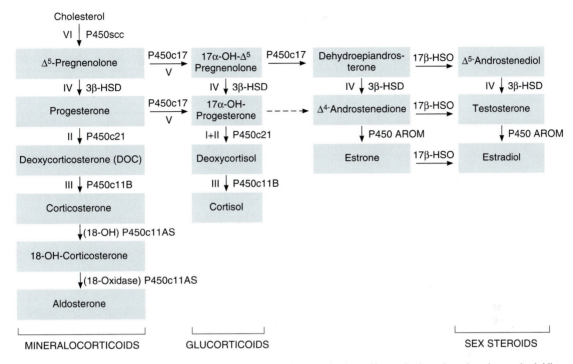

Figure 14–13. A diagrammatic representation of the steroid biosynthetic pathways in the adrenal and gonads. I–VI correspond to enzymes whose deficiency results in congenital adrenal hyperplasia. (OH, hydroxy or hydroxylase; 3β-HSD, 3β-hydroxysteroid dehydrogenase and Δ^5-isomerase; 17β-HSO, 17β-hydroxysteroid oxidoreductase (dehydrogenase); P450scc, cholesterol side-chain cleavage, previously termed 20,22 desmolase; P450c21, 21-hydroxylase; P450c17, 17-hydroxylase; P450arom, aromatase. P450c17 also mediates 17,20-lyase activity; P450c11AS (allosterone synthetase) mediates 18-hydroxylase and 18-oxidase reactions; P450c11B mediates 11-hydroxylation of deoxycortisol to cortisol and DOC to corticosterone. The dashed arrow indicates that this reaction may not occur in humans. (See also Figures 9–4, 12–2, and 13–4.) (Modified and reproduced, with permission, from Conte FA, Grumbach MM: Pathogenesis, classification, diagnosis, and treatment of anomalies of sex. In: *Endocrinology*. DeGroot L [editor]. Grune & Stratton, 1989.)

12 weeks of gestation, high fetal androgen levels lead to a varying degree of labioscrotal fusion and clitoral enlargement in the female fetus; exposure to androgen after 12 weeks induces clitoromegaly alone. In the male fetus, no abnormalities in the external genitalia are evident at birth, but the phallus may be enlarged. These patients produce sufficient amounts of aldosterone to prevent the signs and symptoms of mineralocorticoid deficiency, though they may have a defect in mineralocorticoid synthesis as evidenced by an elevated plasma renin level. Virilization continues after birth in untreated patients. This results in rapid growth and bone maturation as well as the physical signs of excess androgen secretion (eg, acne, seborrhea, increased muscular development, premature development of pubic or axillary hair, and phallic enlargement). True (central) precocious puberty can occur following initiation of glucocorticoid therapy in affected children with peripubertal bone ages.

Mild defects in P450c21 (21-hydroxylase) activity have been reported. Patients can be symptomatic (late-onset or nonclassic) or asymptomatic ("cryptic"

form). These mild forms of P450c21 hydroxylase deficiency are HLA-linked, as is "classic" P450c21 hydroxylase deficiency; however, they occur much more frequently than the classic form of the disease. It has been postulated that "nonclassic" P450c21 hydroxylase deficiency is the most common autosomal recessive disorder, affecting about one in 100 persons of all ethnic groups but having an incidence two to three times higher in Hispanics and Ashkenazi Jews. Females with late-onset P450c21 hydroxylase deficiency have normal female genitalia at birth and do not have an electrolyte abnormality. Mild virilization occurs later in childhood and adolescence, resulting in the premature development of pubic or axillary hair, slight clitoral enlargement, menstrual irregularities, acne, hirsutism, polycystic ovary syndrome, and an advanced bone age. Affected males have normal male genitalia at birth, rapid growth, and advanced skeletal maturation. Later in childhood, they exhibit premature growth of pubic or axillary hair, sexual precocity with inappropriately small testes, and increased muscular development. While tall as children, they end up as short adults due to ad-

Table 14–5. Clinical manifestations of the various types of congenital adrenal hyperplasia.

Enzymatic Defect	StAR[1]		3β-Hydroxysteroid Dehydrogenase		P-450c17 (17α-Hydroxylase)		P-450c11 (11β-Hydroxylase)		P-450c21 (21α-Hydroxylase)	
Type	VI		IV		V		III		II and I	
Chromosomal	XX	XY	XX	XY	XX	XY	XX	XY	XX	XY
External genitalia	Female	Female	Female (clitori-megaly)[1]	Ambig-uous	Female	Female or am-biguous	Ambig-uous[2]	Male	Ambig-uous[1]	Male
Postnatal virilization	– (Sexual infantilism at puberty)		±	Mild to moder-ate	– (Sexual infantilism at puberty)		+		+	
Addisonian crises	+		±		–		–		+ in 80% (type II)	
Hypertension	–		–		+		+		–	

[1]StAR: Steroidogenic acute regulatory protein. StAR deficiency leads secondarily to P450scc deficiency.
[2]Normal female in late-onset and "cryptic" forms.

vanced bone maturation and premature epiphysial fusion. Asymptomatic individuals who have the same biochemical abnormalities as patients with mild forms of P450c21 hydroxylase deficiency have been detected by hormonal testing of families in which there is at least one member with symptoms.

B. P450c21 Hydroxylase Deficiency With Virilization and Salt Loss: The salt-losing variant of P450c21 hydroxylase deficiency accounts for about 80% of patients with classic 21-hydroxylase deficiency and involves a more severe deficit of P450c21 hydroxylase, which leads to impaired secretion of both cortisol and aldosterone. This results in electrolyte and fluid losses after the fifth day of life and, as a consequence, hyponatremia, hyperkalemia, acidosis, dehydration, and vascular collapse. Masculinization of the external genitalia of affected females tends to be more severe than that found in patients with simple P450c21 hydroxylase deficiency. Affected males may have macrogenitosomia.

The diagnosis of P450c21 hydroxylase deficiency should always be considered (1) in patients with ambiguous genitalia who have a 46,XX karyotype (and are thus female pseudohermaphrodites); (2) in apparent cryptorchid males; (3) in any infant who presents with shock, hypoglycemia, and chemical findings compatible with adrenal insufficiency; and (4) in males and females with signs of virilization prior to puberty, including premature adrenarche. In the past, the diagnosis of P450c21 hydroxylase deficiency was based on the finding of elevated levels of 17-ketosteroids and pregnanetriol in the urine. Although still valid and useful, urinary steroid determinations have been replaced by the simpler and more cost-effective measurement of plasma 17-hydroxyprogesterone, androstenedione and testosterone levels.

The concentration of plasma 17-hydroxyproges-

terone is elevated in umbilical cord blood but rapidly decreases into the range of 1–2 μg/L (3–6 nmol/L) by 24 hours after delivery. In premature infants and in stressed full-term newborns, the levels of 17-hydroxyprogesterone are higher than those observed in nonstressed full-term infants. In patients with P450c21 hydroxylase deficiency, the 17-hydroxyprogesterone values usually range from 30 to 40 μg/L (90–1200 nmol/L), depending on the age of the patient and the severity of P450c21 hydroxylase deficiency. Patients with mild P450c21 hydroxylase deficiency, ie, late-onset and cryptic forms, may have borderline basal 17-hydroxyprogesterone values, but they can be distinguished from heterozygotes by the magnitude of the 17-hydroxyprogesterone response to the parenteral administration of ACTH.

Salt losers may be ascertained clinically or by chemical evidence of hyponatremia and hyperkalemia on a regular infant diet. In these patients, aldosterone levels in both plasma and urine are low in relation to the serum sodium concentration, while plasma renin activity is elevated. Breast milk and many infant formulas have a low concentration of sodium.

HLA typing, measurement of amniotic fluid 17-hydroxyprogesterone levels, and chorionic villus biopsy with HLA typing and gene analysis have been used in the prenatal diagnosis of affected fetuses. Data indicate that prenatal therapy with dexamethasone given to the mother early in pregnancy can lessen the genital ambiguity seen in affected newborn females.

Heterozygosity has been ascertained by HLA typing in informative families and by the use of ACTH-induced rises in plasma 17-hydroxyprogesterone levels. Measurement of plasma 17-hydroxyprogesterone levels using heel-stick capillary blood specimens blotted onto paper has been shown to be a useful and valid screening tool for the diagnosis of 21-hydroxy-lase deficiency in newborn infants.

C. P450c11 Hydroxylase Deficiency: (Viril-ization with hypertension.) Classic P450c11 hydrox-ylase deficiency is rare; however, it is the second most common form of CAH, representing 5–8% of all cases. It occurs in 1:100,000 births in persons of European ancestry. However, in Middle Eastern people, it is much more common, occurring in 1:7000–1:5000 births. In the classic patient, a defect in 11-hydroxylation leads to decreased cortisol levels with a consequent increase in ACTH and the hyper-secretion of 11-deoxycorticosterone and 11-deoxy-cortisol in addition to adrenal androgens. Marked heterogeneity in the clinical and hormonal manifesta-tions of this defect has been described, including mild, late-onset, and even "cryptic" forms. Patients with this form of adrenal hyperplasia classically ex-hibit virilization secondary to increased androgen production and hypertension related to increased 11-deoxycorticosterone secretion. Plasma renin activity is either normal or suppressed. The hypertension is not invariable; it occurs in approximately two-thirds of patients and may be associated with hyperkalemic alkalosis.

Two P450c11 hydroxlyase genes have been local-ized to the long arm of chromosome 8: *P450c11*β and *P450c11AS*. Similar to 21-hydroxylase, these two genes are 95% homologous. *P450c11*β encodes the enzyme for 11-hydroxylation and is expressed in the zona fasciculata and reticularis and is ACTH-de-pendent. It primarily mediates 11-hydroxylation of 11-deoxycortisol to cortisol and DOC to corticos-terone. It has about one-twelfth the capacity of P450c11AS for 18-hydroxylation and does not oxi-dize 18-hydroxycorticosterone to aldosterone. *P450c11AS* encodes the angiotensin-dependent isozyme aldosterone synthetase and is only expressed in the zona glomerulosa, where it mediates 11-hy-droxylation, 18-hydroxylation, and 18 oxidation. Mutations, deletions, and gene duplications can pro-duce a wide variety of clinical manifestations from virilization and hypertension (P450c11β deficiency) to isolated salt wasting (P450c11AS-aldosterone syn-thetase deficiency) to glucocorticoid remedial hyper-tension (due to fusion of the ACTH-dependent regu-latory region of the 11-hydroxylase gene with the coding region of aldosterone synthetase). Both the gene encoding *P450c11*β and *P450c11AS* genes are located on chromosome 8 and thus are not linked to HLA. ACTH stimulation tests have thus far failed to demonstrate a consistent biochemical abnormality in obligate heterozygotes.

The diagnosis of P450c11β-hydroxylase defi-ciency can be confirmed by demonstration of ele-vated plasma levels of 11-deoxycortisol and 11-de-oxycorticosterone and increased excretion of their metabolites in urine (mainly tetrahydro-11-deoxycor-

tisol) either in the basal state or after the administra-tion of ACTH.

D. Type IV—3β-Hydroxysteroid Dehydroge-nase Deficiency: (Male or female pseudohermaph-roditism and adrenal insufficiency.) See below.

E. Type V—P450c17 Deficiency: (Male pseu-dohermaphroditism, sexual infantilism, hypertension and hypokalemic alkalosis.) See below.

F. Type VI—StAR Deficiency: (Congenital lipoid adrenal hyperplasia, male pseudohermaphro-ditism, sexual infantilism, and adrenal insufficiency.) See below.

Treatment

Treatment of patients with adrenal hyperplasia may be divided into acute and chronic phases. In acute adrenal crises, a deficiency of both cortisol and aldosterone results in hypoglycemia, hyponatremia, hyperkalemia, hypovolemia, acidosis, and shock. If the patient is hypoglycemic, an intravenous bolus of glucose, 0.25–0.5 g/kg (maximum 25 g) should be administered. If the patient is in shock, an infusion of normal saline (20 mL/kg) may be given over the first hour; thereafter, replacement of glucose, fluid, and electrolytes is calculated on the basis of deficits and standard maintenance requirements. Hydrocortisone sodium succinate, 50 mg/m^2, should be given as a bolus and another 50–100 mg/m^2 added to the infu-sion fluid over the first 24 hours of therapy. If hy-ponatremia and hyperkalemia are present, 0.05–0.1 mg of fludrocortisone by mouth may be given along with the intravenous saline and hydrocortisone. Since hydrocortisone has mineralocorticoid activity, it may suffice to correct the electrolyte abnormality along with the saline. In extreme cases of hyponatremia, hyperkalemia, and acidosis, sodium bicarbonate and a cation exchange resin (eg, sodium polystyrene sul-fonate) may be needed.

Once the patient is stabilized and a definitive diag-nosis has been arrived at by means of appropriate steroid studies, the patient should receive mainte-nance doses of glucocorticoids to permit normal growth, development, and bone maturation (hydro-cortisone, approximately 12–18 mg/m^2/d by mouth in three divided doses). The dose of hydrocortisone must be titrated in each patient, depending on steroid hormone levels in plasma and urine, linear growth, bone maturation, and clinical signs of steroid over-dose or of virilization. Salt losers need treatment with mineralocorticoid (fludrocortisone, 0.05–0.2 mg/d by mouth) and added dietary salt (1–3 g/d). The dose of mineralocorticoid should be adjusted so that the elec-trolytes and blood pressure, as well as the plasma renin activity, are in the normal range. (See also Chapters 9 and 10.)

Patients with ambiguous external genitalia should have plastic repair before age 1 year. Clitoral reces-sion or clitoroplasty—*not clitoridectomy!*—is indicated. Of major importance to the family with an affected child is the assurance that the child will grow and develop into a normal adult. In patients with the most common form of adrenal hyperplasia—21-hydroxylase deficiency—fertility in males and feminization, menstruation and fertility in females can be expected with adequate treatment. Long-term psychologic guidance and support by the physician for the patient and family is essential.

Adrenal rests in the testes of males with P450c21 hydroxylase deficiency (especially salt losers) may enlarge under the stimulus of ACTH and be mistaken for testicular neoplasms. These adrenal rests are often bilateral and are made up of cells that appear indistinguishable from Leydig cells histologically except that they lack Reinke crystalloids. The rests are usually seen in noncompliant or undertreated patients. To prevent this complication as well as the risk of adrenal crisis, pituitary basophil hyperplasia, and adrenal carcinoma, continuous treatment with a glucocorticoid (and, if indicated, a mineralocorticoid) is recommended even in adult males.

P450 AROMATASE DEFICIENCY

Recently, a new form of androgen-induced female pseudohermaphroditism has been defined that is due to aromatase deficiency. Mutations in the gene encoding P450arom result in defective placental conversion of C_{19} steroids to estrogens leading to exposure of the fetus to excessive amounts of testosterone and masculinization of the external genitalia of the female fetus. Virilization of the mother during gestation can also occur. At puberty, defective aromatase activity in the gonads leads to pubertal failure, hypergonadotropic hypogonadism, polycystic ovaries, mild virilization, tall stature, and osteoporosis. A striking delay in bone age occurs despite increased concentrations of plasma testosterone, supporting the concept that estrogens rather than androgens are the major sex steroids affecting bone maturation and bone turnover in females as well as males. The diagnosis of aromatase deficiency is suggested by the finding of the above clinical picture and elevated plasma androstenedione and testosterone levels in the face of low estrogen levels.

MATERNAL ANDROGENS & PROGESTOGENS

Masculinization of the external genitalia of a female infant can occur if the mother is given testosterone, other androgenic steroids, or certain synthetic progestational agents during pregnancy. After the 12th week of gestation, exposure results in clitoromegaly alone. Norethindrone, ethisterone, norethynodrel, and medroxyprogesterone acetate have all been implicated in masculinization of the female fetus. Nonadrenal female pseudohermaphroditism can occur as a consequence of maternal ingestion of danazol, the 2,3-*d*-isoxazole derivative of 17α-ethinyl testosterone. In rare instances, masculinization of a female fetus is due to a virilizing maternal ovarian or adrenal tumor, congenital virilizing adrenal hyperplasia in the mother, or a luteoma of pregnancy.

The diagnosis of female pseudohermaphroditism arising from transplacental passage of androgenic steroids is based on exclusion of other forms of female pseudohermaphroditism and a history of drug exposure. Surgical correction of the genitalia, if needed, is the only therapy necessary.

Nonadrenal female pseudohermaphroditism can be associated with imperforate anus, renal anomalies, and other malformations of the lower intestine and urinary tract. Sporadic as well as familial cases have been reported.

MALE PSEUDOHERMAPHRODITISM

Male pseudohermaphrodites have gonads that are testes, but the genital ducts or external genitalia, or both, are not completely masculinized. Male pseudohermaphroditism can result from deficient testosterone secretion as a consequence of (1) defective testicular differentiation (testicular dysgenesis), (2) impaired secretion of testosterone or anti-müllerian hormone, (3) failure of target tissue response to testosterone and dihydrotestosterone or anti-müllerian hormone, and (4) failure of conversion of testosterone to dihydrotestosterone. (See also Chapter 12.)

Testicular Unresponsiveness to hCG & LH

Male sexual differentiation is dependent upon the production of testosterone by fetal Leydig cells. Leydig cell testosterone secretion is under the influence of placental hCG during the critical period of male sexual differentiation and, thereafter, fetal pituitary LH during gestation.

The finding of normal male sexual differentiation in XY males with anencephaly, apituitarism, or congenital hypothalamic hypopituitarism suggests that male sex differentiation in the human occurs independently of the secretion of fetal pituitary gonadotropins.

Absence, hypoplasia, or unresponsiveness of Leydig cells to hCG-LH results in deficient testosterone production and, consequently, male pseudohermaphroditism. The extent of the genital ambiguity is a function of the degree of testosterone deficiency, and the phenotype has ranged from extreme forms with female external genitalia to milder forms with micropenis and to males with normal male genitalia and hypergonadotropic hypogonadism at puberty. A small number of patients with absent, hypoplastic, or unresponsive Leydig cells due to a mutation in the gene encoding the LH-hCG receptor have been reported as well as an animal model, the "vet" rat. In most of the patients thus far reported, the defect resulted in female-appearing genitalia and a short blind-ending vagina. Müllerian duct regression was complete. Basal gonadotropin levels as well as GnRH-evoked responses were elevated in postpubertal patients. Plasma 17α-hydroxyprogesterone, androstenedione, and testosterone levels were low, and hCG elicited little or no response in testosterone or its precursors. In two siblings with the extreme phenotype of this syndrome, a homozygous missense mutation in exon 11 of the LH receptor gene was found. This mutation resulted in an alanine to proline change in the sixth transmembrane domain of the LH receptor and a nonfunctional receptor. Other mutations affecting LH binding, G protein activation, and postsynthesis transport are possible and may be found in other patients with this syndrome. Treatment depends on the age at diagnosis and the extent of masculinization. A female sex assignment has usually been chosen in patients with female-appearing genitalia.

Inborn Errors of Testosterone Biosynthesis

Figure 14–14 demonstrates the major pathways in testosterone biosynthesis in the gonads; each step is associated with an inherited defect that results in testosterone deficiency and, consequently, male pseudohermaphroditism (see also Chapter 12). Steps 1, 2, and 3 are enzymatic deficiencies that occur in both the adrenals and gonads and result in defective synthesis of both corticosteroids and testosterone. Thus, they represent forms of congenital adrenal hyperplasia.

A. StAR Deficiency and Congenital Lipoid Adrenal Hyperplasia: (Male pseudohermaphroditism, sexual infantilism and adrenal insufficiency.) This is a very early defect in the synthesis of all steroids affecting the conversion of cholesterol to Δ^5-pregnenolone and results in severe adrenal and gonadal deficiency. The *P450scc* gene has been isolated, cloned, and localized to chromosome 15. However, thus far, molecular analysis of this gene has not revealed a defect in affected patients with this syndrome. Mutations in a steroidogenic acute regulatory

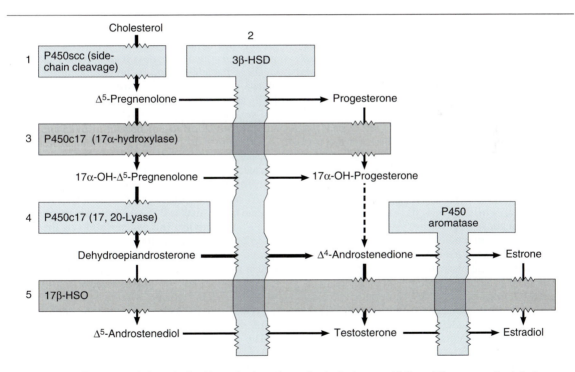

Figure 14–14. Enzymatic defects in the biosynthetic pathway for testosterone. All five of the enzymatic defects cause male pseudohermaphroditism in affected males. Although all of the blocks affect gonadal steroidogenesis, those at steps 1, 2, and 3 are associated with major abnormalities in the biosynthesis of glucocorticoids and mineralocorticoids in the adrenal. Patients with apparent P450scc deficiency have a mutation in StAR (steroidogenic acute regulatory protein), a protein necessary for the transport of cholesterol from outer to inner mitochondrial membrane where P450scc resides. (OH, hydroxy; 3β-HSD, 3β-hydroxysteroid dehydrogenase; 17β-HSO, 17β-hydroxysteroid oxidoreductase (dehydrogenase). Chemical names for enzymes are shown with traditional names in parentheses. (See also Figure 12–2.) (Modified and reproduced, with permission, from Conte FA, Grumbach MM: Pathogenesis, classification, diagnosis, and treatment of anomalies of sex. In: *Endocrinology.* DeGroot L [editor]. Grune & Stratton, 1989.)

protein (StAR) that is necessary for the transport of cholesterol from the outer to the inner mitochondrial membrane, the site of P450scc, have been identified in patients with the clinical syndrome of congenital lipoid adrenal hyperplasia. StAR is expressed in the adrenals and gonads but not in the placenta; hence, placental synthesis of progesterone, which is required to maintain pregnancy in humans, is apparently not affected. A mutation in the *P450scc* gene resulting in a deficit of side chain cleavage enzymatic activity most likely would be lethal, as it is essential for progesterone synthesis by the human fetoplacental unit.

Affected males have female or, rarely, ambiguous external genitalia with a blind vaginal pouch and hypoplastic male genital ducts but no müllerian derivatives; the genitalia of affected females are normal. Large lipid-laden adrenals that displace the kidneys downward may be demonstrated by intravenous urography, abdominal ultrasonography, or CT scan. Death in early infancy from adrenal insufficiency is not uncommon. The diagnosis is confirmed by the lack of or low levels of all C_{21}, C_{19}, and C_{18} steroids in plasma and urine and an absent response to ACTH and hCG stimulation. Treatment involves replacement with appropriate doses of glucocorticoids and mineralocorticoids.

B. 3β-Hydroxysteroid Dehydrogenase- and Δ⁵-Isomerase Deficiency: (Male or female pseudohermaphroditism and adrenal insufficiency.) 3β-Hydroxysteroid dehydrogenase and Δ^5-isomerase deficiency is an early defect in steroid synthesis that results in inability of the adrenals and gonads to convert 3β-hydroxy-Δ^5 steroids to 3-keto-Δ^4 steroids. This enzyme is encoded for by a gene on the short arm of chromosome number 1. Recent data indicate that there are two highly homologous genes encoding 3β-hydroxysteroid dehydrogenase on chromosome 1. The type I 3β-hydroxysteroid dehydrogenase gene is expressed in the placenta and peripheral tissues, while type II is expressed in the adrenals and gonads. 3β-Hydroxysteroid dehydrogenase is not a cytochrome P450 enzyme, and it requires NAD⁺ as a cofactor. Mutations causing frame shifts, stops, and missense have been reported in the type II gene in affected patients. This defect in its complete form results in a severe deficiency of aldosterone, cortisol, testosterone, and estradiol secretion. Males with this defect are incompletely masculinized, and females have mild clitoromegaly. Salt loss and adrenal crises usually occur in early infancy in affected patients. Affected males may experience normal male puberty but often have prominent gynecomastia. Patients with a mild non-salt-losing form of 3β-hydroxysteroid dehydrogenase deficiency have been described as well as late-onset patients presenting with only premature pubarche. These patients were shown to have elevated Δ^5 steroids as well as mutations in the 3β-hydroxysteroid type II gene.

The diagnosis of 3β-hydroxysteroid dehydrogenase deficiency is based on finding elevated concentrations of Δ^5-pregnenolone, Δ^5-17α-hydroxypregnenolone, dehydroepiandrosterone (DHEA) and its sulfate, and other 3β-hydroxy-Δ^5 steroids in the plasma and urine of patients with a consistent clinical picture. 3-keto-Δ^4 steroids, ie, 17-hydroxyprogesterone and androstenedione, may be elevated due to peripheral conversion of 3β-hydroxy-Δ^5 to 3-keto-Δ^4 steroids by the enzyme encoded by the type 1 gene. The diagnosis of 3β-hydroxysteroid dehydrogenase deficiency may be facilitated by detecting abnormal levels of serum Δ^5-17α-hydroxypregnenolone and dehydroepiandrosterone (DHEA) and its sulfates as well as abnormal ratios of Δ^5 to Δ^4 steroids after intravenous administration of 0.25 mg of synthetic ACTH. It can be confirmed by detecting a mutation in the type II β-hydroxysteroid dehydrogenase Δ^5 isomerase gene. Suppression of the increased plasma and urinary 3β-hydroxy-Δ^5 steroids by the administration of dexamethasone distinguishes 3β-hydroxysteroid dehydrogenase deficiency from a virilizing adrenal tumor. Treatment of this condition is similar to that of other forms of adrenal hyperplasia (see above).

C. P450c17 Deficiency, 17α-Hydroxylase Deficiency: (Male pseudohermaphroditism, sexual infantilism, hypertension, and hypokalemic alkalosis.) A defect in 17α-hydroxylation in the zona fasciculata of the adrenal and in the gonads results in impaired synthesis of 17-hydroxyprogesterone and 17-hydroxypregnenolone and, consequently, cortisol and sex steroids. The secretion of large amounts of corticosterone and deoxycorticosterone (DOC) leads to hypertension, hypokalemia, and alkalosis. Increased DOC secretion with resultant hypertension produces suppression of renin and, consequently, decreased aldosterone secretion.

A single gene on chromosome 10 encodes both adrenal and testicular P450c17 hydroxylase as well as 17,20-lyase activity. This enzyme catalyzes the 17-hydroxylation of pregnenolone and progesterone to 17-hydroxypregnenolone and 17-hydroxyprogesterone as well as the scission (lyase) of 17-hydroxypregnenolone to the c19 steroid—dehydroepiandrosterone—in the adrenal cortex and gonads. Mutations affecting 17-hydroxylase activity have included stop codons, frame shifts, deletions, and missense substitutions.

The clinical manifestations result from the adrenal and gonadal defect. Affected XX females have normal development of the internal ducts and external genitalia but manifest sexual infantilism with elevated gonadotropin concentrations at puberty. Affected males have impaired testosterone synthesis by the fetal testes, which results in female or ambiguous genitalia. At adolescence, sexual infantilism, low renin hypertension, and often hypokalemia are the hallmarks of this defect.

The diagnosis of 17-hydroxylase deficiency

should be suspected in XY males with female or ambiguous genitalia or XX females with sexual infantilism who also manifest hypertension associated with hypokalemic alkalosis. High levels of progesterone, Δ^5-pregnenolone, DOC, corticosterone, and 18-hydroxycorticosterone in plasma and increased excretion of their urinary metabolites establish the diagnosis. Plasma renin activity and aldosterone secretion are diminished in these patients.

Note: The following errors affect testosterone and estrogen biosynthesis in the gonads primarily.

D. P450c17 Deficiency (17,20-Lyase Deficiency): The enzyme P450c17 mediates the 17-hydroxylation of pregnenolone and progesterone to 17-hydroxypregnenolone and 17-hydroxyprogesterone as well as the scission of the $C_{17,20}$ bond to yield DHEA. In the human, the scission of 17-hydroxyprogesterone to androstenedione has not yet been demonstrated. Rare patients are reported to have a putative defect primarily in the scission of the C_{21} steroids to C_{19} steroids, which results in a defect in testosterone synthesis and subsequently pseudohermaphroditism in the male and impaired sex steroid synthesis and secretion in the affected 46,XX female. One putative case of isolated 17,20-lyase deficiency studied by molecular analysis is a compound heterozygote for mutations in the carboxyl terminal end of the *P450c17* gene. In expression vectors, both 17-hydroxylase activity and 17,20-lyase activity are reduced by the mutations. The finding of Wolffian ducts associated with female external genitalia in these patients is as yet unexplained. Müllerian derivatives were absent as a result of the secretion of anti-müllerian hormone by the fetal testes.

Patients with 17,20-lyase deficiency have low circulating levels of testosterone, androstenedione, DHEA, and estradiol. The diagnosis can be confirmed by demonstration of an increased ratio of 17-hydroxy C_{21} steroids to C_{19} steroids (testosterone, DHEA, Δ^5-androstenediol, and androstenedione) after stimulation with ACTH or hCG and by DNA analysis of the *P450c17* gene.

E. 17β-Hydroxysteroid Oxidoreductase (Dehydrogenase) Deficiency: The last step in testosterone and estradiol biosynthesis by the gonads involves the reduction of androstenedione to testosterone and estrone to estradiol. 17-Hydroxysteroid oxidoreductase is an NADPH-dependent microsomal enzyme. Two genes are found in tandem on the long arm of chromosome 17. They are 89% homologous. One gene appears to be a pseudogene because of the presence of a stop codon. A third gene has been found on chromosome 9q22. This gene is expressed primarily in the testes, and its product is 23% homologous to the other 17β-hydroxysteroid oxidoreductase enzyme. This enzyme utilizes NADPH as a cofactor and catalyzes the reduction of androstenedione to testosterone. Mutations in this gene have been described in male pseudohermaphrodites. At birth, males with a deficiency of the enzyme 17-hydroxy-

steroid oxidoreductase have female or mildly ambiguous external genitalia resulting from testosterone deficiency during male differentiation. They have male duct development, absent müllerian structures with a blind vaginal pouch, and inguinal or intra-abdominal testes. Dissociation of 17-hydroxylase and 17,20-lyase activity of the enzyme has been demonstrated by site directed mutagenesis of the gene in both the rat and human. Two male pseudohermaphrodites with missense mutations of arginine 347-histidine, and arginine 358-glycine in the *P450c17* gene have been reported. These homozygous missense mutations resulted in measurable 17-hydroxylase activity but absent 17,20-lyase activity as assessed by steroid levels. These two males each had a microphallus, perineal hypospadias, a bifid scrotum, and a blind vaginal pouch. At puberty, progressive virilization with clitoral hypertrophy occurs, often associated with the concurrent development of gynecomastia. Plasma gonadotropin, androstenedione, and estrone levels are elevated, whereas testosterone and estradiol concentration are relatively low. A putative late-onset form of 17-hydroxysteroid oxidoreductase deficiency has been reported in a small number of postadolescent males with gynecomastia and normal male genitalia.

17-Hydroxysteroid oxidoreductase deficiency should be included in the differential diagnosis of (1) male pseudohermaphrodites with absent müllerian derivatives who have no abnormality in glucocorticoid or mineralocorticoid synthesis; and (2) male pseudohermaphrodites who virilize at puberty, especially if they also exhibit gynecomastia. The diagnosis of 17-hydroxysteroid oxidoreductase deficiency is confirmed by the demonstration of inappropriately high plasma levels of estrone and androstenedione and increased ratios of plasma androstenedione to testosterone and estrone to estradiol before and after stimulation with hCG.

Management of the patients, as of those with other forms of male pseudohermaphroditism, depends on the age at diagnosis and the degree of ambiguity of the external genitalia. In the patient assigned a male gender identity, plastic repair of the genitalia and testosterone augmentation of phallic growth prepubertally as well as testosterone replacement therapy at puberty is indicated. In patients reared as females (the usual case), the appropriate treatment is castration, followed by estrogen replacement therapy at puberty.

Defects in Androgen-Dependent Target Tissues

The complex mechanism of action of steroid hormones at the cellular level has recently been clarified (Figure 14–15).

Free testosterone enters the target cells and undergoes 5α reduction to dihydrotestosterone. Dihydrotestosterone binds to the intracellular androgen receptor, inducing a conformational change that

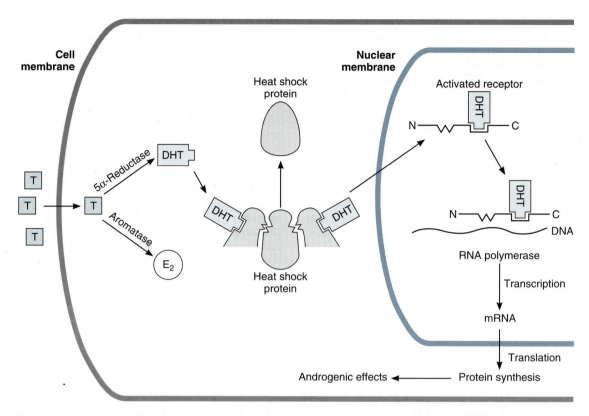

Figure 14–15. Diagrammatic representation of the putative mechanism of action of testosterone on target cells. Testosterone (T) enters the cells, where it is either 5α-reduced to dihydrotestosterone (DHT) or aromatized to estradiol. Dihydrotestosterone enters the nucleus, where it binds to the androgen receptor and "activates" it with release of the heat shock protein. The activated androgen receptor complex then binds as a dimer (not shown) to specific hormone response elements of the DNA and initiates transcription, translation, and protein synthesis, with consequent androgenic effects. (See also Figure 12–3.) (Reproduced, with permission, from Grumbach MM, Conte FA: Disorders of sex differentiation. In: *Williams Textbook of Endocrinology,* 8th ed. Wilson JD, Foster DW [editors]. Saunders, 1992.)

facilitates the release of heat shock protein, nuclear transport, dimerization, and binding to the specific hormone response elements of DNA. It initiates transcription, translation, and protein synthesis that leads to androgenic actions. A lack of androgen effect at the end organ and, consequently, male pseudohermaphroditism may result from abnormalities in 5α-reductase activity, transformation of the steroid-receptor complex, receptor binding of dihydrotestosterone, receptor-ligand complex binding to DNA, transcription, exportation, or translation.

End-Organ Resistance to Androgenic Hormones (Androgen Receptor Defects)

A. Syndrome of Complete Androgen Resistance and Its Variants (Testicular Feminization): The syndrome of complete androgen resistance (testicular feminization) is characterized by a 46,XY karyotype, bilateral testes, absent or hypoplastic wolffian ducts, female-appearing external genitalia with a hypoplastic clitoris and labia minora,

a blind vaginal pouch, and absent or rudimentary müllerian derivatives (33%). At puberty, female secondary sexual characteristics develop, but menarche does not ensue. Pubic and axillary hair is usually sparse and in one-third of patients is totally absent. Affected patients are taller than average females. Some patients have a variant form of this syndrome and exhibit slight clitoral enlargement. These patients may exhibit mild virilization in addition to the development of breasts and a female habitus.

Androgen resistance during embryogenesis prevents masculinization of the external genitalia and differentiation of the wolffian ducts. Secretion of anti-müllerian hormone by the fetal Sertoli cells leads to regression of the müllerian ducts. Thus, affected patients are born with female external genitalia and a blind vaginal pouch. At puberty, androgen resistance results in augmented LH secretion with subsequent increases in testosterone and estradiol. Estradiol arises from peripheral conversion of testosterone and androstenedione as well as from direct secretion by the testes. Androgen resistance coupled with increased testicular estradiol secretion and conversion of androgens to estrogens result in the development of female secondary sexual characteristics at puberty.

The androgen receptor gene is located on the X chromosome between Xq11 and Xq13. The gene is composed of eight exons, A–H. Exon A encodes the amino terminal end of the androgen receptor protein and is thought to play a role in transcription. Exons B and C code for the DNA binding zinc finger of the androgen receptor protein. The 5′ portion of exon D is called the hinge region and plays a role in nuclear targeting. Exons E–H specify the carboxyl terminal portion of the androgen receptor, which is the androgen binding domain (Figure 14–16).

Patients with complete androgen resistance have been found to be heterogeneous with respect to dihydrotestosterone binding to the androgen receptor. Receptor-negative and receptor-positive individuals with qualitative defects such as thermolability, instability, and impaired binding affinity as well as individuals with presumed normal binding have been described. Analysis of the androgen receptor gene has shed light on the pathogenesis of the heterogeneity in receptor studies found in patients with complete androgen resistance. Patients with the receptor-negative form of complete androgen resistance have been found to have primarily point mutations or substitutions in exons E–H, which code for the androgen-binding domain of the receptor. The majority of the mutations are familial in nature. Other defects such

as deletions, mutations in a splice donor site, and point mutations causing premature termination codons are less common in this group of patients. Mutations in exon C (which encodes the DNA-binding segment of the androgen receptor) is associated with normal binding of androgen to the receptor but inability of the ligand-receptor complex to bind to DNA and thus to initiate mRNA transcription. These mutations result in receptor-positive complete androgen resistance. The phenotype of the affected patient does not correlate as well with the receptor studies but does correlate with the transcriptional activity of the ligand-androgen receptor complex.

The diagnosis of complete androgen resistance can be suspected from the clinical features. Before puberty, the presence of testis-like masses in the inguinal canal or labia in a phenotypic female suggests the diagnosis. Postpubertally, the patients present with primary amenorrhea, normal breast development, and absent or sparse pubic or axillary hair. Pelvic examination or ultrasound confirms the absence of a cervix and uterus.

The complete and incomplete forms (Reifenstein's syndrome) of androgen resistance must be distinguished from other forms of male pseudohermaphroditism due to androgen deficiency or to 5α-reductase deficiency. Unfortunately, there is no readily available in vivo assay for androgen sensitivity. The diagnosis is suggested by the clinical picture, the family history, and the presence of elevated basal and hCG-induced testosterone levels with normal levels of

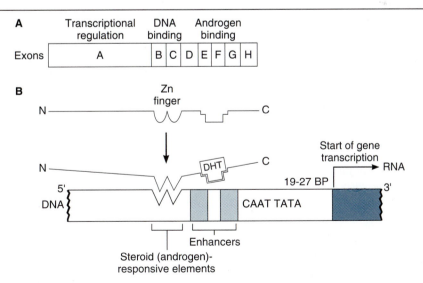

Figure 14–16. *A:* Diagrammatic representation of the androgen receptor gene divided into its nine exons. Exon A codes for the NH₂-terminal domain and regulates transcription. Exons B and C code for two zinc fingers. Exons D–H code for the androgen-binding domain of the receptor. *B:* The organization of a steroid-responsive gene. Ligand binding activates the receptor, and it binds to the steroid response elements of the gene (as a dimer; not shown). Enhancers as well as a CAAT and a TATA box are present. Gene transcription begins 19–27 base pairs downstream of the TATA box. (Reproduced, with permission, from (Reproduced, with permission, from Grumbach MM, Conte FA: Disorders of sex differentiation. In: *Williams Textbook of Endocrinology,* 8th ed. Wilson JD, Foster DW [editors]. Saunders, 1992.)

DHT. A lack of decrease in sex hormone-binding globulin (SHBG) levels after a short course of the anabolic steroid stanozolol has been suggested as a biologic test for androgen resistance. However, little or no confirmatory data on this assay has yet been reported. Also one would expect that some patients with incomplete androgen resistance might respond to this test in somewhat the same way as normal individuals. It has been suggested that an elevated anti-müllerian hormone level is a marker of androgen resistance and androgen deficiency. Abnormalities in androgen binding and mutational analysis as well as studies of transactivation are all diagnostic, but they are time-consuming, labor-intensive, and not universally available. In the infant with ambiguous genitalia in whom the sex of rearing is in question, we have used a trial of testosterone enanthate in oil, 25 mg intramuscularly monthly for 3 months, as a predictive test of androgen responsiveness and future phallic growth before finally deciding on a sex of rearing.

Therapy of patients with complete androgen resistance involves affirmation and reinforcement of their female gender identity. Castration, either prior to or after puberty, is indicated because of the increased risk of gonadal neoplasms with age. Estrogen replacement therapy is required at the age of puberty in orchidectomized patients. In most cases, vaginal reconstructive surgery is not required.

B. Syndrome of Incomplete Androgen Resistance and Its Variants (Reifenstein's Syndrome): Patients with incomplete androgen resistance manifest a wide spectrum of phenotypes as far as the degree of masculinization is concerned. The external genitalia at birth can range from ambiguous, with a blind vaginal pouch, to hypoplastic male genitalia. Müllerian duct derivatives are absent and wolffian duct derivatives present, but they are usually hypoplastic. At puberty, virilization recapitulates that seen in utero and is generally poor; pubic and axillary hair as well as gynecomastia are usually present. The most common phenotype postpubertally is the male with perineoscrotal hypospadias and gynecomastia. Axillary and pubic hair are normal. The testes remain small and exhibit azoospermia as a consequence of germinal cell arrest. As in the case of patients with complete androgen resistance, there are elevated levels of plasma LH, testosterone, and estradiol. However, the degree of feminization in these patients despite high estradiol levels is less than that found in the syndrome of complete androgen resistance.

Androgen receptor studies in these patients have usually shown quantitative or qualitative abnormalities in androgen binding. It would be expected that mutations which lead to partial reduction of androgen action would result in incomplete virilization. As previously noted, the best correlation to phenotype is the degree of impairment of transcriptional activity of the ligand-androgen receptor complex. A wide variety of androgen receptor gene mutations can result

in the same phenotype, and a specific mutation may not always be associated with the same phenotype in all affected patients. In general, point mutations that result in more conservative amino acid substitutions are more likely to result in partial rather than complete androgen resistance.

Androgen Resistance in Men With Normal Male Genitalia

Partial androgen resistance has been described in a group of infertile men who have a normal male phenotype but may exhibit gynecomastia. Unlike other patients with androgen resistance, some of these patients have normal plasma LH and testosterone levels. Infertility in otherwise normal men may be the only clinical manifestation of androgen resistance. However, infertility may not always be associated with androgen resistance. A family has been described in which there were five males with gynecomastia, all of them with a small phallus. Plasma testosterone levels were elevated, and a subtle qualitative abnormality in ligand binding was noted. Fertility was documented in four of the five males. These patients represent the mildest form of androgen resistance presently documented.

Defects in Testosterone Metabolism by Peripheral Tissues; 5α-Reductase Deficiency (Pseudovaginal Perineoscrotal Hypospadias)

The defective conversion of testosterone to dihydrotestosterone produces a unique form of male pseudohermaphroditism (Figure 14–17). Phenotypically, these patients may vary from those with a microphallus to patients with pseudovaginal perineoscrotal hypospadias. At birth, in the most severely affected patients, ambiguous external genitalia are manifested by a small hypospadiac phallus bound down in chordee, a bifid scrotum, and a urogenital sinus that opens onto the perineum. A blind vaginal pouch is present, opening either into the urogenital sinus or onto the urethra, immediately behind the urethral orifice. The testes are either inguinal or labial. Müllerian structures are absent, and the wolffian structures are well-differentiated. At puberty, affected males virilize; the voice deepens, muscle mass increases, and the phallus enlarges. The bifid scrotum becomes rugose and pigmented. The testes enlarge and descend into the labioscrotal folds, and spermatogenesis may ensue. Gynecomastia is notably absent in these patients. Of note is the absence of acne and the presence of temporal hair recession and hirsutism. A remarkable feature of this form of male pseudohermaphroditism in some cultural isolates has been the reported change in gender identity from female to male at puberty.

After the onset of puberty, patients with 5α-reductase deficiency have normal to elevated testosterone

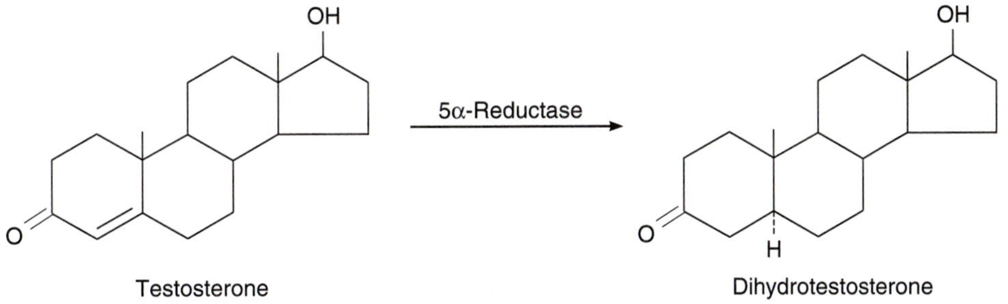

Figure 14–17. Metabolism of testosterone.

levels and slightly elevated plasma concentrations of LH. As expected, plasma dihydrotestosterone is low, and the testosterone:dihydrotestosterone ratio is abnormally high. Apparently, lack of 5α reduction of testosterone to dihydrotestosterone in utero during the critical phases of male sex differentiation results in incomplete masculinization of the urogenital sinus and external genitalia, while testosterone-dependent wolffian structures are normally developed. Partial and mild forms of 5α-reductase deficiency have been described. These patients can present with hypospadias or microphallus (or both).

5α-Reductase deficiency is transmitted as an autosomal recessive trait, and the enzymatic defect exhibits genetic heterogeneity. There are two classes of affected individuals: those with absent enzyme activity and those with a measurable but unstable enzyme. Two genes catalyze the conversion of testosterone to dihydrotestosterone, and they are termed type I and type II. The type I enzyme is not expressed in the fetus but is expressed in skin, especially from puberty onward. The type II isoenzyme is the enzyme found in fetal genital skin, male accessory glands, and the prostate. In patients with 5α-reductase deficiency, the isozyme with a pH 5.5 optimum is deficient (type II). The gene encoding this enzyme contains five exons and is localized to chromosome 2, band p23. A variety of mutations are reported including deletions, nonsense, splicing defects, and the more common missense mutations. Two-thirds of patients are homozygous for a single mutation, while the remainder are compound heterozygotes. It has been suggested that the marked virilization noted at puberty as opposed to its absence in utero may be the result of the expression and function of the type I gene at puberty and, consequently, the generation of sufficient amounts of DHT by peripheral conversion to induce phallic growth and other signs of masculinization.

5α-Reductase deficiency should be suspected in male pseudohermaphrodites with a blind vaginal pouch and in males with hypospadias or microphallus. The diagnosis can be confirmed by demonstration of an abnormally high plasma testosterone:dihydrotestosterone ratio, either under basal conditions or after hCG stimulation. Other confirmatory findings, especially in

newborns, include an increased $5\beta:5\alpha$ ratio of urinary C_{19} and C_{21} steroid metabolites. One can also examine the level of 5α-reductase activity in cultures of genital skin and the degree of conversion of infused labeled testosterone to dihydrotestosterone in vivo.

The early diagnosis of this condition is particularly critical. In view of the natural history of this disorder, a male gender assignment may be considered, and dihydrotestosterone (if available) or high-dose testosterone therapy should be initiated in order to augment phallic size. Repair of hypospadias should be performed as soon as possible in infancy. In patients who are diagnosed after infancy in whom gender identity is unequivocally female, prophylactic orchiectomy and estrogen substitution therapy may still be considered the treatment of choice until further experience with this biochemical entity and sex reversal in our culture is available.

Dysgenetic Male Pseudohermaphroditism (Ambiguous Genitalia Due to Dysgenetic Gonads)

Defective gonadogenesis of the testes results in ambiguous development of the genital ducts, urogenital sinus, and external genitalia. Patients with 45,X/46,XY mosaicism, structural abnormalities of the Y chromosome, and forms of XY gonadal dysgenesis manifest defective gonadogenesis and thus defective virilization. These disorders are classified under disorders of gonadal differentiation but are included also as a subgroup of male pseudohermaphroditism. 46,XY gonadal dysgenesis has been associated with deletion and mutation of the *SRY* gene on the Y chromosome, duplication of the DSS region of the X chromosome, and chromosome 9p– or 10q– deletions.

Male pseudohermaphroditism can occur in association with degenerative renal disease and hypertension as well as with Wilms' tumor (Denys-Drash syndrome). In this syndrome, both the kidneys and the testes are dysgenetic, and a predisposition for renal neoplasms exists. Patients with the Wilms' tumor-aniridia-genital anomalies and mental retardation (WAGR), have been described. These patients exhibit various forms of ambiguous or hypoplastic male genitalia, including bifid scrotum, hypospadias, and cryptorchidism. Recent data indicate that the Denys-Drash and WAGR syndromes are due to heterozygous mutations (Denys-Drash) or deletions (WAGR) involving the Wilms tumor repressor gene, *WT-1* on chromosome 11.

A mutation in SF-1 has not been reported in humans; however, as adduced from the mouse SF-1 knockout experiment, one would expect a 46,XY patient to have no gonads and female sex differentiation including müllerian duct derivatives. The adrenals would be absent, resulting in adrenal crises in infancy. At puberty, sexual infantilism with low plasma gonadotropins would be expected.

Testicular Regression Syndrome (Vanishing Testes Syndrome; XY Agonadism; Rudimentary Testes Syndrome; Congenital Anorchia)

Cessation of testicular function during the critical phases of male sex differentiation can lead to various clinical syndromes depending on when testicular function ceases. At one end of the clinical spectrum of these heterogeneous conditions are the XY patients in whom testicular deficiency occurred prior to 8 weeks of gestation, which results in female differentiation of the internal and external genitalia—so-called XY gonadal dysgenesis.

At the other end of the spectrum are the patients with "anorchia" or "vanishing testes" in which the testes are lost later in gestation. These patients have perfectly normal male differentiation of their internal and external structures, but gonadal tissue is absent. The diagnosis of anorchia should be considered in all cryptorchid males. Administration of chorionic gonadotropin, 1000–2000 units per m^2 injected intramuscularly every other day for 2 weeks (total of seven injections), is a useful test of Leydig cell function. In the presence of normal Leydig cell function, there is a rise in serum testosterone from concentrations of less than 20 ng/dL (0.69 nmol/L) to over 200 ng/dL (6.9 nmol/L) in prepubertal males. In infants under 4 years of age and children over 10 years of age, plasma FSH levels are a sensitive index of gonadal integrity. The gonadotropin response to a 100 µg intravenous injection of GnRH can also be used to diagnose the absence of gonadal feedback on the hypothalamus and pituitary. In agonadal children, GnRH elicits a rise in LH and FSH levels that is greater than that achieved in prepubertal children with normal gonadal function. Patients with high gonadotropin levels and no testosterone response to chorionic gonadotropin usually lack recognizable testicular tissue at surgery. Recent data indicate that both anti-müllerian hormone and inhibin levels may be useful in ascertaining the absence of functioning Sertoli cells and, hence, presumed anorchia.

Persistent Müllerian Duct Syndrome (Defects in the Synthesis, Secretion, or Response to Anti-müllerian Hormone)

Patients have been described in whom normal male development of the external genitalia has occurred but in whom the müllerian ducts persist. The retention of müllerian structures can be ascribed to failure of the Sertoli cells to synthesize anti-müllerian hormone and to an end-organ defect in the response of the duct to anti-müllerian hormone. This condition is transmitted as an autosomal recessive trait. The gene for anti-müllerian hormone has been cloned and mapped to chromosome 19, and mutations in the anti-müllerian gene have been reported. More recently, the gene encoding the anti-müllerian receptor has been isolated, and patients with mutations in the AMH receptor have been described. In these patients müllerian ducts are present despite the presence of normal to high levels of AMH in plasma. Therapy involves removal of the müllerian structures.

Environmental Chemicals

An increase in disorders of development and function of the urogenital tract in males has been noted over the past 50 years. It has been hypothesized that this increased incidence of reproductive abnormalities observed in human males is related to increasing exposure in utero to "estrogens" found in the diet both naturally and as a result of chemical contamination. Recently, it has been demonstrated that *p,p'*-DDE (dichlordiphenyldichloroethylene)—the major and persistent DDT metabolite—binds to the androgen receptor and inhibits androgen action in developing rodents. Further studies on the levels as well as the risks to humans of environmental chemicals are necessary before abnormalities of the reproductive tract can be ascribed to these agents.

UNCLASSIFIED FORMS OF ABNORMAL SEXUAL DEVELOPMENT IN MALES

Hypospadias

Hypospadias occurs as an isolated finding in 1:300 newborn males. It is often associated with ventral contraction and bowing of the penis, called chordee. Deficient virilization of the external genitalia of the male fetus implies subnormal Leydig cell function in utero, end-organ resistance, or an inappropriate temporal correlation of the rise in fetal plasma testosterone and the critical period for tissue response. Although in most patients there is little reason to suspect these mechanisms, recent reports in a small number of patients have suggested that simple hypospadias can be associated with an abnormality (or competitive inhibition) of the androgen receptor, the nuclear localization of the ligand-receptor complex, an aberration in the maturation of the hypothalamic-pituitary-gonadal axis, and 5α-reductase deficiency. Further studies are necessary to determine the prevalence and role of these abnormalities in the pathogenesis of simple hypospadias. Nonendocrine factors that affect differentiation of the primordia may be found in a variety of genetic syndromes. A study of 100 patients with hypospadias reported one patient to be an XX female with congenital adrenal hyperplasia; five had sex chromosome abnormalities; and one had the incomplete form of XY gonadal dysgenesis. Nine affected males were the product of pregnancies in which the mother had taken progestational compounds during the first trimester. Thus, a presumed pathogenetic mechanism was found in 15% of patients.

Microphallus

Microphallus without hypospadias can result from a heterogeneous group of disorders, but by far the most common cause is fetal testosterone deficiency; more rarely, 5α-reductase deficiency or mild defects in the androgen receptor are implicated. In the human male fetus, testosterone synthesis by the fetal Leydig cell during the critical period of male differentiation (8–12 weeks) is under the influence of placental hCG. After midgestation, fetal pituitary LH modulates fetal testosterone synthesis by the Leydig cell and, consequently, affects the growth of the differentiated penis. Thus, males with congenital hypopituitarism as well as isolated gonadotropin deficiency and "late" fetal testicular failure can present with normal male differentiation and microphallus at birth (phallus < 2 cm in length). Patients with hypothalamic hypopituitarism or pituitary aplasia may also have midline craniofacial defects, hypoglycemia, and giant cell hepatitis. After appropriate evaluation of anterior pituitary function (ie, determination of the plasma concentration of GH, ACTH, cortisol, TSH, thyroxine, and gonadotropins), stabilization of the patient with hormone replacement should be achieved. Thereafter, all patients with microphallus should receive a trial of testosterone therapy before definitive gender assignment is made. Patients with fetal testosterone deficiency as a cause of microphallus—whether due to gonadotropin deficiency or to a primary testicular disorder—respond to 25–50 mg of testosterone enanthate intramuscularly monthly for 3 months with a mean increase of 2 cm in phallic length (Figure 14–18). In the rare patient in whom a trial of testosterone therapy does not result in an increase in phallic size due to an intrinsic penis defect, castration and assignment of a female gender may then be a prudent course to follow.

Complete absence of the phallus is a rare anomaly. The urethra may open on the perineum or into the rectum. Assignment of a female gender, castration, and plastic repair of the genitalia and urethra are appropriate in these cases.

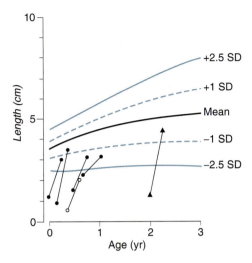

Figure 14–18. The response in phallic length to a 3-month course of testosterone in six patients with microphallus. Patients were under 2 years of age. Each patient was given 25 mg of testosterone enanthate in oil intramuscularly monthly for 3 months. Lines set off with solid triangles and open boxes indicate two patients who subsequently underwent a second course of testosterone therapy. (Reproduced, with permission, from Burstein S, Grumbach MM, Kaplan SL: Early determination of androgen-responsiveness is important in the management of microphallus. Lancet 1979;2:983.)

UNCLASSIFIED FORMS OF ABNORMAL SEXUAL DEVELOPMENT IN FEMALES

Congenital absence of the vagina occurs in 1:5000 female births. It can be associated with müllerian derivatives that vary from normal to absent. Ovarian function is usually normal. Therapy may involve plastic repair of the vagina.

Müllerian agenesis may be associated with renal aplasia (an absent kidney) and cervicothoracic somite dysplasia ("MURCS").

MANAGEMENT OF PATIENTS WITH INTERSEX PROBLEMS

Choice of Sex

The goal of the physician in management of patients with ambiguous genitalia is to establish a diagnosis and to assign a sex for rearing that is most compatible with a well-adjusted life and sexual adequacy. Once the sex for rearing is assigned, the gender role is reinforced by the use of appropriate surgical, hormonal, or psychologic measures. Except in female pseudohermaphrodites, ambiguities of the genitalia are caused by lesions that almost always make the

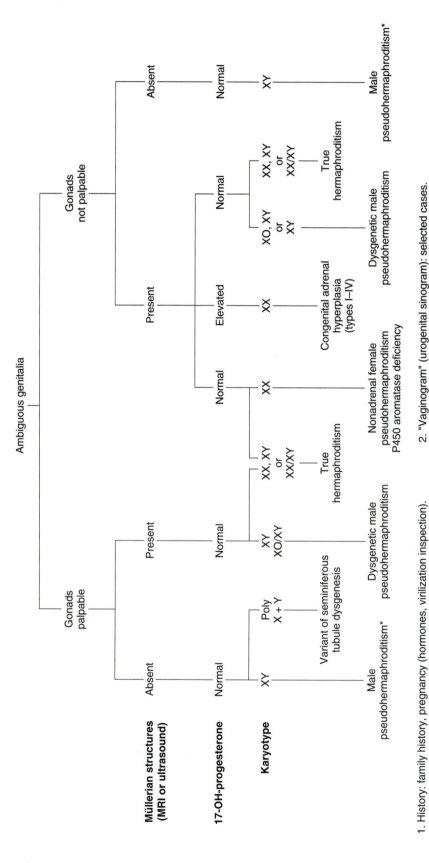

Figure 14–19. Steps in the diagnosis of intersexuality in infancy and childhood. Step 1 involves initial work-up and provisional diagnosis. Step 2 is utilized in selected cases. (Reproduced, with permission, from Grumbach MM, Conte FA: Disorders of sex differentiation. In: *Williams Textbook of Endocrinology*, 8th ed. Wilson JD, Foster DW [editors]. Saunders, 1992.)

1. History: family history, pregnancy (hormones, virilization inspection).
   Palpation of inguinal region and labioscrotal folds; rectal examination.
   Karyotype analysis.
   Initial studies: plasma 17-hydroxyprogesterone, androstenedione,
      dehydroepiandrosterone, testosterone, and dihydrotestosterone.
   Serum electrolytes.
   Sonogram or MRI of kidneys, ureters, and pelvic contents.
   Provisional diagnosis.

2. "Vaginogram" (urogenital sinogram): selected cases.
   Endoscopy, laparotomy, gonadal biopsy: restricted to male
      pseudohermaphrodites, true hermaphrodites, and selected
      instances of nonadrenal female pseudohermaphroditism.
   *Plasma 17-hydroxyprogesterone levels may be modestly
      elevated in patients with P450c11 (type III) and 3β-
      hydroxysteroid dehydrogenase deficiency (type IV) and are
      "low" in patients with P450c17 (type V) and P450scc
      deficiency (type V).

518

patient infertile. In recommending male sex assignment, the adequacy of the size of the phallus should be the most important consideration.

The steps in the diagnosis of intersexuality are set forth in Figure 14–19.

Reassignment of sex in infancy and childhood is always a difficult psychosocial problem for the patient, the parents, and the physicians involved. While easier in infancy than after 2 years of age, it should only be undertaken after deliberation and with provision for long-term medical and psychiatric supervision and counseling.

It is desirable to initiate plastic repair of the external genitalia prior to 6–12 months of age. In children raised as females, the clitoris should be salvaged, if possible, by clitoroplasty or clitoral recession; clitoridectomy is to be avoided. Reconstruction of a vagina, if necessary, can be deferred until adolescence.

Removal of the gonads in children with Y chromosome material and gonadal dysgenesis should be performed at the time of initial repair of the external genitalia, because gonadoblastomas, seminomas, and germinomas can occur during the first decade.

In a patient with complete androgen resistance, the gonads may be left in situ (provided they are not situated in the labia majora) to provide estrogen until late adolescence. The patient may then undergo prophylactic castration, having had her female identity reinforced by normal feminization at puberty. However,

it is reasonable to remove the gonads prepubertally, especially if herniorrhaphy is necessary. In this circumstance, sex steroid replacement therapy at the time of puberty is indicated.

In patients with incomplete androgen resistance reared as females or in patients with errors of testosterone biosynthesis in whom some degree of masculinization occurs at puberty, gonadectomy should be performed prior to puberty.

Cyclic estrogen and progestin are used in individuals reared as females in whom a uterus is present. In males, virilization is achieved by the administration of a repository preparation of testosterone.

Sex is not a single biologic feature but the sum of many morphogenetic, functional, and psychologic potentialities. The physician should not express to the parent or child any doubts about the sex of rearing. Chromosomal and gonadal sex are secondary considerations; the sex of rearing is paramount. With proper surgical reconstruction, hormone substitution, and continuing psychologic support and reinforcement of the sex of rearing, the individual whose psychosexual gender is discordant with chromosomal sex need not have any psychologic catastrophes as long as the sex of rearing is accepted with conviction by the family and others during the critical early years. These individuals should reach adulthood as well-adjusted men or women capable of normal sexual interaction, though usually not of procreation.

REFERENCES

Aittomaki K et al: Mutation in the follicle-stimulating hormone receptor gene causes hereditary hypergonadotrophic ovarian failure. Cell 1995;82:954.

Andersson S et al: Molecular genetics and pathophysiology of 17β-hydroxysteroid dehydrogenase 3 deficiency. J Clin Endocrinol Metab 1996;81:130.

Ballabio A, Willard HF: Mammalian X-chromosome inactivation and the XIST gene. Curr Opin Genet Dev 1992; 2:439.

Bardoni B et al: A dosage sensitive locus at chromosome Xp21 is involved in male to female sex reversal. Nature Genet 1994;7:497.

Behringer RR: The in vivo role of müllerian-inhibiting substance. Curr Top Dev Biol 1994;29:171.

Berkovitz GD et al: Clinical and pathologic spectrum of 46,XY gonadal dysgenesis: Its relevance to the understanding of sex differentiation. Medicine 1991;70:375.

Berkovitz GD et al: The role of the sex-determining region of the Y chromosome (SRY) in the etiology of 46,XX true hermaphroditism. Hum Genet 1992;88:411.

Bose HS et al. The physiology and genetics of congenital lipoid adrenal hyperplasia. N Eng J Med 1996;335:1870.

Conte FA et al: A syndrome of female pseudohermaphroditism, hypergonadotrophic hypogonadism, and multicystic ovaries associated with missense mutations in the gene encoding aromatase (P450arom). J Clin Endocrinol Metab 1994;78:1287.

da Silva SM et al: Sox9 expression during gonadal development implies a conserved role for the gene in testis differentiation in mammals and birds. Nature Genet 1996;14:62.

Donahoue PA et al: Congenital adrenal hyperplasia. In: *The Metabolic and Molecular Bases of Inherited Disease,* 7th ed. Scriver CR et al (editors). McGraw-Hill, 1995.

Fechner PY et al: Report of a kindred with X-linked (or autosome dominant sex linked) 46,XY partial gonadal dysgenesis. J Clin Endocrinol Metab 1993;76:1248.

Ferguson-Smith MA, Goodfellow PN: SRY and primary sex reversal syndromes. In: *The Metabolic and Molecular Bases of Inherited Disease,* 7th ed. Scriver CR et al (editors). McGraw-Hill, 1995.

Geissler WM et al: Male pseudohermaphroditism caused by mutations of testicular 17β-hydroxysteroid dehydrogenase 3. Nature Genet 1994;7:34.

Goodfellow P, Lovell-Badge R: SRY and sex determination in mammals. Ann Rev Genet 1993;27:71.

Griffen JE, Wilson JD: The androgen resistance syndromes: Steroid 5α reductase 2 deficiency, testicular feminization and related syndromes. In: *The Metabolic and Molecular Bases of Inherited Disease,* 7th ed. Scriver CR et al (editors). McGraw-Hill, 1995.

Grumbach MM, Conte FA: Disorders of sex differentiation. In: *Williams Textbook of Endocrinology,* 8th ed. Wilson JD, Foster DW (editors). Saunders, 1992.

Hadjiathanasiou CG et al: True hermaphroditism: Genetic variants and clinical management. J Pediatr 1994;125:738.

Harada N et al: Biochemical and molecular genetic analyses on placental aromatase (P450arom) deficiency. J Biol Chem 1992;267:4781.

Harly VR et al: DNA binding activity of recombinant SRY from normal males and XY females. Science 1992;255:453.

Hawkins JR et al: Mutational analysis of SRY: Nonsense and missense mutations in XY sex reversal. Hum Genet 1992;88:471.

Hawkins JR. Sex determination. Hum Molec Genet 1994;3:1463.

Hibi I, Takano K (editors): *Basic and Clinical Approach to Turner Syndrome.* International Congress Series 1014, Amsterdam, Excerpta Medica, 1993.

Imbeau S et al: Insensitivity to anti-müllerian hormone due to a mutation in the human anti-müllerian hormone receptor. Nature Genet 1995;11:382.

Imbeau S et al: A 27 base-pair deletion of the anti-müllerian Type II receptor gene is the most common cause of the persistent müllerian duct syndrome. Hum Mol Genet 1996;5:1269.

Josso N et al: An enzyme linked immunoassay for anti-müllerian hormone: A new tool for the evaluation of testicular function in infants and children. J Clin Endocrinol Metab 1990;70:23.

Knebelmann B et al: Anti-Müllerian hormone Bruxelles: A nonsense mutation associated with the persistent Müllerian duct syndrome. Proc Natl Acad Sci USA 1991;88:3767.

Koopman P et al: Male development of chromosomally female mice transgenic for SRY. Nature 1991;351:117.

Kreidberg JA et al: WT-1 is required in early kidney development. Cell 1993;74:679.

Kremer H et al: Male pseudohermaphroditism due to a homozygous missense mutation of the luteinizing hormone receptor gene. Nature Genet 1994;9:160.

Labrie F et al: Structure, regulation and role of 3β-hydroxysteroid dehydrogenase, 17β-hydroxysteroid dehydrogenase and aromatase enzymes in the formation of sex steroids in classical and peripheral intracrine tissues. Bailliere's Clin Endocrinol Metab 1994;8:451.

Lin D et al: Role of steroidogenic acute regulatory protein in adrenal and gonadal steroidogenesis. Science 1995;267:1828.

Luo X et al: A cell specific receptor is essential for adrenal and gonadal development and sexual differentiation. Cell 1994;77:481.

Mendonca BB et al: Mutation in 3β-hydroxysteroid dehydrogenase type II associated with pseudohermaphroditism in males and premature pubarche or cryptic expression in females. J Mol Endocrinol 1994;12:119.

Miller WL: Genetics, diagnosis and management of 21-hydroxylase deficiency. J Clin Endocrinol Metab 1994;78:241.

Moore CCD, Grumbach MM: Sex determination and gonadogenesis: A transcription cascade of sex chromosome and autosomal genes. Semin Perinatol 1992;16:266.

Morel Y, Miller W: Clinical and molecular genetics of congenital adrenal hyperplasia due to 21-hydroxylase deficiency. Adv Genet 1991;20:1.

Morishima A et al: Aromatase deficiency in male and female siblings caused by a novel mutation and the physiological role of estrogens. J Clin Endocrinol Metab 1995;80:3689.

Pelletier J et al: Germline mutations in the Wilms tumor suppressor gene are associated with abnormal urogenital development in Denys-Drash syndrome. Cell 1991;67:437.

Petit C et al: An abnormal terminal X-Y interchange accounts for most but not all cases of human XX maleness. Cell 1987;49:595.

Quigley CA et al: Androgen receptor defects: Historical, clinical and molecular properties. Endocr Rev 1995;6:271.

Pontiggia A et al: Sex-reversing mutations affect the architecture of SRY-DNA complexes. EMBO J 1994;13:6115.

Russell DW, Wilson JD: Steroid 5α-reductase: Two genes/two enzymes. Ann Rev Biochem 1994;63:25.

Schafer AJ: Sex determination and its pathology in man. Adv Genet 1995;33:275.

Simard J et al: Molecular basis of human 3 beta-hydroxysteroid dehydrogenase deficiency. J Steroid Biochem Mol Biol 1995;53:127.

Speiser PW et al: Disease expression and molecular genotype in congenital adrenal hyperplasia due to 21-hydroxylase deficiency. J Clin Invest 1992;90:584.

Thigpen AE et al: Molecular genetics of steroid 5α-reductase deficiency. J Clin Invest 1992;90:799.

Van Niekerk WA: *True Hermaphroditism.* Harper & Row, 1974.

Wagner T et al: Autosomal sex reversal and campomelic dysplasia. Cell 1994;79:1111

Wilson JD et al: Steroid 5α-reductase deficiency. Endocr Rev 1993;14:577.

Yanese T et al: 17α-Hydroxylase/17,20-lyase deficiency: From clinical investigation to molecular definitions. Endocr Rev 1991;12:91.

Yanese T et al: Molecular basis of apparent isolated 17,20-lyase deficiency: Compound heterozygous mutations in the C-terminal region (Arg(496) → Cys, Gln(461) → Stop) actually cause combined 17α-hydroxylase/17,20-lyase deficiency. Biochem Biophys Acta 1992;1139:275.

Yanese T: 17α-Hydroxylase/17,20-lyase defects. J Steroid Biochem Mol Biol 1995;53:153.

Zanaria E et al: An unusual member of the hormone receptor superfamily responsible for X-linked adrenal hypoplasia congenita. Nature 1994;372:635.

Puberty

15

Dennis Styne, MD

Puberty is best considered as one stage in the continuing process of growth and development that begins during gestation and continues until the end of reproductive life. After an interval of childhood quiescence, the hypothalamic pulse generator increases activity in the peripubertal period, leading to increased secretion of pituitary gonadotropins and, subsequently, gonadal sex steroids that bring about secondary sexual development, the pubertal growth spurt, and fertility. Historical records show that the age at onset of particular stages of puberty in boys and girls in Western countries has steadily declined over the last several hundred years; this is probably due to improvements in socioeconomic conditions, nutrition, and, therefore, the general state of health during that period. However, this trend ceased during the last 5 decades in developed societies, suggesting the attainment of optimal conditions to allow puberty to begin at a genetically determined age.

Many endogenous and exogenous factors can alter age at onset of puberty. Moderate obesity may be associated with an earlier onset, while severe obesity may delay puberty. Chronic illness and malnutrition often delay puberty. There is a significant concordance of age at menarche between mother-daughter pairs and within ethnic populations, indicating the influence of genetic factors.

ACRONYMS USED IN THIS CHAPTER	
AASH	Adrenal androgen-stimulating hormone
ACTH	Adrenocorticotropic hormone
cAMP	Cyclic adenosine monophosphate
DHEA	Dehydroepiandrosterone
DHEAS	Dehydroepiandrosterone sulfate
FSH	Follicle-stimulating hormone
GH	Growth hormone
GnRH	Gonadotropin-releasing hormone
hCG	Human chorionic gonadotropin
hGH	Human growth hormone
ICMA	Immunochemiluminometric assay
IRMA	Immunoradiometic assay
LH	Luteinizing hormone
PRL	Prolactin
PSA	Prostate-specific antigen
RIA	Radioimmunoassay
SHBG	Sex hormone-binding globulin
TSH	Thyroid-stimulating hormone (thyrotropin)

PHYSIOLOGY OF PUBERTY

Physical Changes Associated With Puberty

Descriptive standards proposed by Tanner for assessing pubertal development in males and females are in wide use. They focus attention on specific details of the examination and make it possible to objectively record subtle progression of secondary sexual development that may otherwise be overlooked.

A. Female Changes: The first sign of puberty in the female, as noted in longitudinal studies, is an increase in growth velocity that heralds the beginning of the pubertal growth spurt; girls are not usually examined frequently enough to demonstrate this change

in clinical practice, so breast development is the first sign of puberty noted by most examiners. Breast development (Figure 15–1) is stimulated chiefly by ovarian estrogen secretion, though other hormones also play a part. The size and shape of the breasts may be determined by genetic and nutritional factors, but the characteristics of the stages in Figure 15–1 are the same in all females. Standards are available for the change in nipple plateau diameter during puberty: Nipple diameter changes little from stages B1 to B3 (mean of 3–4 mm); but it enlarges substantially in subsequent stages (mean of 7.4 mm at stage B4 to 10 mm at stage B5), presumably as a result of estrogen secretion at the time of menarche. Other features

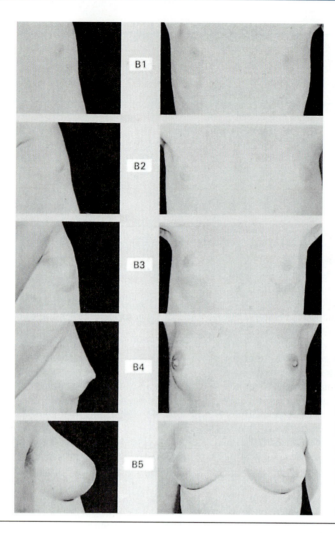

Figure 15–1. Stages of breast development, according to Marshall and Tanner. (Photographs from van Wieringen JC et al, 1971; with permission.) *Stage B1:* Preadolescent; elevation of papilla only. *Stage B2:* Breast bud stage; elevation of breast and papilla as a small mound, and enlargement of areolar diameter. *Stage B3:* Further enlargement of breast and areola, with no separation of their contours. *Stage B4:* Projection of areola and papilla to form a secondary mound above the level of the breast. *Stage B5:* Mature stage; projection of papilla only, owing to recession of the areola to the general contour of the breast. (Reproduced, with permission, from Marshall WA, Tanner JM: Variations in the pattern of pubertal changes in girls. Arch Dis Child 1969;44:291.)

reflecting estrogen action include enlargement of the labia minora and majora, dulling of the vaginal mucosa from its prepubertal reddish hue, and production of a clear or slightly whitish vaginal secretion prior to menarche. Pubic hair development (Figure 15–2) is determined chiefly by adrenal and ovarian androgen secretion. Breast development and growth of pubic hair usually proceed at similar rates, but because discrepancies in rates of advancement are possible, it is best to stage breast development separately from pubic hair progression.

Uterine size and shape change with pubertal development as reflected by ultrasonographic studies; with prolonged estrogen stimulation, the fundus:cervix ratio increases, leading to a bulbous form, and the uterus elongates from less than 3 cm to 5 cm or more. Ovaries enlarge with puberty from a volume of less than 1 mL to 2–10 mL. Ultrasonographers can determine the developmental stage of the uterus and ovaries by comparing the results with established standards.

B. Male Changes: The first sign of normal puberty in boys is usually an increase in the size of the testes to over 2.5 cm in the longest diameter, excluding the epididymis: this is equivalent to a testicular volume of greater than 4 mL. Most of the increase in testicular size is due to seminiferous tubular development secondary to stimulation by FSH, with a smaller component due to Leydig cell stimulation by LH. Thus, if only Leydig cells are stimulated, as in an hCG-secreting tumor, the testis does not grow as large as in normal puberty. Pubic hair development is caused by adrenal and testicular androgens and is classified separately from genital development, as noted in Figure 15–3. A recent longitudinal study of over 500 boys suggests adding a stage 2a to the classic five stages of pubertal development. Stage 2a indicates the absence of pubic hair in the presence of a testicular volume of 3 mL or more. Further pubertal development occurred in 82% of the subjects in stage 2a after the passage of 6 months: thus, reaching stage 2a would allow the examiner to reassure a patient that

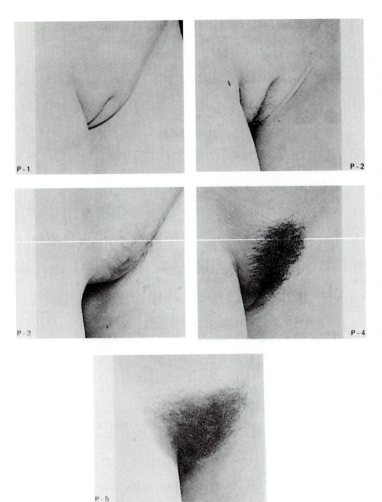

Figure 15–2. Stages of female pubic hair development, according to Marshall and Tanner. (Photographs from van Wieringen JC et al, 1971; with permission.) **Stage P1:** Preadolescent; the vellus over the pubes is no further developed than that over the anterior abdominal wall, ie, no pubic hair. **Stage P2:** Sparse growth of long, slightly pigmented, downy hair, straight or only slightly curled, appearing chiefly along the labia. This stage is difficult to see on photographs. **Stage P3:** Hair is considerably darker, coarser, and curlier. The hair spreads sparsely over the junction of the pubes. **Stage P4:** Hair is now adult in type, but the area covered by it is still considerably smaller than in most adults. There is no spread to the medial surface of the thighs. **Stage P5:** Hair is adult in quantity and type, distributed as an inverse triangle of the classic feminine pattern. Spread is to the medial surface of the thighs but not up the linea alba or elsewhere above the base of the inverse triangle. (Reproduced, with permission, from Marshall WA, Tanner JM: Variations in the pattern of pubertal changes in girls. Arch Dis Child 1969;44:291.)

further spontaneous development is likely. The appearance of spermatozoa in early morning urinary specimens (spermarche) occurs at a mean chronologic age of 13.4 years or a similar bone age; this usually occurs at gonadal stage 3–4 and pubic hair stage 2–4. If puberty starts at an earlier or later chronologic age, the age of spermarche changes accordingly with reference to chronologic age although spermarche occurs in such patients at the same range of gonadal or pubic hair stages. Remarkably, spermaturia is more common earlier in puberty than later, suggesting that sperm are directly released into the urine early in puberty while ejaculation may be responsible for the presence of sperm in the urine of older children.

Boys are reported with spermaturia and no secondary sexual development.

Thus, boys are reproductively mature prior to physical maturity and certainly prior to psychologic maturity!

C. Age at Onset: Although American data are sparse, the limits of onset of normal secondary sexual development in 98.8% of North American children (ie, mean ± 2.5 SD) are accepted as 8–13 years for girls and 9–14 years for boys. A graphic representation of the stages of pubertal development for British children is shown in Figure 15–4; North American and British boys develop at about the same ages, but 6 months should be subtracted from these figures to correct for North American girls. African-American boys develop chronologically in somewhat the same way as white boys, but African-American girls develop earlier than white girls. (African-American girls have a mean age at menarche 0.3 years younger than white girls.) Late onset of pubertal development may indicate hypothalamic, pituitary, or gonadal failure. The time from onset of puberty to complete adult development is also of importance; delays in reaching subsequent stages may indicate any type of hypogonadism. Girls complete secondary sexual development in 1.5–6 years, with a mean of 4.2 years; and boys in 2–4.5 years, with a mean of 3.5 years.

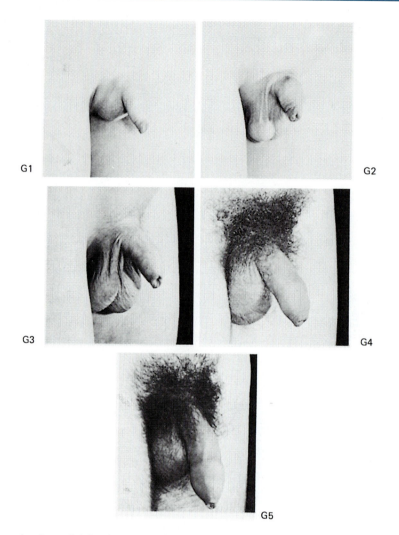

Figure 15–3. Stages of male genital development and pubic hair development, according to Marshall and Tanner. (Photographs from van Wieringen JC et al, 1971; with permission.) **Genital:** *Stage G1:* Preadolescent. Testes, scrotum, and penis are about the same size and proportion as in early childhood. *Stage G2:* The scrotum and testes have enlarged, and there is a change in the texture and some reddening of the scrotal skin. *Stage G3:* Growth of the penis has occurred, at first mainly in length but with some increase in breadth; further growth of testes and scrotum. *Stage G4:* Penis further enlarged in length and girth with development of glans. Testes and scrotum further enlarged. The scrotal skin has further darkened. *Stage G5:* Genitalia adult in size and shape. No further enlargement takes place after stage G5 is reached. **Pubic hair:** *Stage P1:* Preadolescent. The vellus is no further developed than that over the abdominal wall, ie, no pubic hair. *Stage P2:* Sparse growth of long, slightly pigmented, downy hair, straight or only slightly curled, appearing chiefly at the base of the penis. *Stage P3:* Hair is considerably darker, coarser, and curlier and spreads sparsely laterally. *Stage P4:* Hair is now adult in type, but the area it covers is still considerably smaller than in most adults. There is no spread to the medial surface of the thighs. *Stage P5:* Hair is adult in quantity and type, distributed as an inverse triangle. Spread is to the medial surface of the thighs but not up the linea alba or elsewhere above the base of the inverse triangle. Most men will have further spread of pubic hair. (Modified and reproduced, with permission, from Marshall WA, Tanner JM: Variations in the pattern of pubertal changes in boys. Arch Dis Child 1970;45:13.)

D. Growth Spurt: The striking increase in growth velocity in puberty (pubertal growth spurt) is under complex endocrine control. Hypothyroidism decreases or eliminates the pubertal growth spurt. The amplitude of growth hormone secretion in-

creases in puberty, as does production of IGF-1; peak serum IGF-1 concentrations are reached about 1 year after peak growth velocity, and serum IGF-1 levels remain above normal adult levels for up to 4 years thereafter. GH and sex steroids are important in the

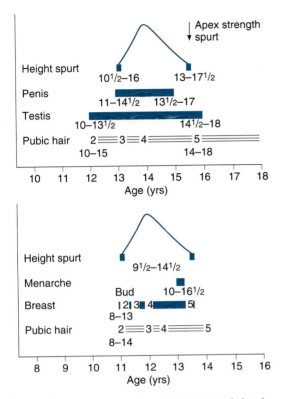

Figure 15–4. Sequence of secondary sexual development in British males *(top)* and females *(bottom)*. The range of ages is indicated. (Reproduced, with permission, from Marshall WA, Tanner JM: Variations in the pattern of pubertal changes in boys. Arch Dis Child 1970;45:13.)

pubertal growth spurt; when either or both are deficient, the growth spurt is decreased or absent. Sex steroids indirectly stimulate IGF-1 production by increasing the secretion of GH and also directly stimulate IGF-1 production in cartilage. Estrogen has recently been shown to be the most important factor in stimulating maturation of the chondrocytes and osteoblasts, ultimately leading to epiphysial fusion. Patients with estrogen receptor defects and aromatase deficiency were recently reported in spite of the fact that, in the past, such abnormalities were thought to be lethal. The patient with estrogen receptor deficiency was tall, with continued growth past the age of 20 years in spite of a remarkable retardation of skeletal maturation. The patient with aromatase deficiency also had a lack of appropriate maturation of bone age. With exogenous estrogen administration, the bone age advanced and a growth spurt occurred. This 46,XX individual had virilized genitalia at birth and further virilization at a pubertal age with the additional feature of multicystic ovaries. The patient, in spite of high serum testosterone concentrations, had elevated FSH and LH in the absence of estrogen production. Skeletal density is also decreased in both

conditions. These patients demonstrate the key role played by estrogen in advancing bone age and bringing about the cessation of growth by epiphysial fusion as well as the importance of estrogen in increasing bone density.

It is essential to realize that a pubertal growth spurt occurring in a young patient with precocious puberty may increase the growth rate sufficiently to mask the presence of coexisting GH deficiency. This situation may occur, for example, in a child with a brain tumor causing precocious puberty treated with radiation that decreases GH secretion.

In girls, the pubertal growth spurt begins in early puberty and is mostly completed by menarche. In boys, the pubertal growth spurt occurs toward the end of puberty, at an average age 2 years older than in girls. Total height attained during the growth spurt in girls is about 25 cm; in boys, it is about 28 cm. The mean adult height differential of 12 cm between men and women is due in part to heights already attained before onset of the pubertal growth spurt and in part to the height gained during the spurt.

E. Changes in Body Composition: Changes in body composition are also prominent during pubertal development. Prepubertal boys and girls start with equal lean body mass, skeletal mass, and body fat, but at maturity men have approximately 1½ times the lean body mass, skeletal mass, and muscle mass of women, while women have twice as much body fat as men.

F. Other Changes of Puberty: Other changes that are characteristic of puberty are mediated either directly or indirectly by the change in sex steroids. Bone density increases during normal pubertal development. Seborrheic dermatitis may appear at this age. The mouth flora changes, and periodontal disease, rare in childhood, may appear at this stage. Insulin resistance intensifies in adolescents with insulin-dependent diabetes mellitus; this may be partly related to the increased GH levels.

Endocrine Changes From Fetal Life to Puberty

Pituitary gonadotropin secretion is controlled by the hypothalamus, which releases pulses of gonadotropin-releasing hormone (GnRH) into the pituitary-portal system to reach the anterior pituitary gland. Control of GnRH secretion is exerted by a "hypothalamic pulse generator" in the arcuate nucleus. It is sensitive to feedback control from sex steroids and inhibin, a gonadal protein product that controls the frequency and amplitude of gonadotropin secretion during development in both sexes and during the progression of the menstrual cycle in females (see Chapter 13). Individual GnRH neurons have an intrinsic pulsatility that may be the basis of the pattern of GnRH secretion.

In males, luteinizing hormone (LH) stimulates the Leydig cells to secrete testosterone, while follicle-stimulating hormone (FSH) stimulates the Sertoli cells to produce inhibin. Inhibin feeds back to inhibit FSH. Inhibin is also released in a pulsatile pattern, but concentrations do not change with pubertal progression. In females, FSH stimulates the granulosa cells to produce estrogen and the follicles to secrete inhibin, while LH appears to play a minor role in the endocrine milieu until menarche, when it triggers ovulation and later stimulates the theca cells to secrete androgens (see Chapters 12 and 13).

A. Fetal Life: The concept of the continuum of development between the fetus and the adult is well illustrated by the changes that occur in the hypothalamic-pituitary-gonadal axis. Gonadotropins are demonstrable in fetal pituitary glands and serum during the first trimester. The pituitary content of gonadotropins rises to a plateau at mid gestation. Serum concentrations of LH and FSH rise to a peak at mid gestation and then gradually decrease until term. During the first half of gestation, hypothalamic GnRH content also increases, and the hypophysial-portal circulation achieves anatomic maturity. These data are compatible with a theory of early unrestrained GnRH secretion stimulating pituitary gonadotropin secretion, followed by the appearance of factors that inhibit GnRH release and decrease gonadotropin secretion after mid gestation. Since the male fetus has measurable serum testosterone concentrations but lower serum gonadotropin concentrations than the female fetus, negative feedback inhibition of gonadotropin secretion by testosterone appears operative after mid gestation.

B. Changes at Birth: At term, serum gonadotropin concentrations are suppressed, but with postnatal clearance of high circulating estrogen concentrations, negative inhibition is reduced and postnatal peaks of serum LH and FSH are measurable several months after birth. Serum testosterone concentrations may be increased to midpubertal levels during the several months after birth in normal males. While episodic peaks of serum gonadotropins may occur until 2 years of age, serum gonadotropin concentrations are low during later years in normal childhood.

C. The Juvenile Pause or the Mid-Childhood Nadir of Gonadotropin Secretion: While serum gonadotropin concentrations are low in mid childhood, sensitive assays indicate that pulsatile secretion occurs and that the onset of puberty is heralded more by an increase in amplitude of secretory events than in frequency. Patients with gonadal failure—such as those with the syndrome of gonadal dysgenesis (Turner's syndrome)—demonstrate an exaggeration of the normal pattern of gonadotropin secretion, with exceedingly high concentrations of serum LH and FSH during the first several years of life (see Chapter 14). Such patients show that negative feedback inhibition is active during childhood; without sex steroid or inhibin secretion to exert inhibition, serum gonadotropin values are greatly elevated. During mid childhood, normal individuals and patients with primary hypogonadism have lower serum gonadotropin levels than they do in the neonatal period, but the range of serum gonadotropin concentrations in hypogonadal patients during mid childhood is still higher than that found in healthy children of the same age. The decrease in serum gonadotropin concentrations in primary hypogonadal children during mid childhood is incompletely understood but has been attributed to an increase in the central nervous system inhibition of gonadotropin secretion during these years.

D. Peripubertal Gonadotropin Increase: Prepubertal children demonstrate a circadian rhythm of LH and FSH secretion with a circadian rhythm of sex steroid secretion lagging behind the gonadotropin rhythm, the delay presumably due to the time necessary for biosynthesis. Thus, the changes that are described below which occur at puberty do not arise *de novo* but are based upon preexisting patterns of endocrine secretion. In the peripubertal period, endogenous GnRH secretion increases in amplitude and frequency during the early hours of sleep and serum testosterone and estrogen concentrations rise several hours later, suggesting that biosynthesis or aromatization occurs during the period of delay—a pattern that differs from the prepubertal period mainly in the increased amplitude of the secretion encountered in puberty (Figure 15–5). As puberty progresses in both sexes, the peaks of serum LH and FSH occur more often during waking hours; and, finally, in late puberty, the peaks occur at all times, eliminating the diurnal variation. Thus, daytime samples of blood for determination of serum gonadotropin concentrations are of less value during early puberty because such sampling misses these nighttime peaks.

During the peripubertal period of endocrine change prior to secondary sexual development, gonadotropin secretion becomes less sensitive to negative feedback inhibition. Before this time, a small dose of exogenous sex steroids virtually eliminates gonadotropin secretion, while afterward a far larger dose is required to suppress serum FSH and LH. In prepuberty or early puberty, naltrexone, an opioid receptor antagonist, can completely suppress gonadotropin secretion as a consequence of its weak opioid effects, while after mid puberty the anti-opioid effects predominate and gonadotropin secretion increases, demonstrating decrease in sensitivity to opioids with pubertal development.

Most studies of gonadotropin secretion measure gonadotropin concentrations by radioimmunoassay (RIA). However, the biologic activity of LH changes because of alterations in the glycosylation and tertiary structure of gonadotropin molecules; this change may not be reflected in the RIA. Studies comparing immunoassayable LH (I-LH) to bioassayable LH (B-LH) suggest that the ratio of B-LH: I-LH increases with the onset of puberty and that this

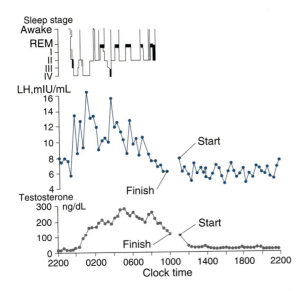

Figure 15–5. Plasma LH and testosterone measured during a 24-hour period in a 14-year-old boy in pubertal stage 2. Samples collected at night are displayed with electroencephalographic sleep stages. (Reproduced, with permission, from Boyar RM et al: Simultaneous augmented secretion of luteinizing hormone and testosterone during sleep. J Clin Invest 1974;54:609.)

tions of gonadal steroids are episodically elevated. This indicates the potential for secretory activity in the neonatal gonad. Later, when gonadotropin secretion decreases in mid childhood, gonadal activity decreases, but testes can still be stimulated by LH or hCG and ovaries by FSH with resulting secretion of gonadal steroids. A new sensitive estradiol assay demonstrates higher values of serum estradiol in prepubertal girls than prepubertal boys, indicating definite basal ovarian activity during the juvenile pause. With the onset of puberty, serum gonadal steroid concentrations progressively increase (Figure 15–6). While sex steroids are secreted in a diurnal rhythm in early puberty, they are bound to sex hormone-binding globulin, and the half-life of sex steroids is longer than that of gonadotropins. Thus, random daytime measurements of serum sex steroids are more helpful in determining pubertal status than random measurements of serum gonadotropins.

ratio may explain the profound endocrine changes of puberty better than the rather small changes in I-LH secretion. Furthermore, bioactive FSH rises early in puberty, perhaps stimulating ovarian activity before most of the rise in LH occurs. Recently, highly sensitive "sandwich" assays (immunoradiometric assay [IRMA]) and immunochemiluminometric assays (ICMA) were developed for gonadotropin determination. They can be used to indicate the state of pubertal development by the use of basal samples without the necessity for GnRH testing. Elevated LH values (> 0.3 IU/L) determined by third-generation assays in random blood samples are highly predictive of elevated peak GnRH-stimulated LH and therefore indicate the onset of central precocious puberty or normal puberty. These third-generation assays further reflect the remarkable logarithmic increase in spontaneous LH secretion in the latest stages of prepuberty and earliest stages of puberty as the testicular volume increases from 1 mL to 10 mL; these increases in serum LH are far greater proportionately than those found in the last stages of pubertal development. The magnitude of increase in serum testosterone is also greater in the early stages of puberty and correlates with the increase in serum LH during this same period of early pubertal development.

E. Sex Steroid Secretion: Sex steroid secretion is correlated with the development of gonadotropin secretion. During the postnatal period of episodic gonadotropin secretion, plasma concentra-

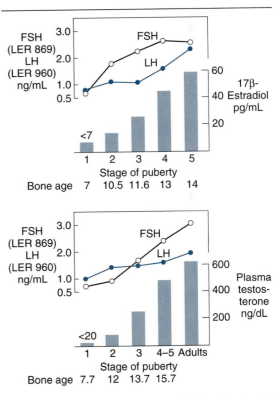

Figure 15–6. Mean plasma LH, FSH, and estradiol (girls) or testosterone (boys) correlated with stage of puberty and bone age. LER 869 and LER 960 are the reference standards for FSH and LH, respectively. The values reported here in ng/mL would be reported as mIU/mL in most laboratories. The conversion factors are as follows: for FSH (LER 869), 1 ng = 3 mIU; for LH (LER 960), 1 ng = 7.8 mIU. (Reproduced, with permission, from Grumbach MM: Onset of puberty. In: *Puberty.* Berenberg SR [editor]. H.E. Stenfert Kroese. Copyright © 1975 by Martinus Nijhoff.)

Most (97–99%) of the circulating estradiol and testosterone is associated with sex hormone-binding globulin (SHBG). The free hormone is the active fraction, but SHBG modulates the activity of the total testosterone and estradiol. Prepubertal boys and girls have equal concentrations of SHBG, but because testosterone decreases SHBG and estrogen increases SHBG, adult males have only half the concentration of SHBG than that of adult females. Thus, SHBG amplifies androgen effect in men; while adult men have 20 times the amount of plasma testosterone that adult women have, adult men have 40 times the amount of free testosterone that adult women have (see Chapter 12).

F. GnRH Stimulation: The use of intravenous GnRH has further clarified the pattern of pubertal development (Figure 15–7). When GnRH is administered to children under 2 years of age, pituitary secretion of LH and FSH increases markedly. During the juvenile pause, the period of low basal gonadotropin secretion (age 2 to age 9 or 10 years), exogenous GnRH has less effect on LH release. By the peripubertal period, 100 µg of intravenous GnRH induces a rise in LH concentrations of more than 15.6 mIU/mL in boys and girls, and this response continues until adulthood; this is the pubertal response. There is no significant change in the magnitude of FSH secretion after GnRH with the onset of puberty, though females at all ages release more FSH than males.

Gonadotropins are released in secretory spurts in response to endogenous GnRH, which itself is secreted episodically about every 90–120 minutes in response to a central nervous system "pulse generator." Individual GnRH-containing neurons in culture secrete GnRH in a pulsatile manner with an intrinsic rhythm. GnRH can be administered to patients in episodic boluses that mimic the natural secretory episodes. A prepubertal subject without significant gonadotropin peaks will demonstrate the normal pubertal pattern of episodic secretion of gonadotropins after only a few days of such exogenously administered GnRH boluses. Hypogonadotropic patients, who in the basal state do not have great secretory episodes of gonadotropin release, may be converted to a pattern of normal adult episodic gonadotropin secretion by this method of pulsatile GnRH administration. Varying the timing of pulsatile GnRH administration can regulate the ratio of FSH to LH just as the frequency of endogenous hypothalamic GnRH release shifts during the menstrual cycle and puberty to naturally alter this ratio. Increasing the frequency of GnRH pulses increases the LH:FSH ratio; an increased ratio is characteristic of midcycle and peripubertal dynamics. Alternatively, if GnRH is administered continuously rather than in pulses or if long-acting superactive analogs of GnRH are given, a brief period of increased gonadotropin secretion is followed by LH and FSH suppression. This phenomenon is responsible for the therapeutic effects of

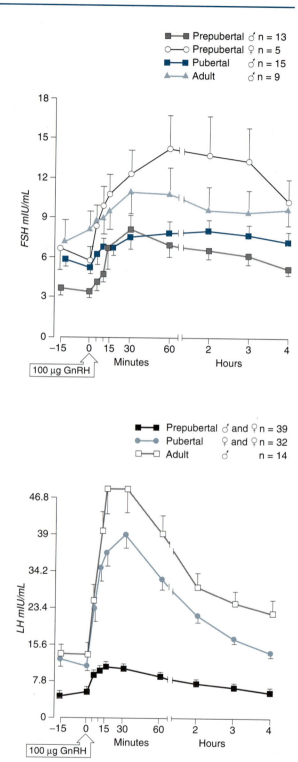

Figure 15–7. The changes in plasma FSH *(top)* and LH *(bottom)* after GnRH was administered in prepubertal, pubertal, and adult subjects. (Modified and reproduced, with permission, from Grumbach MM et al: *Control of the Onset of Puberty.* Grumbach MM, Grave GD, Mayer FE [editors]. Wiley, 1974.)

GnRH analogs in conditions such as central precocious puberty.

Ovulation and Menarche

The last stage in hypothalamic-pituitary development is the onset of positive feedback, leading to ovulation and menarche. After mid puberty, estrogen in the right amount at the right time can stimulate gonadotropin release just as it can suppress gonadotropin secretion in other situations. The frequency of pulsatile GnRH release increases during the normal menstrual cycle and raises the ratio of LH to FSH secretion. This stimulates the ovary to produce estrogen and leads to the midcycle LH surge that causes ovulation. Administration of pulsatile GnRH by programmable pump can be used to bring about fertility in patients with hypothalamic GnRH deficiency by mimicking this natural pattern. However, even if the midcycle surge of gonadotropins is present, ovulation may not occur during the first menstrual cycles; 90% of menstrual cycles are anovulatory in the first year after menarche, and it is not until 4–5 years after menarche that the percentage of anovulatory cycles decreases to less than 20%. However, it is clear that the first cycles after menarche may be ovulatory. In the USA, the mean age at menarche is 12.8 years ± 1.2 years (mean ± 1 SD). Menarche is closely correlated with a skeletal age of 13 years (see Chapter 6).

Thus, just as in boys, girls may become fertile and pregnant prior to physical maturity.

Adrenarche

While the hypothalamic-pituitary axis has been well characterized in recent years, our understanding of the mechanism of control of adrenal androgen secretion is still somewhat rudimentary. The adrenal cortex secretes the weak androgens dehydroepiandrosterone (DHEA), its sulfate, dehydroepiandrosterone sulfate (DHEAS), and androstenedione in increasing amounts beginning at about 6–7 years of age in girls and 7–8 years of age in boys (Table 15–1). A continued rise in adrenal androgen secretion persists until late puberty. Thus, adrenarche (the secretion of adrenal androgens) occurs years before gonadarche (the secretion of gonadal sex steroids). The observation that patients with Addison's disease, who do not secrete adrenal androgens, and patients with premature adrenarche, who secrete increased amounts of adrenal androgens at an early age, usually enter gonadarche at a normal age suggests that age at adrenarche does not significantly influence age at gonadarche. Furthermore, patients treated with a GnRH agonist to suppress gonadotropin secretion progress through adrenarche despite their suppressed gonadarche. Measurements of urinary 17-ketosteroids reflect principally adrenal androgen secretion and not secretion of testosterone or its metabolites. Thus, urinary 17-ketosteroid levels rise considerably at adrenarche but need not do so at gonadarche.

Miscellaneous Metabolic Changes

The onset of puberty is associated with many changes in laboratory values that are either directly or indirectly caused by the rise of sex steroid concentrations. Thus, in boys, hematocrit rises and HDL concentrations fall as a consequence of increasing testosterone. The latter effect causes older boys and men to have a higher risk of arteriosclerotic coronary artery disease than females. In both boys and girls, alkaline phosphatase rises during the pubertal growth spurt. Serum IGF-1 concentrations rise with the growth spurt, but IGF-1 is more closely correlated with sex steroid concentration than with growth rate.

Table 15–1. Mean serum concentrations of DHEAS during childhood.[1]

	Boys		Girls	
	(μg/dL)	(μmol/L)	(μg/dL)	(μmol/L)
Chronologic age (years)				
1–6	15.4 ± 6.8	0.53 ± 0.23	24.7 ± 11.1	0.86 ± 0.38
6–8	18.8 ± 4.1	0.65 ± 0.14	30.4 ± 7.6	1.05 ± 0.26
8–10	58.6 ± 10.1	2.03 ± 0.35	117.3 ± 41.7	4.06 ± 1.44
10–12	126.4 ± 28.0	4.38 ± 0.97	112.7 ± 16.4	3.90 ± 0.57
12–14	133.4 ± 22.2	4.62 ± 0.77	168.9 ± 19.3	5.85 ± 0.67
14–16	264.3 ± 19.4	9.15 ± 0.67	253.5 ± 41.3	8.78 ± 1.43
16–20	264.1 ± 61.8	9.14 ± 2.14	232.5 ± 49.8	8.05 ± 1.72
Bone age (years)				
1–6	16.6 ± 6.1	0.57 ± 0.21	2.5 ± 2.5	0.09 ± 0.09
6–8	36.3 ± 6.7	1.25 ± 0.23	27.2 ± 9.6	0.94 ± 0.33
8–10	57.4 ± 8.5	1.98 ± 0.29	. . .	. . .
10–12	125.0 ± 22.7	4.33 ± 0.79	112.9 ± 27.6	3.91 ± 0.96
12–14	214.9 ± 30.1	7.44 ± 1.04	159.7 ± 26.3	5.53 ± 0.91
14–16	403.4 ± 99.4	14.00 ± 3.44	261.0 ± 45.0	9.04 ± 1.56
16–20	. . .	. . .	145.3 ± 32.2	5.03 ± 1.12

[1]Modified and reproduced, with permission, from Reiter EO, Fuldauer LG, Root AW: *J Pediatr* 1977;**90**:766.

IGF-1 levels peak 1 year after peak growth velocity is reached and remain elevated for 4 years thereafter even though growth rate is decreasing. Prostate-specific antigen (PSA) is measurable after the onset of puberty in boys and provides another biochemical indication of pubertal onset.

DELAYED PUBERTY OR ABSENT PUBERTY (Sexual Infantilism)

Any girl of 13 or boy of 14 years of age with no signs of pubertal development falls more than 2.5 SD below the mean and is considered to have delayed puberty (Table 15–2). By this definition, 0.6% of the healthy population are classified as having **constitutional delay** in growth and adolescence. These normal patients need reassurance rather than treatment and will ultimately progress through the normal stages of puberty, albeit later than their peers. The examining physician must make the sometimes difficult decision about which patients older than these guidelines are constitutionally delayed and which have organic disease.

Constitutional Delay in Growth & Adolescence

A patient with delayed onset of secondary sexual development who has a history of being shorter than age-matched peers but who consistently maintains a normal growth velocity for bone age and whose skeletal development is delayed more than 2 SD from the mean is likely to have constitutional delay in puberty (Figure 15–8). These patients are at the older end of the distribution curve of age at onset of puberty. A family history of a similar pattern of development in a parent or sibling supports the diagnosis. The subject is usually thin as well. Studies suggest that disproportionately poor growth of the spine in constitutional delay in growth and adolescence relative to increased growth of the legs leads to a noticeable disproportion (lowering) of the upper to lower segment ratio; the disproportion is said to be an indicator of better final height attainment in this group. In many cases, even if they show no physical signs of puberty at the time of examination, the initial elevation of gonadal sex steroids has already begun, or their plasma LH response to intravenous GnRH is pubertal (a rise in LH of > 15.6 mIU/mL). These results suggest that secondary sexual development will commence within 6 months. However, in some cases, observation for endocrine or physical signs of puberty must continue for a period of months or years before the diagnosis is made. Generally, signs of puberty will appear after the patient reaches a skeletal age of 11 years (girls) or 12 years (boys). Patients with constitutional delay in adolescence will almost always manifest secondary sexual development by 18 years of chronologic age, though there is one reported case of spontaneous puberty occurring at 25 years of age. (This patient may have had Kallmann's syndrome; see below and Chapter 5.) Adrenarche is characteristically delayed—along with gonadarche—in constitutional delay in puberty.

Hypogonadotropic Hypogonadism

The absent or decreased ability of the hypothalamus to secrete GnRH or of the pituitary gland to secrete LH and FSH leads to hypogonadotropic hypogonadism. This classification denotes an irreversible condition requiring replacement therapy. If the pituitary deficiency is limited to gonadotropins, patients are usually close to normal height for age—in contrast to the shorter patients with constitutional delay. Bone age is usually not delayed in childhood but does not progress normally after the patient reaches the age at which sex steroid secretion ordinarily increases and normally stimulates maturation of the bone age. If GH deficiency accompanies gonadotropin deficiency, severe short stature will result.

A. Central Nervous System Disorders:

1. Tumors–A tumor involving the hypothalamus or pituitary gland can interfere with hypothalamic-pituitary-gonadal function as well as the control of GH, ACTH, TSH, PRL, and vasopressin secretion. Thus, delayed puberty may be a manifestation of a central nervous system tumor accompanied by any or all of the following: GH deficiency, secondary hypothyroidism, secondary adrenal insufficiency, hyperprolactinemia, and diabetes insipidus. The combination of anterior and posterior pituitary deficiencies

Table 15–2. Classification of delayed puberty.

Constitutional delay in growth and adolescence
Hypogonadotropic hypogonadism
 Central nervous system disorders
  Tumors
  Other acquired disorders
  Congenital disorders
 Isolated gonadotropin deficiency
 Multiple pituitary hormonal deficiencies
 Miscellaneous disorders
  Prader-Willi syndrome
  Laurence-Moon, Bardet-Biedl syndromes
  Chronic disease
  Weight loss
  Anorexia nervosa
  Increased physical activity in female athletes
  Hypothyroidism
Hypergonadotropic hypogonadism
 Males
  Klinefelter's syndrome
  Other forms of primary testicular failure
  Anorchia or cryptorchism
 Females
  Turner's syndrome
  Other forms of primary ovarian failure
 Pseudo-Turner's syndrome
 XX and XY gonadal dysgenesis

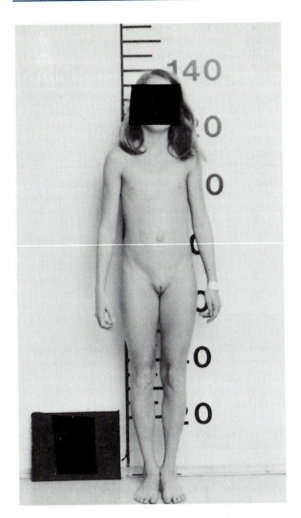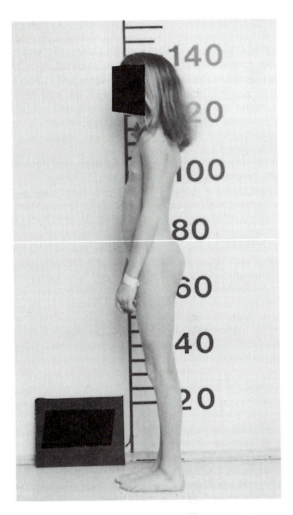

Figure 15–8. 13⁴/₁₂ years old girl with constitutional delay in growth and puberty. History revealed a normal growth rate but short stature at all ages. Physical examination revealed a height of 138 cm (–4.5 SD) and a weight of 28.6 kg (–3 SD). The patient had early stage 2 breast development, with 1 cm of glandular tissue on the right breast and 2 cm on the left breast. The vaginal mucosa was dulled, and there was no pubic hair. Karyotype was 46,XX. Bone age was 10 years. After administration of GnRH, LH rose from 14.8 to 37.4 mIU/mL (from 1.9 to 4.8 ng/mL) and FSH from 11.7 to 20.1 mIU/mL (from 3.9 to 6.7 ng/mL). Estradiol was 40 pg/mL. She has since spontaneously progressed through pubertal development. (Reproduced, with permission, from Styne DM, Kaplan SL: Pediatr Clin North Am 1979;26:123.)

acquired after birth makes it imperative that a hypothalamic-pituitary tumor be ruled out.

Craniopharyngioma is the most common type of hypothalamic-pituitary tumor leading to delay or absence of pubertal development. This neoplasm originates in Rathke's pouch but may develop into a suprasellar tumor. The peak age incidence of craniopharyngioma is between 6 and 14 years. Presenting symptoms may include headache, visual deficiency, growth failure, polyuria, and polydipsia; presenting signs may include visual defects, optic atrophy, or papilledema. Clinical manifestations may reflect gonadotropin, thyroid, and GH deficiency. Laboratory evaluation may reveal any type of anterior or posterior pituitary deficiencies. Bone age is often retarded at the time of presentation.

Calcification in the suprasellar region is the hallmark of craniopharyngiomas; 80% of cases will have calcifications on lateral skull x-ray, and a higher percentage will show this on CT scan. The tumor often presents a cystic appearance on CT or MRI scan and at the time of surgery may contain dark, cholesterol-laden fluid. The rate of growth of craniopharyngiomas is quite variable—some are indolent and some are quite aggressive. Small intrasellar tumors may be resected by transsphenoidal surgery; larger ones require partial resection and radiation therapy (see Chapter 5).

Extrasellar tumors that involve the hypothalamus and produce sexual infantilism include germinomas, gliomas (sometimes with neurofibromatosis), and astrocytomas (see Chapter 5). Intrasellar tumors such as chromophobe adenomas are quite rare in children compared to adults. Hyperprolactinemia—with or without a diagnosed microadenoma or galactorrhea—may delay the onset or progression of puberty; with therapy to decrease prolactin concentrations, puberty progressed in reported cases.

2. Other acquired central nervous system disorders–Other acquired central nervous system disorders may lead to hypothalamic-pituitary dysfunction. Granulomatous diseases such as Hand-Schüller-Christian disease or histiocytosis X, when involving the hypothalamus, most frequently lead to diabetes insipidus, but any other hypothalamic defect may also occur including gonadotropin deficiency. Tuberculous or sarcoid granulomas, other postinfectious inflammatory lesions, vascular lesions, and trauma more rarely cause hypogonadotropic hypogonadism.

3. Developmental defects–Developmental defects of the central nervous system may cause hypogonadotropic hypogonadism or other types of hypothalamic dysfunction. Cleft palate or other midline anomalies may also be associated with hypothalamic dysfunction. Optic dysplasia is associated with small, hypoplastic optic disks and, in some patients, absence of the septum pellucidum on pneumoencephalography, CT scanning, or MRI; associated hypothalamic deficiencies are often present. Optic hypoplasia or dysplasia must be differentiated from optic atrophy; optic atrophy implies an acquired condition and may indicate a hypothalamic-pituitary tumor. Both anterior and posterior pituitary deficiencies may occur with congenital midline defects or acquired defects. Early onset of such a combination suggests a congenital defect, while late onset more strongly indicates a neoplasm.

4. Radiation therapy–Central nervous system radiation therapy involving the hypothalamic-pituitary area can lead to hypogonadotropic hypogonadism with onset at 6–18 months (or longer) after treatment. Growth hormone is more frequently affected than gonadotropin secretion, and growth hormone deficiency occurs with as little as an 18-Gy dose of therapy. Other hypothalamic deficiencies such as gonadotropin deficiency, hypothyroidism, and hyperprolactinemia occur more often with higher doses up to or exceeding 40 Gy.

B. Isolated Hormonal Deficiency: Patients who have isolated deficiency of gonadotropins but normal GH secretion tend to be of normal height for age until the teenage years but will lack a pubertal growth spurt. They have eunuchoid proportions of increased span for height and decreased upper to lower segment ratios. Their skeletal development will be delayed for chronologic age during the teenage years, and they will continue to grow after an age when normal adolescents stop growing.

Kallmann's syndrome is the most common form of isolated gonadotropin deficiency (Figure 15–9). Gonadotropin deficiency in these patients is associated with hypoplasia or aplasia of the olfactory lobes and hyposmia or anosmia; remarkably, they may not notice that they have no sense of smell, though olfactory testing will reveal it. GnRH-containing neurons fail to migrate from the olfactory placode (where they originate) to the medial basal hypothalamus in Kallmann's syndrome. This is a familial syndrome of variable manifestations in which anosmia may occur with or without hypogonadism in a given member of a kindred. Kallman's syndrome is due to gene deletions in the region of Xp22.3, causing the absence of the *KAL* gene, which appears to code for an adhesion molecule. There is an association of Kallmann's syndrome with X-linked ichthyosis due to steroid sulfatase deficiency, mental retardation, and chondrodysplasia punctata. Associated abnormalities in Kallmann's syndrome may affect the kidneys and bones, and patients may have undescended testes, gynecomastia, and obesity. Ultimate height is normal, though patients are delayed in reaching adult height.

Other cases of hypogonadotropic hypogonadism may occur sporadically or via an autosomal recessive pattern without anosmia. X-linked congenital adrenal hypoplasia is associated with hypogonadotropic hypogonadism; glycerol kinase deficiency and muscular dystrophy have been linked to this syndrome. Some hypogonadal patients lack only LH secretion and have spermatogenesis without testosterone production (fertile eunuch syndrome); others lack only FSH.

C. Idiopathic Hypopituitary Dwarfism: Patients with congenital GH deficiency have early onset of growth failure (Figure 15–10); this feature distinguishes them from patients with GH deficiency due to hypothalamic tumors, who usually have late onset of growth failure. Even without associated gonadotropin deficiency, untreated GH-deficient patients often have delayed onset of puberty associated with their delayed bone ages. With appropriate hGH therapy, however, onset of puberty occurs at a normal age. Patients who have combined GH and gonadotropin deficiency do not undergo puberty even when bone age reaches the pubertal stage. Idiopathic hypopituitarism is usually sporadic but may follow an autosomal recessive or X-linked inheritance pattern. Birth injury or breech delivery is a common feature of the neonatal history of patients with idiopathic hypopituitarism (breech delivery being more common in the history of affected males).

The syndrome of microphallus (due to congenital gonadotropin deficiency) and neonatal hypoglycemic seizures (due to congenital ACTH deficiency, GH deficiency, or both) must be diagnosed and treated early to avoid mental retardation. Patients with this syndrome will not undergo spontaneous pubertal de-

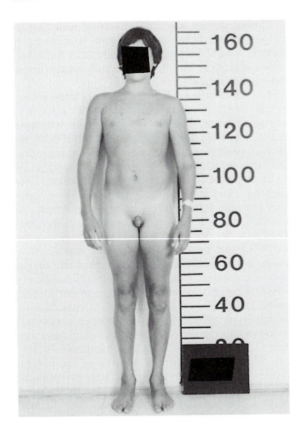 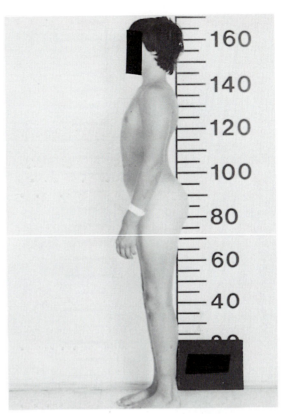

Figure 15–9. Boy 15^{10}⁄$_{12}$ years old with Kallmann's syndrome. His testes were originally undescended, but they descended into the scrotum after human chorionic gonadotropin treatment was given. His height was 163.9 cm (–1.5 SD), and the US:LS ratio was 0.86 (eunuchoid). The penis was 6.3 × 1.8 cm. Each testis was 1 × 2 cm. Plasma LH was not detectable and rose to 5.6 mIU/mL after administration of 100 µg of GnRH; FSH rose from 3.6 to 7.2 mIU/mL. Testosterone did not change from 17 ng/dL. He had no ability to smell standard odors. (Reproduced, with permission, from Styne DM, Grumbach MM: *Reproductive Endocrinology.* Yen SSC, Jaffe RB [editors]. Saunders, 1978.)

velopment. Testosterone in low doses (testosterone enanthate, 25 mg intramuscularly every month for three doses) can increase the size of the penis in infants diagnosed with congenital hypopituitarism without significantly advancing the bone age. Males with isolated GH deficiency can also have microphallus; the penis will enlarge to some degree with hGH therapy in these patients. It is important to note that microphallus due to hypopituitarism is medically treatable, and sex reversal usually need not be considered (see Chapter 14).

D. Miscellaneous Disorders:

1. Prader-Willi syndrome—Prader-Willi syndrome occurs sporadically and is associated with fetal and infantile hypotonia, short stature; poor feeding in infancy but insatiable hunger later, leading to massive obesity; characteristic facies with almond-shaped eyes, small hands and feet after infancy, mental retardation, and emotional instability in patients of either sex; delayed menarche in females; and micropenis and cryptorchism in males. Osteoporosis is common in these patients during the teenage years,

and sex steroid replacement, when indicated, may help. Behavioral modification may improve the usual pattern of rampant weight gain. About 50% of patients have deletion or translocation of chromosome 15, and the affected chromosome is usually the paternally derived one. Fluorescent in situ hybridization for the area of the chromosome is available from laboratories for diagnosis.

2. Laurence-Moon and Bardet-Biedl syndromes—These autosomal recessive conditions are characterized by obesity, short stature, mental retardation, and retinitis pigmentosa. Hypogonadotropic hypogonadism and primary hypogonadism have variously been reported in affected patients. A distinction between Laurence-Moon and Bardet-Biedl syndromes may be made, with the latter demonstrating polydactyly and obesity while the former was characterized by paraplegia.

3. Chronic disease and malnutrition—A delay in sexual maturation may be due to chronic disease or malnutrition. For example, children with intractable asthma have delayed pubertal development

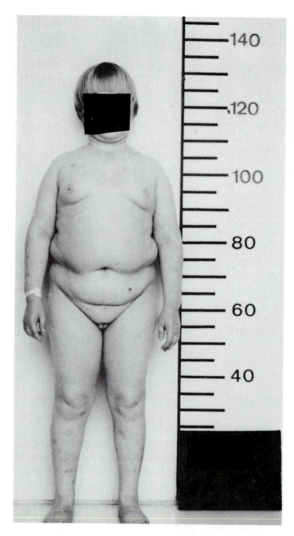

Figure 15–10. Twenty-year-old male with congenital deficiency of GH, GnRH, TSH, and ACTH. Height was 8 SD below the mean, and the phallus was 2 × 1 cm. Bone age was 10 years, and the sella turcica was small on lateral skull x-ray. LH was 1.56 mIU/mL and rose only to 4.68 mIU/mL after administration of 100 μg of GnRH. Testosterone was less than 10 ng/dL and did not rise after administration of GnRH. (Reproduced, with permission, from Styne DM, Grumbach MM: *Reproductive Endocrinology.* Yen SSC, Jaffe RB [editors]. Saunders, 1978.)

leading to short stature during the teenage years, though they ultimately reach an appropriate height. Children with other chronic diseases may not fare so well in long-term follow-up; eg, HIV infection in adolescence causes poor growth and pubertal progression. Weight loss to less than 80% of ideal weight caused by disease or voluntary dieting may result in gonadotropin deficiency; weight gain toward the ideal usually restores gonadotropin function.

Chronic disease may have effects on sexual maturation separate from nutritional state. For example, there is a high incidence of hypothalamic hypogonadism in thalassemia major even with regular transfusion and chelation therapy.

4. Anorexia nervosa–Anorexia nervosa involves weight loss associated with significant psychologic disorder. Patients are usually girls who have a disturbed body image and exhibit typical behavior such as avoidance of food and induction of regurgitation after ingestion. Weight loss may be so severe as to cause a fatal complication such as immune dysfunction, fluid and electrolyte imbalance, or circulatory collapse. Primary or secondary amenorrhea is a classic finding in these patients and has been correlated with the degree of weight loss, though there is evidence that patients with anorexia nervosa may cease to menstruate before their substantial weight loss is exhibited. Other endocrine abnormalities in anorexia nervosa include elevated serum growth hormone and decreased IGF-1 (these are characteristic of any type of starvation), decreased serum triiodothyronine, decreased serum 1,25-dihydroxyvitamin D_3 and elevated 24,25-hydroxyvitamin D_3 levels. Weight gain to the normal range for height, however, does not ensure immediate resumption of menses. There is an increased incidence of anorexia nervosa in ballet dancers or ballet students; the incidence of scoliosis and mitral valve insufficiency is also increased in these patients. Functional amenorrhea may also occur in women of normal weight, some of whom demonstrate evidence of psychologic stress. Decreased LH response to GnRH administration, impaired monthly cycles of gonadotropin secretion, and retention of a diurnal rhythm of gonadotropin secretion are found in anorexia nervosa patients, patterns which indicate a reversion to an earlier stage of endocrine puberty.

5. Increased physical activity–Girls who regularly participate in strenuous athletics, ballet dancing, etc, may have delayed thelarche, delayed menarche, and irregular or absent menstrual periods; this effect is not always related to less than ideal weight. Since such amenorrheic patients may resume menses while temporarily bedridden, increased physical activity and not decreased weight appears to be the cause of the amenorrhea. Statistical analysis of mothers' ages at menarche and the type of sport pursued by their daughters indicates that late maturation of gymnasts may be referable to a familial tendency to late menarche allowing the girl to continue gymnastics rather than gymnastic activity acting as the primary cause of late menarche. However, there are disturbing studies indicating that intensive gymnastics training at an early age leads to a decrease in ultimate stature.

6. Hypothyroidism–Hypothyroidism can delay all aspects of growth and maturation, including puberty and menarche. Galactorrhea may occur in severe primary hypothyroidism due to concomitant elevation of serum prolactin. With thyroxine therapy, catch-up growth and resumed pubertal development and menses will occur. Conversely, severe primary hypothyroidism may be associated with precocious puberty and galactorrhea (due to elevated serum prolactin) in some patients (Van Wyk-Grumbach syndrome). There is evidence that TSH can stimulate FSH receptors, leading to estrogen secretion.

Hypergonadotropic Hypogonadism

Primary gonadal failure is heralded by elevated gonadotropin concentration due to the absence of negative feedback effects of gonadal sex steroids. The most common causes of hypergonadotropic hypogonadism are associated with karyotypic and somatic abnormalities, but isolated gonadal failure can also present with delayed puberty without other physical findings. When hypergonadotropic hypogonadism is present in patients with a Y chromosome (genetic males or conditions noted below), testicular dysgenesis must be considered in the differential diagnosis. The risk of testicular cancer rises in testicular dysgenesis. (Testicular cancer in normal boys is rare; for example, the incidence in Scandinavia is 0.5 per 100,000 in childhood.)

A. Syndrome of Seminiferous Tubule Dysgenesis (Klinefelter's Syndrome): (See Chapters 12 and 14.) The most common form of primary testicular failure is Klinefelter's syndrome (47,XXY karyotype), with an incidence of 1:1000 males. Before puberty, patients with Klinefelter's syndrome have decreased upper segment:lower segment ratios, small testes, and an increased incidence of developmental delay and personality disorders. Onset of puberty is not usually delayed, because Leydig cell function is characteristically less affected than seminiferous tubule function in this condition and testosterone is adequate to stimulate pubertal development. Serum gonadotropin levels rise to castrate concentrations after the onset of puberty; the testes become firm and are rarely larger than 3.5 cm in diameter. After the onset of puberty, there are histologic changes of seminiferous tubule hyalinization and fibrosis, adenomatous changes of the Leydig cells, and impaired spermatogenesis. Gynecomastia is common, and variable degrees of male secondary sexual development are found.

Other forms of male hypergonadotropic hypogonadism are found with 46,XX/47,XXY, 48,XXYY, 48,XXXY, and 49,XXXXY karyotypes. Phenotypic males are described with 46,XX karyotypes and some physical features of Klinefelter's syndrome (see Chapter 14).

B. Other Forms of Primary Testicular Failure: Patients surviving treatment for malignant diseases form a growing category of patients with testicular failure. Chemotherapy—primarily with alkylating agents—or radiation therapy directed to the gonads may lead to gonadal failure; injury is more likely if treatment is given during puberty than if it occurs in the prepubertal period. A recent report indicated normal pubertal development in boys treated prepubertally with polychemotherapy, though they demonstrated elevated peak serum LH and elevated basal and peak serum FSH after GnRH as well as a high incidence of decreased or absent sperm counts; this indicates that prepubertal status does not protect a child against testicular damage from chemotherapy and that normal physical development may hide significant endocrine and reproductive damage.

The "Sertoli cell only" syndrome (germinal cell aplasia) is a congenital form of testicular failure manifested by azoospermia and elevated FSH concentrations but generally normal secondary sexual characteristics, normal testosterone concentrations, and no other anomalies. Patients with Down's syndrome may have elevated LH and FSH levels even in the presence of normal testosterone levels, suggesting some element of primary gonadal failure.

C. Cryptorchism or Anorchia: Phenotypic males with a 46,XY karyotype but no palpable testes have either cryptorchism or anorchia. Cryptorchid males should produce a rise in testosterone levels > 2 ng/mL 72 hours after intramuscular administration of 2000 units of chorionic gonadotropin, and the testes may descend during 2 weeks of treatment with 2000 units given three times a week. Patients with increased plasma testosterone levels in response to chorionic gonadotropin administration but without testicular descent have cryptorchism; their testes should be surgically brought into the scrotum to decrease the likelihood of further testicular damage due to the elevated intra-abdominal temperature and to guard against the possibility of undetected tumor formation. Cryptorchid testes may demonstrate congenital abnormalities and may not have normal function even if brought into the scrotum early in life. Furthermore, the descended testis in a unilaterally cryptorchid boy may itself show abnormal histologic features; such patients have a 69% incidence of decreased sperm counts. Thus, unilateral cryptorchid patients can be infertile even if they received early treatment of their unilateral cryptorchism. In addition, patients undergoing orchiopexy may sustain subtle damage to the vas deferens, leading to the later production of antibodies to sperm that may result in infertility.

It is important to determine if any testicular tissue is present in a boy with no palpable testes, since unnoticed malignant degeneration of the tissue is a possibility. The diagnosis of anorchia may be pursued by ultrasound or MRI, laparotomy or laparoscopic examination, or by the endocrine evaluation noted above. Furthermore, the presence of antimüllerian factor in a young child indicates the presence of testicular tissue, although during puberty antimüllerian factor becomes nondetectable and this test cannot be employed. The presence of normal basal gonadotropin levels in a prepubertal boy without palpable testes suggests the presence of testicular tissue even if the testosterone response to hCG is low, while the presence of elevated gonadotropin levels without any testosterone response to hCG suggests anorchia. Except for the absence of testes, patients with anorchia have normal infantile male genital development, including wolffian duct formation and müllerian duct regression. The testes were presumably present in these patients early in fetal life during sexual differentiation but degenerated after the 13th week of gestation for unknown reasons ("vanishing testes syndrome") (see Chapter 12).

D. Syndrome of Gonadal Dysgenesis (Turner's Syndrome): (See Chapters 13 and 14.) 45,X gonadal dysgenesis is associated with short stature, female phenotype with sexual infantilism, and a chromatin-negative buccal smear. Patients have "streak" gonads consisting of fibrous tissue without germ cells. Other classic but variable phenotypic features include micrognathia, "fish" mouth (downturned corners of the mouth), ptosis, low-set or deformed ears, a broad shield-like chest with the appearance of widely spaced nipples, hypoplastic areolae, a short neck with low hairline and webbing of the neck (pterygium colli), short fourth metacarpals, cubitus valgus, structural anomalies of the kidney, extensive nevi, hypoplastic nails, and vascular anomalies of the left side of the heart (most commonly coarctation of the aorta). The medical history of patients with the syndrome of gonadal dysgenesis will often reveal small size at birth, lymphedema of the extremities most prominent in the newborn period, and loose posterior cervical skin folds. (The terms "Bonnevie-Ullrich syndrome" and "infant Turner's syndrome" have been applied to this neonatal appearance.) Affected patients often have a history of frequent otitis media with conductive hearing loss. Intelligence is normal, but there is often impaired spatial orientation. Patients have no pubertal growth spurt and reach a mean final height of 143 cm. Short stature is a classic feature of Turner's syndrome but not of other forms of hypergonadotropic hypogonadism that occur without karyotypic abnormalities. GH function is usually normal in Turner's syndrome, and the cause of short stature is not known. However, studies suggest that hGH treatment improves growth rate in affected girls (see Chapter 14). Pubic hair may appear late and is usually sparse in distribution owing to the absence of any ovarian secretions; thus, adrenarche progresses in Turner's syndrome even in the absence of gonadarche. Autoimmune thyroid disease (usually hypothyroidism) is common in Turner's syndrome, and determination of thyroid function and thyroid antibody levels is important in evaluation of these patients.

Serum gonadotropin concentrations in Turner's syndrome are extremely high between birth and age 4 years. They decrease toward the normal range in prepubertal patients and then rise again to castrate levels after age 10 years. (See Chapter 14.)

Sex chromatin-positive variants of gonadal dysgenesis include 45,X/46,XX, 45,X/47,XXX, and 45,X/46,XX/47,XXX mosaicism with chromatin-positive buccal smears. Patients with these karyotypes may resemble patients with the classic syndrome of gonadal dysgenesis, or they may have fewer manifestations and normal or nearly normal female phenotypes. Streak gonad formation is not invariable; some patients have had secondary sexual development, and menarche and (rarely) even pregnancy have been reported. Patients with Turner's syndrome have benefited from in vitro fertilization techniques. After exogenous hormonal preparation, a fertilized ovum (possibly her sister's ovum fertilized by the patient's male partner, or an extra fertilized ovum from another couple undergoing in vitro fertilization) can be introduced into the patient's uterus, and the pregnancy is then brought to term by exogenous hormone administration.

Sex chromatin-negative variants of the syndrome of gonadal dysgenesis have karyotypes with 45,X/46,XY mosaicism. Physical features vary; some patients have the features of classic Turner's syndrome, while others may have ambiguous genitalia or even the features of phenotypic males. Gonads are dysgenetic but vary from streak gonads to functioning testes. These patients are at risk for gonadoblastoma formation. Since gonadoblastomas may secrete androgens or estrogens, patients with gonadoblastoma may virilize or feminize as though they had functioning gonads, confusing the clinical picture. Gonadoblastomas may demonstrate calcification on abdominal x-ray. Malignant germ cell tumors may arise in dysgenetic testes, and orchiectomy is generally indicated. In some mosaic patients with one intact X chromosome and one chromosomal fragment, it is difficult to determine whether the fragment is derived from an X chromosome or a Y chromosome; present research into appropriate markers for the chromosome or for the presence of testis-determining factor will probably in future allow diagnosis of patients at risk for such complications. At present, the use of Y chromosome-specific DNA probes may identify such patients at risk.

E. Other Forms of Primary Ovarian Failure: Ovaries appear to be more resistant to damage from the chemotherapy used in the treatment of malignant disease than are testes. Nonetheless, ovarian failure can occur with medical therapy. Damage is common if the ovaries are not surgically "tacked" out of the path of the beam in abdominal radiation therapy. Premature menopause has also been described in otherwise healthy girls owing to the presence of antiovarian antibodies; patients with Addison's disease may have autoimmune oophoritis as well as adrenal failure. A sex steroid biosynthetic defect due to 17α-hydroxylase (P450c17) deficiency will be manifested as sexual infantilism and primary amenorrhea in a phenotypic female (regardless of genotype) with hypokalemia and hypertension. The patient with 17α-hydroxylase deficiency may have ovaries or testes and still present as a phenotypic female.

F. Pseudo-Turner's Syndrome (Noonan's Syndrome, Ullrich's Syndrome, Male Turner's Syndrome): Pseudo-Turner's syndrome is associated with manifestations of Turner's syndrome such as webbed neck, ptosis, short stature, cubitus valgus, and lymphedema, but other clinical findings such as a normal karyotype, triangular facies, pectus excavatum, right-sided heart disease, and an increased incidence of mental retardation differentiate these patients from those with Turner's syndrome. Males may have undescended testes and variable degrees of germinal cell and Leydig cell dysfunction. Pseudo-Turner's syndrome follows an autosomal dominant pattern of inheritance with incomplete penetrance.

G. Familial and Sporadic Forms of 46,XX or 46,XY Gonadal Dysgenesis: These forms of gonadal dysgenesis are characterized by structurally normal chromosomes and streak gonads or partially functioning gonads. If there is some gonadal function, 46,XY gonadal dysgenesis may present with ambiguous genitalia or virilization at puberty. If no gonadal function is present, patients appear as phenotypic sexually infantile females. Patients with 46,XY gonadal dysgenesis and dysgenetic testes should undergo gonadectomy to eliminate the possibility of malignant germ cell tumor formation.

H. Primary Amenorrhea Associated With Normal Secondary Sexual Development: If a structural anomaly of the uterus or vagina interferes with the onset of menses but the endocrine milieu remains normal, the patient presents with primary amenorrhea in the presence of normal breast and pubic hair development. A transverse vaginal septum will seal the uterine cavity from the vaginal orifice,

leading to the retention of menstrual flow—as may an imperforate hymen. The Rokitansky-Küster-Hauser syndrome combines congenital absence of the vagina with abnormal development of the uterus, ranging from a rudimentary bicornuate uterus that may not open into the vaginal canal to a virtually normal uterus; surgical repair may be possible in patients with minimal anatomic abnormalities, and fertility has been reported. Associated abnormalities include major urinary tract anomalies and spinal or other skeletal disorders. The rarest anatomic abnormality in this group is absence of the uterine cervix in the presence of a functional uterus.

Male pseudohermaphroditism is an alternative cause of primary amenorrhea if a patient has achieved thelarche. The syndrome of complete androgen resistance leads to female genitalia and phenotype without axillary or pubic hair development in the presence of pubertal breast development (syndrome of testicular feminization; see Chapter 14).

Differential Diagnosis of Delayed Puberty (Table 15–3)

Patients who do not begin secondary sexual development by age 13 (girls) or age 14 (boys) and patients who do not progress through development on a timely basis (girls should menstruate within 5 years after breast budding; boys should reach stage 5 pubertal development 4½ years after onset) should be evaluated for hypogonadism. The yield of diagnosable conditions is quite low in children younger than these ages, but many patients and families will request evaluation well before these limits. Without significant sign or symptoms of disorders discussed above, it is best to resist evaluation until these ages in most cases.

If the diagnosis is not obvious on the basis of physical or historical features, the differential diagnostic process begins with determination of whether plasma gonadotropins are (1) elevated owing to primary gonadal failure or (2) decreased owing to secondary or tertiary hypogonadism or constitutional de-

Table 15–3. Differential diagnosis of delayed puberty.

	Serum Gonadotropins	Serum Gonadal Steroids	Miscellaneous
Constitutional delay in growth and adolescence	Prepubertal (low)	Low	Patient usually has short stature for chronologic age but appropriate height and growth rate for bone age. Adrenarche and gonadarche are delayed.
Hypogonadotropic hypogonadism	Prepubertal (low)	Low	Patient may have anosmia (Kallmann's syndrome) or other associated pituitary hormone deficiencies. If gonadotropin deficiency is isolated, patient usually has normal height and growth rate. Adrenarche may be normal in spite of absent gonadarche (serum DHEA sulfate may be pubertal).
Hypergonadotropic hypogonadism	Elevated	Low	Patient may have abnormal karyotype and stigmas of Turner's or Klinefelter's syndrome.

layed puberty. If plasma gonadotropins are low, the differential diagnosis rests between hypogonadotropic hypogonadism and constitutionally delayed puberty. A patient with constitutional delay may have a characteristic history of short stature for age with normal growth velocity for bone age and a family history of delayed but spontaneous puberty. The patient's mother may have had late onset of menses, or the father may have begun to shave late or continue growing after high school. Not all patients with constitutional delay are so classic, and gonadotropin-deficient patients may have some features similar to those of constitutional delay in adolescence. Determination of the rise in LH after administration of GnRH is helpful in differential diagnosis; secondary sexual development usually follows within 6 months after conversion to a pubertal LH response to GnRH. Frequent nighttime sampling (every 20 minutes through an indwelling catheter) to determine the amplitude of peaks of LH secretion during sleep is an alternative to GnRH testing but quite cumbersome. Unfortunately, the results of GnRH infusions or nighttime sampling are not always straightforward. Patients may have pubertal responses to exogenous GnRH but may not spontaneously secrete adequate gonadotropins to allow secondary sexual development. In females with amenorrhea, the frequency and amplitude of gonadotropin secretion may not change to allow monthly menstrual cycles. The retention of a diurnal rhythm of gonadotropin secretion (normal in early puberty) into late puberty interferes with pubertal progression. In males, a morning serum testosterone concentration over 50 ng/dL indicates the likelihood of pubertal development within 6 months. Other methods of differential diagnosis between constitutional delay and hypogonadotropic hypogonadism have been proposed but are complex or are not definitive.

Clinical observation for signs of pubertal development and laboratory evaluation for the onset of rising levels of sex steroids may have to continue until the patient is 18 years of age before the diagnosis is definite. In most cases, if spontaneous pubertal development is not noted by 18 years of age, the diagnosis is gonadotropin deficiency. Of course, the presence of neurologic impairment or other endocrine deficiency should immediately lead to investigation for central nervous system tumor or congenital defect in a patient with delayed puberty. CT or MRI scanning may be helpful in this situation.

Treatment of Delayed Puberty

A. Constitutional Delay in Growth and Adolescence:

1. Psychologic support–Patients with constitutional delay in growth and adolescence should be counseled that normal pubertal development will occur spontaneously. Peer pressure and teasing can be oppressive. While the majority of these patients will do quite well, severe depression must be treated appropriately, since short patients with pubertal delay have become suicidal. In some cases it helps to excuse the patient from physical education class, as the lack of development is most apparent in the locker room.

2. Sex steroids–Teenagers who are so embarrassed about short stature and lack of secondary sexual development as to have significant psychologic problems may require special help if they have passed the ages of 13 years for girls or 14 years for boys. The following treatment can be given: (1) for girls, a 3-month course of conjugated estrogen (0.3 mg) or ethinyl estradiol (5–10 mg) given orally each day; (2) for boys, a 3-month course of testosterone enanthate (100 mg) given intramuscularly once every 28 days for three doses. This treatment will elicit noticeable secondary sexual development and a slight increase in stature. The low doses recommended do not advance bone age and have not significantly changed final height. Such low-dose sex steroid treatment is claimed to promote spontaneous pubertal development after sex steroid therapy is discontinued, but a recent study suggests that it is those boys who are on the brink of further pubertal development who are most likely to achieve a growth response to androgen therapy. A short course of therapy may improve patients' psychologic outlook and allow them to await spontaneous pubertal development with greater confidence. Continuous gonadal steroid replacement in these patients is not indicated, as it will advance bone age and lead to epiphysial fusion and a decrease in ultimate stature; however, after a 3- to 6-month break to observe spontaneous development, another course of therapy may be offered.

B. Permanent Hypogonadism: Once a patient has been diagnosed as having delayed puberty due to permanent primary or secondary hypogonadism, replacement therapy must be considered.

Males with hypogonadism may be treated with testosterone enanthate intramuscularly every month, gradually increasing the dosage from 100 mg to 300 mg every 28 days. Frequent erections or priapism may occur if the higher dose is used initially. Oral halogenated testosterone or methylated testosterone is not recommended because of the risk of hepatocellular carcinoma or cholestatic jaundice. A testosterone patch may provide an alternative to intramuscular testosterone enanthate.

Testosterone therapy may not cause adequate pubic hair development, but patients with secondary or tertiary hypogonadism may benefit from hCG administration with increased pubic hair growth resulting from endogenous androgen secretion in addition to the exogenous testosterone.

Therapy with oxandrolone has been suggested as a method of increasing secondary sexual development and increasing growth without advancing skeletal development; such claims have not been sufficiently well documented to justify a preference for oxandrolone therapy over low-dose depo-testosterone. Furthermore, testosterone, which can be aromatized, increases the generally low endogenous growth hormone secretion in constitutional delayed puberty to normal, while oxandrolone, which cannot be aromatized, does not increase growth hormone secretion (see Chapter 12).

Females may be treated with ethinyl estradiol (increasing from 5 mg/d to 10–20 mg/d depending upon clinical results) or conjugated estrogens (0.3 or 0.625 mg/d) on days 1–21. Ten milligrams of medroxyprogesterone acetate are then added on days 12–21 after physical signs of estrogen effect are noted and breakthrough bleeding occurs (and always within 6 months after initiating estrogen). Neither hormone is administered from day 22 to the end of the month to allow regular withdrawal bleeding (see Chapter 13).

C. Coexisting GH Deficiency: The treatment of patients with coexisting GH deficiency requires consideration of their bone age and amount of growth left before epiphysial fusion; if they have not yet received adequate treatment with growth hormone, sex steroid therapy may be kept in the lower range or even delayed to optimize final adult height. The goal is to allow appropriate pubertal changes to support psychologic development and to allow the synergistic effects of combined sex steroids and GH without fusing the epiphyses prematurely.

Constitutional delayed puberty may be associated with decreased growth hormone secretion in 24-hour profiles of spontaneous secretion or in stimulated testing. Growth hormone secretion increases when pubertal gonadal steroid secretion rises, so decreased GH secretion in this condition should be considered temporary. Growth hormone therapy is not proved to increase final height in patients with constitutional delay in puberty and normal height predictions; some studies have shown an increased growth rate in the first year of such therapy, with a decreasing growth rate thereafter. Nonetheless, true growth hormone-deficient patients may have delayed puberty due to the growth hormone deficiency or to coexisting gonadotropin deficiency. Therefore, deciding whether a pubertal patient has temporary or a permanent GH deficiency can be difficult; previous observation may indicate a long history characteristic of constitutional delay in adolescence, while a recent decrease in growth rate may suggest the onset of a brain tumor or other cause of hypopituitarism.

D. The Syndrome of Gonadal Dysgenesis: In the past, patients with the syndrome of gonadal dysgenesis were frequently not given estrogen replacement until after age 13 years, for fear of compromising final height. It has now been demonstrated that low-dose estrogen therapy (5–10 mg of ethinyl estradiol orally) can be administered to allow feminization and improve psychologic status at 12–13 years of age without decreasing final height in these patients. Low-dose estrogen will increase growth velocity, while high-dose estrogen suppresses it; even if growth velocity is increased, however, final height is not increased with such estrogen treatment. Treatment of Turner's syndrome with GH may be successful in increasing adult stature according to several different international studies (see Chapter 14).

E. Bone Mass: Most bone mass accrues during the second decade, and disorders of puberty may affect the process. Delayed puberty in males causes decreased bone density when the subjects are tested as adults. A range of defects in girls such as anorexia nervosa, athletics-induced delayed puberty, and Turner's syndrome also cause decreased bone density. Unfortunately, the use of testosterone in males and estrogen and progesterone in girls is not clearly proved to reverse this process sufficiently to allow normal adult bone mass. There are, however, data which look promising in males which demonstrate a short-term increase in bone density with testosterone therapy. Increased ingestion of dairy products containing calcium or calcium supplementation may be helpful in hypogonadal or constitutionally delayed patients as well as in normal children, but no long-term follow-up is available to prove the efficacy of this therapy either.

PRECOCIOUS PUBERTY (Sexual Precocity)

The appearance of secondary sexual development before the age of 8 years in girls and 9 years in boys is greater than 2.5 SD below the mean age at onset of puberty and constitutes precocious sexual development (Table 15–4). When the cause is premature activation of the hypothalamic-pituitary axis, the diag-

---

Table 15–4. Classification of precocious puberty.

Complete (true) precocious puberty
  Constitutional
  Idiopathic
  Central nervous system disorders
  Following androgen exposure
Incomplete precocious puberty
  Males
    Gonadotropin-secreting tumors
    Excessive androgen production
    Premature Leydig and germinal cell maturation
  Females
    Ovarian cysts
    Estrogen-secreting neoplasms
  Males and females
    Severe hypothyroidism
    McCune-Albright syndrome
Sexual precocity due to gonadotropin or sex steroid
  exposure
Variation in pubertal development
  Premature thelarche
  Premature menarche
  Premature pubarche
  Adolescent gynecomastia

nosis is **complete (true) precocious puberty;** if ectopic gonadotropin secretion occurs in boys or autonomous sex steroid secretion occurs in either sex, the diagnosis is **incomplete precocious puberty.** In all forms of sexual precocity, there is an increase in growth velocity, somatic development, and skeletal maturation. When unchecked, this rapid epiphysial development may lead to tall stature during the early phases of the disorder but to short final stature because of early epiphysial fusion. Plasma IGF-1 values may be elevated for age but more appropriate for pubertal stage in the untreated state.

Complete (True) Precocious Puberty
(Figure 15–11)

A. Constitutional Complete (True) Precocious Puberty: Children who demonstrate isosexual precocity at an age more than 2.5 SD below the mean may simply represent the lower reaches of the distribution curve of age at onset of puberty; often there is a familial tendency toward early puberty. True precocious puberty is rarely reported to be due to an autosomal dominant or (in males) X-linked autosomal dominant trait.

B. Idiopathic Complete (True) Precocious Puberty: Affected children with no familial tendency toward early development and no organic disease may be considered to have idiopathic precocious puberty. Electroencephalographic abnormalities or other evidence of neurologic dysfunction such as epilepsy or developmental delay may be found in these patients. Pubertal development may follow the normal course in these patients or may wax and wane. Gonadotropin and sex steroid concentrations and response to GnRH are similar to those found in normal pubertal subjects. In idiopathic true precocious puberty, as in all forms of true isosexual precocity, testicular enlargement in boys should be the first sign; in girls, breast development, or rarely, pubic hair appearance may be first. Girls present with idiopathic precocious puberty more commonly than boys.

C. Central Nervous System Disorders:

1. Tumors—Central nervous system tumor as a cause of precocious puberty is more common in boys than in girls. Optic gliomas or hypothalamic gliomas, astrocytomas, ependymomas, and other central nervous system tumors may cause precocious puberty by interfering with neural pathways that inhibit GnRH secretion. A survey of children with neurofibromatosis type I found 46% of patients with optic gliomas and neurofibromatosis had precocious puberty, but no patients with neurofibromatosis that did not have optic gliomas demonstrated precocious puberty. Remarkably, craniopharyngiomas, which are known to cause delayed puberty, can also trigger precocious pubertal development. Hamartomas of the tuber cinereum contain GnRH and neurosecretory

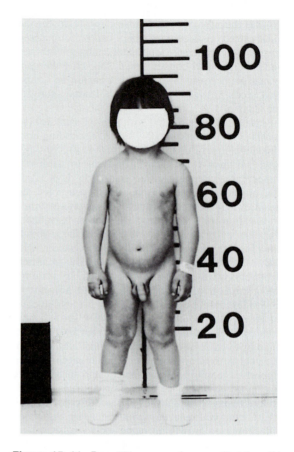

Figure 15–11. Boy, 2⁵/₁₂ years of age, with idiopathic true precocious puberty. By 10 months of age, he had pubic hair and phallic and testicular enlargement. At 1 year of age, his height was 4 SD above the mean; the phallus was 10 × 3.5 cm; each testis was 2.5 × 1.5 cm. Plasma LH was 14.8 mIU/mL and rose to 65.5 mIU/mL after administration of 100 μg of GnRH. Plasma testosterone was 416 ng/dL. At the time of the photograph, he had been treated with medroxyprogesterone acetate for 1½ years, with reduction of his rapid growth rate and decreased gonadotropin and testosterone secretion. His height was 95.2 cm (> 2 SD above mean height for his age); plasma testosterone was 7 ng/dL, and after 100 μg of GnRH, plasma LH rose from 7 to 17.9 mIU/mL. (Reproduced, with permission, from Styne, DM, Grumbach MM: *Reproductive Endocrinology.* Yen SSC, Jaffe RB [editors]. Saunders, 1978.)

cells such as are found in the median eminence; they may cause precocious puberty by secreting GnRH. With improved methods of imaging the central nervous system, hamartomas, with their characteristic radiographic appearance, are now being more frequently diagnosed in patients who were previously thought to have idiopathic precocious puberty. These tumors do not grow and so pose no increasing threat to the patients. Surgery is a dangerous alternative to GnRH therapy owing to the location of the hamartoma and is not indicated for the control of precocious puberty, as hamartomas respond readily to GnRH agonist therapy. Radiation therapy is indicated in radiosensitive tumors such as germinomas and craniopharyngiomas, where complete surgical extirpation is impossible.

Tumors or other abnormalities of the central nervous system may cause growth hormone deficiency in association with precocious puberty. This may also occur after irradiation therapy for such tumors. Such patients will grow much faster than isolated growth hormone-deficient patients but slower than children with classic precocious puberty. Often the growth hormone deficiency will be unmasked after successful treatment of precocious puberty. This combination must be considered during the diagnostic process. (See also Chapter 5.)

2. Other causes of true precocious puberty–Infectious or granulomatous conditions such as encephalitis, brain abscess, postinfectious (or postsurgical or congenital) suprasellar cysts, sarcoidosis, and tuberculous granulomas of the hypothalamus cause true precocious puberty. Suprasellar cysts and hydrocephalus are conditions that cause precocious puberty that are particularly amenable to surgical correction. Brain trauma may be followed by either precocious or delayed puberty. Radiation therapy for acute lymphoblastic leukemia is characteristically associated with hormonal deficiency, but an increasing number of cases are reported of precocious puberty occurring after such therapy; higher doses of radiation may be more likely to cause gonadotropin-releasing hormone deficiency, and lower doses down to 18 Gy may lead to central precocious puberty. Epilepsy and developmental delay are associated with central precocious puberty in the absence of a central nervous system anatomic abnormality.

D. Virilizing Syndromes: Patients with long-untreated virilizing adrenal hyperplasia who have advanced bone ages may manifest precocious puberty after the adrenal hyperplasia is controlled with glucocorticoid suppression. Children with virilizing tumors or those given long-term androgen therapy may follow the same pattern when the androgen source is removed. Advanced maturation of the hypothalamic-pituitary-gonadal axis appears to occur with any condition causing excessive androgen secretion and advanced skeletal age.

Incomplete Precocious Puberty

A. Males: Male patients may manifest premature sexual development in the absence of hypothalamic-pituitary maturation from either of two causes: (1) ectopic or autonomous endogenous secretion of hCG or LH or iatrogenic exogenous administration of chorionic gonadotropin, which can stimulate Leydig cell production of testosterone; or (2) autonomous endogenous secretion of androgens from the testes or adrenal glands or from iatrogenic exogenous administration of androgens. (In females, secretion of hCG will not by itself cause secondary sexual development.)

1. Gonadotropin-secreting tumors–These include hepatomas or hepatoblastomas of the liver as well as teratomas or choriocarcinoma of the mediastinum, gonads, retroperitoneum, or pineal gland and germinomas of the central nervous system. The testes are definitely enlarged but not to the degree found in central precocious puberty.

2. Autonomous androgen secretion–Secretion of androgens can occur because of inborn errors of adrenal enzyme function, as in 21-hydroxylase (P450c21) or 11β-hydroxylase (P450c11β) deficiency, virilizing adrenal carcinomas, interstitial cell tumors of the testes, or premature Leydig and germinal cell maturation. Newly recognized forms of late-onset congenital adrenal hyperplasia, generally of the 21-hydroxylase deficiency form, may occur years after birth with no congenital or neonatal manifestations of virilization. Adrenal rest tissue may be found in the testes as a vestige of the embryonic common origin of these two organs; in states of ACTH excess, primarily congenital adrenal hyperplasia, adrenal rests can enlarge and secrete adrenal androgens (see Chapter 14).

In all forms of incomplete male isosexual precocity, FSH is not elevated, and since the seminiferous tubules are not stimulated, the testes do not enlarge as much as in complete sexual precocity. If incomplete sexual precocity is due to a testicular tumor, the testes may be large, asymmetric, and irregular in contour. Symmetric bilateral moderate enlargement of the testes suggests familial gonadotropin-independent premature maturation of Leydig and germinal cells, which is a sex-limited dominant condition. The testes are somewhat smaller in this condition than in true precocious puberty but are still over 2.5 cm in diameter.

In boys with **familial gonadotropin-independent premature Leydig and germinal cell maturation,** plasma testosterone levels are in the pubertal range but plasma gonadotropin levels and the LH response to exogenous GnRH are in the prepubertal range because autonomous testosterone secretion suppresses endogenous GnRH release. The cause of this sex-limited dominant condition lies in a constitutive activation of the LH receptor causing increased cyclic adenosine monophosphate (cAMP) production in the absence of LH leaving the LH receptor "on"; mutations have been reported in the receptor in several gene abnormalities in different families (eg, Asp578 → Gly or Met571 → Ile—and no doubt many other defects will be found). The differential diagnosis rests between testosterone-secreting tumor of the adrenal, testosterone-secreting Leydig cell neoplasm, and premature Leydig and germinal cell maturation.

B. Females: Female patients with incomplete isosexual precocity have a source of excessive estrogens. In all cases of autonomous endogenous estrogen secretion or exogenous administration, serum LH and FSH levels should be low.

1. Follicular cysts–If follicular cysts are large enough, they can secrete sufficient estrogen to cause breast development and even vaginal withdrawal bleeding; some girls have recurrent cysts that lead to several episodes of vaginal bleeding. Patients with cysts may have levels of serum estrogen high enough to mimic a tumor. Larger follicular cysts can twist on their pedicles and become infarcted, causing symptoms of acute abdomen in addition to the precocious estrogen effects.

2. Granulosa or theca cell tumors–These tumors of the ovaries secrete estrogen and are palpable in 80% of cases. Gonadoblastomas found in streak gonads, lipoid tumors, cystadenomas, and ovarian carcinomas are rare ovarian sources of estrogens or androgens.

3. Adrenal rest tissue–Adrenal rest tissue has long been known to cause testicular enlargement and androgen secretion in boys, particularly with the increased ACTH secretion of congenital adrenal hyperplasia. Recently, however, a girl with an ovarian adrenal rest was reported to have hypertension, precocious puberty, Cushing's syndrome, and ovarian enlargement.

4. Exogenous estrogen administration–Ingestion of estrogen-containing substances or even cutaneous absorption of estrogen can cause feminization in children. Epidemics of gynecomastia and precocious thelarche in Puerto Rico and Italy have variously been attributed to ingestion of estrogen-contaminated food, estrogens in the environment, or undetermined causes. One outbreak of gynecomastia in boys and precocious thelarche in girls in Bahrain was traced to a cow given continuous estrogen treatment by its owner to ensure uninterrupted milk production.

5. Virilization in girls–Excess androgen effect can be caused by premature adrenarche or more significant pathologic conditions such as congenital or nonclassical adrenal hyperplasia or adrenal or ovarian tumors. P450c20 adrenal hyperplasia can be diagnosed on the basis of elevated serum 17-hydroxyprogesterone concentrations in the basal or ACTH-stimulated state (other adrenal metabolites may be elevated depending upon the defect under investigation). Both adrenal and ovarian tumors generally secrete testosterone, while adrenal tumors secrete DHEA as well. The source of the tumor may be difficult to differentiate if it produces only testosterone; MRI or CT scanning may be inadequate to diagnose the tumor's organ of origin, and selective venous sampling may be needed.

C. Males and Females:

1. McCune-Albright syndrome–McCune-Albright syndrome is classically manifested as a triad of irregular *café au lait* spots, fibrous dysplasia of long bones with cysts, and precocious puberty. However, cases have been reported that also included hyperthyroidism, adrenal nodules with Cushing's syndrome, acromegaly, hyperprolactinemia, hyperparathyroidism, hypophosphatemic hyperphosphaturic rickets, or autonomous endogenous functioning ovarian cysts in girls. Precocious puberty may be complete or incomplete; longitudinal study suggests that some patients start with incomplete precocious puberty and progress to complete precocious puberty. Long-term follow-up of McCune-Albright patients reveals a high incidence of pathologic fractures and orthopedic deformities due to the bone cysts, as well as hearing impairment due to the thickening of the temporal area of the skull. One patient had a mutation of the Arg201 of exon 8 of the G protein alpha subunit that stimulates cAMP formation; this leads to decreased G protein and increased adenylyl cyclase activity leading to the increased endocrine activity. This defect originates in somatic rather than germ cells and manifests irregularly through the body.

2. Hypothyroidism–Severe untreated hypothyroidism can be associated with sexual precocity and galactorrhea (Van Wyk-Grumbach syndrome); treatment with thyroxine will correct hypothyroidism, halt precocious puberty and galactorrhea, and lower PRL levels. The cause of this syndrome was postulated to be increased gonadotropin secretion associated with the massive increase in TSH secretion. Recent investigations demonstrated that TSH can act on FSH receptors, causing gonadotropic effects due to elevated serum TSH concentrations.

Variations in Pubertal Development

A. Premature Thelarche: The term "premature thelarche" denotes unilateral or bilateral breast enlargement without other signs of androgen or estrogen secretion of puberty. Patients are usually under 3 years of age; the breast enlargement may regress within months or remain until actual pubertal development occurs at a normal age. Areolar development and vaginal mucosal signs of estrogen effect are usually absent. Premature thelarche may be caused by brief episodes of estrogen secretion from ovarian cysts. Plasma estrogen levels are usually low in this disorder, perhaps because blood samples are drawn after the initiating secretory event. Classically, premature thelarche is self-limited and does not lead to central precocious puberty. However, there are reports of progression to central precocious puberty in a minority of cases, perhaps due to incorrect initial diagnosis or perhaps due to a true relationship between the conditions.

B. Premature Menarche: In rare cases, girls may begin to menstruate at an early age without showing other signs of estrogen effect. An unproved theory suggests that they may be manifesting increased uterine sensitivity to estrogen. In most subjects, menses stop within 1–6 years, and normal pubertal progression occurs thereafter.

C. Premature Adrenarche: The term "premature adrenarche" denotes the early appearance of pubic or axillary hair without other signs of virilization or puberty. This nonprogressive disorder is compatible with a normal age at onset of other signs of puberty. It is more common in girls than in boys and usually is found in children over 6 years of age. Plasma and urinary DHEAS are elevated to stage 2 pubertal levels, which are higher than normally found in this age group. Bone and height ages may be slightly advanced for chronologic age. Patients may have abnormal electroencephalographic tracings without other signs of neurologic dysfunction. The presenting symptoms of late-onset adrenal hyperplasia may be similar to those of premature adrenarche, and the differential diagnosis may require ACTH stimulation testing (see Chapter 9).

D. Adolescent Gynecomastia: Seventy-five percent of boys have transient unilateral or bilateral gynecomastia, usually beginning in stage 2 or 3 of puberty and regressing about 2 years later. Serum estrogen and testosterone concentrations are normal, but the estradiol:testosterone ratio may be elevated and SHBG concentrations may be high. Reassurance is usually all that is required, but some severely affected patients with extremely prominent breast development will require reduction mammoplasty if psychologic distress is extreme. Some pathologic conditions such as Klinefelter's and Reifenstein's syndromes and the syndrome of incomplete androgen resistance are also associated with gynecomastia; these disorders should be clearly differentiated from the gynecomastia of normal puberty in males.

Differential Diagnosis of Precocious Puberty

The history and physical examination should be directed toward one of the diagnostic possibilities discussed above. Serum gonadotropin and sex steroid concentrations are determined in order to distinguish gonadotropin-mediated secondary sexual development (serum gonadotropin and sex steroid levels elevated) from autonomous endogenous secretion or exogenous administration of gonadal steroids (serum gonadotropin levels suppressed and sex steroid levels elevated).

New commercial immunoassays are said to more clearly indicate the onset of increased gonadotropin secretion with only a basal unstimulated sample. Furthermore, these new assays, when applied to urinary collections, are reported to clearly indicate the onset of pubertal or precocious pubertal development, eliminating the need for serum sampling. In the past, a GnRH test was required to confirm an increase in LH secretion at puberty because of the overlap of pubertal and prepubertal values of LH in the basal state. It is not yet clear that these new assays will replace the GnRH test in the diagnosis of disorders of puberty.

If serum LH (or hCG) levels are quite high in a boy or a pregnancy screening test is positive, the likely diagnosis is an extrapituitary hCG-secreting tumor. If no abdominal source of hCG is found, MRI of the head with particular attention to the hypothalamic-pituitary area is indicated to evaluate the possibility of a germinoma of the pineal gland.

If serum sex steroid levels are very high and gonadotropin levels are low, an autonomous source of gonadal steroid secretion must be assumed. If plasma gonadotropin and sex steroid levels are in the pubertal range, the most likely diagnosis is complete precocious puberty. In such patients, the GnRH test will usually result in a rise in LH levels compatible with normal puberty and will thus confirm the diagnosis (Table 15–5).

Differentiation between premature thelarche and central precocious puberty is usually accomplished by physical examination, but determination of serum estradiol or gonadotropins may be invoked. The evaluation of uterine size by ultrasound may also be useful as premature thelarche causes no increase in uterine volume while central precocious puberty does; ovarian size determination is a less useful method of distinguishing between the two possibilities. As noted above, some girls first thought to have precocious thelarche are reported to progress to complete precocious puberty; there is no way to distinguish girls who will progress from those who will not.

The onset of true or complete precocious puberty may indicate the presence of a hypothalamic tumor. Boys more often than girls have central nervous system tumors associated with complete precocious puberty. Skull x-rays are not usually helpful, but CT or MRI scanning is indicated in children with true precocious puberty. The present generation of CT and MRI scanners can make thin cuts through the hypothalamic-pituitary area with good resolution; small hypothalamic hamartomas are now being diagnosed more frequently. Generally, MRI is preferable to CT scan for the determination of central nervous system lesions causing central precocious puberty; the use of contrast may help to exclude central nervous system lesions.

Treatment of Precocious Puberty

A. Complete Precocious Puberty: In the past, medical treatment of true precocious puberty utilized medroxyprogesterone acetate or cyproterone acetate, progestational agents that reduce gonadotropin secretion by negative feedback.

However, current treatment for precocious puberty due to a central nervous system lesion is much more effective. Chronic administration of highly potent and long-acting analogs of GnRH has been shown to down-regulate GnRH receptors and reduce pituitary

Table 15–5. Differential diagnosis of precocious puberty.

	Serum Gonadotropin Concentrations	LH Response to GnRH	Serum Sex Steroid Concentrations	Gonadal Size	Miscellaneous
Complete (true) precocious puberty	Pubertal.	Pubertal pattern.	Pubertal values.	Normal pubertal enlargement of testes in males.	CT or MRI scan of head to rule out a central nervous system tumor.
Incomplete precocious puberty **Males** Gonadotropin-secreting tumor	High hCG or LH (positive pregnancy test).	High basal LH that does not rise with GnRH.	High or pubertal values.	Slight to moderate enlargement of testes.	Hepatic tumor must be considered. CT or MRI scan of head if gonadotropin-secreting central nervous system tumor suspected.
Leydig cell tumor	Prepubertal (low).	Prepubertal or suppressed pattern.	Extremely high testosterone.	Irregular asymmetric enlargement of testes.	
Gonadotropin-independent sexual precocity with premature Leydig and germinal cell maturation	Prepubertal (low).	Prepubertal or suppressed pattern.	Pubertal or higher values.	Testes larger than 2.5 cm but smaller than expected for stage of pubertal development.	Often found in sex-limited dominant patterns.
Females Granulosa cell tumor (follicular cysts may be similar to presentation)	Prepubertal (low).	Prepubertal or suppressed pattern.	Extremely high estradiol.	Ovarian enlargement on physical, CT, or sonographic examination.	Granulosa cell tumor is usually palpable on rectal examination.
Follicular cyst	Prepubertal (low).	Prepubertal pattern of LH. FSH secretion may rise above normal range.	Estradiol may be normally low or quite high, depending upon the stage of cyst formation or regression.	Cysts may be visible on sonogram.	Withdrawal bleeding may occur when estrogen levels decrease. Cysts may recur.

gland response to GnRH, thereby causing decreased secretion of gonadotropin and sex steroids and rapidly stopping the progression of signs of sexual precocity. This suppressive effect is reversed after therapy is discontinued. Treatment of idiopathic precocious puberty and precocious puberty caused by hamartomas of the tuber cinereum, neoplasms of the central nervous system, or long-term androgen exposure has been successful.

The GnRH agonists were originally given by daily subcutaneous injection or intranasal insufflation; the successful use of these agents in microcapsules that are injected every 3 weeks or in depot preparations has now made treatment much easier and has improved compliance. Numerous agents with varying potencies are used. Because of these differing potencies, it is possible that patients may only be partially suppressed inadvertently, and their response to

GnRH may therefore be only partially suppressed. Such a patient may appear to have arrested pubertal development while actually secreting low but significant levels of sex steroids, so that bone age is advancing while the growth rate is decreased. Side effects have generally been limited to allergic skin reactions and elevation of immunoglobulins directed to the agent. However, at least one child manifested a significant anaphylactic reaction to an injection. The FDA has approved histrelin, a GnRH agonist administered on a daily basis, and leuprolide acetate, a long-acting GnRH agonist, administered every 28 days. The dose of leuprolide is 3.37 mg subcutaneously if body weight is 20 kg or more or 1.87 mg if body weight is less than 20 kg. Individual monitoring is essential to ascertain gonadotropin suppression.

GnRH agonists are the preferred treatment for true precocious puberty to decrease sexual maturation and decrease growth rate and skeletal maturation. Growth velocity decreases within 6 months after the start of therapy, and rapid bone age advancement decreases to a rate below the increase in chronologic age. Without therapy, final height in patients with central precocious puberty approaches 152 cm in girls and 155–164 cm in boys. With correct dosage and early initiation of GnRH agonist therapy, final height is improved in numerous reports of long-term follow-up in patients with central precocious puberty. The first patients treated with GnRH agonists have recently reached final height: The girls have a mean height of 157 cm and the boys a mean height of 164 cm—a definite improvement over the untreated state. The worst height prognosis is in children with an early diagnosis of precocious puberty who are not treated. The best outcomes of therapy are noted when diagnosis and therapy are achieved early, and as earlier diagnosis is made in children with central precocious puberty and earlier therapy is offered, better results are expected in the future. Menarche is reported after the discontinuation of therapy in girls, indicating a reversion to normal pubertal endocrine function after GnRH agonist treatment. Mild central precocious puberty may not require GnRH agonist therapy. Patients without significant elevation of serum estrogen or IGF-1 and who have a predicted height appropriate for family who have slowly progressing variants may achieve an appropriate final height without therapy.

Psychologic support is important for patients with sexual precocity. The somatic changes or menses will frighten some children and may make them the object of ridicule. These patients do not experience social maturation to match their physical development, though their peers, teachers, and relatives will tend to treat them as if they were older because of their large size. Thus, supportive counseling must be offered to both patient and family. Evidence indicates that children with precocious puberty are more often sexually abused, so appropriate precautions are necessary.

B. Incomplete Precocious Puberty: Treatment of the disorders discussed above under incomplete precocious puberty is directed toward the underlying tumor or abnormality rather than toward the signs of precocious puberty. If the primary cause is controlled, signs of sexual development will be halted in progression or may even regress.

Males with familial Leydig and germ cell maturation will not initially respond to GnRH agonist therapy, but some have improved with medroxyprogesterone acetate. Boys were successfully treated with ketoconazole, an antifungal agent that can block 17,20-lyase and therefore decrease testosterone production. After initial control with ketoconazole, the boys developed true precocious puberty, because prolonged exposure to androgens matured their hypothalamic-pituitary axis; treatment with a GnRH agonist then effectively halted this pubertal progression. Another successful therapy for this condition is a combination of testolactone (an aromatase inhibitor) and spironolactone (which acts as an anti-androgen). Long-term follow-up demonstrated some decrease in menses and improvement in growth patterns and bone age advancement, though some escape from control, necessitating the addition of a GnRH agonist, which then suppressed pubertal development. Girls with recurrent estrogen-secreting ovarian cyst formation may have a decreased incidence of cysts with medroxyprogesterone acetate therapy, and a GnRH agonist may also be effective in such cases. Surgical removal of such ovarian cysts may be unnecessary if such medical therapy is first utilized.

Precocious thelarche or adrenarche requires no treatment, as both are self-limited benign conditions. No therapy has been reported for premature menarche, and none may be indicated. Severe, persistent cases of adolescent gynecomastia have been treated successfully by testolactone and dihydrotestosterone heptanoate, though surgical removal of breast tissue is often necessary.

REFERENCES

General

Arisaka O et al: Effect of testosterone on bone density and bone metabolism in adolescent male hypogonadism. Metabolism 1995;44:419.

Chan GM, Hoffman K, McMurry M: Effects of dairy products on bone and body composition in pubertal girls. J Pediatr 1995;126:551.

Goji K: Twenty-four-hour concentration profiles of gonadotropin and estradiol (E2) in prepubertal and early pubertal girls: The diurnal rise of E2 is opposite the nocturnal rise of gonadotropin. J Clin Endocrinol Metab 1993;77:1629.

Goji K, Tanikaze S: Spontaneous gonadotropin and testosterone concentration profiles in prepubertal and pubertal boys: Temporal relationship between luteinizing hormone and testosterone. Pediatr Res 1993;34:229.

Grumbach MM, Styne DM: Puberty: Ontogeny, neuroendocrinology, physiology, and disorders. In: *Williams Textbook of Endocrinology,* 8th ed. Wilson JD, Foster DW (editors). Saunders, 1992.

Hergenroeder AC: Bone mineralization, hypothalamic amenorrhea, and sex steroid therapy in female adolescents and young adults. J Pediatr 1995;126:683.

Manasco PK et al: Ontogeny of gonadotropin, testosterone, and inhibin secretion in normal boys through puberty based on overnight serial sampling. J Clin Endocrinol Metab 1995;80:2046.

Neely EK et al: Normal ranges for immunochemiluminometric gonadotropin assays. J Pediatr 1995;127:40.

Nysom K et al: Spermaturia in two normal boys without other signs of puberty. Acta Paediatr 1994;83:520.

Vieira JG: Serum levels of prostate-specific antigen in normal boys throughout puberty. J Clin Endocrinol Metab 1994;78:1185.

Klein KO et al: Estrogen levels in childhood determined by an ultrasensitive recombinant cell bioassay. J Clin Invest 1994;94:2475.

Styne DM, Grumbach MM: Puberty in the male and female: Its physiology and disorders. In: *Reproductive Endocrinology,* 3rd ed. Yen SSC, Jaffe RB (editors). Saunders, 1992.

Styne DM: The testes. In: *Pediatric and Adolescent Endocrinology.* Sperling M (editor). Saunders, 1992.

Physical Changes Associated With Puberty

Attie KM et al: The pubertal growth spurt in eight patients with true precocious puberty and growth hormone deficiency: Evidence for a direct role of sex steroids. J Clin Endocrinol Metab 1990;71:975.

Bayley N, Pinneau SF: Tables for predicting adult height from skeletal age: Revised for use with the Greulich-Pyle standards. J Pediatr 1952;40:423.

Greulich WW, Pyle SI: *Radiographic Atlas of Skeletal Development of the Hand and Wrist,* 2nd ed. Stanford Univ Press, 1959.

Harlan WR, Harlan EA, Grillo GP: Secondary sex characteristics of girls 12 to 17 years of age: The U.S. Health Examination Survey. J Pediatr 1980;96:1074.

Harlan WR et al: Secondary sex characteristics of boys 12 to 17 years of age: The U.S. Health Examination Survey. J Pediatr 1979;95:293.

Marshall WA, Tanner JM: Variations in the pattern of pubertal changes in boys. Arch Dis Child 1970;45:13.

Marshall WA, Tanner JM: Variations in the pattern of pubertal changes in girls. Arch Dis Child 1969;44:291.

Rohn RD: Nipple (papilla) development in puberty: Longitudinal observations in girls. Pediatrics 1987; 79:745.

Smith EP et al: Estrogen resistance caused by a mutation in the estrogen-receptor gene in a man. N Engl J Med 1994;331:1056.

Tanner JM et al: The adolescent growth spurt of boys and girls of the Harpenden Growth Study. Ann Hum Biol 1976;3:109.

Van Wieringen JC et al: Growth Diagrams 1965 Netherlands: Second National Survey on 0–24 Year Olds. Groningen, Netherlands Institute for Preventive Medicine NO Leiden, Wolters-Noordhoff Publishing, 1971.

Endocrine Changes From Fetal Life to Puberty

Harris DA et al: Somatomedin-C in normal puberty and in true precocious puberty before and after treatment with a potent LRF agonist: Evidence for an effect of estrogen and testosterone on somatomedin-C concentrations. J Clin Endocrinol Metab 1985;61:152.

Kirkland R et al: Decrease in plasma high-density lipoprotein cholesterol levels at puberty in boys with delayed adolescence: Correlation with plasma testosterone levels. JAMA 1987;257:502.

Sklar CA et al: Human chorionic gonadotropin-secreting pineal tumor: Relation to pathogenesis and sex limitation of sexual precocity. J Clin Endocrinol Metab 1981;53:656.

Reiter EO, Fuldauer VG, Root AW: Secretion of the adrenal androgen, dehydroepiandrosterone sulfate, during normal infancy, childhood, and adolescence, in sick infants and in children with endocrinologic abnormalities. J Pediatr 1977;90:766.

Delayed Puberty & Sexual Infantilism

Attanasio A et al: Final height and long-term outcome after growth hormone therapy in Turner syndrome: Results of a German multicentre trial. Horm Res 1995;43:147.

Connors MH, Styne DM: Familial functional anorchism: A review of etiology and management. J Urol 1985; 133:1049.

Curtis J et al: The endocrine outcome after surgical removal of craniopharyngiomas. Pediatr Neurosurg 1994;21(Suppl 1):24.

Gertner JM et al: Delayed somatic growth and pubertal development in human immunodeficiency virus-infected hemophiliac boys. Hemophilia Growth and Development Study. J Pediatr 1994;124:896.

Grumbach MM, Conte FA: Disorders of sexual differentiation. In: *Williams Textbook of Endocrinology,* 8th ed. Wilson JD, Foster DW (editors). Saunders, 1992.

Mustieles C et al: Male gonadal function after chemotherapy in survivors of childhood malignancy. Med Pediatr Oncol 1995 24:347.

Thomsett MJ et al: Endocrine and neurologic outcome in childhood craniopharyngioma: Review of effect of treatment in 42 patients. J Pediatr 1980;97:728.

Van Dop C et al: Isolated gonadotropin deficiency in boys: Clinical characteristics and growth. J Pediatr 1987;111:684.

Sexual Precocity

Anasti JN et al: A potential novel mechanism for precocious puberty in juvenile hypothyroidism. J Clin Endocrinol Metab 1995;80:276.

Bar A et al: Bayley-Pinneau method of height prediction in girls with central precocious puberty: Correlation with adult height. J Pediatr 1995;126:955.

Brauner R et al: Adult height in girls with idiopathic true precocious puberty. J Clin Endocrinol Metab 1994; 79:415.

Egli CA et al: Pituitary gonadotropin-independent male-limited autosomal dominant sexual precocity in nine generations: Familial testotoxicosis. J Pediatr 1985; 106:33.

Feuillan PP, Jones J, Cutler GB: Long-term testolactone therapy for precocious puberty in girls with the McCune-Albright syndrome. J Clin Endocrinol Metab 1993;77:647.

Habiby R et al: Precocious puberty in children with neurofibromatosis type 1. J Pediatr 1995;126:364.

Holland FJ: Gonadotropin-independent precocious puberty. Endocrinol Metab Clin North Am 1991;20:191.

Kornreich L et al: Central precocious puberty: Evaluation by neuroimaging. Pediatr Radiol 1995;25:7.

Laue L et al: Genetic heterogeneity of constitutively activating mutations of the human luteinizing hormone receptor in familial male-limited precocious puberty. Proc Natl Acad Sci U S A. 1995;92:1906.

Lee PA, Van Dop C, Migeon CJ: McCune-Albright syndrome: Long-term follow-up. JAMA 1986;256:2980.

Neely EK et al: Spontaneous serum gonadotropin concentrations in the evaluation of precocious puberty. J Pediatr 1995;127:47.

Paul D et al: Long-term effect of gonadotropin-releasing hormone agonist therapy on final and near-final height in 26 children with true precocious puberty treated at a median age of less than 5 years. J Clin Endocrinol Metab 1995;80:546.

Robben SG et al: Idiopathic isosexual central precocious puberty: Magnetic resonance findings in 30 patients. Br J Radiol 1995;68:34.

Styne DW et al: Treatment of true precocious puberty with a potent luteinizing hormone-releasing factor agonist: Effect on growth, sexual maturation, pelvic sonography, and the hypothalamic-pituitary-gonadal axis. J Clin Endocrinol Metab 1985;61:142.

Wheeler MD, Styne DM: Diagnosis and management of precocious puberty. Pediatr Clin North Am 1990;37:1255.

Yano K et al: A new constitutively activating point mutation in the luteinizing hormone/choriogonadotropin receptor gene in cases of male-limited precocious puberty. J Clin Endocrinol Metab 1995;80:1162.

16

The Endocrinology of Pregnancy

Robert N. Taylor, MD, PhD, & Mary C. Martin, MD

Throughout pregnancy, the fetal-placental unit secretes protein and steroid hormones into the mother's bloodstream, and these apparently or actually alter the function of every endocrine gland in her body. Both clinically and in the laboratory, pregnancy can mimic hyperthyroidism, Cushing's disease, pituitary adenoma, diabetes mellitus, and polycystic ovary syndrome.

The endocrine changes associated with pregnancy are adaptive, allowing the mother to nurture the developing fetus. Although maternal reserves are usually adequate, occasionally, as in the case of gestational diabetes or hypertensive disease of pregnancy, a woman may develop overt signs of disease as a direct result of pregnancy.

Aside from creating a satisfactory maternal environment for fetal development, the placenta serves as an endocrine gland as well as a respiratory, alimentary, and excretory organ. Measurements of fetal-placental products in the maternal serum provide one means of assessing the health of the developing fetus. This chapter will consider the changes in maternal endocrine function in pregnancy and during parturition as well as fetal endocrine development. The chapter concludes with a discussion of some endocrine disorders complicating pregnancy.

CONCEPTION & IMPLANTATION

Fertilization

In fertile women, ovulation occurs approximately 12–16 days after the onset of the previous menses. The ovum must be fertilized within 24–48 hours if conception is to result. For about 48 hours around ovulation, cervical mucus is copious, nonviscous, and slightly alkaline and forms a gel matrix that acts as a filter and conduit for sperm. Following intercourse, sperm that are to survive penetrate the cervical mucus within minutes and can remain viable there until the mucus character changes, approximately 24 hours following ovulation. Sperm begin appearing in the outer third of the uterine tube (the ampulla) 5–10 minutes after coitus and continue to

ACRONYMS USED IN THIS CHAPTER	
ACTH	Adrenocorticotropic hormone
CBG	Corticosteroid-binding globulin
CST	Contract stress test
DHEA	Dehydroepiandrosterone
DOC	Deoxycorticosterone
EGF	Epidermal growth factor
FGF	Follicle-stimulating hormone
FSH	Gonadotropin-releasing hormone
GDM	Gestational diabetes mellitus
GH	Growth hormone
GnRH	Gonadotropin-releasing hormone
hCG	Human chorionic gonadotropin
hCGnRH	Human chorionic gonadotropin-releasing hormone
hCS	Human chorionic somatomammotropin
hPL	Human placental lactogen
IDM	Infants of diabetic mothers
IGFs	Insulin-like growth factors
LH	Luteinizing hormone
L/S	Lecithin/sphingomyelin (ratio)
NST	Nonstress test
PDGF	Platelet-derived growth factor
PRL	Prolactin
RDS	Respiratory distress syndrome
SHBG	Sex hormone-binding globulin
TBG	Thyroid hormone-binding globulin
TRH	Thyrotropin-releasing hormone
TSH	Thyroid-stimulating hormone (thyrotropin)
TSI	Thyroid-stimulating immunoglobulin

migrate to this location from the cervix for about 24–48 hours. Of the 200×10^6 sperm that are deposited in the vaginal fornices, only approximately 200 reach the distal uterine tube. Fertilization normally occurs in the ampulla.

Implantation

Implantation in the uterus does not occur until 6 or 7 days later, when the conceptus is a blastocyst. In most pregnancies, the dates of ovulation and implantation are not known. Weeks of gestation ("gestational age") are by convention calculated from the first day of the last menstrual period. Within 24 hours after implantation, or at about 3 weeks of gestation, human chorionic gonadotropin (hCG) is detectable in maternal serum. Under the influence of increasing hCG production, the corpus luteum continues to secrete steroid hormones in increasing quantities. Without effective implantation and subsequent hCG production, the corpus luteum survives for only about 14 days following ovulation.

Symptoms & Signs of Pregnancy

Breast tenderness, fatigue, nausea, absence of menstruation, softening of the uterus, and a sustained elevation of basal body temperature are all attributable to hormone production by the corpus luteum and developing placenta.

Ovarian Hormones of Pregnancy

The hormones produced by the corpus luteum include progesterone, 17-hydroxyprogesterone, and estradiol. The indispensability of the corpus luteum in early pregnancy has been demonstrated by ablation studies, in which luteectomy or oophorectomy before 42 days of gestation results in precipitous decreases in levels of serum progesterone and estradiol, followed by abortion. Exogenous progesterone will prevent abortion, proving that progesterone alone is required for maintenance of early pregnancy. After about the seventh gestational week, the corpus luteum can be removed without subsequent abortion, owing to increasing progesterone production by the placenta.

Because the placenta does not produce appreciable amounts of 17-hydroxyprogesterone, this steroid provides a marker of corpus luteum function. As shown in Figure 16–1, the serum concentrations of estrogens and total progesterone exhibit a steady increase, but the concentration of 17-hydroxyprogesterone rises and then declines to low levels that persist for the duration of the pregnancy. The decline of corpus luteum function occurs despite the continued production of hCG; in fact, corpus luteum production of 17-hydroxyprogesterone declines while hCG is still rising to maximal levels. Whether this is due to down-regulation of corpus luteal hCG receptors is not known.

Another marker of corpus luteum function is the polypeptide hormone relaxin, a protein with a molec-

ular mass of about 6000. It is similar in its tertiary structure to insulin. Relaxin becomes detectable at about the same time as hCG begins to rise, and it maintains a maximum maternal serum concentration of about 1 ng/mL during the first trimester. The serum concentration then falls approximately 20% and is constant for the remainder of the pregnancy.

Pharmacologically, relaxin ripens the cervix, softens the pubic symphysis, and acts synergistically with progesterone to inhibit uterine contractions. A major physiologic role for relaxin in human gestation has not been established. Luteectomy after 7 weeks of gestation does not interfere with gestation in spite of undetectable relaxin levels. Extraluteal production of relaxin by the decidua and placenta has been demonstrated, however, and local effects may be exerted without alteration of systemic hormone concentrations.

FETAL-PLACENTAL-DECIDUAL UNIT

The function of the placenta is to establish effective communication between the mother and the developing fetus while maintaining the immune and genetic integrity of both individuals. Initially, the placenta functions autonomously. By the end of the first trimester, however, the fetal endocrine system is sufficiently developed to influence placental function and to provide some hormone precursors to the placenta. From this time, it is useful to consider the conceptus as the fetal-placental unit.

The fetal-placental unit will be considered in three separate but related categories: as sources of secretion of protein and steroid hormones into the maternal circulation; as participants in the control of fetal endocrine function, growth, and development; and as a selective barrier governing the interaction between fetal and maternal systems.

Within 7 days after fertilization, implantation begins. The trophoblast invades the endometrium, and two layers of developing placenta can be demonstrated. Columns of invading cytotrophoblasts anchor the placenta to the endometrium. The differentiated syncytiotrophoblast, also derived from precursor cytotrophoblasts, is in direct contact with the maternal circulation. The syncytiotrophoblast is the major source of hormone production, containing the cellular machinery needed for synthesis, packaging, and secretion of both steroid and polypeptide hormones.

The decidua is the endometrium of pregnancy. Recent investigation has shown that the decidual cells are capable of synthesizing a variety of polypeptide hormones, including prolactin (PRL), relaxin, and a variety of paracrine factors, in particular IGF-binding protein 1. The role of the decidua as an endocrine organ has not been established, but its role as a source of prostaglandins during labor is certain (see Endocrine Control of Parturition, below).

SYSTEM	HORMONE	PATTERN	AVERAGE PEAK CONCENTRATION (TIME)
Placenta and corpus luteum	Progesterone	Rises to term.	190 ng/mL (552 nmol/L) (term)
	17-Hydroxy-progesterone	Peaks at 5 weeks, then declines.	6 ng/mL (19 nmol/L) (5 weeks)
Adrenal	Cortisol	Increases to 3 times prepregnancy values at term.	300 ng/mL (0.83 µmol/L) (term)
	Aldosterone	Plateaus at 34 weeks with small rise near term.	100 ng/mL (277 nmol/L) (term)
	DOC	Increases to 10 times prepregnancy value at term.	1200 pg/mL (3.48 nmol/L) (term)
Thyroid	Total T_4	Increases during first trimester, then plateaus.	150 ng/mL (193 pmol/L)
	Free T_4	Unchanged.	30 pg/mL (38.6 pmol/L)
	Total T_3	Increases during first trimester, then plateaus.	2 ng/mL (3.1 nmol/L)
	Free T_3	Unchanged.	4 pg/mL (5.1 pmol/L)

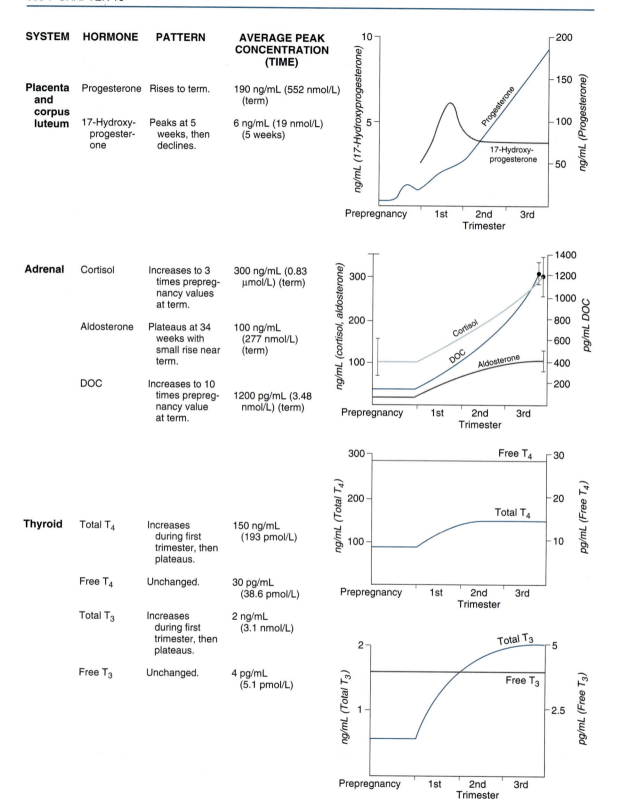

Figure 16–1. Maternal serum hormone changes during pregnancy.

SYSTEM	HORMONE	PATTERN	AVERAGE PEAK CONCENTRATION (TIME)
Anterior pituitary	GH	Unchanged.	
	LH, FSH	Low, basal levels.	
	ACTH	Unchanged.	
	TSH	Unchanged.	
	PRL	Rise to term.	≈200 ng/mL (200 µg/L) (term)
Placental proteins	hCG	Peaks at 10 weeks, then decreases to a lower plateau.	5 µg/mL (5µg/L) (end of first trimester)
	hPL	Rises with placental weight.	5–25 µg/mL (5–25 µgl/L) (term)
Fetoplacental estrogens	Estriol	Increases to term.	15–17 ng/mL (55–62 nmol/L) (term)
	Estradiol	Increases to term.	12–15 ng/mL (42–52 nmol/L) (term)
	Estrone	Increases to term.	5–7 ng/mL (18.5–26 nmol/L) (term)
Fetoplacental androgens	Testosterone	Rises to 10 times pre-pregnancy values.	≈2000 pg/mL (6.9 nmol/L) (term)
	DHEA	Falls during pregnancy.	5 ng/mL (17.3 nmol/L) (pre-pregnancy)
	Androstenedione	Small increase.	2.6 ng/mL (9.0 nmol/L) (term)

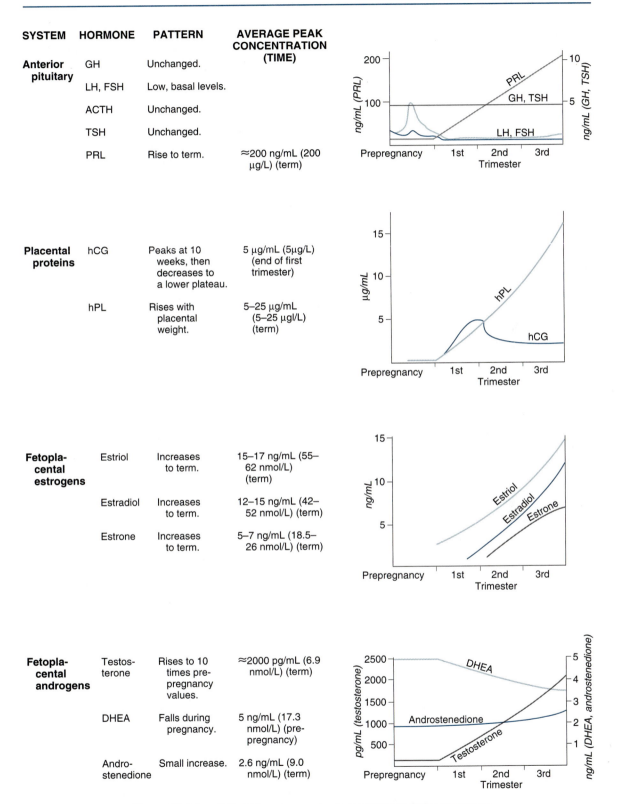

Figure 16–1 (cont'd). Maternal serum hormone changes during pregnancy.

Modern methods of screening for fetal chromosomal aneuploidy, particularly trisomy 21 (Down's syndrome), utilize circulating biochemical markers. Screening by maternal age alone (> 35 years) led to the prenatal identification of only about 25% of aneuploid fetuses. As an aneuploid chromosome complement affects both fetal and placental tissues, their protein and steroid products have been evaluated. A combination of alpha-fetoprotein, hCG, and unconjugated estriol concentrations, secreted into and measured in maternal serum between 15 and 18 weeks' gestation, can be used to detect fetal Down's syndrome with a sensitivity and specificity greater than 90%. Thus, generalized prenatal screening can be offered to pregnant women of all ages with low false-positive rates and a low rate of amniocentesis.

POLYPEPTIDE HORMONES

Human Chorionic Gonadotropin

The first marker of trophoblast differentiation and the first measurable product of the placenta is chorionic gonadotropin (hCG). hCG is a glycoprotein consisting of about 237 amino acids. It is quite similar in structure to the pituitary glycoproteins in that it consists of two chains: an alpha chain, which is species-specific; and a beta chain, which determines receptor interaction and ultimate biologic effect. The alpha chain is identical in sequence to the alpha chains of the hormonal glycoproteins TSH, FSH, and LH. The beta chain has significant sequence homology with LH but is not identical; of the 145 amino acids in β-hCG, 97 (67%) are identical to those of β-LH. In addition, the placental hormone has a carboxyl terminal segment of 30 amino acids not found in the pituitary LH molecule. Carbohydrate constitutes approximately 30% by weight of each subunit. Sialic acid alone accounts for 10% of the weight of the molecule and confers a high degree of resistance to degradation and consequently a long plasma half-life of about 24 hours. Despite limited primary sequence similarity, α and β subunits of hCG have complementary three-dimensional crystal structures and extensive subunit interfaces.

In the early weeks of pregnancy, the concentration of hCG doubles every 1.7–2 days, and serial measurements provide a sensitive index of early trophoblast function. Maternal plasma hCG peaks at about 100,000 mIU/mL during the tenth gestational week and then declines gradually to about 10,000 mIU/mL in the third trimester. Peak concentrations correlate temporally with the establishment of maternal blood flow in the intervillous space (Figure 16–1).

These characteristics of hCG all contribute to the possibility of diagnosing pregnancy several days before any symptoms occur or a menstrual period has been missed. Without the long plasma half-life of hCG (24 hours), the tiny mass of cells comprising the blastocyst could not produce sufficient hormone to be detected in the peripheral circulation within 24 hours of implantation. Antibodies to the unique β-carboxyl terminal segment of hCG do not cross-react significantly with any of the pituitary glycoproteins. As little as 5 mIU/mL (1 ng/mL) of hCG in plasma can be detected without interference from the higher levels of LH, FSH, and TSH.

Like its pituitary counterpart LH, hCG is luteotropic, and the corpus luteum has high-affinity receptors for hCG. The stimulation of increased amounts of progesterone production by corpus luteum cells is driven by increasing concentrations of hCG. Steroid synthesis can be demonstrated in vitro and is mediated by the cAMP system. hCG has been shown to enhance placental conversion of maternal low-density lipid cholesterol to pregnenolone and progesterone.

The concentration of hCG in the fetal circulation is less than 1% of that found in the maternal compartment. However, there is evidence that fetal hCG is an important regulator of the development of the fetal adrenal and gonad during the first trimester.

hCG is also produced by trophoblastic neoplasms such as hydatidiform mole and choriocarcinoma, and the concentration of hCG or its beta subunit is used as a tumor marker, for diagnosis, and for monitoring the success or failure of chemotherapy in these disorders. Women with very high hCG levels due to trophoblastic disease may become clinically hyperthyroid and revert to euthyroidism as hCG is reduced during chemotherapy.

Human Placental Lactogen

A second placental polypeptide hormone, also with homology to a pituitary protein, is termed placental lactogen (hPL) or chorionic somatomammotropin (hCS). hCS is detectable in the early trophoblast, but detectable serum concentrations are not reached until 4–5 gestational weeks. hCS is a protein of about 190 amino acids whose primary, secondary, and tertiary structures are similar to those of growth hormone (GH). The two molecules cross-react in immunoassays and in some receptor and bioassay systems. However, hCS has only some of the biologic activities of GH. Like GH, hCS is diabetogenic, but it has minimal growth-promoting activity as measured by standard GH bioassays. hCS also shares many structural features with prolactin (PRL).

The physiologic role of hCS during pregnancy remains controversial, and normal pregnancy without detectable hCS production has been reported. Although not clearly shown to be a mammotropic agent, hCS contributes to altered maternal glucose metabolism and mobilization of free fatty acids; causes a hyperinsulinemic response to glucose loads; appears to directly stimulate pancreatic islet insulin secretion; and contributes to the peripheral insulin resistance characteristic of pregnancy. Factors that regulate the synthesis or release of hCS from the syncytiotrophoblast have not been fully determined, but prolonged fasting and insulin-induced hypoglycemia raise hCS concentrations. hCS production is roughly proportionate to placental mass. Actual production rates may reach as much as 1–1.5 g/d. The disappearance curve shows multiple components but yields a serum half-life of 15–30 minutes. Serum hCS concentration had been proposed as an indicator of the continued health of the placenta, but the range of normal values is wide, and serial determinations are necessary. hCS determinations have largely been replaced by biophysical profiles, which are more sensitive indicators of fetal jeopardy.

Other Chorionic Peptide Hormones & Growth Factors

Other chorionic peptides have been identified, but their functions have not yet been defined. One of these proteins is a glycoprotein with partial sequence and functional homology to TSH. Its existence as a separate entity from hCG has been debated in the literature, with some reports suggesting that chorionic TSH is a protein with a molecular weight of about 28,000, structurally different from hCG, with weak thyrotropic activity. Similarly, ACTH-like, lipotropin-like, and endorphin-like peptides have been isolated from placenta, but they have low biologic potency and undetermined physiologic roles. A chorionic FSH-like protein has also been isolated from placenta but has not yet been detected in plasma. Good evidence exists that the cytotrophoblast produces a human chorionic gonadotropin-releasing hormone (hCGnRH) that is biologically and immunologically indistinguishable from the hypothalamic GnRH. The release of hCG from the syncytiotrophoblast may be under the direct control of this factor, in a fashion analogous to the hypothalamic control of anterior pituitary secretion of gonadotropins. Preliminary evidence is also available for similar paracrine control of syncytiotrophoblastic release of TSH, somatostatin, and corticotropin by analogous cytotrophoblastic releasing hormones. Activin, inhibin, corticotropin-releasing factor, and multiple peptide growth factors, including fibroblast growth factor (FGF), epidermal growth factor (EGF), platelet-derived growth factor (PDGF), and the insulin-like growth factors (IGFs)—and many of their cognate receptors—have all been isolated from placental tissue. Placental EGF and the related TGFα have been suggested to play a role in fetal growth.

STEROID HORMONES

In contrast to the impressive synthetic capability exhibited in the production of placental proteins, the placenta does not appear to have the capability to synthesize steroids de novo. All steroids produced by the placenta are derived from maternal or fetal precursor steroids.

No tissue, however, even remotely approaches the syncytiotrophoblast in its capacity to efficiently interconvert steroids. This activity is demonstrable even in the early blastocyst, and by the seventh gestational week, when the corpus luteum has undergone relative involution, the placenta becomes the dominant source of steroid hormones.

Progesterone

The placenta relies on maternal cholesterol as its substrate for progesterone production. Fetal death has no immediate influence on progesterone production, suggesting that the fetus is a negligible source of substrate. Enzymes in the placenta cleave the cholesterol side chain, yielding pregnenolone, which in turn is partially isomerized to progesterone; 250–350 mg of progesterone is produced daily by the third trimester, and most enters the maternal circulation. The maternal plasma concentration of progesterone rises progressively throughout pregnancy and appears to be independent of factors that normally regulate steroid synthesis and secretion. Whereas exogenous hCG increases progesterone production in pregnancy, hypophysectomy has no effect. Administration of ACTH or cortisol does not influence progesterone concentrations, nor does adrenalectomy or oophorectomy do so after 7 weeks.

Progesterone is necessary for establishment and maintenance of pregnancy. Insufficient corpus luteum production of progesterone may contribute to failure of implantation, and luteal phase deficiency is implicated in some cases of infertility and recurrent pregnancy loss. Furthermore, progesterone contributes to maintaining a relatively quiescent state of the myometrium. In some animals, such as the rabbit or sheep, labor is heralded by a decrease in progesterone concentration, and the administration of progesterone in these species can delay labor indefinitely. Progesterone also may act as an immunosuppressive agent in some systems and inhibits T cell-mediated tissue rejection. Thus, high local concentrations of progesterone may contribute to immunologic tolerance by the uterus of invading embryonic trophoblast tissue.

Estrogens

Estrogen production by the placenta also depends on circulating precursors, but in this case both fetal and maternal steroids are important sources. Most of the estrogens are derived from fetal androgens, primarily dehydroepiandrosterone sulfate (DHEA sulfate). Fetal DHEA sulfate, produced mainly by the fetal adrenal, is converted by placental sulfatase to the free dehydroepiandrosterone (DHEA) and then, through enzymatic pathways common to steroid-producing tissues, to androstenedione and testosterone.

These androgens are finally aromatized by the placenta to estrone and estradiol, respectively.

The greater part of fetal DHEA sulfate is metabolized to produce a third estrogen: estriol. While serum estrone and estradiol concentrations are increased during pregnancy about 50-fold over their maximal prepregnancy values, estriol increases approximately 1000-fold. The key step in estriol synthesis is 16α-hydroxylation of the steroid molecule (Figure 13–4). The substrate for the reaction is primarily fetal DHEA sulfate, and the vast majority of the production of the 16α-hydroxy-DHEA sulfate occurs in the fetal adrenal and liver, not in maternal or placental tissues. The final steps of desulfation and aromatization to estriol occur in the placenta. Maternal serum or urinary estriol measurements, unlike measurements of progesterone or hCS, reflect fetal as well as placental function. Normal estriol production, therefore, reflects the integrity of fetal circulation and metabolism as well as adequacy of the placenta. Rising serum or urinary estriol concentrations are the best available biochemical indicator of fetal well-being (Figure 16–1). When estriol is assayed daily, a significant drop (> 50%) may be a sensitive early indicator of fetal jeopardy.

There are some circumstances in which altered estriol production does not signal fetal compromise but is instead the result of congenital derangements or iatrogenic intervention. Maternal estriol remains low in pregnancies with placental sulfatase deficiency and in cases of fetal anencephaly. In the first case, DHEA sulfate cannot be hydrolyzed; in the second, little fetal DHEA is produced because fetal adrenal stimulation by ACTH is lacking. Maternal administration of glucocorticoids inhibits fetal ACTH and lowers maternal estriol. Administration of DHEA to the mother during a healthy pregnancy increases estriol production. Antibiotic therapy can reduce estriol levels by interfering with bacterial glucuronidases and maternal reabsorption of estriol from the gut. Estetrol, an estrogen metabolite with a fourth hydroxyl at the 15 position, is unique to pregnancy.

Cases of aromatase deficiency and estrogen receptor mutations indicate that estrogen action is not mandatory for the maintenance of pregnancy. Homozygous mutant mice with disrupted estrogen receptor genes undergo apparently normal blastocyst, fetal, and placental development. This observation has been corroborated by a clinical case of a spontaneous missense mutation of the estrogen receptor in a man.

MATERNAL ADAPTATION TO PREGNANCY

As a successful "parasite," the fetal-placental unit manipulates the maternal "host" for its own gain but normally avoids imposing excessive stress that would jeopardize the "host" and thus the "parasite"

itself. The prodigious production of polypeptide and steroid hormones by the fetal-placental unit directly or indirectly results in physiologic adaptations of virtually every maternal organ system. These alterations are summarized in Figure 16–2. Most of the commonly measured maternal endocrine function tests are radically changed. In some cases, true physiologic alteration has occurred; in others, the changes are due to increased production of specific serum binding proteins by the liver or to decreased serum levels of albumin. Additionally, some hormonal changes are mediated by altered clearance rates owing to increased glomerular filtration, decreased hepatic excretion of metabolites, or metabolic clearance of steroid and protein hormones by the placenta. The changes in endocrine function tests are summarized in Table 16–1. Failure to recognize normal pregnancy-induced alterations in endocrine function tests can lead to unnecessary diagnostic tests and therapy that may be seriously detrimental to mother and fetus.

Maternal Pituitary Gland

The mother's anterior pituitary gland hormones have little influence on pregnancy after implantation has occurred. The gland itself enlarges by about one-third, with the major component of this increase being hyperplasia of the lactotrophs in response to the high plasma estrogens. PRL, the product of the lactotrophs, is the only anterior pituitary hormone that rises progressively during pregnancy, with contributions from both the anterior pituitary and the decidua. In spite of the high serum concentrations, pulsatile release of PRL and nocturnal and food-induced increases persist. Hence, the normal neuroendocrine regulatory mechanisms appear to be intact. Pituitary ACTH and TSH secretion remain unchanged. Serum FSH and LH fall to the lower limits of detectability and are unresponsive to GnRH stimulation. GH concentrations are not significantly different from nonpregnant levels, but pituitary response to provocative testing is markedly altered. GH response to hypoglycemia and arginine infusion is enhanced in early pregnancy but thereafter becomes depressed. Established pregnancy can continue in the face of hypophysectomy, and in women hypophysectomized prior to pregnancy, induction of ovulation and normal pregnancy can be achieved with appropriate replacement therapy. In cases of primary pituitary hyperfunction, the fetus is not affected.

Maternal Thyroid Gland

The thyroid becomes palpably enlarged during the first trimester, and a bruit may be present. Thyroid iodide clearance and ^{131}I uptake (which are clinically contraindicated in pregnancy) have been shown to be increased. These changes are due in large part to the increased renal clearance of iodide, which causes a relative iodine deficiency. While total serum thyrox-

SYSTEM	PARAMETER	PATTERN
Cardiovascular	Heart rate	Gradually increases 20%.
	Blood pressure	Gradually decreases 10% by 34 weeks, then increases to prepregnancy values.
	Stroke volume	Increases to maximum at 19 weeks, then plateaus.
	Cardiac output	Rises rapidly by 20%, then gradually increases an additional 10% by 28 weeks.
	Peripheral venous distention	Progressive increase to term.
	Peripheral vascular resistance	Progressive decrease to term.
Pulmonary	Respiratory rate	Unchanged.
	Tidal volume	Increases by 30–40%.
	Expiratory reserve	Gradual decrease.
	Vital capacity	Unchanged.
	Respiratory minute volume	Increases by 40%.
Blood	Volume	Increases by 50% in second trimester.
	Hematocrit	Decreases slightly.
	Fibrinogen	Increases.
	Electrolytes	Unchanged.
Gastrointestinal	Sphincter tone	Decreases.
	Gastric emptying time	Increases.

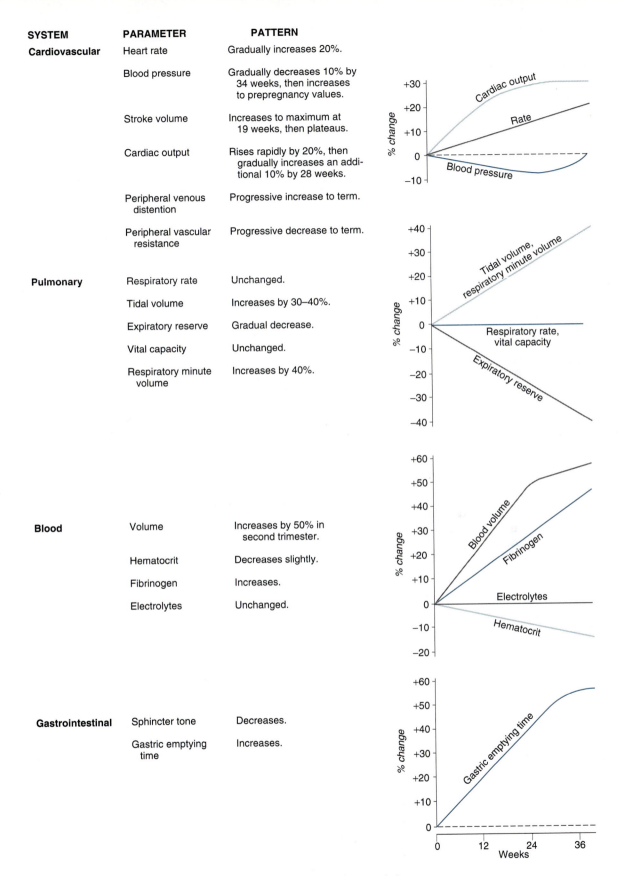

Figure 16–2. Maternal physiologic changes during pregnancy.

555

SYSTEM	PARAMETER	PATTERN
Renal	Renal flow	Increases 25–50%.
	Glomular filtration rate	Increases early, then plateaus.
Weight	Uterine weight	Increases from about 60–70 g to about 900–1200 g.
	Body weight	Average 11-kg (25-lb) increase.

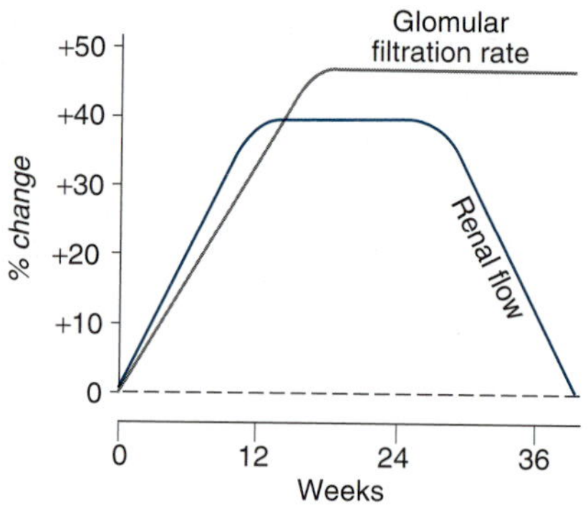

Figure 16–2 (cont'd). Maternal physiologic change during pregnancy.

ine is elevated as a result of increased thyroid hormone-binding globulin (TBG), free thyroxine and triiodothyronine are normal (Figure 16–1). High circulating concentrations of hCG, particularly asialo-hCG, appear to contribute to the thyrotropic action of the placenta in early pregnancy.

Table 16–1. Effect of pregnancy on endocrine function tests.

	Test	Result
Pituitary FSH, LH	GnRH stimulation	Unresponsive from third gestational week until puerperium.
GH	Insulin tolerance test	Response increases during the first half of pregnancy and then is blunted until the puerperium.
	Arginine stimulation	Hyperstimulation during the first and second trimesters, then suppression
TSH	TRH stimulation	Response unchanged.
Pancreas Insulin	Glucose tolerance	peak glucose increases, and glucose concentration remains elevated longer.
	Glucose challenge	Insulin concentration increases to higher peak levels
	Arginine infusion	Insulin response is blunted in mid to late pregnancy
Adrenal Cortisol	ACTH infusion	Exaggerated cortisol and 17-hydroxycorticosterone responses
	Metyrapone	Diminished response
Mineralo-corticoids	ACTH infusion	No DOC response
	Dexamethasone suppression	No DOC response

Maternal Parathyroid Gland

The net calcium requirement imposed by fetal skeletal development is estimated to be about 30 g by term. This is met by hyperplasia of the parathyroid glands and elevated serum levels of parathyroid hormone. The maternal serum calcium concentration declines to a nadir at 28–32 weeks, largely owing to the hypoalbuminemia of pregnancy. Ionized calcium is maintained at normal concentrations throughout pregnancy.

Maternal Pancreas

The nutritional demands of the fetus require alteration of maternal metabolic homeostatic control, which results in both structural and functional changes in the maternal pancreas. The size of pancreatic islets increases, and insulin-secreting β cells undergo hyperplasia. Basal levels of insulin are lower or unchanged in early pregnancy but increase during the second trimester. Thereafter, pregnancy is a hyperinsulinemic state, with resistance to the peripheral metabolic effects of insulin. The increased concentration of insulin has been shown to be a result of increased secretion rather than decreased metabolic clearance. The measured half-life for insulin is unchanged in pregnant women. The effects of pregnancy on the pancreas can be mimicked by appropriate treatment with estrogen, progesterone, hCS, and corticosteroids.

Pancreatic production of glucagon remains responsive to usual stimuli and is suppressed by glucose loading, although the degree of responsiveness has not been well evaluated.

The major role of insulin and glucagon is the intracellular transport of nutrients, specifically glucose, amino acids, and fatty acids. These concentrations are regulated during pregnancy for fetal as well as maternal needs, and the pre- and postfeeding levels cause pancreatic responses that act to support the fetal economy. Insulin is not transported across the placenta but rather exerts its effects on transportable metabolites. During pregnancy, peak insulin secretion in response to meals is accelerated, and glucose tolerance curves are characteristically altered. Fasting glucose levels are maintained at low normal levels. Excess carbohydrate is converted to fat, and fat is readily mobilized during decreased caloric intake.

Amino acid metabolism is also altered during pregnancy at the expense of maternal needs. Because alanine, the key amino acid for gluconeogenesis, is preferentially transported to the fetus, maternal hypoglycemia leads to lipolysis.

The normal result of pregnancy, then is to reduce glucose levels modestly but to reserve glucose for fetal needs while maternal energy requirements are met increasingly by the peripheral metabolism of fatty acids. These changes in energy metabolism are beneficial to the fetus and innocuous to the mother with an adequate diet. Even modest fasting, however, causes ketosis, which is potentially injurious to the fetus.

Maternal Adrenal Cortex

A. Glucocorticoids: Plasma cortisol concentrations increase to three times nonpregnant levels by the third trimester. Most of the increase can be accounted for by a doubling of corticosteroid-binding globulin (CBG). The increased estrogen levels of pregnancy account for the increase in CBG, which, in turn, is sufficient to account for decreased catabolism of cortisol by the liver. The result is a doubling of the half-life of plasma cortisol. The actual production of cortisol by the zona fasciculata also is increased in pregnancy. The net effect of these changes is an increase in plasma free cortisol, which is approximately doubled by late pregnancy. Whether this increase is mediated through ACTH or by other mechanisms is not known. In spite of cortisol concentrations approaching those found in Cushing's syndrome, diurnal variation in plasma cortisol is maintained. The elevated free cortisol probably contributes to the insulin resistance of pregnancy and possibly to the appearance of striae, but most signs of hypercortisolism do not occur in pregnancy. It is possible that high progesterone levels act as a glucocorticoid antagonist and prevent some cortisol effects.

B. Mineralocorticoids and the Renin-Angiotensin System: Serum aldosterone is markedly elevated in pregnancy. The increase is due to an eight- to tenfold increased production of aldosterone by the zona glomerulosa and not to increased binding or decreased clearance. The peak in aldosterone production is reached by mid pregnancy and is maintained until delivery. Renin substrate is increased owing to the influence of estrogen on hepatic synthesis, and renin also is increased.

The increases in both renin and renin substrate inevitably lead to increases in renin activity and angiotensin. In spite of these dramatic changes, normal pregnant women show few signs of hyperaldosteronism. There is no tendency to hypokalemia or hyper-

natremia, and blood pressure at mid pregnancy—when changes in the aldosterone-renin-angiotensin system are maximal—tends to be lower than in the nonpregnant state.

Although the quantitative aspects of this apparent paradox are not fully understood, a qualitative explanation is possible. Progesterone is an effective competitive inhibitor of mineralocorticoids in the distal renal tubules. Exogenous progesterone (but not synthetic progestins) is natriuretic and potassium-sparing in intact humans, whereas it has no effect in adrenalectomized subjects not receiving mineralocorticoids. Progesterone also blunts the response of the kidney to exogenous aldosterone—thus, the increases in renin and aldosterone may simply be an appropriate response to the high gestational levels of progesterone. The concomitant increase in angiotensin II as a result of increased plasma renin activity apparently does not normally result in hypertension, because of diminished sensitivity of the maternal vascular system to angiotensin. Even during the first trimester, exogenous angiotensin provokes less of a rise in blood pressure than in the nonpregnant state.

It is clear that the high levels of renin, angiotensin, and aldosterone in pregnant women are subject to the usual feedback controls, because they respond appropriately to changes in posture, dietary sodium, and water loading and restriction in qualitatively the same way as they do in nonpregnant women. Finally, in patients with preeclampsia, the most common form of pregnancy-related hypertension, serum renin, aldosterone, and angiotensin levels are lower than in normal pregnancy, thus ruling out any primary role for the renin-angiotensin system in this disorder. Production of the mineralocorticoid 11-deoxycorticosterone (DOC) rises throughout pregnancy, and plasma levels six to ten times normal are achieved by term. In contrast to the nonpregnant state, DOC production in pregnancy is unaffected by ACTH or glucocorticoid administration. The source of DOC appears to be conversion of progesterone to DOC in peripheral tissue. DOC is not elevated in hypertensive disorders of pregnancy.

C. Androgens: In normal pregnancy, the maternal production of androgens is slightly increased. The most important determinant of plasma levels of specific androgens, however, appears to be whether or not the androgen binds to sex hormone-binding globulin (SHBG). Testosterone, which binds avidly to SHBG, increases to the normal male range by the end of the first trimester, but free testosterone levels are actually lower than in the nonpregnant state. Dehydroepiandrosterone sulfate (DHEA sulfate) does not bind significantly to SHBG, and plasma concentrations of DHEA sulfate actually decrease during pregnancy. The desulfation of DHEA sulfate by the placenta and the conversion of DHEA sulfate to estrogens by the fetal-placental unit also are important factors in its increased metabolic clearance.

FETAL ENDOCRINOLOGY

Because of the inaccessibility of the fetus, much of our information about fetal endocrinology is derived indirectly. Most early studies of fetal endocrinology relied upon observations of infants with congenital disorders or inferences from ablation studies or acute manipulation in experimental animals. The development of effective cell culture methods, sensitive immunoassays, and the ability to achieve stable preparations of chronically catheterized monkey fetuses have increased our understanding of the dynamics of intrauterine endocrine events.

Study of the fetal endocrine system is further complicated by the multiplicity of sources of the various hormones. The fetus is exposed to maternal and placental hormones as well as to those it produces itself. Amniotic fluid contains a variety of hormones of mixed fetal and maternal origin, and these hormones are of uncertain importance. Study of the isolated fetus, even if possible, would thus be of little physiologic relevance.

A final pitfall in the study of fetal endocrine systems relates to the process of development itself. Inferences from the behavior of adult endocrine systems are not transferable to the fetus, because target organs, receptors, modulators, and regulators develop at different times. Thus, the role of a particular hormone in the fetal economy at any one point in gestation may bear little or no relationship to its role in postnatal life.

Dating of events in fetal development is usually given in "fetal weeks," which begin at the time of ovulation and fertilization. Thus, fetal age is always 2 weeks less than gestational age.

Human fetal growth is influenced by endocrine and hemodynamic factors that dictate the partitioning of nutrients between the mother and the conceptus. The main metabolic substrates for fetal and placental growth are glucose, lactate, amino acids, and lipids. A variety of placental transport proteins regulate the partitioning of these nutrients. In addition, placental hormones such as hPL, GH-variant, and IGF-1 and IGF-2 are secreted into the maternal and fetal circulations where they modulate energy metabolism and fetal growth.

The endocrine system is among the first to develop in fetal life. Differentiation of the gonads is crucial for normal male sexual development and reproductive potential. Primary testis differentiation begins with development of the Sertoli cells at 8 weeks' gestation. The testis-determining factor on the Y chromosome directs the differentiation of the Sertoli cells which are the sites of müllerian-inhibiting substance (MIS) synthesis. MIS, a member of the TGFβ family of growth factors, specifically triggers the ipsilateral resorption of the müllerian tract in males. Embryonic androgen production begins in the developing Leydig cells at about 10 weeks, coinci-dent with the peak production of placental hCG. The ovarian counterpart in the female is smaller and less differentiated at this stage of embryonic life. Oogonia mitosis is active and steroid-producing theca cell precursors are identifiable at 20 weeks. This corresponds with peak gonadotropin levels from the fetal pituitary. Activin and inhibin peptide subunits are expressed in the midtrimester human testis but not in the midtrimester human ovary. In contrast to the male fetus, ovarian steroid production is not essential for female phenotypic development (see Chapter 14).

Fetal Anterior Pituitary Hormones

The characteristic anterior pituitary cell types are discernible as early as 8–10 fetal weeks, and all of the hormones of the adult anterior pituitary are extractable from the fetal adenohypophysis by 12 weeks. Similarly, the hypothalamic hormones thyrotropin-releasing hormone (TRH), gonadotropin-releasing hormone (GnRH), and somatostatin are present by 8–10 weeks. The direct circulatory connection between hypothalamus and pituitary develops later, with capillary invasion initially visible at about 16 weeks.

The role of the fetal pituitary in organogenesis of various target organs during the first trimester appears to be negligible. None of the pituitary hormones are released into the fetal circulation in large quantities until after 20 fetal weeks. Even growth hormone (GH) appears not to be influential, and in fact total absence of GH is consistent with normal development at birth. Development of the gonads and adrenals during the first trimester appears to be directed by hCG rather than by fetal pituitary hormones.

During the second trimester, there is a marked increase in secretion of all of the anterior pituitary hormones, which coincides with maturation of the hypophysial portal system. Observations include a marked rise in production of GH and an increase in fetal serum TSH, with a concomitant increase in fetal thyroidal iodine uptake. Gonadotropin production also increases, with the female achieving higher FSH levels in both pituitary and serum than does the male. The fetal gonadotropins do not direct the events of early gonadal development but are essential for normal development of the differentiated gonads and external genitalia. ACTH rises significantly during the second trimester and assumes an increasing role in directing the maturation of the differentiated adrenal, as shown by the anencephalic fetus, in which the fetal zone of the adrenal undergoes atrophy after 20 weeks. Fetal PRL secretion also increases after the 20th fetal week, but the functional significance of this hormone, if any, is unknown.

During the third trimester, maturation of feedback systems modulating hypothalamic release signals causes serum concentrations of all of the pituitary hormones except PRL to decline.

Fetal Posterior Pituitary Hormones

Vasopressin and oxytocin are demonstrable by 12–18 weeks in the fetal posterior pituitary gland and correlate with the development of their sites of production, the supraoptic and paraventricular nuclei. The hormone content of the gland increases toward term, with no evidence of feedback control.

During labor, umbilical artery oxytocin is higher than umbilical vein oxytocin. It has been suggested that the fetal posterior pituitary may contribute to the onset or maintenance of labor.

Fetal Thyroid Gland

The thyroid gland develops in the absence of detectable TSH. By 12 weeks the thyroid is capable of iodine-concentrating activity and thyroid hormone synthesis.

During the second trimester, TRH, TSH, and free T_4 all begin to rise. The maturation of feedback mechanisms is suggested by the subsequent plateau of TSH at about 20 fetal weeks. Fetal T_3 and reverse T_3 do not become detectable until the third trimester. The hormone produced in largest amount throughout fetal life is T_4, with the metabolically active T_3 and its inactive derivative, reverse T_3, rising in parallel to T_4 during the third trimester. At birth, conversion of T_4 to T_3 becomes demonstrable.

The development of thyroid hormones occurs independently of maternal systems, and very little placental transfer of thyroid hormone occurs in physiologic concentrations. This prevents maternal thyroid disorders from affecting the fetal compartment but also prevents effective therapy for fetal hypothyroidism through maternal supplementation. Goitrogenic agents such as propylthiouracil are transferred across the placenta and may induce fetal hypothyroidism and goiter.

The function of the fetal thyroid hormones appears crucial to somatic growth and for successful neonatal adaptation.

Fetal Parathyroid Gland

The fetal parathyroid is capable of synthesizing parathyroid hormone by the end of the first trimester. However, the placenta actively transports calcium into the fetal compartment, and the fetus remains relatively hypercalcemic throughout gestation. This contributes to a suppression of parathyroid hormone, and fetal serum levels in umbilical cord have been reported to be low or undetectable. Fetal serum calcitonin levels are elevated, enhancing bone accretion. Fetal vitamin D levels reflect maternal levels but do not appear to be significant in fetal calcium metabolism.

Fetal Adrenal Cortex

The fetal adrenal differs anatomically and functionally from the adult gland. The cortex is identifiable as early as 4 weeks of fetal age, and by the seventh week, steroidogenic activity can be detected in the inner zone layers.

By 20 weeks, the adrenal cortex has increased to a mass that is considerably larger than its relative postnatal size. During gestation, it occupies as much as 0.5% of total body volume, and most of this tissue is composed of a unique fetal zone that subsequently regresses or is transformed into the definitive (adult) zone during the early neonatal period. The inner fetal zone is responsible for the majority of steroids produced during fetal life and comprises 80% of the mass of the adrenal. During the second trimester, the inner fetal zone continues to grow, while the outer zone remains relatively undifferentiated. At about 25 weeks, the definitive (adult) zone develops more rapidly, ultimately assuming the principal role in steroid synthesis during the early postnatal weeks. This transfer of function is accompanied by involution of the fetal zone, which is completed during the first months of neonatal life.

Fetal Gonads

The testis is a detectable structure by about 6 fetal weeks. The interstitial or Leydig cells, which synthesize fetal testosterone, are functional at this same stage. The maximal production of testosterone coincides with the maximal production of hCG by the placenta; binding of hCG to fetal testes with stimulation of testosterone release has been demonstrated. Other fetal testicular products of importance are the reduced testosterone metabolite dihydrotestosterone and müllerian-inhibiting substance. Dihydrotestosterone is responsible for development of the external genital structures, whereas müllerian-inhibiting substance prevents development of female internal structures.

Little is known about fetal ovarian function. By 7–8 weeks of intrauterine life, the ovaries become recognizable, but their importance in fetal physiology has not been established, and the significance of the steroids produced by the ovaries remains unclear.

ENDOCRINE CONTROL OF PARTURITION

During the last few weeks of normal pregnancy, two processes herald approaching labor. Uterine contractions, usually painless, become increasingly frequent, and the lower uterine segment and cervix become softer and thinner, a process known as effacement, or "ripening." Although false alarms are not uncommon, the onset of true labor is usually fairly abrupt, with the establishment of regular contractions every 2–5 minutes, leading to delivery in less than 24 hours. There is a huge literature describing the physiologic and biochemical events that occur during human labor, but the key inciting event has eluded detection. For sheep, it is the fetus that controls the onset of labor. The initial measurable event is an increase in fetal plasma cortisol, which, in turn, alters placental steroid production, resulting in a drop in progesterone. Cortisol reliably induces labor in sheep, but in humans, glucocorticoids do not induce labor and there is no clear drop in plasma progesterone prior to labor. Furthermore, exogenous progesterone does not prevent labor in humans.

The difficulty in identifying a *single* initiating event in human labor suggests that there is more than one. Approaching the matter in a different way, one could ask: What are the factors responsible for maintenance of pregnancy, and how can they fail?

Sex Steroids

Progesterone is essential for maintenance of early pregnancy, and withdrawal of progesterone leads to termination of pregnancy. Progesterone causes hyperpolarization of the myometrium, decreasing the amplitude of action potentials and preventing effective contractions. In various experimental systems, progesterone decreases alpha-adrenergic receptors, stimulates cAMP production, and inhibits oxytocin receptor synthesis. Progesterone also inhibits estrogen receptor synthesis, promotes the storage of prostaglandin precursors in the decidua and fetal membranes, and stabilizes the lysosomes containing prostaglandin-synthesizing enzymes. Estrogen opposes progesterone in these actions and may have an independent role in ripening the uterine cervix and promoting uterine contractility. Thus, the estrogen:progesterone ratio may be an important parameter. In a small series of patients, an increase in the estrogen:progesterone ratio has been shown to precede labor. Thus, for some individuals, a drop in progesterone or an increase in estrogen may initiate labor. The cause of the change in steroids may be placental maturation or a signal from the fetus, but there are not data to support either thesis. It has been shown that an increase in the estrogen:progesterone ratio increases the number of oxytocin receptors and myometrial gap junctions; this finding may explain the coordinate, effective contractions that characterize true labor as opposed to the nonpainful, ineffective contractions of false labor.

Oxytocin

Oxytocin infusion is commonly used to induce or augment labor. Both maternal and fetal oxytocin levels increase spontaneously during labor, but neither has been convincingly shown to increase prior to labor. Data in animals suggest that oxytocin's role in initiation of labor is due to increased sensitivity of the uterus to oxytocin rather than increased plasma concentrations of the hormone. Even women with diabetes insipidus are able to deliver without oxytocin augmentation; thus a maternal source of the hormone is not indispensable.

Prostaglandins

Prostaglandin $F_{2\alpha}$ administered intra-amniotically or intravenously is an effective abortifacient as early as 14 weeks of gestation. Prostaglandin E_2 administered by vagina will induce labor in most women in the third trimester. The amnion and chorion contain high concentrations of arachidonic acid, and the decidua contains active prostaglandin synthetase. Prostaglandins are almost certainly involved in maintenance of labor once it is established. They also probably are important in initiating labor in some circumstances, such as in amnionitis or when the membranes are "stripped" by the physician. They probably are part of the "final common pathway" of labor.

Prostaglandin synthetase inhibitors abolish premature labor, but their clinical usefulness has been restricted by their simultaneous effect of closing the ductus arteriosus, which can lead to fetal pulmonary hypertension.

Catecholamines

Catecholamines with α_2-adrenergic activity cause uterine contractions, whereas β_2-adrenergics inhibit labor. Progesterone increases the ratio of beta receptors to alpha receptors in myometrium, thus favoring continued gestation. There is no evidence that changes in catecholamines or their receptors initiate labor, but it is likely that such changes help sustain labor once initiated. The beta-adrenergic drug ritodrine has proved to be a valuable agent in the management of premature labor. Alpha-adrenergic agents have not been useful in inducing labor, because of their cardiovascular side effects.

Nitric Oxide

Uterine smooth muscle may also be affected by nitric oxide (NO), which may act as a uterine smooth muscle relaxant. Some laboratory findings suggest that uterine NO production decreases at term and that inhibitors of NO synthesis might some day be used to initiate or augment human labor.

ENDOCRINOLOGY OF THE PUERPERIUM

Extirpation of any active endocrine organ leads to compensatory changes in other organs and systems. Delivery of the infant and placenta causes both immediate and long-term adjustment to loss of the pregnancy hormones. The sudden withdrawal of fetal-placental hormones at delivery permits determination of their serum half-lives and some evaluation of their effects on maternal systems.

Physiologic & Anatomic Changes

Some of the physiologic and anatomic adjustments that take place after delivery are hormone-dependent, whereas others are themselves responsible for hormonal changes. For example, major readjustments of the cardiovascular system occur in response to the normal blood losses associated with delivery and to loss of the low-resistance placental shunt. By the third postpartum day, blood volume is estimated to decline to about 84% of predelivery values. These cardiovascular changes influence renal and liver clearance of hormones.

Reproductive Tract Changes

The uterus decreases progressively in size at the rate of about 500 g/wk and continues to be palpable abdominally until about 2 weeks postpartum, when it reoccupies its position entirely within the pelvis. Nonpregnant size and weight (60–70 g) are reached by 6 weeks. The reversal of myometrial hypertrophy occurs with a decrease in size of individual myometrial cells rather than by reduction in number. Uterine discharge also changes progressively during this period, with the mixture of fresh blood and decidua becoming a serous transudate and then ceasing in 3–6 weeks.

The endometrium, which is sloughed at the time of delivery, regenerates rapidly; by the seventh day, there is restoration of surface epithelium, except at the placental site. By the second week after delivery, the endometrium resembles normal proliferative-phase endometrium, except for the characteristic hyalinized decidual areas. The earliest documented appearance of a secretory endometrium occurred on day 44 in one series of daily biopsies. These rapid regenerative changes do not apply to the area of placental implantation, which requires much longer for restoration and retains pathognomonic histologic evidence of placentation indefinitely.

The cervix and vagina also recover rapidly from the effects of pregnancy, labor, and delivery. The cervix regains tone over the first week; by 6 weeks postpartum, it usually exhibits complete healing of trauma sustained at the time of delivery. Histologically, involution may continue beyond 6 weeks, with stromal edema, leukocytic infiltration, and glandular hyperplasia still apparent. Similarly, the vagina regains muscular tone following delivery, and rugae appear as early as 3 weeks. However, in women who nurse, the vaginal mucosa may remain atrophic for months, sometimes resulting in dyspareunia and a watery discharge.

Endocrine Changes

A. Steroids: With expulsion of the placenta, the steroid levels decline precipitously, their half-lives being measured in minutes or hours. As a consequence of continued low-level production by the corpus luteum, progesterone does not reach basal prenatal levels as rapidly as does estradiol. Plasma progesterone falls to luteal-phase levels within 24 hours after delivery but to follicular-phase levels only after several days. Removal of the corpus luteum results in a fall to follicular levels within 24 hours. Estradiol reaches follicular-phase levels within 1–3 days after delivery.

B. Pituitary Hormones: The pituitary gland, which enlarges during pregnancy owing primarily to an increase in lactotrophs, does not diminish in size until after lactation ceases. Secretion of FSH and LH continues to be suppressed during the early weeks of the puerperium, and stimulus with bolus doses of GnRH results in subnormal release of LH and FSH. Over the ensuing weeks, responsiveness to GnRH gradually returns to normal, and most women exhibit follicular-phase serum levels of LH and FSH by the third or fourth postpartum week.

C. Prolactin: Serum prolactin (PRL), which rises throughout pregnancy, falls with the onset of labor and then exhibits variable patterns of secretion depending upon whether breast feeding occurs. Delivery is associated with a surge in PRL, which is followed by a rapid fall in serum concentrations over 7–14 days in the nonlactating mother.

In nonlactating women, the return of normal cyclic function and ovulation may be expected as soon as the second postpartum month, with the initial ovulation occurring at an average of 9–10 weeks postpartum. In lactating women, PRL usually causes a persistence of anovulation. Surges of PRL are believed to act on the hypothalamus to inhibit GnRH secretion. Administration of exogenous GnRH during this time induces normal pituitary responsiveness, and occasional ovulation may occur spontaneously even during lactation. The average time for ovulation in women who have lactated for at least 3 months is about 17 weeks. The percentage of nonlactating women who have resumed menstruation increases linearly up to 12 weeks, by which time 70% will have restored menses. In contrast, the linear increase for lactating women exhibits a much shallower slope, and 70% of lactating women will have menstruated by about 36 weeks.

Lactation

Development of the breast alveolar lobules occurs throughout pregnancy. This period of mammogenesis requires the concerted participation of estrogen, progesterone, PRL, GH, and glucocorticoids. hPL may also play a role but is not indispensable. Milk secretion in the puerperium is associated with further enlargement of the lobules, followed by synthesis of milk constituents such as lactose and casein.

Lactation requires PRL, insulin, and adrenal steroids. It does not occur until unconjugated estrogens fall to nonpregnant levels at about 36–48 hours postpartum.

PRL is essential to milk production. Its action involves induced synthesis of large numbers of PRL receptors; these appear to be autoregulated by PRL, since PRL increases receptor levels in cell culture and since bromocriptine, a PRL inhibitor, causes a decrease in both PRL and its receptors. In the absence of PRL, milk secretion does not take place; but even in the presence of high levels of PRL during the third trimester, milk secretion does not take place until after delivery, owing to the blocking effect of high levels of estrogen.

Galactopoiesis, or the process of continued milk secretion, is also dependent upon the function and integration of several hormones. Evidence from GH-deficient dwarfs and hypothyroid patients suggests that GH and thyroid hormone are not required.

Milk secretion requires the additional stimulus of emptying of the breast. A neural arc must be activated for continued milk secretion. Milk ejection occurs in response to a surge of oxytocin, which induces a contractile response in the smooth muscle surrounding the gland ductules. Oxytocin release is occasioned by stimuli of a visual, psychologic, or physical nature that prepare the mother for suckling.

ENDOCRINE DISORDERS & PREGNANCY

PREGNANCY & PITUITARY ADENOMAS

In women of reproductive age, small tumors of the anterior pituitary are not uncommon (see also Chapter 5). While most are nonfunctional and asymptomatic, the most common symptom of pituitary microadenomas is amenorrhea, frequently accompanied by galactorrhea. In the past, few affected women became pregnant, but now most can be made to ovulate and to conceive with the aid of clomiphene citrate, menotropins and hCG, or bromocriptine. Before ovulation is induced in any patient, serum PRL should be determined. If it is elevated, the sella turcica should be evaluated by magnetic resonance imaging (MRI) or by high-resolution CT scanning with contrast. About 10% of women with secondary amenorrhea will be found to have adenomas, while 20–50% of women with amenorrhea and galactorrhea will have detectable tumors.

The effect of pregnancy on pituitary adenomas depends on the size of the adenoma. Among 215 women with microadenomas (< 10 mm in diameter), fewer than 1% developed progressive visual field defects, 5% developed headaches, and none experienced more serious neurologic sequelae. Of 60 patients who had macroadenomas and became pregnant, 20% developed abnormal changes in their visual fields or other neurologic signs, usually in the first half of their pregnancies. Many of these required therapy. Monitoring of patients with known PRL-secreting adenomas during pregnancy is primarily based on clinical examination. The normal gesta-

tional increase in PRL may obscure the increase attributable to the adenoma, and radiographic procedures are undesirable in pregnancy.

Visual disturbances are usually experienced as "clumsiness" and are objectively found to be due to visual field changes. The most frequent findings is bitemporal hemianopia, but in advanced cases the defect can progress to concentric contraction of fields and enlargement of the blind spot.

Since the pituitary normally increases in size during pregnancy, headaches are common and bitemporal hemianopia not uncommon in patients with adenomas. These changes almost always revert to normal after delivery, so that aggressive therapy for known pituitary adenomas is not indicated except in cases of rapidly progressive visual loss.

Management

Management of the pregnant woman with a small adenoma includes early ophthalmologic consultation for formal visual field mapping and repeat examinations once a month or every other month throughout pregnancy.

If visual field disturbances are minimal, pregnancy may be allowed to proceed to term. If symptoms become progressively more severe and the fetus is mature, labor should be induced. If symptoms are severe and the fetus is immature, management may consist of transsphenoidal resection of the adenoma or medical treatment with bromocriptine. While bromocriptine inhibits both fetal and maternal pituitary PRL secretion, it does not affect decidual PRL secretion. Bromocriptine appears not to be teratogenic, and no adverse fetal effects have been reported. In most cases it is probably preferable to surgery. Radiation therapy should not be used in pregnancy.

Management of PRL-secreting tumors in women who want to become pregnant is controversial. Surgical resection by surgeons with experience in transsphenoidal procedures results in reduction of PRL levels and resumption of normal ovulation in 60–80% of women with microadenomas and 30–50% of women with macroadenomas. The incidence of recurrence is at least 10–15% and will probably increase with further follow-up. Bromocriptine is usually well tolerated and is successful in achieving normal menstrual cycles and lowering PRL levels in 40–80% of patients. Bromocriptine also causes a marked decrease in tumor size, but the original size of the tumor is usually regained within days or weeks after discontinuing therapy. In the case of large tumors, combined medical and surgical management may often be appropriate. Radiation therapy has an important role in arresting growth of tumors that are resistant to other management, particularly large tumors that involve the cavernous sinuses and tumors that secrete both GH and PRL (see Chapter 5).

Lymphocytic adenohypophysitis is an enigmatic autoimmune inflammation of the pituitary that classically occurs in women in late pregnancy or during the puerperium. The clinical presentation is difficult to distinguish from that of a large prolactin-secreting adenoma. Expectant conservative medical management with corticosteroids is sometimes possible, with vigilant postpartum observation to prevent consequences of pituitary insufficiency.

Prognosis & Follow-Up

There appears to be no increase in obstetric complications associated with pituitary adenomas, and no fetal jeopardy. The rate of prematurity increases in women with tumors requiring therapy, but this is probably due to aggressive intervention rather than to spontaneous premature labor.

The postpartum period is characterized by rapid relief of even severe symptoms, with less than 4% of untreated tumors developing permanent sequelae. In some cases, tumors improve following pregnancy, with normalization or lowering of PRL relative to prepregnancy values. Management should include radiography and assessment of PRL levels 4–6 weeks after delivery. There are no contraindications to breast-feeding.

PREGNANCY & BREAST CANCER

Breast cancer complicates one in 1500–5000 pregnancies. Only one-sixth of breast cancers occur in women of reproductive age, but of these, one in seven is diagnosed during pregnancy or the puerperium. Pregnancy and breast cancer have long been considered such an ominous combination that only one in 20 young women who have had breast cancer have later become pregnant. It now appears, however, that pregnancy has little effect on growth of breast cancer, though it presents problems of detection and management of the cancer.

Influence of Pregnancy on Breast Cancer

Pregnancy is not an etiologic factor in breast cancer. Indeed, there is good evidence that pregnancy at an early age actually reduces the risk of developing mammary cancer, and multiple pregnancies may also make the disease less likely. Moreover, contemporary concepts of the rate of tumor growth suggest that a tumor becomes clinically evident only 8–10 years after its inception. Thus, a tumor cannot arise and be discovered during the same pregnancy. In view of the increased glandular proliferation and blood flow and marked increase in lymph flow that occur during pregnancy, it could be argued that pregnancy accelerates the appearance of previously subclinical diseases, but this has not been demonstrated.

Probably the most important influence of pregnancy on breast cancer is the delay it may cause in making the diagnosis and starting therapy. In some series, the interval between initial symptoms and treatment was 6–7 months longer than in the absence of pregnancy. The increased density of the breasts in pregnancy makes small masses less apparent; and even when masses are found, both the patient and the physician are apt to attribute them to expected physiologic changes in pregnancy. Larger tumors may be misdiagnosed as galactoceles, and inflammatory carcinoma in the puerperium is liable to be misdiagnosed as mastitis.

At the time of diagnosis, 60% of pregnancy-associated breast cancers have metastasized to regional lymph nodes, and an additional 20% have distant metastases. Stage for stage, however, survival rates following appropriate therapy are comparable to those achieved in nonpregnant patients. Termination of pregnancy, either by abortion or by early delivery, does not influence maternal survival.

Pregnancy After Treatment for Cancer

Pregnancy following definitive treatment of breast cancer has no adverse effect on survival. Indeed, women who become pregnant following stage I or II breast cancer have a somewhat better 5-year survival rate than matched controls who did not become pregnant but who survived at least as long as their match before becoming pregnant.

Women who have had breast cancer are frequently advised to avoid pregnancy for 5 years. Because most fertile women with breast cancer are in their mid 30s, such a plan virtually precludes pregnancy. Because pregnancy is not known to influence the rate of cancer recurrence, the only reasons for proscribing pregnancy are to avoid the possibility that management of a recurrence will be complicated by the pregnancy or to avoid the problem of producing motherless children. For a couple strongly desiring pregnancy, these risks may become acceptable in a much shorter time than 5 years, especially if the original lesion was small and the spread of disease minimal.

Estrogen Receptors in Breast Cancer

Determinations of soluble estrogen and progesterone receptors are frequently used in breast cancer to predict whether the tumor is likely to respond to endocrine therapy. There is also evidence that the presence of estrogen receptor-positive tumors is correlated with a lower risk of early recurrence. In the pregnant patient, however, high progesterone levels inhibit estrogen and progesterone receptor synthesis, and high levels of both hormones cause their receptors to become tightly associated with the nuclear fraction. Thus, when soluble receptors are quantified, all breast cancers arising in pregnancy appear to be receptor-negative, making such measurements in pregnancy at best worthless and at worst dangerously misleading. The introduction of immunohistochemical assays, which allow identification of occupied nuclear receptors, may lead to a more reliable assessment.

Early Diagnosis

It is clear that early diagnosis of breast cancer in pregnancy gives the best chance of improved survival. Self-examination should be encouraged in spite of the anxiety it will cause, and thorough breast examinations should be performed periodically throughout pregnancy, not just at the initial examination. Even mildly suspicious lesions should be investigated if they persist for 1–2 weeks; waiting for a lesion to grow before further investigation is not acceptable practice. If a woman has discovered a small mass, her assessment should be accepted even if the physician cannot feel the mass by the usual techniques. Small lesions that would otherwise be missed can often be felt if soap and water are used for lubrication. Cytologic examination of fine-needle aspirates is probably the best technique for investigating discrete lesions. If any question persists, ultrasonography or low-dose mammography should be employed. Unless one is very experienced with evaluating early breast carcinomas, consultation with a surgical oncologist is always in order.

Treatment of Breast Cancer in Pregnancy

Once the diagnosis of cancer is made, the patient must be treated surgically without delay. In view of the large percentage of patients with positive nodes, the procedure should be one that provides adequate sampling of the axillary nodes, such as modified radical mastectomy. Simple mastectomy with axillary irradiation should be avoided. Therapeutic abortion is not routinely indicated. If, on the basis of surgical staging, adjuvant therapy is considered advisable, the decision must be made either to terminate the pregnancy by abortion or early delivery or to postpone therapy. Since delay in treatment is the principal known reason for the poorer prognosis of breast cancer in pregnancy, delivery should be accomplished as soon as there is a substantial probability of good fetal outcome—usually at 32–34 weeks. Many of the drugs used in cytotoxic therapy of breast carcinoma are contraindicated in pregnancy. Radiation can be given with appropriate shielding, but the dose to the fetus will not be negligible.

HYPERTENSIVE DISORDERS OF PREGNANCY

Hypertension associated with pregnancy is generally categorized as chronic, in which elevated blood pressures antedate the pregnancy or are clinically recognized prior to the 20th week, or gestational, when the onset is beyond 20 weeks of gestation. If the latter is complicated by proteinuria and generalized edema, the triad is referred to as preeclampsia. When seizures accompany this syndrome, the condition is termed eclampsia. The incidence of preeclampsia is about 7%. Women at highest risk include primigravidas under 18 years old, multiparous women over 35 years old, and women with twin gestations, diabetes, hydramnios, pregnancy obesity, or prepregnancy hypertension. As many as half of women with prepregnancy hypertension develop exacerbations of hypertension in the third trimester.

Course of Hypertension in Pregnancy

In normal pregnancies, as well as those complicated by mild essential hypertension, diastolic blood pressure decreases 10–15 mm Hg in the second trimester. Hypertensive patients first seen at that time may be mistakenly identified as having preeclampsia when the blood pressure again increases in the third trimester. Clinically, preeclampsia usually appears after the 32nd week of gestation and, most frequently, during labor. In severe cases, especially those complicated by essential hypertension, acute rises in blood pressure may occur as early as 26 weeks. If hypertension appears in the first or early second trimester, it is associated either with gestational trophoblastic disease or an underlying disorder such as an acute flare-up of lupus nephritis. Occasionally, the onset of hypertension is recognized during the 24 hours following delivery.

In normal pregnancies, all of the components of the renin-angiotensin-aldosterone system are markedly elevated. In pregnancies complicated by chronic hypertension or preeclampsia, these components are slightly reduced toward normal nonpregnant levels, suggesting an appropriate feedback response. The most consistent finding in women with preeclampsia is the increased sensitivity to vasopressor agents compared to women with normal pregnancy. In pregnancies destined to be complicated by preeclampsia, an *increase* in arteriolar response to angiotensin that becomes statistically significant by 18–22 weeks of gestation–long before changes in blood pressure are detectable. The cause of this increase in vascular sensitivity to angiotensin is not known. Considerable evidence suggests that dyslipidemia and endothelial cell dysfunction may explain many of the pathophysiologic features of preeclampsia.

Symptoms & Signs

Signs of preeclampsia include a rise in diastolic pressure by 15 mm Hg or more over first trimester values, and proteinuria exceeding 500 mg daily. Symptoms include headaches, visual disturbances, and epigastric pain. Eclampsia may occur even with mild elevation of blood pressure and is associated with a maternal mortality rate as high as 10%. Deaths occur most frequently from cerebral hemorrhage, renal failure, disseminated intravascular coagulopathy, acute pulmonary edema, or hepatic failure. The fetal perinatal mortality rate is in excess of 30%, and the risk of perinatal morbidity due to hypoxia is even higher.

Treatment of Preeclampsia

The only definitive therapy for preeclampsia is delivery. If a modest increase in blood pressure first occurs in association with proteinuria at 32–36 weeks of gestation, bed rest, preferably in the left lateral decubitus position, is frequently effective in temporarily inducing diuresis and controlling progression of the disease, thus gaining time for the developing fetus. If labor occurs or induction of labor is attempted, parenteral magnesium sulfate should be used to prevent seizures and should be continued for 24 hours following delivery. Moderate hypertension need not be treated with antihypertensive agents; however, diastolic blood pressure above 120 mm Hg must be controlled to reduce the risk of intracranial hemorrhage. The agent of choice is hydralazine, 5 mg intravenously at 15- to 20-minute intervals, until the diastolic pressure is approximately 100 mm Hg. If hydralazine is unsuccessful, diazoxide or nitroprusside may be used, but these agents are rarely required. Recent trials indicate that low-dose aspirin can prevent the development of preeclampsia in high-risk situations. Reduction of the thromboxane: prostacyclin ratio at the platelet:endothelial cell interface appears to be the protective mechanism.

Treatment of Chronic Hypertension

Women with chronic hypertension who become pregnant require special management. Roberts's recommendations are probably the best:

(1) Diastolic pressures under 100 mm Hg should not be treated. However, if a woman is receiving antihypertensive therapy when first seen in pregnancy, therapy should be continued. If she is taking propranolol, consideration may be given to switching to a more specific β_1-antagonist such as metoprolol or atenolol. The rare patient who has been taking ganglionic blockers should receive another form of therapy instead. Owing to a transient decrease in blood volume and placental perfusion associated with thiazide diuretics, use of these agents should usually not be initiated during pregnancy; however, if a woman is already receiving such therapy, it may be continued.

(2) Diastolic pressures above 100 mm Hg discovered during pregnancy call for antihypertensive management. Initial therapy should be with methyldopa, 250 mg orally at bedtime. This may be increased 1 g twice daily as required. If unacceptable drowsiness lasting more than 2–3 days occurs, the dosage may be reduced, and hydralazine, beginning at 10 mg orally twice daily and increasing up to 100 mg twice daily, may be added. If hydralazine is not tolerated, prazosin may be gradually added to the methyldopa therapy.

(3) Accelerated hypertension at any stage of gestation should be managed with bed rest and, if necessary, intravenous hydralazine. Unless diastolic pressure can be reduced to 110 mm Hg promptly, delivery should be performed regardless of gestational age.

Prognosis

The prognosis for hypertensive cardiovascular disease in later life in women with pregnancy-related hypertension depends on the type of disorder. Preeclampsia in the young primigravida is not associated with an increased risk of hypertension in later pregnancies or in later life. By contrast, transient hypertension (late-gestation hypertension without proteinuria) is associated with an increased risk of chronic hypertension in later life.

HYPERTHYROIDISM IN PREGNANCY

Pregnancy mimics hyperthyroidism. There is thyroid enlargement, increased cardiac output, and peripheral vasodilation. Owing to the increase in thyroid hormone-binding globulin (TBG), total serum thyroxine is in the range expected for hyperthyroidism. Free thyroxine, the free thyroxine index, and TSH levels, however, remain in the normal range (see Chapter 7).

True hyperthyroidism complicates one or two per 1000 pregnancies. The most common form of hyperthyroidism during pregnancy is Graves' disease. Hyperthyroidism is associated with an increased risk of premature delivery (11–25%) and may modestly increase the risk of early abortion. In Graves' disease, thyroid-stimulating immunoglobulin (TSI), a 7S immune gamma globulin, crosses the placenta and may cause fetal goiter and transient neonatal hyperthyroidism, but these effects rarely jeopardize the fetus.

Treatment

The treatment of maternal hyperthyroidism is complicated by pregnancy. Radioiodides are strictly contraindicated. Iodide therapy can lead to huge fetal goiter and is contraindicated except as acute therapy to prevent thyroid storm before thyroid surgery. All antithyroid drugs cross the placenta and may cause fetal hypothyroidism and goiter or cretinism in the newborn. However, propylthiouracil in doses of 300 mg/d or less has been shown to be reasonably safe, although even at low doses about 10% of newborns will have a detectable goiter. Propranolol has been used to control maternal cardiovascular symptoms but may result in fetal bradycardia, growth retardation, premature labor, and neonatal respiratory depression. Partial or total thyroidectomy, especially in the second trimester, is a reasonably safe procedure except for the risk of premature labor.

A. Propylthiouracil: A reasonable plan of management is to begin therapy with propylthiouracil in doses high enough to bring the free T_4 index into the mildly hyperthyroid range and then to taper the dose gradually. Giving thyroxine along with propylthiouracil in the hope that it will cross the placenta in sufficient quantities to prevent fetal hypothyroidism is not effective and serves only to increase the amount of propylthiouracil required. If the maintenance dose of propylthiouracil is above 300 mg/d, serious consideration should be given to partial thyroidectomy.

B. Propranolol: Propranolol may be used transiently to ameliorate cardiovascular symptoms while control is being achieved.

Management of Newborn

Newborns should be observed carefully. In infants of mothers given propylthiouracil, even equivocal evidence of hypothyroidism is an indication for thyroxine replacement therapy. Neonatal Graves' disease, which may present as late as 2 weeks after delivery, requires intensive therapy (see Chapter 7).

HYPOTHYROIDISM IN PREGNANCY

Hypothyroidism is uncommon in pregnancy, since most women with the untreated disorder are oligoovulatory. As a practical matter, women taking thyroid medication at the time of conception should be maintained on the same or a slightly larger dose throughout pregnancy, whether or not the obstetrician believes thyroid replacement was originally indicated. Physiologic doses of thyroid are innocuous, but maternal hypothyroidism may be hazardous to the developing fetus. The correlation between maternal and fetal thyroid status is poor, and hypothyroid mothers frequently deliver euthyroid infants. The strongest correlation between maternal and newborn hypothyroidism occurs in areas where endemic goiter due to iodide deficiency is common. In these regions, dietary iodide supplementation in addition to thyroid hormone treatment of the mother may be of the greatest importance in preventing cretinism.

DIABETES MELLITUS & PREGNANCY

John L. Kitzmiller, MD

Hormone & Fuel Balance During Normal Pregnancy

Pregnancy produces major changes in the homeostasis of all metabolic fuels and in this way affects the management of diabetes. Plasma concentrations of glucose in the **postabsorptive state** (distant from meals) decline during pregnancy, because of increasing placental uptake of glucose and alanine and a limitation on hepatic glucose production due to decreased substrate. Therefore, fasting hypoglycemia is more common during pregnancy. Gluconeogenesis could be limited by a relative lack of the major substrate alanine. The plasma concentration of alanine has been shown in some studies to be lower during pregnancy, probably as a result of placental uptake and a restraint on proteolysis. Although fat deposition is accentuated in early pregnancy, lipolysis is enhanced by human placental lactogen (hPL) later in gestation, and more glycerol and free fatty acids are released in the postabsorptive state. Ketogenesis is thus accentuated in the postabsorptive state during pregnancy, probably secondary to increased provision of substrate free fatty acids and hormonal effects on the maternal liver cells.

The balance of metabolic fuels is also different in the **fed state** during pregnancy. Despite hyperinsulinism in normal pregnancy, there is a 50–70% reduction in net insulin-mediated glucose disposal by the third trimester. The insulin resistance can be identified in both peripheral tissues and the liver. The result is somewhat higher maternal blood glucose levels in nondiabetic subjects. The contra-insulin effects of gestation have been related to hPL, progesterone, cortisol, and prolactin. The disappearance in plasma of administered insulin is not greater during pregnancy, despite the presence of placental insulin receptors and degrading enzymes. Glucagon is well suppressed by glucose during pregnancy, and secretory responses of glucagon to amino acids are not increased above nonpregnant levels. After meals, more glucose is converted to triglyceride in pregnant compared with nonpregnant animals, which would tend to conserve calories and enhance fat deposition. Insulin resistance during pregnancy apparently does not extend to the lipogenic and antilipolytic effects of the hormone.

Overview of Diabetes During Pregnancy

Diabetic pregnant women have been classified on the basis of duration and severity of diabetes (Table 16–2). A classification system (White) was originally used for prognosis of perinatal outcome and to determine obstetric management. Because the perinatal mortality rate has declined dramatically for many reasons in women in all classes, the system is now used mainly to describe and compare populations of diabetic pregnant women. However, certain characteristics of patients are still pertinent. The risk of complications is minimal if gestational diabetes is well controlled by diet alone, and these patients may be otherwise managed as normal pregnant women. Class B patients, whose insulin dependence is of recent onset, will probably have residual islet B cell

Table 16–2. Classification of diabetes during pregnancy (Priscilla White).

Class	Characteristics	Implications
Gestational diabetes	Abnormal glucose tolerance during pregnancy; postprandial hyperglycemia during pregnancy.	Diagnosis before 30 weeks' gestation important to prevent macrosomia. Treat with diet adequate in calories to prevent maternal weight loss. Goal is postprandial blood glucose <130 mg/dL (7.2 mmol/L) at 1 hour or <105 mg/dL (5.8 mmol/L) at 2 hours. If insulin is necessary, manage as in classes B, C, and D.
A	Chemical diabetes diagnosed before pregnancy; managed by diet alone; any age at onset.	Management as for gestational diabetes.
B	Insulin treatment or oral hypoglycemic agent used before pregnancy; onset at age 20 or older; duration <10 years.	Some endogenous insulin secretion may persist. Fetal and neonatal risks same as in classes C and D, as is management; can be type I or II.
C	Onset at age 10–20, or duration 10–20 years.	Insulin-deficient diabetes of juvenile onset; type 1.
D	Onset before age 10, or duration >20 years, or chronic hypertension (not preeclampsia), or background retinopathy (tiny hemorrhages).	Fetal macrosomia or intrauterine growth retardation possible. Retinal microaneurysms, dot hemorrhages, and exudates may progress during pregnancy, then regress after delivery.
F	Diabetic nephropathy with proteinuria.	Anemia and hypertension common; proteinuria increases in third trimester, declines after delivery. Fetal intrauterine growth retardation common; perinatal survival about 90% under optimal conditions; bed rest necessary.
H	Coronary artery disease.	Serious maternal risk.
R	Proliferative retinopathy.	Neovascularization, with risk of vitreous hemorrhage or retinal detachment; laser photocoagulation useful; abortion usually not necessary. With active process of neovascularization, prevent bearing-down efforts.

function, and control of hyperglycemia may be easier than in class C or D patients. Finally, the most complicated and difficult pregnancies occur in women with renal, retinal, or cardiovascular disease.

The hormonal and metabolic effects of pregnancy are associated with increased risks of both hypoglycemic reactions and ketoacidosis. Increasing amounts of insulin are usually required to control hyperglycemia throughout gestation.

If diabetes is poorly controlled in the first weeks of pregnancy, the risks of spontaneous abortion and congenital malformation of the infant are increased. Later in pregnancy, polyhydramnios is also common in women with poorly controlled diabetes and may lead to preterm delivery. Fetal hypoxia may develop in the third trimester if diabetic control has been inadequate. Careful fetal monitoring must be used to prevent stillbirth. The high incidence of fetal macrosomia (birth weight > 90th percentile for gestational age) increases the potential for traumatic vaginal delivery; primary cesarean deliveries are more common in these cases. Fetal intrauterine growth retardation may occur in diabetic women with vascular disease.

Neonatal risks linked to maternal glycemic control include respiratory distress syndrome, hypoglycemia, hyperbilirubinemia, hypocalcemia, and poor feeding. Although these problems are usually limited to the first days of life, excess glucose and beta-hydroxybutyrate levels in utero have been related to diminished performance on psychomotor testing during childhood development. However, diabetic women have a 97–98% chance of delivering a healthy child if they adhere to a program of careful management and surveillance.

In the following sections, the convention used for designating the number of weeks of gestation is the number of weeks from the last menstrual period.

Gestational Diabetes (GDM)

The hormonal and metabolic changes of pregnancy result in the diagnosis of glucose intolerance during the second half of gestation in 2–4% of pregnant women. Criteria for diagnosis are given in Table 16–3. Gestational diabetes may result from inadequate insulin response to carbohydrate load, from excessive resistance to the action of insulin, or from both. Once the diagnosis has been made, the patient should be placed on a diabetic diet modified for pregnancy: 25–35 kcal/kg ideal weight, 40–55% carbohydrate, 20% protein, and 25–40% fat. Calories are distributed over three meals and three snacks (Table 16–4). The goal of therapy is not weight reduction but prevention of both fasting and postprandial hyperglycemia. If 1-hour or 2-hour postprandial glu-

Table 16–3. Diagnosis of gestational diabetes.

Screening with glucose loading test:
  Indications: (1) Screen all gravidas or (2) screen all gravidas who are overweight[1] or over 25 years of age (misses 10% of cases) plus all gravidas with glycosuria, a family history of diabetes in parents, sibling, aunts, or uncles), or a history of still-birth or macrosomic infants (misses 40% of cases).
  Procedure: Give 50 g of glucose by mouth at 24–26 weeks of gestation.[2] Measure plasma glucose 1 hour later. If value exceeds 130 mg/dL (7.2 mmol/L), give the oral glucose tolerance test.
Oral glucose tolerance test:
  Procedure: Give 100 g of glucose by mouth. Normal values for venous plasma glucose are as follows:

	NDDG[3]	C and C,S[4]
Fasting	105 mg/dL (5.8 mmol/L)	95 mg/dL (5.3 mmol/L)
1	190 mg/dL (10.5 mmol/L)	180 mg/dL (10.0 mmol/L)
2	165 mg/dL (9.2 mmol/L)	155 mg/dL (8.6 mmol/L)
3	145 mg/dL (8.0 mmol/L)	140 mg/dL (7.7 mmol/L)

[1]Overweight = height under 165 cm with weight over 68 kg (< 5 ft 5 in, > 150 lb) in first trimester; height over 156 cm with weight over 81 kg (> 5 ft 5 in, > 180 lb) in first trimester.
[2]Screen at 12–14 weeks for women at high risk of gestational diabetes; if negative, repeat at 24–26 weeks. If glucose loading test is done fasting, threshold of 140 mg/dl (7.7 mmol/L) is used.
[3]National Diabetes Data Group's modification of O'Sullivan's original criteria.
[4]O'Sullivan's criteria adapted for current methodology of measurement by Carpenter and Coustan, experimentally validated by Sacks.

cose values are consistently greater (respectively) than 130 or 105 mg/dL (7.2 or 5.8 mmol/L), therapy is begun with human insulin, and the patient is managed as if insulin-dependent.

The risk of developing overt diabetes later in life is influenced by body weight and the need for insulin treatment in pregnancy. Follow-up studies indicate that 5–15% of nonobese women with GDM will need treatment in 5–20 years, compared to 35–50% of gestational diabetic women with a body weight greater than 120% of ideal. This suggests the possibility of preventive benefits of achieving weight loss after pregnancy and lactation. All patients with GDM should undergo a 75-g 2-hour glucose tolerance test at 6–10 weeks after delivery to guide future medical management. Diagnostic criteria for the nonpregnant state are presented in Table 16–5. (See also Chapter 18.)

Table 16–4. Management of diet for patients with gestational diabetes.

(1) Assess present pattern of food consumption.
(2) Balance calories with optimal weight gain.
  (a) Caloric intake: 25–35 kcal/kg ideal weight.
  (b) Weight gain: 0.45 kg (1 lb) per month during the first trimester; 0.2–0.35 kg (0.5–0.75 lb) per week during the second and third trimesters.
(3) Distribute calories and carbohydrates over 3 meals and 3 snacks; evening snack to include complex carbohydrate and at least one meat exchange.
(4) Use food exchanges to assess the amount of carbohydrate, protein, and fat:
  (a) Carbohydrate: 40–55% of calories or ≥ 150 g/d.
  (b) Protein: 20% of calories or ≥74 g/d.
  (c) Fat: 25–40% of calories.
(5) Emphasize high-fiber, complex carbohydrate foods.
(6) Identify individual glycemic responses to certain foods.
(7) Tailor eating plans to personal needs.

Insulin Management

The goal of insulin therapy during pregnancy is to prevent both fasting and postprandial hyperglycemia and to avoid debilitating hypoglycemic reactions. Maternal hyperglycemia and fetal hyperinsulinemia are associated with fetal macrosomia and delayed lung maturation. Most experts believe that one should aim for fasting plasma glucose levels below 105 mg/dL (5.8 mmol/L) and postprandial levels below 140 mg/dL (7.8 mmol/L). Self-monitoring of capillary blood glucose at home with glucose oxidase strips and portable reflectance colorimeters has proved a reliable means of helping patients monitor the course of therapy. Since glycosylated hemoglobin correlates with mean daily capillary blood glucose over a few weeks during pregnancy, sequential measurement will provide another indicator of long-term control. Yet because insulin dosage must be frequently adjusted up or down during the metabolically dynamic state of pregnancy, capillary blood glucose must be measured several times each day to assist in the "fine-tuning" of insulin management.

Most pregnant diabetic patients will require at least two injections of about a 1:2 mixture of regular and intermediate insulin each day in order to prevent fasting and postprandial hyperglycemia. The usual practice is to give two-thirds of the insulin before breakfast and one-third before supper (Table 16–6). More stringent regimens of administering regular subcutaneous insulin three times a day before meals and NPH at bedtime, or continuously with a portable insulin pump, may be necessary to achieve normoglycemia in some women.

Hypoglycemic reactions are more frequent and sometimes more severe in early pregnancy. Therefore, patients with established diabetes must keep glucagon on hand, and a member of the household

Table 16–5. National Diabetes Data Group diagnostic criteria for diabetes mellitus in nonpregnant women.[1]

Diagnosis	Fasting	Two Hours
Normal	<115 mg/dL (<6.4 mmol/L)	<140 mg/dL (<7.8 mmol/L)
Impaired glucose tolerance	>115 mg/dL and <140 mg/dL	>140 mg/dL and <200 mg/dL
Diabetes	≥140 mg/dL (≥7.8 mmol/L)	≥200 mg/dL (≥11.1 mmol/L)

[1]Test consists of giving 75 g glucose load and then measuring venous plasma glucose.
[2]The National Diabetes Data Group also requires one intervening value ≥200 mg/dL between fasting and 2 hours for the diagnosis of diabetes after pregnancy.

must be instructed in the technique of injection. Hypoglycemic reactions have not been associated with fetal death or congenital anomalies, but they pose a risk to maternal cerebral function.

Fetal Development & Growth

Major congenital anomalies are those which may severely affect the life of the individual or require major surgery for correction. The incidence of major congenital anomalies in infants of diabetic mothers (IDM) is 6–12%, compared with 2% in infants of a nondiabetic population. Since perinatal deaths due to stillbirth and respiratory distress syndrome (RDS) have declined in pregnancies complicated by diabetes, the proportion of fetal and neonatal deaths ascribed to congenital anomalies has risen to 50–80%. The types of anomalies most common in IDM and their presumed time of occurrence during embryonic development are listed in Table 16–7. It is apparent that any intervention to reduce the incidence of major congenital anomalies must be applied very early in pregnancy. The finding that the excess risk of anomalies is associated with the group of diabetic women with elevated glycosylated hemoglobin early in pregnancy suggests that poor diabetic control is related to the risk of major congenital anomalies in their infants. Protocols of intensive diabetic management instituted prior to conception and continued through early pregnancy have resulted in significant reduction in the frequency of anomalies. This means that primary care physicians treating diabetic women of reproductive age must evaluate them for the possibility of becoming pregnant and inform them of the risks of unplanned pregnancies related to the level of hyperglycemia.

Ultrasonography in the first half of pregnancy confirms the dating of gestation and may detect neural tube defects (anencephaly, meningomyelocele) that occur with a higher than normal incidence in infants of poorly controlled diabetic mothers. The physician should also screen all insulin-dependent pregnant women for elevated serum alpha-fetoprotein levels at 14–16 weeks of gestation that may suggest less severe cases of neural tube defects, eg, spina bifida. Later in pregnancy at 18–22 weeks, sophisticated ultrasonographic examinations are used to detect congenital heart defects or other severe anomalies. Subsequent examinations at 26 and 36 weeks measure fetal growth and well-being.

Many fetuses of poorly controlled diabetic mothers are large for dates, ie, macrosomic infants with increased fat stores, increased length, and increased abdomen-to-head or thorax-to-head ratios. The hypothesis that fetal macrosomia results from the causal chain of maternal hyperglycemia → fetal hyperglycemia → fetal hyperinsulinemia → fetal macrosomia has been confirmed by clinical and experimental studies. Macrosomic IDM have significantly higher concentrations of C peptide in their cord sera or amniotic fluid (representing endogenous insulin secre-

Table 16–6. Illustration of use of home blood glucose monitoring to determine insulin dosage during pregnancy.

Self-Monitored Capillary Blood Glucose		Insulin Doses
Fasting blood glucose	148 mg/dL (8.2 mmol/L)	14 units regular, 28 units intermediate
1 h after breakfast	206 mg/dL (11.4 mmol/L)	
1 h after lunch	152 mg/dL (8.4 mmol/L)	
1 h after supper	198 mg/dL (11.0 mmol/L)	9 units regular, 10 units intermediate
2–4 AM	142 mg/dL (7.9 mmol/L)	

Suggested changes based on pattern of blood glucose values over 2–3 days: slight increases in presupper intermediate insulin to control fasting blood glucose next day, in morning regular insulin to control postbreakfast glucose, and in presupper regular insulin to control postsupper hypoglycemia. Dose of morning intermediate insulin is adequate to control early afternoon blood glucose. When dose of presupper intermediate insulin is increased, patient should test to detect and prevent nocturnal hypoglycemia. One-hour postprandial testing is advised to detect the probable peaks of glycemic excursions. Patient should also test when symptoms of hypoglycemia appear.

Table 16–7. Congenital malformations in infants of diabetic mothers.[1]

	Ratio of Incidences Diabetic vs Control Group	Latest Gestational Age for Occurrence (Weeks After Menstruation)
Caudal regression	252	5
Anencephaly	3	6
Spina bifida, hydrocephalus, or other central nervous system defects	2	6
Cardiac anomalies	4	
Transposition of great vessels		7
Ventricular septal defect		8
Atrial septal defect		8
Anal/rectal atresia	3	8
Renal anomalies	5	
Agenesis	6	7
Cystic kidney	4	7
Ureter duplex	23	7
Situs inversus	84	6

[1]Modified and reproduced, with permission, from Kucera J: Rate and type of congenital anomalies among offspring of diabetic women. *J Reprod Med* 1971;7:61; and Mills JL, Baker L, Goldman AS: Malformations in infants of diabetic mothers occur before the seventh gestational week: Implications for treatment. Diabetes 1979;**28**:292.

tion) than do IDM with birth weights appropriate for gestational age. Monkey fetuses with insulin-releasing pellets implanted in utero become macrosomic. In human pregnancy, the determinants of fetal hyperinsulinemia may not be simply maternal hyperglycemia, however. Other metabolic substrates that cross the placenta and are insulinogenic (eg, branched-chain amino acids) may play a role in fetal macrosomia, and transplacental lipids could contribute to fat deposition.

The degree of maternal glycemia is related to birth weights of IDM, as adjusted for gestational age. This suggests that prevention of maternal hyperglycemia throughout pregnancy may reduce the incidence of macrosomia. The glycemic threshold for fetal macrosomia seems to be *postprandial* peak values above 130—140 mg/dL. On the other hand, average peak postprandial blood sugar levels below 110 mg/dL are associated with insufficient fetal growth and small-for-dates infants, which may also induce complications in the neonatal period.

Polyhydramnios is an excess volume of amniotic fluid (> 1000 mL, often > 3000 mL). It may cause severe discomfort or premature labor and is most often associated with fetal macrosomia. The excess volume of amniotic fluid was not related to the concentration of glucose or other solutes in amniotic fluid or to excess fetal urine output as measured by change in bladder size by means of ultrasonography. Additional possible factors in causation of polyhydramnios in diabetic pregnancies include fetal swallowing, decidual and amniotic fluid PRL, and as yet unknown determinants of the complicated multicompartmental intrauterine transfer of water. However, diuretics do little to mobilize excessive amniotic fluid. Polyhydramnios is rare in women with well-controlled diabetes.

In contrast to fetal macrosomia, the fetus of a woman with diabetes of long duration and vascular disease may suffer intrauterine growth retardation. This problem is apparently related to inadequate uteroplacental perfusion. All body diameters may be below normal on ultrasonographic measurements, and oligohydramnios is common.

Obstetric Management

Not long ago the incidence of apparently sudden intrauterine fetal demise in the third trimester of diabetic pregnancies was at least 5%. Since the risk increased as pregnancies approached term, preterm delivery was instituted but the incidence of neonatal deaths from respiratory distress syndrome (RDS) increased. Curiously, the cause of stillbirth was usually not obvious. The risk was greater with poor diabetic control, and the incidence of fetal death exceeded 50% with ketoacidosis. Some instances of fetal demise were associated with preeclampsia, which is a common complication of diabetic pregnancy. Fetal death was also associated with pyelonephritis, which is now largely prevented by screening for and treating asymptomatic bacteriuria. Other than these known risk factors, one can speculate that fetal distress was related to (1) a combination of relative fetal hypoxia and hyperglycemia or (2) fetal myocardial dysfunction.

Advances during the past decade have led to techniques for detecting fetal hypoxia and preventing stillbirth. The infrequency of fetal movement as noted in fetal activity determinations (< 4/h) may indicate fetal jeopardy. More quantitative studies of fetal activity patterns using ultrasonography are now available.

Maternal estriol assays were also used for fetal evaluation, based on the knowledge that placental production of estriol is dependent on precursors from the fetal adrenals. It was demonstrated that the maternal 24-hour urine estriol level correlates with the mass of the fetal-placental unit and that a 40% or greater drop in maternal plasma or urinary estriol level usually preceded fetal demise in pregnancies complicated by diabetes. However, estriol monitoring was somewhat nonspecific and has been replaced by biophysical assessment.

The primary mode of fetal assessment is antepartum fetal heart rate monitoring. The presence of fetal heart rate (FHR) accelerations and good long-range variability on the nonstress test (NST) and the absence of late decelerations (lower FHR persists after the contraction subsides) on the contraction stress test (CST) almost always suggests that the fetus is well oxygenated and has a low risk of dying within several days. However, the predictive value of normal test results is only valid for a short duration in diabetic women with unstable metabolic control or hypertension. Generally, the NST and CST are sensitive screening tests, and abnormal results in these tests of FHR monitoring will overestimate the diagnosis of fetal distress. Therefore, some authorities require that additional evidence of fetal jeopardy (by biophysical ultrasonographic assessment) be obtained before intervention in preterm pregnancies can be recommended.

In the past, all insulin-dependent diabetic patients were usually admitted to the hospital at 36 weeks' gestation or earlier for fetal monitoring and careful control of diabetes. However, normotensive women achieving very good control (fasting blood glucose about 100 mg/dL, 1-hour postprandial blood glucose < 140 mg/dL) with self-monitoring of blood glucose levels have no excess risk of fetal hypoxia and do not require antepartum admission to the hospital.

Unless maternal or fetal complications arise, the goal for the termination of pregnancy should be 39–41 weeks, in order to reduce neonatal morbidity from preterm deliveries. On the other hand, the obstetrician may wish to induce labor before 39 weeks if there is concern about increasing fetal weight. Before a preterm delivery decision is made, fetal pulmonary maturity should be determined. The standard test for pulmonary maturity is the lecithin/sphingomyelin (L/S) ratio, in which a value greater than 2 indicates a low risk for respiratory distress syndrome. However, in pregnancies complicated by diabetes, many authors have reported a false-positive rate of 6–12% with L/S values between 2 and 3. The reason for the discrepancy may be related to low surfactant apoprotein production due to fetal hyperinsulinemia. The lowest risk for respiratory distress syndrome is attained by delaying delivery (if possible) until the L/S ratio becomes abnormally high (> 3.5). The false-negative rate for L/S ratios of 1.5–2.0 is at least 50% in nondiabetic pregnancies (ie, delivery occurs within 72 hours, but respiratory distress syndrome does not develop). Other amniotic fluid assays (eg, measurement of phosphatidylglycerol) can be used to evaluate the risk for respiratory distress syndrome. If phosphatidylglycerol is present in the amniotic fluid, the risk is low even if the L/S ratio is below 3.5.

Once fetal lung maturity is likely, the route of delivery must be selected based on the usual obstetric indications. If the fetus seems large (> 4200 g) on clinical and ultrasonographic or CT pelvimetric examination, cesarean section probably should be performed because of the possibility of shoulder dystocia and permanent deformity from birth trauma. Otherwise, induction of labor is reasonable, because maternal and peripartum risks are fewer following vaginal delivery. Once labor is under way, continuous fetal heart rate monitoring must be performed. Maternal blood glucose levels > 150 mg/dL are associated with intrapartum fetal distress problems.

Insulin Management for Labor & Delivery

The diabetic parturient may be unusually sensitive to insulin during active labor and delivery, and insulin shock is possible if delivery occurs sooner than anticipated and a high dose of subcutaneous intermediate insulin was previously administered. Protocols for continuous low-dose intravenous insulin administration during labor or prior to cesarean delivery are now used to achieve stringent control of blood glucose in order to reduce the incidence of intrapartum fetal distress and neonatal metabolic problems (Table 16–8). A cord blood glucose level at delivery correlates positively with the higher maternal levels, and there does not seem to be an upper limit on placental transfer of glucose. During labor, maternal plasma glucose can usually be kept below 100 mg/dL (5.6 mmol/L) with 1–2 units of regular insulin and 7.5 g of dextrose given intravenously every hour. If cesarean section is necessary, insulin management is similar, and infants do equally well with general, spinal, or epidural anesthesia. Nonetheless, the anesthesiologist should be cautioned against the administration of copious glucose-containing intravenous solutions.

Neonatal Morbidity

Planning for the care of IDM should begin prior to delivery, with participation by the pediatrician or

Table 16–8. Intrapartum insulin infusion.

Capillary Glucose (mg/dL)	Insulin Rate[1] (units/h)
< 70	0.0
71–90	0.5
91–110	1.0
111–130	2.0
131–150	3.0
151–170	4.0
171–190	5.0
> 190	Call MD

[1]With blood glucose < 130 mg/dL, infusion should be 5% dextrose in lactated Ringer's solution at a rate of 125 mL/h; if blood glucose ≥ 130 mg/dL, use lactated Ringer's without dextrose until blood glucose declines.

neonatologist in decisions about timing and management of delivery. In complicated cases, the pediatrician must be in attendance to learn about antenatal problems, to assess the need for resuscitation, to identify major congenital anomalies, and to plan initial therapy for the sick IDM.

Infants of poorly controlled diabetic mothers have an increased risk of RDS compared with infants of matched nondiabetic mothers. Possible reasons include abnormal production of pulmonary surfactant or connective tissue changes leading to decreased pulmonary compliance. However, in recent years, the incidence of RDS has declined from 24% to 5%, probably related to better maternal control, selected use of the L/S ratio, and delivery of most infants at term (see above). The diagnosis of RDS is based on clinical signs (grunting, retraction, respiratory rate > 60/min), typical findings on chest x-ray (diffuse reticulogranular pattern and air bronchogram), and an increased oxygen requirement (to maintain the PaO_2 at 50–70 mm Hg) for more than 48 hours with no other identified cause of respiratory difficulty (heart disease, infection). Survival of infants with RDS has dramatically improved as a result of advances in ventilation therapy and intrapulmonary administration of surfactant.

Hypoglycemia is common in the first 48 hours after delivery of previously hyperglycemic mothers and is defined as blood glucose below 30 mg/dL (1.7 mmol/L) regardless of gestational age. The symptomatic infant may be lethargic rather than jittery, and hypoglycemia may be associated with apnea, tachypnea, cyanosis, or seizures. Hypoglycemia has been related to elevated fetal insulin levels during and after delivery. Nevertheless, IDM may also have deficient catecholamine and glucagon secretion, and the hypoglycemia may be related to diminished hepatic glucose production and oxidation of free fatty acids. The pediatrician attempts to prevent hypoglycemia in "well" infants with early feedings of 10% dextrose in water by bottle or gavage by 1 hour of age. If this is not successful, treatment with intravenous dextrose solutions is indicated. There are usually no long-term sequelae of episodes of neonatal hypoglycemia.

Other frequent problems in infants of diabetic mothers include hypocalcemia (< 7 mg/dL [1.75 mmol/ L]), hyperbilirubinemia (> 15 mg/dL [256 μmol/L]), polycythemia (central hematocrit > 70%), and poor feeding. Further investigation is necessary to determine the cause of these problems. Better control of the maternal diabetic state in the future should reduce their incidence.

REFERENCES

General

Burrow GN, Ferris TF (editors): *Medical Complications During Pregnancy,* 4th ed. Saunders, 1995.

Cedard L, Firth A (editors): *Placental Signals: Autocrine and Paracrine Control of Pregnancy.* Univ Rochester Press, 1992.

Glasser SR, Mulholland J, Psychoyos A: Endocrinology of Embryo-endometrium Interactions. Plenum, 1994.

Haig D: Genetic conflicts in human pregnancy. Q Rev Biol 1995;68:495.

Jaffe RB: Endocrine-metabolic alterations induced by pregnancy. In: *Reproductive Endocrinology: Physiology, Pathophysiology, and Clinical Management,* 3rd ed. Yen SSC, Jaffe RB (editors). Saunders, 1991.

Jovanovic-Peterson L, Peterson CM (editors): Endocrine disorders in pregnancy. Endocrinol Metab Clin North Am 1995; 24:1.

O'Leary P et al: Longitudinal assessment of changes in reproductive hormones during normal pregnancy. Clin Chem 1991;37:667.

Tulchinsky D, Little AB (editors): *Maternal-Fetal Endocrinology,* 2nd ed. Saunders, 1994.

Chorionic Proteins & Pregnancy Tests

Lin LS, Roberts VJ, Yen SS: Expression of human gonadotropin-releasing hormone receptor gene in the placenta and its functional relationship to human chorionic gonadotropin secretion. J Clin Endocrinol Metab 1995;80:580.

Meuris S, Nagy AM et al: Temporal relationship between the human chorionic gonadotrophin peak and the establishment of intervillous blood flow in early pregnancy. Hum Reprod 1995;10:947.

O'Connor JF et al: Recent advances in the chemistry and immunochemistry of human chorionic gonadotropin: Impact on clinical measurements. Endocr Rev 1994; 15:650.

Petraglia F: Placental neurohormones secretion and physiological implications. Mol Cell Endocrinol 1991;78:C109.

Szilagyi A, Benz R, Rossmanith WG: The human first-term placenta in vitro: Regulation of hCG secretion by GnRH and its antagonist. Gynecol Endocrinol 1992;6:293.

Than GN, Bohn H, Szabo DG: *Advances in Pregnancy-Related Protein Research: Functional and Clinical Applications.* CRC Press, 1993.

Ovarian Proteins

Bryant-Greenwood GD, Schwabe C: Human relaxin: Chemistry and biology. Endocr Rev 1994;15:5.

Goldsmith LT, Weiss G, Steinetz BG: Relaxin and its role in pregnancy. Endocrinol Metab Clin North Am 1995; 24:171.

Wathen NC et al: Relaxin levels in amniotic fluid, extra amniotic coelomic fluid, and maternal serum in early human pregnancy. Early Hum Dev 1995;43:71.

Steroid Hormones

Conley AJ, Mason JI: Placental steroid hormones. Ballieres Clin Endocrinol Metab 1990;4:249.

Donaldson A et al: Changes in concentrations of cortisol, dehydroepiandrosterone sulfate and progesterone in fetal and maternal serum during pregnancy. Clin Endocrinol 1991;35(4):447.

Korach KS: Insights from the study of animals lacking functional estrogen receptor. Science 1994;266:1524.

Partsch CJ et al: The steroid hormone milieu of the undisturbed human fetus and mother at 16–20 weeks gestation. J Clin Endocrinol Metab 1991;73(5):969.

Pepe GJ, Albrecht ED: Actions of placental and fetal adrenal steroid hormones in primate pregnancy. Endocr Rev 1995;16:608.

Fetal Endocrinology

Cheng KY et al: A prospective evaluation of a second-trimester screening test for fetal Down syndrome using maternal serum alpha fetoprotein, hCG, and unconjugated estriol. Obstet Gynecol 1993;81:72.

de Zegher F et al: The prenatal role of thyroid hormone evidenced by fetomaternal Pit-1 deficiency. J Clin Endocrinol Metab 1995;80:3127.

Evain-Brion D: Hormonal regulation of fetal growth. Horm Res 1994;42:20.

Gluckman PD: The endocrine regulation of fetal growth in late gestation: The role of insulin-like growth factors. J Clin Endocrinol Metab 1995;80:1047.

Hercz P et al: Quantitative comparison of serum steroid and peptide hormone concentrations in male and female fetuses in the maternal-fetoplacental system during the 28th–40th weeks of pregnancy. Eur J Obstet Gynecol Reprod Biol 1989;30:201.

Kratzer PG et al: First-trimester aneuploidy screening using serum human chorionic gonadotropin (hCG) free α hCG and progesterone. Prenat Diag 1991;11:751.

Porterfield SP, Hendrich CE: The role of thyroid hormones in prenatal and neonatal neurological development: Current perspectives. Endocr Rev 1993;14:94.

Rabinovici J, Jaffe RB: Development and regulation of growth and differentiated function in human and subhuman primate fetal gonads. Endocr Rev 1990;11:532.

Thorpe-Beeston JG, Nicolaides KH: Fetal thyroid function. Fetal Diagn Ther 1993;8:60.

Waddell BJ: The placenta as hypothalamus and pituitary: Possible impact on maternal and fetal adrenal function. Reprod Fertil Dev 1993;5:479.

Parturition

Chwalisz K, Garfield RE: Antiprogestins in the induction of labor. Ann N Y Acad Sci 1994;734:387.

Downing SJ, Hollingsworth M: Action of relaxin on uterine contractions: A review. J Reprod Fertil 1993;99:275.

Neulen J. Breckwoldt M: Placental progesterone, prostaglandins and mechanisms leading to initiation of parturition in the human. Exper Clin Endocrinol 1994;102:195.

Olson DM, Mijovic JE, Sadowsky DW: Control of human parturition. Semin Perinatol 1995;19:52.

Steer PJ: The endocrinology of parturition in the human. Baillieres Clin Endocrinol Metab 1990;4:333.

Thorburn GD: The placenta, PGE_2 and parturition. Early Hum Dev 1992;29:63.

Verhaeghe J, Bouillon R: Calciotropic hormones during reproduction. J Steroid Biochem Mol Biol 1992;41:469.

Puerperium and Lactation

Crowley WR, Armstrong WE: Neurochemical regulation of oxytocin secretion in lactation. Endocr Rev 1992;13:33.

McNeilly AS: Lactational amenorrhea. Emerg Med Clin North Am 1993;22:59.

McNeilly AS, Tay CC, Glasier A: Physiological mechanisms underlying lactational amenorrhea. Ann N Y Acad Sci 1994 Feb 18;709:145.

Pituitary Adenomas

Barbieri RL, Ryan KJ: Bromocriptine: Endocrine pharmacology and therapeutic applications. Fertil Steril 1983;39:727.

Johnston DG et al: Hyperprolactinemia: Long-term effects of bromocriptine. Am J Med 1983;75:868.

Marshall JR: Pregnancy in patients with prolactin-producing pituitary tumors. Clin Obstet Gynecol 1980;23:453.

Breast Cancer & Pregnancy

Petrek JA: Breast cancer and pregnancy. Monogr Natl Cancer Inst 1994;16:113.

Petrek JA, Dukoff R, Rogatko A: Prognosis of pregnancy-associated breast cancer. Cancer 1991;67:869.

Saunders CM, Baum M: Breast cancer and pregnancy: A review. J R Soc Med 1993;86(3):162.

Hypertensive Disorders

Broughton Pipkin F: The hypertensive disorders of pregnancy. Br Med J 1995;311:609.

de Groot CJM, Taylor RN: New insights into the etiology of preeclampsia. Ann Med 1993;25:243.

Roberts JM: Pregnancy-related hypertension. In: *Maternal-Fetal Medicine: Principles and Practice.* Creasy RK, Resnick R (editors). Saunders, 1984.

Hyperthyroidism in Pregnancy

Becks GP, Burrow GN: Thyroid disease and pregnancy. Med Clin North Am 1991;75:121.

Burrow GN, Fisher DA, Larsen PR: Maternal and fetal thyroid function. N Engl J Med 1994;331:1072.

Glinoer D et al: Regulation of maternal thyroid during pregnancy. J Clin Endocrinol Metab 1990;71(2):276.

Diabetes Mellitus & Pregnancy

Bochner CJ et al: Early third trimester ultrasound screening in gestational diabetes to determine the risk of macrosomia and labor dystocia at term. Am J Obstet Gynecol 1987;157:703.

Carpenter MW, Coustan DR: Criteria for screening tests of gestational diabetes. Am J Obstet Gynecol 1982;144:768.

Cheney C, Shragg P, Hollingsworth D: Demonstration of heterogeneity in gestational diabetes by a 400 kcal breakfast meal tolerance test. Obstet Gynecol 1985;65:17.

Chew EY et al: Metabolic control and progression of retinopathy. Diabetes Care 1995;18:631.

Cousins L: Pregnancy complications among diabetic women. Obstet Gynecol Surv 1987;42:140.

Coustan DR et al: Maternal age and screening for gestational diabetes: A population-based study. Obstet Gynecol 1989;73:557.

Coustan DR et al: Should the fifty-gram, one-hour plasma glucose screening test be administered in the fasting or fed state? Am J Obstet Gynecol 1986;154:1031.

Coustan DR, Berkowitz RL, Hobbins JC: Tight metabolic control of overt diabetes in pregnancy. Am J Med 1980;68:845.

Fuhrmann K et al: Prevention of congenital malformations in infants of insulin-dependent diabetic mothers. Diabetes Care 1983;6:219.

Greene MF et al: Prematurity among insulin-requiring diabetic gravid women. Am J Obstet Gynecol 1989;161:106.

Jovanovic L, Peterson CM: Optimal insulin delivery for the pregnant diabetic patient. Diabetes Care 1982;5 (Suppl 1):24.

Jovanovic-Peterson L et al: Maternal postprandial glucose levels and infant birth weight: The diabetes in early pregnancy study. Am J Obstet Gynecol 1991;164:103.

Kimmerle R et al: Pregnancies in women with diabetic nephropathy: Longterm outcome for mother and child. Diabetologia 1995;38:227.

Kitzmiller JL et al: Diabetic nephropathy and perinatal outcome. Am J Obstet Gynecol 1981;141.

Kitzmiller JL et al: Measurement of fetal shoulder width with computed tomography in diabetic women. Obstet Gynecol 1987;70:941.

Kitzmiller JL et al: Preconception care of diabetes glycemic control prevents congenital anomalies. JAMA 1991;265:731.

Kitzmiller JL: Sweet success with diabetes: The development of insulin therapy and glycemic control for pregnancy. Diabetes Care 1993;16(Suppl 3):107.

Klein BEK, Moss SE, Klein R.: Effect of pregnancy on progression of diabetic retinopathy. Diabetes Care 1990;13:34.

Landon MB et al: Neonatal morbidity in pregnancy complicated by diabetes mellitus: Predictive value of maternal glycemic profiles. Am J Obstet Gynecol 1987;156:1089.

Landon MO, Langer O, Gabbe SG: Fetal surveillance in pregnancies complicated by insulin-dependent diabetes mellitus. Am J Obstet Gynecol 1992;617:617.

Langer O et al: Gestational diabetes: Insulin requirements in pregnancy. Am J Obstet Gynecol 1987;157:669.

Magee MS et al: Influence of diagnostic criteria on the incidence of gestational diabetes and perinatal morbidity. JAMA 1993;269:609.

Miadovnik M et al: Elevated maternal glycohemoglobin in early pregnancy and spontaneous abortion among insulin-dependent diabetic women. Am J Obstet Gynecol 1985;153:439.

Miller E et al: Elevated maternal hemoglobin A_{1c} in early pregnancy and major congenital anomalies in infants of diabetic mothers. N Engl J Med 1981;304:1331.

Mills JL, Baker L, Goldman AS: Malformations in infants of diabetic mothers occur before the seventh gestational week: Implications for treatment. Diabetes 1979;28:292.

Mueller-Heubach E et al: Lecithin/sphingomyelin ratio in amniotic fluid and its value for the prediction of neonatal respiratory distress syndrome in pregnant diabetic women. Am J Obstet Gynecol 1978;130.

Norton M, Kitzmiller JL, Buchanan T: The endocrine pancreas and maternal metabolism. In: *Maternal-Fetal Endocrinology,* 2nd ed. Tulchinsky DT, Ryan KJ (editors). Saunders, 1980.

O'Sullivan JB et al: Medical treatment of the gestational diabetic. Obstet Gynecol 1974;43:817.

O'Sullivan JB: Body weight and subsequent diabetes mellitus. JAMA 1982;248:949.

Reece E et al: Diabetic nephropathy: Pregnancy performance and fetomaternal outcome. Am J Obstet Gynecol 1988;159:56.

Reece EA et al: Coronary artery disease in diabetic pregnancies. Am J Obstet Gynecol 1986;154:150.

Rizzo T et al: Correlations between antepartum maternal metabolism and intelligence of offspring. N Engl J Med 1991;325:911.

Sacks DA et al: Do the current standards for glucose tolerance testing in pregnancy represent a valid conversion of O'Sullivan's original criteria? Am J Obstet Gynecol 1989;161:638.

Silverman BL et al: Fetal hyperinsulinism and impaired glucose tolerance in adolescent offspring of diabetic mothers. Diabetes Care 1995;18:611.

White P: Diabetes mellitus in pregnancy. Clin Perinatol 1974;1:331.

Regulatory Peptides of the Gut

17

Sean J. Mulvihill, MD, & Haile T. Debas, MD

The origins of gastrointestinal endocrinology can be traced to experiments performed by William Bayliss and Ernest Starling at University College in London in 1902. These physiologists showed that acidification of the duodenum or denervated jejunum stimulated exocrine pancreatic secretion in anesthetized dogs. Furthermore, intravenous injection of an extract of jejunal—but not ileal—mucosa similarly stimulated pancreatic secretion. They postulated the presence of a chemical messenger, which they termed "secretin," within the duodenal and jejunal mucosa. Starling later went on to define chemical messengers as substances "carried from the organ where they are produced to the organ where they affect by means of the bloodstream." He called these messengers "hormones," a word suggested by William Hardy. Thus began the physiologic era of gastrointestinal endocrinology, in which hormones such as gastrin, secretin, and cholecystokinin were discovered through their physiologic actions. Only later were these substances isolated and characterized.

Since the early 1970s, in what could be termed the "biochemical era" of gastrointestinal endocrinology, about 30 new peptides have been described through biochemical purification of extracts of gastrointestinal mucosa. The discovery that many of these peptides are located in the central nervous system and in enteric neurons—in addition to being found in specialized endocrine cells of the gastrointestinal tract—has led to the concept of a brain-gut axis (see below). Recently, recombinant DNA technology has been used to identify gastrointestinal peptides in the absence of physiologic or biochemical information, initiating a "molecular era." The presence of calcitonin gene-related peptide (CGRP) in many neural tissues, including those of the gut, was identified in this manner after examination of the calcitonin gene suggested the presence of a second peptide sequence.

The physiologic importance of many of the newly discovered peptides is unclear. Unlike the hormonal components of other systems, in which specific kinds of endocrine cells are concentrated into distinct organs, those of the gut are widely dispersed. Furthermore, disease states attributable to disorders of gut endocrine cells are rare, and there are no known deficiency states. In other endocrine organs, such as the thyroid and adrenal, disorders of function have provided natural models for physiologic study, but this is uncommon in the gastrointestinal tract.

ACRONYMS USED IN THIS CHAPTER	
ACTH	Adrenocorticotropic hormone
APUD	Amine precursor uptake and decarboxylation
CCK	Cholecystokinin
CGRP	Calcitonin gene-related peptide
CRH	Corticotropin-releasing hormone
DNA	Deoxyribonucleic acid
ECL	Enterochromaffin-like
ENS	Enteric nervous system
GH	Growth hormone
GIP	Glucose-dependent insulin-releasing peptide (gastric inhibitory peptide)
GLP-1	Glucagon-like peptide-1
GRH	Growth hormone-releasing hormone
GRP	Gastrin-releasing peptide
5-HIAA	5-Hydroxyindoleacetic acid
MEN	Multiple endocrine neoplasia
MSH	Melanocyte-stimulating hormone
NPY	Neuropeptide Y
NSE	Neuronal-specific enolase
PHI	Peptide histidine isoleucine
PHM	Peptide histidine methionine
PP	Pancreatic polypeptide
PRL	Prolactin
PTH	Parathyroid hormone
PYY	Peptide YY
TRH	Thyrotropin-releasing hormone
VIP	Vasoactive intestinal polypeptide

Modes of Gut Peptide Delivery (Table 17–1)

Gastrointestinal peptides are delivered to their sites of action in three main ways: Some circulate in the bloodstream in order to reach the target cell (**endocrine delivery**); some are released into the interstitial fluid and affect nearby cells (**paracrine delivery**); and still others, within neurons, act as neurotransmitters or neuromodulators (**neurocrine delivery**). A few peptides act to stimulate or inhibit further function of the cell of origin (**autocrine delivery**) (Figure 17–1; see also Chapter 1). Some peptides have more than one mode of delivery. For example, somatostatin has an endocrine function, is present in neurons, and also exercises paracrine actions in the gastric body and antrum. Because of their various modes of delivery, it may be preferable to refer to these substances as regulatory peptides rather than as hormones.

To prove that a substance has a possible endocrine function in the gastrointestinal tract, two criteria must be met: (1) blood levels of the substance must rise after a meal, and (2) infusion of the substance at a rate that reproduces postprandial blood levels must elicit a physiologic response from the target organ. Only a handful of peptides meet these criteria in the gastrointestinal tract: gastrin, for stimulation of gastric acid and pepsin secretion; secretin, for stimulation of pancreatic bicarbonate secretion; cholecystokinin (CCK), for stimulation of gallbladder contraction and pancreatic enzyme secretion; somatostatin, for inhibition of gastric acid secretion; and glucose-dependent insulinotropic peptide (also known as gastric inhibitory peptide; GIP), for stimulation of insulin release. Most gut peptides serve as neurocrine or paracrine agents. It has been difficult to prove that these agents have important regulatory activities on digestive processes because of the difficulty in measuring the concentrations of these locally acting agents at their presumed sites of action and replicating these levels in experimental models.

Cellular Mechanisms of Action

The actions of most gastrointestinal peptide hormones are mediated by membrane-bound receptors. Receptor complementary DNAs (cDNAs) for some gut peptide receptors have been cloned, allowing identification of primary structural information. These receptors are proteins whose synthesis is subject to regulation, often by the hormone itself. In the best-studied examples, such as gastrin, CCK, and somatostatin, receptor concentrations are down-regulated by high plasma levels of the hormone. This may be due to alterations in synthesis, function, internalization, or degradation of the receptor. Hormone-receptor affinity can be quantified by measurement of binding in the presence of varying concentrations of the hormone. There is some evidence, particularly in the case of CCK, that there may be two classes of receptor-one with low affinity and high capacity and one with high affinity and low capacity.

Binding to cell membrane receptors activates one of two major intracellular pathways and stimulates cell function. These pathways have been termed second messengers (see Chapter 3). The effects of some

Table 17–1. Gastrointestinal hormones

	Mode of Delivery[1]			
	Endocrine	Neurocrine	Paracrine	Major Action
Gastrin	+	(+)	−	Gastric acid and pepsin secretion.
CCK	+	+	−	Pancreatic enzyme secretion, gallbladder contraction.
Secretin	+	−	−	Pancreatic bicarbonate secretion.
GIP	+	−	−	Enhances glucose-mediated insulin release. Inhibits gastric acid secretion.
VIP	−	+	(+)	Smooth muscle relaxation. Stimulates pancreatic bicarbonate secretion.
Motilin	+	−	−	Initiates interdigestive intestinal motility.
Somatostatin	+	+	+	Numerous inhibitory effects.
PP	+	−	(+)	Inhibits pancreatic bicarbonate and protein secretion.
Enkephalins	−	+	(+)	Inhibition of gut motility.
Substance P	−	+	(+)	Smooth muscle contraction
GRP	−	+	(+)	Stimulates release of gastrin and CCK.
Neurotensin	+	−	(+)	Vasodilation.
Enteroglucagon	(+)	(+)	(+)	Incretin, mucosal mitogen.
PYY	+	−	(+)	Inhibits pancreatic bicarbonate and protein secretion.
NPY	−	+	−	Inhibits pancreatic bicarbonate and protein secretion.
CGRP	−	+	−	Stimulates acid secretion and somatostatin release

[1]( ) denotes inconclusive evidence.

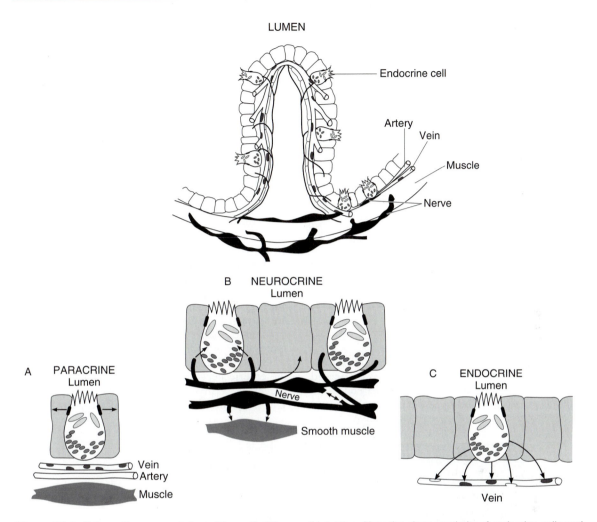

Figure 17–1. Schematic representation of the wall of the small intestine. Note the close proximity of endocrine cells and nerves to mucosal cells, blood vessels, and smooth muscle. Anatomically, local release of hormone by endocrine cells or nerves could affect secretion and absorption (mucosal cells), motility (muscle), and blood flow (blood vessels). *A:* Paracrine delivery—release of a messenger locally to affect adjacent cells. *B:* Neurocrine delivery—release of messenger by nerves to affect mucosal cells, other endocrine cells, or smooth muscle of both small intestine and blood vessels. *C:* Endocrine delivery—release of messenger into the blood to act as a circulating hormone.

hormones (eg, gastrin, CCK, and the neurotransmitter acetylcholine) are due to the release of intracellular calcium from stores in rough endoplasmic reticulum. Other peptides, such as secretin, vasoactive intestinal polypeptide (VIP), glucagon, and the paracrine substance histamine, activate adenylyl cyclase, the enzyme responsible for catalyzing the conversion of ATP to cyclic AMP (cAMP). These two second messenger systems, intracellular calcium and cAMP, are distinct in their early steps but may cause similar changes in intracellular processes. For example, in the parietal cell, histamine, acting through the generation of intracellular cAMP, and acetylcholine, acting through the release of intracellular calcium, both stimulate the H^+-K^+ ATPase in canalicular

membranes, resulting in the secretion of H^+ into the extracellular space.

Structure of Gastrointestinal Peptide Hormones

Most gut regulatory substances are polypeptides. Notable exceptions include histamine, acetylcholine, nitric oxide, and serotonin. Many exhibit structural homology, which allows them to be grouped into families (Table 17–2). Most of these peptides are probably synthesized as precursor molecules, with posttranslational processing to their active forms. The amino acid sequence for most gut peptides is now known, and in many instances the gene sequence has also been determined.

Table 17–2. Gastrointestinal peptide families.

Family	Peptides
Gastrin	Gastrin CCK
Secretin	Secretin VIP PHI PHM Glucagon GIP
PP	PP PYY NPY
Tachykinin	Substance P Neuromedins Neurokinins
Others	Motilin Neurotensin Somatostatin GRP Galanin

Distribution of Gut Peptides

Gut peptides are located both in specialized endocrine cells and in neurons widely dispersed throughout the gastrointestinal tract. The endocrine cells are distinguished by a clear cytoplasm and prominent basal acidophilic granules. Most gut endocrine cells are triangular, with a broad base and narrow apex, usually with a brush border facing the intestinal lumen (Figure 17–2). In enteric neurons, gut peptides probably act as neurotransmitters, or neurocrine agents. The bodies of enteric neurons are located within the gut wall, usually in the submucosal or myenteric plexus, from which their pathways extend to cells of the mucosa, smooth muscle, blood vessels, and other endocrine cells. It is estimated that the gut contains between 80 million and 100 million neurons. This enteric nervous system (ENS) is best thought of as a third division of the autonomic nervous system. Table 17–3 summarizes the distribution of gut peptides in their respective cells.

Brain-Gut Axis

Many of the peptides originally isolated from the gut are also found in the brain, and vice versa (Table 17–4). This observation led to the concept of a brain-gut axis. In the central nervous system, gut peptides are thought to be important in the regulation of bodily functions such as satiety (CCK, NPY) and thermoregulation (bombesin). Furthermore, neurons of the central nervous system interact with those of the enteric nervous system to influence digestive processes. Many of these neurons are peptidergic. This interaction occurs via both afferent and efferent

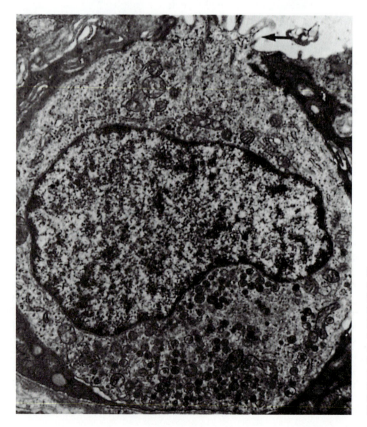

Figure 17–2. Typical endocrine cell of the gut. The arrow points to the brush border, which is at the cell apex and is open to the lumen of the gut. Granules at the cell base contain a peptide messenger, which in this cell is gastrin (G cell). (Reproduced, with permission, from Lechago J: Endocrine cells of the gastrointestinal tract and their pathology. Pathol Annu 1978;13:329.)

Table 17–3. Distribution of gastrointestinal hormones.[1]

	Endocrine Cell[2]	Localization	Localized in Gut Nerves
Gastrin	G	Gastric antrum, duodenum	No
CCK	I	Duodenum, jejunum	Yes
Secretin	S	Duodenum, jejunum	No
GIP	K	Small bowel	No
VIP	D_1	Pancreas	Yes
Motillin	EC_2	Small bowel	No
Substance P	EC_1	Entire gastrointestinal tract	Yes
Neurotensin	N	Ileum	No
Somatostatin	D	Stomach, duodenum, pancreas	Yes
Enkephalins	. . .	Stomach, duodenum, gallbladder	Yes
GRP	. . .	Stomach, duodenum	Yes
PP	D_2F	Pancreas	No
Enterogluca-gon	A	Pancreas	No
	L	Small intestine	
PYY	. . .	Small intestine, colon	No
CGRP	. . .	Entire gastrointestinal tract	Yes
NPY	. . .	Small intestine	Yes

[1]Note that several peptides are found both in nerves and in endocrine cells. VIP has been found only in nerves and is probably not present in endocrine cells.
[2]Endocrine cells identified with a specific hormone are identified by a letter. EC = enterochromaffin cell. The cells containing enkephalins and PYY have yet to be named.

Table 17–4. Peptides found in the brain and gut (brain-gut axis).

Originally Found in Brain	Originally Found in Gut
Substance P	CCK
Thyrotropin-releasing hormone (TRH)	Gastrin
	Secretin
Somatostatin	VIP
Enkephalins	Glucagon
CGRP	PHI
Corticotropin-releasing hormone (CRH)	PP
	PYY
	NPY
	Bombesin
	GRP
	Neurotensin
	Insulin

pathways and involves vagal and spinal neurons. Neurons of the enteric nervous system exert local control over digestive processes, including absorption, secretion, motility, immune function, and blood flow. It is likely that the pathophysiology of some poorly understood conditions, such as the irritable bowel syndrome, are the result of abnormalities of regulation of gut function by the enteric nervous system and central nervous system.

APUD Concept

The cytochemical and ultrastructural characteristics of gastrointestinal endocrine cells were described by Pearse in 1966. These cells are similar in their ability to produce peptide hormones and biogenic amines (epinephrine, norepinephrine, dopamine, and serotonin) and to actively absorb amine precursors and convert them to amines. It was speculated that the uptake of 5-hydroxytryptophan and conversion of 5-hydroxytryptamine (serotonin) was linked to the production of peptide hormones. Most of the cells possessing these characteristics are found in the gut or central nervous system (hypothalamus, pituitary axis, and pineal gland), but they are also present in the thyroid (calcitonin cell), parathyroid, and placenta. Pearse referred to them as APUD cells from their characteristic amine handling (amine precursor uptake and decarboxylation). It was postulated that APUD cells originated from the primitive neural crest. It has now been shown that these cells actually have their origins from gut endoderm. Regardless of their origin, it is clear that the endocrine cells of the gut are remarkably similar to other cells of the hypothalamic-pituitary axis and to neurons within the gut wall.

GASTRIN

In 1905, Edkins discovered a potent gastric acid secretagogue in extracts of antral mucosa and named it "gastrin." Initially, it was not possible to exclude the possibility that the extract contained histamine, another secretagogue, but by the early 1960s Gregory et al isolated, sequenced, and synthesized gastrin from antral mucosa.

Biochemistry & Distribution

Gastrin exists in three known biologically active forms of 14, 17, and 34 amino acids (Figure 17–3). They are also known as "mini gastrin," "little gastrin," and "big gastrin," respectively. The biologically active portion of the gastrin molecule is the 14-amino-acid carboxyl terminal residue. This sequence is identical in all three forms. Gastrin is secreted in an inactive form with a glycine extension at the carboxyl terminal. Conversion into the active form requires the presence of a deaminizing enzyme. The tyrosine in the sixth position from the carboxyl ter-

The gastrin-cholecystokinin family

Gastrin 17 II:

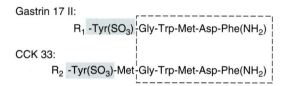

CCK 33:

Figure 17–3. Gastrin and cholecystokinin possess identical carboxyl terminal pentapeptides. However, the tyrosine is seven amino acids from the carboxyl end of CCK and must be sulfated for maximal potency. The tyrosine is six positions from the carboxyl end in gastrin and need not be sulfated for maximal potency. R_1 and R_2 represent the amino terminal sequences for gastrin and CCK.

minal may be nonsulfated (gastrin-I) or sulfated (gastrin-II).

The genes encoding for gastrin have been characterized in several species. In the pig, a precursor cDNA to gastrin corresponds to an mRNA sequence of 312 nucleotides, which codes for a preprogastrin of 104 amino acids. The corresponding human mRNA codes for a preprogastrin of 101 amino acids. The entire human gene, which includes two introns, is 4100 base pairs long.

Ninety percent of gastrointestinal gastrin is found in G cells of the gastric antrum. G17 accounts for most of the gastrin at this site. Most of the remainder of gastrointestinal tract gastrin is in the duodenum. Although immunoreactive gastrin and its mRNA are present in fetal pancreas, expression of gastrin is lost at term. This embryologic finding, however, may explain the presence of gastrinomas in the pancreas. Gastrin has been identified in the central nervous system.

Measurement & Release

Measurement of the serum concentration of gastrin is widely available by radioimmunoassay. Fasting levels average between 21 and 105 pg/mL (10–50 pmol/L) and increase by 42–84 pg/mL (20–40 pmol/L) 30–60 minutes postprandially. The main stimulants for gastrin release are partially digested proteins, peptides, and amino acids, while carbohydrates and fats are ineffective. Minor stimulants of gastrin release include calcium, beer, wine, and coffee. Gastrin release is inhibited by somatostatin during antral acidification. Substantial inhibition occurs at pH 2.5, and release is abolished at pH 1.0.

Vagal stimulation by electrical current, insulin hypoglycemia, or injection of 2-deoxyglucose stimulates gastrin release. This pathway is mediated by neurons of the enteric nervous system using GRP as a neurotransmitter. The observation that cholinergic blockade with atropine enhances meal-stimulated gastrin release suggests the presence of a vagal inhibitory mechanism. This is mediated by paracrine release of somatostatin from antral D cells.

Actions

The main actions of gastrin that occur at physiologic levels are stimulation of gastric acid secretion and parietal cell growth. Gastrin evokes acid secretion indirectly by release of histamine from enterochromaffin-like (ECL) cells in the gastric mucosa and directly by activation of specific cell-surface gastrin receptors. The former action appears to be the dominant mechanism. The trophic effects of gastrin have been observed in vitro and in vivo and appear to involve polyamine synthesis. Prolonged hypergastrinemia is associated with enterochromaffin-like cell hyperplasia and, occasionally, ECL cell carcinoid tumors.

Other gastric effects of gastrin include stimulation of mucosal blood flow and pepsin release. It is not known whether these effects are directly due to gastrin or secondary to increased acid secretion. Several other actions have been ascribed to gastrin, such as contraction of the lower esophageal sphincter and gallbladder, but they are not seen at physiologic concentrations.

CHOLECYSTOKININ

In 1928, Ivy and Oldberg observed that instillation of fat into the small intestine caused the gallbladder to contract. They postulated a hormonal mechanism and named the mediator "cholecystokinin" (CCK). In the early 1940s, Harper and Raper discovered a substance in extracts of duodenal mucosa that stimulated the secretion of enzyme-rich juice by the pancreas and called it "pancreozymin." In 1964, Jorpes et al found that increasing purification of a single extract from porcine small intestine proportionately increased its potency for both gallbladder contraction and pancreatic enzyme secretion, indicating that the two actions were properties of a single hormone. In 1968, Mutt and Jorpes reported the amino acid sequence of what we now know as CCK.

Biochemistry & Distribution

CCK exists in several molecular forms containing 58, 39, 33, and 8 amino acids (Figure 17–3). The carboxyl terminal octapeptide sequences are identical for all molecular forms. Like gastrin, CCK is probably synthesized as a precursor, with CCK39 and CCK33 representing progressive steps in the creation of CCK8. All of the biologic activity of CCK is contained in this terminal octapeptide. The human gene for CCK consists of a sequence of 345 base pairs that codes for a preprocholecystokinin of 115 amino acids. Sulfation of the tyrosine moiety in position 7 from the carboxyl terminal is necessary for full biologic potency. CCK has considerable structural homology with gastrin.

CCK is located in the duodenum and proximal jejunum within the mucosal I cell (Table 17–3). It is also found in the central nervous system, in neurons of the myenteric plexus of the intestine, and in nerves supplying the pancreas, urinary bladder and uterus. CCK8 is the major molecular form in neurons, while CCK33 is the major circulating form.

Measurement & Release

Development of a radioimmunoassay for CCK has been difficult, because antibodies directed at the carboxyl terminal tend to cross-react with gastrin, while those directed at the amino terminal tend to miss small molecular weight forms, such as CCK8. The available radioimmunoassays and an in vitro bioassay using dispersed pancreatic acini demonstrate fasting CCK levels of about 3.9 ng/mL (1 pmol/L) and postprandial levels of 20–40 ng/mL (5–10 pmol/L). The half-life of CCK in blood is short (2.5–7 minutes).

Release of CCK is stimulated by digested intraduodenal protein and fat. The aromatic amino acids phenylalanine and tryptophan are particularly potent stimulants. Fatty acids require dispersion into micelles and chain lengths of nine or more carbon atoms to be effective. The mechanism of stimulation of CCK release appears to involve a low-molecular-weight trypsin-sensitive peptide that has been termed CCK-releasing factor. A second stimulatory factor (monitor peptide) appears to be present in pancreatic juice. CCK release is inhibited by somatostatin.

Actions

The two major actions of CCK are stimulation of gallbladder contraction and pancreatic enzyme secretion. Gallbladder contraction is an endocrine effect, but at least in the rat, CCK stimulates pancreatic exocrine secretion via both endocrine and neurocrine pathways. CCK also has potent trophic effects on pancreatic acini both in vitro and in vivo. CCK causes relaxation of the sphincter of Oddi via an indirect neural mechanism involving release of VIP and NO. CCK delays gastric emptying via an indirect action on sensory neurons. At pharmacologic doses, CCK increases small intestinal and colonic motility. CCK induces satiety in several species, including humans. This effect is mediated by CCK-A receptors on vagal afferent neurons.

SECRETIN

Secretin is the prototypical gastrointestinal hormone. Bayliss and Starling in 1902 demonstrated that jejunal acidification or intravenous injection of extracts of jejunal mucosa stimulated secretion of water and bicarbonate from the pancreas. Secretin was purified by Jorpes and Mutt in 1961, and its amino acid sequence was identified in 1966.

Biochemistry & Distribution

Unlike most other gastrointestinal peptides, secretin has been identified in only one 27-amino-acid form. The entire secretin molecule is necessary for full biologic activity. Secretin has structural similarities to glucagon, GIP, VIP, peptide histidine isoleucine (PHI), and peptide histidine methionine (PHM). These peptides are known as the secretin family (Table 17–2). The secretin gene consists of 813 base pairs. Secretin is found in S cells in the duodenum and proximal jejunum and in the central nervous system. The secretin receptor has been cloned. It is a 427 amino acid protein with seven transmembrane domains coupled to G-proteins.

Measurement & Release

Measurement of secretin has been difficult because the molecule is highly unstable and lacks a tyrosine residue for iodination. The latter problem has been solved by iodination under conditions that label histidine or by using a synthetic secretin analog in which tyrosine has been substituted for one of the other amino acids. Immunoassays for secretin show fasting serum values of 3–15 pg/mL (1–5 pmol/L), increasing to about 30 pg/mL (10 pmol/L) with stimulation. The half-life of secretin in blood is 3–7.5 minutes.

The only known stimulus for secretin release is duodenal acidification, which causes an increase in serum levels within minutes. This effect may be mediated by a secretin-releasing peptide. The threshold for secretin release is a duodenal pH of less than 4.5. Infusion of bile salt into the duodenum also causes a small increase in serum levels of secretin. Other substances such as fats, alcohols, glucose, and amino acids do not release secretin if the pH of the duodenum is kept constant. Neither vagotomy nor atropine alters the secretin response to intraduodenal acid. Vagotomy may indirectly affect secretin release by elevating duodenal pH. Somatostatin inhibits secretin release and action.

Actions

The main action of secretin is stimulation of pancreatic bicarbonate and water secretion. Infusion of secretin intravenously to mimic physiologic levels produces a corresponding increase in pancreatic water and bicarbonate secretion, supporting a physiologic effect. CCK markedly potentiates the effect of secretin on pancreatic secretion. Although pharmacologic doses of secretin inhibit meal-stimulated gastrin release and gastric acid secretion, these effects are not seen at physiologic levels of secretin.

SOMATOSTATIN

Somatostatin was first isolated from the hypothalamus, where it was found to inhibit the release of GH. Somatostatin was subsequently found in large amounts in both the brain and the gut. It is the preeminent inhibitory peptide of the gastrointestinal tract.

Biochemistry & Distribution

Somatostatin is a cyclic peptide with two naturally occurring forms of 14 and 28 amino acids (Figure 18–7). An eight-amino-acid analog has been synthesized (octreotide) that preserves the biologic activity of somatostatin and has a longer serum half-life. Somatostatin is widely distributed in both the central nervous system and the gastrointestinal tract. In the gastrointestinal tract, somatostatin is most prominent in endocrine cells within the mucosa of the gastric antrum, in the D cells of the pancreatic islets, and in neurons of the myenteric plexus.

The gene sequence for human somatostatin codes for a 116-amino-acid preprosomatostatin molecule on chromosome 3. Posttranslational processing occurs at both the amino- and carboxyl terminal regions. The sequence of the tetradecapeptide somatostatin is strongly conserved among species. Expression of somatostatin mRNA in the foregut occurs early in gestation and precedes morphologic differentiation of the D cell. At least five somatostatin receptor subtypes have been identified. Functional studies suggest that these receptor subtypes differ in their distribution and effects on signal transduction pathways.

Measurement & Release

Fasting somatostatin plasma concentrations average less than 2.35 ng/dL (< 10 pmol/L), with increases of 2.35–7.1 ng/dL (10–30 pmol/L) postprandially. The main stimulant for somatostatin release is ingestion of protein and fat in a meal. In the antrum, somatostatin release is reciprocally linked with gastrin release. Cholinergic stimulation increases gastrin release and suppresses somatostatin release. Conversely, antral acidification inhibits gastrin release and stimulates somatostatin release. This reciprocal regulation of release of gastrin and somatostatin is also seen at the level of mRNA expression. Somatostatin itself inhibits its release from the D cell, an example of autocrine regulation.

Actions

Somatostatin has broad inhibitory activity in the gut. It inhibits the release and action of numerous gut peptides, including gastrin, CCK, secretin, VIP, motilin, GIP, insulin, and glucagon. It has potent inhibitory effects on gut secretion, including gastric acid, pancreatic enzymes and bicarbonate, and intestinal fluid and electrolytes. Somatostatin at higher doses inhibits gut motility and gallbladder contraction. At lower doses, however, somatostatin initiates the migratory motor complex and increases the rate of gastric emptying. Somatostatin inhibits mesenteric blood flow and reduces portal pressures, even in patients with portal hypertension, but it has no significant systemic hemodynamic effects. Finally, somatostatin has antitrophic effects in both normal tissues, particularly the pancreas, and some neoplastic tissues.

Somatostatin is unique among gut peptides in that evidence is available to support delivery to the target cell by endocrine, paracrine, neurocrine, and autocrine routes. Postprandial elevations in plasma somatostatin, for example, are sufficient to inhibit gastric and pancreatic exocrine secretion. The evidence for a paracrine function for somatostatin is indirect and is based on the morphology of somatostatin-containing D cells and their proximity to target cells in sites such as the gastric antrum and the pancreatic islet. The presence of somatostatin in neurons in the gut wall and the inhibitory action of somatostatin on myenteric plexus acetylcholine release and intestinal motility support its role as a neurotransmitter. Finally, recent evidence supports the autocrine regulation of somatostatin release in the D cell.

Clinical Uses

Octreotide has found a clinical role in the management of patients with metastatic gut endocrine tumors, secretory diarrhea, enterocutaneous fistula, and a variety of unusual conditions such as the postgastrectomy dumping syndrome.

BOMBESIN & GASTRIN-RELEASING PEPTIDE

Bombesin, a peptide found in the skin, brain, and gut of frogs, shares biologic activity with mammalian gastrin-releasing peptide (GRP). The ten carboxyl terminal amino acid sequences of GRP and bombesin are nearly identical, accounting for their similar physiologic actions.

Biochemistry & Distribution

Bombesin, a 14-amino-acid polypeptide, belongs to a group of homologous amphibian peptides (litorin, ranatensin, and alytensin) found to influence gut motility and secretion. Bombesin has not been identified in mammals, but GRP, a 27-amino-acid polypeptide with strong structural homology, has been isolated from mammalian gut and brain. The human GRP gene has been cloned from a patient with carcinoid tumor metastatic to the lungs. It encodes a precursor molecule of 148 amino acids, termed preproGRP, which undergoes posttranslational processing to the active 27-amino-acid form. Recently, the GRP gene has been identified in frog gut extracts, and sequence analysis reveals that it codes for a precursor peptide distinct from that encoded by the frog bombesin gene. GRP is found throughout the gut and in the brain in neurons. It is most concentrated in the antral and duodenal mucosa. The receptor for GRP has been cloned and its amino acid sequence determined. GRP receptors are found on gastric G cells, gut smooth muscle cells, and pancreatic acinar cells.

Measurement & Release

Little or no change in plasma GRP concentrations occurs postprandially. In anesthetized pigs, marked release of GRP occurs in the venous outflow of the stomach in response to electrical vagal stimulation. The neuronal origin, mechanism of release, and low plasma levels of GRP support its function as a neurotransmitter. Gene expression of antral-but not fundic-GRP is increased by fasting and acid inhibition.

Actions

The main physiologic action of GRP is stimulation of gastrin release from antral G cells. Paradoxically, in the gastric fundus, GRP-containing neurons appear to inhibit parietal cell acid secretion indirectly via the release of somatostatin. At pharmacologic doses, GRP stimulates pancreatic exocrine secretion via a mechanism independent of CCK. Additionally, GRP stimulates smooth muscle contraction in the gallbladder, duodenum, and stomach. GRP has mitogenic effects in vitro and is a potent autocrine stimulant of growth of certain tumors, including small-cell lung cancer. In the brain, it may play a role in thermoregulation and pain perception. In animals and humans, GRP induces satiety.

CALCITONIN GENE-RELATED PEPTIDE

Biochemistry & Distribution

Calcitonin gene-related peptide (CGRP) is a 37-amino-acid peptide produced by alternative processing of the calcitonin gene. Two CGRP-encoding genes and four highly homologous CGRPs have been described. CGRP is widely distributed in neurons of the central, peripheral, and enteric nervous systems. It is found throughout the gut, especially in sensory neurons. CGRP is commonly colocalized with substance P.

Measurement & Release

CGRP immunoreactivity may be measured in plasma, but it probably functions as a neurotransmitter. It is released by electrical stimulation and by specific sensory neuron stimulation with agents such as capsaicin.

Actions

CGRP probably plays an important role in the gut as a sensory neurotransmitter. Actions ascribed to CGRP in the gastrointestinal tract include inhibition of gastric and pancreatic secretion and smooth muscle contraction. Furthermore, CGRP stimulates somatostatin and acetylcholine release and increases mucosal blood flow. CGRP may have important effects in gastric mucosal cytoprotection.

GASTRIC INHIBITORY PEPTIDE

Biochemistry & Distribution

Gastric inhibitory peptide (GIP) is a 42-amino-acid polypeptide with a structure similar to those of secretin, glucagon, and VIP. The human GIP cDNA encodes for a 153-amino-acid preproGIP with a predicted molecular weight of 17,100. GIP and its mRNA are found in mucosal K cells in the duodenum, jejunum, and ileum.

Measurement & Release

Basal levels of GIP are in the range of 250 pg/mL (50 pmol/L). GIP release is stimulated by ingestion of food, with a peak of approximately 1000 pg/mL (200 pmol/L) occurring 60 minutes postprandially. The most potent stimuli for release of GIP are intraluminal glucose, triglycerides, and amino acids. Release of GIP may also be modulated by adrenergic stimulation, calcium, and glucagon. The half-life of GIP in plasma is about 20 minutes.

Actions

Originally, GIP was identified by its inhibitory effect on acid secretion. The main physiologic action of GIP, however, is to increase the insulin response to glucose in the presence of elevated blood glucose levels. This has prompted some to suggest that GIP be renamed glucose-dependent insulinotropic polypeptide. GIP may function as an "incretin," enhancing insulin release and glucose disposal during intestinal absorption of glucose when compared with intravenous administration of glucose. GIP also inhibits gastrin release and gastric acid secretion, but it is unlikely that these effects occur at physiologic levels of the hormone. The amino terminal portion of the molecule is essential for the effect on insulin, and the carboxyl terminal portion is essential for the gastric effect. GIP in physiologic doses inhibits absorption of fluid and electrolytes by the ileal mucosa, but the importance of this is not known.

VASOACTIVE INTESTINAL POLYPEPTIDE

Biochemistry & Distribution

Vasoactive intestinal polypeptide (VIP) was first isolated in 1970 by Said and Mutt from porcine small intestine. VIP is colocalized on a gene with peptide histidine isoleucine (PHI). VIP is a basic 28-amino-acid peptide with strong homology to PHI, pituitary adenylyl cyclase-activating polypeptide, secretin, glucagon, GIP, and growth hormone-releasing factor. In addition, it has a close structural relationship to helospectin and helodermin, which occur in the venom of Gila monsters. This suggests that, as a highly conserved molecule, it has important biologic activity.

VIP is distributed in a wide range of neurons in the gut, the central nervous system, and the urogenital tract. It is not present in gut endocrine cells except in lower vertebrates. It probably functions as a neurocrine agent, and its presence in neurons with processes extending to mucosal cells, smooth muscle, and blood vessels suggests that VIP affects local secretion, motility, and blood flow. Some myenteric VIPergic neurons also express nitric oxide (NO) synthase.

Measurement & Release

Fasting serum levels of VIP are low (< 33 pg/mL or 10 pmol/L) and do not increase significantly postprandially, compatible with its function as a neurotransmitter. VIP concentrations in venous effluent from the gut increase with electrical stimulation, esophageal distention, and mechanical stimulation of intestinal mucosa.

Actions

The most important physiologic actions of VIP are probably relaxation of the lower esophageal sphincter, receptive relaxation of the gastric fundus, and relaxation of the anal sphincter. Additionally, VIP increases gut blood flow and is responsible for penile erection. When infused intravenously, VIP inhibits pentagastrin and histamine-stimulated gastric acid and pepsin secretion. It stimulates lipolysis, glycogenolysis, and secretion by the small intestine and pancreas. The action of VIP is mediated by stimulatory G proteins and activation of adenylyl cyclase.

GALANIN

Biochemistry & Distribution

Galanin is a recently characterized 29-amino-acid peptide found in both the central nervous system and the gastrointestinal tract. It does not have structural similarity to any other gut peptides. In the gut, galanin is found in neurons of the myenteric and submucosal plexuses. It is commonly colocalized with VIP. An mRNA encoding a 124-amino-acid preprogalanin has been described.

Measurement & Release

Antibodies for estimation of galanin concentration by radioimmunoassay are available. Circulating levels are low. Galanin is released by neural stimulation, and increased concentrations are seen in venous drainage from the intestine and pancreas.

Actions

The physiologic role of galanin is unclear. Reported actions include inhibition of postprandial release of neurohumoral substances such as insulin, neurotensin, somatostatin, and pancreatic polypeptide. Additionally, galanin inhibits intestinal motility. This effect may be indirect, via inhibition of release of the excitatory neurotransmitters acetylcholine and substance P. Minor effects include inhibition of acid and pancreatic secretion.

SUBSTANCE P

Substance P was discovered by Von Euler and Gaddum in 1931 and was the first peptide found in both brain and gut. Little further research was done on substance P until 1970, when Chang and Leeman isolated and purified it from the brain.

Biochemistry & Distribution

Substance P is an 11-amino-acid polypeptide of the tachykinin family (Table 17–2). The gene encoding substance P has been cloned and sequenced. Distinct mRNA sequences have been identified coding for substance P and two other tachykinins known as neurokinin A (also called substance K or neuromedin L) and neurokinin B (also called neuromedin K). Substance P is distributed throughout the body in tissues of neural crest origin. In the gut, substance P is localized in neurons. It appears especially important as a neurotransmitter substance in small-diameter, unmyelinated sensory C fibers and in motor neurons of the myenteric plexus. Three tachykinin receptors have been cloned (NK_1, NK_2, and NK_3), all of which are of the seven-transmembrane domain class. Substance P and its receptor are up-regulated in some inflammatory conditions in the intestine.

Measurement & Release

Substance P is released from enteric neurons in response to electrical stimulation, serotonin, and CCK. This release is inhibited by somatostatin. The normal serum concentration of substance P is about 91 pg/mL (70 pmol/L), most of which is of enteric origin. Substance P is not released into the blood except in disease states (eg, carcinoid syndrome and dumping syndrome).

Actions

The major gastrointestinal actions of substance P are stimulation of smooth muscle contraction and epithelial secretion. In the circulatory system, substance P causes marked vasodilation, probably due to release of secondary mediators. Substance P has marked stimulatory effects on the gut immune response and probably plays a pathophysiologic role in inflammatory conditions of the gut.

ENKEPHALINS

The enkephalins are neuropeptides closely related to other central nervous system opiate peptides, the α-, β-, and γ-endorphins. The endorphins and enkephalins bind to opiate receptors found in the brain and gut.

Biochemistry & Distribution

The two gastrointestinal enkephalins, met-enkephalin and leu-enkephalin, are pentapeptides differing only at the terminal carboxyl residue. Three distinct genes have been identified that code for opiate peptides. The pro-opiomelanocortin gene gives rise to ACTH, MSH, and α-endorphin. Its expression in the enteric nervous system is poorly understood. A second gene (preproenkephalin) codes for precursor molecules of met-enkephalin and leu-enkephalin. There is direct evidence of synthesis of these peptides within myenteric neurons in the gut. A third gene (preprodynorphin) codes for precursor molecules of dynorphin, α-neoendorphin, and leu-enkephalin. Enkephalins are widely distributed in neurons throughout the gastrointestinal tract.

Measurement & Release

Enkephalins are rapidly destroyed in blood, which makes it unlikely that they act as circulating hormones. The normal stimulus for the release of enkephalins is unclear. It is likely that they function as neurocrine or paracrine agents within the gut wall. Specific and nonspecific degrading enzymes have been found in the interstitial fluid and lymphatic channels of the gut.

Actions

The main actions of enkephalins in the gastrointestinal tract are inhibition of gut motility, stimulation of sphincter tone, and inhibition of mucosal secretion. Opioid receptors have been identified on smooth muscle cells isolated from the circular muscle layer of the gut but appear to be absent on cells from the longitudinal layer. In vitro, enkephalins cause dose-dependent contraction of smooth muscle cells and inhibit acetylcholine release from myenteric plexus neurons.

NEUROTENSIN

Neurotensin was discovered accidentally during isolation of substance P from the hypothalamus when a fraction of the extract was found to produce vasodilation and hypotension. The term "neurotensin" derives from its neurologic origin and its hypotensive properties.

Biochemistry & Distribution

Neurotensin is a 13-amino-acid polypeptide found extensively in nerve cells in the central nervous system. In the gut, it is located in endocrine N cells of the ileum and is almost absent from nerve fibers. The carboxy terminal segment of the molecule is responsible for its biologic activity. The neurotensin gene encodes for a 170-amino-acid precursor molecule containing both neurotensin and an allied molecule, neuromedin N.

Measurement & Release

Basal neurotensin serum levels by radioimmunoassay average 1–5 pmol/L. The main stimulant for the release of neurotensin is intraluminal fat, leading to increases of up to 20 pmol/L in serum. An exaggerated postprandial release of neurotensin has been reported to occur in patients with dumping syndrome.

Actions

The physiologic role of neurotensin is not known, but pharmacologic gastrointestinal actions include inhibition of gastric acid secretion, stimulation of pancreatic protein and bicarbonate secretion, stimulation of colonic motility, and inhibition of gastric and small intestinal motility. Additionally, neurotensin has trophic effects on gastric, small bowel, and colonic mucosa. Central nervous system neurotensin may participate in gastric mucosal cytoprotection. Neurotensin binds to mast cells, and since many of its effects are histamine-like (ie, hypotension, hypoglycemia, increased vascular permeability, smooth muscle contraction), neurotensin may act by releasing histamine.

MOTILIN

Biochemistry & Distribution

Motilin is a 22-amino-acid peptide found mainly in endocrine cells in the mucosa of the duodenum and proximal jejunum. Some immunoassays have purportedly shown localization of motilin within enterochromaffin cells, though this finding has been disputed. Motilin-like immunoreactivity has been identified in the brain, especially the pituitary and pineal glands. The human motilin gene encodes a 114-amino-acid prepromotilin molecule on chromosome 6. The entire molecule appears necessary for full biologic activity.

Measurement & Release

Motilin is released into the blood in cyclic fashion in the fasting state. Its release corresponds to phase III of the cyclic migratory motor complex; however, the mechanism of regulation of motilin release is unclear. Motilin release is inhibited by somatostatin.

Actions

Motilin was first identified by its ability to stimulate gastric motility. Its main action appears to be induction of myoelectric complexes in the antroduodenal region which propagate distally. This action is mimicked by the macrolide antibiotic erythromycin. In vitro, motilin causes contraction of duodenal, ileal, colonic, and gallbladder smooth muscle. Other pharmacologic properties include stimulation of pepsin and of pancreatic and chloride secretion.

PANCREATIC POLYPEPTIDE FAMILY

Biochemistry & Distribution

The pancreatic polypeptide family consists of three peptides: pancreatic polypeptide (PP), peptide YY (PYY), and neuropeptide Y (NPY). All three are 36-amino-acid peptides with strong structural similarities. PP and PYY are localized in endocrine cells of the gut, mainly in the pancreas and colon, respectively. NPY is found both in the brain and in enteric neurons. NPY is commonly colocalized with norepinephrine. The genes for PP, PYY, and NPY have been characterized.

Measurement & Release

Both PP and PYY appear to have endocrine function and are released postprandially. NPY appears to function as a neuropeptide. PP release is strongly stimulated by protein and by cholinergic stimulation. Release of PYY is stimulated by intestinal fat.

Actions

The major physiologic action of PP is inhibition of pancreatic bicarbonate and protein secretion. Minor effects include relaxation of the gallbladder. PYY inhibits gastric motility and acid secretion and, in dogs, pancreatic secretion. The mechanism of PYY action on motility probably involves inhibition of cholinergic neurotransmission and activation of inhibitory G proteins. NPY is a potent vasoconstrictor and inhibits acetylcholine release. In the central nervous system, NPY potently stimulates food intake.

ENTEROGLUCAGON

Biochemistry & Distribution

The best-known form of glucagon is a 29-amino-acid peptide found mainly in the pancreatic A cells. A number of other enteroglucagons exist in the gut, including glicentin, glucagon-like peptide 1 (GLP-1), and oxyntomodulin. All are coded for by the same gene sequence. GLP-1 is derived from the carboxyl terminal portion of preproglucagon, whereas glicentin and oxyntomodulin are present in the amino terminal region. The enteroglucagons are found in intestinal L cells.

Measurement & Release

Measurement of serum levels of enteroglucagon is imprecise, owing to the presence of multiple molecular forms and cross-reactivity of antibody assays with pancreatic glucagon. Intestinal carbohydrate and fat are the most important stimulants of enteroglucagon release.

Actions

The intestinal forms of glucagon are much less potent than pancreatic glucagon in the regulation of hepatic glucose production. GLP-1 enhances insulin release and functions as an incretin. Enteroglucagons inhibit gastric acid secretion. It has been postulated that enteroglucagon is a trophic factor for small intestinal mucosa.

ABNORMALITIES OF REGULATORY PEPTIDES IN DISEASES OF THE GASTROINTESTINAL TRACT

Although gastrointestinal peptides are clearly important in the regulation of digestion, their role in disease states of the gut is less clear. A variety of tumors have been identified that secrete large quantities of gut hormones and produce definable clinical syndromes. These so-called neuroendocrine tumors of the gut have provided important clues to the physiologic actions of peptides. It is strongly suspected that abnormalities of regulation by the enteric nervous system underlie several motility disorders of the gut. More recently, evidence has been obtained supporting the concept that abnormalities of gut regulatory peptides play important roles in the pathogenesis of inflammatory bowel disease.

DUODENAL ULCER

Although patients with duodenal ulcer secrete more acid than do subjects without duodenal ulcer, fasting serum gastrin levels and the number of antral G cells are normal. Meal-stimulated gastrin release, however, is greater than normal in these patients, and inhibition of gastrin release by antral acidification is diminished. These two findings are attributable to the bacterium *Helicobacter pylori,* which infects the antral mucosa in virtually all patients with duodenal ulcer.

Evaluation of Hypergastrinemia

Several causes of basal hypergastrinemia have been described. In the evaluation of a patient with recurrent duodenal ulcer, one should measure gastrin levels, and if hypergastrinemia is present, these conditions should be considered.

A. Gastrinoma: Patients with gastrinoma have unregulated secretion of large amounts of gastrin by a tumor. The result is excessive acid secretion and severe ulcer disease. Evaluation and treatment are discussed in some detail later in this chapter.

B. Hypercalcemia: Patients with hypercalcemia may secrete increased amounts of gastrin and gastric acid. In patients with hyperparathyroidism, removal of a parathyroid adenoma with return of the serum calcium level to normal usually returns serum gastrin and gastric acid secretion to normal. However, the relationship between hypercalcemia and duodenal ulcer disease is not close, and in general, if severe duodenal ulcer disease is present in a patient with hyperparathyroidism, the cause is more likely to be gastrinoma (as part of multiple endocrine neoplasia [MEN] syndrome type I) than a direct effect of hypercalcemia (see Chapter 24).

C. Massive Small Bowel Resection: Following massive small bowel resection, patients often have acid hypersecretion and hypergastrinemia. The pathophysiology of the hypergastrinemia is unclear, but the disorder may be due to loss of an enterogastrone (a hormone from the intestine that inhibits gastrin release and gastric acid secretion). The increased acid secretion that follows enterectomy usually subsides within a few months, so that treatment with H_2 blocking agents is usually sufficient.

D. Renal Failure: Renal failure may be accompanied by hypergastrinemia and gastric hyperacidity, probably because of decreased catabolism of the large molecular forms of gastrin by the diseased kidneys. Treatment consists of antacids and H_2 blocking agents.

E. Gastric Outlet Obstruction: Hypergastrinemia in association with gastric outlet obstruction is related to antral distention. Tube decompression of the stomach usually results in a return of gastrin levels to normal.

F. Antral G Cell Hyperplasia: Rare patients have hypergastrinemia from hyperactivity of the G cells, a condition referred to as antral G cell hyperplasia. Treatment consists of H_2 blocking agents or antrectomy.

G. Retained Antrum Syndrome: If, in the course of a distal gastrectomy, antral tissue adjacent to the pylorus is left intact and reconstruction of gastrointestinal continuity is made by a Billroth II gastrojejunostomy, hypergastrinemia may occur as a result of lack of acid inhibition of G cell secretion. This syndrome is rare now that the factors regulating gastrin secretion are widely known.

MOTILITY DISORDERS OF THE GASTROINTESTINAL TRACT

Achalasia is characterized by abnormal or absent peristalsis in the body of the esophagus, a high resting lower esophageal pressure, and absence of relaxation of the sphincter with swallowing. Immunochemical staining of the sphincter reveals decreased or absent VIPergic neurons in the myenteric plexus. In view of the known relaxant effects of VIP on the lower esophageal sphincter, it is likely that achalasia represents an acquired disorder of sphincteric VIPergic innervation.

Hirschsprung's disease is due to congenital absence of neural ganglia in the distal colon and internal anal sphincter. The affected colon is contracted and aperistaltic. The proximal colon dilates as a consequence of chronic partial obstruction. The concentration of VIP as well as the number of nerves containing VIP are greatly decreased in the contracted colonic segment. This absence of the relaxing effects of VIP probably results in the tonic contracted state.

Infantile hypertrophic pyloric stenosis is a congenital tonic contraction of the pyloric sphincteric muscle, leading to gastric outlet obstruction. Nitric oxide synthase, which produces the relaxant substance nitric oxide, is absent in pyloric muscle from afflicted infants, and genetically altered mice lacking the neuronal nitric oxide synthase gene develop a disorder remarkably similar to the human condition. These findings suggest that pyloric stenosis is a disease of the inhibitory neurons of the pyloric sphincter.

Chronic intestinal pseudo-obstruction is a poorly characterized disorder of intestinal motility which clinically simulates obstruction in the absence of any mechanical cause. Abnormalities of myenteric ganglia and intestinal nerve fibers have been described, but the defects are not uniform among patients. It is likely, however, that abnormalities of enteric neuron function are responsible for the motility defect.

Irritable bowel syndrome. Evidence is accumulating that patients with irritable bowel syndrome have heightened sensitivity of gut afferent neurons. Rectal balloon distention, for example, results in more pain in patients with irritable bowel syndrome than in controls. It is possible that this heightened sensitivity to luminal stimuli initiates reflex arcs, resulting in the diarrhea and gut hypermotility characteristic of irritable bowel syndrome. A similar heightened sensitivity of visceral afferent neurons may play a role in the pathophysiology of noncardiac chest pain and nonulcer dyspepsia.

Other motility disorders suspected of being due to abnormalities of regulation by gut peptides include biliary dyskinesia, gastric dysrhythmias, and Chagas' disease.

INFLAMMATORY BOWEL DISEASE

Recently, it has been noted that gut peptides have effects on immune function and conversely that immune regulators such as cytokines affect gut function. Several links between abnormalities of the enteric nervous system and inflammatory conditions of the gut have been identified. Rectal concentrations of VIP, for example, are increased in patients with Crohn's disease, while receptors for other gut peptides, such as substance P, are up-regulated in Crohn's disease and ulcerative colitis. Cytokines such as IL-6 and novel neuropeptides, such as the trefoil peptides, are overexpressed in these conditions. These findings have led to the concept that gut regulatory peptides may play a role in the pathophysiology of inflammatory conditions of the gut. .

NEUROENDOCRINE TUMORS OF THE GUT

Neuroendocrine tumors of the gut may be found in the pancreas, the bowel wall, or the retroperitoneum. They are known by the general term "apudomas" and probably arise from pleuripotential stem cells. Many gut endocrine tumors secrete more than one peptide, but they are named after the one responsible for the clinical manifestations.

The diagnosis of a neuroendocrine tumor of the gut is first suspected by the clinical history and physical examination. Biochemical confirmation of the diagnosis is made by measurement of the hormonal marker in the blood or urine. Radiologic staging of the tumor with CT scan or MRI of the abdomen is used to identify hepatic metastases or (rarely) the primary tumor. The primary tumors are usually small, and efforts at preoperative localization have been disappointing. It now appears that operative exploration and complementary use of intraoperative sonography are the most efficient approach to localization. In general, tumor excision is the preferred treatment. When resection is not possible, palliation of the hormonal syndrome can generally be achieved with the somatostatin analog octreotide. In selected cases, systemic chemotherapy, hepatic chemoembolization, or hepatic resection of metastases is valuable.

MULTIPLE ENDOCRINE NEOPLASIA SYNDROMES

Wermer's syndrome (or multiple endocrine neoplasia [MEN] type I) is an autosomal dominant inherited condition manifested by tumors of the pancreas, pituitary, and parathyroid glands. MEN type IIa, also known as **Sipple's syndrome,** consists of medullary carcinoma of the thyroid, pheochromocytoma, and hyperparathyroidism (see Chapter 24). The tumors are always multiple and diffuse in both MEN type I and MEN type IIa. Screening of afflicted families through the use of specific DNA probes linked to MEN is now feasible.

ZOLLINGER-ELLISON SYNDROME

Zollinger-Ellison syndrome is characterized by virulent peptic ulceration associated with gastric acid hypersecretion and a gastrin-producing tumor (gastrinoma). Gastrinomas usually occur in the pancreas or duodenum. The tumors may be as small as 2–3 mm and are often difficult to find. When associated with MEN type I, they are nearly always multiple. Gastrinomas should be viewed as malignant tumors. Even though the histologic appearance may be benign, 50% of patients present with lymph node or liver metastases.

Most patients with gastrinoma present with symptoms of peptic ulcer disease recalcitrant to histamine H_2 receptor antagonist therapy. Hemorrhage, perforation, and obstruction are common complications. Patients with multiple duodenal ulcers, jejunal ulcers, or recurrent ulcers following treatment for *Helicobacter pylori* infection or previous acid-reductive surgery should be suspected of having gastrinoma. About 5% of patients with gastrinoma have only diarrhea as their presenting symptom. If gastrinoma is suspected, the diagnosis should be confirmed by measurement of fasting serum gastrin levels. Normal fasting gastrin concentrations are less than 200 pg/mL (95 pmol/L). In gastrinoma, levels usually exceed 500 pg/mL (238 pmol/L). Patients with borderline gastrin values (200–500 pg/mL [95–238 pmol/L]) should have a secretin provocative test. After administration of secretin, 2 units/kg as a bolus, an increase in the serum gastrin level of 200 pg/mL or more within 15 minutes is diagnostic of gastrinoma. The secretin stimulation test is useful to differentiate gastrinoma from hypergastrinemia due to gastric outlet obstruction, retained antrum after Billroth II gastrojejunostomy, and antral gastrin cell hyperplasia (Table 17–5).

Efforts to localize gastrinomas preoperatively have been disappointing. Computed tomography of the abdomen should be performed to exclude the presence of liver metastases. Selective angiography and transhepatic portal vein blood sampling can sometimes demonstrate the pancreatic tumor, but misleading results are common. Endoscopic ultrasonography is a promising new technique, but its value is as yet unproved. Similarly, radioisotope scintigraphy using a labeled analog of somatostatin may prove to be useful localization technique. Currently, however, careful exploration by an experienced surgeon, intraoperative endoscopy with duodenal transillumination, and intraoperative ultrasonography of the pancreas is the most efficient localization strategy. Recent studies suggest that over 90% of gastrinomas can be identified intraoperatively with these methods.

In the absence of known liver metastases or MEN type I, virtually all patients with gastrinoma should be explored with the intent of curative excision of the tumor. This approach results in 5-year survival rates

Table 17–5. Hormones that may affect acid secretion or duodenal pH.

Action	Stimulation	Inhibition
Acid secretion	Gastrin CCK	VIP GIP Somatostatin Secretin
Gastrin release	Dombesin GRP	Secretin Somatostatin VIP GIP Glucagon
Pancreatic bicarbonate secretion	CCK Secretin VIP	PP Somatostatin
Delay of gastric emptying of acid into duodenum	CCK	

over 90% for completely resected patients. Tumor recurrence is reported in about half of patients in long-term follow-up studies. Total gastrectomy, formerly a mainstay of therapy, is reserved now only for noncompliant patients with unresectable tumors. Inhibition of acid secretion for palliation in unresectable patients is best achieved with omeprazole, which acts to inhibit the parietal cell H^+-K^+ ATPase. Omeprazole has proved to be superior to histamine H_2 receptor antagonists such as cimetidine, ranitidine, and famotidine. The goal of medical therapy is reduction of basal acid output to less than 10 mmol/h. The long-acting somatostatin analog octreotide inhibits gastrin release, gastric acid secretion, and diarrhea in patients with gastrinoma. It has occasional application in patients refractory to histamine H_2 receptor antagonists or omeprazole.

VIPOMA

VIPoma (also known as pancreatic cholera or the Verner-Morrison syndrome) is characterized by profuse watery diarrhea, marked fecal loss of potassium and bicarbonate, hypokalemia, and low or absent gastric acid secretion. Severe metabolic acidosis may be present. The syndrome is due to intestinal secretion of fluid and electrolytes in response to elevated circulating levels of VIP, usually from an islet cell tumor of the pancreas. In children, and rarely in adults, the tumor is a retroperitoneal ganglioneuroma. While most of the pancreatic tumors are malignant, the ganglioneuromas tend to be benign.

When VIPoma is suspected from the clinical presentation, the diagnosis is confirmed by measurement of fasting VIP serum levels by radioimmunoassay. Localization of the tumor is best accomplished with computed tomography, which may identify the primary tumor in the pancreas or retroperitoneum and

exclude liver metastases. As with gastrinomas, occult tumors are best approached with thorough intraoperative exploration aided by intraoperative sonography.

The optimal treatment for VIPoma is surgical resection, which is possible in about 50% of patients. Palliative therapy includes cytotoxic chemotherapy (usually streptozocin plus fluorouracil), indomethacin, and a somatostatin analog.

GLUCAGONOMA

Glucagonomas are characterized by a migratory necrolytic dermatitis (usually involving the legs and perineum), weight loss, stomatitis, hypoaminoacidemia, anemia, and mild diabetes mellitus. Visual scotomas and changes in visual acuity have been reported in some cases. The age range is 20–70 years, and the condition is more common in women. The diagnosis is usually suspected from the distinctive skin lesion; in fact, the presence of a prominent rash in a patient with diabetes mellitus should be enough to raise suspicions. Confirmation of the diagnosis depends on demonstration of elevated serum glucagon levels. It may be possible to demonstrate the tumor by arteriography or CT scanning.

Glucagonomas arise from A_2 cells in the pancreatic islets. About 25% are benign and confined to the pancreas. The remainder have metastasized by the time of diagnosis, most often to the liver, lymph nodes, adrenal glands, or vertebrae. A few cases have been the result of islet cell hyperplasia. Most tumors are large enough to be localized by computed tomography.

Surgical removal of the primary lesion and metastases is indicated if technically feasible. Even if it is not possible to remove all of the tumor deposits, considerable palliation may result from subtotal removal. Streptozocin, dacarbazine, and somatostatin analogs are effective palliative agents for unresectable lesions. The clinical course generally parallels changes in serum levels of glucagon in response to therapy.

CARCINOID TUMORS & CARCINOID SYNDROME

Carcinoids are the most common of the gut endocrine tumors. They arise throughout the gut from the gastroesophageal junction to the anus, and a few are found in extraintestinal sites such as the bronchus and ovary. Their malignant potential depends both on size and on location. For example, fewer than 10% of the appendiceal or rectal carcinoids—but 30% of ileal and 60% of colonic carcinoids—are malignant. Carcinoids have been categorized as foregut (bronchus and stomach), midgut (small intestine and colon), or hindgut (rectum) tumors. Hindgut carcinoids synthesize no specific by-products, and they do not stain with silver salts (ie, they are argentaffin- and argyrophil-negative). Foregut carcinoids secrete 5-hydroxytryptophan and are argentaffin-negative and argyrophil-positive. Midgut tumors secrete 5-hydroxytryptamine (serotonin) and are both argentaffin- and argyrophil-positive.

Carcinoid syndrome is caused by the systemic release of substances from carcinoid tumors. The syndrome is also occasionally caused by other tumors, such as oat cell carcinoma and medullary carcinoma of the thyroid. Because the humoral substances liberated by carcinoids are metabolized by the liver, the presence of the syndrome implies either a primary lesion draining into the systemic circulation or hepatic metastasis from a gastrointestinal lesion. The distribution of primary tumors in the carcinoid syndrome is as follows: ileum (45%), bronchus (30%), ovary (10%), stomach (5%), and other sites rarely. Fortunately, only 1% of patients with a gastrointestinal carcinoid manifest the carcinoid syndrome.

Clinical Features

The most common symptoms of the carcinoid syndrome are flushing of the head and neck and diarrhea. The flushing attacks last a few minutes and may be accompanied by hypotension. The attacks may be provoked by emotional stress, ingestion of particular foods, and straining at stool. Diarrhea is often severe and may be debilitating. It appears that the diarrhea is due to serotonin, whereas the flushing is due to release of tachykinins from the tumor. About 35% of patients develop endocardial fibrosis of the tricuspid and pulmonary valves. Retroperitoneal fibrosis, arthritis, and bronchial asthma also occur but less frequently.

Diagnosis

The diagnosis of carcinoid syndrome is biochemically confirmed by the measurement of elevated levels of a metabolite of serotonin, 5-hydroxyindoleacetic acid (5-HIAA), in the urine. Measurements of serotonin, histamine, prostaglandin, and bradykinin levels in blood are less reliable. Staging of the tumor consists of a chest radiograph and CT scan of the abdomen. Radionuclide scanning using radiolabeled octreotide has promise, in early series, of high sensitivity in identifying occult primary and metastatic deposits. Small bowel contrast studies and arteriography help to localize primary gastrointestinal carcinoid tumors. In selected patients, echocardiography should be performed to assess valvular fibrosis.

Treatment

Where feasible, localized carcinoid tumors should be resected. In the most common situation, small tumors of the appendix may be treated with appendectomy alone. Tumors involving the cecum at the base of the appendix or those greater than 2 cm in size should be treated with right hemicolectomy to encompass regional lymph node drainage. Patients with carcinoid syndrome occasionally require operation for resection of ileal primary tumors causing obstruction. Selected patients benefit from hepatic resection for tumor debulking. In gastric carcinoid tumors arising in the setting of atrophic gastritis and hypergastrinemia, local excision should be combined with antrectomy to control the mitogenic effect of gastrin.

Palliation of the symptoms of carcinoid syndrome is best achieved with the long-acting analog of somatostatin, octreotide. This is successful in about 80% of patients. Octreotide is useful also for management of life-threatening carcinoid crisis. Other agents, such as methysergide, cyproheptadine, and diphenoxylate with atropine (Lomotil), have been largely been replaced by octreotide for symptomatic management of these patients.

Cytotoxic chemotherapy should be considered for patients with rapidly progressive tumors, for those with urinary excretion of 5-HIAA greater than 150 mg/d, and for those with carcinoid-induced valvular heart disease. The most widely used regimen consists of streptozocin plus fluorouracil. Other agents with potential antitumor activity include doxorubicin and alpha-interferon. Hepatic artery chemoembolization has produced long-lasting palliation in a few patients.

Prognosis

The 5-year survival rate for patients with metastases is 20%. However, the cure rate for surgical resection of localized disease is good. If only regional nodes are involved, the 5-year survival rate is 65%; if the tumor is locally invasive without lymph node involvement, the 5-year survival rate is 95%. The 5-year survival rates associated with different tumor sites are 99% for appendix, 87% for lung, 50% for small intestine and colon, and 83% for rectum and rectosigmoid.

MISCELLANEOUS TUMORS

Other islet cell tumors have been reported that produce pancreatic polypeptide, somatostatin, neurotensin, vasopressin, a GH-releasing factor, ACTH, and MSH. Of these, the pancreatic polypeptide-secreting tumors (PPomas) have been the most common. Since PP produces few (if any) symptoms, the clinical manifestations in patients with PPomas have been chiefly due to direct effects of the tumor (eg, abdominal pain, weight loss). The tumor is malignant in 50% of cases. Treatment consists of tumor resection.

Somatostatinomas are rare tumors characterized by diabetes mellitus (usually mild), diarrhea and malabsorption, and dilation of the gallbladder (usually with cholelithiasis). High levels of calcitonin and IgM have been present in the serum in some patients.

The syndrome results from secretion of somatostatin by an islet cell tumor of the pancreas, which in most cases is malignant and accompanied by hepatic metastases. The diagnosis may be made by recognizing the clinical syndrome and measuring increased concentrations of somatostatin in the serum. In most cases, however, the somatostatin syndrome has been unsuspected until histologic evidence of metastatic islet cell carcinoma has been obtained. Surgery is indicated if the disease is localized. More often, chemotherapy or chemoembolization is the only treatment possible.

CLINICAL USES OF GUT PEPTIDES

Gastrointestinal peptides have been increasingly used in diagnosis and management of both gastrointestinal and nongastrointestinal conditions. These applications stem from basic knowledge of the physiology of the substances.

DIAGNOSTIC USES

Gut peptides are useful in diagnosis of a number of conditions. This use includes provocative testing, such as the stimulation of release of gastrin from gastrinomas by secretin, and functional tests, such as measurement of pentagastrin-stimulated acid secretion. In radiology, glucagon is widely used to reduce spasm during gastrointestinal procedures such as endoscopic retrograde cholangiopancreatography and hypotonic duodenography. Glucagon is similarly an aid during colonoscopy or duodenoscopy. The gallbladder contraction induced by cholecystokinin has been utilized as a test of gallbladder function in CCK scintigraphy, in which incomplete emptying suggests gallbladder disease. Emerging radionuclide imaging procedures involve the administration of radiolabeled analogs of somatostatin or VIP intravenously to detect occult neoplasms. The frequent presence of somatostatin or VIP receptors on a wide variety of cancers allows detection of lesions unseen by conventional imaging methods.

THERAPEUTIC USES

Octreotide, the long-acting analog of somatostatin, has proved useful in the management of a variety of conditions, including palliation of symptoms in patients with metastatic gut endocrine tumors, inhibition of fluid output in enterocutaneous fistula, control of massive secretory diarrhea, and prevention of postprandial symptoms in patients with severe dumping syndrome. Octreotide inhibits mesenteric blood flow and reduces portal vein pressure in cirrhotics and, in some studies, reduces variceal bleeding in a way comparable to vasopressin. Although octreotide is generally well tolerated, gallstones develop in at least 15% of patients during long-term treatment.

REFERENCES

General

Debas HT, Mulvihill SJ: Neuroendocrine design of the gut. Am J Surg 1991;161:243.

Guillemin R. The language of polypeptides and the wisdom of the body. Physiologist 1985;28:391.

Le Douarin NM: On the origin of pancreatic endocrine cells. Cell 1988;53:169.

Walsh J: Gastrointestinal hormones: Past, present, and future. Gastroenterology 1993;104:653.

Gastrin

Freston JW et al: Effects of hypochlorhydria and hypergastrinemia on structure and function of gastrointestinal cells: A review and analysis. Dig Dis Sci 1995; 40(2 Suppl):50S.

Gittes GK, Rutter WJ, Debas HT: Initiation of gastrin expression during the development of the mouse pancreas. Am J Surg 1993;165:23.

Kopin AS et al: Expression cloning and characterization of the canine parietal cell gastrin receptor. Proc Natl Acad Sci U S A 1992;89:3605.

Prinz C et al: Gastrin effects on isolated rat enterochromaffin-like cells in primary culture. Am J Physiol 1994;267:G663.

Walsh JH: Physiology and pathophysiology of gastrin. Mt Sinai J Med 1992;59:117.

Cholecystokinin

Ballinger AB, Clark ML: L-Phenylalanine releases cholecystokinin (CCK) and is associated with reduced food intake in humans: Evidence for a physiologic role of CCK in control of eating. Metabolism 1994;43:735.

Deschenes RJ et al: Cloning and sequence analysis of a cDNA encoding rat preprocholecystokinin. Proc Natl Acad Sci U S A 1984;81:726.

Li Y, Owyang C: Endogenous cholecystokinin stimulates pancreatic enzyme secretion via vagal afferent pathway in rats. Gastroenterology 1994;107:525.

Liddle RA: Regulation of cholecystokinin secretion by intraluminal releasing factors. Am J Physiol 1995; 269(3 Part 1):G319.

Nelson MT, Debas HT, Mulvihill SJ: Vagal stimulation of rat exocrine pancreatic secretion occurs via multiple mediators. Gastroenterology 1993;105:221.

Secretin

Chung I et al: Dual inhibitory mechanism of secretin action on acid secretion in totally isolated, vascularly perfused rat stomach. Gastroenterology 1994;107: 1751.

Gyr K et al: Plasma secretin and pancreatic response to various stimulants including a meal. Am J Physiol 1984;246:G535.

Ishihara T et al: Molecular cloning and expression of a cDNA encoding the secretin receptor. EMBO J 1991; 10:1635.

Mutt V, Jorpes J, Magnusson S: Structure of porcine secretin: The amino acid sequence. Eur J Biochem 1970;15:513.

Somatostatin

Gittes GK, Rutter WJ: Onset of cell-specific gene expression in the developing mouse pancreas. Proc Natl Acad Sci U S A 1992;89:1128.

Reisine T, Bell GI: Molecular properties of somatostatin receptors. Neuroscience 1995;67:777.

Shen LP, Rutter WJ: Sequence of the human somatostatin I gene. Science 1984;224:168.

Bombesin and Gastrin-Releasing Peptide

Dimaline R et al: Functional control of gastrin releasing peptide (GRP) mRNA in rat stomach. FEBS Lett 1992;301:291.

Gutzwiller JP et al: Effect of intravenous human gastrin-releasing peptide on food intake in humans. Gastroenterology 1994;106:1168.

Hajri A et al: Gastrin-releasing peptide: In vivo and in vitro growth effects on an acinar pancreatic carcinoma. Cancer Res 1992;52:3726.

Nagalla SR et al: Gastrin-releasing peptide (GRP) is not mammalian bombesin: Identification and molecular cloning of a true amphibian GRP distinct from amphibian bombesin in Bombina orientalis. J Biol Chem 1992;267:6916.

Schubert ML et al: Regulation of acid secretion by bombesin/GRP neurons of the gastric fundus. Am J Physiol 1991;260:G156.

Terashima H, Debas HT, Bunnett NW: Effects of cholecystokinin and gastrin antagonists on pancreatic exocrine secretion stimulated by gastrin-releasing peptide. Pancreas 1992;7:212.

Calcitonin Gene-Related Peptide

Gray JL et al: A role for calcitonin gene-related peptide in protection against gastric ulceration. Ann Surg 1994;219:58.

Morris HR et al: Isolation and characterization of human calcitonin gene-related peptide. Nature 1984;308:746.

Muff R, Born W, Fischer JA: Calcitonin, calcitonin gene-related peptide, adrenomedullin and amylin: Homologous peptides, separate receptors and overlapping biological actions. Eur J Endocrinol 1995; 133:17.

Gastric Inhibitory Polypeptide

Brown JC: Gastric inhibitory polypeptide. Monogr Endocrinol 1982;24:1.

Kieffer TJ et al: Release of gastric inhibitory polypeptide from cultured canine endocrine cells. Am J Physiol 1994;267:E489.

Lacroix A et al: Gastric inhibitory polypeptide-dependent cortisol hypersecretion: A new cause of Cushing's syndrome. N Engl J Med 1992;327:974.

Vasoactive Intestinal Polypeptide

Biancani P, Walsh J, Behar J: Vasoactive intestinal polypeptide: A neurotransmitter for esophageal sphincter relaxation. J Clin Invest 1984;73:963.

Ghatei MA et al: Distribution, molecular characterization of pituitary adenylate cyclase-activating polypeptide and its precursor encoding messenger RNA in human and rat tissues. J Endocrinol 1993;136:159.

Grider JR et al: Stimulation of nitric oxide from muscle cells by VIP: Prejunctional enhancement of VIP release. Am J Physiol 1992;262:G774.

Itoh N et al: Human preprovasoactive intestinal polypeptide contains a novel PHI-27-like peptide, PHM-27. Nature 1983;304:547.

Krejs G et al: Effect of VIP infusion in water and ion transport in the human jejunum. Gastroenterology 1980;78:722.

Sreedharan SP et al: Cloning and expression of the human vasoactive intestinal peptide receptor. Proc Natl Acad Sci U S A 1991;88:4986.

Galanin

Kaplan LM et al: Tissue-specific expression of the rat galanin gene. Proc Natl Acad Sci U S A 1988;85:1065.

Mulholland MW, Schoeneich S, Flowe K: Galanin inhibition of enteric cholinergic neurotransmission: Guanosine triphosphate-binding protein interactions with adenylate cyclase. Surgery 1992;112:195.

Rattan S: Role of galanin in the gut. Gastroenterology 1991;100:1762.

Substance P

Bowden JJ et al: Direct observation of substance P-induced internalization of neurokinin 1 (NK1) receptors at sites of inflammation. Proc Natl Acad Sci U S A 1994;91:8964.

Garland AM et al: Agonist-induced internalization of the substance P (NK1) receptor expressed in epithelial cells. Biochem J 1994;303(Part 1):177.

Huber O et al: Tachykinins contract the circular muscle of the human esophageal body in vitro via NK2 receptors. Gastroenterology 1993;105:981.

Nawa H et al: Nucleotide sequences of cloned cDNAs for two types of bovine brain substance P precursor. Nature 1983;306:32.

Enkephalins

Ambinder RF, Schuster MM: Endorphins: New gut peptides with a familiar face. Gastroenterology 1979;77: 1132.

Nakanishi S et al: Nucleotide sequence of cloned cDNA for bovine corticotropin—lipotropin precursor. Nature 1979;278:423.

Polak J et al: Enkephalin-like immunoreactivity in the human gastrointestinal tract. Lancet 1972;1:972.

Neurotensin

Evers BM et al: Characterization of promoter elements required for cell-specific expression of the neurotensin/neuromedin N gene in a human endocrine cell line. Mol Cell Biol 1995;15:3870.

Evers BM et al: Neurotensin stimulates growth of colonic mucosa in young and aged rats. Gastroenterology 1992;103:86.

Motilin

Poitros P et al: Motilin-independent ectopic fronts of the interdigestive myoelectric complex in dogs. Am J Physiol 1980;239:215.

Sarna SK et al: Gastrointestinal motor effects of erythromycin in humans. Gastroenterology 1991;101:1488.

Pancreatic Polypeptide Family

Adrian TE et al: Human distribution and release of a putative new gut hormone, peptide YY. Gastroenterology 1985;89:1070.

Okumura T, Pappas TN, Taylor IL: Pancreatic polypeptide microinjection into the dorsal motor nucleus inhibits pancreatic secretion in rats. Gastroenterology 1995;108:1517.

Takeuchi T, Yamada T: Isolation of a cDNA clone encoding pancreatic polypeptide. Proc Natl Acad Sci U S A 1985;82:1536.

Tatemoto K: Isolation and characterization of peptide YY (PYY), a candidate gut hormone that inhibits pancreatic exocrine secretion. Proc Natl Acad Sci U S A 1982;79:2514.

Enteroglucagon

Wang L et al: Glucagon-like peptide-1 is a physiologic incretin in rat. J Clin Invest 1995;95:417.

Hormonal Abnormalities in Diseases
of the Gastrointestinal Tract

Bieligk S, Jaffe BM: Islet cell tumors of the pancreas. Surg Clin North Am 1995;75:1025.

Debas HT, Mulvihill SJ: Neuroendocrine gut neoplasms: Important lessons from uncommon tumors. Arch Surg 1994;129:965.

Geracioti TD Jr, Liddle RA: Impaired cholecystokinin secretion in bulimia nervosa. N Engl J Med 1988;319:683.

Mayer EA, Raybould HE: Role of visceral afferent mechanisms in functional bowel disorders. Gastroenterology 1990;99:1688.

Vanderwinden JM et al: Nitric oxide synthase activity in infantile hypertrophic pyloric stenosis. N Engl J Med 1992;327:511.

Walsh JH, Peterson WL: The treatment of *Helicobacter pylori* infection in the management of peptic ulcer disease. N Engl J Med 1995;333:984.

Yee LF, Mulvihill SJ: Neuroendocrine disorders of the gut. West J Med 1995;163:454.

Multiple Endocrine Neoplasia Syndromes

Frilling A et al: Multiple endocrine neoplasia type 2. J Molec Med 1995;73:229.

Kraimps JL et al: Hyperparathyroidism in multiple endocrine neoplasia syndrome. Surgery 1992;112:1080.

Larsson C et al: Predictive testing for multiple endocrine neoplasia type I using DNA polymorphisms. J Clin Invest 1992;89:1344.

Neumann HP et al: Consequences of direct genetic testing for germline mutations in the clinical management of families with multiple endocrine neoplasia, type II. JAMA 1995;274:1149.

Zollinger-Ellison Syndrome

Ellison EC: Forty-year appraisal of gastrinoma: Back to the future. Ann Surg 1995;222:511.

Fraker DL et al: Surgery in Zollinger-Ellison syndrome alters the natural history of gastrinoma. Ann Surg 1994;220:320.

Meko JB, Norton JA: Management of patients with Zollinger-Ellison syndrome. Annu Rev Med 1995;46:395.

Metz DC et al: Control of gastric acid hypersecretion in the management of patients with Zollinger-Ellison syndrome. World J Surg 1993;17:468.

Weber HC et al: Determinants of metastatic rate and survival in patients with Zollinger-Ellison syndrome: A prospective long-term study. Gastroenterology 1995;108:1637.

VIPoma

Kane M, O'Dorisio T, Krejs G: Production of secretory diarrhea by intravenous infusion of vasoactive intestinal polypeptide. N Engl J Med 1983;309:1482.

Mekhjian HS, O'Dorisio TM: VIPoma syndrome. Semin Oncol 1987;14:282.

Rood RP et al: Pancreatic cholera syndrome due to a vasoactive intestinal polypeptide-producing tumor: Further insights into the pathophysiology. Gastroenterology 1988;94:813.

Yasunami Y et al: In vitro release of vasoactive intestinal polypeptide and pancreatic polypeptide from human VIPoma cells and its inhibition by somatostatin analogue (SMS 201-995). Surgery 1994;115:713.

Glucagonoma

Edney JA et al: Glucagonoma syndrome is an underdiagnosed clinical entity. Am J Surg 1990;160:625.

Fehmann HC, Strowski M, Goke B: Functional characterization of somatostatin receptors expressed on hamster glucagonoma cells. Am J Physiol 1995;268(1 Part 1):E40.

Leichter SB: Clinical and metabolic aspects of glucagonoma. Medicine 1980;59:100.

Stacpoole PW: The glucagonoma syndrome: Clinical features, diagnosis, and treatment. Endocr Rev 1981;76:125.

Carcinoid Tumors & Carcinoid Syndrome

Basson MD et al: Biology and management of the midgut carcinoid. Am J Surg 1993;165:288.

Codd JE, Drozda J, Merjavy J: Palliation of carcinoid heart disease. Arch Surg 1987;122:1076.

Gouzi JL et al: Indications for right hemicolectomy in carcinoid tumors of the appendix. Surg Gynecol Obstet 1993;176:543.

Kvols LK et al: Treatment of the malignant carcinoid syndrome: Evaluation of a long-acting somatostatin analogue. N Engl J Med 1986;315:663.

Moertel CG et al: Streptozocin-doxorubicin, streptozocin-fluorouracil, or chlorozotocin in the treatment of advanced islet-cell carcinoma. N Engl J Med 1992;326:519.

Norheim I et al: Malignant carcinoid tumors: An analysis of 103 patients with regard to tumor localization, hormone production, and survival. Ann Surg 1986; 206: 115.

Que FG et al: Hepatic resection for metastatic neuroendocrine carcinomas. Am J Surg 1995;169:36.

Thomas RM et al: Gastric carcinoids: An immunohistochemical and clinicopathologic study of 104 patients. Cancer 1994;73:2052.

Miscellaneous Tumors

Krejs GJ et al: Somatostatinoma syndrome: Biochemical, morphologic and clinical features. N Engl J Med 1979;301:285.

Sawady J et al: Somatostatin-producing neuroendocrine tumor of the ampulla (ampullary somatostatinoma): evidence of prosomatostatin production. Am J Clin Pathol 1992; 97:411.

Strodel WE et al: Pancreatic polypeptide-producing tumors: Silent lesions of the pancreas? Arch Surg 1984; 119:508.

Vinik AI et al: Somatostatinomas, PPomas, neurotensinomas. Semin Oncol 1987;14:263.

Clinical Uses of Gut Peptides

Harris AG et al: Consensus statement: Octreotide dose titration in secretory diarrhea. Diarrhea Management Consensus Development Panel. Dig Dis Sci 1995;40: 1464.

Mulvihill SJ: Perioperative use of octreotide in gastrointestinal surgery. Digestion 1993;54(Suppl 1):33.

Olsen JO et al: Somatostatin receptor imaging of neuroendocrine tumors with indium-111 pentetreotide (Octreoscan). Semin Nucl Med 1995;25:251.

Redfern JS, Fortuner WJ 2nd: Octreotide-associated biliary tract dysfunction and gallstone formation: Pathophysiology and management. Am J Gastroenterol 1995;90:1042.

Pancreatic Hormones & Diabetes Mellitus

18

John H. Karam, MD

I. THE ENDOCRINE PANCREAS

The pancreas is made up of two functionally different organs: the **exocrine pancreas,** the major digestive gland of the body; and the **endocrine pancreas,** the source of insulin, glucagon, somatostatin, and pancreatic polypeptide. Whereas the major role of the products of the exocrine pancreas (the digestive enzymes) is the processing of ingested foodstuffs so that they become available for absorption, the hormones of the endocrine pancreas modulate every other aspect of cellular nutrition from rate of adsorption of foodstuffs to cellular storage or metabolism of nutrients. Dysfunction of the endocrine pancreas or abnormal responses to its hormones by target tissues result in serious disturbances in nutrient homeostasis, including the important clinical syndromes grouped under the name of **diabetes mellitus.**

ANATOMY & HISTOLOGY

The endocrine pancreas consists of 0.7–1 million small endocrine glands—the islets of Langerhans—scattered within the glandular substance of the exocrine pancreas. The islet volume comprises 1–1.5% of the total mass of the pancreas and weighs about 1–2 g in adult humans.

At least four cell types—A, B, D, and F—have been identified in the islets (Table 18–1). These cell types are not distributed uniformly throughout the pancreas. The F cell, which secretes pancreatic polypeptide (PP), has been found primarily in islets in the posterior portion (posterior lobe) of the head, a discrete lobe of the pancreas separated from the anterior portion by a fascial partition. This lobe originates in the primordial ventral bud as opposed to the dorsal bud. The posterior lobe receives its blood supply from the superior mesenteric artery; the remainder of the pancreas derives most of its blood flow from the celiac artery.

ACRONYMS USED IN THIS CHAPTER	
ADA	American Diabetes Association
ADH	Antidiuretic hormone (vasopressin)
ATP	Adenosine triphosphate
cAMP	Cyclic adenosine monophosphate
CBMW	Capillary basement membrane width
CCK	Cholecystokinin
DCCT	Diabetes control and complications trial
DNA	Deoxyribonucleic acid
FDA	Food and Drug Administration
GH	Growth hormone
GI	Glycemic index
GIP	Gastric inhibitory polypeptide
GLP-1	Glucagon-like peptide-1
GLP-2	Glucagon-like peptide 2
HDL	High-density lipoprotein(s)
HLA	Human leukocyte antigen
IDDM	Insulin-dependent diabetes mellitus
MODY	Maturity-onset diabetes of the young
NIDDM	Non-insulin-dependent diabetes mellitus
NPH	Neutral protamine Hagedorn
PP	Pancreatic polypeptide
RNA	Ribonucleic acid
UGDP	University Group Diabetes Program
VLDL	Very low density lipoprotein(s)

Islets in the posterior lobe area consist of 80–85% F cells, 15–20% B cells, and less than 0.5% glucagon-producing A cells. The pancreatic polypeptide cell volume varies with age and sex—the volume tends to be larger in men and in older persons. In contrast to the posterior lobe, the PP-poor islets located in the tail,

Table 18–1. Cell types in pancreatic islets of Langerhans.

Cell types	Approximate Percentage of Islet Volume		Secretory Products
	Dorsally Derived (Anterior Head, Body, Tail)	**Ventrally Derived (Posterior Portion of Head)**	
A cell (α)	10%	< 0.5%	Glucagon, proglucagon, glucagon-like peptides (GLP-1 and GLP-2)
B cell (β)	70–80%	15–20%	Insulin, C peptides, proinsulin, amylin, γ-aminobutyric acid (GABA)
D cell (δ)	3–5%	< 1%	Somatostatin
F cell (PP cell)	< 2%	80–85%	Pancreatic polypeptide

body, and *anterior* portion of the head of the pancreas, arising from the embryonic dorsal bud, contain predominantly insulin-secreting B cells (70–80% of the islet cells), with approximately 20% of the cells being glucagon-secreting A cells and about 3–5% D cells that produce somatostatin. A typical islet from this part of the pancreas is depicted in Figure 18–1.

Islet Vascularization

The islets are richly vascularized, receiving five to ten times the blood flow of a comparable portion of exocrine pancreatic tissues. The direction of the blood flow within the islet has been postulated to play a role in carrying insulin secreted from the central region of

an islet to its peripheral zone~ where the insulin modulates and decreases glucagon release from A cells which are mainly located in the periphery of islets.

HORMONES OF THE ENDOCRINE PANCREAS

1. INSULIN

Biosynthesis

The human insulin gene is located on the short arm of chromosome 11. A precursor molecule, **preproinsulin,** a long-chain peptide of MW 11,500, is

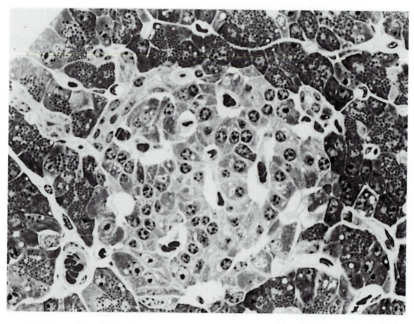

Figure 18–1. Photomicrograph of a section of the pancreas. In the islet of Langerhans, A cells appear mainly in the periphery as large cells with dark cytoplasm. Some D cells are also present in the periphery, while the central core is composed chiefly of B cells. (Reproduced, with permission, from Junqueira LC, Carneiro J, Long JA: *Basic Histology,* 7th ed. Lange, 1992.)

produced by DNA/RNA-directed synthesis in the rough endoplasmic reticulum of pancreatic B cells (Figure 18–2). It is cleaved by microsomal enzymes to **proinsulin** (MW about 9000) almost immediately after synthesis. Proinsulin (Figure 18–3) is transported to the Golgi apparatus, where packaging into clathrin-coated secretory granules takes place. Maturation of the secretory granule is associated with loss of the clathrin coating and conversion of proinsulin into **insulin** and a smaller connecting peptide, or **C peptide,** by proteolytic cleavage at two sites along the peptide chain. Normal mature (uncoated) secretory granules contain insulin and C peptide in equimolar amounts and only small quantities of proinsulin, a small portion of which consists of partially cleaved intermediates.

Biochemistry

Proinsulin (Figure 18–3) consists of a single chain of 86 amino acids, which includes the A and B chains of the insulin molecule plus a connecting segment of 35 amino acids. Converting enzymes (probably trypsin-like and carboxypeptidase-B-like proteases) cleave off two pairs of dibasic amino acids (three arginines and one lysine) from the proinsulin molecule as shown in Figure 18–3. The result is a 51-amino-acid insulin molecule and a 31-amino-acid residue, the C peptide.

A small amount of proinsulin produced by the pancreas escapes cleavage and is secreted intact into the bloodstream, along with insulin and C peptide. Most anti-insulin sera used in the standard immunoassay for insulin cross-react with proinsulin; about 3–5% of immunoreactive insulin extracted from human pancreas is actually proinsulin. Because proinsulin is not removed by the liver, it has a half-life three to four times that of insulin. This allows proinsulin to accumulate in the blood, where it accounts for 12–20% of the circulating immunoreactive "insulin" in the basal state in humans. Human proinsulin has about 7–8% of the biologic activity of insulin. The kidney is the principal site of proinsulin degradation.

Of the two major split proinsulin products, the one split at arginine 32–33 of the major proinsulin-like molecule present in plasma, far exceeding the barely detectable 65–66 split product. In control subjects, concentrations of proinsulin and 32–33 split proinsulin after an overnight fast averaged 2.3 and 2.2 pmol/L, respectively, with corresponding postprandial rises to 10 and 20 pmol/L.

C peptide, the 31-amino-acid residue (MW 3000) formed during cleavage of insulin from proinsulin,

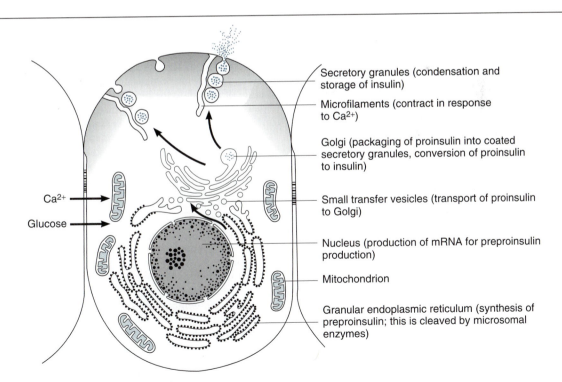

Figure 18–2. Structural components of the pancreatic B cell involved in glucose-induced biosynthesis and release. Schematic representation of secretory granular alignment on microfilament "tracks" that contract in response to calcium. (Based on data presented by Orci L: A portrait of the pancreatic B cell. Diabetologia 1974;10:163.) (Modified and reproduced, with permission, from Junqueira LC, Carneiro J, Long JA: *Basic Histology,* 5th ed. Lange, 1986.)

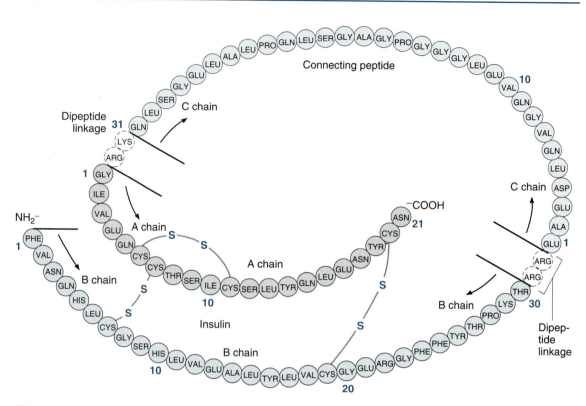

Figure 18–3. Structure of human proinsulin C peptides and insulin molecules connected at two sites by dipeptide links.

has no known biologic activity. It is released from the B cells in equimolar amounts with insulin. It is not removed by the liver but is degraded or excreted chiefly by the kidney. It has a half-life three to four times that of insulin. In the basal state after an overnight fast, the average concentration of C peptide may be as high as 1000 pmol/L.

Insulin is a protein consisting of 51 amino acids contained within two peptide chains: an A chain, with 21 amino acids; and a B chain, with 30 amino acids. The chains are connected by two disulfide bridges as shown in Figure 18–3. In addition, there is an intrachain disulfide bridge that links positions 6 and 11 in the A chain. The molecular weight of human insulin is 5808.

Human insulin differs only slightly in amino acid composition from the two mammalian insulins, which have been used for therapeutic insulin replacement. Pork insulin differs from human by only one amino acid—alanine instead of threonine at the carboxyl terminus of the B chain (position B 30). Beef insulin differs by three amino acids—alanine instead of threonine at A 8 as well as the B 30 position and valine instead of isoleucine at A 10.

Endogenous insulin has a circulatory half-life of 3–5 minutes. It is catabolized chiefly by insulinases in liver, kidney, and placenta. Approximately 50% of insulin is removed in a single pass through the liver.

Secretion

The human pancreas secretes about 40–50 units of insulin per day in normal adults. The basal concentration of insulin in the blood of fasting humans averages 10 μU/mL (0.4 ng/mL, or 69 pmol/L). In normal control subjects, insulin seldom rises above 100 μU/mL (690 pmol/L) after standard meals. There is an increase in peripheral insulin concentration beginning 8–10 minutes after ingestion of food and reaching peak concentration in peripheral blood by 30–45 minutes. This is followed by a rapid decline in postprandial plasma glucose concentration, which returns to baseline values by 90–120 minutes (Figure 18–4).

Basal insulin secretion, which occurs in the absence of exogenous stimuli, is the quantity of insulin secreted in the fasting state. Although it is known that plasma glucose levels below 80–100 mg/dL (4.4–5.6 mmol/L) do not stimulate insulin release, it has also been demonstrated that the presence of glucose is necessary (in in vitro systems) for most other known regulators of insulin secretion to be effective.

Stimulated insulin secretion is that which occurs in response to exogenous stimuli. In vivo, this is the response of the B cell to ingested meals. Glucose is the most potent stimulant of insulin release. The perfused rat pancreas has demonstrated a biphasic release of insulin in response to glucose (Figure 18–5). When the glucose concentration in the system is increased

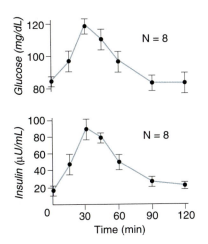

Figure 18–4. Plasma glucose and insulin response to a standard 530-kcal breakfast in normal subjects.

passive diffusion, which is facilitated by a specific membrane protein termed glucose transporter-2. By virtue of its relatively low affinity for glucose, this protein more effectively facilitates transport of glucose during the hyperglycemia after meals than at the lower levels of blood glucose during an overnight fast. There is a body of data suggesting that *metabolism* of glucose is essential in stimulating insulin release. Indeed, agents such as 2-deoxyglucose that inhibit the metabolism of glucose interfere with release of insulin. The rate-limiting step in glucose metabolism by the pancreatic B cell appears to be the phosphorylation of glucose by the low-affinity enzyme glucokinase.

Insulin release has been shown to require calcium. It has been proposed that mature insulin-containing granules in the B cell attach linearly to microtubules that contract after exposure to high intracellular calcium, thereby ejecting the granules (Figure 18–2). The following effects of glucose on calcium ion movement have been demonstrated: (1) Calcium uptake is increased by glucose stimulation of the B cell. (2) Calcium efflux from the cell is retarded by some action of glucose. (3) Mobilization of calcium from mitochondrial compartments occurs secondary to cAMP induction by glucose.

cAMP is another important modulator of insulin release. As mentioned above, glucose has been shown to directly induce cAMP formation. Furthermore, many nonglucose stimuli to insulin release are

suddenly, an initial short-lived burst of insulin release occurs (the **early phase**); if the glucose concentration is held at this level, the insulin release gradually falls off and then begins to rise again to a steady level (the **late phase**). However, sustained levels of high glucose stimulation ($\geq$ 4 hours in vitro or > 24 hours in vivo) results in a reversible desensitization of the B cell response to glucose but not to other stimuli.

Glucose is known to enter the pancreatic B cell by

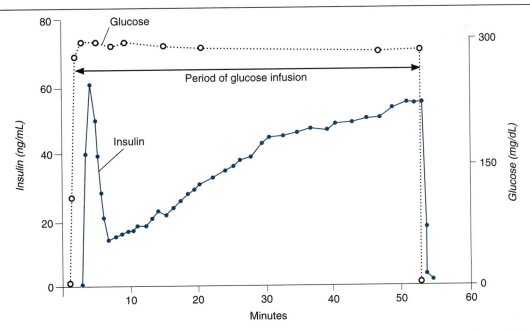

Figure 18–5. Multiphasic response of the in vitro perfused pancreas during constant stimulation with glucose. (Modified from Grodsky GM et al: Further studies on the dynamic aspects of insulin release in vitro with evidence for a two-compartmental storage system. Acta Diabetol Lat 1969;6[Suppl 1]:554.)

known to increase intracellular cAMP. Elevations of cAMP, however, will not stimulate insulin release in the absence of glucose.

Other factors involved in the regulation of insulin secretion are summarized in Table 18–2. These factors can be divided into three categories: **direct stimulants,** which are known to stimulate insulin release directly; **amplifiers,** which appear to potentiate the response of the B cell to glucose; and **inhibitors.** The action of the amplifier substances, many of which are gastrointestinal hormones stimulated by ingestion of meals, explains the observation that insulin response to an ingested meal is greater than the response of intravenously administered substrates.

Insulin Receptors & Insulin Action

Insulin action begins with binding of insulin to a receptor on the surface of the target cell membrane. Many cells of the body appear to have specific cell surface insulin receptors. In fat, liver, and muscle cells, binding of insulin to these receptors is associated with the biologic response of these tissues to the hormone. These receptors bind insulin rapidly, with high specificity and with an affinity high enough to bind picomolar amounts.

It has recently been demonstrated that insulin receptors are membrane glycoproteins composed of two subunits, a larger alpha subunit (MW 130,000), which extends extracellularly and is involved in binding the insulin molecule, and a smaller beta subunit (MW 90,000), which is predominantly cytoplasmic and contains a tyrosine kinase that becomes activated during insulin binding and results in autophosphorylation of the beta subunit itself. After insulin is bound to its receptor, a number of insulin-receptor complexes are internalized. However, it remains controversial whether these internalized complexes contribute to further action of insulin or whether they limit continued insulin action by exposing insulin to intracellular scavenger lysosomes.

Two models for insulin action have been pro-posed. One involves a cascade of phosphorylations emanating from the activated kinase region that induces an intracellular compartment of proteins, including the glucose transporter-4 (see below), transferrin, the low-density lipoprotein receptor, and the insulin-like growth factor II (IGF-II) receptor, to move to the cell surface. When these proteins, which are sequestered intracellularly during the postabsorptive period, move to the cell surface during feeding they facilitate transport of nutrients into insulin target tissues and can promote growth by giving circulating IGF-II access to a cell surface receptor. Within this model, genetic defects distal to the insulin receptor could result in "postreceptor" insulin resistance. Possible defects include abnormalities in the enzymes responsible for phosphorylation of the glucose transporter protein, mutation of the glucose transporter itself, or abnormalities in its processing. Moreover, abnormalities in phosphatase enzymes might account for a delay in the normal restoration of the insulin receptor to its surface membrane locus, resulting in resistance to the further action of insulin. A second model invokes the hydrolysis of a membrane glycolipid by insulin-stimulated phospholipase C activity. Potential "second messengers" such as inositol monophosphate, or diacylglycerol may mediate the intracellular response to insulin, with diacylglycerol promoting intracellular phosphorylations by activating protein kinase C (see Chapter 3 and Figure 3–7).

Abnormalities of insulin receptors—in concentration, affinity, or both—will affect insulin action. **"Down-regulation"** is a phenomenon in which the number of insulin receptors is decreased in response to chronically elevated circulating insulin levels, probably by increased intracellular degradation. When insulin levels are low, on the other hand, receptor binding is up-regulated. Conditions associated with high insulin levels and lowered insulin binding to the receptor include obesity, high intake of carbohydrates, and (perhaps) chronic exogenous overinsulinization. Conditions associated with low insulin levels and increased insulin binding include exercise and fasting. The presence of excess amounts of cortisol decreases insulin binding to the receptor, although it is not clear if this is a direct effect of the hormone itself or one that is mediated through accompanying increases in the insulin level.

Metabolic Effects of Insulin

The major function of insulin is to promote **storage of ingested nutrients.** Although insulin directly or indirectly affects the function of almost every tissue in the body, the discussion here will be limited to a brief overview of the effects of insulin on the three major tissues specialized for energy storage: liver, muscle, and adipose tissue. In addition, the **paracrine effects** of insulin will be discussed briefly. The section on hormonal control of nutrient metabolism (see below) presents a detailed discussion of the ef-

Table 18–2. Regulation of insulin release in humans.

Stimulants of insulin release
  Glucose, mannose
  Leucine
  Vagal stimulation
  Sulfonylureas
Amplifiers of glucose-induced insulin release
  1. Enteric hormones:
      Glucagon-like peptide I (7–37)
      Gastrin inhibitory peptide
      Cholecystokinin
      Secretin, gastrin
  2. Neural amplifiers: beta-adrenergic stimulation
  3. Amino acids: arginine
Inhibitors of insulin release
  Neural: alpha-adrenergic effect of catecholamines
  Humoral: somatostatin
  Drugs: diazoxide, phenytoin, vinblastine, colchicine

fects of insulin and glucagon on the regulation of intermediary metabolism.

A. Paracrine Effects: The effects of the products of endocrine cells on surrounding cells are termed "paracrine" effects, in contrast to actions that take place at sites distant from the secreting cells, which are termed "endocrine" effects (Chapter 1). Paracrine effects of the B and D cells on the close-lying A cells (Figure 18–1) are of considerable importance in the endocrine pancreas. The first target cells reached by insulin are the pancreatic A cells at the periphery of the pancreatic islets. In the presence of insulin, A cell secretion of glucagon is reduced. In addition, somatostatin, which is released from D cells in response to most of the same stimuli that provoke insulin release, also acts to inhibit glucagon secretion.

Because glucose stimulates only B and D cells (whose products then inhibit A cells) whereas amino acids stimulate glucagon as well as insulin, the type and amounts of islet hormones released during a meal depend on the ratio of ingested carbohydrate to protein. The higher the carbohydrate content of a meal, the less glucagon will be released by any amino acids absorbed. In contrast, a predominantly protein meal will result in relatively greater glucagon secretion, because amino acids are less effective at stimulating insulin release in the absence of concurrent hyperglycemia but are potent stimulators of A cells.

B. Endocrine Effects: (Table 18–3.)

1. Liver—The first major organ reached by insulin via the bloodstream is the liver. Insulin exerts its action on the liver in two major ways:

Table 18–3. Endocrine effects of insulin.

Effects on liver
Anabolic effects:
  Promotes glycogenesis
  Increases synthesis of triglycerides, cholesterol, and
    VLDL.
  Increases protein synthesis
Anticatabolic effects:
  Inhibits glycogenolysis.
  Inhibits ketogenesis.
  Inhibits gluconeogenesis.
Effects on muscle
Promotes protein synthesis:
  Increases amino acid transport.
  Stimulates ribosomal protein synthesis.
Promotes glycogen synthesis:
  Increases glucose transport.
  Enhances activity of glycogen synthetase.
  Inhibits activity of glycogen phosphorylase.
Effects on fat
Promotes triglyceride storage:
  Induces lipoprotein lipase, making fatty acids available
    for absorption into fat cells.
  Increases glucose transport into fat cells, thus increasing
    availability of α-glycerol phosphate for triglyceride syn-
    thesis.
  Inhibits intracellular lipolysis.

a. Insulin promotes anabolism—Insulin promotes glycogen synthesis and storage at the same time it inhibits glycogen breakdown. These effects are mediated by changes in the activity of enzymes in the glycogen synthesis pathway (see below). The liver has a maximum storage capacity of 100–110 g of glycogen, or approximately 440 kcal of energy.

Insulin increases both protein and triglyceride synthesis and VLDL formation by the liver. It also inhibits gluconeogenesis and promotes glycolysis through its effects on enzymes of the glycolytic pathway.

b. Insulin inhibits catabolism—Insulin acts to reverse the catabolic events of the postabsorptive state by inhibiting hepatic glycogenolysis, ketogenesis, and gluconeogenesis.

2. Muscle—Insulin promotes protein synthesis in muscle by increasing amino acid transport as well as by stimulating ribosomal protein synthesis. In addition, insulin promotes glycogen synthesis to replace glycogen stores expended by muscle activity. This is accomplished by increasing glucose transport into the muscle cell, enhancing the activity of glycogen synthetase, and inhibiting the activity of glycogen phosphorylase. Approximately 500–600 g of glycogen is stored in the muscle tissue of a 70-kg man, but because of the lack of glucose 6-phosphatase in this tissue, it cannot be used as a source of blood glucose. except by indirectly supplying the liver with lactate for conversion to glucose.

3. Adipose tissue—Fat, in the form of triglyceride, is the most efficient means of storing energy. It provides 9 kcal per gram of stored substrate, as opposed to the 4 kcal/g generally provided by protein or carbohydrate. In the typical 70-kg man, the energy content of adipose tissue is about 100,000 kcal.

Insulin acts to promote triglyceride storage in adipocytes by a number of mechanisms: (I) It induces the production of lipoprotein lipase (this is the lipoprotein lipase that is bound to endothelial cells in adipose tissue and other vascular beds), which leads to hydrolysis of triglycerides from circulating lipoproteins. (2) By increasing glucose transport into fat cells, insulin increases the availability of α-glycerol phosphate, a substance used in the esterification of free fatty acids into triglycerides. (3) Insulin inhibits intracellular lipolysis of stored triglyceride by inhibiting intracellular lipase (also called "hormone-sensitive lipase").

Glucose Transporter Proteins

Glucose oxidation is a major source of energy for many cells of the body and is especially essential for brain function. Since cell membranes are impermeable to hydrophilic molecules such as glucose, all cells require carrier proteins to transport glucose across the lipid bilayers into the cytosol. While the intestine and kidney have an energy dependent Na^+-glucose cotransporter, all other cells have non-energy-dependent transporters that facilitate diffusion of glucose from a higher concentration to a lower concentration across cell membranes. At least five "facilitative glucose transporters" have been described, and these have different affinities for glucose. They have been termed GLUT 1, GLUT 2, GLUT 3, GLUT 4, and GLUT 5, with the numbers designating the order of their identification (Table 18–4).

GLUT 1 is present in all human tissues. It appears to mediate basal glucose uptake, since it has a very high affinity for glucose and therefore is able to transport glucose at relatively low concentrations as found in the basal state. For this reason, it is an important component of the brain vascular system (blood-brain barrier) to ensure adequate transport of plasma glucose into the central nervous system. GLUT 3, which is also found in all tissues, is the major glucose transporter on the neuronal surface. It also has a very high affinity for glucose and is responsible for transferring glucose from the cerebrospinal fluid into neuronal cells.

In contrast, GLUT 2 has a very low affinity for glucose and seems to act as a transporter only when plasma glucose levels are relatively high, such as postprandially. It is the major transporter of glucose in the pancreatic B cell and hepatic cells, so that diffusion of glucose into these cells is facilitated only when hyperglycemia exists. This prevents hepatic uptake of glucose or inappropriate insulin discharge during the basal state or during fasting.

GLUT 4 is found in two major insulin target tissues: skeletal muscle and adipose tissue. It appears to be sequestered mainly within an intracellular compartment of these cells and thus is not able to function as a glucose transporter until a signal from insulin results in translocation of GLUT 4 to the cell membrane, where it facilitates glucose entry into these storage tissues after a meal.

GLUT 5 is expressed on the brush border of human small intestine cells, and its biochemical properties suggest that it is mainly a fructose transporter. Since a large fraction of calories is derived from fructose, this relatively high-affinity transporter is responsible for its absorption as well as its uptake by liver cells and spermatozoa, where it is also highly expressed.

Islet Amyloid Polypeptide (IAPP), or Amylin

IAPP, or amylin, is a recently identified peptide made up of 37 amino acids which is stored with insulin in the pancreatic B cell, but only in a low ratio of one molecule of amylin to 100 of insulin. It is cosecreted with insulin in response to glucose and other B cell stimulators. Amylin's function has not been determined, but it appears to produce amyloid deposits in pancreatic islets of most patients with type II diabetes of long duration. These amyloid deposits are insoluble fibrillar proteins (containing mainly amylin as well as its precursor peptide) which encroach upon and may even occur within pancreatic B cells. There have been reports of amylin producing insulin resistance when administered to animals in supraphysiologic doses, but evidence currently available does not support this activity in humans. Islets of nondiabetic elderly persons often contain some amyloid deposits indistinguishable from those in diabetics but to a much lesser extent. This observation—as well as the failure to detect mutations of amylin in type II diabetes—suggests that the extensive deposition of amyloid in islets of patients with type II diabetes is a consequence of their disordered and hyperstimulated islet function rather than a direct genetic effect that produces an abnormal amylin molecule.

2. GLUCAGON

Biochemistry

Pancreatic glucagon, whose gene is located on human chromosome 2, is a single-chain polypeptide consisting of 29 amino acids with a molecular weight of 3485 (Figure 18–6). It is synthesized in the A cells on the islets of Langerhans and derived from a large 160-amino-acid precursor molecule that is five to six times larger than glucagon. Within this proglucagon molecule are several other peptides connected in tandem: glicentin-related peptide, glucagon, glucagon-like peptide 1 (GLP-1), and glucagon-like peptide 2 (GLP-2). The combination of glicentin-related peptide with glucagon consists of 69 amino acids and comprises the hormone glicentin, which is predominantly secreted from the intestine and not the pan-

Table 18–4. Human glucose transporters.

Name	Major Sites of Expression	Affinity for Glucose[1]	Chromosomal Location of Gene
GLUT 1	Brain vasculature, red blood cells, all tissues	High (Km = 1 mmol/L)	1
GLUT 2	Liver, pancreatic B cell; serosal surfaces of gut and kidney	Low (Km 15–20 mmol/L)	3
GLUT 3	Brain neurons; also found in all tissues	High (Km < 1 mmol/L)	12
GLUT 4	Muscle, fat cells	Medium (Km = 2.5–5 mmol/L)	17
GLUT 5	Jejunum, liver, spermatozoa	Medium (Km = 6 mmol/L)	1

[1]Km represents the level of blood glucose at which the transporter has reached one-half of its maximum capacity to transport glucose. It is inversely proportionate to the affinity.

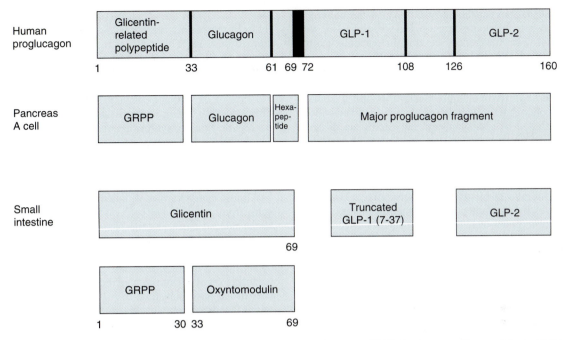

Figure 18–6. Tissue-specific secretory products of human proglucagon. (GLP-1, glucagon-like peptide-1; GLP-2, glucagon-like peptide-2; GRPP, glicentin-related polypeptide.)

creas (Figure 18–6). Both GLP-1 and GLP-2 increase after meals. An endogenous truncated derivative of GLP-1, with the first six of its 37 amino acids absent (GLP-1 [7–37]), is an extremely potent stimulator of pancreatic B cells and is felt to be the major physiologic gut factor ("incretin") which potentiates glucose-induced insulin secretion after meals. It is released by small intestinal L cells of the duodenum during mixed meals and is several times more potent than glucagon itself as an insulinotropic secretagogue, whereas intact GLP-1 (1–37) and GLP-2 do not stimulate insulin secretion. In healthy humans, the average fasting plasma immunoreactive glucagon level is 75 pg/mL (25 pmol/L). Only 30–40% of this is actually pancreatic glucagon, the remainder being a heterogeneous composite of higher-molecular-weight molecules with glucagon immunoreactivity such as proglucagon, glicentin, truncated GLP-1, and GLP-2. The circulation half-life of pancreatic glucagon is 3–6 minutes. Glucagon is mainly removed by the liver and kidney.

Secretion

Glucagon secretion is inhibited by glucose—in contrast to the effect of glucose on insulin secretion. There are conflicting data about whether the effect of glucose is a direct one on the A cell or whether it is mediated via release of insulin or somatostatin, both of which are known to inhibit the A cell directly (see above).

In addition, since γ-aminobutyric acid (GABA) is released by B cells and its receptors have recently been detected on A cells, GABA may participate in the inhibition of A cells during B cell stimulation.

Many amino acids stimulate glucagon release, although there are differences in their ability to do so. Some, such as arginine, release both glucagon and insulin; others (eg, alanine) stimulate primarily glucagon release. Leucine, a good stimulant for insulin release, does not stimulate glucagon. Other substances that promote glucagon release are catecholamines, the gastrointestinal hormones (cholecystokinin [CCK], gastrin, and gastric inhibitory polypeptide [GIP]), and glucocorticoids. Both sympathetic and parasympathetic (vagal) stimulation promote glucagon release; this is especially important in augmenting the response of the A cell to hypoglycemia. High levels of circulating fatty acid are associated with suppression of glucagon secretion.

Action of Glucagon

In contrast to insulin, which promotes energy storage in a variety of tissues, glucagon is a humoral mechanism for making energy available to the tissues between meals, when ingested food is not available for absorption. Glucagon stimulates the breakdown of stored glycogen, maintains hepatic output of glucose from amino acid precursors (gluconeogenesis), and promotes hepatic output of ketone bodies from fatty acid precursors (ketogenesis). The liver, because of its geographic proximity to the pancreas, represents the major target organ for glucagon, with portal vein glucagon concentrations reaching as high as 300–500 pg/mL (100–166 pmol/L). Binding of glucagon to its receptor on hepatocytes results in activation of adenylyl cyclase and generation of cAMP, which both promotes glycogenolysis and stimulates gluconeogenesis. Uptake of alanine by liver cells is facilitated by glucagon, and fatty acids are directed away from reesterification to triglycerides and toward ketogenic pathways (see below). It is unclear whether physiologic levels of glucagon affect tissues other than the liver.

The ratio of insulin to glucagon affects key target tissues by mediating phosphorylation or dephosphorylation (either or both) of key enzymes affecting nutrient metabolism. In addition, this ratio increases or decreases actual quantities of certain enzymes, thereby controlling the flux of these nutrients into or out of storage (see also Chapter 17.)

3. SOMATOSTATIN

The gene for somatostatin is on the long arm of chromosome 3. It codes for a 116-amino-acid peptide, preprosomatostatin, from whose carboxyl terminal is cleaved the hormone somatostatin, a 14-amino-acid cyclic polypeptide with a molecular weight of 1640 (Figure 18–7). It is present in D cells at the periphery of the human islet (Figure 18–1). It was first identified in the hypothalamus and owes its name to its ability to inhibit release of growth hormone (pituitary somatotropin). Since that time, somatostatin has been identified in a number of tissues, including many areas of the brain, the gastrointestinal tract, and the pancreas. In the central nervous system and the pancreas, somatostatin-14 predominates, but approxi-

mately 5–10% of the somatostatin-like immunoreactivity in the brain is due to a 28-amino-acid peptide, somatostatin-28. This consists of an amino terminal region of 14 amino acids and a carboxyl terminal segment containing somatostatin-14. In small intestine, the larger molecule is more prevalent, with 70–75% of the hormone having 28 amino acids and only 25–30% being somatostatin-14. In contrast, pancreatic D cells synthesize only somatostatin-14. The larger peptide somatostatin-28 is ten times more potent than somatostatin-14 in inhibiting growth hormone and insulin, whereas somatostatin-14 is more effective on inhibition of glucagon release.

Almost every known stimulator of release of insulin from pancreatic B cells also promotes somatostatin release from D cells. This includes glucose, arginine, gastrointestinal hormones, and tolbutamide. The importance of circulating somatostatin is unclear, since a major role of this peptide may be as a paracrine regulator of the pancreatic islet and the tissues of the gastrointestinal tract (Chapter 17). Physiologic levels of somatostatin in humans seldom exceed 80 pg/mL (49 pmol/L). The metabolic clearance of exogenously infused somatostatin in humans is extremely rapid; the half-life of the hormone is less than 3 minutes.

Recently, molecular cloning has demonstrated the existence of at least five somatostatin receptors (SSTR1–5) which are G protein-coupled receptors with seven membrane-spanning domains. They vary in size from 364 to 418 amino acids (with 105 amino acids invariant) and are found in the central nervous system and in a wide variety of peripheral tissues including the pituitary gland, the small intestine, and the pancreas. These receptors act by activating tyrosine phosphatase, which by dephosphorylating proteins interferes with the secretory process. Inhibition of insulin secretion is due to binding of SSTR5,

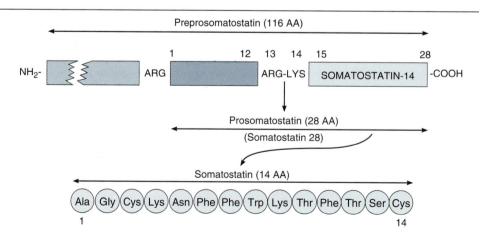

Figure 18–7. Amino acid sequence of somatostatin and its cleavage from dibasic amino acid residue in prosomatostatin and preprosomatostatin.

whereas inhibition of growth hormone release is due to effects of SSTR2. This explains why an analog of somatostatin, octreotide, which has a much greater affinity for SSTR2 than for SSTR5, can be so effective in correcting growth hormone excess without much of an effect on carbohydrate tolerance when used to treat acromegaly.

Somatostatin acts in several ways to restrain the movement of nutrients from the intestinal tract into the circulation. It prolongs gastric emptying time, decreases gastric acid and gastrin production, diminishes pancreatic exocrine secretion, decreases splanchnic blood flow, and retards xylose absorption. Neutralization of circulating somatostatin with antisomatostatin serum is associated with enhanced nutrient absorption in dogs. This implies that at least some of the effects of somatostatin are truly endocrine, as opposed to the paracrine effects discussed earlier.

4. PANCREATIC POLYPEPTIDE

Pancreatic polypeptide (PP) is found in F cells located chiefly in islets in the posterior portion of the head of the pancreas. PP is a 36-amino-acid peptide with a molecular weight of 4200. Little is known about its biosynthesis. Circulating levels of the peptide increase in response to a mixed meal; however, intravenous infusion of glucose or triglyceride does not produce such a rise, and intravenous amino acids cause only a small increase. Vagotomy abolishes the response to an ingested meal.

In healthy subjects, basal levels of PP average 24 ± 4 pmol/L and may become elevated owing to a variety of factors including old age, alcohol abuse, diarrhea, chronic renal failure, hypoglycemia, or inflammatory disorders. Values above 300 pmol/L are found in most patients with pancreatic endocrine tumors such as glucagonoma or VIPoma and in all patients with tumors of the pancreatic F cell. As many as 20% of patients with insulinoma and one-third of those with gastrinomas also have pancreatic polypeptide plasma concentrations of greater than 300 pmol/L.

The physiologic action of PP is unknown. It is discussed further in Chapter 17.

II. DIABETES MELLITUS

Clinical diabetes mellitus is a syndrome of disordered metabolism with inappropriate hyperglycemia due either to an absolute deficiency of insulin secretion or a reduction in the biologic effectiveness of insulin (or both).

CLASSIFICATION

Traditionally, diabetes has been classified according to the patient's age at onset of symptoms (juvenile-onset versus adult-onset). In 1979, the NIH Diabetes Data Group recommended that diabetes mellitus be classified into one of two major types according to dependence on exogenous insulin: **insulin-dependent** (type I) or **non–insulin-dependent** (type II) diabetes mellitus (Table 18–5).

The above "therapeutic" classification is far from satisfactory. The term "type II" implies a single type of disorder even though patients who are not dependent on insulin therapy to sustain life represent a variety of heterogeneous disorders, including all diabetic conditions that are not type I diabetes. Furthermore, many patients whose diabetes is not "insulin-dependent" may be managed with insulin therapy by their physicians yet are still identified as being "non-insulin-dependent." Likewise, occasional young adults with a classic onset of diabetic ketoacidosis associated with islet cell antibodies may enter remissions during which insulin therapy is discontinued, rendering them "non-insulin-dependent" despite an evident pathogenetic mechanism characteristic of patients with IDDM. These inadequacies of the current "therapeutic" classifications have led to semantic confusion about whether type II patients can become type I patients and vice versa.

With the establishment of an autoimmune pathogenesis for clinical type I diabetes and immunoassays to detect islet cell antibodies, the classification of diabetes should be based on etiologic rather than therapeutic criteria.

One possibility would be "immune-dependent diabetes mellitus" as one type, with all the other types being termed "nonimmune-dependent diabetes mellitus," so that we can retain the acronyms IDDM and NIDDM.

TYPE I: INSULIN-DEPENDENT (IMMUNE-DEPENDENT) DIABETES MELLITUS (IDDM)

Type I is a severe form of diabetes mellitus and is associated with ketosis in the untreated state. About 10–20% of diabetics in North America and Europe are of the insulin-dependent type. It is most common in young individuals but occurs occasionally in nonobese adults. It is a catabolic disorder in which circulating insulin is virtually absent, plasma glucagon is elevated, and the pancreatic B cells fail to respond to all known insulinogenic stimuli. In the absence of insulin, the three main target tissues of insulin (liver,

Table 18–5. Clinical classification of diabetes mellitus.[1]

Terminology and Estimated Prevalence	Ketosis	Islet Cell Antibodies	HLA Association	Treatment
INSULIN-DEPENDENT DIABETES (IDDM; type I) (10–20% of all diabetics)	Marked	Usually present at onset	Yes	1. Insulin 2. Diet
NON-INSULIN-DEPENDENT DIABETES (NIDDM; type II) (80–90% of all diabetics) Nonobese (15% of NIDDM patients)	Absent	Absent	No	1. Eucaloric diet alone or– 2. Diet plus sulfonylurea, metformin, or insulin
Obese (85% of NIDDM patients)	Absent	Absent	No	1. Weight reduction 2. Hypocaloric diet plus sulfonylureas, metformin, or insulin for symptomatic control only
SECONDARY DIABETES: Diabetes mellitus and impaired glucose tolerance secondary to or associated with other conditions, eg, pancreatic disease, drug toxicity, endocrine disorders, genetic disease, insulin receptor abnormalities with acanthosis nigricans.				Treatment varies according to the specific condition. In general, removal or correction of offending agent if possible, diet, and insulin are the foundations of treatment. See text for details.

[1]Gestational diabetes is discussed in Chapter 16.

muscle, and fat) not only fail to appropriately take up absorbed nutrients but continue to deliver glucose, amino acids, and fatty acids into the bloodstream from their respective storage depots. Furthermore, alterations in fat metabolism lead to the production and accumulation of ketones. This inappropriate persistence of the fasted state postprandially can be reversed by the administration of insulin.

Genetics of Type I Diabetes

Studies in monozygotic twins suggest that genetic influences are less marked in type I diabetes than in type II diabetes. Only 30–40% of identical twins of type I diabetic patients will develop the disease. This also suggests that an environmental factor is required for induction of diabetes in these cases. In contrast, the identical twin of a type II diabetic is much more prone to develop diabetes within a year of onset of the disease in the sibling.

Type I diabetes is believed to result from an infectious or toxic environmental insult to the pancreatic B cells in genetically predisposed persons whose aggressive immune system destroys pancreatic B cells while overcoming the invasive agent. Environmental factors that have been associated with altered pancreatic islet cell function include viruses (mumps, rubella, coxsackievirus B4), toxic chemical agents such as vacor (a nitrophenylurea rat poison), and other destructive cytotoxins such as hydrogen cyanide from spoiled tapioca or cassava root.

Type I diabetes is strongly associated with an increased frequency of certain HLA antigens. Genes coding for these antigens are on the short arm of chromosome 6. They consist of the class I genes, termed A, B, and C, whose protein biosynthesis

products are found on the surfaces of all body cells except red blood cells and sperm; and class II genes, termed D, located closer to the centromere of chromosome 6. These latter genes code for the class II antigens expressed on the surfaces of macrophages and B lymphocytes. These antigens are glycoproteins that allow the immune system to distinguish other body cells from foreign invaders such as viruses, bacteria, or fungi. The predominant HLA antigens associated with type I diabetes vary in different racial groups. Thus, HLA-B8, -B15, -B18, -Cw3, -DR3, and -DR4 occur with increased frequency on leukocytes of Caucasian diabetics, whereas of the above, only HLA-DR3 and -DR4 appear to be correlated with type I diabetes in Asians, Africans, and Latin-Americans. Either HLA-DR3 or -DR4 occurs in about 95% of Caucasian type I diabetics, compared with 45–50% of Caucasian controls. It has been shown that HLA-DQ genes are even more specific markers of susceptibility to type I diabetes, since a particular variety (HLA-DQw3.2) is invariably found in the HLA-DR4 patients with type I diabetes while a "protective" gene (HLA-DQw3.1), which has an aspartic acid encoded in region 57 of the HLA-DQ beta chain, is prevalent in the HLA-DR4 controls. Moreover, HLA-DR2, which is generally protective against type I diabetes, seems to be so by virtue of its linkage to HLA-DQ genes which express antigens containing aspartic acid at position 57 of their beta chains.

It remains a mystery why people with certain HLA types are predisposed to development of type I diabetes. The concept of an autoimmune destruction of pancreatic B cells with selective loss of immune tolerance is supported by evidence that immune suppression therapy interrupts progression to insulin deficiency in a number of newly diagnosed IDDM patients. Moreover, extensive infiltration with both helper and cytotoxic T lymphocytes is present in the islets of children who just developed IDDM, and their serum contains autoantibodies against structural and secretory proteins of the pancreatic B cells before the onset of IDDM and for some time after diagnosis.

On the strength of the above evidence, a theory for autoimmune B cell destruction has been proposed based on molecular mimicry, wherein the immune system mistakenly targets B cell proteins that share homologies with certain viral peptides. The efficiency of presenting certain proteins depends on the composition of the class II antigens on the surface of the antigen-presenting cells (macrophages). Maximum susceptibility to IDDM was found when a certain HLA-DQ gene was present that expressed on the macrophage surface both a "nonaspartic" amino acid at position 57 on the DQ beta chain and an arginine at position 52 on the DQ alpha chain. Structural analysis of the DQ protein suggested that this configuration facilitated presentation of certain antigens to the immune system, whereas either an aspartic acid in the DQ beta chain at the 57 position or a "nonarginine" at the DQ alpha chain at the 52 position interfered with efficient presentation of certain peptides such as those found during the processing of coxsackie B4 viruses.

Circulating islet cell autoantibodies, virtually absent in nondiabetics, have been detected in as many as 85% of type I diabetics tested in the first few weeks after onset of diabetes. Moreover, when sensitive immunoassays are used, up to 60% of these patients also have detectable antibodies to insulin prior to receiving insulin therapy, and these are especially prevalent with an onset of disease in childhood. The high prevalence of these islet cell and insulin autoantibodies in type I diabetes, as well as in certain of their siblings who later develop overt diabetes, supports the concept that autoimmune mechanisms may contribute significantly to progressive B cell destruction.

Most of the islet cell antibodies are directed against glutamic acid decarboxylase (GAD), an enzyme localized within pancreatic B cells. This enzyme has isoforms with molecular weights of 65,000 and 67,000 which are also found in central nervous system "inhibitory" neurons that secrete γ-aminobutyric acid. Evidence that a rare neurologic condition, "stiff man syndrome," was associated with an autoimmune destruction of neurons containing GAD—and that these patients' sera also had islet cell antibodies—led to the discovery that antibodies to GAD made up the bulk of antibodies previously described in IDDM as being against a 64-kDa antigen in pancreatic B cells. The concept of "molecular mimicry" is supported by the recent finding that part of the protein component of the coxsackie B4 virus contains a sequence of 24 amino acids with considerable homology to GAD.

Manifestations of stiff man syndrome have not been reported in patients with IDDM even though their islet cell antibodies contain a major component that reacts in vitro with GAD-containing neurons. The blood-brain barrier may have some protective effect against neuronal damage of a degree that might cause stiff man syndrome in IDDM. However, investigations are in progress to see if autoimmunity to GAD plays a role in some severe forms of peripheral neuropathy.

Another candidate for the molecular mimicry hypothesis is bovine serum albumin, which has a region of homology with a B cell surface protein, p69. Children who were exclusively breast-fed as infants had a statistically lower incidence of IDDM than those who received cow's milk. Moreover, 142 Finnish children with newly diagnosed IDDM had high titers of antibodies against bovine albumin, in contrast to much lower levels in a control population of children. It is postulated that immature gut enzymes in infants permit absorption of peptide fragments of bovine albumin that induce immune responses which attack B cell protein p69. However, subsequent failure to demonstrate cellular immunity to bovine albumin, despite humoral immunity, has weakened support for this antigen as a primary initiator of B cell destruction in IDDM.

A genetic link to chromosome 11 has been identified in type I diabetes. Population studies of a polymorphic DNA locus flanking the 5' region of the insulin gene on chromosome 11 revealed a slight, but statistically significant linkage between IDDM and this genetic locus in a Caucasian population of type I diabetics. This polymorphic locus does not seem either to encode a protein or to affect insulin gene expression, but it may represent a marker for a linked gene relating to B cell replication such as IGF-2, which is contiguous with the insulin gene on chromosome 11, or to some other linked gene whose function influences susceptibility to type I diabetes. The established genetic association with the HLA region of chromosome 6 contributes much more (about 40%) to the genetic susceptibility to IDDM than does this locus flanking the insulin gene on chromosome 11, which contributes about 10%. The recommended nomenclature for these two known susceptibility gene associations are *IDDM1* for the HLA region and *IDDM2* for the insulin gene region.

Immunosuppression in the Treatment of Recent-Onset Type I Diabetes

Since the destruction of B cells in type I diabetes is a progressive, immune-mediated process, several clinical trials with immunosuppressive therapy at the onset of type I diabetes are in progress. Unfortunately, their outcomes have so far been disappointing. Although some reduction or elimination of insulin requirement has been observed, most subjects manifest continued carbohydrate intolerance while being exposed to considerable risk from the adverse effects of immunosuppressive drugs. Cyclosporine, as a result of its substantial nephrotoxicity and nonspecific immunosuppression, is not recommended for the treatment of patients with newly diagnosed IDDM.

More specific strategies for immunosuppression, such as the use of monoclonal antibodies against particular T cell products, may reduce the hazards of long-term immunotherapy.

Some nonimmunosuppressive therapeutic modalities under investigation include probucol, which tends to quench free radicals that have been implicated as a means of T lymphocyte cytotoxicity, and nicotinamide, an inhibitor of poly(ADP-ribose) synthetase, an enzyme whose repair of DNA injury tends to deplete the cell of its vital supply of NAD. Daily exposure to insulin antigen has been shown to delay or prevent the onset of IDDM in a special strain of prediabetic mice as well as in a small pilot study in nondiabetic humans at high risk to develop IDDM (an first-degree relative with IDDM, positive islet cell antibodies, and a blunted insulin release to glucose). Because of these encouraging findings, a large-scale multicenter Diabetes Prevention Trial (DPT-1) has begun under the auspices of the National Institutes of Health to test low-dose insulin injections in nondiabetic relatives of people with IDDM, who are at high risk to develop IDDM themselves (having islet cell antibodies and a low serum insulin response to a glucose load). Up to 80,000 first-degree relatives are being screened to recruit 830 volunteers needed for the study. Volunteers with *high* risk (antibody titer and a low serum insulin response) will be assigned to a control group or to a group receiving 0.25 units of ultralente insulin per kilogram of body weight given in divided doses. Volunteers at *intermediate* risk, who have islet cell antibodies and also insulin autoantibodies but normal serum insulin responses to glucose loading, will be randomly assigned to a control group or to a group receiving oral insulin.

TYPE II: NON-INSULIN-DEPENDENT (NON-IMMUNE-DEPENDENT) DIABETES MELLITUS (NIDDM)

Type II diabetes, which comprises a heterogeneous group of the milder forms of diabetes, occurs predominantly in adults but may occasionally have its onset in childhood.

Type II diabetes is defined mainly in negative terms. It is a nonketotic form of diabetes which is not linked to HLA markers on the sixth chromosome and is not associated with islet cell autoantibodies. The patients are not dependent on exogenous insulin therapy to sustain life—thus the name, non-insulin-dependent diabetes mellitus. An element of tissue insensitivity to insulin has been noted in most NIDDM patients. Possible mechanisms for this are shown in Table 18–6.

Syndrome X (Insulin Resistance Syndrome)

Several investigators speculate that type II diabetes may represent only one facet of a syndrome caused by insulin resistance. They have noted that the well-established association of **hyperglycemia, hyperinsulinemia, dyslipidemia,** and **hypertension,** which leads to coronary artery disease and stroke, may result from a genetic defect producing insulin resistance, particularly when obesity aggravates the degree of insulin resistance. They propose that impaired action of insulin predisposes to hyperglycemia, which in turn induces hyperinsulinemia. If this hyperinsulinemia is of insufficient magnitude to correct the hyperglycemia, type II diabetes will be manifested. They feel that this excessive insulin level increases sodium retention by renal tubules, thereby contributing to or causing hypertension; an increased VLDL production in the liver, leading to hypertriglyceridemia (and consequently a low HDL-cholesterol level), has also been attributed to hyperinsulinism. Moreover, they propose that high insulin levels can stimulate endothelial and vascular smooth muscle cell proliferation—by virtue of the hormone's action on growth factor receptors—to initiate atherosclerosis.

While there is full agreement on an association of the above disorders, the mechanism of their interrelationship remains speculative and open to experimental investigation. Controversy persists about whether or not hypertension is caused by hyperinsulinism, since these two manifestations, which often coexist in whites, are not highly associated in American blacks or Pima Indians. Moreover, patients with hy-

---

Table 18–6. Factors reducing response to insulin.

Prereceptor inhibitors: Insulin antibodies
Receptor inhibitors:
  Insulin receptor autoantibodies
  "Down-regulation" of receptors by hyperinsulinism:
    Primary hyperinsulinism (B cell adenoma)
    Hyperinsulinism, secondary to a postreceptor defect (obesity, Cushing's syndrome, acromegaly, pregnancy) or prolonged hyperglycemia (diabetes mellitus, post-glucose tolerance test)
Postreceptor influences:
  Poor responsiveness of principal target organs: obesity, hepatic disease, muscle inactivity
  Hormonal excess: glucocorticoids, growth hormone, oral contraceptive agents, progesterone, human chorionic somatomammotropin, catecholamines, thyroxine

perinsulinism due to an insulinoma are generally normotensive, and there is no reduction of blood pressure after surgical removal of the insulinoma restores normal insulin levels. Australian epidemiologists prefer to group these disorders together as a syndrome, without necessarily implying that hyperinsulinism is etiologically responsible for the other components. They suggest the acronym CHAOS to signify coronary artery disease, hypertension, adult-onset diabetes, obesity, and stroke. The main value of grouping these disorders as a syndrome, regardless of its nomenclature, is to remind physicians that the therapeutic goals are not only to correct hyperglycemia but also to manage the elevated blood pressure and hyperlipidemia that result in considerable cardiovascular morbidity as well as cardiovascular deaths in these patients. It also raises awareness that indiscriminate therapeutic use of high doses of exogenous insulin may conceivably have adverse effects on a patient's risk profile for cardiovascular disease if the hypothesis behind the insulin resistance syndrome is substantiated. Finally, it reminds physicians that when choosing antihypertensive agents or lipid-lowering drugs to manage one of the components of this syndrome, their possible untoward effects on other components of the syndrome should be carefully considered. For example, physicians aware of this syndrome are less likely to prescribe antihypertensive drugs that raise lipids (diuretics, beta-blockers) or that raise blood sugar (diuretics). Likewise, they will refrain from prescribing drugs that correct hyperlipidemia but increase insulin resistance with aggravation of hyperglycemia (niacin).

Subgroups of Type II Diabetes

Type II diabetics can be distributed on the basis of body weight into obese or nonobese subtypes. Currently, it is impossible to identify diagnostic characteristics that allow further clear-cut separation into more specific subtypes. Circulating insulin levels are presently considered too variable to be of use in classification.

Among this "non-type I" group are a wide assortment of heterogeneous disorders. These include rare instances in which a defective insulin gene produces a biologically inadequate abnormal insulin or a proinsulin that is not transformed to insulin in the B cell. Receptor blocks to insulin action have been demonstrated in some cases. In most patients with type II diabetes, the cause of the disorder is presently undefined although both a defect in insulin secretion and a defect in insulin action at the postreceptor level are generally present.

Obese NIDDM

Up to 85% of type II diabetics are obese. These patients have an insensitivity to endogenous insulin that is positively correlated with the presence of an abdominal distribution of fat, producing an abnor-

mally high waist to hip ratio. In addition, distended adipocytes and overnourished liver and muscle cells may also resist the deposition of additional glycogen and triglycerides in their storage depots. Hyperplasia of pancreatic B cells is often present and probably accounts for the normal or exaggerated insulin responses to glucose and other stimuli seen in the milder forms of this disease. In more severe cases, secondary (but potentially reversible) failure of pancreatic B cell secretion may result after exposure to prolonged fasting hyperglycemia. This phenomenon has been called "desensitization." It is selective for glucose, and the B cell recovers sensitivity to glucose stimulation once the sustained hyperglycemia is corrected by any form of therapy, including diet therapy, sulfonylureas, and insulin.

A major cause of the observed resistance to insulin in target tissues of obese patients is believed to be a postreceptor defect in insulin action. This is associated with overdistended storage depots and a reduced ability to clear nutrients from the circulation after meals. Consequent hyperinsulinism can further enhance insulin resistance by down-regulation of insulin receptors. Furthermore, when hyperglycemia becomes sustained, a specific glucose transporter protein in insulin target tissue also becomes down-regulated after continuous activation. This contributes to further defects in postreceptor insulin action, thereby aggravating the hyperglycemia.

When overfeeding is corrected so that storage depots become less saturated, the cycle is interrupted. Insulin sensitivity improves and is further normalized by a reduction in both the hyperinsulinism and the hyperglycemia.

Nonobese NIDDM

Approximately 15% of patients with NIDDM are nonobese diabetics. In most of these patients, impaired insulin action at the postreceptor level and an absent or delayed early phase of insulin release in response to glucose can be demonstrated. However, other insulinogenic stimuli, such as acute infusion of amino acids, intravenous tolbutamide, or intramuscular glucagon, often remain effective in eliciting acute insulin release.

The hyperglycemia in patients with nonobese NIDDM often responds to dietary therapy or to oral hypoglycemic agents. Occasionally, insulin therapy is required to achieve satisfactory glycemic control even though it is not needed to prevent ketoacidosis.

While most nonobese NIDDM patients cannot be subclassified, several discrete subtypes are suggested in a small proportion of patients on the basis of genetic characteristics:

A. NIDDM Occurring in Late Childhood or Young Adulthood:

1. Autosomal dominant nonobese NIDDM– A specific subclass of nonobese NIDDM includes patients with "maturity-onset diabetes of the young"

(MODY, or Mason type). These patients have mild hyperglycemia with onset in late childhood or young adulthood. Their strong family history of a mild form of diabetes occurring in one parent and in one-half of the parent's offspring suggests an autosomal dominant transmission. In a large proportion of families with this syndrome, mutations of the glucokinase gene on chromosome 7 have been incriminated. Over 26 mutations of this gene have now been identified in a variety of families with MODY, including Europeans, blacks, Japanese, and Hispanics. The most detailed reports describe 32 French families with MODY in whom 18 families had 16 different mutations of the glucokinase gene. Ten of these mutations resulted in an amino acid substitution, three resulted in a truncated protein, and three affected RNA processing of glucokinase.

A reduction in glucokinase activity within the pancreatic B cell is critical in determining the threshold of plasma glucose at which the B bell secretes insulin, since glucokinase is thought to act as a glucose sensor. In those families with mutations of glucokinase, mild hyperglycemia began during childhood, while in the 14 French families without detectable glucokinase mutations, hyperglycemia was not observed until after puberty.

In a large kindred in Michigan consisting of more than 285 individuals over five generations, 40 subjects with MODY were found to have an as yet unidentified genetic defect traced to the long arm of chromosome 20, where it is tightly linked to the adenosine deaminase gene. This mutation, which has been termed MODY 1, results in a syndrome generally characterized by more insulin deficiency and greater hyperglycemia than in families having glucokinase deficiencies. Consequently, a greater number of these families with chromosome 20 defects have chronic diabetic complications comparable in degree to those experienced by adults with NIDDM and often fare better with exogenous insulin replacement. This is in contrast to families with glucokinase mutations who in many instances have only mild hyperglycemia, a lower incidence of microvascular complications, and less need for insulin therapy.

A recently identified locus on the long arm of chromosome 12 has been identified as predisposing to a form of MODY in five families in the USA, Europe, and Japan. This has been termed MODY 3 in contrast to MODY 1, which was first identified, and MODY 2, which is the only one of the three whose mutated gene product, glucokinase, has been well characterized (Table 18–7).

2. Type II diabetes of early onset–A high familial prevalence of type II diabetes has been noted in patients whose age at onset of mild diabetes is 25–40 years. Epidemiologic studies suggest that this familial prevalence is due to inheritance of diabetogenic genes from both parents (homozygous state). When only one parent passes on the diabetogenic

Table 18–7. Maturity-onset diabetes of the young (MODY).

Syndrome	Mutation	Chromosome
MODY 1	Unknown; locus near gene for adenosine deaminase	20q
MODY 2	Glucokinase gene (16 different mutations (identified)	7p
MODY 3	Unknown	12q

gene (heterozygous state), its later expression as clinical diabetes may require additional genetic or environmental factors (eg, aging, obesity). Thus, two heterozygous parents may or may not each develop diabetes after age 40 years, but as many as 75% of their offspring are at high risk of developing diabetes, with as many as 25% of them becoming diabetic before age 40 years.

3. Diabetes mellitus associated with a mutation of mitochondrial DNA–Since sperm do not contain mitochondria, only the mother transmits mitochondrial genes to her offspring. Diabetes due to a mutation of mitochondrial DNA that impairs the transfer of leucine into mitochondrial proteins has been described in 22 Japanese families involving 52 individuals. Most patients have a mild form of maternally transmitted diabetes that responds to oral hypoglycemic agents, although four persons have a nonimmune form of IDDM. As many as 63% of patients with this subtype of diabetes have a hearing loss, and a smaller proportion (15%) had a syndrome of myopathy, encephalopathy, lactic acidosis, and stroke-like episodes (MELAS).

B. Mutant Insulins: Despite awareness of this disorder over the past 12 years, only eight families have been identified as having abnormal circulating forms of insulin. In three of these families, there is impaired cleavage of the proinsulin molecule; in the other five families, abnormalities of the insulin molecule itself have been reported (Table 18–8).

Analysis of the insulin gene, circulating insulin, and clinical features of family members in these cases indicates that individuals with mutant insulin are heterozygous for this defect, with both a normal and an abnormal insulin molecule being equally ex-

Table 18–8. Mutant insulins and proinsulins.

	Amino Acid Substitution
Insulin Chicago (USA)	B 25 (Phe → Leu)
Insulin Los Angeles (USA)	B 24 (Phe → Ser)
Insulin Wakayama (Japan) I, II, III (three families)	A 3 (Val → Leu)
Proinsulin Tokyo (Japan)	Arg 65 (Arg → His)
Proinsulin Boston (USA)	Arg 65 (Arg → ?)
Proinsulin Providence (USA)	B 10 (His → Asp)

pressed. However, because the abnormal insulin binds to receptors poorly, it has very low biologic activity and accumulates in the blood to exceed the concentration of the normal insulin. This decreased removal rate of mutant insulin results in hyperinsulinemia after overnight fasting and a subnormal molar ratio of C peptide to immunoreactive insulin. Diabetes mellitus may or may not be present in association with mutant insulin, depending on the concentration and bioactivity of circulating normal and abnormal insulins and on the insulin responsiveness of peripheral tissues. Since there is no obvious resistance to insulin in any of these cases, it appears that abnormal insulin does not interfere with binding of normal insulin to receptors; therefore, a feature of this syndrome is the normal response to exogenously administered insulin.

1. Abnormalities of the proinsulin molecule–A partially cleaved intermediate of proinsulin comprising up to 90% of circulating insulin immunoreactivity has been described in two families, one from Japan and one from Boston. Both families seem to have similar defects, with the arginine in position 65 being replaced by histidine and thereby interfering with cleavage of the C peptide from the A chain of insulin. However, mild diabetes mellitus was present only in the three affected members of the family from Japan; it was not present in 17 affected members of the large kindred in Boston, despite a similar mutation of the insulin gene.

In a third family, hyperproinsulinemia was reported in five members. Although one of the five members (a 12-year-old girl) had borderline glucose intolerance, the other four had normal blood glucose levels. In this family, a mutation in the insulin gene coding for histidine at B 10 results in substitution of an aspartic acid, inducing a conformational change that prevents conversion of proinsulin to insulin.

2. Abnormalities of the insulin molecule– Genetic defects in insulin synthesis have resulted in substitutions of leucine for phenylalanine at position B 25 ("insulin Chicago") and serine for phenylalanine at position B 24 ("insulin Los Angeles"). (See Figure 18–3.) The observation that there was loss of a normal restriction endonuclease cleavage site in the area of the insulin gene coding for B 24 and B 25 phenylalanine was used in conjunction with results of high-performance liquid chromatographic analysis of circulating insulin to establish the nature of the mutant insulin in affected family members. Glucose tolerance ranged from normal to overtly diabetic in affected individuals, who were generally nonobese and had subnormal molar ratios of C peptide to immunoreactive insulin.

In Japan, a mutant insulin with a substitution of leucine for the normal valine at A 3 was initially described in Wakayama but was subsequently identified in the adjacent Osaka region in two other families who had no documented relationship.

With improved screening techniques becoming available such as the polymerase chain reaction, more cases of mutation of the insulin gene will undoubtedly be detected. However, from present experience it is unlikely that patients with this defect will make up more than a very small fraction of the NIDDM population.

"NIDDM" Diabetics Who May Be Type I Diabetics in Remission

The current classification of diabetes mellitus has been widely accepted throughout the world, but its deficiencies are apparent in many cases. A subgroup that has been difficult to place in the current "therapeutic" classification is made up of those type I diabetics who remain in temporary remission for up to 2 years. A history of ketoacidosis with the finding of islet cell autoantibodies at the onset of the diabetes— and an HLA pattern that includes HLA-B8, -B15, -DR3, or -DR4—would indicate that these patients have type I diabetes from an etiologic standpoint even though they may be temporarily not "insulin-dependent."

Moreover, it is possible that a number of adult-onset diabetic patients, particularly when not obese, may represent an early stage of type I diabetes due to autoimmune destruction of enough pancreatic B cells to make them hyperglycemic but not necessarily insulin-dependent. In one study, as many as 16% of a group of adult-onset diabetics in a British clinic population who were classified as NIDDM were found to be positive for islet cell antibodies. With the availability of more convenient radioimmunoassays for islet cell antibodies, such as those for antibodies against glutamic acid decarboxylase, it will be possible to screen many more populations of adult diabetics. This will be particularly useful in ethnic groups who are prone to autoimmune disease and in whom IDDM is prevalent. This might permit earlier identification of those patients with immune-induced partial B cell destruction who may thus be more likely to fail sulfonylureas and to require insulin therapy.

SECONDARY DIABETES

As noted in Table 18–5, there is a diverse group of disorders characterized by the association of diabetes with another condition. Only a few of the many types of secondary diabetes will be discussed here.

Pancreatic Disease

Surgical removal of the pancreas, pancreatic disease due to chronic alcoholism, and other forms of pancreatitis are associated with many of the clinical characteristics of insulin-dependent diabetes mellitus, because the primary abnormality is insulin deficiency. There is, however, a greater tendency to develop insulin-induced hypoglycemia, probably because of the concomitant lack of the counterregulatory hormone glucagon. At least two-thirds of the pancreas must be destroyed to develop the clinical syndrome. It is usually associated with exocrine pancreatic insufficiency as well.

Drug Toxicity

Many drugs are associated with carbohydrate intolerance or frank diabetes mellitus. Some act by interfering with insulin release from the B cells (thiazides, phenytoin), some by inducing insulin resistance (glucocorticoids, oral contraceptive pills), and some by causing B cell destruction (pentamidine).

While calcium channel blockers as well as clonidine are potent inhibitors of glucose-induced insulin release from in vitro preparations of pancreatic B cells, the inhibitory concentrations required are quite high and are not generally achieved during standard antihypertensive therapy with these agents in humans.

Endocrine Disorders

Excess production of certain hormones—growth hormone (acromegaly), glucocorticoids (Cushing's syndrome or disease), catecholamines (pheochromocytoma), glucagon (glucagonoma), or pancreatic somatostatin (somatostatinoma)—can produce the syndrome of NIDDM by a number of mechanisms. In all but the last instance (somatostatinoma), peripheral responsiveness to insulin is impaired. In addition, excess of catecholamines or somatostatin decreases insulin release from B cells.

Insulin-Resistant Diabetes With Acanthosis Nigricans

Patients with the rare syndrome of extreme insulin resistance associated with acanthosis nigricans can be divided into two groups on the basis of clinical and laboratory manifestations. **Group A** consists of younger women with androgenic features (hirsutism, amenorrhea, polycystic ovaries) in whom insulin receptors are deficient in number. With development of newer molecular biology methods using polymerase chain reaction analysis, as many as 25 different mutations of the insulin receptor have been characterized. When patients with type A insulin resistance have two mutant alleles, they tend to be more insulin-resistant than when only one mutant allele is present. **Group B** consists of older people, mostly women, in whom immunologic disease is suspected. They have a high erythrocyte sedimentation rate, DNA autoantibodies, and a circulating immunoglobulin that binds to insulin receptors, thereby reducing their affinity for insulin.

In both of the above groups, carbohydrate tolerance may at times be normal, and in most cases ketoacidosis does not develop despite severe insulin resistance and diabetes. Occasionally, spontaneous remission of insulin resistance and diabetes occurs, particularly in the group A patients. In neither of the above groups is insulin therapy very effective. Acanthosis nigricans seems to be a consequence of very high circulating levels of insulin binding to insulin-like growth factor receptors on epidermal and melanin-containing cutaneous cells.

Other Forms of Secondary Diabetes

Other rare diseases associated with insulin receptor or postreceptor abnormalities include leprechaunism, ataxia-telangiectasia, Prader-Willi syndrome, and certain forms of myotonic dystrophy.

Wolfram's syndrome is a rare autosomal recessive disease which in its complete form includes optic atrophy, diabetes insipidus, neural deafness, and a nonimmune form of pancreatic B cell death resulting in insulin deficiency and diabetes mellitus. It has recently been found to be associated with a genetic mutation on the short arm of chromosome 4 and an increased frequency of HLA-DR2 antigen.

CLINICAL FEATURES OF DIABETES MELLITUS

The principal clinical features of the two major types of diabetes mellitus are listed for comparison in Table 18–9.

TYPE I DIABETES (IDDM)

IDDM patients present with a characteristic symptom complex, as outlined below. An absolute deficiency of insulin results in excessive accumulation of circulating glucose and fatty acids, with consequent hyperosmolality and hyperketonemia. The severity of the insulin deficiency and the acuteness with which the catabolic state develops determine the intensity of the osmotic and ketotic excess.

Table 18–9. Clinical features of diabetes at diagnosis.

	Diabetes Type I (IDDM)	Diabetes Type II (NIDDM)
Polyuria and thirst	++	+
Weakness or fatigue	++	+
Polyphagia with weight loss	++	−
Recurrent blurred vision	+	++
Vulvovaginitis or pruritus	+	++
Peripheral neuropathy	+	++
Nocturnal enuresis	++	−
Often asymptomatic	−	++

Clinical Features

A. Symptoms: Increased urination is a consequence of osmotic diuresis secondary to sustained hyperglycemia. This results in a loss of glucose as well as free water and electrolytes in the urine. Nocturnal enuresis due to polyuria may signal the onset of diabetes in very young children. Thirst is a consequence of the hyperosmolar state, as is blurred vision, which often develops as the lenses and retinas are exposed to hyperosmolar fluids.

Weight loss despite normal or increased appetite is a common feature of IDDM when it develops subacutely over a period of weeks. The weight loss is initially due to depletion of water, glycogen, and triglyceride stores. Chronic weight loss due to reduced muscle mass occurs as amino acids are diverted to form glucose and ketone bodies.

Lowered plasma volume produces dizziness and weakness due to postural hypotension when sitting or standing. Total body potassium loss and the general catabolism of muscle protein contribute to the weakness.

Paresthesias may be present at the time of diagnosis of type I diabetes, particularly when the onset is subacute. They reflect a temporary dysfunction of peripheral sensory nerves and usually clear as insulin replacement restores glycemic levels closer to normal; thus, their presence suggests neurotoxicity from sustained hyperglycemia.

When insulin deficiency is severe and of acute onset, the above symptoms progress in an accelerated manner. Ketoacidosis exacerbates the dehydration and hyperosmolality by producing anorexia, nausea, and vomiting, thus interfering with oral fluid replacement. As plasma osmolality exceeds 330 mosm/L (normal, 285–295 mosm/L), impaired consciousness ensues. With progression of acidosis to a pH of 7.1 or less, deep breathing with a rapid ventilatory rate (Kussmaul respiration) occurs as the body attempts to eliminate carbonic acid. With worsening acidosis (to pH 7.0 or less), the cardiovascular system may be unable to maintain compensatory vasoconstriction; severe circulatory collapse may result.

B. Signs: The patient's level of consciousness can vary depending on the degree of hyperosmolality. When insulin deficiency develops relatively slowly and sufficient water intake is maintained to permit renal excretion of glucose and appropriate dilution of extracellular sodium chloride concentration, patients remain relatively alert and physical findings may be minimal. When vomiting occurs in response to worsening ketoacidosis, dehydration progresses and compensatory mechanisms become inadequate to keep plasma osmolality below 330 mosm/L. Under these circumstances, stupor or even coma may occur. Evidence of dehydration in a stuporous patient, with rapid deep breathing and the fruity breath odor of acetone, suggests the diagnosis of diabetic ketoacidosis.

Postural hypotension indicates a depleted plasma volume; hypotension in the recumbent position is a serious prognostic sign. Loss of subcutaneous fat and muscle wasting are features of more slowly developing insulin deficiency. In occasional patients with slow, insidious onset of insulin deficiency, subcutaneous fat may be considerably depleted. An enlarged liver, eruptive xanthomas on the flexor surface of the limbs and on the buttocks, and lipemia retinalis indicate that chronic insulin deficiency has resulted in chylomicronemia, with circulating triglycerides elevated usually to over 2000 mg/dL (Chapter 20).

TYPE II DIABETES (NIDDM)

NIDDM patients also present with characteristic signs and symptoms. The presence of obesity or a strongly positive family history of mild diabetes also suggests a high risk for the development of type II diabetes.

Clinical Features

A. Symptoms: The classic symptoms of polyuria, thirst, recurrent blurred vision, paresthesias, and fatigue are manifestations of hyperglycemia and osmotic diuresis and are therefore common to both forms of diabetes. However, many patients with type II diabetes have an insidious onset of hyperglycemia and may be relatively asymptomatic initially. This is particularly true in obese patients, whose diabetes may be detected only after glycosuria or hyperglycemia is noted during routine laboratory studies. Chronic skin infections are common. Generalized pruritus and symptoms of vaginitis are frequently the initial complaints of women with NIDDM. Diabetes should be suspected in women with chronic candidal vulvovaginitis as well as in those who have delivered large infants (> 9 lb, or 4.1 kg) or have had polyhydramnios, preeclampsia, or unexplained fetal losses. Occasionally, a man with previously undiagnosed diabetes may present with impotence.

B. Signs: Nonobese patients with this mild form of diabetes often have no characteristic physical findings at the time of diagnosis. Obese diabetics may have any variety of fat distribution; however, diabetes seems to be more often associated in both men and women with localization of fat deposits on the upper part of the body (particularly the abdomen, chest, neck, and face) and relatively less fat on the appendages, which may be quite muscular. This centripetal fat distribution has been termed "android" and is characterized by a high waist to hip ratio. It differs from the more centrifugal "gynecoid" form of obesity, in which fat is localized more in the hips and thighs and less in the upper parts of the trunk. Refined radiographic techniques of assessing abdominal fat distribution with CT scans has documented that a "visceral" obesity, due to accumulation of fat in the omental and mesenteric regions, correlates with insulin resistance, whereas fat predominantly in subcutaneous tissues of the abdomen has little, if any, association with insulin insensitivity. Mild hypertension may be present in obese diabetics, particularly when the "android" form of obesity is predominant. In women, candidal vaginitis with a reddened, inflamed vulvar area and a profuse whitish discharge may herald the presence of diabetes.

LABORATORY FINDINGS IN DIABETES MELLITUS

Tests of urine glucose and ketone bodies as well as whole blood or plasma glucose measured in samples obtained under basal conditions and after glucose administration are very important in evaluation of the diabetic patient. Tests for glycosylated hemoglobin have proved useful in both initial evaluation and in assessment of the effectiveness of therapeutic management. In certain circumstances, measurements of insulin or C peptide levels and levels of other hormones involved in carbohydrate homeostasis (eg, glucagon, GH) may be useful. In view of the increased risk of atherosclerosis in diabetics, determination of serum cholesterol (including its beneficial HDL fraction) and triglycerides may be helpful. From these three measurements, an estimate of LDL-cholesterol can be made. (See Chapter 20.)

URINALYSIS

Glycosuria

Several problems are associated with using urine glucose as an index of blood glucose, regardless of the method employed. First of all, the glucose concentration in bladder urine reflects the blood glucose at the time the urine was formed. Therefore, the first voided specimen in the morning contains glucose that was excreted throughout the night and does not reflect the morning blood glucose at all. Some improvement in the correlation of urine glucose to blood glucose can be obtained if the patient "double voids"—that is, empties the bladder completely, discards that sample, and then urinates again about one-half hour later, testing only the second specimen for glucose content. However, difficulty in completely emptying the bladder (large residual volumes), problems in understanding the instructions, and the inconvenience impair the usefulness of this test. Self-monitoring of blood glucose has replaced urine glucose testing in most patients with IDDM and in many patients with NIDDM (particularly those receiving insulin therapy).

Several commercial products are available for determining the presence and amount of glucose in urine. The older and more cumbersome bedside assessment of glycosuria with Clinitest tablets has generally been replaced by the dipstick method, which is rapid, convenient, and glucose-specific. This method consists of paper strips (Clinistix, Tes-Tape) impregnated with enzymes (glucose oxidase and hydrogen peroxidase) and a chromogenic dye that is colorless in the reduced state. Enzymatic generation of hydrogen peroxide oxidizes the dye to produce colors whose intensity depends on the glucose concentration. These dipsticks are sensitive to as little as 0.1% glucose (100 mg/dL) but do not react with the smaller amounts of glucose normally present in urine. The strips are subject to deterioration if exposed to air, moisture, and extreme heat and must be kept in tightly closed containers except when in use. False-negative results may be obtained in the presence of alkaptonuria and when certain substances such as salicylic acid or ascorbic acid are ingested in excess. All of these false-negative results occur because of the interference of strong reducing agents with oxidation of the chromogen.

Differential Diagnosis of Glycosuria

Although glycosuria reflects hyperglycemia in over 90% of patients, two major classes of nondiabetic glycosuria must be considered:

A. Nondiabetic Glycosuria Due to Glucose: This occurs when glucose appears in the urine despite a normal amount of glucose in the blood. Disorders associated with abnormalities in renal glucose handling include Fanconi's~syndrome (an autosomal dominant genetic disorder), dysfunction of the proximal renal tubule, and a benign familial disorder of the renal tubule manifest only by a defect in renal glucose reabsorption (occurs predominantly in males).

In addition, glycosuria is relatively common in pregnancy as a consequence of the increased load of glucose presented to the tubules by the elevated glomerular filtration rate during pregnancy. As many as 50% of pregnant women normally have demonstrable sugar in the urine, especially after the first trimester. This sugar is almost always glucose except during the late weeks of pregnancy, when lactose may be present (see below).

B. Nondiabetic Glycosuria Due to Sugars Other Than Glucose: Occasionally, a sugar other than glucose is excreted in the urine. Lactosuria during the late stages of pregnancy and the period of lactation is the most common example. Much rarer are other conditions in which inborn errors of metabolism allow fructose, galactose, or a pentose (1-xylose) to be excreted in the urine. Testing the urine with glucose-specific strips will help differentiate true glucosuria from other glycosurias.

Ketonuria

In the absence of adequate insulin, three major "ketone bodies" are formed and excreted into the urine: β-hydroxybutyric acid, acetoacetic acid, and acetone (see also Serum Ketone Determinations, below). Commercial products are available to test for the presence of ketones in the urine. Acetest tablets, Ketostix, and Keto-Diastix utilize a nitroprusside reaction that measures only acetone and acetoacetate. Therefore, these tests can be misleading if β-hydroxybutyric acid is the predominant metabolite present. Ketostix and Keto-Diastix have short shelf-lives once the containers are opened and thus may give false-negative results.

Other conditions besides diabetic ketoacidosis may cause ketone bodies to appear in the urine; these include starvation, high-fat diets, alcoholic ketoacidosis, fever, and other conditions in which metabolic requirements are increased.

Proteinuria

Proteinuria as noted on a routine dipstick examination of the urine is often the first sign of renal complications of diabetes. If proteinuria is detected, a 24-hour urine collection should be analyzed to quantify the degree of proteinuria (normal individuals excrete < 30 mg of protein per day) and the rate of urinary creatinine excretion; at the same time, serum creatinine levels should be determined so that the creatinine clearance (an estimate of the glomerular filtration rate) can be calculated. In some cases, heavy proteinuria (3–5 g/d) develops later, along with other features of the nephrotic syndrome such as edema, hypoalbuminemia, and hypercholesterolemia.

Microalbuminuria

Urinary albumin can now be detected in microgram concentrations using a radioimmunoassay method that is more sensitive than the dipstick method, whose minimal detection limit is 0.3–0.5%. Conventional 24-hour urine collections, in addition to being inconvenient for patients, also show wide variability of albumin excretion, since several factors such as sustained upright posture, dietary protein, and exercise tend to increase albumin excretion rates. For these reasons, many clinics prefer to screen patients with a timed *overnight* urine collection beginning at bedtime, when the urine is discarded and the time recorded. The collection is ended at the time the bladder is emptied the next morning, and this urine, as well as any other urine voided overnight, is assayed for albumin. Normal subjects excrete less than 15 μg/min during overnight urine collections; values between 20 and 200 μg/min or higher represent abnormal microalbuminuria, which may be an early predictor of the development of diabetic nephropathy.

BLOOD GLUCOSE TESTING

Normal Values

The normal fasting *whole blood* glucose varies from 60 to 110 mg/dL (3.3–6.1 mmol/L). Plasma or serum levels are 10–15% higher because structural components of blood cells are absent, so that more glucose is present per unit volume. Thus, the normal range of fasting plasma or serum glucose is 70–120 mg/dL (3.9–6.7 mmol/L). Plasma or serum glucose measurements are more frequently used clinically because they are independent of the hematocrit, more closely approach the glucose level in the interstitial tissue spaces, and lend themselves to automated analytic procedures. Whole blood glucose determinations are used in spot testing of glucose in emergency situations and also in the procedures for self-monitoring of capillary blood glucose, a technique that has become widely accepted in the management of diabetes mellitus (see below).

The accepted normal range of blood or plasma glucose requires a correction for age of 1 mg/dL (0.056 mmol/L) per year of age past 60. Thus, fasting plasma glucose in elderly nondiabetics will range from 80 to 150 mg/dL (4.4–8.3 mmol/L).

Venous Blood Samples

Samples should be collected in tubes containing sodium fluoride, which prevents glycolysis in the blood sample that would artifactually lower the measured glucose level. If such tubes are not available, samples must be centrifuged within 30 minutes of collection and the plasma or serum stored at 4 °C.

The laboratory methods regularly used for determining plasma glucose utilize enzymatic methods (such as glucose oxidase or hexokinase), colorimetric methods (such as *o*-toluidine), or automated methods. The automated methods utilize reduction of copper or iron compounds by reducing sugars in dialyzed serum. They are convenient but are not specific for glucose, since they react with other reducing substances (which are elevated in azotemia or with high ascorbic acid intake).

Capillary Blood Samples

There are several paper strip (glucose oxidase) methods for measuring capillary whole blood glucose. All have been adapted for use with portable, battery-operated reflectance meters that give a digital readout. One test strip kit, Chemstrip bG, provides a color chart for visual comparison and estimation of the blood glucose range. First-generation reflectance meters required exact timing by the operator as well as careful removal of all traces of blood from the strip prior to reading of the color. Second-generation devices (eg, One Touch II, Glucometer Encore, Accu-Chek Easy, Exac Tech, etc) have eliminated these two potential sources of technical error by providing automatic timing and allowing quantitation without removal of the blood. To monitor their own blood glucose levels, patients must prick their fingers with a 21-gauge lancet (eg, Monolet), a procedure that can be facilitated by a small plastic trigger device (eg, Autolet, Penlet). Recently, an ultrafine 28-gauge lancet (Becton Dickinson) has become available, which reduces discomfort while providing an adequate blood drop for measurement. With proper instruction in technique, patients can obtain accurate and reliable measurements of their own blood glucose levels, which are indispensable to the proper long-term management of their diabetes. These methods are also of great value to health care professionals in the bedside management of seriously ill hospitalized diabetic patients.

Third-generation devices are presently in the developmental stage. They represent a noninvasive method relying on infrared absorption spectra which allow quantitation of glycemia flowing through capillary beds of the finger or earlobe. Present pilot models are relatively large and expensive, but they appear to be accurate and have the great advantage of eliminating painful finger sticks. Developmental goals are directed toward smaller, less expensive devices with which patients can perform self-monitoring of blood glucose.

SERUM KETONE DETERMINATIONS

As noted above in the section on ketonuria, there are three major ketone bodies: β-hydroxybutyrate (often the most prevalent in diabetic ketoacidosis), acetoacetate, and acetone. The same testing materials used for determining urine ketones may be used to measure serum (or plasma) ketones. However, whereas urine readily penetrates "intact" Acetest tablets, more viscous fluids such as serum or plasma do not have access to the bulk of the tablet unless it is first crushed. When a few drops of serum are placed on a crushed Acetest tablet, the appearance of a purple color indicates the presence of ketones. A strongly positive reaction in undiluted serum correlates with a serum ketone concentration of at least 4 mmol/L. It must be kept in mind that Acetest tablets (as well as Ketostix and Keto-Diastix) utilize the nitroprusside reaction, which measures only acetoacetate and acetone. Specific enzymatic techniques are available to quantitate each of the ketone acids, but these techniques are cumbersome and not necessary in most clinical situations.

GLYCOSYLATED HEMOGLOBIN ASSAYS

Glycohemoglobin is produced by a ketoamine reaction between glucose and the amino terminal

amino acid of both beta chains of the hemoglobin molecule. The major form of glycohemoglobin is hemoglobin A_{1c}, which normally comprises only 4–6% of total hemoglobin. The remaining glycohemoglobins (2–4% of total hemoglobin) contain phosphorylated glucose or fructose and are termed hemoglobin A_{1a} and A_{1b}, respectively. The hemoglobin A_{1c} fraction is abnormally elevated in diabetics with chronic hyperglycemia and appears to correlate positively with metabolic control. Specific assays for hemoglobin A_{1c} are technically less convenient than assays for total glycohemoglobin and offer little advantage for clinical purposes. Therefore, many laboratories measure the sum of these three glycohemoglobins and report it simply as hemoglobin A_1 or "glycohemoglobin."

The glycosylation of hemoglobin is dependent on the concentration of blood glucose. The reaction is not reversible, so that the half-life of glycosylated hemoglobin relates to the life span of red cells (which normally circulate for up to 120 days). Thus, glycohemoglobin generally reflects the state of glycemia over the preceding 8–12 weeks, thus providing a method of assessing chronic diabetic control. A glycosylated hemoglobin close to the normal range (5–8%) would reflect good control during the preceding 2–3 months, whereas a glycosylated hemoglobin in the range of 12–15% would reflect poor control during the same period.

Conditions Interfering With Glycohemoglobin Measurements (Table 18–10)

The most common laboratory error in measuring glycohemoglobins occurs when chromatographic methods measure an acutely generated intermediary aldimine in blood (prehemoglobin A_{1c}), which fluctuates directly with the prevailing blood glucose level. This artifact can falsely elevate glycohemoglobin by as much as 1–2% during an episode of acute hyperglycemia. It can be eliminated either by washing the red blood cells with saline prior to assay or by dialyzing the hemolysate prior to chromatography. Other substances that falsely elevate "glycohemoglobin" are carbamoylated hemoglobin and hemoglobin F; the former is seen in association with uremia, and

Table 18–10. Factors interfering with chromatographic measurement of glycohemoglobins.

Substances causing falsely high values:
  Prehemoglobin A_{1C} (reversible aldimine intermediate)
  Carbamoylated hemoglobin (uremia)
  Hemoglobin F
Conditions causing falsely low values:
  Hemoglobinopathies (hemoglobins C, D, and S)
  Reduced life span of erythrocytes:
    Hemorrhage of therapeutic phlebotomies
    Hemolytic disorders

the latter circulates in some adults with genetic or hematologic disorders. In these cases, more intricate methodology such as thiobarbituric acid colorimetry or isoelectric focusing is required to distinguish hemoglobin A_{1c} from the interfering substance.

Hemoglobinopathies such as those associated with hemoglobin C, D, and S will cause falsely low values, since their glycosylated products elute only partially from chromatographic columns. In addition, these hemoglobinopathies are often associated with hemolytic anemias that shorten the life span of red blood cells, thereby further lowering glycohemoglobin measurements. Falsely low values are also seen in patients with chronic or acute blood loss from hemorrhage or phlebotomies and in diabetic patients with hemochromatosis; under these conditions, measurements of glycohemoglobin are not valid for assessment of diabetic therapy.

Glycohemoglobin assays suffer from the lack of universally available reference standards. However, in a reliable laboratory where reversible aldimines (prehemoglobin A_{1c}) are routinely removed prior to chromatography, they are useful in assessing the effectiveness of diabetic therapy and particularly helpful in evaluating the reliability of a patient's self-monitoring records of urine or blood glucose values. A glycosylated hemoglobin test has been evaluated for diagnostic screening purposes, and while the test is generally too insensitive to rule out impaired glucose tolerance, a value above the normal range is generally a specific indicator of diabetes mellitus.

When abnormal hemoglobins or hemolytic states affect the interpretation of glycohemoglobin results or when a narrower time frame is required, eg, when ascertaining glycemic control at the time of conception in a diabetic woman who has recently become pregnant, serum fructosamine assays offer some advantage. Serum fructosamine is formed by nonenzymatic glycosylation of serum proteins (predominantly albumin). Since serum albumin has a much shorter half-life than hemoglobin, serum fructosamine generally reflects the state of glycemic control for only the preceding 2 weeks. In most circumstances, however, glycohemoglobin assays remain the preferred method for assessing long-term glycemic control in diabetic patients.

CAPILLARY MORPHOMETRY

The basement membrane of capillaries from skeletal muscle tissue of the quadriceps area is abnormally thickened in adults with overt spontaneous diabetes (fasting hyperglycemia of 140 mg/dL [7.8 mmol/L] or more). Capillary morphometry appears to be less discriminatory in diabetic children, being normal in as many as 60% of those below age 18. Evidence of the reversibility of capillary basement membrane thickening after near-normalization of glycemia with intensive therapy suggests that this thickening in diabetes is a consequence of long-term hyperglycemia, although the rapidity and severity of its progression may vary according to an individual's genetic predisposition.

LIPOPROTEINS IN DIABETES

Levels of circulating lipoprotein are dependent on normal levels and action of insulin, just as is the plasma glucose. In type I diabetes, moderately deficient control of hyperglycemia is associated with only a slight elevation of LDL cholesterol and serum triglycerides and little if any changes in HDL cholesterol. Once the hyperglycemia is corrected, lipoprotein levels are generally normal. However, in obese patients with type II diabetes, a distinct "diabetic dyslipidemia" is characteristic of the insulin resistance syndrome. Its features are a high serum triglyceride level (300–400 mg/dL), a low HDL cholesterol (less than 30 mg/dL), and a qualitative change in LDL particles producing a smaller dense LDL whose membrane carries supranormal amounts of free cholesterol. Since a *low* HDL cholesterol is a major feature predisposing to macrovascular disease, the term "dyslipidemia" has preempted the previous label of "hyperlipidemia," which mainly described the elevated triglycerides. Measures designed to correct this obesity and hyperglycemia, such as exercise, diet, and hypoglycemic therapy, are the treatment of choice for diabetic dyslipidemia, and in occasional patients in which normal weight was achieved all features of the lipoprotein abnormalities cleared. Since primary disorders of lipid metabolism may coexist with diabetes, persistence of lipid abnormalities after restoration of normal weight and blood glucose should prompt a diagnostic workup and possible pharmacotherapy of the lipid disorder. Chapter 20 discusses these matters in detail.

DIAGNOSIS OF DIABETES MELLITUS

SIMPLE DIAGNOSTIC TEST BY FASTING PLASMA GLUCOSE

A fasting plasma glucose value above 140 mg/dL (7.8 mmol/L) on more than one occasion establishes the diagnosis of diabetes mellitus. The sample for fasting plasma glucose is best drawn in the morning after an overnight fast.

ORAL GLUCOSE TOLERANCE TEST

An oral glucose tolerance test is only rarely indicated, since the criteria for a positive test are still poor, being based on a nonhospitalized group of active young people who are not really comparable to any bedridden, ill, or aging population. In the past, oral glucose tolerance testing led to the overdiagnosis of diabetes. The much more rigid criteria currently recommended (see interpretation, below) should alleviate this tendency for overdiagnosis and improve the utility of the test.

If the fasting plasma glucose is between 120 and 140 mg/dL, an oral glucose tolerance test may be considered, especially in men with impotence or women who have delivered infants above 9 lb (4.1 kg) birth weight or have had recurrent vaginal yeast infections.

Preparation for Test

In order to optimize insulin secretion and effectiveness, especially when patients have been on a low-carbohydrate diet, a minimum of 150–200 g of carbohydrate per day should be included in the diet for 3 days preceding the test. The patient should eat nothing after midnight prior to the test day.

Testing Procedure

Adults are given 75 g of glucose in 300 mL of water; children are given 1.75 g of glucose per kilogram of ideal body weight. The glucose load is consumed within 5 minutes. Blood samples for plasma glucose are obtained at 0, 30, 60, 90, and 120 minutes after ingestion of glucose.

Interpretation

An oral glucose tolerance test is normal if the fasting venous plasma glucose value is less than 115 mg/dL (6.4 mmol/L), the 2-hour value falls below 140 mg/dL (7.8 mmol/L), and the value in none of the samples exceeds 200 mg/dL (11.1 mmol/L). A 2-hour value of greater than 200 mg/dL (11.1 mmol/L) in addition to one other value greater than 200 mg/dL (11.1 mmol/L) is diagnostic of diabetes mellitus. The diagnosis of "impaired glucose tolerance" is reserved for values between the upper limits of normal and those values diagnostic for diabetes. False-positive results may occur in patients who are malnourished at test time, bedridden, or afflicted with an infection or severe emotional stress. Diuretics, oral contraceptives, glucocorticoids, excess thyroxine, phenytoin, nicotinic acid and some of the psychotropic drugs may also cause false-positive results.

INSULIN LEVELS

To measure insulin levels during the glucose tolerance test, serum or plasma must be separated within 30 minutes after collection of the specimen and frozen prior to assay. Normal immunoreactive insulin levels range from 5–20 μU/mL in the fasting state, reach 50–130 μU/mL at 1 hour, and usually return to levels below 30 μU/mL by 2 hours. Insulin levels are rarely of clinical usefulness during glucose tolerance testing for the following reasons: When fasting glucose levels exceed 120 mg/dL (6.7 mmol/L), B cells generally have reduced responsiveness to further degrees of hyperglycemia regardless of the type of diabetes. When fasting glucose levels are below 120 mg/dL (6.7 mmol/L), late hyperinsulinism may occur as a result of insulin resistance in type II diabetes; however, it also may occur even in mild forms or in the early phases of type I diabetes when sluggish early insulin release results in late hyperglycemia that may stimulate excessive insulin secretion at 2 hours.

INTRAVENOUS GLUCOSE TOLERANCE TEST

The intravenous glucose tolerance test is performed by giving a rapid infusion of glucose followed by serial plasma glucose measurements to determine the disappearance rate of glucose per minute. The disappearance rate reflects the patient's ability to dispose of a glucose load. Perhaps its most widespread present use is to screen siblings at risk for type I diabetes to determine if autoimmune destruction of B cells has reduced peak early insulin responses (at 1–5 minutes after the glucose bolus) to levels below the normal lower limit of 40 μU/mL. It has also been used to evaluate glucose tolerance in patients with gastrointestinal abnormalities (such as malabsorption). Caution should be used in clinical interpretation of the results, because the test bypasses normal glucose absorption and associated changes in gastrointestinal hormones that are important in carbohydrate metabolism. Furthermore, the test is relatively insensitive, and adequate criteria for diagnosis of diabetes have not been established for the various age groups.

Preparation for Test

Preparation is the same as for the oral glucose tolerance test (see above).

Testing Procedure

Intravenous access is established and the patient is given a bolus of 50 g of glucose per 1.7 m^2 body surface area (or 0.5 g/kg of ideal body weight) as a 25% or 50% solution over 2–3 minutes. Timing begins with injection. Samples for plasma glucose determination are obtained from an indwelling needle in the opposite arm at 0, 10, 15, 20, and 30 minutes. The plasma glucose values are plotted on semilogarithmic paper against time. K, a rate constant that reflects the rate of fall of blood glucose in percent per minute, is calculated by determining the time necessary for the glucose concentration to fall by one-half ($t_{1/2}$) and using the following equation:

$$K \text{ (glucose)} = (0.693/t_{1/2}) \times 100$$

The average K value for a nondiabetic patient is approximately 1.72% per minute; this value declines with age but remains above 1.3% per minute. Diabetic patients almost always have a K value of less than 1% per minute.

Careful attention to venous access is essential, since leakage or infiltration of this hypertonic solution into subcutaneous tissues can cause considerable discomfort which can last for several days.

TREATMENT OF DIABETES MELLITUS

Rational therapy of diabetes requires the application of principles derived from current knowledge concerning both the nature of the particular type of diabetes and the mechanism of action, efficacy, and safety of the available treatment regimens: diet, oral hypoglycemic drugs, and insulin.

A fundamental controversy regarding whether microangiopathy is related exclusively to the existence and duration of hyperglycemia or whether it reflects a separate genetic disorder has recently been resolved by the findings of the Diabetes Control and Complications Trial, which confirmed the beneficial effects of intensive therapy to achieve improved glycemic control in IDDM (see below).

The Diabetes Control & Complications Trial (DCCT)

In September 1993, a long-term randomized prospective study involving 1441 type I diabetic patients in 29 medical centers reported that "near" normalization of blood glucose resulted in a delay in the onset and a major slowing of the progression of established microvascular and neuropathic complications of diabetes during an up to 10-year follow-up period.

The patients were divided into two equal study groups. Approximately half of the total group had no detectable diabetic complications (prevention trial), whereas mild background retinopathy was present in the other half (intervention trial). Some patients in the latter group had slightly elevated microalbuminuria and mild neuropathy, but no one with serious diabetic complications was enrolled in the trial. Multiple insulin injections (66%) or insulin pumps (34%) were used in the intensively treated group, who were trained to modify their therapy in response to fre-

quent glucose monitoring. The conventionally treated group used no more than two insulin injections, and clinical well-being was the goal with no attempt to modify management based on glycated hemoglobin or glucose results. Patients were between the ages of 13 and 19 years, with an average age of 27 years, and half of the subjects were women.

In the intensively treated subjects, a mean glycated hemoglobin of 7.2% (normal, < 6%) and a mean blood glucose of 155 mg/dL were achieved, whereas in the conventionally treated group glycated hemoglobin averaged 8.9%, with an average blood glucose of 225 mg/dL. Over the study period, which averaged 7 years, there was an approximately 60% reduction in risk of diabetic retinopathy, nephropathy, and neuropathy in the intensively treated group.

Intensively treated patients had a threefold greater risk of serious hypoglycemia as well as a greater tendency toward weight gain. However, there were no deaths from hypoglycemia in any subjects in the DCCT study, and no evidence of posthypoglycemic neurologic damage was detected.

The general consensus of the American Diabetes Association is that intensive insulin therapy associated with comprehensive self-management training should become standard therapy in most type I patients after the age of puberty. Exceptions include those with advanced renal disease and the elderly, since in these groups the detrimental risks of hypoglycemia outweigh the benefit of tight glycemic control. In children under age 7 years, the extreme susceptibility of the developing brain to damage from hypoglycemia contraindicates attempts at tight glycemic control, particularly since diabetic complications do not seem to occur until some years after the onset of puberty.

While patients with NIDDM were not studied in the DCCT, there is no reason to believe that the effects of better control of blood glucose levels would not also benefit this group. The eye, kidney, and nerve abnormalities are quite similar in both types of diabetes, and it is likely that similar underlying mechanisms apply. However, because weight gain may be greater in obese NIDDM patients receiving intensive insulin therapy—and because of an increased prevalence of macrovascular disease in older patients with NIDDM, in whom hypoglycemia may be more hazardous—The ADA feels that common sense and clinical judgment on an individual basis should determine whether tight glycemic control is appropriate in NIDDM.

A preliminary report describes a prospective randomized multicenter trial of 153 obese NIDDM men with an average age of 60 years who responded poorly to diet and sulfonylurea therapy. The trial was conducted at five VA hospitals over a 30-month period as follows: Stepwise intensification of insulin therapy (three or four injections per day) in 75 men was compared with a standard regimen of one or, if necessary, no more than two injections of insulin daily in 78 patients matched for obesity, smoking status, lipid profile, and number of known cardiovascular complications. A consistently lower glycohemoglobin was achieved in the intensively treated group (7.2% versus 9.5%) over the final year of the pilot study with insulin doses of 100–200 units/d (as compared with an average of 60 units/d in the standard group). It is of interest that there were only five severe hypoglycemic reactions with intensive therapy, in contrast to the DCCT trial in IDDM patients, which had a rate 20 times greater. Furthermore, there was no weight gain as a consequence of intensive insulin therapy in these obese men, nor were there any adverse effects on blood pressure. Lipid profiles showed no changes in major cholesterol patterns, but there was a slight fall in triglycerides in both groups. Six fatal cardiac events were distributed equally among the two groups. However, 61 new cardiovascular events occurred in 40 patients during the study and seemed to concentrate more in the intensively treated patients, though there was no temporal association with hypoglycemia in either the fatal or new cardiovascular events.

The investigators conclude that a long-term expanded trial is needed to further assess the risk-benefit ratio of intensified treatment of hyperglycemia in NIDDM patients requiring insulin.

The recommendations of the Executive Committee of the American Diabetes Association are to try to restore known metabolic derangements to normal in an attempt to retard (if not prevent) the progression of microvascular disease. One should aim at simulating a normal physiologic status by administering insulin in such a manner as to provide a continuous low basal level of circulating insulin and produce an eight- to tenfold rise in plasma insulin concentration with the average meal. Care should be taken to avoid administration of excessive insulin that might induce hypoglycemia. To achieve these goals, the patient, in cooperation with the physician, must learn to make adjustments in diet, exercise, and, if indicated, hypoglycemic agents.

AVAILABLE TREATMENT REGIMENS

1. DIET

A proper diet remains a fundamental element of therapy in all patients with diabetes. However, in over half of cases, diabetics fail to follow their diet. The reasons include unnecessary complexity of dietary instructions and poor understanding of the goals of dietary control by the patient and physician.

Revised ADA Recommendations

In 1994, the American Diabetes Association released a position statement on medical nutrition therapy that replaced the calculated ADA diet formula of the past with suggestions for an individually tailored dietary prescription based on metabolic, nutritional, and lifestyle requirements. They contend that the concept of one diet for "diabetes" and prescription for an "ADA diet" no longer can apply to both major types of diabetes. In their medical nutrition therapy recommendations for persons with type II diabetes, the 55–60% carbohydrate content of previous "ADA" diets have been reduced considerably because of the tendency of high carbohydrate intake to cause hyperglycemia, hypertriglyceridemia, and a lowered HDL cholesterol. In obese type II patients, glucose and lipid goals join weight loss as the focus for therapy. These patients are advised to limit their carbohydrate intake by substituting noncholesterologenic monounsaturated oils such as olive oil, rapeseed (canola) oil or the oils in nuts and avocados. This maneuver is also indicated in type I patients on intensive insulin regimens in whom near-normoglycemic control is less achievable on diets higher in carbohydrate content. In these patients, the ratio of carbohydrate to fat will vary among individuals in relation to their glycemic responses, insulin regimens, and exercise patterns.

The new recommendations for both types of diabetes continue to limit cholesterol to 300 mg daily and advise a daily protein intake of 10–20% total calories. They suggest that saturated fat be no higher than 8–9% of total calories with a similar proportion of polyunsaturated fat and that the remainder of the caloric needs be made up of an individualized ratio of monounsaturated fat and of carbohydrate containing 20–35 g dietary fiber. Previous recommendations of polyunsaturated fat supplements as part of a prudent diabetic diet have been revised because of their potential hazards. Polyunsaturated fatty acids appear to promote oxidation of LDL and lower HDL cholesterol, both of which may contribute to atherogenesis; furthermore, in large quantities during supplementation, they may promote carcinogenesis. Poultry, veal, and fish continue to be recommended as a substitute for red meats for keeping saturated fat content low. Stearic acid is the least cholesterologenic saturated fatty acid, since it is rapidly converted to oleic acid— in contrast to palmitic acid (found in animal fat as well as coconut oil), which is a major substrate for cholesterol formation. In contrast to previous recommendations, the present ADA position statement adduces no evidence that reducing protein intake below 10% of total caloric intake (about 0.8 g/kg/d) is of any benefit in patients with nephropathy with renal impairment, and in fact the investigators feel it may be detrimental.

Exchange lists for meal planning can be obtained from the American Diabetes Association (ADA; 1660 Duke Street, Alexandria, Virginia 22314) and its affiliate associations or from the American Dietetic Association (430 North Michigan Avenue, Chicago 60611).

Prescribing the Diet

A. Type I Diabetes (IDDM): In type I diabetes, total calories are calculated to maintain ideal body weight. In the typical patient, insulin is administered at least twice a day, often as a mixture of a short-acting and an intermediate-acting insulin. Meals should be adjusted accordingly in an effort to match food intake with insulin action. Breakfast should be eaten within ½–1 hour after the morning insulin dose (especially if short-acting insulin is administered at this time). A carbohydrate snack should be eaten 3 hours later and lunch no later than 5 hours after the morning insulin dose. A midafternoon carbohydrate snack is given 7–8 hours after the morning insulin. Dinner should follow the second injection by ½–1½ hours, depending on whether a short-acting insulin is administered at this time. A bedtime snack containing protein as well as carbohydrate should be given 3 hours after the evening insulin in order to provide a slow influx of carbohydrate from metabolized protein during most of the night. When multiple insulin injections are prescribed, greater flexibility with regard to timing of meals is possible.

B. Type II Diabetes (NIDDM): In type II diabetes, patients are often at least mildly obese. Treatment requires a vigorous program to achieve weight reduction. A fall in fasting blood sugar may follow caloric restriction prior to any significant weight loss. Weight reduction is an elusive goal that can be achieved and maintained only by close supervision of the obese patient and a supervised exercise program. The total amount of calories prescribed must take into account the patient's ideal body weight, lifestyle, and activity level. A diet consisting of no more than 600 kcal daily may be appropriate for a sedentary patient who is overweight, but a mildly active person can lose weight on a diet of up to 1400 kcal.

A recent discovery of an obesity (*ob*) gene in mice and its homolog in humans has led to the development of a commercial gene product, leptin, which when given parenterally reduces fat tissue in both obese and normal mice. Clinical trials in human obesity are pending, though preliminary data as yet show no evidence of mutations of this gene in human obese patients (Chapter 21).

Special Considerations in Dietary Control

A. Dietary Fiber: Plant components such as cellulose, gum, and pectin are indigestible by humans and are termed dietary "fiber." **Insoluble fibers** such as cellulose or hemicellulose, as found in bran, tend to increase intestinal transit time and may have beneficial effects on colonic function. In contrast, **soluble fibers** such as gums and pectins, as found in beans, oatmeal, or apple skin, tend to decrease gastric and intestinal transit so that glucose absorption is slower and hyperglycemia is diminished. Although the ADA diet does not require insoluble fiber supplements such as added bran, it recommends foods such as oatmeal, cereals, and beans with relatively high soluble fiber content as stable components of the diet in diabetics. High soluble fiber content in the diet may also have a favorable effect on blood cholesterol levels.

B. Glycemic Index: Quantitation of the relative glycemic contribution of different carbohydrate foods has formed the basis of a "glycemic index" (GI), in which the area of blood glucose (plotted on a graph) generated over a 3-hour period following ingestion of a test food containing 50 g of carbohydrate is compared with the area plotted after giving a similar quantity of reference food such as glucose or white bread:

$$GI = \frac{\text{Blood glucose area of test food}}{\text{Blood glucose area of reference food}} \times 100$$

White bread is preferred to glucose as a reference standard because it is more palatable and has less tendency to slow gastric emptying by high tonicity, as happens when glucose solution is used.

Differences in GI were noted in normal subjects and diabetics when various foods were compared. In comparison to white bread, which was assigned an index of 100, the mean GI for other foods was as follows: baked potato, 135; table sugar (sucrose), 86; spaghetti, 66; kidney beans, 54; ice cream, 52; and lentils, 43. Some investigators have questioned whether the GI for a food ingested alone is meaningful, since the GI may become altered considerably by the presence of fats and protein when the food is consumed in a mixed meal.

Further studies of the reproducibility of the GI in the same person and the relation of a particular food's GI to its insulinotropic action on pancreatic B cells are needed before the utility of the GI in prescribing diabetic diets can be appropriately assessed. At present, however, it appears that small amounts of sucrose—particularly when taken with high-fiber substances such as cereals or whole-grain breads—may have no greater glycemic effects than comparable portions of starch from potatoes, rice, or bread.

C. Sweeteners: The nonnutritive sweetener **saccharin** is widely used as a sugar substitute (Sweet N'Low) and continues to be available in certain foods and beverages despite recent warnings by the FDA about its potential long-term bladder carcinogenicity. A committee of the National Academy of Sciences recommended restrictions in the use of saccharin in children and pregnant women. The panel felt that physicians might be best suited to determine on an individual basis its comparative benefit versus risk for patients with diabetes or obesity.

Aspartame (NutraSweet) may prove to be the safest sweetener for use in diabetics; it consists of two major amino acids, aspartic acid and phenylalanine, which combine to produce a nutritive sweetener 180 times as sweet as sucrose. A major limitation is its heat lability, which precludes its use in baking or cooking.

Other sweeteners such as sorbitol and fructose have recently gained popularity. Except for acute diarrhea induced by ingestion of large amounts of sorbitol-containing foods, their relative risk has yet to be established. **Fructose** represents a "natural" sugar substance that is a highly effective sweetener which induces only slight increases in plasma glucose levels and does not require insulin for its utilization. However, because of potential adverse effects of large amounts of fructose (up to 20% of total calories) on raising serum cholesterol and LDL cholesterol, the ADA feels it may have no overall advantage as a sweetening agent in the diabetic diet. This does not preclude, however, ingestion of fructose-containing fruits and vegetables or fructose-sweetened foods in moderation.

D. Starch Blockers: The FDA has decided that enzymatic antagonists of amylase and sucrase (alpha-glucosidase inhibitors) can no longer be classified as "foods" but must be classified as drugs. At present, clinical trials are in progress to ascertain the efficacy and safety of these substances in reducing postprandial hyperglycemia in diabetes. They have not proved effective as an adjunct to weight reduction in the management of obesity.

2. ORAL HYPOGLYCEMIC DRUGS

Two major types of oral hypoglycemic drugs are commonly used in the United States: the sulfonylureas and the biguanides. The modes of action of the two types are quite different. Sulfonylureas remain the most widely prescribed oral drugs for treating hyperglycemia. However, in December 1994, the United States Food and Drug Administration gave approval to a member of the biguanide family, metformin, for clinical use. In contrast to sulfonylureas, which work by stimulating the pancreas to secrete more insulin, metformin lowers hyperglycemia by other mechanisms and is an "insulin-sparing" drug that does not cause weight gain in treated diabetic patients. For these reasons, it has been advocated as a first-line drug for obese diabetics with the insulin-resistance syndrome as well as for use in combination with a sulfonylurea in patients responding poorly to a sulfonylurea alone. The FDA feels that metformin has met satisfactory standards of safety after several years of clinical trials in the United States and over 20 years of use in more than 70 countries worldwide. Its tendency to cause lactic acidosis is only one-tenth that of phenformin, another biguanide, which was taken off the market in 1977 in the USA as well as in many other countries. A third class of drugs, the starch blocker, Acarbose, was recently approved for use by the FDA (see below).

Sulfonylureas

This group of drugs contains a sulfonic acid-urea nucleus that can be modified by chemical substitutions to produce agents that have similar qualitative actions but differ widely in potency. The proposed mechanisms of action of the sulfonylureas include (1) augmentation of insulin release from pancreatic B cells and (2) potentiation of insulin's action on its target cells.

A. Mechanism of Action: Specific receptors on the surface of pancreatic B cells bind sulfonylureas in the rank order of their insulinotropic potency (glyburide with the greatest affinity and tolbutamide with the least). It has been shown that activation of these receptors closes potassium channels, resulting in depolarization of the B cell. This depolarized state permits calcium to enter the cell and actively promote insulin release (Figure 18–8). Controversy persists, however, about whether this well-documented insulinotropic action during acute administration is sufficient to explain adequately the hypoglycemic effect of sulfonylureas during chronic therapy. Additional extrapancreatic effects of sulfonylureas, such as their potentiation of the peripheral effects of insulin at the receptor or postreceptor level, have been invoked to account for their continued effectiveness during long-term treatment despite a lack of demonstrable increase in insulin secretion. However, several clinical trials have failed to demonstrate any therapeutic benefit on long-term glycemic control when sulfonylureas are added to insulin therapy in the patient with IDDM. These observations suggest that in vitro evidence for a potentiation by sulfonylureas of the peripheral effects of insulin may have little clinical relevance.

B. Indications: Sulfonylureas are not indicated in ketosis-prone type I diabetic patients, since these drugs require functioning pancreatic B cells to produce their effect on blood glucose. Moreover, clinical trials show no benefit from the use of sulfonylureas as an adjunct to insulin replacement in type I diabetic patients. The sulfonylureas seem most appropriate for use in the nonobese patient with mild maturity-onset diabetes whose hyperglycemia has not responded to diet therapy. In obese patients with mild diabetes and slight to moderate peripheral insensitivity to levels of circulating insulin, the primary emphasis should be on weight reduction. When hyperglycemia in obese diabetics has been more severe, with consequent impairment of pancreatic B cell function, sulfonylureas may improve glycemic control until concurrent measures such as diet, exercise, and weight reduction can sustain the improvement without the need for oral drugs.

C. Sulfonylureas Currently Available in the USA: (Table 18–11.)

1. Tolbutamide (Orinase)—Tolbutamide is supplied in tablets of 250 and 500 mg. It is rapidly oxidized in the liver to an inactive form. Because its du-

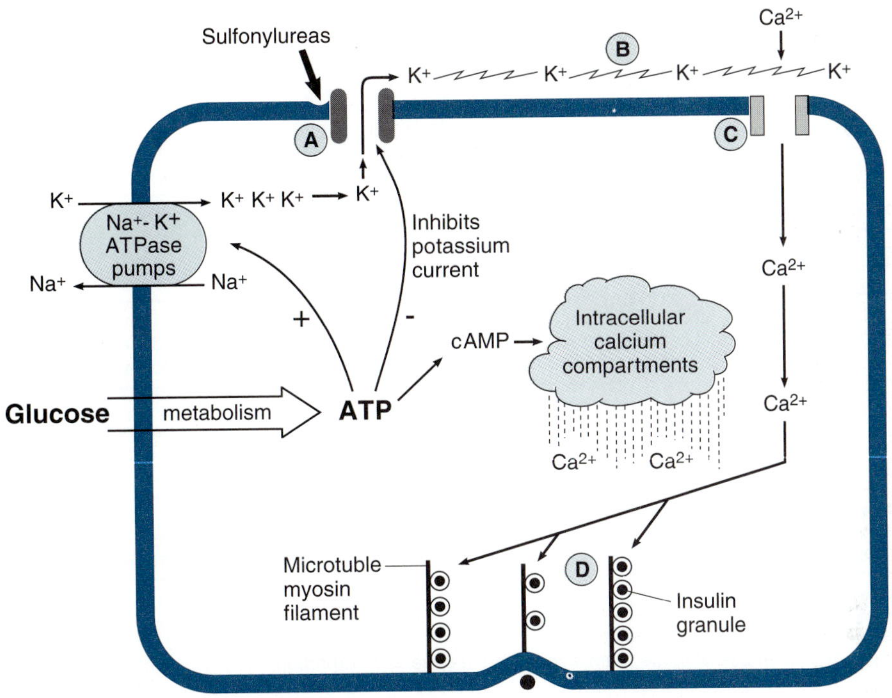

Figure 18–8. Proposed mechanism for sulfonylurea stimulation of insulin release by the pancreatic B cell. Energy-dependent pumps maintain a high intracellular concentration of potassium (K^+). In the resting B cell, K^+ diffuses from the cell through non-energy-dependent potassium channels (A). This current of potassium ions generates an electrical potential that polarizes the resting cell membrane (B) and closes a voltage-gaited calcium channel (C), thereby preventing extracellular calcium from entering the cell. When sulfonylureas bind to a specific receptor on the potassium channel (or when glucose metabolism generates ATP), the potassium channel closes. This depolarizes the cell, allowing calcium to enter and cause microtubules to contract (D), moving insulin granules to the cell surface for emeiocytosis. (Modified and reproduced, with permission, from Karam JH: Type II diabetes and syndrome X. Endocrinol Metab Clin North Am 1992;21:339.)

ration of effect is short (6–10 hours), it is usually administered in divided doses (eg, 500 mg before each meal and at bedtime). The usual daily dose is 1.5–3 g; some patients, however, require only 250–500 mg daily. Acute toxic reactions such as skin rashes are rare. Because of its short duration of action, which is independent of renal function, tolbutamide is probably the safest agent to use in elderly patients in whom hypoglycemia would be a particularly serious risk. Prolonged hypoglycemia has been reported rarely, mainly in patients receiving certain drugs (eg, warfarin, phenylbutazone, or sulfonamides) that compete with sulfonylureas for hepatic oxidation, resulting in maintenance of high levels of unmetabolized active sulfonylureas in the circulation.

2. Chlorpropamide (Diabinese)–This drug is supplied in tablets of 100 and 250 mg. It has a half-life of 32 hours and a duration of action of up to 60 hours. It is slowly metabolized by the liver, with approximately 20–30% excreted unchanged in the urine. Since the metabolites retain hypoglycemic activity, elimination of the biologic effect is almost completely dependent on renal excretion, so that its use is contraindicated in patients with renal insufficiency. The average maintenance dose is 250 mg daily (range, 100–500 mg), given as a single dose in the morning. Chlorpropamide is a potent agent, and prolonged hypoglycemic reactions are more common than with tolbutamide and other shorter-acting oral hypoglycemic agents. This is particularly of concern in elderly patients who may gradually develop impaired renal clearance with aging putting them at greater risk of developing prolonged hypoglycemia on chlorpropamide therapy. For this reason, the drug should not be prescribed to people over 65 years of age. Doses in excess of 500 mg/d increase the risk of cholestatic jaundice, which does not occur with the usual dose of 250 mg or less. About 15% of patients taking chlorpropamide develop a facial flush when they drink alcohol, and occasionally they may develop a full-blown disulfiram-like reaction, with nausea, vomiting, weakness, and even syncope. There appears to be a genetic predisposition to the development of this reaction.

Table 18–11. Oral antidiabetic drugs.

Drug	Tablet Size	Daily Dose	Duration of Action
Tolbutamide (Orinase)	250 and 500 mg	0.5–2 g in 2 or 3 divided doses	6–12 hours
Tolazamide* (Tolinase)	100, 250, and 500 mg	0.1–1 g as single dose or in 2 divided doses	Up to 24 hours
Acetohexamide* (Dymelor)[1]	250 and 500 mg	0.25–1.5 g as single dose or in 2 divided doses	8–24 hours
Chlorpropamide* (Diabinese)[1]	100 and 250 mg	0.1–0.5 g as single dose	24–72 hours
Glyburide* (Diaβeta, Micronase) (Glynase)	1.25, 2.5, and 5 mg 1.5, 3, and 6 mg	1.25–20 mg as single dose or in 2 divided doses 1.5–18 mg as single dose or in 2 divided doses.	Up to 24 hours Up to 24 hours
Glipizide (Glucotrol) (Glucotrol XL)	5 and 10 mg 5 and 10 mg	2.5–40 mg as single dose or in 2 divided doses on an empty stomach. Up to 20 or 30 mg daily as a single dose.	6–12 hours Up to 24 hours
Glimeperide (Amaryl)	1, 2, and 4 mg	1–4 mg as single dose.	Up to 24 hours
Metformin (Glucophage)	500 and 850 mg	1–2.55 g. One tablet with meals 2 or 3 times daily.	7–12 hours
Acarbose (Precose)	50 and 100 mg	75–300 mg in 3 divided doses with first bite of food.	4 hours

*Generic available.
[1]There has been a decline in use of these formulations. In the case of chlorpropamide, the decline is due to its numerous side effects (see text).

Other side effects of chlorpropamide include water retention and the development of hyponatremia, effects that are mediated through an ADH mechanism. The hyponatremia is generally a benign condition with sodium values between 125 and 130 meq/L, but occasional cases of symptomatic hyponatremia with sodium concentrations below 125 meq/L have been reported, particularly when concomitant diuretic therapy is being used. Chlorpropamide stimulates ADH secretion and also potentiates its action at the renal tubule. Its antidiuretic effect is somewhat unusual, since three other sulfonylureas (acetohexamide, tolazamide, and glyburide) appear to facilitate water excretion in humans.

Since other sulfonylureas have now become available with comparable potency but without the disadvantages of depending solely on renal excretion or of causing water retention and alcohol flushing, there presently is less need to choose chlorpropamide when prescribing sulfonylurea therapy in NIDDM patients.

3. Tolazamide (Tolinase)–Tolazamide is supplied in tablets of 100, 250, and 500 mg. The average daily dose is 200–1000 mg, given in one or two doses. It is comparable to chlorpropamide in potency but is devoid of disulfiram-like or water-retaining effects. Tolazamide is more slowly absorbed than the other sulfonylureas, with effects on blood glucose not appearing for several hours. Its duration of action may last up to 20 hours, with maximal hypoglycemic effect occurring between the fourth and 14th hours. Tolazamide is metabolized to several compounds

that retain hypoglycemic effects. If more than 500 mg/d is required, the dose should be divided and given twice daily. Doses larger than 1000 mg/d do not improve the degree of glycemic control.

4. Acetohexamide (Dymelor)–This agent is supplied in tablets of 250 and 500 mg. Its duration of action is about 10–16 hours (intermediate in duration of action between tolbutamide and chlorpropamide). The usual daily dose is 250–1500 mg given in one or two doses. Liver metabolism is rapid, but an active metabolite is produced and excreted by the kidney.

5. Second-generation sulfonylureas–In April, 1984, the FDA approved two potent sulfonylurea compounds, glyburide and glipizide. These agents have similar chemical structures, with cyclic carbon rings at each end of the sulfonylurea nucleus; this causes them to be highly potent (100-fold more potent than tolbutamide). The drugs should be used with caution in patients with cardiovascular disease as well as in elderly patients, in whom hypoglycemia would be especially dangerous. Neither glyburide nor glipizide should be prescribed to patients with hepatic or renal impairment, since a reduced clearance of these drugs from the blood would greatly increase the risk of hypoglycemia.

Diabetic patients who have not responded to tolbutamide or even tolazamide often—but not always—respond to the more potent first-generation sulfonylurea, chlorpropamide, or to either of the second-generation sulfonylureas. Unfortunately, substantial glycemic benefit has not always resulted when a maximum therapeutic dose of chlorpropamide has been replaced with that of a second-generation drug in NIDDM patients whose glucose control has been unsatisfactory. In 1994, standard forms of both glyburide and glipizide became available as generic medications.

a. Glyburide (glibenclamide)–Glyburide is supplied in tablets containing 1.25, 2.5, and 5 mg. The usual starting dose is 2.5 mg/d, and the average maintenance dose is 5–10 mg/d given as a single morning dose. If patients are going to respond to glyburide, they generally do so at doses of 10 mg/d or less, given once daily. If they fail to respond to 10 mg/d, it is uncommon for an increase in dosage to result in improved glycemic control. Maintenance doses higher than 20 mg/d are not recommended and may even worsen hyperglycemia. Glyburide is metabolized in the liver into products with such low hypoglycemic activity that they are considered clinically unimportant unless renal excretion is compromised. Although assays specific for the unmetabolized compound suggest a plasma half-life of only 1–2 hours, the biologic effects of glyburide clearly persist for 24 hours after a single morning dose in diabetic patients.

A recently marketed Press Tab formulation of "micronized" glyburide, which apparently increases its bioavailability, is now available in "bent" tablet sizes of 1.5 mg, 3 mg, and 6 mg. These are easy to break in half with very mild pressure at the angle of the bend in the tablet. However, there is some question as to its bioequivalency as compared with nonmicronized formulations, so that the FDA recommends careful monitoring to reiterate dosage when switching from standard glyburide doses or from other sulfonylurea drugs.

Glyburide does not cause water retention, as chlorpropamide does, and even slightly enhances free water clearance. Glyburide has few adverse effects other than its potential for causing hypoglycemia. It is particularly hazardous in patients over 65 years of age, in whom serious, protracted, and even fatal hypoglycemia can occur even with relatively small daily doses. Drugs with a shorter half-life, eg, tolbutamide or possibly glipizide, are preferable in the treatment of type II diabetes in the elderly patient.

b. Glipizide (glydiazinamide)–Glipizide is supplied in tablets containing 5 and 10 mg. For maximum effect in reducing postprandial hyperglycemia, this agent should be ingested 30 minutes before breakfast, since rapid absorption is delayed when the drug is taken with food. The recommended starting dose is 5 mg/d, with up to 15 mg/d given as a single daily dose. When higher daily doses are required, they should be divided and given before meals. The maximum recommended dose is 40 mg/d.

At least 90% of glipizide is metabolized in the liver to inactive products, and only a small fraction is excreted unchanged in the urine. Glipizide therapy is contraindicated in patients who have hepatic or renal impairment and who would therefore be at high risk for hypoglycemia, but because of its lower potency and shorter half-life, it is preferable to glyburide in elderly patients.

Recently, a new formulation of glipizide has been marketed as Glucotrol-XL in 5 mg and 10 mg tablets. The medication is enclosed in a nonabsorbable shell that contains an osmotic compartment which expands slowly, thereby slowly pumping out the glipizide in a sustained manner. It provides extended release during transit through the gastrointestinal tract, with greater effectiveness in lowering of prebreakfast hyperglycemia than the shorter-duration immediate-release standard glipizide tablets. However, this formulation appears to have sacrificed its lesser propensity for severe hypoglycemia compared with longer-acting glyburide without showing any demonstrable therapeutic advantages over glyburide, which presently can be obtained as a generic drug.

c. Glimeperide–This sulfonylurea has recently completed clinical trials and was approved in January 1966 by the FDA for "once-daily use as monotherapy or in combination with insulin to lower blood glucose in diabetes patients who cannot control their glucose level through diet and exercise." Glimeperide achieves blood glucose lowering with the lowest dose of any sulfonylurea compound. A single daily dose of 1 mg/d has been shown to be effective, and the maximal recommended dose is 4 mg. Glimiperide has a long duration of effect with a half-life of 5 hours, allowing once-daily administration, which improves compliance. It is completely metabolized by the liver to relatively inactive metabolic products. Further experience will be required to determine whether any efficacy and safety advantages favor its use over other less expensive generic forms of sulfonylureas.

Biguanides

Unlike sulfonylureas, the biguanides (Table 18–11) do not require functioning pancreatic B cells for reduction of hyperglycemia. Use of **phenformin** was discontinued in the USA because of its association with the development of lactic acidosis in patients with coexisting liver or kidney disease. Also of note was lack of documentation of any long-term efficacy of this drug in treating diabetes. Biguanides continue to be used in many countries throughout the world. **Metformin,** a biguanide reported to be less likely to produce lactic acidosis, has generally replaced phenformin in the treatment of diabetics.

Metformin (1,1-dimethylbiguanide hydrochloride) was introduced in France in 1957 as an oral agent for therapy of type II diabetes, either alone or in conjunction with sulfonylureas. It received FDA approval in 1995 for use in the United States and is marketed under the brand name Glucophage.

A. Clinical Pharmacology: The exact mechanism of action of metformin remains unclear. It reduces both the fasting level of blood glucose and the degree of postprandial hyperglycemia in patients with type II diabetes but has no effect on fasting blood glucose in normal subjects. Metformin does not stimulate insulin action, yet it is particularly effective in reducing hepatic gluconeogenesis. Other proposed mechanisms include a slowing down of gastrointestinal absorption of glucose and increased glucose uptake by skeletal muscle, which have been reported in some but not all clinical studies. Because of its very high concentration in intestinal cells after oral administration, metformin increases glucose-to-lactate turnover in these cells, and this also contributes to its action in reducing hyperglycemia.

Metformin has a half-life of 1½–3 hours, is not bound to plasma proteins, and is not metabolized in humans, being excreted unchanged by the kidneys.

B. Indications and Dosage: Metformin may be used as an adjunct to diet for the control of hyperglycemia and its associated symptomatology in patients with type II diabetes, particularly those who are obese or are not responding optimally to maximal doses of sulfonylureas. A side benefit of metformin therapy is its tendency to improve both fasting and postprandial hyperglycemia and hypertriglyceridemia in obese diabetics without the weight gain associated with insulin or sulfonylurea therapy. For this reason—and because of its ability to correct hyperglycemia while having an insulin-sparing action—metformin has particular potential in treating patients with the insulin resistance syndrome (syndrome X). Metformin is not indicated for patients with type I diabetes and is contraindicated in diabetics with renal insufficiency, since failure to excrete this drug would produce high blood and tissue levels of metformin that would stimulate lactic acid overproduction. Likewise, patients with hepatic insufficiency or abusers of ethanol should not receive this drug since lactic acid production from the gut and other tissues, which rises during metformin therapy, could result in lactic acidosis when defective hepatocytes cannot remove the lactate or when alcohol-induced reduction of nucleotides interferes with lactate clearance. Finally, metformin is contraindicated in patients with cardiorespiratory insufficiency, since they have a propensity to develop hypoxia which would aggravate the lactic acid production already occurring from metformin therapy. The "age" cutoff for prescribing metformin has not been defined and remains relative to the overall health of the patient, but generally there is concern that after the age of 65–70 years, the potential for progressive impairment of renal function or development of a cardiac event while taking metformin raises the risk enough to outweigh the benefits of prescribing metformin to the elderly patient with NIDDM.

Metformin is dispensed as 500 mg or 850 mg tablets, and the dosage range is from 500 mg to a maximum of 2.55 g daily, with the lowest possible effective dose being recommended. It is important that metformin be taken with meals to reduce minor gastrointestinal upsets. A common schedule would be to begin with a single 500-mg tablet given with breakfast for several days, and if this is tolerated without gastrointestinal discomfort to add a second 500-mg tablet with the evening meal if hyperglycemia persists. If further dosage increases are required, after 1 week an additional 500-mg tablet can be added to be taken with the midday meal, or the larger tablet (850 mg) can be prescribed twice daily or even three times daily (maximum recommended dose) if needed. Divided dosage is necessary because ingestion of more than 850 mg at any one time is seldom tolerated because of gastrointestinal side effects.

C. Adverse Reactions: The most frequent side effects of metformin are gastrointestinal symptoms (anorexia, nausea, vomiting, abdominal discomfort, diarrhea), which occur in up to 20% of patients. These effects are dose-related, tend to occur at onset of therapy, and often are transient. However, in 3–5% of patients, therapy may have to be discontinued because of persistent diarrheal discomfort. Absorption of vitamin B_{12} appears to be reduced during chronic metformin therapy, and annual screening of serum B_{12} levels and red blood cell parameters has been encouraged by the manufacturer to determine the need for B_{12} injections.

Hypoglycemia does not occur with therapeutic doses of metformin, which permits its description as a "euglycemic" or "antihyperglycemic" drug rather than an oral hypoglycemic agent. Dermatologic or hematologic toxicity is rare.

Lactic acidosis (see below) has been reported as a side effect but is uncommon with metformin in contrast to phenformin, and almost all reported cases have involved subjects with associated risk factors that should have contraindicated its use (renal, hepatic, or cardiorespiratory insufficiency, alcoholism, advanced age).

Alpha-Glucosidase Inhibitors

A third class of oral antihyperglycemic drugs are the competitive inhibitors of intestinal brush border alpha-glucosidases. A representative of this class, acarbose, received FDA approval in December 1995. It tends to reduce postprandial hyperglycemia by reducing the rate of absorption of most carbohydrates such as starches, dextrins, maltose, and sucrose (but not lactose, which has a beta linkage). Acarbose is an oligosaccharide analog that binds 1000 times more avidly to the intestinal disaccharidases than do products of carbohydrate digestion or sucrose. This competitive inhibition of alpha-glucosidase limits the rise of glucose after meals and results in an insulin-sparing action. When used to treat hyperglycemic patients, its overall effect is slight, with a reduction of HbA_{1c} of only 0.5–1%, and a reduction of postprandial hyperglycemia by 30–50%. The principal adverse effect, seen in 20–30% of patients, is flatulence. This is caused by undigested carbohydrate reaching the lower bowel, where gases are produced by bacterial flora. In 3% of cases, troublesome diarrhea occurs. This gastrointestinal discomfort tends to discourage excessive carbohydrate consumption and promotes improved compliance of NIDDM patients to their diet prescriptions. The recommended starting dose of acarbose is 50 mg twice daily, gradually increasing to 100 mg three times daily. For maximal benefit on postprandial hyperglycemia, acarbose should be given with the first mouthful of food ingested. When acarbose is given alone, there is no risk of hypoglycemia. However if combined with insulin or sulfonylureas, it might increase risk of hypoglycemia from these agents. A slight rise in hepatic aminotransferases has been noted in clinical trials (5% versus 2% in placebo controls, and particularly with doses greater than 300 mg/d). This generally returns to normal on stopping this drug.

Insulin Sensitizers (Thiazolidinediones)

A new class of oral hypoglycemic agents is undergoing clinical trials. Troglitazone, a member of this group, appears to improve the action of insulin in the liver, skeletal muscle, and adipose tissue in vitro by a mechanism that has not yet been defined. It corrects hyperglycemia and hyperinsulinemia in type II diabetes and improves glucose tolerance and corrects hyperinsulinemia in obese subjects. However, it will not be available for clinical use until its long-term efficacy and safety are established.

Efficacy & Safety of Oral Hypoglycemic Agents

The University Group Diabetes Program (UGDP) reported that the number of deaths due to cardiovascular disease in diabetic patients treated with tolbutamide or phenformin was excessive when compared to either insulin-treated patients or to patients receiving placebos. Controversy persists about the validity of the conclusions reached by the UGDP because of the heterogeneity of the population studied, its preponderance of obese subjects, and certain features of the experimental design, such as the use of a fixed dose of oral drug and lack of control for cigarette smoking. At present, a warning label outlining their cardiovascular risk is inserted in each packet of sulfonylureas and metformin dispensed. However, the American Diabetes Association has withdrawn its original support for the UGDP conclusions.

3. INSULIN

Insulin is indicated for type I diabetics as well as for those type II diabetics whose hyperglycemia does not respond to diet therapy and oral hypoglycemic drugs.

Insulin replacement in patients with type I diabetes has been less than optimal because it is not possible to completely reproduce the normal physiologic pattern of insulin secretion into the portal vein. The problem of achieving optimal insulin delivery remains unsolved with the present state of technology. Subcutaneous injections do not reproduce the physiologic patterns of insulin secretion; however, with the help of appropriate modifications of diet and exercise and careful monitoring of capillary blood glucose levels at home, it is possible to achieve acceptable control of blood glucose by using multiple injections of short- and intermediate-acting insulins. In some patients, a portable insulin infusion pump may be required for optimal control.

With the development of highly purified human insulin preparations, immunogenicity has been markedly reduced, thereby decreasing the incidence of therapeutic complications such as insulin allergy, immune insulin resistance, and localized lipoatrophy at the injection site.

Characteristics of Currently Available Insulin Preparations

Commercial insulin preparations differ with regard to the animal species from which they are obtained; their purity, concentration, and solubility; and their time of onset and duration of biologic action (Table 18–12 and Figure 18–9). In 1995, approximately 30 different formations of insulin were available in the USA.

A. Species of Insulin: Because the supply of human or pork insulin is still too limited to satisfy the demand for insulin in the USA, many commercial insulins are composed of mixtures of beef and pork insulin. Beef insulin, which differs by three amino

Table 18–12. Summary of bioavailability characteristics of the insulins.

	Insulin Type	Onset	Peak Action	Duration
Short-acting	Insulin lispro Regular, Velosulin	5–15 minutes 15–30 minutes	1–1.5 hours 1–3 hours	3–4 hours 5–7 hours
Intermediate-acting	Lente, NPH	2–4 hours	8–10 hours	18–24 hours
Long-acting	Ultralente	4–5 hours	8–14 hours	25–36 hours

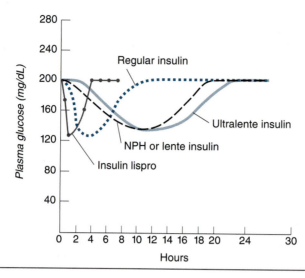

Figure 18–9. Extent and duration of action of various types of insulin (in a fasting diabetic). Duration of action is extended considerably when the dose of a given insulin formulation increases above the average therapeutic doses depicted here. (Modified, with permission, from Katzung BG [editor]: *Basic & Clinical Pharmacology,* 2nd ed. Lange, 1985.)

acids from human insulin, is more antigenic than pork insulin, which differs from human insulin by just one amino acid. The standard preparation of Iletin I (Lilly) is a mixture of 70% beef and 30% pork insulin, whereas the highly purified Iletin II insulins are available as pork insulin. Human insulin is now produced by recombinant DNA techniques, and most insulin-producing companies are converting their insulin production to this type of insulin as availability of animal sources continues to diminish. Human insulin prepared by the recombinant DNA method in *E coli* is available for clinical use as Humulin (Lilly) and dispensed as either Regular (R), NPH (N), or Lente (L). Human insulin made by recombinant DNA methods using yeast is marketed as Novolin and as Velosulin by Novo Nordisk. Novolin-R is a rapid-acting soluble form of human insulin. Novolin-L is a zinc suspension with an intermediate duration of action similar to that of Novolin-N, which is an isophane suspension of human insulin with protamine. Since human insulin tends to be slightly more hydrophilic than beef insulin, an ultralente formulation of human insulin with the required degree of insolubility has been introduced, but questions persist about whether it has the same slow and sustained release as beef ultralente, which unfortunately is no longer manufactured. The cost of human insulin is approximately 1¼ times the cost of standard beef or pork insulin but slightly less than the cost of purified pork insulin.

B. Purity of Insulin: Improvements in purification techniques with Sephadex gel columns have reduced or eliminated contamination with proteins having molecular weights greater than that of insulin (eg, proinsulin). Although these contaminants were biologically inactive, they were capable of inducing anti-insulin antibodies. The degree of purification in which proinsulin contamination is greater than 10

ppm but less than 25 ppm justifies their present labeling as "standard insulin" and is the main form of animal insulin produced in the USA by Eli Lilly as Iletin I (Table 18–13). When the proinsulin content is reduced to less than 10 ppm, manufacturers are entitled by FDA regulations to label the insulin "purified." The Eli Lilly products highly purified from pork pancreas are called Iletin II, whereas all human insulins as well as Novo Nordisk pork insulins are also highly purified.

The more highly purified insulins currently in use preserve their potency quite well; therefore, refrigeration while in use is not necessary. During travel, reserve supplies of insulin can be readily transported for weeks without significant loss of potency provided they are protected from extremes of heat or cold.

Concentrations of Insulin (Table 18–13)

At present, insulins in the USA are available only in a concentration of 100 units/mL (U100); all are dispensed in 10-mL vials. To accommodate children and the occasional adult who may require small quantities of insulin, "low-dose" (0.5 mL and 0.3-mL) disposable insulin syringes have been introduced so that U100 insulin can now be measured accurately in doses as low as 1 or 2 units. This has eliminated the need for lower concentrations of insulin and has resulted in the phasing out of all U40 insulins in the United States. For use in rare cases of severe insulin resistance in which large quantities of insulin are required, a limited supply of U500 (500 units/mL) regular insulin is available from Lilly (pork, Iletin II).

Bioavailability Characteristics

Three principal types of insulin are available: (1) short-acting insulin, with rapid onset of action; (2)

Table 18–13. Insulin preparations available in the USA.[1]

Preparation	Special Source	Concentration
SHORT-ACTING INSULINS		
Standard[2]		
Regular Iletin I (Lilly)	Beef and pork	U100
"Purified"[3]		
Regular (Novo Nordisk)[4]	Pork or human	U100
Regular Humulin (Lilly)	Human	U100
Regular Iletin II (Lilly)	Pork	U100, U500[5]
Velosulin (Novo Nordisk)[6]	Pork or human	U100
Humalog (Lilly)	Recombinant DNA	U100
INTERMEDIATE-ACTING INSULINS		
Standard[2]		
Lente Iletin I (Lilly)	Beef and pork	U100
NPH Iletin I (Lilly)	Beef and pork	U100
"Purified"[3]		
Lente Humulin (Lilly)	Human	U100
Lente Iletin II (Lilly)	Pork	U100
Lente (Novo Nordisk)[4]	Pork or human	U100
NPH Humulin (Lilly)	Human	U100
NPH Iletin II (Lilly)	Pork	U100
NPH (Novo Nordisk)	Pork or human	U100
PREMIXED INSULINS (% NPH/% REGULAR)		
Novolin 70/30 (Novo Nordisk)	Human	U100
Humulin 70/30 and 50/50 (Lilly)	Human	U100
LONG-ACTING INSULINS		
"Purified"[3]		
Ultralente Humulin (Lilly)	Human	U100

[1]These agents are all available without prescription except for Humalog (Lilly).
[2]Greater than 10 but less than 25 ppm proinsulin.
[3]Less than 10 ppm proinsulin.
[4]Novo Nordisk human insulins are termed Novolin R, L, and N.
[5]U500 available only as pork insulin.
[6]Velosulin contains phosphate buffer, which favors its use in infusion pumps but precludes its being mixed with lente insulin.

intermediate-acting; and (3) long-acting, with slow onset of action (Table 18–12). Short-acting (unmodified) insulin is a crystalline zinc insulin with a neutral pH in soluble form; it is dispensed as a clear solution. All other commercial insulins have been specifically modified to obtain more prolonged action. They are dispensed as opaque suspensions at neutral pH with either protamine (derived from fish sperm) in phosphate buffer (NPH) or varying concentrations of zinc in acetate buffer (ultralente and lente insulins), rendering the insulin insoluble. These preparations are designed for subcutaneous use. Semilente preparations are no longer available in the United States because of the more favorable bioavailability features of regular insulin.

As noted above, conventional insulin therapy relies on combinations of short-acting and either intermediate-acting or long-acting insulin. The characteristics of these various insulins are discussed below and summarized in Table 18–13 and Figure 18–9. It is important to recognize that values given for time of onset of action, peak effect, and duration of action are only approximate ones and that there is great variability in these parameters from patient to patient and even in a given patient depending on the size of the dose, the site of injection, the degree of exercise, the avidity of circulating anti-insulin antibodies, and other less well defined variables.

A. Short-Acting Insulins (Regular Insulin): Regular insulins (Regular Iletin I or II, or Humulin [Lilly], Novolin-R [Novo Nordisk], Velosulin [Novo Nordisk]) are short-acting, soluble crystalline zinc insulins whose hypoglycemic effect appears within 15 minutes after subcutaneous injection, peaks at 1–3 hours, and lasts for about 5–7 hours when usual quantities, eg, 5–15 units, are administered. Regular insulin is the only type that can be administered intravenously or used in continuous subcutaneous infusion pumps. It is particularly useful in the treatment of diabetic ketoacidosis and when the insulin requirement is changing rapidly, such as after surgery or during acute infections.

Regular insulin produced by Novo Nordisk and Lilly is dispensed without a buffer. When it is used in reservoirs or infusion pumps, stability is improved when regular insulin is buffered with disodium phosphate (Velosulin).

Insulin lispro—Humalog (Lilly)—is a human insulin analog of recombinant DNA origin that contains the same amino acids as human insulin except that proline at position 28 and lysine at position 29 on the insulin B chain are reversed. This switching results in an insulin molecule that resists formation of hexamers and tends to remain in monomeric form, thereby promoting a more rapid rate of absorption from subcutaneous injection sites.

B. Intermediate-Acting Insulins:

1. Lente insulin–This is a mixture of 30% short-acting (Lente Iletin I and II and Humulin-L [Lilly] and Novolin-L [Novo Nordisk]) with 70% ultralente insulin. Its onset of action is delayed to 2–4 hours, and its peak response is generally reached in about 8–10 hours. Because its duration of action is often less than 24 hours (with a range of 18–24 hours), most patients require at least two injections daily to maintain a sustained insulin effect. The supernatant of the lente suspension contains an excess of zinc ions, which may precipitate regular insulin if it is added to lente.

2. NPH (neutral protamine Hagedorn, or isophane) insulin–(NPH Iletin I and II or Humulin-N [Lilly], Novolin-N [Novo Nordisk].) NPH is an intermediate-acting insulin in which the onset of action is delayed by combining two parts of soluble crystalline zinc insulin with one part protamine zinc insulin. The mixture is reported to have equivalent concentrations of protamine and insulin, so that neither is in excess ("isophane"). The peak action and duration of action of NPH insulin are similar to those of lente insulin, however, in contrast to lente insulin, regular insulin retains its solubility and independent rapid action when mixed with NPH.

Flocculation of suspended particles may occasionally "frost" the sides of a bottle of NPH insulin or "clump" within bottles from which multiple small doses are withdrawn over a prolonged period. This instability is a rare phenomenon and might occur less frequently if NPH human insulin were refrigerated when not in use and if bottles were discarded after 1 month of use. Patients should be vigilant for early signs of frosting or clumping of the NPH insulin, because it indicates a pronounced loss of potency. Several cases of diabetic ketoacidosis have been reported in IDDM patients who had been inadvertently injecting this denatured insulin.

C. Long-Acting Insulin: Ultralente insulin—Iletin I Ultralente and Ultralente Humulin (Lilly)—is a relatively insoluble crystal of zinc and insulin suspended in an acetate buffer. Its onset of action is quite delayed, with peak effects at 8–14 hours and a duration of action of up to 36 hours. Beef insulin is less soluble than pork insulin, producing larger crystals and thus assuring a prolonged action. Beef insulin

has thus been preferred in producing the ultralente insulins. Unfortunately, the Novo Nordisk Company has discontinued their monospecies beef ultralente; thus, a slightly more soluble ultralente formulation made with human insulin (Humulin U [Lilly]) is the only ultralente insulin available in the USA. Because of its less sustained action compared with beef ultralente, it is generally recommended that the daily dose of Humulin Ultralente be split into two equal doses given every 12 hours. This is needed in type I patients to achieve basal insulin levels throughout the 24 hours which are comparable to that achieved in normal subjects by basal endogenous secretion or by the overnight infusion rate programmed into insulin pumps. Ultralente is increasingly used in association with multiple preprandial injections of regular insulin in an attempt to establish optimal control in IDDM patients.

D. Insulin Mixtures: Since intermediate insulins require several hours to reach adequate therapeutic levels, their use in type I patients requires supplements of regular insulin preprandially. It is well established that insulin mixtures containing increased proportions of lente to regular insulins may retard the rapid action of admixed regular insulin. The excess zinc in lente insulin binds the soluble insulin and partially blunts its action, particularly when a relatively small proportion of regular insulin is mixed with lente (eg, 1 part regular to 1½ or more parts lente). NPH preparations do not contain excess protamine and so do not delay absorption of admixed regular insulin. They are therefore preferable to lente when mixtures of intermediate and regular insulins are prescribed. For convenience, regular or NPH insulin may be mixed together in the same syringe and injected subcutaneously in split dosage before breakfast and supper. It is recommended that the regular insulin be withdrawn first, then the NPH insulin. No attempt should be made to mix the insulins in the syringe, and the injection is preferably given immediately after the syringe is loaded. Stable premixed insulins (70% NPH and 30% regular or 50% of each) are available as a convenience to patients who have difficulty mixing insulin because of visual problems or insufficient manual dexterity. These include Novolin 70:30 (Novo Nordisk) and Humulin 70:30 and 50:50 (Lilly).

E. Insulin Analogs: Among the many variables affecting the absorptive kinetics of insulin, an important one seems to be the property of insulin molecules of aggregating in hexameric form when formulated at pharmacologic concentrations. This causes lag periods of up to 30 minutes before insulin absorption is initiated from a subcutaneous depot site and results in a prolonged profile of absorption because the U100 injected regular insulin must be diluted more than 1000-fold by tissue fluids before it becomes monomeric and more readily absorbable into the circulation. The Eli Lilly Company has developed a monomeric insulin analog wherein two amino acids near the terminal end of the B chain have been reversed in position. Proline at position B28 has been switched to B29, with lysine moving from B29 to B28, and this analog has been termed "insulin lispro" (Humalog). The FDA approved insulin lispro in August 1996 after clinical trials demonstrated a favorable profile of rapid absorption after subcutaneous injection, excellent biologic activity in vivo, relatively low immunogenicity, and safety. However, pending further experience, it is the only insulin formulation requiring a medical prescription before it can be dispensed.

Methods of Insulin Administration

A. Insulin Syringes and Needles: Disposable plastic syringes with needles attached are available in 1-mL, 0.5-mL, and 0.3-mL sizes. Their finely honed 27- or 28-gauge attached needles have greatly reduced the pain of injections. They are light, not susceptible to damage, and convenient when traveling. Moreover, their clear markings and tight plungers allow accurate measurement of insulin dosage. In cases where very low insulin doses are prescribed, specially calibrated 0.3-mL and 0.5-mL disposable syringes facilitate accurate measurement of U100 insulin in doses up to 50 units. These "low-dose" syringes have become increasingly popular because it is now recommended that diabetics not take more than 50 units of insulin in a single injection except in the rare instance of extreme insulin resistance. Several reports indicate that "disposable" syringes may be reused until blunting of the needle occurs (usually after three to five injections). Wiping the needle with a clean alcohol swab, reapplying the needle guard, and refrigeration after use appear to maintain adequate sterility to avoid infection. A concern, however, arises from a report that flecks of silicone may become suspended in insulin bottles into which disposable syringes have been repeatedly inserted; the silicone flecks seem to reduce the activity of the insulin.

B. Sites for Injection: Any part of the body covered by loose skin can be used as an injection site, including the abdomen, thighs, upper arms, flanks, and upper outer quadrants of the buttocks. In general, regular insulin is absorbed more rapidly from upper regions of the body such as the deltoid area or the abdomen rather than from the thighs or buttocks. Exercise appears to facilitate insulin absorption when the injection site is adjacent to the exercising muscle. Rotation of sites continues to be recommended to avoid delayed absorption when fibrosis or lipohypertrophy occurs owing to repeated use of a single site. However, considerable variability of absorption rates from different sites, particularly with exercise, may contribute to the instability of glycemic control in certain IDDM patients if injection sites are rotated indiscriminately over different areas of the body. Consequently, diabetologists recommend limiting injection sites to a single region of the body and rotating sites within that region. It is possible that some of the stability of glycemic control achieved by infusion pumps may be related to the constancy of the site of infusion from day to day. For most patients the abdomen is the recommended site for injection, since it provides a considerable area in which to rotate sites and there may be less variability of absorption with exercise than when the thigh or deltoid areas are used.

C. Insulin Delivery Systems: Efforts to administer insulin by "closed loop" systems (glucose-controlled insulin infusion systems [Biostator]) have been successful in acute situations such as diabetic ketoacidosis or during surgery. However, chronic use is precluded by the bulkiness of the computerized pump and by the need for continuous aspiration of blood for the external glucose sensor that activates the appropriate insulin or glucose infusion.

Several small portable "open loop" devices for the delivery of insulin are on the market. These devices contain an insulin reservoir and a pump programmed to deliver regular insulin subcutaneously; they do not contain a glucose sensor. With improved methods for self-monitoring of *blood* glucose at home (see below), these pump systems have become very useful for managing some diabetic patients. However, there have been occasional reports of acute complications, such as infection at the catheter site and ketoacidosis due to kinking of the tube attached to the insulin reservoir. At present, conventional methods of insulin administration, with multiple subcutaneous injections of mixtures of a rapid and either an intermediate-acting or long-acting insulin, can provide glycemic control almost as effectively as the open loop systems in most patients with IDDM who self-monitor their blood glucose levels accurately and regularly. However, occasional patients continue to have extreme lability of blood glucose control and frequent hyperglycemia after overnight fasting despite meticulous compliance with a regimen of multiple subcutaneous injections of insulin. In these cases, switching over to the appropriate use of continuous subcutaneous insulin infusion pumps has achieved improved glycemic control. Currently, the results of clinical trials have been encouraging regarding the usefulness of implantable insulin pumps that deliver insulin intraperitoneally under control of a programmed radio signal activated by the subject in response to information obtained from periodic self-monitoring of capillary blood glucose concentrations.

To facilitate treatment of patients who are adhering to a regimen of multiple preprandial injections of regular insulin that supplement a single injection of long-acting insulin delivered by a conventional syringe, portable **pen injectors** have been introduced. These pen-sized devices (Novo-Pen, Insuject) contain cartridges of U100 regular human insulin and retractable needles and eliminate the need to carry an insulin bottle and syringes during the day.

Intranasally administered soluble insulin is rapidly absorbed when given along with a detergent substance to facilitate adsorption. Preliminary clinical trials have demonstrated its efficacy in reducing postprandial hyperglycemia in insulin-dependent diabetics. However, its absorption is limited to less than 10% of the administered nasal dose. This reduces its cost-effectiveness, and most manufacturers have discontinued clinical trials until more progress is made in improving its bioavailability.

Pancreatic islet cells have been successfully transplanted in genetically similar strains of rodents with experimental diabetes; however, this approach has not yet been successful in humans because of difficulties in preparing and maintaining viable islets and because of immunologic rejection of the tissue. Similarly, **whole pancreas transplants** have generally proved unsatisfactory in treating the insulin-dependent (type I) patient because of the present hazards of prolonged antirejection therapy. However, when a renal transplant is required in an IDDM patient with end-stage renal disease and the kidney is from a nonliving donor, the pancreas from the same donor is often transplanted simultaneously and with good results.

STEPS IN THE MANAGEMENT OF THE DIABETIC PATIENT

Diagnostic Examination

A. History and Physical Examination: A complete history is taken and physical examination is performed for diagnostic purposes and to rule out the presence of coexisting or complicating disease. Nutritional status should be noted, particularly if catabolic features such as progressive weight loss are present despite a normal or increased food intake. The family history should include not only the incidence but also the age at onset of diabetes in other members of the family, and it should be noted whether affected family members were obese and whether they required insulin. Other factors that increase cardiovascular risk, such as a smoking history, presence of hypertension or hyperlipidemia, or oral contraceptive pill use should be documented.

A careful physical examination should include baseline height and weight, pulse rate, and blood pressure. If obesity is present, it should be characterized as to its distribution and a waist to hip ratio should be recorded. All peripheral arterial pulses should be examined, noting whether bruits or other signs of atherosclerotic disease are present. Neurologic and ophthalmologic examinations should be performed, with emphasis on investigation of abnormalities that may be related to diabetes, such as neo-

vascularization of the retina or stocking/glove sensory loss in the extremities.

B. Laboratory Diagnosis: (See also Laboratory Findings in Diabetes Mellitus, above.) Laboratory diagnosis should include documentation of the presence of fasting hyperglycemia (plasma glucose > 140 mg/dL [7.7 mmol/L]) or postprandial (post-glucose tolerance test) values consistently above 200 mg/dL (11.1 mmol/L). An attempt should be made to characterize the diabetes as IDDM or NIDDM, based on the clinical features present and on whether or not ketonuria accompanies the glycosuria. With current emphasis on home blood glucose monitoring, laborious attempts to document the renal threshold for glucose are no longer necessary in the initial evaluation of diabetic patients, particularly since "double-voided" urine specimens are difficult to obtain and since acceptable control of glycemia now allows only rare episodes of glycosuria.

Other baseline laboratory measurements that should be made part of the record include either glycohemoglobin or hemoglobin A_{1c}, total and HDL cholesterol, plasma triglycerides, electrocardiogram, chest x-ray, complete blood count, complete urinalysis, and renal function studies (serum creatinine, blood urea nitrogen, and, if possible, creatinine clearance).

Patient Education & Self-Management Training

Education is the most important task of the physician who provides care to diabetic patients. It must be remembered that education is necessary not only for newly diagnosed diabetic patients and their families but also for patients with diabetes of any duration who may never have been properly educated about their disorder or who may not be aware of advances in diabetes management. The "teaching curriculum" should include explanations of the nature of diabetes, its potential acute and chronic complications, and information on how these complications can be prevented or at least recognized and treated early. The importance of self-monitoring of blood glucose should be emphasized, particularly in all insulin-requiring diabetic patients, and instructions on proper testing and on recording of data should be provided. Patients should be trained in self-management and taught to use algorithms to adjust the timing and quantity of their insulin dose, food, and exercise in response to their recorded blood glucose values, so that optimal blood glucose control is achieved. Patients must be helped to accept the fact that they have diabetes; until this difficult adjustment has been made efforts to cope with the disorder are likely to be futile. Counseling should be directed at avoidance of extremes such as compulsive rigidity or self-destructive neglect. All patients should be made aware of community agencies (Diabetes Association chapters, etc.) that serve as resources for continuing education.

A. Diet Instruction: All diabetic patients should receive individual instruction on diet, as described earlier in this chapter. Unrestricted diets are not advised for insulin requiring diabetics. Until new methods of insulin replacement are available to provide more normal patterns of insulin delivery in response to metabolic demands, multiple small feedings restricted in simple sugars will continue to be recommended.

B. Insulin: Give the patient an understanding of the actions of the various insulins and the methods of administration of insulin. Since infections, particularly pyogenic ones with fever and toxemia, provoke a marked increase in insulin requirements, patients must be taught how to appropriately administer supplemental regular insulin as needed to correct hyperglycemia during infections. Patients and their families or friends should also be taught to recognize signs and symptoms of hypoglycemia and how to institute appropriate therapy for hypoglycemic reactions (see Acute Complications of Diabetes Mellitus, below).

C. Oral Hypoglycemic Agents: Information must be provided on the principles of hypoglycemic therapy (including information about time of onset, peak action, and duration of action of any pharmacologic agent being used). Patients should be made aware of the maximum recommended dose of the sulfonylureas that they are taking and should learn to inquire about possible drug interactions whenever any new medications are added to their regimens.

D. Effect of Exercise: Exercise increases the effectiveness of insulin, and regular daily moderate exercise is an excellent means of improving utilization of fats and carbohydrates in diabetic patients. A judicious balance of the size and frequency of meals with moderate regular exercise can often stabilize the insulin dosage in diabetics who tend to slip out of control easily. Strenuous exercise, however, can precipitate hypoglycemia in an unprepared patient, and diabetics must therefore be taught to reduce their insulin dosage or take supplemental carbohydrate in anticipation of strenuous activity. Injection of insulin into a site farthest away from the muscles most involved in exercise may help meliorate exercise-induced hypoglycemia, since insulin injected to exercising muscle is much more rapidly mobilized. With more knowledge regarding the relationship between caloric intake and expenditure and insulin requirements, the patient can become liberated from much of the regimentation imposed by the disorder.

E. Good Hygiene: All diabetic patients must receive adequate instruction on personal hygiene, especially with regard to care of the feet (see p 626), skin, and teeth.

F. Infections: Infections with fever and severe illness provoke the release of high levels of insulin antagonists that will bring about a marked increase in insulin requirements. It is essential to limit the period of infection, since infection raises the blood glucose level and this, in turn, can impair the general defense mechanisms that the body uses against bacterial and even viral organisms. Thus, the early and sufficient use of bactericidal antibiotics is imperative. Type I diabetics must be taught how to supplement the regimen with regular insulin if persistent glycosuria and ketonuria occur—especially if associated with infection. Patients must understand that insulin therapy should never be withheld in the presence of gastric upset and vomiting if glycosuria with ketonuria is present. When food intake is limited by nausea or vomiting, the patient should take ginger ale, apple juice, or grape juice in small sips and should notify the physician in case supplemental intravenous fluids might be required.

G. Self-Monitoring: Patients in whom labile diabetes is difficult to control should receive instructions on techniques for self-monitoring of blood glucose (see below). They should be encouraged to keep careful records of their glucose measurements and instructed on appropriate measures to correct for emerging patterns of hyperglycemia as well as to prevent recurrent episodes of hypoglycemia. Self-monitoring instructs patients on the glycemic effects of specific foods and exercise and alleviates. the likelihood of unexpected episodes of severe hypoglycemia. Moreover, when combined with an appropriate algorithm for therapy so that patients can respond appropriately to the various effects of glycemia, self-monitoring allows for greater flexibility in life-style and enables patients to be more fully in control of their diabetes.

H. Identification Bracelet: All patients receiving hypoglycemic therapy should wear a Medic-Alert bracelet or necklace that clearly states that insulin or an oral sulfonylurea drug is being taken. A card in the wallet or purse is less useful, since legal problems may arise if a victim's person and belongings are searched without permission. (Information on how to obtain a Medic-Alert identification device can be obtained from the Medic-Alert Foundation, PO Box 1009, Turlock, CA 95380.)

I. Restrictions on Occupation: Certain occupations potentially hazardous to the diabetic patient or others will continue to be prohibited (eg, piloting airplanes, operating cranes).

Avoidance of Stress & Emotional Turmoil

Prevention of psychologic turmoil is of great importance in the control of diabetes, particularly when the disease is difficult to stabilize. One reason blood glucose control in diabetics may be particularly sensitive to emotional upset is that their pancreatic A cells are hyperresponsive to physiologic levels of epinephrine, producing excessive levels of glucagon with consequent hyperglycemia.

Specific Therapy

Treatment must be individualized depending on the specific needs of each patient. Certain general principles of management pertaining to each type of diabetes are outlined below.

A. Type I Diabetes (IDDM): IDDM patients require replacement therapy with exogenous insulin. This should be instituted under conditions of an individualized diabetic diet with multiple feedings and normal daily activities so that an appropriate dosage regimen can be developed.

At the onset of diabetes, many type I patients recover some pancreatic B cell function and may temporarily need only low doses of exogenous insulin to supplement their own endogenous insulin secretion. This is known as the "honeymoon period." Within 8 weeks to 2 years, however, most of these patients show either absent or negligible pancreatic B cell function. At this point, these patients may be instructed to take a "conventional" regimen of two injections of insulin mixtures (a short-acting combined with intermediate-acting NPH insulin). Alternatively, if more flexibility with meal intervals and exercise is desired, multiple preprandial small injections of regular insulin may be prescribed along with a bedtime injection of long-acting or intermediate-acting insulin. (See Table 18–14 for advantages and disadvantages of various insulin regimens.) Self-monitoring of blood glucose levels is the recommended means of

determining the adjustment of insulin dosage and the modulation of food intake and exercise in type I diabetes.

1. Conventional insulin therapy (split doses of insulin mixtures)–A conventional insulin regimen in a 70-kg patient taking 2200 kcal divided into six feedings might be 10 units of regular and 10 units of NPH insulin in the morning and 8 units of regular and 8 units of NPH insulin in the evening. The morning blood glucose level gives a measure of the effectiveness of NPH insulin administered the previous evening; the noon level reflects the effects of the morning regular insulin; and the 5 PM and 9 PM levels represent the effects of the morning NPH and the evening regular insulins, respectively. A properly educated patient should be taught to adjust insulin dosage by observing the pattern of recorded self-monitored blood glucose levels and correlating it with the approximate duration of action and the time of peak effect after injection of the various insulin preparations (Figure 18–9). Adjustments should be made gradually, preferably not more often than every 2 or 3 days if possible.

Certain caveats should be kept in mind regarding insulin treatment. Considerable variations in absorption and bioavailability exist, even when the same dose is injected in the same region on different days in the same individual. Such variation often can be minimized by injecting smaller quantities of insulin

Table 18–14. Advantages and disadvantages of various insulin regimens in treatment of type I diabetes.

Regimen	Advantages	Disadvantages
Single injection of NPH or Lente	Convenience only	Poor hyperglycemic control or nocturnal hypoglycemia. Requires frequent feedings to avoid hypoglycemia if acceptable control attempted. Inflexible feeding schedules. Variability of absorption of large doses predisposes to hypoglycemia, which is common. Because of these disadvantages, this regimen is not recommended.
Conventional split dose of mixture (regular and NPH twice daily)	Relatively convenient. Controls postprandial glycemia at breakfast and dinner.	Prebreakfast hyperglycemia is common. Increased risk of nocturnal hypoglycemia in attempt to control prebreakfast hyperglycemia. Variability of absorption due to relatively large NPH doses to last overnight.
Three injections (mixture of regular and NPH in the morning, regular at dinner, NPH at bedtime)	Controls postprandial glycemia at breakfast and dinner. Can prevent prebreakfast hyperglycemia with less risk of nocturnal hypoglycemia. Less variability of absorption of NPH, since lower doses are injected to last overnight.	Less convenient. Lunch schedule is relatively inflexible as to time and quantity to avoid hypoglycemia from morning NPH. Dinner schedule cannot be delayed without extra feedings.
Four injections (regular before meals and NPH, Lente, or Ultralente at bedtime) or subcutaneous infusion of regular insulin with pump	Controls postprandial glycemia. Allows flexibility of meal schedules and quantity. Less variability of absorption of small doses of insulins given more frequently. Tight glycemic control is possible with least risk of hypoglycemia.	Relatively inconvenient. Pumps are expensive and are generally less convenient than multiple injections and add risk of skin infections and pump failures.

at each dose and consequently using multiple doses. Also, a given insulin dose may undergo considerable differences in pharmacokinetics in different individuals, either because of insulin antibodies that bind insulin with different avidity, or for other as yet unknown reasons.

2. Intensive multiple-dose insulin therapy— While split doses of insulin mixtures daily have improved the quality of glycemic control as compared to single injections of intermediate insulin in type I diabetics, blood glucose values throughout the day are often not optimal, and nocturnal hypoglycemia may result from attempts to achieve prebreakfast euglycemia. In cases in which conventional split doses of insulin mixtures cannot maintain near-normalization of blood glucose without hypoglycemia (particularly at night), multiple injections of insulin may be required. An increasingly popular regimen consists of reducing or omitting the evening dose of intermediate insulin and adding a portion of it at bedtime. For example, 10 units of regular insulin mixed with 10 units of NPH insulin might be prescribed in the morning, 8–10 units of regular insulin before the evening meal, and 6 units of NPH at bedtime.

To further reduce variation in absorption kinetics, which is aggravated when ratios of insulin in mixtures are altered on different days, a multiple injection regimen that avoids mixing insulin has been devised. The patient administers small doses of regular insulin more frequently (eg, four times a day) along with a longer-acting insulin, eg, NPH or ultralente insulin, to provide basal levels of insulin during the postabsorptive state. Since beef insulin is no longer available as ultralente, the less sustained-acting ultralente made with human insulin generally requires two injections at 12-hour intervals (eg, 10 units every 12 hours in a 60- to 70-kg person). To avoid precipitation of the prebreakfast regular insulin, the morning ultralente dose should be injected separately rather than mixed with the dose of regular insulin.

Both of these multiple-dose regimens give greater flexibility regarding meal patterns and content than conventional therapy with split doses of insulin mixtures and are helpful in reducing the frequency and severity of hypoglycemia in patients attempting near-normalization of blood glucose.

3. Intensive insulin therapy using insulin pumps—Several types of portable battery-operated "open loop" devices have been marketed to deliver insulin continuously (see Methods of Insulin Administration, above). These generally infuse insulin through a needle or catheter implanted subcutaneously in the abdomen. A basal infusion rate of regular insulin is provided over a 24-hour period, and this is augmented by a bolus of regular insulin prior to meals. In addition, since insulin requirements appear to increase slightly in the early dawn period in the majority of patients with type I diabetes, most pumps also have adjustable basal rates that can be programmed to rise automatically at 6 AM. Unbuffered regular insulins such as Humulin-R, Iletin I and II, or Novolin-R have been associated with frequent blockage of pump tubing due to precipitation of the insulin. Accordingly, only insulin buffered with phosphate such as Velosulin has been recommended for use in insulin infusion pumps. The FDA has qualified its recent approval for insulin lispro by suggesting that it not be used in insulin pumps until further clinical trials are completed to ascertain its efficacy and safety for use in pumps.

The use of pumps requires knowledgeable and compliant patients who can be depended on to monitor their blood glucose levels as often as four times daily. The indwelling needle or catheter should be changed every 48 hours to reduce the risk of infection, and patients should be alert for symptoms of sudden deterioration of glycemic control, due to pump blockage, pump failure, or leakage of insulin from the tubing. The selection of dosage is usually based on providing 40–50% of the estimated daily dose of insulin as the basal infusion rate and the remaining amount divided as intermittent boluses given prior to meals to control postprandial metabolism. For example, in a 70-kg patient requiring 40–45 units of insulin a day, 20 units of regular insulin would be administered as a basal infusion of 0.8 unit/h, with the remaining units administered as follows: 7–8 units before breakfast, 5–6 units before lunch, 6–8 units before supper, and 0–2 units prior to a bedtime snack. The results of blood glucose monitoring as well as the extent of physical activity and dietary intake will all contribute to fine-tuning the proper dosage of insulin administered at various meals and basally.

4. Selection of patients for intensive insulin therapy—Patient selection is difficult, and exact criteria are controversial. Patients should be highly motivated and willing to monitor their blood glucose levels several times daily and record the results. They should not have impaired adrenergic responses to hypoglycemia, as is often seen with autonomic neuropathy, since this reduces their awareness of being hypoglycemic and increases the risk of severe hypoglycemic episodes. Finally, if nonproliferative ("background") or proliferative retinopathy is present, intensive insulin—therapy should be initiated slowly and with careful attention to possible progression of retinal disease (see Ophthalmologic Complications, below).

5. Self-monitoring of blood glucose levels— Glycemic self-monitoring should be considered a *means* of achieving near-normal blood glucose control rather than being an *end in itself*. This implies that diabetic patients must be educated to make appropriate behavioral adjustments in their diet, activity, timing of insulin injections, etc, based on their preprandial capillary blood glucose measurements, in order to achieve the desired level of blood glucose

GUIDELINES FOR INTENSIVE INSULIN THERAPY

DATE:_____ IDDM Patients:_____

YOUR BASIC DAILY DOSE OF INSULIN

• Inject regular insulin 30 minutes before meals or as directed by your physician.[1]

INSULIN	BREAKFAST	LUNCH	DINNER	BEDTIME[2]
Regular	_____	_____	_____	_____
NPH	_____	_____	_____	_____

BLOOD GLUCOSE TESTING

The goal of insulin therapy is to lower your blood glucose levels to just above normal values. Here are some acceptable targets to aim for. Keep a daily record of your blood glucose concentrations. Test _4_ times daily.

TEST TIME	ACCEPTABLE BLOOD GLUCOSE TARGET[3]	
Fasting (first morning test before breakfast)	95 to 140 mg/dL	_____
Before meals	95 to 140 mg/dL	_____
Two hours after meals	Less than 180 mg/dL	_____

SUPPLEMENTING YOUR BASIC INSULIN DOSE - REGULAR INSULIN

Once your basic dose of insulin has been established, you will learn to adjust your dose based upon blood glucose measurements before meals.

Supplement your basic insulin dose with regular insulin as indicated:

If your glucose before the meal is in the following range:

2 units less	_70 - 85_ mg/dL[4]
1 unit less	_85 - 95_ mg/dL
no change	_95 - 140_ mg/dL
1 unit extra	_141 - 180_ mg/dL
2 units extra	_181 - 220_ mg/dL
3 units extra	_221 - 260_ mg/dL
4 units extra[5]	_261 - 300_ mg/dL
For glucose greater than 300	Check the urine for ketones. If POSITIVE call physician.

SIGNATURE: _____   DATE: _____

Figure 18–10. Guidelines for intensive insulin therapy in patients with IDDM.

control. Knowledge of the level of blood glucose has been particularly helpful at bedtime in ascertaining the need for supplementary feedings to avoid nocturnal hypoglycemia. Unfortunately, either because of the expense of paper strips or the inconvenience involved, as many as half of adults with IDDM do not self-monitor their blood glucose levels.

Self-monitoring of blood glucose levels is helpful in managing diabetes in all patients on insulin therapy, and especially in the following groups: patients with brittle diabetes; patients who are attempting ideal glycemic control, such as during pregnancy; and patients with impaired or absent early warning of hypoglycemic episodes. Self-monitoring is useful in educating patients about the glycemic effects of specific foods in their diet and reduces the likelihood of unexpected episodes of severe hypoglycemia in insulin-treated diabetics.

There are three essential elements to self-monitoring of blood glucose: (1) obtaining the blood specimen, (2) applying the specimen to enzyme-impregnated strips capable of discriminating the glucose level, and (3) reading the glucose level from the test strip. Each of these will be discussed briefly.

The patient may obtain a capillary blood sample from the fingertip by means of a lancet designed for this purpose. The patient should be taught how to clean the site and how to rapidly pierce the skin to obtain a drop of blood. Automatic spring-loaded devices such as the Autolet or Penlet are useful in simplifying the finger-pricking technique and ensuring an adequate blood sample.

The drop of blood is then applied to the appropriate area of an enzyme-impregnated strip or disposable platform of a glucose meter. It is important to follow the instructions for each type of strip.

Chemstrip bG results can be visually interpreted by comparing the colors obtained on the strip with the color chart supplied by the manufacturer. For most patients, who prefer more exact results, devices with automated digital readouts are available to quantitate the color changes. The second-generation meters are more compact and have the distinct advantage of automatically timing the entire reaction as well as obviating the need to wipe off the strip, thereby reducing the potential for technical error. Most of these devices are comparable in their cost, portability, and ease of use. However, each has a unique disposable platform or paper strip which is relatively expensive and cannot be used in other devices. Various models also differ according to whether they include an electronic memory, averaging capability, and printout function with personal computers. The physician should learn the advantages and disadvantages of these devices and help the patient make an appropriate choice.

Initially, blood glucose levels should be checked at least four times a day in patients with type I diabetes. Generally, these measurements are taken before each meal and at bedtime. In an adult with IDDM receiving multiple daily injections of insulin, a standard premeal dose of regular insulin should be prescribed (eg, 4–7 units) guidelines for raising or lowering this dose appropriately by 1 or more units depending on the level of the premeal capillary blood glucose. Figure 18–10 is such a program used at the University of California in San Francisco. A basic schedule of premeal injection of regular insulin as well as morning and bedtime NPH insulin is ordered, as well as suggested adjustment of the premeal insulin dose according to the premeal blood sugar. This insulin dose adjustment is given in conjunction with

Footnote 1: Doses depend on body size, exercise patterns, food consumption, and general sensitivity to insulin. This is an example of a regimen for a 70-kg adult IDDM patient receiving six feedings per day with average carbohydrate intake and limited exercise:

Insulin	Breakfast	Lunch	Dinner	Bedtime
Regular	8 units	7 units	10 units	—
NPH	2 units	—	—	8 units

Footnote 2: Regular insulin is generally not recommended at bedtime. However, if blood glucose exceeds 300 mg/dL, 2 or 3 units of regular insulin may precede a bedtime snack. Adjustments of bedtime NPH insulin depends on prebreakfast blood glucose values. If they are between 141 and 180 mg/dL for three mornings, add 1 unit NPH to the basic bedtime dose, or if 181–250 mg/dL, add 2 units NPH.

Footnote 3: In patients with hypoglycemia unawareness, autonomic neuropathy, advanced age, or with cardiac or cerebral atherosclerosis, blood glucose targets should be adjusted upward appropriately. Pregnant patients may require downward adjustment of target glucose values (Chapter 16).

Footnote 4: If blood glucose is less than 70 mg/dL, no insulin is given until 30 minutes after a carbohydrate snack, when blood glucose is rechecked to ascertain insulin dosage.

Footnote 5: If extra (or reduced) insulin is consistently needed at a given time period, appropriate adjustments should be made in either the basic insulin dose, food consumption, or exercise during the interval *prior* to the time the unsatisfactory blood glucose measurement is generated.

other measures to modulate glycemic responses to the meal—such as altering the time interval after injecting the insulin or modifying the quantities or the order of ingestion of foodstuffs. Patients should be urged to review their recorded patterns of glycemic measurements over a 2- to 3-day period in relation to insulin dose, food intake, and exercise and to make *prospective* changes in their program when appropriate to correct for deficiencies in the therapeutic regimen. Once glycemic levels are brought into an acceptable range, the patient should continue to check blood glucose levels at least twice daily. In addition, patients should be taught to check their blood glucose level whenever they develop symptoms that could represent a hypoglycemic episode. All blood glucose levels and their timing and corresponding insulin doses should be recorded in an organized fashion and brought with the patient for physician review during regularly scheduled check-ups; such personal blood glucose logs are commercially available.

6. Management of early morning hyperglycemia in IDDM patients—

a. Etiology and diagnosis—One of the more difficult therapeutic problems in managing patients with IDDM is determining the proper adjustment of insulin dose when the early morning blood glucose level is high before breakfast. Prebreakfast hyperglycemia is sometimes due to the **Somogyi effect,** in which nocturnal hypoglycemia evokes a surge of counterregulatory hormones to produce high blood glucose levels by 7 AM. If this is the case, lowering the evening dose of intermediate insulin is indicated. However, a more common cause of prebreakfast hyperglycemia is the **waning of circulating insulin levels,** which requires use of more (rather than less) intermediate insulin in the evening. These two phenomena are not mutually exclusive and can occur together to produce a greater magnitude of hyperglycemia in affected patients with IDDM. A third phenomenon—the **"dawn phenomenon"**—has been reported to occur in as many as 75% of IDDM patients and in the majority of NIDDM patients and normal subjects as well. It is characterized by a reduced tissue sensitivity to insulin between 5 AM and 8 AM (dawn), and apparently is evoked by spikes of growth hormone released hours before, at onset of sleep. When the "dawn phenomenon" occurs alone, it may produce only mild hyperglycemia in the early morning; however, when it is associated with either or both of the other phenomena, it can further aggravate the hyperglycemia (Table 18–15). Diagnosis of the cause of prebreakfast hyperglycemia can be facilitated by asking the patient to self-monitor blood glucose levels at 3 AM in addition to monitoring at the usual times, bedtime and 7 AM. When this was done, the Somogyi effect was found to be much less prevalent and of lower magnitude as a cause of prebreakfast hyperglycemia than had been previously suspected. In insulin-treated patients, serum levels of free immunoreactive insulin (particularly in the basal or low ranges) are difficult to quantitate accurately because of technical interference. In specialized research laboratories, however, these levels have been measured in hospitalized patients with prebreakfast hyperglycemia (Table 18–15).

b. Treatment—When a particular pattern emerges from monitoring blood glucose levels at 10 PM, 3 AM, and 7 AM, appropriate therapeutic measures can be taken. Prebreakfast hyperglycemia due to the Somogyi effect can be treated by either reducing the dose of intermediate insulin, giving a portion of it at bedtime, or supplying more food at bedtime. When the "dawn phenomenon" alone is present, shifting a portion of the intermediate insulin from dinnertime to bedtime often suffices; or when insulin pumps are used, the basal infusion rate can be stepped up appropriately (eg, from 0.8 unit/h to 1 unit/h) from 6 AM until breakfast. Finally, in cases in which the circulating insulin level is waning, either increasing the evening insulin dose or, preferably, shifting it from dinnertime to bedtime (or both) may be efficacious. A bedtime dose of NPH made from animal insulin provides more sustained overnight insulin levels than

Table 18–15. Typical patterns of overnight blood glucose levels and serum free immunoreactive insulin levels in prebreakfast hyperglycemia due to various causes in patients with IDDM.

	Blood Glucose Levels (mg/dL)			Serum Free Immunoreactive Insulin Levels (μU/mL)		
	10 PM	3 AM	7 AM	10 PM	3 AM	7 AM
Somogyi effect	90	40	200	High	Slightly high	Normal
"Dawn phenomenon"	110	110	150	Normal	Normal	Normal
Waning of circulating insulin levels plus "dawn phenomenon"	110	190	220	Normal	Low	Low
Waning of circulating insulin levels plus "dawn phenomenon" plus Somogyi effect	110	40	380	High	Normal	Low

human NPH and thus may be helpful for managing refractory prebreakfast hyperglycemia.

B. Type II Diabetes (NIDDM): The principles of therapy are less well defined in this heterogeneous group of diabetic patients than is the case with type I diabetes. Therapeutic recommendations are based upon the relative contributions of B cell insufficiency and insulin insensitivity in individual patients. With prolonged duration of NIDDM, deposits of amyloid accumulate in islets and encroach on pancreatic B cells, resulting in progressive diminution of insulin-secretory capacity.

1. The obese patient–The most common type of diabetic patient is the obese diabetic with insulin insensitivity. Characteristically, obese patients compensate for their insulin resistance with increased basal levels of circulating insulin and are capable of responding to a glucose load with hypersecretion of insulin. However, as hyperglycemia progresses, the insulin response to a glucose load decreases. This refractoriness of the B cell may be partially reversed with therapeutic correction of the hyperglycemia and seems to be selectively related to the hyperglycemic stimulation, since other B cell-stimulating agents such as sulfonylureas, arginine, and glucagon still provoke rapid insulin release.

a. Weight reduction–One of the primary modes of therapy in the obese type II diabetic patient is weight reduction. Normalization of glycemia can be achieved by reducing adipose stores, with consequent restoration of tissue sensitivity to insulin. A combination of caloric restriction, increased exercise, modification of behavior, and consistent reinforcement of good eating habits is required if a weight reduction program is to be successful. Knowledge of the symptoms of diabetes and an understanding of the risks and complications of diabetes often increase the patient's motivation for weight reduction. Even so, significant weight loss is seldom achieved and even more difficult to maintain in the morbidly obese patient. Weight control is variable in moderately obese patients depending on the enthusiasm of the therapist and the motivation of the patient.

b. Hypoglycemic agents–Hypoglycemic agents, including insulin as well as the oral hypoglycemic drugs are generally *not* indicated for long-term use in the obese patient with mild diabetes. A weight reduction program can be disrupted by real or imagined hypoglycemic reactions when insulin therapy is used, and weight gain is quite common in the insulin-treated obese diabetic patient. Metformin, an insulin-sparing agent and one that does not increase weight or provoke hypoglycemia, offers obvious advantages over insulin or sulfonylureas in treating hyperglycemia in obese patients.

If metformin therapy (combined with a weight reduction regimen) is inadequate to control symptoms of hyperglycemia (eg, nocturia, blurred vision, or candidal vulvovaginitis), a sulfonylurea should be added. If this combination of metformin and sulfonylurea is ineffective in achieving appropriate glycemic control, insulin therapy may be necessary, directed at elimination of symptoms rather than restoration of euglycemia. Use of oral agents or insulin to supplement a weight reduction program should be for a limited period (weeks or months) to ameliorate hyperglycemic symptoms until sufficient weight reduction has occurred to keep the patient symptom-free.

2. The nonobese patient–In the nonobese NIDDM diabetic with moderately severe hyperglycemia, pancreatic B cells are refractory to glucose stimulation. Peripheral insulin resistance is also detectable but is considerably less intense than in obese diabetics who have a comparable degree of hyperglycemia; it is also of less therapeutic import, since insulin-treated nonobese patients do not generally need an excessive dosage of insulin.

a. Diet–If hyperglycemia is mild (fasting blood glucose levels of < 200 mg/dL [11.1 mmol/L]), normal metabolic control can occasionally be restored by a diet devoid of simple sugars and with calories calculated to maintain ideal body weight. Restriction of saturated fats and cholesterol is also strongly advised. An individualized diet with a recommended exchange list should be prescribed for these nonobese NIDDM patients.

b. Oral hypoglycemic agents–When diet therapy alone is not sufficient to correct hyperglycemia, a trial of oral hypoglycemic drugs is indicated to supplement the dietary regimen. In the nonobese NIDDM patient, sulfonylureas are generally the first-line oral drug of choice, and metformin is added later if glycemic control is inadequate. The controversies raised by the UGDP (see Efficacy and Safety of Oral Hypoglycemic Agents, above) apply mainly to obese patients with relatively mild diabetes (who represented the great majority of patients in that study), and there are few data on which to base an assessment of the risk-benefit ratio of sulfonylureas or metformin (or both) in nonobese patients with fasting hyperglycemia above 140 mg/dL (7.8 mmol/L). Therefore, once their efficacy is demonstrated in these patients and since there is no evidence suggesting harm to them, it seems reasonable to continue the use of sulfonylureas or metformin (or both) as long as they remain effective in controlling hyperglycemia. The degree of control to aim for remains arbitrary at present; however, data from the United Kingdom and from studies of Pima Indians suggest that maintaining postprandial plasma glucose levels below 200 mg/dL (11.1 mmol/L) seems to spare NIDDM patients from increased risk of severe retinopathy or vascular complications. Once the dosage of sulfonylurea reaches the upper recommended limit in a compliant patient without maintaining plasma glucose below 200 mg/dL (11.1 mmol/L) throughout the day, a trial of combined therapy with metformin is indicated. If this is ineffective, insulin therapy is indicated.

c. Insulin–When sulfonylureas fail and NIDDM patients require insulin to control their hyperglycemia, various insulin regimens may be effective. Although reliance on a single morning injection of insulin is not recommended in type I diabetes, there are some NIDDM patients with enough residual insulin secretion to get by satisfactorily on a single daily injection of 20–25 units of NPH or lente insulin before breakfast. If hyperglycemia persists on this regimen—or if hypoglycemia occurs before lunch or dinner—a number of alternatives are available. The most popular insulin regimen under these circumstances is to use a split dose of a fixed 70:30 mixture of NPH:regular insulin, which can be started as 18–20 units before breakfast and 10–15 units before dinner, and this can be adjusted appropriately depending on target blood glucoses at 7 AM and 5 PM. If more than 50 units per day does not achieve satisfactory glycemic control, these patients may benefit from more intensive multiple-injection regimens as described for IDDM. Many nonobese patients with mild insulinopenia can have their glycohemoglobin levels brought into the normal range with relatively small doses of insulin and without provoking nocturnal hypoglycemia. Patients with more severe insulinopenia may require split doses of insulin.

d. Therapeutic combinations of sulfonylureas with insulin–Both nonobese and obese NIDDM patients usually show a modest glycemic improvement with a regimen combining sulfonylurea drugs and insulin, but this improvement can generally be achieved with insulin therapy alone. At present, there is no overall consensus regarding how these agents should be combined. One proposed regimen adds a bedtime intermediate-acting insulin to reduce excessive nocturnal hepatic glucose output in NIDDM patients who are responding poorly on maximal doses of sulfonylureas. A recent double-blind trial in a group of obese type II patients who failed sulfonylureas demonstrated that a regimen of bedtime NPH insulin (mean dose of 40–50 units) plus a maximum dose of glipizide (20 mg twice daily) was able to produce near-normoglycemia during a 1-year study. Many diabetologists, however, prefer to stop oral agents if they are ineffective and switch over to insulin therapy alone. In the case of NIDDM patients requiring excessive amounts of insulin (> 100 units/d), it is considered a reasonable option to add metformin or sulfonylureas (or both) to improve glycemic control rather than to prescribe inordinately high insulin doses.

In IDDM patients, the absence of glycemic improvement or reduction in insulin dose when sulfonylureas are added to the insulin regimen suggests that the predominant effect of sulfonylureas is their insulinotropic action, and that any effect on potentiation of insulin action is limited to in vitro systems and of little clinical importance. In NIDDM patients, observations of an improvement in insulin action during sulfonylurea therapy need not be a direct "extrapancreatic" effect but could be explained by improved endogenous insulin release, since other means of reducing hyperglycemia (eg, diet therapy or insulin administration) have been equally effective in decreasing Insulin resistance.

Immunopathology of Insulin Therapy

At least five molecular classes of insulin antibodies are produced during the course of insulin therapy: IgA, IgD, IgE, IgG, and IgM. Even though the use of highly purified pork and human insulins has considerably reduced the immunogenicity of insulin, many diabetics continue to be treated with mixed beef-pork insulins (Table 18–13). These beef-containing insulins usually induce antibodies to insulin after about 2–3 weeks of therapy. Human insulin is much less antigenic than beef insulin, but because of its hexameric presentation at therapeutic injection doses, it is also treated as a foreign substance by the immune system and results in detectable—albeit low—titers of insulin antibodies in most patients.

A. Insulin Allergy: Insulin allergy, a hypersensitivity reaction of the immediate type, is a rare condition in which local or systemic urticaria occurs immediately after insulin injection. This reaction is due to histamine release from tissue mast cells sensitized by adherence of IgE antibodies to their surface. In severe cases, anaphylaxis can occur. The appearance of a subcutaneous nodule at the site of insulin injection, occurring several hours after the injection and lasting for up to 24 hours, has been attributed to an IgG-mediated complement-binding Arthus reaction. Because sensitivity was often due to noninsulin protein contaminants, the highly purified insulins have markedly reduced the incidence of insulin allergy, especially of the local variety. When allergy to beef insulin is present, a species change (eg, to pure pork insulin or to human insulin) may correct the problem, although in rare cases allergic reactions persist even to injected human insulin.. Antihistamines, corticosteroids, and even desensitization may be required, especially for systemic hypersensitivity in an insulin-dependent patient. A commercial kit containing various dilutions of pure beef or pure pork insulin for allergy testing and insulin desensitization is available from the Eli Lilly Company, although requests for its use have greatly diminished, as more human insulins are being prescribed from the outset of insulin therapy.

B. Immune Insulin Resistance: Except for some patients initially treated with highly purified pork or human insulin, all patients who receive insulin develop a low titer of circulating IgG antibodies to insulin, and this neutralizes to a small extent the rapid action of insulin. In some diabetic patients with a history of intermittent exposure to insulin therapy—and especially those with some degree of tissue insensitivity to insulin (such as obese NIDDM patients)—a high titer of circulating IgG antibodies to insulin develops. This results in extremely high insulin requirements, often to more than 200 units/d. This frequently is a self-limited condition and may clear spontaneously after several months. However, in cases where the circulating antibody is specifically more reactive to beef insulin, switching to a less antigenic highly purified pork insulin or human insulin may make possible a dramatic reduction in insulin dosage or at least may shorten the duration of immune resistance. In NIDDM patients, whose excessive circulating insulin antibodies do not completely neutralize endogenous (human) insulin, the foreign insulin can be discontinued and the patient maintained on oral sulfonylureas combined with diet therapy. Owing to the usual effectiveness of human insulin in treating this syndrome, immunosuppressive therapy with high doses of glucocorticoids is no longer required.

C. Lipodystrophy at Injection Sites: Rarely, a disfiguring atrophy of subcutaneous fatty tissue occurs at the site of insulin injection. Although the cause of this complication is obscure, it seems to represent a form of immune reaction, particularly since it occurs predominantly in females and is associated with lymphocyte infiltration in the lipoatrophic area. This complication has become even less common since the development of highly purified insulin preparations of neutral pH. Injection of highly purified preparations of insulin directly into the atrophic area often results in restoration of normal contours.

Lipohypertrophy, on the other hand, is not a consequence of immune responses; rather, it seems to be due to the pharmacologic effects of depositing insulin in the same location repeatedly. It can occur with purified insulins and is best treated with localized liposuction of the hypertrophic areas by an experienced plastic surgeon. It is prevented by rotation of injection sites.

ACUTE COMPLICATIONS OF DIABETES MELLITUS

HYPOGLYCEMIA

Hypoglycemic reactions (see below and Chapter 19) are the most common complications that occur in insulin-treated diabetic patients. They may also occur in patients taking oral sulfonylureas, especially older patients or those with impaired liver or kidney function treated with long-acting and highly potent agents such as chlorpropamide or glyburide. Hypoglycemia

may result from delay in taking a meal or from unusual physical exertion without supplemental calories or a decrease in insulin dose.

Clinical Features

Signs and symptoms of hypoglycemia may be divided into those resulting from neuroglycopenia (insufficient glucose for normal central nervous system function leading to confusion and coma) and those resulting from stimulation of the autonomic nervous system. There is great variation in the pattern of hypoglycemic signs and symptoms from patient to patient; however, individual patients tend to experience the same pattern from episode to episode. In older diabetics, in patients with frequent hypoglycemic episodes, and in those with diabetic autonomic neuropathy, autonomic responses may be blunted or absent, so that hypoglycemia may be manifested only by signs and symptoms of neuroglycopenia. The gradual onset of hypoglycemia with intermediate-acting or long-acting insulin also makes recognition more difficult in older patients.

A. Neuroglycopenia: Signs and symptoms of neuroglycopenia include mental confusion with impaired abstract and, later, concrete thought processes; this may be followed by bizarre antagonistic behavior. Stupor, coma, and even death may occur with profound hypoglycemia. Full recovery of central nervous system function does not always occur if treatment is delayed.

B. Autonomic Hyperactivity: Signs and symptoms of autonomic hyperactivity can be both adrenergic (tachycardia, palpitations, sweating, tremulousness) and parasympathetic (nausea, hunger). Except for sweating, most of the sympathetic symptoms of hypoglycemia are blunted in patients receiving beta-blocking agents for angina or hypertension. Though not absolutely contraindicated, these drugs must be used with great caution in insulin-requiring diabetics.

C. Counterregulatory Responses to Hypoglycemia: (Table 18–16.)

1. Normal counterregulation—When plasma glucose is acutely lowered in normal subjects by intravenous insulin, a rapid surge of both glucagon and epinephrine acts to counterregulate the hypoglycemia. The hormonal responses tend to begin after plasma glucose falls below 70 mg/dL (3.9 mmol/L). If they fail to correct the decline of plasma glucose, symptoms of autonomic hyperactivity usually become apparent once plasma glucose falls below 60 mg/dL (3.3 mmol/L). Plasma glucagon is considered the first line of defense against acute hypoglycemia, while the role of epinephrine and the sympathetic system is to provide a backup system. The latter helps to restore euglycemia and serves as an alarm system to warn the subject of the urgent need for carbohydrate intake in case the counterregulatory response is inadequate to prevent the poten-

Table 18–16. Counterregulatory responses to hypoglycemia.

Normal Counterregulation	Defective Counterregulation in Type I Diabetes[1]
Glucagon rises rapidly to 3–5 times baseline after insulin-induced hypoglycemia, provoking hepatic glycogenolysis.	Glucagon response to insulin-induced hypoglycemia is lost after onset of type I diabetes.
Adrenergic discharge (1) raises hepatic glucose output by glycogenolysis and (2) provides warning to subject of impending hypoglycemic crisis.	Blunted or absent adrenergic response may occur as a result of— (1) Neural damage with (a) advanced age or (b) autonomic neuropathy (2) Neural dysfunction (iatrogenic) from (a) frequent hypoglycemia or (b) human insulin therapy (?)

[1]Type II diabetics are less well characterized for their defective counterregulation as regards glucagon loss but appear to have the same frequency and causes of adrenergic loss as type I diabetics.

tially disastrous consequences of life-threatening neuroglycopenia.

2. Defective counterregulation in diabetes– For unexplained reasons, patients with type I diabetes uniformly lose their ability to secrete glucagon in response to acute insulin-induced hypoglycemia (but not in the presence of amino acids in protein-containing meals) within a few years after developing diabetes. After that time, they are solely dependent upon triggered autonomic adrenergic responses to counteract an impending hypoglycemic crisis as well as for early warning. It is well documented that with advanced age these autonomic responses may be blunted considerably, and in diabetic patients with clinical autonomic neuropathy as a complication of diabetes they may be absent. In these circumstances, reduced awareness of hypoglycemia can lead to potentially life-threatening sequelae from neuroglycopenic convulsions or coma.

3. "Iatrogenic" autonomic failure–Cryer has proposed that frequent and recurrent hypoglycemic episodes such as may be encountered in patients receiving intensive insulin therapy to achieve normoglycemia may result in failure of the sympathetic nervous system to respond to hypoglycemia. Adaptation of the central nervous system to recurrent hypoglycemic episodes is associated with increased glucose transport into the brain despite subnormal levels of plasma glucose. This results from up-regulation of glucose transporter I at the blood-brain barrier induced by recurrent hypoglycemia. The threshold for recognizing hypoglycemia is thereby altered, so that much lower plasma glucose levels are needed to trigger an autonomic response—and by the time this occurs, cognition may already be impaired in some cases, with onset of neuroglycopenia. That this adaptation and autonomic failure is a consequence of chronic hypoglycemia and not diabetes is evidenced by reports of patients with insulinomas who had chronic recurrent episodes of hypoglycemia of which they often were unaware. These were patients who had loss of epinephrine responses and symptoms during acute insulin-induced hypoglycemia and whose symptoms and adrenergic responses during repeat

testing returned to normal after euglycemia had been restored following resection of the insulinomas. This documented reversibility of the syndrome of hypoglycemia unawareness due to chronic hypoglycemia has exciting implications for therapy of those diabetic patients whose unawareness may be iatrogenic as a result of recurrent hypoglycemia during attempts at normalization of blood glucose with intensive insulin therapy.

4. Human insulin and hypoglycemic awareness–In 1987, a preliminary report contended that hypoglycemia unawareness became more prevalent in diabetics transferred from beef-pork to human insulin. Although occasional studies gave support to this claim, most investigators failed to find evidence for a detrimental effect of human insulin on recognition of hypoglycemia. There is some evidence that many of the anecdotal reports of loss of hypoglycemic awareness after changing from animal to human insulin may be a consequence of an increased number of hypoglycemic episodes. The latter may occur on switching from animal to human insulin if the switch is made at equivalent or nearly equivalent dosages without taking the precaution of using a lower human insulin dose to compensate for the reduced neutralization of the injected insulin by preexisting anti-beef or anti-pork insulin antibodies. Another possible cause of more frequent hypoglycemic episodes is the inclination of patients and their physicians to attempt tighter glycemic control when switching from animal to human insulin as part of a general upgrading of diabetes care. As evidenced by the results of the Diabetes Control and Complications Trial (DCCT), the risk of frequent hypoglycemic episodes is greatly increased when "normalization" of the blood glucose is attempted with present suboptimal methods of insulin delivery, and this was independent of the species of insulin used in the DCCT. Although the controversy has not been completely resolved, most authorities do not recommend restricting the use of human insulin because of fear of hypoglycemia.

D. Management of Hypoglycemic Unawareness: (Table 18–17.) Avoiding recurrent hypogly-

Table 18–17. Hypoglycemic "unawareness" in insulin-dependent diabetes mellitus.

I. **Sleeping patient (nocturnal hypoglycemia)**
II. **Hypoglycemia with unawareness while awake—**
   A. **Manifestations:**
     1. Without detectable neuroglycopenia:
       a. Adaptation to chronic hypoglycemia (increased brain glucose transporter I)
     2. With neuroglycopenia:
       a. Maladaptation to hypoglycemia
   B. **Mechanisms:**
     1. Defective autonomic response:
       a. Due to diabetic autonomic neuropathy
       b. Iatrogenic
         i. Frequent hypoglycemia
         ii. Human insulin therapy (?)
   C. **Management:**
     1. Identify patients at risk and reevaluate glycemic goals
     2. Advise frequent self-monitoring of blood glucose
     3. Learn to detect subtle symptoms of neuroglycopenia
     4. Avoid recurrent hypoglycemia
     5. Frequent snacks should be prescribed
     6. Multiple small doses of insulin may be needed
     7. Injectable glucagon made available to family

cemia is the main principle of therapy to restore hypoglycemic awareness. Many insulin-treated diabetics have nocturnal episodes of hypoglycemia of which they are often unaware. These may be detected only with screening by capillary blood testing at least once a week at 2–3 AM. If such episodes do occur, appropriate reduction of evening insulin doses or an increase in the amount of food taken as a snack at bedtime should be advised.

When hypoglycemic unawareness occurs while the patient is awake, two patterns of presentation have been described. In some cases, patients appear perfectly alert with no obvious neuroglycopenia or adrenergic symptoms when a scheduled preprandial capillary blood glucose measurement indicates a level below 40 or 50 mg/dL (2.2 or 2.7 mmol/L). This suggests some degree of adaptation with probable provision of increased glucose transporter-1 proteins among brain capillaries to provide minimum requirements of glucose to the brain despite the hypoglycemia. These patients are at increased risk, however, of developing severe neuroglycopenia if hypoglycemia progresses.

In the second pattern of presentation, patients exhibit neuroglycopenia and progress to require assistance for recovery without having had any awareness of the impending crisis. This form of unawareness is life-threatening and requires immediate measures to prevent recurrences.

When either of these patterns of hypoglycemic unawareness presents while the patient is awake, careful evaluation for autonomic neuropathy with reduced or absent adrenergic responses is indicated.

Evidence for this condition consists of orthostatic hypotension or a fixed heart rate measured during a change in position, during respiration, or after a Valsalva maneuver.

If autonomic neuropathy is detected, glycemic target goals should be appropriately raised by lowering the daily insulin dosage and ensuring that it is administered in multiple small doses, which have a more predictable pharmacokinetic pattern than do larger depot injections. To further lower the risk of severe hypoglycemic episodes, the frequency of self-monitoring of blood glucose should be increased to provide awareness of glycemic status at regular intervals, and patients should be trained to detect subtle signs or symptoms of autonomic responses they might otherwise overlook.

In patients without obvious autonomic neuropathy who have lost awareness to hypoglycemia, special efforts should be made to avoid hypoglycemia for weeks or months in order to reverse central nervous system adaptation to recurrent hypoglycemia. This can be done by increasing the frequency of self-monitoring of blood glucose, raising the mean blood glucose level to be targeted, eating frequent small snacks, and reducing the size of insulin doses at any one injection.

Treatment

All of the manifestations of hypoglycemia are rapidly relieved by glucose administration. Because of the danger of insulin reactions, diabetic patients should carry packets of table sugar or a candy roll at all times for use at the onset of hypoglycemic symptoms. Tablets containing 3 g of glucose are available. The educated patient soon learns to take the amount of glucose needed to correct symptoms without ingesting excessive quantities of orange juice or candy, which can provoke very high glycemic levels. Family members or friends of the patient should be provided with a glucagon emergency kit (Lilly), which contains a syringe, diluent, and a 1-mg ampule of glucagon that can be injected intramuscularly if the patient is found unconscious; these kits are available by prescription. Detailed instructions in the use of glucagon are an essential part of the diabetic education program. An identification Medic Alert bracelet, necklace, or card in the wallet or purse should be carried by every diabetic receiving hypoglycemic drug therapy. The telephone number for the Medic Alert Foundation International in Turlock, California, is 800-ID-ALERT.

A. The Conscious Patient: Patients with symptoms of hypoglycemia who are conscious and able to swallow should eat or drink orange juice, glucose tablets, or any sugar-containing beverage or food except pure fructose (which does not cross the blood-brain barrier).

B. The Unconscious Patient: In general, oral feeding is contraindicated in stuporous or unconscious patients. The preferred treatment is 50 mL of 50% glucose solution given rapidly over 3–5 minutes. If trained personnel are not available to administer intravenous glucose, the treatment of choice is for a family member or friend to administer 1 mg of glucagon intramuscularly (see above), which will usually restore the patient to consciousness within 10–15 minutes; the patient should then be given an oral form of sugar to ingest. If glucagon is not available, small amounts of honey, syrup, or glucose gel can be rubbed into the buccal mucosa. Rectal administration of syrup or honey (30 mL per 500 mL of warm water) has also been used effectively.

COMA

Coma is a *medical emergency* calling for immediate evaluation to determine its cause so that proper therapy can be started. There are several causes of coma that result directly from diabetes mellitus or its treatment. When evaluating a comatose diabetic patient, these must be considered *in addition* to the myriad causes included in the differential diagnosis of coma (cerebrovascular accidents, head trauma, intoxication with alcohol or other drugs, etc).

Etiologic Classification of Diabetic Coma

The causes of coma resulting directly from diabetes mellitus or its treatment include the following:

A. Hyperglycemic Coma: Hyperglycemic coma may be associated with either severe insulin deficiency (diabetic ketoacidosis) or with mild to moderate insulin deficiency (hyperglycemic, hyperosmolar, nonketotic coma).

B. Hypoglycemic Coma: This results from excessive doses of insulin or oral hypoglycemic agents (see above).

C. Lactic Acidosis: Lactic acidosis in diabet-

ics is particularly apt to occur in association with severe tissue anoxia, sepsis, or cardiovascular collapse.

Emergency Management of Coma

The standard approach to *any comatose patient* is outlined below. Prompt action is required.

(1) Establish an airway.

(2) Establish intravenous access. About 30 mL of blood should be drawn and sent for complete blood count, serum electrolyte determinations, renal function and liver function tests, and blood glucose measurements.

(3) Administer 50 mL of 50% dextrose in water to all comatose patients, unless bedside monitoring of blood glucose shows hyperglycemia.

(4) Administer 1 ampule (0.4 mg) of naloxone intravenously and 100 mg of thiamine intravenously.

Diagnosis of Coma

After emergency measures have been instituted, a careful history (from family, friends, paramedics, etc), physical examination, and laboratory evaluation are required to resolve the differential diagnosis. Patients in deep coma from a hyperosmolar nonketotic state or from hypoglycemia are generally flaccid and have quiet breathing—in contrast to patients with acidosis, whose respirations are rapid and deep if the pH of arterial blood has dropped to 7.1 or below. When hypoglycemia is a cause of the coma, hypothermia is usually present and the state of hydration is usually normal. Although the clinical laboratory remains the final arbiter in confirming the diagnosis, a rapid *estimation* of blood glucose and ketones can be obtained by the use of enzyme-impregnated glucose oxidase strips and crushed Acetest tablets (see Laboratory Findings in Diabetes Mellitus, above). Table 18–18 is a summary of some laboratory abnormalities found in diabetic patients with coma attributable to diabetes or its treatment. The in-

Table 18–18. Summary of some laboratory abnormalities in patients with coma directly attributable to diabetes or its treatment.

	Urine		Plasma			
	Glucose	**Acetone**	**Glucose**	**Bicarbonate**	**Acetone**	**Osmolality**
Hyperglycemia, hyperosmolar coma Diabetic ketoacidosis	++ to ++++	++++	High	Low	++++	+++
Hyperglycemic nonketotic coma	++ to ++++	0 or +[1]	High	Normal or slightly low[2]	0	++++
Hypoglycemia	0[3]	0 or +	Low	Normal	0	Normal
Lactic acidosis	0 to +	0 or +	Normal, low, or high	Low	0 or +	Normal

[1] A small degree of ketonuria may be present if the patient is severely stressed or has not been eating because of illness.
[2] A patient may be acidotic if there is severe volume depletion with cardiovascular collapse or if sepsis is present.
[3] Leftover urine in bladder might still contain sugar from earlier hyperglycemia.

dividual clinical syndromes are discussed in detail on the following pages.

1. DIABETIC KETOACIDOSIS

This acute complication of diabetes mellitus may be the first manifestation of previously undiagnosed type I diabetes or may result from increased insulin requirements in type I diabetes patients during the course of infection, trauma, myocardial infarction, or surgery. It is a life-threatening medical emergency with a mortality rate just under 5%. In all cases, precipitating factors such as infection should be searched for and treated appropriately. Poor compliance, either for psychological reasons or because of inadequate patient education, is probably the most common cause of diabetic ketoacidosis, particularly when episodes are recurrent. In adolescents with type I diabetes, recurrent episodes of severe ketoacidosis often indicate the need for counseling to alter this behavior.

Diabetic ketoacidosis has been found to be one of the more common serious complications of insulin pump therapy, occurring in approximately one per 80 patient months of treatment. Many patients who monitor capillary blood glucose regularly ignore urine ketone measurements, which would signal the possibility of insulin leakage or pump failure before serious illness develops.

Patients with type II diabetes may also develop ketoacidosis under severe stress such as sepsis, trauma, or major surgery.

Pathogenesis

Acute insulin deficiency results in rapid mobilization of energy from stores in muscle and fat depots, leading to an increased flux of amino acids to the liver for conversion to glucose and of fatty acids for conversion to ketones (acetoacetate, β-hydroxybutyrate, and acetone). In addition to this increased availability of precursor, there is a direct effect of the low insulin:glucagon ratio on the liver that promotes increased production of ketones. In response to both the acute insulin deficiency and the metabolic stress of ketosis, the levels of insulin-antagonistic hormones (corticosteroids, catecholamines, glucagon, and GH) are consistently elevated. Furthermore, in the absence of insulin, peripheral utilization of glucose and ketones is reduced. The combination of increased production and decreased utilization leads to an accumulation of these substances in blood, with plasma glucose levels reaching 500 mg/dL (27.8 mmol/L) or more and plasma ketones reaching levels of 8–15 mmol/L or more.

The hyperglycemia causes osmotic diuresis leading to depletion of intravascular volume. As this progresses, impaired renal blood flow reduces the kidney's ability to excrete glucose, and hyperosmolality is worsened. Severe hyperosmolality (> 330 mosm/ kg) correlates closely with central nervous system depression and coma.

In a similar manner, impaired renal excretion of hydrogen ions aggravates the metabolic acidosis that occurs as a result of the accumulation of the ketone acids, β-hydroxybutyrate and acetoacetate. The accumulation of ketones may cause vomiting, which exacerbates the intravascular volume depletion. In addition, prolonged acidosis can compromise cardiac output and reduce vascular tone. The result may be severe cardiovascular collapse with generation of lactic acid, which then adds to the already existent metabolic acidosis.

Clinical Features

A. Symptoms and Signs: As opposed to the acute onset of hypoglycemic coma, the appearance of diabetic ketoacidosis is usually preceded by a day or more of polyuria and polydipsia associated with marked fatigue, nausea, and vomiting. Eventually, mental stupor ensues and can progress to frank coma. On physical examination, evidence of dehydration in a stuporous patient with rapid and deep respirations and the "fruity" breath odor of acetone would strongly suggest the diagnosis. Postural hypotension with tachycardia indicates profound dehydration and salt depletion. Abdominal pain and even tenderness may be present in the absence of abdominal disease, and mild hypothermia is usually present.

B. Laboratory Findings: Four-plus glycosuria, strong ketonuria, hyperglycemia, ketonemia, low arterial blood pH, and low plasma bicarbonate (5–15 meq/L) are typical laboratory findings in diabetic ketoacidosis. Serum potassium is usually normal or slightly elevated (5–8 meq/L) despite total body potassium depletion, because of the shift of potassium from the intracellular to extracellular spaces that occurs in systemic acidosis. The average total body potassium deficit resulting from osmotic diuresis, acidosis, and gastrointestinal losses is about 5–10 meq/kg body weight. Similarly, serum phosphate is elevated (6–7 mg/dL), but total body phosphate is generally depleted. Serum sodium is generally reduced (to about 125–130 meq/L) because severe hyperglycemia pulls cellulose water into the interstitial compartment, thereby diluting the already depleted sodium ions lost by polyuria and vomiting. (For every 100 mg/dL of plasma glucose above normal, serum sodium decreases by 1.6 meq/L.) Serum osmolality can be directly measured by standard tests of freezing-point depression or can be estimated by calculating the molarity of sodium, chloride, and glucose in the serum. A convenient formula for estimating *effective* serum osmolality is as follows (physiologic values in humans are generally between 280–300 mosm/L):

$$\text{mosm/L} = 2[\text{Na}^+] + \frac{\text{glucose (mg/dL)}}{18}$$

These calculated estimates are usually 10–20 mosm/L lower than values recorded by standard cryoscopic techniques. Blood urea nitrogen and serum creatinine are invariably elevated because of dehydration. While urea exerts an effect on freezing point depression as measured in the laboratory, it is freely permeable across cell membranes and therefore not included in calculations of effective serum osmolality. In the presence of keto acids, values from multichannel chemical analysis of serum creatinine may be falsely elevated and therefore quite unreliable. However, most laboratories can correct for these interfering chromogens by using a more specific method if asked to do so.

The nitroprusside reagents (Acetest and Ketostix) used for the bedside assessment of ketoacidemia and ketoaciduria measure only acetoacetate and its by-product, acetone. The sensitivity of these reagents for acetone, however, is quite poor, requiring over 10 mmol/L, which is seldom reached in the plasma of ketoacidotic subjects—although this detectable concentration is readily achieved in urine. Thus, in the plasma of ketotic patients, only acetoacetate is measured by these reagents. The more prevalent β-hydroxybutyrate has no ketone group and is therefore not detected by the conventional nitroprusside tests. This takes on special importance in the presence of circulatory collapse during diabetic ketoacidosis, wherein an increase in lactic acid can shift the redox state to increase β-hydroxybutyrate at the expense of the readily detectable acetoacetate. Bedside diagnostic reagents would then be unreliable, suggesting no ketonemia in cases where β-hydroxybutyric acid is a major factor in producing the acidosis.

In about 90% of cases, serum amylase is elevated. However, this often represents salivary as well as pancreatic amylase and correlates poorly with symptoms of pancreatitis, such as pain and vomiting. Therefore, in patients with diabetic ketoacidosis, an elevated serum amylase does not justify a diagnosis of acute pancreatitis; serum lipase may be useful if the diagnosis of pancreatitis is being seriously considered.

C. Data Recording on a Flow Sheet: The need for frequent evaluation of the patient's status cannot be overemphasized (Figure 18–11). Patients with moderately severe diabetic ketoacidosis (pH < 7.2) are best managed in an intensive care unit. Essential baseline blood chemistries include glucose, ketones, electrolytes, arterial blood gases, blood urea nitrogen, and serum creatinine. Serum osmolality should be estimated and tabulated during the course of therapy.

Typically, the patient with moderately severe diabetic ketoacidosis will have a plasma glucose of 350–900 mg/dL (19.4–50 mmol/L), the presence of serum ketones at a dilution of 1:8 or greater, slight hyponatremia of 130 meq/L, hyperkalemia of 5–8 meq/L, hyperphosphatemia of 6–7 mg/dL, and an el-

evated blood urea nitrogen and creatinine. Acidosis may be severe (pH ranging from 6.9 to 7.2 and bicarbonate ranging from 5 to 15 meq/L); PCO_2 is low (15–20 mm Hg) from hyperventilation.

A comprehensive flow sheet that includes vital signs, serial laboratory data, and therapeutic interventions should be meticulously maintained by the physician responsible for the patient's care (Figure 18–11). Plasma glucose should be recorded hourly and electrolytes and pH at least every 2–3 hours during the initial treatment period. Insulin therapy is greatly facilitated when plasma glucose results are available within a few minutes of sampling. This can be achieved by the use of reflectance colorimeters designed for bedside glucose measurements of capillary blood glucose. With trained personnel, these devices are also sufficiently accurate for use in this situation (see Blood Glucose Testing, above). Fluid intake and output as well as details of insulin therapy and the administration of other medications should also be carefully recorded on the flow sheet.

Treatment

A. Immediate Resuscitation and Emergency Measures: If the patient is stuporous or comatose, immediately institute the emergency measures outlined in the section on coma (see above). Once the diagnosis of diabetic ketoacidosis is established in the emergency room, administration of at least 2 L of normal saline (in an adult patient) in the first 2–3 hours is necessary to help restore plasma volume and stabilize blood pressure while acutely reducing the hyperosmolar state. In addition, by improving renal plasma flow, fluid replacement also restores the renal capacity to excrete hydrogen ions, thereby ameliorating the acidosis as well. Immediately after the initiation of fluid replacement, a rapid bolus of 0.3 unit of regular insulin per kilogram of body weight should be given. This will inhibit both gluconeogenesis and ketogenesis while promoting utilization of glucose and keto acids. If arterial blood pH is 7.0 or less, intravenous bicarbonate may be administered (details of administration are outlined below). Gastric intubation is recommended in the comatose patient to prevent vomiting and aspiration that may occur as a result of gastric atony, a common complication of diabetic ketoacidosis. An indwelling bladder catheter is required in all comatose patients but should be avoided, if possible, in a fully cooperative diabetic patient because of the risk of bladder infection. In patients with preexisting cardiac or renal failure or those in severe cardiovascular collapse, a central venous pressure catheter or a Swan-Ganz catheter should be inserted to evaluate the degree of hypovolemia and to monitor subsequent fluid administration.

B. Specific Measures: Each case must be managed individually depending on the specific ab-

DIABETIC KETOACIDOSIS FLOW SHEET

Name _____

Hospital No. _____

Age _____ Initial weight _____

Initial level of consciousness

_____ Alert
_____ Lethargic
_____ Semicomatose
_____ Comatose

DATE									
TIME									
BLOOD PRESSURE									
PULSE									
BLOOD									
Creatinine									
Blood urea nitrogen									
Glucose									
Acetone									
Hematocrit									
pH									
P_{O_2}									
P_{CO_2}									
Na^+									
K^+									
HCO_3^-									
Cl^-									
URINE									
Volume									
Glucose									
Acetone									
REGULAR INSULIN									
Intravenous									
Intramuscular									
Units									
Hours									
INTRAVENOUS FLUIDS									
Type									
Amount									
HCO_3^-									
Phosphate									
OTHER									

Figure 18–11. Flow sheet for treatment of diabetic ketoacidosis.

normalities present and subsequent response to initial therapy.

1. Insulin—Only regular insulin, and preferably human insulin, should be used in the management of diabetic ketoacidosis. As noted above, a "loading" dose of 0.3 unit/kg body weight of regular insulin is given initially as an intravenous bolus followed by 0.1 unit/kg/h, either continuously infused or injected intramuscularly. Doses of insulin as low as 0.1 unit/kg, given hourly either by slow intravenous drip or intramuscularly, are as effective in most cases as the much higher doses previously recommended, and they appear to be safer. When a continuous infusion of insulin is used, 25 units of regular human insulin should be placed in 250 mL of physiologic saline and the first 50 mL of solution flushed through to saturate the tubing before connecting it to the intravenous line. An I-Vac or Harvard pump provides a reliable infusion rate. The insulin dose should be "piggybacked" into the fluid line so the rate of fluid replacement can be changed without altering the insulin delivery rate. For optimal effects, continuous low-dose insulin infusions should always be preceded by a rapid intravenous loading dose of regular insulin, 0.3 unit/kg, to prime the tissue insulin receptors. If the plasma glucose level fails to fall at least 10% in the first hour, a repeat loading dose is recommended. Rarely, a patient with insulin resistance is encountered; this requires doubling the insulin dose every 2–4 hours if severe hyperglycemia does not improve after the first two doses of insulin and fluid replacement.

Insulin therapy, either as a continuous infusion or as injections given every 1–2 hours, should be continued until arterial pH has normalized.

2. Fluid replacement—In most adult patients, the fluid deficit is 4–5 L. Initially, normal saline is preferred for restoration of plasma volume and, as noted above, should be infused rapidly to provide 1 L/h over the first 1–2 hours. After the first 2 L of fluid have been given, the fluid should be changed to 0.45% saline solution given at a rate of 300–400 mL/h; this is because water loss exceeds sodium loss in uncontrolled diabetes with osmotic diuresis. Failure to give enough volume replacement (at least 3–4 L in 8 hours) to restore normal perfusion is one of the most serious therapeutic shortcomings affecting satisfactory recovery. In the same way, excessive fluid replacement (more than 5 L in 8 hours) may contribute to acute respiratory distress syndrome or cerebral edema. When blood glucose falls to approximately 250 mg/dL, the fluids should be changed to a 5% glucose solution to maintain plasma glucose in the range of 250–300 mg/dL. This will prevent the development of hypoglycemia and reduce the likelihood of cerebral edema, which could result from too rapid decline of blood glucose. Intensive insulin therapy should be continued until the ketoacidosis is corrected.

3. Sodium bicarbonate—The use of sodium bicarbonate in management of diabetic ketoacidosis has been questioned since clinical benefit was not demonstrated in one prospective randomized trial and because of the following potentially harmful consequences: (1) development of hypokalemia from rapid shift of potassium into cells if the acidosis is overcorrected; (2) tissue anoxia from reduced dissociation of oxygen from hemoglobin when acidosis is rapidly reversed (leftward shift of the oxygen dissociation curve); and (3) cerebral acidosis resulting from lowering of cerebrospinal fluid pH. It must be emphasized, however, that these considerations are less important when severe acidosis exists. It is therefore recommended that bicarbonate be administered to diabetic patients in ketoacidosis if the arterial blood pH is 7.0 or less or if hypotension, arrhythmia, or coma is present along with an arterial blood pH of less than 7.1 with careful monitoring to prevent overcorrection.

One to two ampules of sodium bicarbonate (one ampule contains 44 meq/50 mL) should be added to 1 L of 0.45% saline. (*Note:* Addition of sodium bicarbonate to 0.9% saline would produce a markedly hypertonic solution that could aggravate the hyperosmolar state already present.) This should be administered rapidly (over the first hour). It can be repeated until the arterial pH reaches 7.1, but *it should not be given if the pH is 7.1 or greater* since additional bicarbonate would increase the risk of rebound metabolic alkalosis as ketones are metabolized. Alkalosis shifts potassium from serum into cells, which could precipitate a fatal cardiac arrhythmia. As noted earlier, serious consideration should be given to placement of a central venous or Swan-Ganz catheter when administering fluids to severely ill patients with cardiovascular compromise.

4. Potassium—Total body potassium loss from polyuria and vomiting may be as high as 200 meq. However, because of shifts of potassium from cells into the extracellular space as a consequence of acidosis, serum potassium is usually normal to slightly elevated prior to institution of treatment. As the acidosis is corrected, potassium flows back into the cells, and hypokalemia can develop if potassium replacement is not instituted. If the patient is not uremic and has an adequate urine output, potassium chloride in doses of 10–30 meq/h should be infused during the second and third hours after beginning therapy as soon as the acidosis starts to resolve. Replacement should be started sooner if the initial serum potassium is inappropriately normal or low and should be delayed if serum potassium fails to respond to initial therapy and remains above 5 meq/L, as in cases of renal insufficiency. Cooperative patients with only mild ketoacidosis may receive part or all of their potassium replacement orally.

An ECG can be of help in monitoring the patient's potassium status: high peaked T waves are a sign of hyperkalemia, and flattened T waves with U waves are a sign of hypokalemia.

Foods high in potassium content should be prescribed when the patient has recovered sufficiently to take food orally. Tomato juice has 14 meq of potassium per 240 mL, and a medium-sized banana has about 10 meq.

5. Phosphate—Phosphate replacement is seldom required in treating diabetic ketoacidosis. However, if severe hypophosphatemia of less than 1 mg/dL (< 0.35 mmol/L) develops during insulin therapy, a small amount of phosphate can be replaced per hour as the potassium salt. Correction of hypophosphatemia helps to restore the buffering capacity of the plasma, thereby facilitating renal excretion of hydrogen. It also corrects the impaired oxygen dissociation from hemoglobin by regenerating 2,3-diphosphoglycerate. However, three randomized studies in which phosphate was replaced in only half of a group of patients with diabetic ketoacidosis did not show any apparent clinical benefit from phosphate administration. Moreover, attempts to use the phosphate salt of potassium as the sole means of replacing potassium have led to a number of reported cases of severe hypocalcemia with tetany. To minimize the risk of inducing tetany from too rapid replacement of phosphate, the average deficit of 40–50 mmol of phosphate should be replaced intravenously at a rate *no greater than 3–4 mmol/h* in a 60- to 70-kg person. A stock solution (Abbott) provides a mixture of 1.12 g KH_2PO_4 and 1.18 g K_2HPO_4 in a 5-mL single-dose vial (this equals 22 mmol of potassium and 15 mmol of phosphate). One-half of this vial (2.5 mL) should be added to 1 L of either 0.45% saline or 5% dextrose in water. Two liters of this solution, infused at a rate of 400 mL/h, will correct the phosphate deficit at the optimal rate of 3 mmol/h while providing 4.4 meq of potassium per hour. (Additional potassium should be administered as potassium chloride to provide a total of 10–30 meq of potassium per hour, as noted above.) If the serum phosphate remains below 2.5 mg/dL after this infusion, a repeat 5-hour infusion can be given.

It remains controversial whether phosphate replacement is beneficial. Several clinics prohibit its use in the routine treatment of diabetic ketoacidosis, since the risk of inducing hypocalcemia is thought to outweigh its potential benefits. However, potential hazards of phosphate replacement can be greatly reduced by administering phosphate at a rate no greater than 3–4 mmol/h. To prevent errors of overreplacement, phosphate should be administered separately rather than included as a component of potassium replacement.

6. Hyperchloremic acidosis during therapy—Because of the considerable loss of keto acids in the urine during the initial phase of therapy, substrate for subsequent regeneration of bicarbonate is lost and correction of the total bicarbonate deficit is hampered. A portion of the bicarbonate deficit is replaced with chloride ions infused in large amounts as saline to correct the dehydration. In most patients, as the ketoacidosis clears during insulin replacement, a hyperchloremic, low-bicarbonate pattern emerges with a normal anion gap. This is a relatively benign condition that reverses itself over the subsequent 12–24 hours once intravenous saline is no longer being administered.

Prognosis

Insulin and fluid and electrolyte replacement combined with careful monitoring of patients' clinical and laboratory responses to therapy have dramatically reduced the morbidity and mortality rates of diabetic ketoacidosis. However, this complication still represents a potential threat to survival, especially in older people with cardiovascular disease. Even in specialized centers, the mortality rate may approach 5–10%. Therefore, physicians treating diabetic ketoacidosis must not be lured into adopting "cookbook" approaches that lessen their attentiveness to changes in the patient's condition. Signs to be watched for include failure of improvement in mental status after a period of treatment, continued hypotension with minimal urine flow, or prolonged ileus (which may suggest bowel infarction). Laboratory abnormalities to be watched include failure of blood glucose to fall by 80–100 mg/dL during the first hour of therapy, failure to increase serum bicarbonate or arterial pH appropriately, serum potassium above 6 or below 2.8 meq/L, and electrocardiographic evidence of cardiac arrhythmias. Any of these signs call for a careful search for the cause of the abnormality and prompt specific therapy.

Disposition

After recovery and stabilization, patients should receive intensive detailed instructions about how to avoid this potentially disastrous complication of diabetes mellitus. They should be taught to recognize the early symptoms and signs of ketoacidosis.

Urine ketones should be measured in patients with signs of infection or in those using an insulin pump when capillary blood glucose is unexpectedly and persistently high. When heavy ketonuria and glycosuria persist on several successive examinations, supplemental regular insulin should be administered and liquid foods such as lightly salted tomato juice and broth should be ingested to replenish fluids and electrolytes. Patients should be instructed to contact the physician if ketonuria persists, and especially if vomiting develops or if appropriate adjustment of the infusion rate on an insulin pump does not correct the hyperglycemia and ketonuria. In adolescents, recurrent episodes of severe diabetic ketoacidosis often indicate poor compliance with the insulin regimen, and these patients should receive intensive family counseling.

2. HYPERGLYCEMIC, HYPEROSMOLAR, NONKETOTIC STATE

This form of hyperglycemic coma is characterized by severe hyperglycemia, hyperosmolality, and dehydration in the absence of significant ketosis. It occurs in middle-aged or elderly patients with non-insulin-dependent diabetes which is often mild or occult. Lethargy and confusion develop as serum osmolality exceeds 300 mosm/L, and coma can occur if osmolality exceeds 330 mosm/L. Underlying renal insufficiency or congestive heart failure is common, and the presence of either worsens the prognosis. A precipitating event such as pneumonia, cerebrovascular accident, myocardial infarction, burns, or recent operation can often be identified. Certain drugs, such as phenytoin, diazoxide, glucocorticoids, and thiazide diuretics, have been implicated in its development, as have procedures associated with glucose loading, eg, peritoneal dialysis.

Pathogenesis

A partial or relative insulin deficiency may initiate the syndrome by reducing glucose utilization by muscle, fat, and the liver while at the same time inducing hyperglucagonemia and increasing hepatic glucose output. The result is hyperglycemia that leads to glycosuria and osmotic diuresis with obligatory water loss. The presence of even small amounts of insulin is believed to prevent the development of ketosis by inhibiting lipolysis in the adipose stores. Therefore even though a low insulin:glucagon ratio promotes ketogenesis in the liver, the limited availability of precursor free fatty acids from the periphery restricts the rate at which ketones are formed. If a patient is unable to maintain adequate fluid intake because of an associated acute or chronic illness or has suffered excessive fluid loss (eg, from burns or therapy with diuretics), marked dehydration results. As plasma volume contracts, renal insufficiency develops; this, then, limits renal glucose excretion and contributes markedly to the rise in serum glucose and osmolality. As serum osmolality exceeds 320–330 mosm/L, water is drawn out of cerebral neurons, resulting in mental obtundation and coma.

Clinical Features

A. Symptoms and Signs: The onset of the hyperglycemic, hyperosmolar, nonketotic state may be insidious, preceded for days or weeks by symptoms of weakness, polyuria, and polydipsia. A history of reduced fluid intake is common, whether due to inappropriate absence of thirst, gastrointestinal upset, or, in the case of elderly or bedridden patients, lack of access to water. A history of ingestion of large quantities of glucose-containing fluids, such as soft drinks or orange juice, can occasionally be obtained; these patients are usually less hyperosmolar than those in whom fluid intake was restricted. The absence of

toxic features of ketoacidosis may retard recognition of the syndrome and thus delay institution of therapy until dehydration is profound. Because of this delay in diagnosis, the hyperglycemia, hyperosmolality, and dehydration in hyperglycemic, hyperosmolar, nonketotic coma is often more severe than in diabetic ketoacidosis.

Physical examination will reveal the presence of profound dehydration (orthostatic fall in blood pressure and rise in pulse, supine tachycardia or even frank shock, dry mucous membranes, decreased skin turgor). The patient may be lethargic, confused, or comatose. Kussmaul respirations are absent unless the precipitating event for the hyperosmolar state has also led to the development of metabolic acidosis (eg, sepsis or myocardial infarction with shock).

B. Laboratory Findings: Severe hyperglycemia is present, with blood glucose values ranging from 800 to as high as 2400 mg/dL (44.4–133.2 mmol/L). In mild cases, where dehydration is less severe, dilutional hyponatremia as well as urinary sodium losses may reduce serum sodium to about 120–125 meq/L—this protects, to some extent, against extreme hyperosmolality. Once dehydration progresses further, however, serum sodium can exceed 140 meq/L, producing serum osmolalities of 330–440 mosm/L* (normal, 280–295 mosm/L). Ketosis is usually absent or mild; however, a small degree of ketonuria may be present if the patient has not been eating because of illness. Acidosis is not a part of the hyperglycemic, hyperosmolar state, but it may be present (usually lactic acidosis) because of other acute underlying conditions (sepsis, acute renal failure, myocardial infarction, etc). (See Lactic Acidosis, below.)

Treatment

There are some differences in fluid, insulin, and electrolyte replacement in this disorder, as compared to diabetic ketoacidosis. However, in common with the treatment of ketoacidotic patients, careful monitoring of the patient's clinical and laboratory response to therapy is essential.

A. Fluid Replacement: Fluid replacement is of paramount importance in treating nonketotic hyperglycemic coma. If circulatory collapse is present, fluid therapy should be initiated with isotonic saline. In all other cases, initial replacement with hypotonic (usually 0.45%) saline is preferable, because these patients are hyperosmolar with considerable loss of body water and excess solute in the vascular compartment. As much as 4–6 L of fluid may be required in the first 8–10 hours. Careful monitoring of fluid quantity and type, urine output, blood pressure, and pulse is essential. Placement of a central venous pres-

---

*A convenient method for estimating serum osmolality is provided in the section on diabetic ketoacidosis

sure or Swan-Ganz catheter should be strongly considered to guide replacement of fluid, especially if the patient is elderly or has underlying renal or cardiac disease. Because insulin therapy will decrease plasma glucose and therefore serum osmolality, a change to isotonic saline may be necessary at some time during treatment in order to maintain an adequate blood pressure and a urine output of at least 50 mL/h. Once blood glucose reaches 250 mg/dL, 5% dextrose in 0.45% or 0.9% saline solution should be substituted for the sugar-free fluids. When consciousness returns, oral fluids should be encouraged.

B. Electrolyte Replacement: Hyperkalemia is less marked and much less potassium is lost in the urine during the osmotic diuresis of hyperglycemic, hyperosmolar, nonketotic coma than in diabetic ketoacidosis. There is, therefore, less severe total potassium depletion, and less potassium replacement is needed to restore potassium stores to normal. However, because the initial serum potassium usually is not elevated and because it declines rapidly as insulin therapy allows glucose and potassium to enter cells, it is recommended that potassium replacement be initiated earlier than in ketotic patients: 10 meq of potassium chloride can be added to the *initial* liter of fluid administered if the initial serum potassium is not elevated and if the patient is making urine. When serum phosphate falls below 1 mg/dL during insulin therapy, phosphate replacement can be given intravenously with the same precautions as those outlined for ketoacidotic patients (see above). If the patient is awake and cooperative, part or all of the potassium and phosphate replacement can be given orally.

C. Insulin Therapy: In general, less insulin is required to reduce the hyperglycemia of nonketotic patients than is the case for patients in diabetic ketoacidosis. In fact, fluid replacement alone can decrease glucose levels considerably. An initial dose of 15 units of regular insulin given intravenously and 15 units given intramuscularly is usually quite effective in lowering blood glucose. In most cases, subsequent doses need not be greater than 10–25 units every 4 hours. (Insulin should be given intramuscularly or intravenously until the patient has stabilized; it may then be given subcutaneously.) Some patients—especially those who are severely ill because of other underlying diseases—may require continuous intravenous administration of insulin (in a manner similar to that described for ketoacidosis) with careful monitoring, preferably in an intensive care setting.

D. Search for the Precipitating Event: The physician must initiate a careful search for the event that precipitated the episode of hyperglycemic, hyperosmolar, nonketotic coma if it is not obvious after the initial history and physical examination. Chest x-rays and cultures of blood, urine, and other body fluids should be obtained to look for occult sources of sepsis; empiric antibiotic coverage should be considered in the seriously ill patient. Cardiac enzymes and serial ECGs can be ordered to look for evidence of "silent" myocardial infarction.

Prognosis

The overall mortality rate of hyperglycemic, hyperosmolar, nonketotic coma is over ten times that of diabetic ketoacidosis, chiefly because of its higher incidence in older patients, who may have compromised cardiovascular systems or associated major illnesses. (When patients are matched for age, the prognoses of these two forms of hyperosmolar coma are reasonably comparable.)

Disposition

After the patient is stabilized, the appropriate form of long-term management of the diabetes must be determined. This must include patient education on how to recognize situations (gastrointestinal upset, infection) that will predispose to recurrence of hyperglycemic, hyperosmolar, nonketotic coma as well as detailed information on how to prevent the escalating dehydration (small sips of sugar-free liquids, increase in usual hypoglycemic therapy, or early contact with the physician) that culminates in hyperosmolar coma. For a detailed discussion of therapeutic alternatives for type II diabetic patients, see Steps in the Management of the Diabetic Patient (above).

3. HYPOGLYCEMIC COMA

Hypoglycemia is a common complication of insulin replacement therapy in diabetic patients. In most cases, it is detected and treated by patients or their families before coma results. However, it remains the most frequent cause of coma in the insulin-treated diabetic patient. In addition, it can occur in any patient taking oral sulfonylurea drugs, particularly if the patient is elderly, has renal or liver disease, or is taking certain other medications that alter metabolism of the sulfonylureas (eg, phenylbutazone, sulfonamides, or warfarin). It occurs more frequently with the use of long-acting sulfonylureas than when shorter-acting agents are used.

Clinical Findings & Treatment

The clinical findings and emergency treatment of hypoglycemia are discussed at the beginning of this section.

Prognosis

Most patients who arrive at emergency rooms in hypoglycemic coma appear to recover fully; however, profound hypoglycemia or delays in therapy can result in permanent neurologic deficit or even death. Furthermore, repeated episodes of hypoglycemia may have a cumulative adverse effect on intellectual functioning.

Disposition

The physician should carefully review with the patient the events leading up to the hypoglycemic episode. Associated use of other medications, as well as alcohol or narcotics, should be noted. Careful attention should be paid to diet, exercise pattern, insulin or sulfonylurea dosage, and general compliance with the prescribed diabetes treatment regimen. Any factors thought to have contributed to the development of the episode should be identified and recommendations made in order to prevent recurrences of this potentially disastrous complication of diabetes therapy.

If the patient is hypoglycemic from use of a long-acting oral hypoglycemic agent (eg, chlorpropamide or glyburide) or from high doses of a long-acting insulin, admission to hospital for treatment with continuous intravenous glucose and careful monitoring of blood glucose is indicated.

4. LACTIC ACIDOSIS

When severely ill diabetic patients present with profound acidosis but relatively low or undetectable levels of keto acids in plasma, the presence of excessive plasma lactate (> 5 mmol/L) should be considered, especially if other causes of acidosis such as uremia are not present.

Pathogenesis

Lactic acid is the end product of anaerobic metabolism of glucose. Normally, the principal sources of this acid are the erythrocytes (which lack the enzymes for aerobic oxidation), skeletal muscle, skin, and brain. The chief pathway for removal of lactic acid is by hepatic (and to some degree renal) uptake for conversion first to pyruvate and eventually back to glucose, a process that requires oxygen. Lactic acidosis occurs when excess lactic acid accumulates in the blood. This can be the result of overproduction (tissue hypoxia), deficient removal (hepatic failure), or both (circulatory collapse). Lactic acidosis is not uncommon in any severely ill patient suffering from cardiac decompensation, respiratory or hepatic failure, septicemia, or infarction of the bowel or extremities.

With the discontinuance of phenformin therapy in the USA, lactic acidosis in patients with diabetes mellitus has become uncommon, but it still must be considered in the acidotic diabetic if the patient is seriously ill, and especially if the patient is receiving metformin therapy as well.

Clinical Features

A. Symptoms and Signs: The main clinical features of lactic acidosis are marked hyperventilation and mental confusion, which may progress to stupor or coma. When lactic acidosis is secondary to tissue hypoxia or vascular collapse, the clinical presentation is variable, being that of the prevailing catastrophic illness. In the rare instance of idiopathic or spontaneous lactic acidosis, the onset is rapid (usually over a few hours), the cardiopulmonary status is stable, and mentation may be relatively normal.

B. Laboratory Findings: Plasma glucose can be low, normal, or high in diabetic patients with lactic acidosis, but usually it is moderately elevated. Plasma bicarbonate and arterial pH are quite low. An anion gap will be present (calculated by subtracting the sum of the plasma bicarbonate and chloride from the plasma sodium; normal is 12–16 meq/L). Ketones are usually absent from plasma, but small amounts may be present in urine if the patient has not been eating recently. Other causes of "anion gap" metabolic acidosis should be excluded—eg, uremia, diabetic or alcoholic ketoacidosis, and salicylate, methanol, ethylene glycol, or paraldehyde intoxication. In the absence of azotemia, hyperphosphatemia may be a clue to the presence of lactic acidosis.

The diagnosis is confirmed by demonstrating, in a sample of blood that is promptly chilled and separated, a plasma lactate concentration of 6 mmol/L or higher (normal is about 1 mmol/L). Failure to rapidly chill the sample and separate the plasma can lead to falsely high plasma lactate values as a result of continued glycolysis by the red blood cells. Frozen plasma remains stable for subsequent assay.

Treatment

The cornerstone of therapy is aggressive treatment of the precipitating cause. An adequate airway and good oxygenation should be ensured. If hypotension is present, fluids and, if appropriate, pressor agents must be given to restore tissue perfusion. Appropriate cultures and empiric antibiotic coverage should be instituted in any seriously ill patient with lactic acidosis in whom the cause is not immediately apparent. Alkalinization with intravenous sodium bicarbonate to keep the pH above 7.2 has been recommended in the emergency treatment of severe lactic acidosis. However, there is no evidence that the mortality rate is favorably affected by administering bicarbonate and the matter is at present controversial, particularly because of the hazards associated with bicarbonate therapy. Dichloroacetate, an anion that facilitates pyruvate removal by activating pyruvate dehydrogenase, reverses certain types of lactic acidosis in animals and may prove useful in treating lactic acidosis in humans. In a prospective controlled clinical trial involving 252 patients with lactic acidosis, dichloroacetate failed to alter either hemodynamics or survival despite its proved effectiveness in lowering lactate levels and raising arterial pH significantly.

CHRONIC COMPLICATIONS OF DIABETES MELLITUS (Table 18–19)

In most patients with diabetes, a number of pathologic changes occur at variable intervals during the course of the disease. These changes involve the vascular system for the most part; however, they also occur in the nerves, the skin, and the lens.

In addition to the above complications, diabetic patients have an increased incidence of certain types of infections and may handle their infections less well than the general population.

Classifications of Diabetic Vascular Disease

Diabetic vascular disease is conveniently divided into two main categories: microvascular disease and macrovascular disease.

A. Microvascular Disease: Disease of the smallest blood vessels, the capillary and the precapillary arterioles, is manifested mainly by thickening of the capillary basement membrane. Microvascular disease involving the retina leads to diabetic retinopathy, and disease involving the kidney causes diabetic nephropathy. Small vessel disease may also involve the heart, and cardiomegaly with heart failure has been described in diabetic patients with patent coronary arteries.

B. Macrovascular Disease: Large vessel disease in diabetes is essentially an accelerated form of atherosclerosis. It accounts for the increased incidence of myocardial infarction, stroke, and peripheral gangrene in diabetic patients. Just as in the case of atherosclerosis in the general population, the exact cause of accelerated atherosclerosis in the diabetic population remains unclear. Abnormalities in vessel walls, platelets and other components of the clotting system, red blood cells, and lipid metabolism have all been postulated to play a role. In addition, there is evidence that coexistent risk factors such as cigarette smoking and hypertension may be important in determining the course of the disease.

Prevalence of Chronic Complications by Type of Diabetes

Although all of the known complications of diabetes can be found in both types of the disease, some are more common in one type than in the other. Renal failure due to severe microvascular nephropathy is the major cause of death in patients with type I diabetes, whereas macrovascular disease is the leading cause in type II. Although blindness occurs in both types, it occurs more commonly as a result of severe

Table 18–19. Chronic complications of diabetes mellitus.

Eyes
Diabetic retinopathy
  Nonproliferative (background)
  Proliferative
Cataracts
  Subcapsular (snowflake)
  Nuclear (senile)

Kidneys
Intracapillary glomerulosclerosis
  Diffuse
  Nodular
Infection
  Pyelonephritis
  Perinephric abscess
  Renal papillary necrosis
Renal tubular necrosis
  Following dye studies (urograms, arteriograms)

Nervous system
Peripheral neuropathy
  Distal, symmetric sensory loss
  Motor neuropathy
    Foot drop, wrist drop
    Mononeuropathy multiplex (diabetic amyotrophy)
Cranial neuropathy
  Cranial nerves III, IV, VI, VII
Autonomic neuropathy
  Postural hypotension
  Resting tachycardia
  Loss of sweating
  Gastrointestinal neuropathy
    Gastroparesis
    Diabetic diarrhea
  Urinary bladder atony
  Impotence (may also be secondary to pelvic vascular disease)

Skin
Diabetic dermopathy (shin spots)
Necrobiosis lipoidica diabeticorum
Candidiasis
Foot and leg ulcers
  Neurotropic
  Ischemic

Cardiovascular system
Heart disease
  Myocardial infarction
  Cardiomyopathy
Gangrene of the feet
  Ischemic ulcers
  Osteomyelitis

Bones and joints
Diabetic cheirarthropathy
Dupuytren's contracture
Charcot joint

Unusual infections
Necrotizing fasciitis
Necrotizing myositis
Mucor meningitis
Emphysematous cholecystitis
Malignant otitis externa

proliferative retinopathy, vitreous hemorrhages, and retinal detachment in type I disease, whereas macular edema and ischemia or cataracts are the usual cause in type II. Similarly, although diabetic neuropathy is common in both type I and type II diabetes, severe autonomic neuropathy with gastroparesis, diabetic diarrhea, resting tachycardia, and postural hypotension is much more common in type I.

Relationship of Glycemic Control to Development of Chronic Complications

The cause of chronic microvascular complications in diabetic patients has now been resolved. A compelling argument for its being a consequence of impaired metabolic control was initially made by observations in Korean patients who ingested a B cell-toxic rodenticide, vacor, during a suicide attempt and developed persistent diabetes. As many as 44% of these patients developed retinopathy during a 6- to 7-year follow-up of their acquired diabetes, while 28% had clinical proteinuria and more than half showed significant thickening of their quadriceps capillary basement membrane width.

However, in patients with idiopathic diabetes mellitus, the most compelling argument for the view that chronic diabetic complications relate to poor glycemic control is based on the findings of the Diabetes Control and Complications Trial (discussed above). This study of 1441 type I patients over a 7- to 10-year period conclusively demonstrated that near normalization of blood glucose with intensive therapy was able to substantially prevent or delay the development of diabetic retinopathy, nephropathy, and neuropathy.

Genetic Factors in Susceptibility to Development of Chronic Complications of Diabetes

Although no genetic susceptibility genes have been identified as yet, three unrelated observations indicate that roughly 40% of people may be unusually susceptible to the ravages of hyperglycemia or other metabolic sequelae of an inadequate insulin effect.

(1) In one retrospective study of 164 juvenile-onset diabetics with a median age at onset of 9 years, 40% were incapacitated or dead from end-stage renal disease with proliferative retinopathy after a 25-year follow-up, while the remaining subjects were either mildly affected (40%) or had no clinically detected microvascular disease (20%). This study was completed long before the availability of glycemic self-monitoring methodology, so it is unlikely that any of these patients were near optimal glycemic control.

(2) Data from renal transplantation indicate that only about 40% of normal kidneys developed evidence of moderate to severe diabetic nephropathy within 6–14 years of being transplanted into diabetic subjects with end-stage renal failure, whereas as many as 60% were only minimally affected.

(3) Among children under 21 years of age with type I diabetes, 40% had thickening of the capillary basement membrane width (CBMW) of the quadriceps muscle, while 60% had vessels within the normal range. This finding was unrelated to the severity or duration of diabetes and is in contrast to results in

diabetic adults 21 years of age or older, in whom virtually 100% have thickened CBMWs.

These three observations support the hypothesis that while approximately 60% of people suffer only minimal consequences from hyperglycemia and other metabolic hazards of insulin insufficiency, 40% or so suffer severe, potentially catastrophic microvascular complications if the disease is poorly controlled. The genetic mechanisms for this increased susceptibility are as yet unknown but could relate to overproduction or reduced removal of accelerated glycosylation end products in particular tissues. If further studies indicate that the presence of early thickening of the CBMW—found in 40% of children—represents a marker of this susceptibility gene and a predictor of severe microvascular disease, it could justify more intensive insulin therapy in that group to achieve near-normalization of blood glucose. The remaining 60% of less susceptible individuals might then be spared the inconveniences of strict glycemic control as well as the risks of hypoglycemia inherent in present methods of intensive insulin therapy.

SPECIFIC CHRONIC COMPLICATIONS OF DIABETES MELLITUS (Table 18–19)

1. OPHTHALMOLOGIC COMPLICATIONS

Diabetic Retinopathy

For early detection of diabetic retinopathy, adolescent or adult patients who have had type I diabetes for more than 5 years and *all* non-IDDM patients should be referred to an ophthalmologist for examination and follow-up. When hypertension is present in a patient with diabetes, it should be treated vigorously, since hypertension is associated with an increased incidence and accelerated progression of diabetic retinopathy.

A. Pathogenesis and Clinical Features: Two main categories of diabetic retinopathy exist: nonproliferative and proliferative.

Nonproliferative ("background") retinopathy represents the earliest stage of retinal involvement by diabetes and is characterized by such changes as microaneurysms, dot hemorrhages, exudates, and retinal edema. During this stage, the retinal capillaries leak proteins, lipids, or red cells into the retina. When this process occurs in the macula, the area of greatest concentration of visual cells, there will be interference with visual acuity; this is the most common cause of visual impairment in type II diabetes and occurs in up to 18% of these patients over time.

Proliferative retinopathy involves the growth of new capillaries and fibrous tissue within the retina and into the vitreous chamber. It is a consequence of small vessel occlusion, which causes retinal hypoxia; this in turn stimulates new vessel growth. Proliferative retinopathy can occur in both types of diabetes but is more common in type I, developing about 7–10 years after onset of symptoms, with a prevalence of 25% after 15 years' duration. Prior to proliferation of new capillaries, a preproliferative phase often occurs in which arteriolar ischemia is manifested as cotton-wool spots (small infarcted areas of retina). Vision is usually normal until vitreous hemorrhage or retinal detachment occurs. Proliferative retinopathy is a leading cause of blindness in the USA, particularly since it increases the risk of retinal detachment. After 10 years of diabetes, half of all patients have at least some degree of retinopathy, and this proportion increases to more than 80% after 15 years of diabetes.

B. Treatment: Once maculopathy or proliferative changes are detected, panretinal xenon or argon laser photocoagulation therapy is indicated. Destroying retinal tissue with photocoagulation means that surviving tissue receives a greater share of the available oxygen supply, thereby abolishing hypoxic stimulation of new vessel growth. Results of a large-scale clinical trial (the Diabetic Retinopathy Study) have verified the effectiveness of photocoagulation, particularly when recent vitreous hemorrhages have occurred or when extensive new vessels are located near the optic disk.

The best results with photocoagulation are achieved if proliferative retinopathy is detected early. This is best done by obtaining a baseline fluorescein angiogram within 5–10 years after onset of type I diabetes and then repeating this study at intervals of 1–5 years, depending on the severity of the retinal involvement found. Prepubertal children do not develop diabetic retinopathy regardless of the duration of their diabetes. They need not be scheduled for routine ophthalmologic examination until several years after the onset of puberty.

Pituitary ablation, which has been associated with delay in progression of severe retinopathy in the past, is rarely used today because photocoagulation therapy is just as effective and avoids the risks associated with destruction of the pituitary. Occasional cases of rapidly progressive ("florid") proliferative retinopathy in type I adolescent diabetics have been reported in which photocoagulation was less effective than pituitary ablation in preventing blindness.

Cataracts

Two types of cataracts occur in diabetic patients: subcapsular and senile. **Subcapsular cataract** occurs predominantly in type I diabetics, may come on fairly rapidly, and has a significant correlation with the hyperglycemia of uncontrolled diabetes. This type of cataract has a flocculent or "snowflake" appearance and develops just below the lens capsule.

Senile cataract represents a sclerotic change of the lens nucleus. It is by far the most common type of cataract found in either diabetic or nondiabetic adults and tends to occur at a younger age in diabetic patients, particularly when glycemic control is poor.

Two separate abnormalities found in diabetic patients, both of which are related to elevated blood glucose levels, may contribute to the formation of cataracts: (1) glycosylation of the lens protein and (2) an excess of sorbitol, which is formed from the increased quantities of glucose found in the insulin-independent lens. Accumulation of sorbitol leads to osmotic changes in the lens that ultimately result in fibrosis and cataract formation.

Glaucoma

Glaucoma occurs in approximately 6% of persons with diabetes. It is generally responsive to the usual therapy for open-angle disease. Closed-angle glaucoma can result from neovascularization of the iris in diabetics, but this is relatively uncommon except after cataract extraction, when accelerated new vessel growth may occur that involves the angle of the iris and obstructs outflow.

2. RENAL COMPLICATIONS

Diabetic Nephropathy

A. Pathogenesis and Clinical Findings: About 4000 cases of end-stage renal disease due to diabetic nephropathy occur annually among diabetic patients in the USA. This represents about one-fourth of all patients being treated for renal failure. Thickening of capillary basement membranes and of the mesangium of renal glomeruli produces varying degrees of glomerulosclerosis and renal insufficiency. Diffuse glomerulosclerosis is more common than nodular intercapillary glomerulosclerosis (Kimmelstiel-Wilson lesions); both produce heavy proteinuria.

1. Microalbuminuria—New methods of detecting small amounts of urinary albumin have permitted detection of microgram concentrations—in contrast to the less sensitive dipstick strips, whose minimal detection limit is 0.3–0.5%. Conventional 24-hour urine collections, in addition to being inconvenient for patients, also show wide variability of albumin excretion, since several factors such as sustained erect posture, dietary protein, and exercise tend to increase albumin excretion rates. For these reasons, most laboratories prefer to screen patients with a timed overnight urine collection beginning at bedtime, when the urine is discarded and the time noted. Normal subjects excrete less than 15 μg/min during overnight urine collections; values of 20 μg/min or higher are considered to represent abnormal microalbuminuria. Subsequent renal failure can be predicted by urinary albumin excretion rates exceeding 30 μg/min. Increased microalbuminuria correlates with increased levels of blood pressure, and this may explain why increased proteinuria in diabetic patients is associated with an increase in cardiovascular deaths even in the absence of renal failure. Careful glycemic control as well as a low-protein diet (0.8 g/kg/d) may reduce both the hyperfiltration and the elevated microalbuminuria in patients in the early stages of diabetes and those with incipient diabetic nephropathy. Antihypertensive therapy also decreases microalbuminuria, and clinical trials with inhibitors of angiotensin I converting enzyme (eg, enalapril, 20 mg/d) show a reduction of microalbuminuria in diabetic patients even in the absence of hypertension. Although a reduction in mean arterial blood pressure may contribute to this effect even in normotensive patients, the main action of these agents in reducing microalbuminuria is believed to be from a specific dilation of the glomerular efferent arteriole, thereby further reducing glomerular filtration pressure.

2. Progressive diabetic nephropathy–Progressive diabetic nephropathy consists of proteinuria of varying severity, occasionally leading to nephrotic syndrome with hypoalbuminemia, edema, and an increase in circulating betalipoproteins as well as progressive azotemia. In contrast to all other renal disorders, the proteinuria associated with diabetic nephropathy does not diminish with progressive renal failure (patients continue to excrete 10–11 g daily as creatinine clearance diminishes). As renal failure progresses, there is an elevation in the renal threshold at which glycosuria appears.

Hypertension develops with progressive renal involvement, and coronary and cerebral atherosclerosis seems to be accelerated. Once diabetic nephropathy has progressed to the stage of hypertension, proteinuria, or early renal failure, glycemic control is not beneficial in influencing its course. In this circumstance, antihypertensive medications, including ACE inhibitors, and restriction of dietary protein to 0.6 g/kg body weight per day are recommended.

When the serum creatinine reaches 3 mg/dL, consultation with a nephrologist or a diabetologist experienced in the treatment of diabetic nephropathy is recommended. When the serum creatinine reaches 5 mg/dL, consultation with personnel at a center where renal transplantation is performed is indicated.

B. Treatment: Hemodialysis has been of limited success in the treatment of renal failure due to diabetic nephropathy, primarily because of progression of large-vessel disease with resultant death and disability from stroke and myocardial infarction. Growing experience with chronic ambulatory peritoneal dialysis suggests that it may be a more convenient method of providing adequate dialysis with a lower incidence of complications.

Renal transplantation, especially from related donors, is often successful. For patients with compatible donors and no contraindications (such as severe cardiovascular disease), it is the treatment of choice.

Necrotizing Papillitis

This unusual complication of pyelonephritis occurs primarily in diabetic patients. It is characterized by fever, flank pain, pyuria, and sloughing of renal papillae in the urine. It is treated by intravenous administration of appropriate antibiotics.

Renal Decompensation After Radiographic Dyes

The use of radiographic contrast agents in diabetic patients with reduced creatinine clearance has been associated with the development of acute renal failure. Diabetic patients with normal renal function do not appear to be at increased risk for contrast nephropathy. If a contrast study is considered essential, patients with a serum creatinine of 1.5–2.5 mg/dL should be adequately hydrated before the procedure to produce a gentle diuresis of about 75 mL or so per hour. Other nephrotoxic agents such as nonsteroidal anti-inflammatory agents should be avoided. Although it was once believed that newer nonionic contrast agents were less likely to cause acute renal failure in diabetic patients, more recent prospective trials show no difference between these agents and conventional and much less costly ionic radiographic dyes. After the procedure, serum creatinine should be followed closely. Radiographic contrast material should not be given to a patient with a serum creatinine greater than 3 mg/dL unless the potential benefit outweighs the high risk of acute renal failure.

3. NEUROLOGIC COMPLICATIONS (Diabetic Neuropathy)

Peripheral and autonomic neuropathy are the two most common complications of both types of diabetes. Their pathogenesis is poorly understood. Some lesions, such as the acute cranial nerve palsies and diabetic amyotrophy, have been attributed to ischemic infarction of the involved peripheral nerve. The much more common symmetric sensory and motor peripheral neuropathies and autonomic neuropathy are felt to be due to metabolic or osmotic toxicity somehow related to hyperglycemia.

Unfortunately, there is no consistently effective treatment for any of the neuropathies. It remains to be demonstrated definitively whether normalization of blood glucose levels can prevent development and progression of this devastating complication.

Peripheral Sensory Neuropathy

A. Pathogenesis and Clinical Features: Sensory loss is commonly preceded by months or years of paresthesias such as tingling, itching, and increasing pain. The pains can vary from mild paresthesias to severe shooting pains and may be more severe at night. Discomfort of the lower extremities can be incapacitating at times. Radicular pains in the chest and the abdominal area may be extremely difficult to distinguish from pain due to an intrathoracic or intra-abdominal source. Eventually, patients develop numbness, and tactile sensations decrease. The sensory loss is generally bilateral, symmetric, and associated with dulled perception of vibration, pain, and temperature, particularly in the lower extremities, but also evident in the hands. Sensory nerve conduction is delayed in peripheral nerves, and ankle jerks may be absent. Highly sensitive neurothesiometer devices are being utilized to characterize the threshold levels for pain and touch, so that signs of sensory defects can be detected earlier and patients with higher risk for neuropathic foot ulcers can be identified. Because all of these sensory disturbances are made worse by pressure applied to the involved nerves, symptoms may appear first in nerves that are entrapped, such as the median nerve in carpal tunnel syndrome or the nerves around the ankle.

Characteristic syndromes that develop in diabetic patients with sensory neuropathy and are related to their failure to perceive trauma include osteopathy of the distal hand and foot, deformity of the knee or ankle (so-called Charcot joint), and neuropathic ulceration of the foot.

B. Treatment: Amitriptyline (50–75 mg at bedtime) has produced remarkable improvement in the lower extremity pain in some patients with sensory neuropathy. Dramatic relief has often occurred within 48–72 hours. This rapid response is in contrast to the 2 or 3 weeks required for an antidepressive effect. Patients often attribute benefit to their having a full night's sleep after amitriptyline in contrast to many prior sleepless nights occasioned by neuropathic pain. Mild to moderate morning drowsiness is a side effect that generally improves with time or can be lessened by giving the medication several hours before bedtime. This drug should be discontinued if there is no improvement after 4–5 days. Desipramine in doses of 25–150 mg per day has been reported to have the same efficacy for neuropathic leg pains as amitriptyline. These tricyclic drug probably act by directly modulating nociceptive C fibers and their receptors. Other drugs have been used, including carbamazepine and phenytoin, but these are of questionable benefit for leg pain. Capsaicin, a topical irritant, has relieved local nerve pain in some studies; it is dispensed as a cream to be rubbed into the skin over the painful region.

It is essential that diabetic patients with peripheral neuropathy receive detailed instructions in foot care (see p 626). Special custom-made shoes are usually required to redistribute weight evenly over an insensitive foot, particularly when it has been deformed by surgery, by asymptomatic fractures, or by a Charcot joint.

Motor Neuropathy

Symmetric motor neuropathy occurs much less frequently than sensory neuropathy and is associated with delayed motor nerve conduction and muscle weakness and atrophy. Its pathogenesis is presumed to be similar to that of sensory loss. Mononeuropathy develops when there is vascular occlusion of a specific nerve trunk; if more than one nerve trunk is involved, the syndrome of **mononeuritis multiplex** occurs. Motor neuropathy is manifested by an abrupt onset of weakness in a distribution that reflects the nerve involved (eg, peroneal nerve involvement produces foot drop). A surprising number of these motor neuropathies improve after 6–8 weeks. Reversible **cranial nerve palsies** can occur and may present as lid ptosis (cranial nerve III), lateral deviation of the eye (IV), inability to move the eye laterally (VI), or facial paralysis (Bell's palsy) (VII). Acute pain and weakness of thigh muscles bilaterally can occur with progressive wasting and weight loss. This has been termed **diabetic amyotrophy** and is more common in elderly men. Again, the prognosis is good, with recovery of motor function over several months in many cases. In more severe cases with extensive atrophy of limb musculature, this disorder has been termed "malignant cachexia" and mimics the end stages of advanced neoplasia, particularly when depression produces anorexia and weight loss. With this more severe manifestation of diabetic amyotrophy, recovery of muscle function may only be partial.

Autonomic Neuropathy

Neuropathy of the autonomic nervous system is common in patients with diabetes of long duration and can be a very disconcerting clinical problem. It can affect many diverse visceral functions. With autonomic neuropathy, there may be postural hypotension, resting fixed tachycardia, decreased cardiovascular responses to the Valsalva maneuver, gastroparesis, alternating bouts of diarrhea (often nocturnal) and constipation, difficulty in emptying the bladder, and impotence.

Impotence due to neuropathy differs from the psychogenic variety in that the latter may be intermittent (erections occur under special circumstances), whereas diabetic impotence is usually persistent. To distinguish neuropathic or psychogenic impotence from the impotence caused by aortoiliac occlusive disease or vasculopathy, papaverine is injected into the corpus cavernosum. If the blood supply is competent, a penile erection will occur (Chapter 12). Urinary incontinence, with large volumes of residual urine, and retrograde ejaculation can also result from pelvic neuropathy.

Gastroparesis should be a diagnostic consideration in insulin-dependent diabetic patients who develop unexpected fluctuations and variability in their blood glucose levels after meals. Radiographic studies of the stomach and radioisotopic examination of gastric emptying after liquid and solid meals are of diagnostic value in these patients. Involvement of the gastrointestinal system may be manifested by nausea, vomiting, and postprandial fullness (from gastric atony); symptoms of reflux or dysphagia (from esophageal involvement); constipation and recurrent diarrhea, especially at night (from involvement of the small bowel and colon); and fecal incontinence (from anal sphincter dysfunction). Gallbladder function is altered, and this enhances stone formation.

Therapy is difficult and must be directed specifically at each abnormality. Use of Jobst fitted stockings, tilting the head of the bed, and arising slowly from the supine position are useful in minimizing symptoms of **orthostatic hypotension.** Some patients may require the addition of a mineralocorticoid such as fludrocortisone acetate (0.1–0.2 mg twice daily). Metoclopramide has been of some help in treating diabetic gastroparesis over the short term, but its effectiveness seems to diminish over time. It is a dopamine antagonist with central antiemetic effects as well as cholinergic action to facilitate gastric emptying. It can be given intravenously (10–20 mg) or orally (20 mg of liquid metoclopramide) before breakfast and supper. Drowsiness is its major adverse effect. Cisapride in doses of 10 mg three or four times daily is a newer agent that can improve the rate of gastric emptying of both liquid and solids by virtue of its cholinergic and antiserotonin actions. It appears to be better tolerated and to cause fewer central nervous system side effects than metoclopramide, but it may cause troublesome stool frequency in some patients. Bethanechol has also been used for gastroparesis (as well as for an atonic urinary bladder) because of its anticholinergic effects.

Diabetic diarrhea is occasionally aggravated by bacterial overgrowth from stasis in the small intestine, and a trial of broad-spectrum antibiotics may give relief. If this does not help, symptomatic relief can sometimes be achieved with antidiarrheal agents such as diphenoxylate with atropine or loperamide . Clonidine has been reported to lessen diabetic diarrhea, but its tendency to lower blood pressure in those patients who already have some degree of orthostatic hypotension often limits its usefulness. Metamucil and other bulk-providing agents may relieve either the diarrhea or the constipation phases, which often alternate. Beta-lactulose is useful in managing severe constipation. Bethanechol has occasionally improved emptying of the **atonic urinary bladder.** When **impotence** is due to neuropathy, it is usually permanent, and a penile prosthesis should be considered as a therapeutic option in appropriate cases. External vacuum therapy (Erec-Aid System) is a nonsurgical treatment that consists of a suction chamber operated by a hand pump that creates a vacuum around the penis. This draws blood into the corpus cavernosum to produce an erection which is maintained by a specially designed tension ring inserted around the base of the penis and which can be kept in place for up to 20–30 minutes. This approach has met with acceptance by a majority of patients with impotence, while others have preferred surgical implant of a penile prosthesis. Another quite promising noninvasive treatment has recently completed clinical trials which involves instilling a vasodilating prostaglandin directly into the opening of the distal urethra, inducing

a satisfactory erection in neuropathic impotence that can persist for up to an hour. (See Chapter 12.)

Aldose reductase inhibitors have been generally disappointing, with only marginal therapeutic results in either autonomic or peripheral diabetic neuropathy and a relatively high incidence of toxic side effects such as skin rash and neutropenia.

4. CARDIOVASCULAR COMPLICATIONS

Heart Disease

Microangiopathy has recently been recognized to occur in the heart and may explain the existence of congestive cardiomyopathies found in diabetic patients without demonstrable coronary artery disease. Much more commonly, however, heart failure in the diabetic is a consequence of coronary atherosclerosis. Myocardial infarction is three to five times more common in diabetic patients than in age-matched controls and is the leading cause of death in patients with type II diabetes. A loss of the protection against myocardial infarction usually present in women during the age of childbearing is particularly evident in diabetic women. The exact reason for the increased incidence of myocardial infarction in diabetics is not clear. It may be a consequence of hyperlipidemia; abnormalities of platelet adhesiveness or coagulation factors (or both); or hypertension.

Peripheral Vascular Disease

Atherosclerosis is markedly accelerated in the larger arteries. It is often diffuse, with localized enhancement in certain areas of turbulent blood flow, such as at the bifurcation of the aorta or other large vessels. Clinical manifestations of peripheral vascular disease include ischemia of the lower extremities, impotence, and intestinal angina.

The incidence of **gangrene of the feet** in diabetics is 30 times that in age-matched controls. The factors responsible for its development, in addition to peripheral vascular disease, are small vessel disease, peripheral neuropathy with loss of both pain sensation and neurogenic inflammatory responses and secondary infection. In two-thirds of patients with ischemic gangrene, pedal pulses are not palpable. In the remaining one-third who have palpable pulses, reduced blood flow through these vessels can be demonstrated by plethysmographic or Doppler ultrasound examination. Prevention of foot injury is imperative, and certain principles that should be emphasized are outlined on p 626. Agents that reduce peripheral blood flow such as tobacco and propranolol should be avoided. Control of other risk factors such as hypertension is essential. Cholesterol-lowering agents are useful as adjunctive therapy when early ischemic signs are detected and when dyslipidemia is present. Patients should be advised to seek immediate medical care if a diabetic foot ulcer develops. Improvement in peripheral blood flow with endarterectomy and bypass operations is possible in certain patients.

5. SKIN CHANGES

Diabetic dermopathy is characterized by atrophic brown spots on the skin, usually in the pretibial area ("shin spots"). These changes may be a consequence of increased glycosylation of tissue proteins or vasculopathy. Eruptive xanthomas may develop in some poorly controlled diabetics who have marked hypertriglyceridemia. A rare skin complication, necrobiosis lipoidica diabeticorum, occurs predominantly on the shins and is characterized by marked thinning of the skin which allows the subcutaneous vessels to be seen as though through tissue paper. An element of vascular occlusion is generally present.

6. BONE & JOINT COMPLICATIONS

Bone and joint complications are generally attributed to metabolic or vascular sequelae of diabetes of long standing.

Juvenile Diabetic "Cheirarthropathy"

This is a syndrome of chronic progressive stiffness of the hand secondary to contracture and tightening of the skin over the joints. It is characterized by inability to flatten the palms against a flat surface. It usually occurs within 5–6 years after onset of type I diabetes. It is believed to be due to glycosylation of collagen and perhaps other proteins in connective tissue.

Dupuytren's Contracture

This consists of nodular thickening of the palmar fascia of the hand, producing a claw-like deformity. Although not specific to diabetes, when it occurs in a diabetic patient it may be the result of ischemic necrosis and secondary scarring of connective tissue as a consequence of diabetic microangiopathy.

Bone Demineralization

Bone demineralization has been reported to occur with increased frequency in diabetic patients. Bone density, as measured by photon absorption in the forearms, is 10–20% below normal in diabetics as compared to appropriately matched controls. Diabetes mellitus, however, does not seem to be associated with clinically important osteopenia, since there is no increase in the occurrence of skeletal fractures.

Joint Abnormalities

Bursitis, particularly of the shoulders and hips, occurs more frequently than expected in patients with diabetes. Gout also has a higher than expected incidence, especially in obese diabetics.

7. INFECTION

Candidal infections occur more frequently in diabetic patients than in nondiabetic matched controls. Candidal infection can produce erythema and edema of intertriginous areas below the breasts, in the axillas, and between the fingers. It causes vulvovaginitis in most chronically uncontrolled diabetic women with persistent glucosuria and is a frequent cause of pruritus. While antifungal creams containing miconazole or clotrimazole offer immediate relief of vulvovaginitis, recurrence is frequent unless glucosuria is reduced.

There are also several unusual infections that occur almost exclusively in diabetics (eg, emphysematous cholecystitis, mucormycosis, malignant otitis externa and necrotizing papillitis). As noted above, atherosclerosis with peripheral vascular disease is very common in the diabetic population, and the resultant ischemia undoubtedly plays a role in the frequent and severe lower extremity infections seen in these patients.

SURGERY IN THE DIABETIC PATIENT

Surgery represents a stress situation during which most of the insulin antagonists (catecholamines, GH, corticosteroids) are mobilized. In the diabetic patient, this can lead to a worsening of hyperglycemia and perhaps even ketoacidosis. The aim of medical management of diabetics during the perioperative period is to minimize these stress-induced changes. Recommendations for management depend both on the patient's usual diabetic regimen and on the type of surgery (major or minor) to be done.

DIABETICS REGULATED BY DIET ALONE

No special precautions must be taken unless diabetic control is markedly disturbed by the procedure. If this occurs, small amounts of regular insulin twice a day will establish euglycemia in a patient whose food intake is adequate. Human insulin is recommended, since it sensitizes the patient least—ie, anaphylactic complications are very rare, and patients are less likely to be sensitized to the future use of insulin.

DIABETICS TAKING ORAL HYPOGLYCEMIC AGENTS

When oral medications are allowed, these agents should be administered in the usual doses in the perioperative period. Carbohydrates should be supplied orally or by intravenous infusion of dextrose in water, with careful monitoring of blood glucose levels to avoid hypoglycemia or extremes of hyperglycemia. As in the case of diet-controlled diabetes, human insulin can be substituted if symptomatic hyperglycemia or ketosis develops.

DIABETICS TAKING INSULIN

Patients taking insulin represent the only serious challenge to management of diabetes when surgery is necessary. However, with careful attention to changes in the clinical or laboratory picture, most diabetic patients can be managed successfully.

Minor Surgery

For minor surgery requiring only local or spinal anesthesia or intravenous administration of a very transient anesthetic, half of the usual dose of insulin should be given in the morning. The patient should be placed early on the operating room schedule. A constant drip of 5% dextrose in water (at a rate of approximately 5 g of glucose per hour) should be infused, and blood glucose levels should be checked at regular intervals.

Major Surgery

The night before major surgery, a 9 PM bedtime snack is given. Thereafter, the patient should receive nothing by mouth. On the morning of surgery, the usual morning subcutaneous insulin dose is omitted; instead, 10 units of regular insulin is added to 1 L of 5% dextrose in half-normal saline, and this is infused intravenously at a rate of 100–180 mL/h. This will give the patient 1–1.8 units of insulin per hour, which, except in the most severe cases, will generally keep the blood glucose within the range of 100–250 mg/dL (5.5–13.9 mmol/L). The infusion may be continued for several days if necessary. Plasma glucose or blood glucose should be determined every 2–4 hours to be sure metabolic control is adequate. If it is not, adjustments in the ratio of insulin to dextrose in the intravenous solution can be made.

An alternative method which is gaining in popularity consists of separate infusions of insulin and glucose delivered by pumps to permit independent adjustments of each infusion rate depending on hourly variation of blood glucose values. Table 18–20 provides guidelines for management with an insulin drip, and the algorithms are designed to achieve glycemic control in the range of 120–180 mg/dL blood glucose.

After surgery, when the patient has resumed an adequate oral intake, intravenous administration of insulin and dextrose can be stopped. Two hours after discontinuing the intravenous insulin, subcutaneous administration of insulin can be resumed. Insulin needs may vary in the first several days after surgery

Table 18–20. Guidelines for perioperative diabetes management with an intravenous insulin infusion.[1]

- Insulin: Regular (human) 25 units in 250 mL of normal saline (1 unit/10 mL).
- Intravenous infusions of insulin: Flush 50 mL through line before connecting to patient. Piggyback insulin line to the perioperative maintenance fluid line.
- Perioperative maintenance fluid: Fluids must contain 5% dextrose (rate 100 mL/h).
- Blood glucose: Monitor hourly intraoperatively.[2]

Blood Glucose (mg/dL)	Insulin	
	(units/h)	(mL/h)
< 80	0.0	0.0
81–100	0.5	5.0
101–140	1.0	10
141–180	1.5	15
181–220	2.0	20
221–260	2.5	25
261–300	3.0	30
301–340	4.0	40
> 341	5.0	50

- Blood glucose < 80 mg/dL: Stop insulin and administer intravenous bolus of 50% dextrose in water (25 mL). Once blood glucose > 80 mg/dL, restart insulin infusion. It may be necessary to modify the algorithm.
- Decreased insulin needs: Patients treated with diet or oral agents or < 50 units insulin per day, endocrinologic deficiencies.
- Increased insulin needs: Obesity, sepsis, steroid therapy, renal transplant, coronary artery bypass.

[1]Reproduced, with permission, from Gavin LA: Perioperative management of the diabetic patient. Endocrinol Metab Clin North Am 1992;21:457.
[2]Blood glucose value ÷ 100 gives a reasonable estimate of infusion dosage (units/h).

because of continuing postoperative stresses and because of variable caloric intake. In this situation, multiple doses of regular insulin guided by blood glucose determinations can keep the patient in acceptable metabolic control.

PROGNOSIS FOR PATIENTS WITH DIABETES MELLITUS

The period between 10 and 20 years after the onset of type I diabetes seems to be a critical one. If the patient survives this period without fulminating microvascular complications, there is a strong likelihood that reasonably good health will continue. In patients with type I diabetes, the results of the Diabetes Control and Complications Trial have established the benefit of near-normalization of glycemia in preventing or delaying the progression of diabetic microangiopathy. Similar trials of intensive therapy are in progress in the United Kingdom and are being designed in the United States to determine whether a similar benefit occurs in type II diabetes, particularly as regards macrovascular disease as well as microangiopathy. Currently, the prospect for retarding the progression of diabetic eye complications in both types of diabetes is good because of benefits derived from laser photocoagulation. Education as to proper foot care has been immensely valuable in reducing morbidity from diabetic foot problems. Management of hypertension, dyslipidemia, and cessation of cigarette smoking have been of great benefit in preventing or reducing the progression of retinopathy, nephropathy, and atherosclerosis. Newer methods for delivering purified insulins and for self-monitoring blood glucose have improved the overall outlook for patients with diabetes mellitus. However, present methods of insulin delivery remain quite primitive and need much improvement before physiologic insulin secretion is reproduced. Hypoglycemia remains a serious risk in all regimens of intensive insulin therapy attempting normalization of blood glucose. It is clear that the diabetic patient's intelligence, motivation, and awareness of potential complications of the disease are major factors contributing to a successful outcome. In addition, appropriate education of diabetic patients to provide the knowledge, the guidelines, and the tools to help them take charge of their own day-to-day diabetes management is essential to improve the long-term prognosis.

REFERENCES

The Endocrine Pancreas

Atria TE et al: Secretion of pancreatic polypeptide in patients with pancreatic endocrine tumors. N Engl J Med 1986;315:287.

Burant CF et al: Fructose transporter in human spermatozoa and small intestine is GLUT 5. J Biol Chem 1992;267:14523.

Fehman H-C, Goke R, Goke B: Cell and molecular biology of the incretin hormones glucagon-like peptide I and glucose-dependent insulin releasing polypeptide. Endocr Rev 1995;16:390.

Galloway JA et al: Biosynthetic human proinsulin: Review of chemistry, in vitro and in vivo receptor binding, animal and human pharmacology studies, and clinical trial experience. Diabetes Care 1992;15:666.

Goldfine ID, Pilch P: Insulin secretion and action and diabetes mellitus. J Cell Biochem 1992;48:1.

Holst JJ: Glucagonlike peptide 1: A newly discovered hormone. Gastroenterology 1994;107:1848.

Kahn BB: Facilitative glucose transporters: Regulatory mechanisms and dysregulation in diabetes. J Clin Invest 1992;89:1367.

Lefebvre PJ: Glucagon and its family revisited. Diabetes Care 1995;18:715.

Nathan DM et al: Insulinotropic action of glucagonlike peptide-1-(7–37) in diabetic and nondiabetic subjects. Diabetes Care 1992;15:270.

Philippe J: Structure and pancreatic expression of the insulin and glucagon genes. Endocr Rev 1991;12:252.

Pipeleers G: The biosociology of pancreatic B cells. Diabetologia 1987;30:277.

Polonsky KS: The β-cell in diabetes: From molecular genetics to clinical research. Diabetes 1995;44:705.

Resine T, Bell GI: Molecular biology of somatostatin receptors. Endocr Rev 1995;16:427.

Stephens JM, Pilch PF: The metabolic regulation and vesicular transport of GLUT 4, the major insulin responsive glucose transporter. Endocr Rev 1995;16:529.

Swenne I: Pancreatic beta-cell growth and diabetes mellitus. Diabetologia 1992;35:193.

Westermark P et al: Islet amyloid polypeptide A novel controversy in diabetes research. Diabetologia 1992;35:297.

Diagnosis, Classification, & Pathophysiology of Diabetes Mellitus

Atkinson MA et al: Lack of immune responsiveness to bovine serum albumin in insulin-dependent diabetes. N Engl J Med 1993;329:1853.

Bach J-F: Insulin-dependent diabetes mellitus as an autoimmune disease. Endocr Rev 1994;15:516.

Bell GI: Molecular defects in diabetes mellitus. Diabetes 1991;40:413.

Bennett PH: The diagnosis of diabetes: New international classification and diagnostic criteria. Annu Rev Med 1983;34:295.

Bjorntorp P: Metabolic implications of body fat distribution. Diabetes Care 1991;14:1132.

Caro JF: Insulin resistance in obese and nonobese man. J Clin Endocrinol Metab 1991;73:691.

Cavan D, Bain S, Barnett A: The genetics of type I (insulin dependent) diabetes mellitus. J Med Genetics 1992;29:441.

Cerasi E: Insulin deficiency and insulin resistance in the pathogenesis of NIDDM: Is a divorce possible? Diabetologia 1995;38:992.

Clare-Salzer MJ, Tobin AJ, Kaufman DL: Glutamate decarboxylase: An autoantigen in IDDM. Diabetes Care 1992;15:132.

Davies JL et al: A genome-wide search for human type 1 diabetes susceptibility genes. Nature 1994;371:130.

DeFronzo RA, Ferrannini E: Insulin resistance: A multifaceted syndrome responsible for NIDDM, obesity, hypertension, dyslipidemia, and atherosclerotic cardiovascular disease. Diabetes Care 1991;14:173.

Flier JS: Syndromes of insulin resistance: From patient to gene and back again. Diabetes 1992;41:1207.

Froguel P et al: Familial hyperglycemia due to mutations in glucokinase. N Engl J Med 1993;328:697.

Garrow JS: Treatment of obesity. Lancet 1992;340:409.

Howard BV, Howard WJ: Dyslipidemia in noninsulin-dependent diabetes mellitus. Endocr Rev 1994;15:263.

Kadowski T et al: A subtype of diabetes mellitus associated with a mutation of mitochondrial DNA. N Engl J Med 1994;330:962.

Kahn CR: Insulin action, diabetogenes, and the cause of type II diabetes. Diabetes 1994;13:1066.

Karam JH: Type II diabetes and syndrome X: Pathogenesis and glycemic management. Endocrinol Metab Clin North Am 1992;21:329.

Knowler WC et al: Preventing non-insulin-dependent diabetes. Diabetes 1995;44:483.

Leahy JL, Bonner-Weir S, Weir GC: Beta cells dysfunction induced by chronic hyperglycemia: Current ideas on mechanism of impaired glucose-induced insulin secretion. Diabetes Care 1992;15:442.

Muir A, Schatz DA, Maclaren NK: The pathogenesis, prediction, and prevention of insulin-dependent diabetes mellitus. Endocrinol Metab Clin North Am 1992;21:199.

O'Rahilly S, Moller DE: Mutant insulin receptors in syndromes of insulin resistance. Clin Endocrinol 1992;36:121.

Palmer JP: Predicting IDDM: Use of humoral immune markers. Diabetes Reviews 1993;1:104.

Permutt MA, Chiu KC, Tanizawa Y: Glucokinase and NIDDM: A candidate gene that paid off. Diabetes 1992;41:1367.

Ravussin E, Swinburn BA: Pathophysiology of obesity. Lancet 1992;340:404.

Reaven GM: Role of insulin resistance in human disease. Diabetes 1988;37:1595.

Rossini AA et al: Immunopathogenesis of diabetes mellitus. Diabetes Reviews 1993;1:43.

Schade DS et al: The etiology of incapacitating, brittle diabetes. Diabetes Care 1985;8:12.

Solimena M et al: Autoantibodies to GABA-ergic neurons and pancreatic beta cells in stiff-man syndrome. N Engl J Med 1990;332:1555.

Taylor SI et al: Molecular genetics of insulin resistant diabetes mellitus. J Clin Endocrinol Metab 1991;73:1158.

Trucco M: To be or not to be Asp 57, that is the question. Diabetes Care 1992;15:705.

Velho G et al: Primary pancreatic beta-cell secretory defect caused by mutations in glucokinase gene in kindreds of maturity onset diabetes of the young. Lancet 1992;340:444.

Zawalich WS, Kelley GG: The pathogenesis of NIDDM: The role of the pancreatic beta cell. Diabetologia 1995;38:986.

Treatment of Diabetes Mellitus

Abraira C et al: Veterans affairs cooperative study on glycemic control and complications in type II diabetes, results of the feasibility trial. Diabetes Care 1995;18;1113.

Arauz-Pacheco C, Raskin P: Management of hypertension in diabetes. Endocrinol Metab Clin North Am 1992;21:371.

Bailey CJ: Biguanides and NIDDM. Diabetes Care 1992;15:755.

Bolli GB et al: Glucose counterregulation and waning of insulin in the Somogyi phenomenon (posthypoglycemic hyperglycemia). N Engl J Med 1984;311:1214.

Boyd AE III: Sulfonylurea receptors, ion channels, and fruit flies. Diabetes 1988;37:847.

Brange J et al: Monomeric insulins and their experimental and clinical implications. Diabetes Care 1990;13:923.

Bressler R, Johnson D: New pharmacological approaches to therapy of NIDDM. Diabetes Care 1992;15:792.

Brink SJ, Stewart C: Insulin pump treatment in insulin-dependent diabetes mellitus: Children, adolescents, and young adults. JAMA 1986;255:617.

Clarke WL et al: Multifactorial origin of hypoglycemic symptom unawareness in IDDM. Diabetes 1991;40:680.

Cryer PE, Fisher JN, Shamoon H: Hypoglycemia. Diabetes Care 1994;17:734.

Cryer PE: Iatrogenic hypoglycemia as a cause of hypoglycemia-associated autonomic failure in IDDM: A vicious cycle. Diabetes 1992;41:255.

DCCT Research Group: Epidemiology of severe hypoglycemia in the diabetes control and complications trial. Am J Med 1991;90:450.

DCCT Research Group: The effect of intensive treatment of diabetes on the development and progression of long-term complications in insulin-dependent diabetes mellitus. N Engl J Med 1993;329:977.

De Fronzo RA et al: Efficacy of metformin in patients with non-insulin-dependent diabetes mellitus. N Engl J Med 1995;333:541.

Dunn FL: Management of hyperlipidemia in diabetes mellitus. Endocrinol Metab Clin North Am 1992;21:395.

Gavin LA: Perioperative management of the diabetic patient. Endocrinol Metab Clin North Am 1992;21:457.

Genuth S: Management of the adult onset diabetic with sulfonylurea drug failure. Endocrinol Metab Clin North Am 1992;21:351.

Gray H, O'Rahilly S: Toward improved glycemic control in diabetes; what's on the horizon? Arch Intern Med 1995;155:1137.

Groop LC et al: Morning or bedtime insulin combined with sulfonylurea in treatment of NIDDM. Diabetes Care 1992;15:831.

Groop LC: Sulfonylureas in NIDDM. Diabetes Care 1992;15:737.

Halaas JL et al: Weight-reducing effects of the plasma protein encoded by the obese gene. Science 1995;269:543.

Heine RJ et al: Absorption kinetics and action profiles of mixtures of short- and intermediate-acting insulins. Diabetologia 1984;27:558.

Herman LS et al. Therapeutic comparison of metformin and sulfonylurea, alone and in various combinations: A double blind, controlled study. Diabetes Care 1994;17:1100.

Howey DC et al: [Lys (B28), Pro (B29)]-human insulin: A rapidly absorbed analog of human insulin. Diabetes 1994;43:396.

Kang S et al: Subcutaneous insulin absorption explained by insulin's physicochemical properties. Diabetes Care 1991;14:942.

Karam JH: Type II diabetes and syndrome X: Pathogenesis and glycemic management. Endocrinol Metab Clin North Am 1992;21:329.

Lebovitz HE (editor): *Therapy for Diabetes Mellitus and Related Disorders.* American Diabetes Association, 1991.

Little RR et al: Relationship of glycosylated hemoglobin to oral glucose tolerance: Implications for diabetes screening. Diabetes 1988;37:60.

Max MB et al: Effects of desipramine, amitriptyline, and fluoxetine on pain in diabetic neuropathy. N Engl J Med 1992;326:1250.

Mulhauser I et al: Hypoglycemic symptoms and frequency of severe hypoglycemia in patients treated with human and animal insulin preparations. Diabetes Care 1991;14:745.

Nathan DM et al: The clinical information value of the glycosylated hemoglobin assay. N Engl J Med 1984;310:341.

Nolte MS: Insulin therapy in insulin-dependent (type I) diabetes mellitus. Endocrinol Metab Clin North Am 1992;21:281.

Patrick AW, Williams G: The Liverpool symposium on human insulin and hypoglycemia. Diabetic Med 1992;9:579.

Perriello G, De Feo P, Bolli GB: The dawn phenomenon: Nocturnal blood glucose homeostasis in insulin-dependent diabetes mellitus. Diabetic Med 1988;5:13.

Rachman J, Turner RC: Drugs on the horizon for treatment of type 2 diabetes. Diabet Med 1995;12:467.

Robertson RP: Pancreas transplantation in humans with diabetes mellitus. Diabetes 1991;40;1085.

Santiago JV: Intensive management of insulin-dependent diabetes: Risks, benefits, and unanswered questions. J Clin Endocrinol Metab 1992;75:977.

Shank ML, DelPrato S, DeFronzo RA: Bedtime insulin/daytime glipizide: Effective therapy for sulfonylurea failures in NIDDM. Diabetes 1995;44:165.

Tamborlane WV, Amiel SA: Hypoglycemia in the treated diabetic patient: A risk of intensive insulin therapy. Endocrinol Metab Clin North Am 1992;21:313.

Acute Complications of Diabetes Mellitus

Bending JJ, Pickup JC, Keen H: Frequency of diabetic ketoacidosis and hypoglycemic coma during treatment with continuous subcutaneous insulin infusion. Am J Med 1985;79:685.

Cefalu WT: Diabetic ketoacidosis. Crit Care Clin 1991;7:89.

Cohen RD: Lactic acidosis: New perspectives on origins and treatment. Diabetes Rev 1994;2:86.

Ennis ED, Stahl EJ, Kreisberg RA: The hyperosmolar hyperglycemic syndrome. Diabetes Rev 1994;2:115.

Fisher JN, Kitabchi AE: A randomized study of phosphate therapy in the treatment of diabetic ketoacidosis. J Clin Endocrinol Metab 1983;57:177.

Fleckman AM: Diabetic ketoacidosis. Endocrinol Metab Clin North Am 1993;22:181.

Henderson G. The psychosocial treatment of recurrent diabetic ketoacidosis: An interdisciplinary team approach. Diabetes Educator 1991;17:119.

Kitabchi AE, Wall BM: Diabetic ketoacidosis. Med Clin North Am 1995;79:9.

Lorber D: Nonketotic hypertonicity in diabetes mellitus. Med Clin North Am 1995;70:39.

Siperstein MD: Diabetic ketoacidosis and hyperosmolar coma. Endocrinol Metab Clin North Am 1992;21:415.

Wrenn KD et al: The syndrome of alcoholic ketoacidosis. Am J Med 1991;91:119.

Chronic Complications of Diabetes Mellitus

Brownlee M: Glycation products and the pathogenesis of diabetic complications. Diabetes Care 1992;15:1835.

Caputo GM et al: Assessment and management of foot disease in patients with diabetes. N Engl J Med 1994;331:854.

Clark CM, Lee DA: Drug Therapy: Prevention and treatment of the complications of diabetes mellitus. N Engl J Med 1995;332:1210.

Cogan DG et al: Aldose reductase and complications of diabetes. Ann Intern Med 1984;101:82.

Davis MD: Diabetic retinopathy. Diabetes Care 1992;15:1844.

Deckert T et al: Microalbuminuria: Implications for micro- and macrovascular disease. Diabetes Care 1992;15:1181.

Donahue RP, Orchard TJ: Diabetes mellitus and macrovascular complications: An epidemiological perspective. Diabetes Care 1992;15:1141.

Feingold KR et al: Muscle capillary basement membrane width in patients with vacor-induced diabetes mellitus. J Clin Invest 1986;78:102.

Hostetter TH: Diabetic nephropathy: Metabolic versus hemodynamic considerations. Diabetes Care 1992;15:1205.

Klein R, Klein BEK, Moss SE: Epidemiology of proliferative diabetic retinopathy. Diabetes Care 1992;15:1875.

Knowles HC Jr: Long-term juvenile diabetes treated with unmeasured diet. Trans Assoc Am Physicians 1971;84:95.

Markell MS, Friedman EA: Diabetic nephropathy: Management of the end stage patient. Diabetes Care 1992;15:1226.

Mauer SM et al: Long-term study of normal kidneys transplanted into patients with type I diabetes. Diabetes 1989;38:516.

Mogensen CE: Management of diabetic renal involvement and disease. Lancet 1988;1:867.

Parkhouse N, Le Quesne PM: Impaired neurogenic vascular response in patients with diabetes and neuropathic foot lesions. N Engl J Med 1988;318:1306.

Ramsay RC et al: Progression of diabetic retinopathy after pancreas transplantation for insulin-dependent diabetes mellitus. N Engl J Med 1988;318:208.

Raskin P et al: Capillary basement membrane width in diabetic children. Am J Med 1975;58:365.

Rosenbloom AL et al: Limited joint mobility in childhood diabetes: Family studies. Diabetes Care 1983;6:370.

Viberti G et al: Effect of captopril on progression to clinical proteinuria in patients with insulin-dependent diabetes mellitus and microalbuminuria. JAMA 1994;271:275.

Vinik AI et al: Diabetic neuropathies. Diabetes Care 1992;15:1926.

19

Hypoglycemic Disorders

John H. Karam, MD

Circulating plasma glucose concentrations are kept within a relatively narrow range by a complex system of interrelated neural, humoral, and cellular controls. Under the usual metabolic conditions, the central nervous system is wholly dependent on plasma glucose and counteracts declining blood glucose concentrations with a carefully programmed response. This is often associated with a sensation of hunger; and, as the brain receives insufficient glucose to meet its metabolic needs (neuroglycopenia), an autonomic response is triggered to mobilize storage depots of glycogen and fat. Hepatic glycogen reserves directly supply the central nervous system with glucose, which is carried across the blood-brain barrier by a specific glucose transport system, while the mobilization of fatty acids from triglyceride depots provides energy for the large mass of skeletal and cardiac muscle, renal cortex, liver, and other tissues that utilize fatty acids as their basic fuel, thus sparing glucose for use by the tissues of the central nervous system.

PATHOPHYSIOLOGY OF THE COUNTERREGULATORY RESPONSE TO NEUROGLYCOPENIA

The plasma concentration of glucose that will signal the need by the central nervous system to mobilize energy reserves depends on a number of factors, such as the status of blood flow to the brain, the integrity of cerebral tissue, the prevailing arterial level of plasma glucose, the rapidity with which plasma glucose concentration falls, and the availability of alternative metabolic fuels.

A hierarchy of responses has been shown to occur as plasma glucose falls in healthy young volunteers, with hormonal counterregulatory responses being triggered at glucose levels slightly higher than those which induce symptoms of hypoglycemia (Figure 19–1). The first symptoms to appear in healthy people are mediated by autonomic neurotransmitters and occur at plasma glucose levels below 60 mg/dL (3.3 mmol/L). The symptoms consist of tremor, anxiety, palpitations, and sweating, which result from sympa-

thetic discharge; and hunger, which is a consequence of parasympathetic vagal response. Ganglionic blockade and cervical cord section or sympathectomy—but not adrenalectomy—ameliorate these symptoms, indicating that they are due to the release of autonomic neurotransmitters and not to adrenal corticosteroids. As plasma glucose falls below 50 mg/dL (2.8 mmol/L), impaired cognition develops, along with weakness, lethargy, confusion, incoordination and blurred vision.

In elderly people, however, with compromised cerebral blood supply, neuroglycopenic manifestations may be provoked at slightly higher plasma glucose levels. Patients with chronic hyperglycemia, eg, those with poorly controlled insulin-dependent diabetes mellitus, may experience symptoms of neuroglycopenia at considerably higher plasma glucose concentrations than persons without diabetes. This has been attributed to a "down-regulated" glucose transport system across the blood-brain barrier. Conversely, in patients exposed to chronic hypoglycemia—eg, those with an insulin-secreting tumor or those with diabetes who are receiving excessively "tight" glycemic control with an insulin pump—adaptation to recurrent hypoglycemia occurs by "up-regulation" of the glucose transporters, which results in "hypoglycemic unawareness" whereby they show greater tolerance to hypoglycemia without manifesting symptoms (Figure 19–2).

Restoring and maintaining an adequate supply of glucose for cerebral function proceeds by a series of neurogenic events that act directly to raise the plasma glucose concentration and to stimulate hormonal responses that augment the adrenergic mobilization of energy stores (Table 19–1).

Counterregulatory Response to Hypoglycemia

A. Insulin: Endogenous insulin secretion is lowered both by reduced glucose stimulation to the pancreatic B cell and by sympathetic nervous system inhibition from a combination of alpha-adrenergic neural effects and increased circulating catecholamine levels. This reactive insulinopenia facilitates

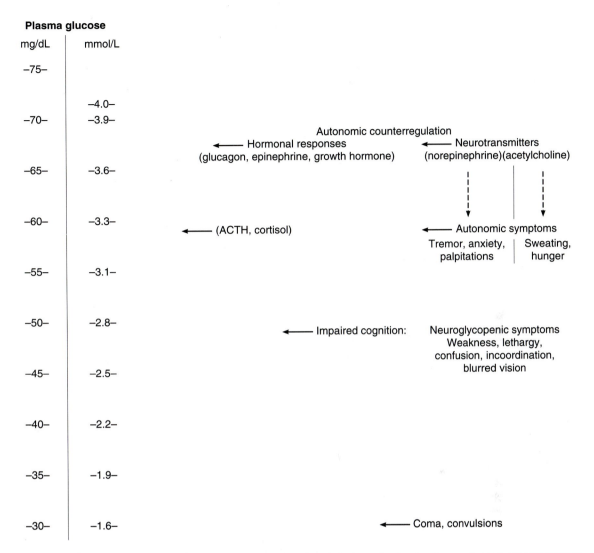

Figure 19–1. Hierarchy of autonomic responses to progressive stepwise reduction in plasma glucose concentration in healthy volunteers. (Adapted from Gerich JE et al: Hypoglycemia unawareness. Endocr Rev 1991;12:356; and from Service FJ: Hypoglycemia disorders. N Engl J Med 1995;332:1144.)

the mobilization of energy from existing energy stores (glycogenolysis and lipolysis), increases hepatic enzymes involved in gluconeogenesis and ketogenesis, and at the same time prevents muscle tissue from consuming the blood glucose being released from the liver (Chapter 18).

B. Catecholamines: Circulating catecholamines—and norepinephrine produced at sympathetic nerve endings—provide muscle tissue with alternative sources of fuel by activating beta-adrenergic receptors, resulting in mobilization of muscle glycogen, and by providing increased plasma free fatty acids from lipolysis of adipocyte triglyceride. Their cardiovascular and other side effects provide a signal that diabetic patients learn to recognize as a warning of their need to rapidly ingest absorbable carbohydrate.

C. Glucagon: Plasma glucagon is released by the beta-adrenergic effects of both sympathetic innervation and circulating catecholamines on pancreatic A cells as well as by the direct stimulation of A cells by the low plasma glucose concentration itself. This glucagon release increases hepatic output of glucose by direct glycogenolysis as well as by facilitating the activity of gluconeogenic enzymes. As shown in Figure 19–3, plasma glucagon appears to be the key counterregulatory hormone affecting recovery from acute hypoglycemia in humans, with the adrenergic-catecholamine response representing a major backup system.

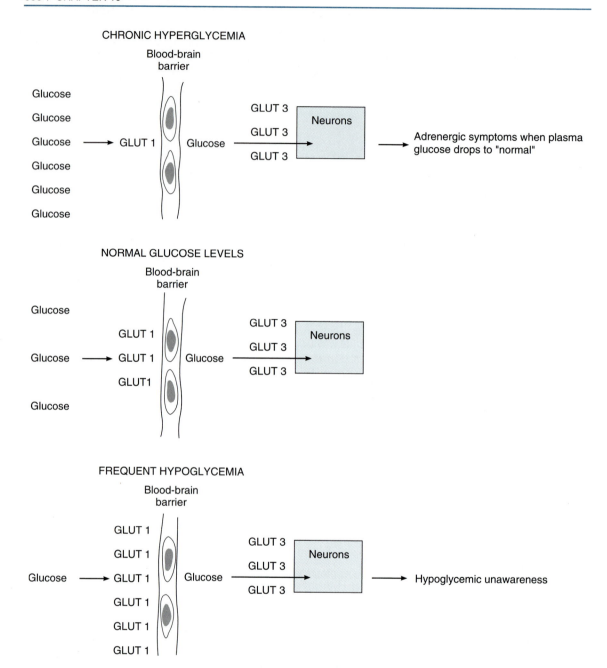

Figure 19–2. Glycemic regulation of glucose transporters. The center panel depicts the normal component of the high-affinity glucose transporter 1 (GLUT 1) on the vascular cells of the central nervous system during euglycemia. An appropriate amount of glucose diffuses across the blood-brain barrier and is then transported into the neurons by another high-affinity glucose transporter, GLUT 3. The upper and lower panels, respectively, show adaptation by either down-regulation of GLUT 1 in the face of chronic hyperglycemia (upper panel) or up-regulation of GLUT 1 in the presence of chronic hypoglycemia. (GLUT 1, glucose transporter 1; GLUT 3, glucose transporter 3.)

D. Corticotropin and Hydrocortisone: Pituitary ACTH is released in association with the sympathetic nervous system stimulation by neuroglycopenia. This results in elevation of plasma cortisol levels, which in turn permissively facilitates lipolysis and actively promotes protein catabolism and conversion of amino acids to glucose by the liver.

E. Growth Hormone: Pituitary growth hormone is also released in response to falling plasma glucose levels. Its role in counteracting hypogly-

Table 19–1. Autonomic nervous system response to hypoglycemia.

Alpha-adrenergic effects
  Inhibition of endogenous insulin release
  Increase in cerebral blood flow (peripheral
    vasoconstriction)

Beta-adrenergic effects
  Hepatic and muscle glycogenolysis
  Stimulation of plasma glucagon release
  Lipolysis to raise plasma free fatty acids
  Impairment of glucose uptake by muscle tissue
  Increase in cerebral blood flow (increase in cardiac output)

Adrenomedullary discharge of catecholamines
  Augmentation of all of the above alpha- and beta-
    adrenergic effects

Cholinergic effects
  Raises level of pancreatic polypeptide
  Increases motility of stomach
  Produces hunger
  Increases sweating

cemia is less well defined, but it is known to antagonize the action of insulin on glucose utilization in muscle cells and to directly activate lipolysis by adipocytes.

F. Cholinergic Neurotransmitters: Acetylcholine is released at parasympathetic nerve endings, and its vagal effects induce the sensation of hunger that signals the need for food to counteract the hypoglycemia. In addition, postsynaptic fibers of the sympathetic nervous system that innervate the sweat glands also release acetylcholine—in contrast to all other sympathetic postsynaptic fibers, which without exception release norepinephrine.

Maintenance of Euglycemia in the Postabsorptive State

Glucose absorption from the gastrointestinal tract ceases by 5–8 hours after a meal. During the "postabsorptive state" immediately following, glucose must be produced endogenously from previously stored nutrients to meet the requirements of the central nervous system. The liver is the central organ involved in this process, producing the 125 mg of glucose per minute required by the brain as well as an additional 25 mg/min for other glucose-dependent tissues—predominantly blood cell elements. This is initially provided by the breakdown of stored hepatic glycogen. However, because these reserves are limited to 80–100 g, they begin to be depleted several hours into the postabsorptive state. Thereafter, hepatic glucose production is augmented by gluconeogenesis—the formation of glucose from amino acids, lactate, and glycerol. These substrates are delivered to the liver

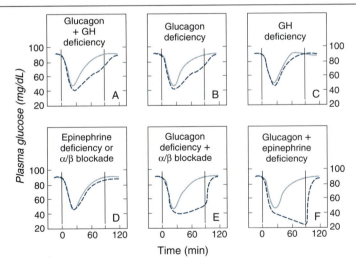

Figure 19–3. Solid lines show changes in plasma glucose that occur in normal subjects in response to insulin administration. Note the rapid recovery of glucose levels mediated by intact counterregulatory mechanisms. The dashed lines show the response to insulin-induced hypoglycemia in patients with deficiencies of the counterregulatory mechanisms induced as follows: **A:** Somatostatin infusion (inhibits both glucagon and growth hormone [GH] release). **B:** Somatostatin infusion plus GH infusion (now with functional isolated glucagon deficiency). **C:** Somatostatin infusion plus glucagon infusion (isolated GH deficiency). Note return of glucose response to normal, implying that glucagon is the main counterregulatory hormone. **D:** Bilateral adrenalectomy, leading to epinephrine deficiency, or infusion of phentolamine plus propranolol (alpha and beta blockers, respectively). Note that such deficiencies cause no major abnormality in response to induced hypoglycemia when glucagon is present. **E and F:** Sympathetic modulation (by phentolamine plus propranolol in **E** and by bilateral adrenalectomy in **F**), which seriously impairs the ability to respond to hypoglycemia in the patient made glucagon-deficient by somatostatin infusion. (Reproduced, with permission, from Cryer PE: Glucose counterregulation in man. Diabetes 1981;30:261.)

from peripheral stores: Muscle and other structural tissues supply amino acids, mainly alanine; blood cell elements supply lactate, the end product of glycolytic metabolism; and adipose tissue supplies glycerol from lipolysis of triglyceride. In addition, oxidation of the free fatty acids released from adipose cells during lipolysis supplies the energy required for gluconeogenesis and provides ketone bodies, acetoacetate, and β-hydroxybutyrate, which can serve as alternative metabolic fuels for the central nervous system during periods of prolonged fasting. Studies have shown that an insulin infusion does not reduce hepatic glucose production if elevated levels of fatty acids are maintained by intravenous administration of a fat emulsion and heparin, suggesting that fatty acids may be the major mediator of gluconeogenesis.

Hormonal changes that begin early in the postabsorptive state regulate the enzymatic steps necessary for hepatic glycogenolysis and gluconeogenesis and ensure the delivery of the necessary substrate (Table 19–2). An appropriate fall in circulating insulin levels with a corresponding rise in glucagon is most important; elevations in the counterregulatory hormones cortisol and growth hormone contribute but are less critical.

In summary, numerous endocrine and metabolic events interact to provide a continuous source of fuel for proper functioning of the central nervous system. Malfunction of any of these mechanisms can lead to symptomatic hypoglycemia.

CLASSIFICATION OF HYPOGLYCEMIC DISORDERS

Symptomatic Hypoglycemia

A clinical classification of the more common causes of symptomatic hypoglycemia in adults is presented in Table 19–3. (Some inborn errors of metabolism that produce hypoglycemia in infants and children are mentioned but will not be discussed in detail in this chapter.) This classification is useful in directing diagnostic considerations.

Table 19–2. Hormonal changes to maintain euglycemia in the postabsorptive state.

Decreased insulin secretion
Increases hepatic glycogenolysis.
Increases lipolysis.
Increases hepatic gluconeogenesis.
Decreases muscle uptake of glucose.

Increased glucagon secretion
Increases hepatic glycogenolysis.
Facilitates hepatic gluconeogenesis.

Increased cortisol secretion
Facilitates lipolysis.
Increases protein catabolism.
Augments hepatic gluconeogenesis.

Table 19–3. Common causes of symptomatic hypoglycemia.

Fasting
  A. With hyperinsulinism:
    Insulin reaction.
    Sulfonylurea overdose.
    Surreptitious insulin or sulfonylurea administration.
    Autoimmune hypoglycemia (idiopathic insulin antibodies, insulin receptor autoantibodies).
    Pentamidine-induced hypoglycemia.
    Pancreatic B cell tumors.
  B. Without hyperinsulinism:
    Severe hepatic dysfunction.
    Chronic renal insufficiency.
    Inanition, ketotic hypoglycemia of childhood.
    Hypocortisolism.
    Alcohol use.
    Nonpancreatic tumors.
    Inborn errors of carbohydrate metabolism (glycogen storage disease, gluconeogenic enzyme deficiencies).

Nonfasting
  Alimentary.
  Functional.
  Occult diabetes.
  Ethanol.
  Leucine sensitivity.
  Hereditary fructose intolerance.
  Galactosemia.
  Newborn infant of diabetic mother.

Symptomatic fasting hypoglycemia is a serious and potentially life-threatening problem warranting thorough evaluation. Conditions that produce inappropriate fasting hyperinsulinism are the most common cause of fasting hypoglycemia in otherwise healthy adults. These include insulin-secreting pancreatic B cell tumors and iatrogenic or surreptitious administration of insulin or sulfonylureas. In patients with illnesses that produce symptomatic fasting hypoglycemia despite appropriately suppressed insulin levels, the clinical picture is dominated by the signs and symptoms of the primary disease, with hypoglycemia often only a late or associated manifestation. This is in contrast to patients with inappropriate hyperinsulinism, who usually appear healthy between hypoglycemic episodes.

Symptoms of nonfasting hypoglycemia in adults, although distressing to the patient, do not imply serious illness or warrant extensive evaluation. Overstimulation of the B cells postprandially as a result of accelerated glucose absorption after rapid gastric emptying may result in too rapid disposal of glucose, with resulting symptoms of sympathetic nervous system hyperactivity (alimentary hypoglycemia). Other than in patients who have had gastric surgery, this diagnosis may be difficult to establish.

Asymptomatic Hypoglycemia

Hypoglycemia may be seen during prolonged fasting, strenuous exercise, or pregnancy or may occur as a laboratory artifact. In normal men, plasma glucose does not fall below 55 mg/dL (3 mmol/L) during a 72-hour fast. However, for reasons that are not clear, normal women may experience a fall to levels as low as 30 mg/dL (1.7 mmol/L) despite a marked suppression of circulating insulin to less than 6 μU/mL. They remain asymptomatic in spite of this degree of hypoglycemia, presumably because ketogenesis is able to satisfy the energy needs of the central nervous system. Basal plasma glucose declines progressively during normal pregnancy, and hypoglycemic levels may be reached during prolonged fasting. This may be a consequence of a continuous fetal consumption of glucose and diminished availability of the gluconeogenic substrate alanine. The cause of these diminished alanine levels in pregnancy is unclear. The greatly increased glucose consumption by skeletal muscle that occurs during prolonged strenuous exercise may lead to hypoglycemia despite increases in hepatic glucose production. Whether the hypoglycemia in this circumstance contributes to fatigue or other symptoms in distance runners is unknown.

In vitro consumption of glucose by blood cell elements may give rise to laboratory values in the hypoglycemic range. This is most commonly seen when an insufficient amount of the metabolic inhibitor sodium fluoride is added to specimens containing increased numbers of leukocytes (as in leukemia and leukemoid reactions).

CLINICAL PRESENTATION OF HYPOGLYCEMIA

Regardless of the cause, hypoglycemia presents certain common features characterized by Whipple's triad: (1) symptoms and signs of hypoglycemia, (2) an associated plasma glucose level of 45 mg/dL (2.5 mmol/L) or less, and (3) reversibility of symptoms upon administration of glucose.

The symptoms and signs of hypoglycemia are the consequences of neuroglycopenia. They vary depending on the degree of hypoglycemia, the age of the patient, and the rapidity of the decline. In diabetic patients treated with insulin, a precipitous fall in plasma glucose from hyperglycemia toward euglycemia may produce neuroglycopenic symptoms.

A. Acute Hypoglycemia: A rapid fall in plasma glucose (> 1 mg/dL/min [> 0.06 mmol/L/min]) to low levels often accompanies conditions associated with arterial hyperinsulinism—a condition that leads to increased peripheral glucose uptake and decreased hepatic glucose output. In diabetics, excessive absorption of exogenous insulin either from overtreatment or from rapid mobilization from an injection site during exercise may be responsible. In nondiabetics, reactive hypersecretion of insulin may be the cause, as in postgastrectomy patients with rapid gastric emptying time. The symptoms include anxiety, tremulousness, and feelings of unnaturalness or detachment.

These are usually accompanied by palpitations, tachycardia, sweating, and hunger and can progress to neurologic sequelae of ataxia, coma, or convulsions. These warning symptoms of hypoglycemia occur even in the absence of adrenal glands and therefore are due to neurogenic responses to hypoglycemia. The autonomic response has probably evolved as more of an alarm than a counterregulatory mechanism, since glucagon is generally sufficient to provide necessary counterregulation to hypoglycemia. In IDDM, however, the adrenergic system becomes of greater importance since the glucagon response to hypoglycemia is lost in most patients (Chapter 18).

B. Subacute and Chronic Hypoglycemia: A relatively slow fall in plasma glucose accompanies conditions caused primarily by a reduction in hepatic glucose output in response to hyperinsulinism (predominantly within the portal vein [insulinoma]), or to the inappropriately sustained effects of long-acting insulin preparations on the liver in the postabsorptive state, or to metabolic derangements of liver functions (eg, alcohol hypoglycemia). Symptoms due to hypoglycemia in patients with these conditions may be less apparent, particularly because symptoms of sympathetic overactivity are usually absent. These patients develop progressive confusion, inappropriate behavior, lethargy, and drowsiness. If the patient does not eat, seizures or coma may develop—though this is not inevitable, and spontaneous recovery can occur. Because these patients are seldom aware of their degree of functional impairment, a history should be obtained from relatives or friends who have observed the episode. Except for hypothermia (often seen during hypoglycemic coma), there are no identifying characteristics on physical examination. Hypoglycemia will often be misdiagnosed as a seizure disorder, transient ischemic attack, or personality disorder.

Documentation of Low Plasma Glucose Values

With the specific laboratory methods now available, it has been arbitrarily decided that fasting hypoglycemia is present when plasma glucose is 45 mg/dL (2.5 mmol/L) or less after an overnight fast (corresponding to a blood glucose level of 40 mg/dL [2.2 mmol/L] or less). In the fasting state, there is no substantial difference between arterial, venous, or capillary blood samples (in contrast to nonfasting hyperglycemia, in which arteriovenous glucose differences may be considerable because of arterial hyperinsulinism and consequent increases in glucose uptake across capillary beds).

The development of glucose oxidase-hydrogen peroxidase paper strips has been of great value for rapid estimation of blood glucose levels, particularly for insulin-treated diabetics undergoing home monitoring. In emergency room or hospital settings, the paper strips are helpful in the differential diagnosis of coma, particularly when used with a reflectance meter, but a sample should also be sent to the laboratory for definitive diagnosis. Although therapeutic decisions to administer glucose can be based on the paper strip results alone in an emergency situation, variability due to exposure to air or aging makes them less dependable as the sole laboratory indicator for a definitive diagnosis of hypoglycemia.

Reversibility of Clinical Manifestations of Hypoglycemia With Treatment

Because prolonged hypoglycemia may cause permanent brain damage and death, prompt recognition and treatment are mandatory. (It is prudent to consider the possibility of hypoglycemic coma in most unconscious patients.)

The goal of therapy is to restore normal levels of plasma glucose as rapidly as possible. If the patient is conscious and able to swallow, glucose-containing foods such as candy, orange juice with added sugar, and cookies should be quickly ingested. Fructose, found in many nutrient low-calorie sweeteners for diabetics, should not be used, because although it can be metabolized by neurons, it is not transported across the blood-brain barrier.

If the patient is unconscious, rapid restoration of plasma glucose must be accomplished by giving 20–50 mL of 50% dextrose intravenously over 1–3 minutes (the treatment of choice) or, when intravenous glucose is not available, 1 mg of glucagon intramuscularly or intravenously. Families or friends of insulin-treated diabetics should be instructed in the administration of glucagon intramuscularly for emergency treatment at home. Attempts to feed the patient or to apply glucose-containing jelly to the oral mucosa should be avoided because of the danger of aspiration.

When consciousness is restored, oral feedings should be started immediately. Periodic blood glucose surveillance after a hypoglycemic episode may be needed for 12–24 hours to ensure maintenance of euglycemia. Prevention of recurrent hypoglycemic attacks depends upon proper diagnosis and management of the specific underlying disorder.

SPECIFIC HYPOGLYCEMIC DISORDERS

SYMPTOMATIC FASTING HYPOGLYCEMIA WITH HYPERINSULINISM

1. INSULIN REACTION

It is not surprising that insulin-treated diabetics make up the bulk of the patient population with symptomatic hypoglycemia. Present methods of insulin delivery rely upon subcutaneous depots of mixtures of soluble and insoluble insulin whose absorption varies with the site of injection and the degree of exercise in surrounding muscles. Variations in physical and emotional stresses can alter the response of patients to insulin, as can the cyclic hormonal changes relating to menstruation. A deficient glucagon response to hypoglycemia in diabetes compounds the problem, as does the lack of awareness of hypoglycemic symptoms in older patients, in those with neuropathy, and in those with recurrent hypoglycemic episodes, who adapt to lower levels of blood glucose without triggering their autonomic alarm system. (See Figure 19–2 and Chapter 18 for further discussion of hypoglycemic unawareness.)

Once the patient's acute hypoglycemic episode is managed, the physician should carefully examine possible correctable factors that may have contributed to the insulin reaction.

Inadequate Food Intake

An insufficient quantity of food or a missed meal is one of the commonest causes of hypoglycemia in insulin-treated diabetics. Until improved insulin delivery systems are available, patients attempting to achieve satisfactory glycemic control should self-monitor their blood glucose levels and eat three regular meals as well as small midmorning, midafternoon, and bedtime snacks, particularly when they are receiving two or more injections of insulin mixtures daily.

Exercise

The insulin-treated diabetic is especially prone to exercise-induced hypoglycemia. In nondiabetics, the enhancement of skeletal muscle glucose uptake (a 20 to 30-fold increase over basal uptake) is compensated for by enhanced hepatic glucose production. This is mediated primarily by a fall in circulating insulin levels consequent to an exercise-induced catecholamine discharge, which inhibits B cell secretion. Such regulation is impossible in the insulin-treated diabetic, whose subcutaneous depot not only continues to release insulin during exercise but also shows an accelerated absorption rate when the injection site is in close proximity to the muscles being exercised. When this occurs, increased levels of circulating insulin compromise the hepatic output of glucose. To prevent hypoglycemia, insulin-treated diabetics must be advised to avoid injections into areas adjacent to muscles most involved in the particular exercise and either to eat supplementary carbohydrate before exercising or to reduce their insulin dose appropriately.

Impaired Glucose Counterregulation in Diabetics

Most patients with insulin-dependent diabetes have a deficient glucagon response to hypoglycemia.

They are thus solely dependent on an adrenergic autonomic response to recover from hypoglycemia and particularly to provide them with symptoms they recognize as a warning of impending hypoglycemia and as a signal to ingest sugar or fruit juice. Some patients, especially those with long-standing diabetes or autonomic neuropathy, lack both a glucagon and an epinephrine response and are virtually defenseless against insulin-induced hypoglycemia. Insulin infusion tests can be used to identify these alterations in glucose counterregulation; however, at present these tests are cumbersome, and their ability to accurately predict which patients will suffer frequent severe and prolonged hypoglycemic episodes is yet to be established. Easier and more reliable methods of identifying such patients are needed. The ability of a patient to spontaneously recover from hypoglycemia may determine whether or not aggressive attempts to maintain euglycemia are associated with undue risk.

Some patients who originally had a normal counterregulatory response to hypoglycemia (except for glucagon) lose this protective response when insulin therapy is intensified to achieve tight control. The mechanisms for this reduction of hormonal response are unknown but may be related to "up-regulated" mechanisms of glucose transport across the blood-brain barrier induced by relatively low circulating blood glucose levels.

Inadvertent or Deliberate Insulin Overdosage in Diabetics

Excessive insulin may be administered inadvertently by patients with poor vision or inadequate instruction or understanding of dosage and injection technique. The widespread use of highly concentrated U100 insulin enhances the likelihood of overdosage with relatively small excesses of administered insulin.

Deliberate overdosage may occur in certain maladjusted patients, particularly adolescents, who wish to gain special attention from their families or escape tensions at school or work.

Miscellaneous Causes of Hypoglycemia in Insulin-Treated Diabetics

A. Stress: Physical stresses—such as intercurrent illnesses, infection, and surgery—or psychic stresses often require an increased insulin dosage to control hyperglycemia. Reduction to prestress doses is necessary to avoid subsequent hypoglycemia when the stresses have abated.

B. Hypocortisolism: In patients with insulin-dependent diabetes who have otherwise unexplained hypoglycemic attacks, reduced insulin requirements may indicate unusual causes (eg, Addison's disease).

C. Diabetic Gastroparesis: Unexplained episodes of postprandial hypoglycemia in insulin-dependent diabetics may be due to delayed gastric emptying consequent to autonomic neuropathy. This diagnosis can be established by appropriate radiologic studies of gastric motility using liquid or solid test meals containing radioisotopic markers.

D. Pregnancy: Pregnancy, with high fetal glucose consumption, decreases insulin requirements in the first trimester.

E. Renal Insufficiency: Renal insufficiency, through impairment of insulin degradation while hepatic gluconeogenesis and food intake are often reduced, also requires a reduction in insulin dosage.

F. Drugs: Numerous pharmacologic agents may potentiate the effects of insulin and predispose to hypoglycemia. Common offenders include ethanol, salicylates, and beta-adrenergic blocking drugs. Beta blockade inhibits fatty acid and gluconeogenic substrate release and reduces plasma glucagon levels; furthermore, the symptomatic response is altered, because tachycardia is blocked while hazardous elevations of blood pressure may result during hypoglycemia in response to the unopposed alpha-adrenergic stimulation from circulating catecholamines and neurogenic sympathetic discharge. However, symptoms of sweating, hunger, and uneasiness are not masked by beta-blocking drugs and remain indicators of hypoglycemia in the aware patient.

Therapy with angiotensin-converting enzyme (ACE) inhibitors increases the risk of hypoglycemia in diabetic patients who are taking insulin or sulfonylureas, presumably because these drugs increase sensitivity to circulating insulin by increasing blood flow to muscle.

2. SULFONYLUREA OVERDOSE

Any of the sulfonylurea drugs may produce hypoglycemia. Chlorpropamide, with its prolonged half-life (35 hours), is a common offender. Older patients—especially those with impaired hepatic or renal function—are particularly susceptible to sulfonylurea-induced hypoglycemia: Liver dysfunction prolongs the hypoglycemic activity of tolbutamide, acetohexamide, and tolazamide, as well as that of the second-generation compounds glyburide and glipizide; renal insufficiency perpetuates the blood glucose-lowering effects of many sulfonylureas, especially chlorpropamide and glyburide. Elderly patients with gradually decreasing creatinine clearance seem to be more at risk for prolonged and severe hypoglycemia when treated with chlorpropamide or glyburide and less so when treated with shorter-acting agents such as tolbutamide or glipizide. In the presence of other pharmacologic agents such as warfarin, phenylbutazone, or certain sulfonamides, the hypoglycemic effects of sulfonylureas may be markedly prolonged.

3. SURREPTITIOUS INSULIN OR SULFONYLUREA ADMINISTRATION (Factitious Hypoglycemia)

Factitious hypoglycemia should be suspected in any patient with access to insulin or sulfonylurea drugs. It is most commonly seen in health professionals and diabetic patients or their relatives. The reasons for selfinduced hypoglycemia vary, with many patients having severe psychiatric disturbances or a need for attention. Inadvertent ingestion of sulfonylureas resulting in clinical hypoglycemia has also been reported, due either to patient error or to a prescription mishap on the part of a pharmacist.

When insulin is used to induce hypoglycemia, an elevated serum insulin level often raises suspicion of an insulin-producing pancreatic B cell tumor. It may be difficult to prove that the insulin is of exogenous origin. The triad of hypoglycemia, high immunoreactive insulin levels, and suppressed plasma C peptide immunoreactivity* is pathognomonic of exogenous insulin administration. Technical difficulties in measuring immunoreactive insulin, caused by the inappropriate presence of circulating antibodies (usually seen only in insulin-treated individuals), will generally support the diagnosis of factitious hypoglycemia. However, the absence of detectable insulin antibodies does not rule out the possibility of exogenous insulin administration, especially with the advent of human insulins with low immunogenicity in humans.

When sulfonylurea abuse is suspected, plasma or urine should be screened for its presence. Hyperinsulinism may not persist despite sustained hypoglycemia from a sulfonylurea overdose.

Treatment of factitious hypoglycemia involves psychiatric therapy and social counseling.

4. AUTOIMMUNE HYPOGLYCEMIA

In recent years, a rare autoimmune disorder has been reported in which patients have circulating insulin antibodies and the paradoxic feature of hypoglycemia. While some of these patients may be surreptitiously administering insulin, in an increasing number of case reports it has not been possible to document exogenous insulin as the inducer of insulin antibodies. Hypoglycemia generally occurs 3–4 hours after a meal and is attributed to a dissociation of insulin-antibody immune complexes, releasing free insulin. This autoimmune hypoglycemia due to accumulation of high titers of antibodies capable of reacting with endogenous insulin has been most commonly reported in methimazole-treated patients with

Graves' disease from Japan but also in patients with lymphoma, multiple myeloma, or lupus syndromes in which paraproteins or antibodies cross-react with insulin.

Hypoglycemia due to insulin receptor autoantibodies is also an extremely rare syndrome, reported in only six patients. All of these patients have also had episodes of insulin-resistant diabetes and acanthosis nigricans. Their hypoglycemia is attributed to an agonistic action of the antibody on the insulin receptor. Balance between the antagonistic and agonistic effects of the antibody determines whether insulin-resistant diabetes or hypoglycemia occurs. Hypoglycemia was found to respond to glucocorticoid therapy but not to plasmapheresis or immunosuppression.

5. PENTAMIDINE-INDUCED HYPOGLYCEMIA

With the increasing use of intravenous pentamidine for treatment of *Pneumocystis carinii* infection in patients with AIDS, more reports of pentamidine-induced hypoglycemia are appearing. The cause of acute hypoglycemia appears to be the drug's lytic effect on B cells, which produces acute hyperinsulinemia in about 10–20% of patients receiving the drug. Physicians treating patients with pentamidine should be aware of the potential complication of acute hypoglycemia, which may be followed later by occasionally persistent insulinopenia and hyperglycemia.

Intravenous glucose should be administered during pentamidine administration and for the period immediately following to prevent or ameliorate hypoglycemic symptoms. Following a complete course of therapy with pentamidine, fasting blood glucose or a subsequent glycohemoglobin should be monitored to assess the extent of pancreatic B cell recovery or residual damage.

6. PANCREATIC B CELL TUMORS

Spontaneous fasting hypoglycemia in an otherwise healthy adult is most commonly due to insulinoma, an insulin-secreting tumor of the islets of Langerhans. Eighty percent of these tumors are single and benign; 10% are malignant (if metastases are identified); and the remainder are multiple, with scattered micro or macroadenomas interspersed within normal islet tissue. (As with some other endocrine tumors, histologic differentiation between benign and malignant cells is difficult, and close follow-up is necessary to ensure the absence of metastases.) Diffuse B cell hyperplasia has rarely been documented as a cause of hypoglycemia in adults.

These adenomas may be familial and have been found in conjunction with tumors of the parathyroid

---

*C peptide, a major portion of the connecting chain in amino acids in proinsulin, remains intact during the conversion of proinsulin to insulin (Chapter 18).

glands and the pituitary (multiple endocrine neoplasia type I). (See Chapter 24.) Ninety-nine percent of them are located within the pancreas and less than 1% in ectopic pancreatic tissue.

These tumors may appear at any age, though they are most common in the fourth to sixth decades. There is no sex predilection.

Clinical Findings

The signs and symptoms are chiefly those of subacute neuroglycopenia rather than adrenergic discharge. The typical picture is that of recurrent central nervous system dysfunction at times of exercise or fasting. The preponderance of neurologic symptoms rather than those commonly associated with hypoglycemia (adrenergic symptoms) often leads to delayed diagnosis following prolonged psychiatric care or treatment for seizure disorders or transient ischemic attacks. Some patients learn to relieve or prevent their symptoms by taking frequent feedings. Obesity may be the result; however, obesity is seen in less than 30% of patients with insulin-secreting tumors.

Diagnosis of Insulinoma

B cell tumors do not reduce secretion in the presence of hypoglycemia, and a serum insulin level of 10 μU/mL or more with concomitant plasma glucose values below 45 mg/dL (2.5 mmol/L) suggests an insulinoma. Other causes of hyperinsulinemic hypoglycemia must be considered, however, such as surreptitious administration of insulin or sulfonylureas.

A. Insulin Assay: Because the insulin radioimmunoassay is crucial in diagnosing insulin-secreting tumors, it is important to be aware of certain limitations in its use. It detects not only human but also beef and pork insulins, and a high level may therefore indicate either endogenous or exogenous insulin. (C peptide measurements are necessary to make this distinction.) In addition, the assay is of no value in patients who have ever taken insulin, as virtually all will have developed low-titer insulin antibodies that will interfere. Falsely low or elevated values will result depending on the method used. Proper collection of samples is also important: If the serum is not separated and then frozen within 1–2 hours, falsely low values will result, because the insulin molecule will undergo proteolytic digestion.

B. Suppression Tests: Failure of endogenous insulin secretion to be suppressed in the presence of hypoglycemia is the hallmark of an insulin-secreting tumor. The most reliable suppression test is the prolonged supervised fast in hospitalized subjects, and this remains the preferred diagnostic maneuver in the workup of suspected insulinomas.

In normal men, the blood glucose value will not fall below 55 mg/dL (3.1 mmol/L) during a 72-hour fast, while insulin levels fall below 10 μU/mL; in

some normal women, however, plasma glucose may fall below 30 mg/dL (1.7 mmol/L) (lower limits have not been established), while serum insulin levels also fall appropriately. (These women remain asymptomatic despite this degree of hypoglycemia, presumably because ketogenesis is able to provide sufficient fuel for the central nervous system.) Calculation of ratios of insulin (in μU/mL) to plasma glucose (in mg/dL) is useful diagnostically. Nonobese normal subjects maintain a ratio of less than 0.25; obese subjects may have an elevated ratio, but hypoglycemia does not occur with fasting. Virtually all patients with insulin-secreting islet cell tumors will have an abnormal insulin:glucose ratio at some time during a 72-hour fast. The majority of these will experience progressive and symptomatic fasting hypoglycemia with associated elevated insulin levels within 24–36 hours and no evidence of ketonuria. However, an occasional patient will not demonstrate hypoglycemia until 72 hours have elapsed. Brisk exercise during the fast may help precipitate hypoglycemia. Once symptoms of hypoglycemia occur, plasma glucose should be obtained and the fast immediately terminated if plasma glucose is below 45 mg/dL (2.5 mmol/L).

C. Stimulation Tests: A variety of stimulation tests with intravenous tolbutamide, glucagon, or calcium have been devised to demonstrate exaggerated and prolonged insulin secretion. However, because insulin-secreting tumors have a wide range of granule content and degrees of differentiation, they are variably responsive to these secretagogues. Thus, absence of an excessive insulin secretory response during any of these stimulation tests does not rule out the presence of an insulinoma. In addition, the tests may be extremely hazardous to patients with responsive tumors by inducing prolonged and refractory hypoglycemia. (None of these secretagogues should be given to a patient when hypoglycemia is present.) The following stimulation tests should be reserved for the difficult case in which results of a prolonged fast are equivocal. They can also be useful for screening when the index of suspicion for an insulin-secreting tumor is low.

1. Tolbutamide stimulation test–One gram of sodium tolbutamide dissolved in 20 mL of distilled water is infused intravenously over 2 minutes. Serum insulin is measured every 5 minutes for 15 minutes; a level exceeding 195 μU/mL during this time suggests an insulin-secreting tumor. However, this response is seen in only 60% or less of patients with insulinomas, and false-positive results may occur (eg, with obesity or hepatic disease). Continuation of the test beyond 15 minutes will uncover additional patients with insulinomas by demonstrating prolonged elevations of insulin; however, hazardous hypoglycemia may result.

2. Glucagon stimulation test–One milligram of glucagon is given intravenously, and serum insulin levels are measured every 5 minutes for 15 minutes. A level exceeding 135 μU/mL suggests an insulin-secreting tumor. However, only about half of patients with insulinomas will demonstrate this hyperinsulinism, and false-positive results may occur. When an exaggerated increase in serum insulin occurs, the hyperglycemic effect of glucagon may be subnormal, and profound hypoglycemia may subsequently develop by 60 minutes.

D. Oral Glucose Tolerance Test: The oral glucose tolerance test is of no value in the diagnosis of insulin-secreting tumors. A common misconception is that patients with insulinomas will have flat glucose tolerance curves, because the tumor will discharge insulin in response to oral glucose. In fact, most insulinomas respond poorly, and curves typical of diabetes are more common. In those rare tumors that do release insulin in response to glucose, a flat curve may result; however, this also can be seen in normal subjects.

E. Euglycemic Clamp: Continuous blood glucose monitoring with feedback-controlled dextrose infusion by an artificial pancreas has been used to demonstrate excessive dextrose requirements to maintain fasting euglycemia in insulinoma patients. This test remains experimental; however, it has the advantage of avoiding hypoglycemia during a supervised fast.

F. Proinsulin Measurements: In contrast to normal subjects, whose proinsulin concentration is less than 20% of the total immunoreactive insulin, patients with insulinoma have elevated levels of proinsulin that represent 30–90% of total immunoreactive insulin. Sensitive new assays for human proinsulin that incorporate specific monoclonal antibodies offer considerable potential in the evaluation of patients with suspected insulinoma.

G. Glycohemoglobin Measurements: Low glycohemoglobin values have been reported in occasional cases of insulinoma, reflecting the presence of chronic hypoglycemia. However, the diagnostic usefulness of glycohemoglobin measurements is limited by the relatively low sensitivity of this test as well as poor accuracy at the lower range of normal in many of the assays. In addition, it is nonspecific for hypoglycemia, with low levels being found in certain hemoglobinopathies and hemolytic states.

H. Tumor Localization Studies:

1. Imaging studies—The diagnosis of an insulin-secreting tumor is dependent on biochemical testing. Since most tumors are too small (80% are < 2 cm) to localize by either ultrasonography, CT scanning, or MRI, a negative result will not be conclusive.

Arteriography is often used for preoperative localization of small tumors. The results are improved if catheterization of small arterial branches and subbranches of the celiac artery (selective and subselective arteriography) is combined with calcium injections, which stimulate insulin release from neoplastic tissue but not from normal islets. Simultaneous measurement of hepatic venous insulin (from a catheter inserted into the hepatic vein) during each selective calcium injection has been reported to help localize small tumors not visible with selective arteriography alone. However, even with these advances, arteriography is seldom helpful enough to outweigh its disadvantages, and it remains a painful and relatively imprecise procedure that exposes insulinoma patients to the risk of hypoglycemia and the discomfort of several hours of invasive and expensive radiography. In most cases, a tumor mass large enough to "blush" on arteriography is large enough for an experienced surgeon to identify by direct visualization or palpation. In addition, false-positive and false-negative results are so common that reliance on operative localization by an experienced surgeon has preempted the use of arteriography in a growing number of medical centers.

Small tumors within the pancreas that are not palpable at laparotomy have been localized using intraoperative ultrasound in which a transducer is wrapped in a sterile rubber glove and passed over the exposed pancreatic surface. *This is at present probably the most effective method of localizing insulinomas.*

2. Transhepatic portal vein sampling—Demonstration of insulin gradients or "step-ups" in insulin concentration in the pancreatic venous effluent can be effective in localizing small insulin-secreting tumors. The procedure entails percutaneous transhepatic portal vein catheterization under local anesthesia with subsequent cannulation of the splenic vein. Samples for insulin assay are obtained along the splenic and portal venous systems in an attempt to show a gradient of 300 μU/mL or more of insulin concentration that would evidence a tumor. Results may be equivocal, however, because of the high rate of blood flow in these venous systems and the consequent dilution of insulin values. In addition, this uncomfortable procedure is not without complications; bile leakage, intraperitoneal hemorrhage, and infection have been reported. This procedure is most helpful when multiple insulinomas are suspected, as in patients with coexisting pituitary or parathyroid tumors who develop hypoglycemia. Since diazoxide would interfere with this test, it should be discontinued for at least 48–72 hours before sampling. An infusion of dextrose may be required, therefore, and patients should be closely monitored during the procedure to avoid hypoglycemia (as well as hyperglycemia, which could affect insulin gradients). Venous sampling is indicated for cases in which hypoglycemia does not respond to diazoxide (see below), so that surgical removal of the insulinoma is therefore mandated. In this instance, only an angiographer with extensive experience in the technique should perform the procedure.

Treatment of Insulinoma

The treatment of choice for insulin-secreting tumors is surgical resection. A flow diagram for the approach to these patients is shown in Figure 19–4.

A. Surgical Treatment: Tumor resection should be performed only by surgeons with extensive experience with removal of islet cell tumors, since these tumors may be small and difficult to recognize. An 85% success rate has been reported without localization procedures if surgeons have prior experience with insulinomas.

1. Preoperative management–

a. Trial of diazoxide–Oral diazoxide, a potent inhibitor of insulin secretion, will maintain euglycemia in most patients with insulin-secreting tumors. Doses of 300–400 mg/d (divided) will usually suffice, but an occasional patient will require up to 800 mg/d. Side effects include edema due to sodium retention (which generally necessitates concomitant thiazide administration), gastric irritation, and mild hirsutism.

b. Selection of patients–Patients who remain euglycemic on diazoxide may be operated on by an experienced surgeon, without attempts at preoperative tumor localization. However, intraoperative ultrasound should be available on call in case an insuli-noma is not palpated after exposure and mobilization of the pancreas. Patients who do not respond to diazoxide or cannot tolerate its side effects are candidates for venous sampling studies in an attempt to localize the tumor preoperatively, since failure to successfully remove the tumor has a poorer prognosis in patients in whom diazoxide therapy is not effective.

2. Treatment during surgery–

a. Glucose need during surgery–An infusion of 5% or 10% dextrose is needed to maintain euglycemia during the surgical procedure. Careful and frequent blood glucose monitoring is needed to determine the infusion rate required in individual patients to avoid hypoglycemia, especially when the insulinoma is being palpated and manipulated prior to removal.

b. Diazoxide–Diazoxide should be administered preoperatively as well as on the day of surgery in patients who are responsive to it, since the drug greatly reduces the need for glucose supplements and the risk of hypoglycemia during surgery while not masking the glycemic rise indicative of surgical cure.

3. Postoperative hyperglycemia–Postoperatively, several days of hyperglycemia may ensue.

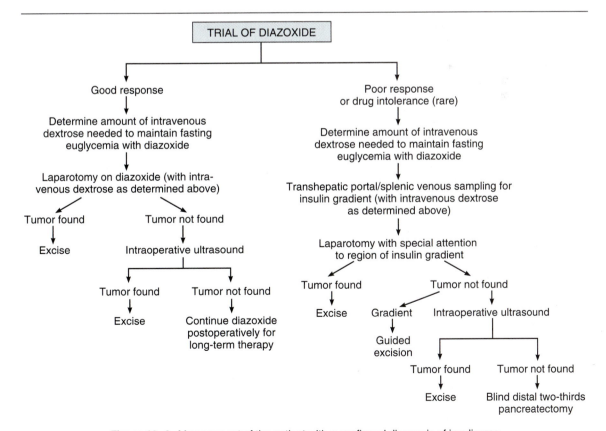

Figure 19–4. Management of the patient with a confirmed diagnosis of insulinoma.

This is due to a combination of factors, including edema and inflammation of the pancreas after surgery, high levels of counterregulatory hormones induced by the procedure, chronic down-regulation of insulin receptors by the previously high circulating insulin levels from the tumor, and perhaps suppression of normal pancreatic B cells by long-standing hypoglycemia. Small subcutaneous doses of regular insulin may be prescribed every 4–6 hours if plasma glucose exceeds 300 mg/dL (16.7 mmol/L), but in most cases pancreatic insulin secretion recovers after 48–72 hours, and very little insulin replacement is required.

4. Failure to find the tumor at operation–In approximately 10% of patients with biochemically demonstrated autonomous insulin secretion, no tumor can be found at exploratory laparotomy. The tumor will most likely be in the head of the pancreas, as this is the most difficult area for the surgeon to mobilize and explore; therefore, blind distal two-thirds pancreatectomy is seldom successful. If intraoperative ultrasound does not identify a tumor, it is best to let the prior response to diazoxide therapy dictate the proper procedure (Figure 19–4). If the patient has responded to diazoxide, this can be continued indefinitely. If the patient has not responded or is intolerant of diazoxide therapy, and if preoperative venous sampling has not been helpful in localizing a tumor, then—and only then—a blind distal two-thirds pancreatectomy should be performed. This procedure has a success rate of only 25%.

B. Medical Treatment: Diazoxide therapy is the treatment of choice in patients with inoperable functioning islet cell carcinomas and in those who are poor candidates for operation. Many patients have been maintained on long-term (> 10 years) diazoxide therapy without apparent ill effects. Hydrochlorothiazide, 25–50 mg daily, should also be prescribed to counteract the edema and hyperkalemia secondary to diazoxide therapy as well as to potentiate its hyperglycemic effect. Frequent carbohydrate feedings (every 2–3 hours) can also be helpful in maintaining euglycemia, though obesity may become a problem.

When patients are unable to tolerate diazoxide because of side effects such as gastrointestinal upset, hirsutism, or edema, a calcium channel blocker such as verapamil (80 mg given orally every 8 hours) may be tried in view of its inhibitory effect on insulin release from insulinoma cells in vitro.

A potent long-acting synthetic octapeptide analog of somatostatin (octreotide) has been used to inhibit release of hormones from a number of endocrine tumors, including inoperable insulinomas, but it has had limited success. Of the five somatostatin receptors (SSTR) that have recently been identified in humans, SSTR2, which predominates in the anterior pituitary, has a much greater affinity for octreotide than

SSTR5, which predominates in the pancreas. This explains why octreotide is much more effective in treating acromegaly than in treating insulinoma, except in the occasional cases where insulinoma cells happen also to express SSTR2. When hypoglycemia persists after attempted surgical removal of the insulinoma and if diazoxide or verapamil is poorly tolerated or ineffective, a trial of 50 μg of octreotide injected subcutaneously twice daily may control the hypoglycemic episodes in conjunction with multiple small carbohydrate feedings.

Streptozocin has proved beneficial in patients with islet cell carcinomas, and effective cytotoxic doses have been achieved without the undue renal toxicity that characterized early experience. Benign tumors appear to respond poorly, if at all.

SYMPTOMATIC FASTING HYPOGLYCEMIA WITHOUT HYPERINSULINISM

1. DISORDERS ASSOCIATED WITH LOW HEPATIC GLUCOSE OUTPUT

Reduced hepatic gluconeogenesis can result from a direct loss of hepatic tissue (acute yellow atrophy from fulminating viral or toxic damage); from disorders reducing amino acid supply to hepatic parenchyma (severe muscle wasting and inanition from anorexia nervosa, chronic starvation, uremia, and glucocorticoid deficit from adrenocortical deficiency); or from inborn errors of carbohydrate metabolism affecting glycogenolytic or gluconeogenic enzymes.

2. ETHANOL HYPOGLYCEMIA

Ethanol impairs hepatic gluconeogenesis but has no effect on hepatic glycogenolysis. In the patient who is imbibing ethanol but not eating, fasting hypoglycemia may occur after hepatic glycogen stores have been depleted (within 8–12 hours of a fast). No correlation exists between the blood ethanol levels and the degree of hypoglycemia, which may occur while blood ethanol levels are declining. It should be noted that ethanol-induced fasting hypoglycemia may occur at ethanol levels as low as 45 mg/dL (10 mmol/L)—considerably below most states' legal standards (80 mg/dL [17.4 mmol/L]) for being "under the influence." Most patients present with neuroglycopenic symptoms, which may be difficult to differentiate from the neurotoxic effects of the alcohol. These symptoms in a patient whose breath smells of alcohol may be mistaken for alcoholic stupor. Intravenous dextrose should be administered promptly to all such stuporous or comatose patients. Because hepatic glycogen stores have been depleted by the time hypoglycemia occurs, parenteral glucagon will not be effective. Adequate food intake during alcohol ingestion will prevent this type of hypoglycemia.

3. NONPANCREATIC TUMORS

A variety of nonpancreatic tumors have been found to cause fasting hypoglycemia. Most are large and mesenchymal in origin, retroperitoneal fibrosarcoma being the classic prototype. However, hepatocellular carcinomas, adrenocortical carcinomas, hypernephromas, gastrointestinal tumors, lymphomas and leukemias, and a variety of other tumors have also been reported.

Laboratory diagnosis depends upon fasting hypoglycemia associated with serum insulin levels below 8 µU/mL. The mechanisms by which these tumors produce hypoglycemia are not entirely clear. None have been unequivocally shown to secrete insulin; thus, true ectopic hyperinsulinemia probably does not exist. Up to 50% of these tumors have been reported to secrete low-molecular-weight peptides with insulin-like activity. These NSILA peptides (so-called because of their nonsuppressible insulin-like activity) include human insulin-like growth factors and some of the somatomedins. Whether further refinement in the assays for these peptides will allow the demonstration of NSILA in all cases of nonpancreatic tumors that are associated with hypoglycemia remains to be seen. Messenger RNA for IGF-2 has been found in high levels in some extrapancreatic tumor tissues. Hypoglycemia in these cases was attributed to a high-molecular-weight form of IGF-2 that was disproportionately present in higher concentration despite normal *total* blood levels of IGF-2 in these patients. Treatment is aimed toward the primary tumor, with supportive therapy using frequent feedings. Diazoxide is ineffective in reversing the hypoglycemia caused by these tumors.

NONFASTING HYPOGLYCEMIA
(Reactive Hypoglycemia)

Reactive hypoglycemia may be classified as early (within 2–3 hours after a meal) or late (3–5 hours). Early (alimentary) hypoglycemia occurs when there is a rapid discharge of ingested carbohydrate into the small bowel followed by rapid glucose absorption and hyperinsulinism. It may be seen after gastrointestinal surgery and is notably associated with the "dumping syndrome" after gastrectomy; occasionally, it is functional and may result from overactivity of the parasympathetic nervous system mediated via the vagus nerve. Late hypoglycemia (occult diabetes) is caused by a delay in early insulin release, which then results in exaggeration of initial hyperglycemia during a glucose tolerance test. As a consequence, an exaggerated insulin response produces late hypo-

glycemia. Early or late hypoglycemia may also occur as a consequence of ethanol's potentiation of the insulin-secretory response to glucose, as when sugar-containing soft drinks are used as mixers to dilute alcohol in beverages (gin and tonic, rum and cola).

1. POSTGASTRECTOMY ALIMENTARY HYPOGLYCEMIA

Reactive hypoglycemia after gastrectomy is a consequence of hyperinsulinism. This results from rapid gastric emptying of ingested food, which produces overstimulation of vagal reflexes and overproduction of beta-cytotropic gastrointestinal hormones, causing arterial hyperinsulinism and consequent acute hypoglycemia. The symptoms are caused by adrenergic hyperactivity in response to the rapidly falling plasma glucose. Treatment is properly directed at avoiding this sequence of events by more frequent feedings with smaller portions of less rapidly assimilated carbohydrate and more slowly absorbed fat or protein. Occasionally, anticholinergic drugs such as propantheline (15 mg orally four times daily) may be useful in reducing vagal overactivity.

2. FUNCTIONAL ALIMENTARY HYPOGLYCEMIA

Early alimentary-type reactive hypoglycemia in a patient who has not undergone surgery is classified as functional. It is most often associated with chronic fatigue, anxiety, irritability, weakness, poor concentration, decreased libido, headaches, hunger after meals, and tremulousness. Whether or not hypoglycemia accounts for these symptoms or occurs at all is difficult to prove.

The usual sequence of events is that the patient presents with a number of nonspecific complaints. Normal laboratory findings and a normal physical examination confirm the initial impression that organic disease is not present, and the symptoms are then attributed to the stresses of modern living. The only form of therapy usually given is reassurance or a mild tranquilizer. When this fails to be of benefit, the patient seeks help elsewhere. Inevitably, the question of hypoglycemia is raised—frequently by the patient, who has heard of the diagnosis from friends or relatives with similar symptoms or has read of it in the lay press. The diagnosis is often supported by the demonstration of hypoglycemia with symptoms during a 5-hour oral glucose tolerance test.

Unfortunately, the precipitation of hypoglycemia with or without symptoms during oral glucose tolerance testing does not distinguish between normal and "hypoglycemic" patients. As many as one-third or more of normal subjects who have never had any symptoms will develop hypoglycemia with or without symptoms during a 5-hour glucose tolerance test. In addition, many patients will develop symptoms in the absence of hypoglycemia. Thus, the test's nonspecificity makes it a highly unreliable tool that is no longer recommended for evaluating patients with suspected episodes of postprandial hypoglycemia. Indeed, the ingestion of a mixed meal did not produce hypoglycemia in 33 patients who had been diagnosed as having reactive hypoglycemia on the basis of oral glucose tolerance testing; this attempt to increase specificity for the diagnosis of reactive hypoglycemia may have resulted in loss of sensitivity.

For increased diagnostic reliability, hypoglycemia should be documented during a spontaneous symptomatic episode in routine daily activity. However, attempts to demonstrate this are almost never successful. Patients should be instructed in the proper use of Chemstrip bG, whose color development is stable enough to allow test strips to be saved and brought to the physician's office for documentation up to 72 hours after the measurement was made. Personality evaluation often discloses hyperkinetic compulsive behavior in thin, anxious patients.

The foregoing discussion should not be taken to imply that functional reactive hypoglycemia does not occur—merely that at present we have no reliable means of diagnosing it. There is no harm (and there is occasional benefit) in reducing or eliminating the content of refined sugars in the patient's diet while increasing the frequency and reducing the size of meals. However, it should not be expected that these maneuvers will cure the asthenia, since the reflex response to hypoglycemia is only a possibly aggravating feature of a generalized primary hyperactivity. Counseling and support and mild sedation should be the mainstays in therapy, with dietary manipulation only an adjunct.

3. LATE HYPOGLYCEMIA (Occult Diabetes)

This condition is characterized by delay in early insulin release from pancreatic B cells, resulting in initial exaggeration of hyperglycemia during a glucose tolerance test. In response to this hyperglycemia, an exaggerated insulin release produces late hypoglycemia 4–5 hours after ingestion of glucose. These patients are usually quite different from those with early hypoglycemia, being more phlegmatic and often obese and frequently having a family history of diabetes mellitus. In the obese, treatment is directed at reduction to ideal weight. These patients often respond to reduced intake of refined sugars with multiple, spaced small feedings high in dietary fiber. They should be considered early diabetics and advised to have periodic medical evaluations.

REFERENCES

Assan R et al: Pentamidine-induced derangements of glucose homeostasis. Diabetes Care 1995;18:47.

Boyle PJ et al: Adaptation in brain glucose uptake following recurrent hypoglycemia. Proc Natl Acad Sci USA 1994;91:9352.

Doherty GM et al: Results of a prospective strategy to diagnose, localize and resect insulinomas. Surgery 1991;110:989.

Doppman JL et al: Localization of insulinomas to regions of the pancreas by intra-arterial stimulation with calcium. Ann Intern Med 1995;123:269.

Fanelli C et al: Long-term recovery from unawareness, deficient counterregulation and lack of cognitive dysfunction during hypoglycemia following institution of rational, intensive insulin therapy in IDDM. Diabetologia 1994;37:1265.

Fischer KF, Lees JA, Newman JH: Hypoglycemia in hospitalized patients: Causes and outcomes. N Engl J Med 1986;315:1245.

Gerich JE et al: Hypoglycemia unawareness. Endocr Rev 1991;12:356.

Grunberger G et al: Factitious hypoglycemia due to surreptitious administration of insulin: Diagnosis, treatment, and long-term follow-up. Ann Intern Med 1988;108:252.

Herings RMC et al: Hypoglycemia associated with use of inhibitors of angiotensin converting enzyme. Lancet 1995;345:1195.

Kahn BB: Facilitative glucose transporters: Regulatory mechanisms and dysregulation in diabetes. J Clin Invest 1992;89:1367.

Klonoff D et al: Hypoglycemia following inadvertent and factitious sulfonylurea overdosages. Diabetes Care 1995;18:563.

Kvols LK et al: Treatment of metastatic islet cell carcinoma with a somatostatin analogue (SMS 201–995). Ann Intern Med 1987;17:162.

Marks V, Teale JD: Tumors producing hypoglycemia. Diabetes Metab Rev 1991;7:79.

Mitrakou A et al: Reversibility of unawareness of hypoglycemia in patients with insulinomas. N Engl J Med 1993;329:834.

Mokan M et al: Hypoglycemia unawareness in IDDM. Diabetes Care 1994;17:1397.

Palardy J et al: Blood glucose measurements during symptomatic episodes in patients with suspected postprandial hypoglycemia. N Engl J Med 1989;321:1421.

Pandit MK et al: Drug-induced disorders of glucose tolerance. Ann Intern Med 1993;118:529.

Perry RR, Vinik AI: Diagnosis and management of functioning islet cell tumors. J Clin Endocrin Metab 1995; 80:2273.

Polansky KS: A practical approach to fasting hypoglycemia. N Engl J Med 1992;326,1020.

Reisine T, Bell GI: Molecular biology of somatostatin receptors. Endocr Rev 1995;16:427.

Service FJ et al: Functioning insulinoma: Incidence, recurrence, and long-term survival of patients. A 60 year study. Mayo Clin Proc 1991;66:771.

Service FJ: Hypoglycemia disorders. N Engl J Med 1995; 332:1144.

Shapiro ET et al: Tumor hypoglycemia: Relationship to high molecular weight insulin-like growth factor-II. J Clin Invest 1990;85:1972.

Towler DA et al: Mechanism of awareness of hypoglycemia: Perception of neurogenic (predominantly cholinergic) rather than neuroglycopenic symptoms. Diabetes 1993;42:1791.

Uchigata Y et al: Insulin autoimmune syndrome (Hirata disease): Clinical features and epidemiology in Japan. Diabetes Res Clin Pract 1994;22:89.

Van Heerden JA et al: Occult functioning insulinomas: Which localizing studies are indicated? Surgery 1992; 112:1010.

20 Disorders of Lipoprotein Metabolism

John P. Kane, MD, PhD, & Mary J. Malloy, MD

The clinical importance of hyperlipoproteinemia derives chiefly from the role of lipoproteins in atherogenesis. However, the greatly increased risk of acute pancreatitis associated with severe hypertriglyceridemia is an additional indication for intervention. Characterization of hyperlipoproteinemia is important for selection of appropriate treatment and may provide clues to underlying primary clinical disorders.

ARTERIOSCLEROSIS

Arteriosclerosis is the leading cause of death in the USA. Abundant epidemiologic evidence establishes the multifactorial character of this disease and indicates that the effects of the multiple risk factors are at least additive. Risk factors that have been convincingly identified for atherosclerosis of the coronary arteries are hyperlipidemia, arterial hypertension, cigarette smoking, diabetes mellitus, physical inactivity, and decreased levels of high-density lipoproteins (HDL) in plasma. Coronary atheromas are complex lesions containing cellular elements, collagen, and lipids. It is clear, however, that the progression of the lesion is chiefly attributable to its content of unesterified cholesterol and cholesteryl esters. It is now firmly established that the cholesterol in the atheroma is delivered to the site by circulating lipoproteins. Epidemiologic evidence indicates that the atherogenic lipoproteins are the low-density (LDL), intermediate-density (IDL), very low density (VLDL), and Lp(a) species, all of which contain the B-100 apolipoprotein. All the apo-B-containing lipoproteins are subject to covalent chemical changes by oxidation, which is mediated by reactive oxygen species in the tissues and perhaps also by lipoxygenases secreted by macrophages in atheromas. Tocopherols (vitamin E) are natural antioxidants that localize in the surface monolayers of lipoproteins, exerting resistance to oxidation. However, increased oxidative stress such as that induced by smoking depletes the tocopherol content of lipoproteins. Oxidation of lipoproteins stimulates their endocytosis via special

scavenger receptors on macrophages and smooth muscle cells, leading to the formation of foam cells. At least four classes of scavenger receptors are recognized. Two are splice variant products of a single gene (class A receptors). Another is a CD36 type protein, and the fourth is an Fc receptor.

In animal models, hypertension is associated with increased access of lipoprotein to the subintimal region. Smoking may accelerate the process of atherogenesis chiefly through its influence on blood platelets, though it is also associated with decreased

---

ACRONYMS USED IN THIS CHAPTER

ACAT	Acyl-CoA:cholesterol acyltransferase
Apo-	Apolipoprotein
CETP	Cholesteryl ester transfer protein
CoA	Coenzyme A
FFA	Free fatty acids
HDL	High-density lipoproteins
HMG-CoA	Hydroxymethylglutaryl-CoA
IDDM	Insulin-dependent diabetes mellitus
IDL	Intermediate-density lipoproteins
LCAT	Lecithin:cholesterol acyltransferase
LDL	Low-density lipoproteins
Lp(a)	A specific high-molecular-weight glycoprotein. Also applies to lipoprotein species containing this protein.
LPL	Lipoprotein lipase
NIDDM	Non-insulin-dependent diabetes mellitus
PDGF	Platelet-derived growth factor
PLTP	Phospholipid transfer protein
VLDL	Very low density lipoproteins

levels of HDL in plasma and accelerates the oxidation of lipoproteins. Increased platelet interaction at sites of damaged endothelium leads to release of platelet-derived growth factor (PDGF), which stimulates migration of cells of smooth muscle origin into the lesion, where they proliferate.

Activated macrophages secrete a number of cytokines that drive an inflammatory and proliferative process. Proteolytic enzymes secreted by macrophages so weaken the atheroma that fissuring and rupture can occur. Exposure of subintimal collagen then attracts platelets, thus stimulating thrombogenesis and precipitating acute coronary events. The inverse relationship between plasma HDL levels and the rate of atherogenesis probably reflects the involvement of at least certain species of HDL in the movement of cholesterol away from the atheroma and in protecting LDL against oxidation.

Reversal of Atherosclerosis

The results of angiographic intervention trials in humans have conclusively shown that physical regression of atherosclerotic lesions occurs with lipid-lowering therapy. Furthermore, several large trials have demonstrated striking reductions in the incidence of new coronary events, in individuals with hyperlipidemia who have had no prior clinical coronary disease (primary prevention) as well as in individuals with antecedent clinical coronary disease (secondary prevention). Thus, timely introduction of hypolipidemic therapy appropriate to the lipid disorder will significantly decrease the incidence of coronary disease and reduce the need for angioplasty, atherectomy, and bypass surgery. In the large intervention trials involving treatment with HMG-CoA reductase inhibitors and with niacin, all-cause mortality has been significantly reduced. Side effects of treatment have been minimal in comparison with the magnitude of this benefit.

The average levels of LDL in plasma in the United States population are considerably higher than in many other nations, where the levels appear to approach the biologic norm for humans. This probably accounts in large part for the markedly higher incidence of coronary disease in industrialized Western nations and suggests that dietary changes that reduce lipoprotein levels toward normal would be beneficial.

OVERVIEW OF LIPID TRANSPORT

The Plasma Lipoproteins

Because all the lipids of plasma are relatively insoluble in water, they are transported in association with proteins. The simplest complexes are those formed between unesterified, or free, fatty acids (FFA) and albumin, which serve to carry the FFA from peripheral adipocytes to other tissues.

The remainder of the plasma lipids are transported in lipoprotein complexes (Table 20–1). All of the major lipoproteins of plasma are spherical, each with a core region containing hydrophobic lipids. The principal core lipids are cholesteryl esters and triglycerides. Triglycerides predominate in the cores of the chylomicrons, which transport newly absorbed lipids from the intestine, and in the cores of the very low density lipoproteins, which originate in the liver. The relative content of cholesteryl ester is increased in remnants derived from these classes of lipoproteins, and cholesteryl esters predominate in the cores of low-density and high-density lipoproteins. Surrounding the core in each type of lipoprotein is a monolayer containing amphophilic (detergent-like) lipids, chiefly phospholipids and unesterified (free) cholesterol. Apolipoproteins, noncovalently bound to the lipids, are mostly located in or on this surface monolayer (Figure 20–1).

B Apolipoproteins

Several lipoproteins contain proteins of very high

Table 20–1. Lipoproteins of human serum.

Lipoprotein	Electrophoretic Mobility in Agarose Gel	Density Interval g/cm³	Predominant Core Lipids	Diameter	Apolipoproteins in Order of Quantitative Importance
High-density (HDL)	Alpha	1.21–1.063	Cholesteryl ester	7.5–10.5 nm	A-I, A-II, C, E, D
Low-density (LDL)	Beta	1.063–1.019	Cholesteryl ester	21.5 nm	B-100
Intermediate-density (IDL)	Beta	1.019–1.006	Cholesteryl ester, triglyceride	25–30 nm	B-100, some C and E
Very low density (VLDL)	Prebeta; some "slow prebeta"	< 1.006	Triglyceride	30–100 nm	B-100, C, E
Chylomicrons	Remain at origin	< 1.006	Triglyceride	60–500 nm	B-48, C, E, A-I, A-II, A-IV
Lp(a)	Prebeta	1.04–1.08	Cholesteryl ester	21–30 nm	B-100, Lp(a)

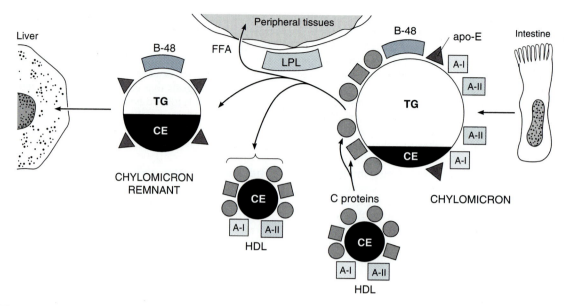

Figure 20–1. Metabolism of chylomicrons. (TG, triglyceride; CE, cholesteryl esters; A-I, A-II, B-48, and C proteins, apolipoproteins.) See text for details.

molecular weight known as the B apolipoproteins, which behave like intrinsic proteins of cell membranes. Unlike the smaller apolipoproteins, the B apolipoproteins do not migrate from one lipoprotein particle to another. The B apolipoproteins of intestinal and hepatic origin are different. VLDL contain the B-100 protein, which is retained in the formation of LDL from VLDL remnants by the liver. The intestinal B protein, B-48, is found in chylomicrons and their remnant particles but is completely absent from LDL. Both forms of apo-B contain a ligand domain for binding to lipoprotein lipase. Apo-B-100 has an additional ligand domain that is conformed as VLDL are transformed into LDL, providing the basis for binding to the LDL receptor.

Other Apolipoproteins

In addition to B-48 and B-100, the following apolipoproteins are present in lipoproteins. (The distribution of these proteins in the different lipoproteins is shown in Table 20–1.)

A. C Apolipoproteins: These are low-molecular-weight (7000–10,000) proteins that equilibrate rapidly among the lipoproteins. There are four distinct species with unique amino acid sequences, designated C-I, C-II, C-III, and C-IV. Apolipoprotein C-II is a requisite cofactor for lipoprotein lipase.

B. E Apolipoproteins: Two normal isoforms (E-3 and E-4) of this MW-35,000 protein are the products of allelic genes. Normal individuals thus may have either or both isoforms, which share with

B-100 protein the property of interacting with certain high-affinity receptors (B-100:E receptors) on cell membranes. Another isoform (E-2) lacks this property. About 15% of people in the USA are heterozygous for E-2.

C. Apolipoprotein A-I: This protein of MW 28,300 is the major apolipoprotein of HDL; it is also present in chylomicrons and is the most abundant of the apolipoproteins of human serum (about 125 mg/dL). It is a cofactor for lecithin:cholesterol acyltransferase (LCAT).

D. Apolipoprotein A-II: This protein of (dimeric) MW 17,400 is an important constituent of HDL. It contains cysteine, which permits the formation of disulfide-bridged dimers with apo-E.

E. D Apolipoprotein: This heavily glycosylated protein of MW 19,000 is involved with LCAT in the centripetal transport of cholesterol.

F. Apolipoprotein A-IV: This protein of MW 46,000 is chiefly associated with chylomicrons.

G. Lp(a) Protein: This high-molecular-weight (200,000–750,000) glycoprotein, which has a high degree of sequence homology with plasminogen, is found as a disulfide-bridged dimer with apo-B-100 in LDL-like species of lipoproteins (Lp(a) lipoproteins).

Absorption of Dietary Fat; Secretion of Chylomicrons

Dietary triglycerides are hydrolyzed in the intestine to β-monoglyceride and fatty acids by pancreatic lipase. This enzyme requires activation by bile acids and a protein cofactor. The partial glycerides and fatty acids form micelles that are absorbed by intestinal epithelial cells. Within these cells, the fatty acids are reesterified with the monoglyceride to form triglycerides. Some dietary cholesterol absorbed with the micelles is esterified by the acyl-CoA:cholesterol acyltransferase (ACAT) system, and some appears as free cholesterol in the surface monolayers of the chylomicrons. Droplets of triglyceride containing small amounts of cholesteryl esters form in the vesicles of the Golgi apparatus. Phospholipids and free cholesterol form a surface monolayer. Some of the phospholipid originates in bile, some is from dietary sources, and some is synthesized by the intestine. Newly synthesized apo-B-48, apo-A-I, and apo-A-II are added, and the nascent chylomicron emerges into the extracellular lymph space (Figure 20–1). Chylomicrons have diameters ranging from about 60 nm to 500 nm. Once in the lymph spaces, the new chylomicron begins to exchange surface components with HDL, acquiring apo-C and apo-E and losing phospholipids. This process continues as the chylomicron is carried via the intestinal lymphatics to the thoracic duct and thence into the bloodstream. Increased triglyceride transport from the intestine results chiefly in an increase of particle diameter of chylomicrons rather than increased numbers of particles.

Formation of Very Low Density Lipoproteins

The liver exports triglycerides to peripheral tissues in the cores of VLDL (Figure 20–2). These triglycerides are synthesized in liver from free fatty acids abstracted from plasma and from fatty acids synthesized de novo. Several major features distinguish VLDL from chylomicrons. The only B apolipoprotein of VLDL is B-100. Whereas the intestine produces only very limited amounts of apo-C, the liver secretes the bulk of these proteins with newly formed VLDL. Upon reaching the plasma, the VLDL acquire still more apo-C from HDL and yield phospholipid in exchange. Release of VLDL by liver is increased by any condition that results in increased flux of FFA to

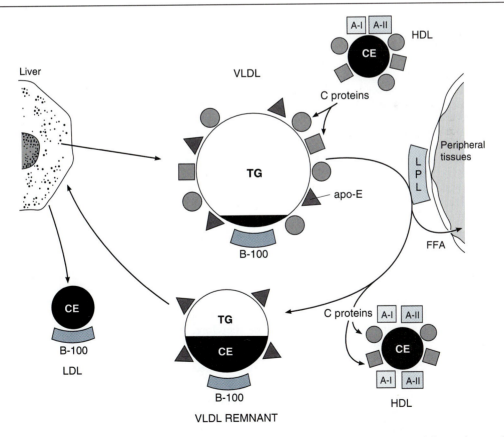

Figure 20–2. Metabolism of VLDL. (TG, triglyceride; CE, cholesteryl esters; A-I, A-II, B-48, and C proteins, apolipoproteins.) See text for details.

liver in the absence of increased ketogenesis. Increased caloric intake, ingestion of ethanol, and the administration of estrogens all greatly stimulate release of VLDL from liver and are important causative factors in clinical disorders resulting in elevated levels of triglycerides in plasma.

Metabolism of Triglyceride-Rich Lipoproteins in Plasma

A. Hydrolysis by Lipoprotein Lipase: Fatty acids derived from the triglycerides of chylomicrons and VLDL are delivered to tissues predominantly through a common pathway involving hydrolysis by the lipoprotein lipase (LPL) system. Most of the FFA derived during hydrolysis of triglycerides by LPL enters tissue directly. The remainder enters the pool of plasma FFA. Lipoprotein lipase is bound to capillary endothelium in heart, skeletal muscle, adipose tissue, mammary gland, and other tissues. The hydrolysis of triglycerides thus takes place within the vascular compartment.

B. Biologic Regulation of Lipoprotein Lipase: When glucose levels in plasma are elevated and the release of insulin is stimulated, LPL activity in adipose tissue increases, and fatty acids derived from triglycerides of circulating lipoproteins are stored. During prolonged fasting, however, LPL activity of adipose tissue falls to undetectable levels, completely preventing storage of fatty acids from VLDL and chylomicrons. Heparin is a cofactor for LPL. When heparin is given intravenously (0.1–0.2 mg/kg), LPL activity is displaced into plasma, permitting its in vitro measurement. Another obligatory cofactor is apo-C-II. Normally, its content in plasma is far in excess of that required for activation of the LPL system.

C. Formation of Lipoprotein Remnants: Hydrolysis by LPL results in depletion of the content of triglycerides in the hydrophobic core of chylomicrons and VLDL, producing a progressive decrease in particle diameter. Lipids from the surface monolayer are transported to HDL. This maintains an appropriate core: monolayer relationship for spheres of smaller diameters. During this process, apo-C and, to a lesser extent, apo-E are transferred to HDL. The products of this series of events are "remnant" lipoproteins containing their original complement of apo-B, a portion of the original amount of apo-E, and little apo-C. Apo-A-I and apo-A-II also leave the particles and become incorporated into HDL. VLDL remnants are 25–30 nm in diameter, and those of chylomicrons are up to 80 nm in diameter. They have lost about 70% of their original complement of triglyceride but are enriched in cholesteryl esters.

D. Fate of Lipoprotein Remnants: Chylomicron remnants are removed from blood quantitatively by high-affinity, receptor-mediated endocytosis in the liver. The receptors appear to include the LDL

(B-100:E) receptors and the related LRP receptors. The endocytosis of chylomicron remnants by both requires the presence of apo-E3 or apo-E4 allele products. The lipid constituents enter hepatic pools, and the B-48 protein is degraded completely. The cholesterol derived from chylomicron remnants is the major mediator of feedback control of cholesterol biosynthesis in liver. Some VLDL remnants are removed from blood via the B-100:E receptors (see below) and are degraded. Those which escape uptake are transformed into LDL. Thus, the rate of removal of VLDL remnants by liver is a determinant of LDL production. The process of formation of LDL involves the removal of essentially all of the residual triglycerides by hepatic lipase present on cell surfaces in the liver. Apo-E appears to be involved in this interaction. LDL particles contain chiefly cholesteryl esters in their cores. They retain the B-100 protein but only traces of other apolipoproteins. In normal individuals, a major fraction of VLDL is converted to LDL, and all of the LDL apo-B comes from VLDL. In certain hypertriglyceridemic states, conversion of VLDL to LDL is decreased.

The fact that LDL originate from the metabolism of VLDL remnants suggests that increases of LDL in plasma can arise from an increased rate of secretion of precursor VLDL as well as from decreased catabolism of LDL. The formation of LDL from VLDL may also contribute to the clinical phenomenon referred to as the "beta shift." This is an increase of LDL (beta-lipoprotein) as hypertriglyceridemia resolves. A classic example of the beta shift occurs temporarily following institution of adequate insulin treatment in uncontrolled diabetes with lipemia. Insulin induces increased lipoprotein lipase activity, resulting in rapid conversion of VLDL to LDL. Because of its longer half-life, the LDL accumulate in plasma. Elevated levels of LDL may persist beyond the time when levels of triglyceride-rich lipoproteins have returned to normal. A similar phenomenon may occur when patients with familial combined hyperlipidemia are treated with fibric acid derivatives.

E. Half-Lives of Lipoproteins: Normally, the half-life of chylomicron apo-B-48 in plasma is 5–20 minutes; that of the apo-B-100 in VLDL is 0.5–1 hour; and that of LDL apo-B-100 is about 2½ days. At triglyceride levels of 800–1000 mg/dL, the lipoprotein lipase mechanism is at kinetic saturation; therefore, increases in the input of triglyceride-rich lipoproteins into plasma at those levels rapidly result in much higher levels.

F. Effect of Dietary Fat Restriction: Individuals consuming a typical North American diet (with about 45% of calories as fat) transport 75–100 g or more of triglyceride per day into plasma in chylomicrons, whereas the liver exports 10–30 g of triglyceride in VLDL. Thus, the flux of triglyceride into plasma can be influenced most acutely by restriction of dietary fat. When the removal mechanisms involving lipoprotein lipase are saturated and plasma triglyceride levels are measured in thousands of milligrams per deciliter, acute restriction of dietary triglyceride intake will usually produce a significant reduction in triglyceride levels. This intervention is important in the lipemic patient with impending pancreatitis. If symptoms suggest that an attack of pancreatitis is imminent, all oral intake should be eliminated, gastric acid secretion should be suppressed with H_2 blockade, and the patient should not be fed by mouth until the symptoms subside and triglyceride levels decrease to less than 800–1000 mg/dL.

Catabolism of Low-Density Lipoproteins

A. Endocytosis via Specific High-Affinity Receptors: The catabolism of LDL appears to proceed by several mechanisms. The best-understood of these is endocytosis mediated by high-affinity receptors on the cell membranes of virtually all nucleated cells but most importantly hepatocytes (Figure 20–3). The receptors bind the apo-B protein of LDL. Because they also bind apo-E, they are called B-100:E receptors. The coated pit regions invaginate into the cell, forming endocytotic vesicles that fuse with lysosomes. The apo-B of the LDL is degraded to amino acids, and the receptor returns to the cell membrane. The cholesteryl esters of the LDL core are hydrolyzed to yield free cholesterol, which is utilized in the production of cell membrane bilayers. Free cholesterol suppresses the activity of hydroxymethylglu-

taryl-CoA (HMG-CoA) reductase, a rate-limiting enzyme in the biosynthetic pathway for cholesterol. Thus, the intake of cholesterol by this pathway decreases the formation of new cholesterol. Cholesterol in excess of need for membrane synthesis is esterified by the acyl-CoA:cholesterol acyltransferase (ACAT) system for storage. In addition to suppression of cholesterol biosynthesis, the entry of cholesterol via the LDL pathway leads to down-regulation of LDL receptors, resulting in decreased uptake and catabolism of LDL. Saturated fats consumed in the diet down-regulate hepatic LDL receptors.

B. Other Pathways: In addition to the high-affinity receptor-mediated pathway of degradation, LDL appear to be catabolized by at least two additional pathways. Macrophages take up chemically or physically altered LDL by a scavenger mechanism that is not subject to feedback control, and a low-affinity process exists in all cells.

Metabolism of High-Density Lipoproteins

When isolated by ultracentrifugation, HDL appear to comprise two major classes: HDL_2 and HDL_3. Similar quantities of HDL_3 are isolated from serum of men and women, but about twice as much HDL_2 is found in serum of premenopausal women. Recent studies indicate that there are as many as ten discrete species of HDL that are obscured by ultracentrifugation. One of these is the 67-kDa prebeta HDL that appears to be the primary acquisitor of cholesterol in

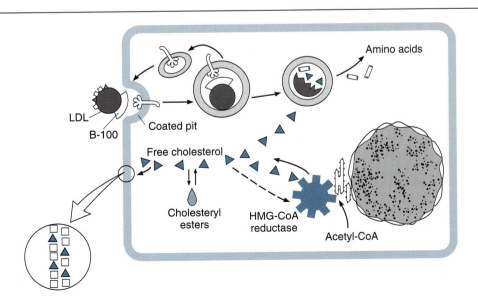

Figure 20–3. Cholesterol homeostasis in the cell. See text for details.

the pathway for retrieval of cholesterol from peripheral tissues.

A. Sources of HDL: Both the liver and intestine produce HDL apolipoproteins, which appear to organize with lipids into the native species of HDL in lymph and plasma. Excess free cholesterol and phospholipids liberated from the surface monolayers of chylomicrons and VLDL as hydrolysis of triglycerides proceeds appear to be transferred to HDL by phospholipid transfer protein (PLTP). Free cholesterol acquired by HDL is esterified by LCAT. This enzyme transfers 1 mol of fatty acid from a lecithin molecule to the hydroxyl group of unesterified cholesterol, forming cholesteryl esters. Lysolecithin, formed by transfer of the fatty acid from lecithin, leaves the lipoprotein complex, binds to albumin, and is transported to various tissues, where it is reacylated to form lecithin. The process of transesterification by LCAT rapidly forms sufficient cholesteryl ester to fill the hydrophobic core region.

LCAT enzyme is secreted by liver. In severe hepatic parenchymal disease, levels of this enzyme in plasma are low and esterification of cholesterol is impeded, leading to the accumulation of free cholesterol in lipoproteins and in membranes of erythrocytes and other cells. Excess free cholesterol in the membranes of erythrocytes transforms them into the target cells classically associated with hepatic disease.

As hydrolysis of triglycerides in chylomicrons and VLDL proceeds, phospholipids and cholesterol are transferred to HDL particles.

B. Metabolic Roles for HDL: Several metabolic roles for HDL are now recognized. These lipoproteins serve as carriers for the C apolipoproteins, transferring them to nascent VLDL and chylomicrons. HDL as well as LDL deliver cholesterol to the adrenal cortex and gonads in support of steroidogenesis. HDL play a major role in the centripetal transport of cholesterol, ie, the transport of surplus cholesterol away from peripheral tissues. Unesterified cholesterol is acquired from the membranes of peripheral tissues by the 67-kDa prebeta HDL particle and is esterified by LCAT, passing through prebeta$_2$ and prebeta$_3$ species before the cholesteryl esters are incorporated into typical HDL particles of alpha electrophoretic mobility. The resulting cholesteryl esters, predominantly cholesteryl linoleate, are then transferred to LDL and to triglyceride-rich lipoproteins. Remnants of chylomicrons and a significant fraction of VLDL remnants and LDL are taken up by liver, providing for transport of the newly formed cholesteryl esters to hepatocytes.

C. Catabolism of HDL: The pathways of catabolism of HDL are not yet known. Radiochemical studies indicate that apo-A-I and apo-A-II are removed from plasma synchronously and that a portion of the degradation occurs in liver and in kidney. Because degradation by perfused rat livers is slower than for the intact animal, it must be presumed that other tissues contribute substantially to the catabolism of HDL.

The Cholesterol Economy

Cholesterol is an essential constituent of the plasma membranes of mammalian cells and of the myelin sheath. It is also required for adrenal and gonadal steroidogenesis and for the production of bile acids by the liver. Virtually all nucleated mammalian cells can synthesize cholesterol, commencing with acetyl-CoA. Formation of HMG-CoA is the initial step. The first committed step, mediated by HMG-CoA reductase, is the formation of mevalonic acid from HMG-CoA. Mevalonic acid is then metabolized via a series of isoprenoid intermediaries to squalene, which cyclizes to form a series of sterols leading to cholesterol. A small amount of the mevalonate is converted eventually to the important isoprenoid substances ubiquinone, dolichol, and isopentenyl pyrophosphate. This pathway also yields the isoprenoid intermediaries geranyl pyrophosphate and farnesyl pyrophosphate that are involved in prenylation of proteins. Prenylation provides an anchor so that proteins such as RAS can bind to membranes. The portion of the pathway leading to cholesterol synthesis is tightly regulated by cholesterol, or some metabolite of cholesterol, which suppresses the activity of HMG-CoA reductase. Thus, cells have the ability to produce cholesterol to the extent that their requirements are not met by that derived from circulating lipoproteins. Cholesteryl esters stored in cells serve as an immediate reserve of cholesterol. Large requirements for cholesterol result from rapid proliferation of cells with attendant need for elaboration of cell membranes. Hepatocytes and intestinal epithelial cells require large amounts of cholesterol for secretion of lipoproteins. In addition, cells are constantly transferring cholesterol to circulating lipoproteins, chiefly HDL. A relatively small amount of cholesterol is lost from the body in desquamated skin and through the loss of intestinal epithelial cells in the stool. Cholesterol is converted to bile acids in liver via a pathway that is initiated by 7α-hydroxylase. About 2% of the bile acids secreted into the intestine are lost in the stool. Activity of 7α-hydroxylase is decreased in hypothyroidism, as is the expression of LDL receptors and hepatic lipase.

Cholesterol is acquired from the diet as well as from endogenous synthesis. Humans, unlike many other species, do not absorb dietary cholesterol quantitatively; however, at normal levels of intake, about one-third of the amount ingested reaches the bloodstream. Most of this cholesterol is transported to liver in chylomicron remnants, leading to suppression of hepatic cholesterogenesis. Recent evidence suggests that individuals may differ substantially in the effect of dietary cholesterol on serum lipoproteins, reflecting in part differences in the efficiency of absorption of cholesterol.

DIFFERENTIATION OF DISORDERS OF LIPOPROTEIN METABOLISM

Laboratory Analyses of Lipids & Lipoproteins

Because chylomicrons normally may be present in plasma up to one hour after a meal, they contribute triglyceride to the total measured during that period, raising the triglyceride concentration to as much as 600 mg/dL (6.9 mmol/L). However, this alimentary lipemia can be substantially prolonged if alcohol is consumed with the meal. Thus, serum lipids and lipoproteins should be measured after a fast of 10–14 hours. If blood glucose is not to be measured, patients may have fruit juice and black coffee with sugar (which provide no triglyceride) for breakfast.

A. Inspection: Much useful information is gained from inspection of the serum, especially before and after overnight refrigeration. As a screening technique, this will identify sera in which triglycerides need to be measured. Opalescence is due to light scattering by large triglyceride-rich lipoproteins. Serum begins to appear hazy when the level of triglycerides reaches 200 mg/dL (2.3 mmol/L), about the point at which clinical significance begins. The presence of chylomicrons is readily detected, because they form a white supernatant layer. A further observation made on serum, which is critical to the detection of the uncommon cases in which binding of immunoglobulins to lipoproteins takes place, is the formation of a curd-like lipoprotein aggregate or a snowy precipitate as serum cools. If one of these disorders is suspected, blood should be kept at 37 °C during the formation of the clot and separation of the serum, because the critical temperatures for precipitation of the cryoglobulin complex may be higher than room temperature.

B. Laboratory Techniques: The cholesterol and triglyceride contents of serum can be measured by several chemical techniques that provide reliable results. These measurements are an essential minimum for differentiation of disorders of lipoprotein metabolism. The usual methods determine unesterified and esterified cholesterol together, so that the reported value is the total content of cholesterol in serum. In most cases, electrophoresis of lipoproteins contributes little additional information; thus, this technique is not a necessary part of the routine laboratory examination. An exception is the identification of lipoproteins found in familial dysbetalipoproteinemia. The best electrophoretic separation of lipoproteins is made in agarose gel. The most complete characterization of a patient's lipoproteins is achieved by measurement of the cholesterol and triglyceride contents and electrophoretic behavior of individual lipoprotein fractions, separated by preparative ultracentrifugation, a technique usually available only in research laboratories. However, the content of high-density lipoproteins can be measured using a technique in which HDL are the only lipoproteins that remain in solution after treatment of the serum with heparin and manganese. Albeit rapid, the results of this technique tend to be unacceptably variable unless rigid quality control is exercised. The prognostic implications of small changes in HDL cholesterol make such controls necessary.

An important determinant of the content of cholesteryl esters in HDL is the amount of triglyceride-rich lipoproteins to which the HDL are exposed in plasma. Triglycerides from these lipoproteins exchange into the core regions of HDL, displacing cholesteryl esters and leading to an inverse logarithmic dependence of HDL cholesterol level upon the plasma triglycerides. Thus, the HDL cholesterol value cannot be interpreted without knowledge of the level of serum triglycerides. For example, a level of HDL that would normally contain 45 mg/dL (1.17 mmol/L) of cholesterol would contain 37 mg/dL (0.96 mmol/L) when the triglycerides were 200 mg/dL (2.3 mmol/L) and 30 mg/dL (0.78 mmol/L) when they reach 500 mg/dL (5.7 mmol/L). In certain forms of hypertriglyceridemia, there is also a moderate decrease in the protein-phospholipid vehicle of HDL, but the principal effect on the measurement of HDL cholesterol levels remains the exchange of triglycerides for cholesteryl esters.

More sophisticated tests of composition of isolated lipoprotein fractions are of use in certain instances. The most important of these is analysis of the ratio of cholesterol to triglycerides by chemical techniques and of the apolipoproteins of VLDL by isoelectric focusing. The latter reveals the absence of the normal isoforms of apo-E, the underlying molecular defect in familial dysbetalipoproteinemia. In this disorder, there is an unusually high content of cholesterol in the VLDL. The apo-E genotype can also be measured by allele-specific oligonucleotide hybridization. Immunoassays are available for a number of apolipoprotein species, but the utility of these measurements, except for Lp(a), in clinical practice remains unclear.

Clinical Differentiation of Abnormal Patterns of Plasma Lipoproteins

A. Preliminary Screening: Serum cholesterol and triglyceride levels are both continuously distributed in the population; therefore, some arbitrary levels must be established to define significant hyperlipidemia. As indicated in the introductory paragraphs, average levels of LDL in Western populations appear to be well above the biologic ideal and are a major etiologic factor underlying the increased incidence of atherosclerotic vascular disease in Western societies. Epidemiologic studies in Europe and the USA have shown that there is a progressive increase in risk of coronary artery disease as levels of serum cholesterol increase. Present evidence would indicate that physicians should at least encourage patients at risk to eat diets low in saturated fats and cholesterol in order to minimize the burden of LDL in plasma.

The National Cholesterol Education Program has developed guidelines for treatment of hypercholesterolemia in adults (Table 20–2). Levels of triglyceride above 200 mg/dL (2.26 mmol/L) merit investigation. One abnormality associated with increased risk of coronary artery disease that will not be detected if only cases with hyperlipidemia are studied is hypoalphalipoproteinemia, or deficiency of HDL. Many of the affected individuals have normal levels of both cholesterol and triglycerides in serum and no clinical stigmas to draw the attention of the physician. The argument has been offered that detection of these individuals is unavailing, because there is little that can currently be done to modify levels of HDL in serum. Appreciation that hypoalphalipoproteinemia is present, however, is important if for no other reason than to underscore the importance of controlling other risk factors and perhaps the avoidance of factors that reduce HDL levels, such as cigarette smoking and the use of some drugs. Niacin and certain other drugs can effect major increases in HDL cholesterol in many of these subjects.

B. Identification of Abnormal Patterns: The second step in investigation of hyperlipidemia is determination of the species of lipoproteins that account for the increased content of lipids in serum. In some cases, multiple species may be involved; in others, qualitative properties of the lipoproteins are of diagnostic importance. After identifying the pattern of the lipoprotein abnormality, the physician must search for underlying disorders that cause secondary hyperlipidemias of similar pattern. Such disorders may be the sole cause of the lipoprotein abnormality or may aggravate primary disorders of lipoprotein metabolism. The differentiation of specific primary disorders usually requires additional clinical and genetic information.

The following diagnostic protocol, based upon initial measurement of cholesterol and triglycerides in serum after a 14-hour fast, supplemented by observation of serum and by additional laboratory measurements where essential, will serve as a practical guide in identifying abnormal patterns of lipoprotein distribution. The term "hyperlipidemia" denotes high levels of any class of lipoprotein; "hyperlipemia" denotes high levels of any of the triglyceride-rich lipoproteins.

Case 1: Serum Cholesterol Levels Increased; Triglycerides Normal

(1) If the serum cholesterol level is modestly elevated (up to 260 mg/dL [6.76 mmol/L]), the HDL cholesterol level should be measured. Hyperalphalipoproteinemia (elevated levels of HDL in serum) may account for the observed increase in serum cholesterol level. Hyperalphalipoproteinemia is usually not associated with disease processes. The LDL cholesterol level in serum (in mg/dL) may be estimated by subtracting the HDL cholesterol level and the estimated cholesterol contribution of VLDL from the total serum cholesterol level. The VLDL cholesterol is approximated as one-fifth of the serum triglyceride level.

$$LDL = TC - \left(\frac{TG}{5} + HDL\right)$$

where LDL = LDL cholesterol
TC = Total cholesterol
TG = Triglycerides
HDL = HDL cholesterol

Calculated values of LDL cholesterol over 130 mg/dL (3.38 mmol/L) are clinically significant. If the patient has arteriosclerosis, levels in excess of 90–100 mg/dL should be considered significant.

(2) Because HDL almost never contribute more than 120 mg/dL (3.12 mmol/L) of cholesterol, serum cholesterol levels in excess of 260 mg/dL (6.76 mmol/L) always represent significant hyperlipidemia. Unless the patient has obstructive hepatic disease, the abnormality may be assumed to be due to an increase in low-density lipoproteins. The abnormal lipoprotein of cholestasis, like LDL, is selectively rich in cholesterol. It can be differentiated because it has gamma mobility on electrophoresis in agarose gel and because it stains metachromatically with Sudan black.

Case 2: Predominant Increase of Triglycerides in Serum; Moderate Increase in Cholesterol Level May Be Present

Here it is apparent that the primary abnormality is an increase in the triglyceride-rich VLDL (hyperpre-

Table 20–2. National Cholesterol Education Program: Adult Treatment Guidelines (1993).

	Total Cholesterol	**LDL Cholesterol**
Desirable	< 200 mg/dL (< 5.2 mmol/L)	< 130 mg/dL (< 3.38 mmol/L)
Borderline to high[1]	200–239 mg/dL (5.2–6.2 mmol/L)	130–159 mg/dL (3.38–4.13 mmol/L)
High	≥ 240 mg/dL (≥ 6.24 mmol/L)	≥ 160 mg/dL (≥ 4.16 mmol/L)

[1]Consider as high if coronary heart disease or more than two risk factors are present.

betalipoproteinemia) or chylomicrons (chylomicronemia), or both (mixed lipemia). Because both VLDL and chylomicrons contain free cholesterol in their surface monolayers and a small amount of cholesteryl ester in their cores, the total cholesterol level in serum may be increased, though to a much smaller extent than is the serum triglyceride level. The contribution of cholesterol in these lipoproteins to the total in serum is about 8–25% of the triglyceride content. Low levels of LDL cholesterol often seen in hypertriglyceridemia may largely offset the increase in cholesterol due to the triglyceride-rich lipoproteins, especially in primary chylomicronemia. A white supernatant layer in serum refrigerated overnight reveals the presence of chylomicrons. Because VLDL and chylomicrons compete as substrates in a common removal pathway, chylomicrons will nearly always be present when triglyceride levels exceed 1000 mg/dL (11.5 mmol/L).

Case 3: Cholesterol and Triglyceride Levels in Serum Both Elevated

This pattern can be the result of either of two abnormal lipoprotein distributions. One of these is a combined increase of VLDL (prebeta-lipoproteins), which provide most of the increase in triglycerides, and LDL (beta-lipoproteins), which account for the bulk of the increase in cholesterol in serum. This pattern is termed combined hyperlipidemia and is one of the three phenotypic patterns encountered in kindreds with the disorder termed familial combined hyperlipidemia. The second distribution is an increase of remnant lipoproteins derived from VLDL and chylomicrons. These lipoprotein particles have been partially depleted of triglyceride by lipoprotein lipase and have been enriched with cholesteryl esters by the LCAT system, such that the total content of cholesterol in serum is similar to that of triglycerides. This pattern is almost always an expression of familial dysbetalipoproteinemia. Differentiation of these two patterns requires application of additional diagnostic tests. Presumptive differentiation can be made with high-quality agarose gel electrophoresis. In combined hyperlipidemia, the prebeta- and beta-lipoprotein bands are both increased in staining intensity, but each has its typical electrophoretic mobility, and they are well resolved from one another. Preparative ultracentrifugation of serum in this disorder shows elevated levels of both VLDL and LDL. In contrast, the remnant particles in dysbetalipoproteinemia are distributed in a "broad beta" pattern that obscures the resolution of beta- and prebeta-lipoprotein bands. A substantial portion of the triglyceride-rich lipoproteins shows beta-electrophoretic mobility after separation from serum in the ultracentrifuge (at a density of 1.006 g/cm³), and they have an increased content of cholesterol. Dysbetalipoproteinemia is usually confirmed by the absence of the E-3 and E-4 isoforms of apo-E.

I. CLINICAL DESCRIPTIONS OF PRIMARY & SECONDARY DISORDERS OF LIPOPROTEIN METABOLISM

THE HYPERTRIGLYCERIDEMIAS

Atherogenicity

Certain triglyceride-rich lipoproteins appear to be atherogenic. There is ample clinical evidence that the remnant lipoproteins of dysbetalipoproteinemia are atherogenic. Whereas patients with primary chylomicronemia have limited atherosclerosis despite extremely high levels of triglycerides in serum, there is clinical evidence in support of the atherogenicity of VLDL of small to moderate particle diameter. Furthermore, VLDL have now been demonstrated in the walls of arteries removed at surgery. Impaired capacity of the VLDL of some individuals to accept cholesteryl esters from the LCAT reaction may also contribute to atherogenesis by impeding centripetal transport of cholesterol.

Cause of Pancreatitis

Very high levels of triglycerides in plasma are associated with risk of acute pancreatitis, probably from the local release of free fatty acids and lysolecithin from lipoprotein substrates in the capillary bed of the pancreas. When the concentrations of these lipids exceed the binding capacity of albumin, they could lyse membranes of parenchymal cells, initiating a chemical pancreatitis. Patients who have had previous attacks of pancreatitis appear to be at higher risk. Many patients with lipemia have intermittent episodes of epigastric pain during which serum amylase does not reach levels commonly considered diagnostic for pancreatitis. This is especially true in patients who have had previous attacks. The observation that these episodes frequently evolve into classic pancreatitis suggests that they represent incipient pancreatic inflammation. The progression of pancreatitis can be prevented by rapid reduction of triglyceride levels in serum, which can usually be accomplished by rigorous restriction of dietary fat and institution of other corrective measures. In more threatening cases, parenteral feeding with glucose may be required for a few days. The clinical course of pancreatitis in patients with lipemia is typical of the general experience with this disease. Fatal hemorrhagic pancreatitis occurs in a few; many develop pseudocysts; and some progress to pancreatic exocrine insufficiency or compromised insulinogenic capacity.

Clinical Signs

When triglyceride levels in serum exceed 3000–4000 mg/dL (34.5–46 mmol/L), light scattering by these particles in the blood lends a whitish cast to the venous vascular bed of the retina, a sign known as **lipemia retinalis.** Markedly elevated levels of VLDL or chylomicrons or triglyceride rich lipoproteins in plasma may be associated with the appearance of **eruptive cutaneous xanthomas.** These lesions, filled with foam cells, appear as yellow morbilliform eruptions 2–5 mm in diameter, often with erythematous areolae. They usually occur in clusters on extensor surfaces such as the elbows, knees, and buttocks. They are transient and usually disappear within a few weeks after triglyceride levels are reduced below 2000–3000 mg/dL (23–34.5 mmol/L).

Effects of Hypertriglyceridemia on Laboratory Measurements

Very high levels of triglyceride-rich lipoproteins may introduce important errors in clinical laboratory measurements. Light scattering from these large particles can cause erroneous results in most chemical determinations involving photometric measurements in spite of corrections for blank values. Amylase activity in serum may be inhibited by triglyceride-rich lipoproteins; hence, lipemic specimens should be diluted for measurement of this enzyme. Because the lipoproteins are not permeable to ionic or polar small molecules, their hydrophobic regions constitute a second phase in plasma. When the volume of this phase becomes appreciable, electrolytes (measured by flame photometry) and other hydrophilic species in serum will be underestimated with respect to their true concentration in plasma water. A practical rule for correcting these values is as follows: for each 1000 mg/dL (11.5 mmol/L) of triglyceride in serum, the measured concentrations of all hydrophilic molecules and ions should be adjusted upward by 1%.

PRIMARY HYPERTRIGLYCERIDEMIA

1. DEFICIENCY OF LIPOPROTEIN LIPASE OR ITS COFACTOR

Clinical Findings

A. Symptoms and Signs: Because the clinical expressions of these defects are identical, they will be considered together. Both appear to be transmitted as autosomal recessive traits. On a typical North American diet, lipemia is usually severe (serum triglyceride levels of 2000–25,000 mg/dL) (23–287.5 mmol/L). Hepatomegaly and splenomegaly are frequently present. Foam cells laden with lipid are found in liver, spleen, and bone marrow. Splenic infarct has been described and may be a source of abdominal pain. Hypersplenism with anemia, granu-

locytopenia, and thrombocytopenia can occur. Recurrent epigastric pain and overt pancreatitis are frequently encountered. Eruptive xanthomas may be present. These disorders are present from birth and may be recognized in early infancy or may go unnoticed until an attack of acute pancreatitis occurs or lipemic serum is noted on blood sampling as late as middle age. Patients with these disorders are classically not obese and have normal carbohydrate metabolism, unless pancreatitis impairs insulinogenic capacity. Estrogens intensify the lipemia by stimulating production of VLDL by liver. Therefore, in pregnancy and lactation or during the administration of estrogenic steroids, the risk of pancreatitis increases.

B. Laboratory Findings: These patients have a preponderance of chylomicrons in serum such that the infranatant layer of serum refrigerated overnight may be nearly clear. Many have a moderate increase in VLDL, however, and in pregnant women or those receiving estrogens, a pattern of mixed lipemia is usually present. Levels of low-density lipoproteins in serum are decreased, probably representing the predominant catabolism of VLDL by pathways that do not involve the production of LDL. Levels of HDL are also decreased. A presumptive diagnosis of these disorders can be made by restricting the oral intake of fat to 10–15 g/d for 3–5 days. The triglyceride level of plasma drops precipitously, usually reaching 200–600 mg/dL (2.3–6.9 mmol/L) within 3–4 days. Confirmation of deficiency of lipoprotein lipase is obtained by measurement in vitro of the lipolytic activity of plasma prepared from blood drawn 10 minutes after heparin, 0.2 mg/kg, is injected intravenously. Analysis of lipolysis is carried out with and without 0.5 mol/L sodium chloride, which inhibits lipoprotein lipase but does not suppress the activity of other plasma lipases, including hepatic lipase. Classically, the lipolytic activity of plasma is very low and is similar in the saline-inhibited and saline-uninhibited incubates. Absence of the cofactor protein of LPL, apo-C-II, is the counterpart of deficiency of LPL and can be demonstrated most readily by electrophoresis or isoelectric focusing of the proteins of VLDL.

Treatment

Treatment of primary chylomicronemia is entirely dietary. Intake of fat should be reduced to 10% or less of total calories. In an adult, this represents 15–30 g/d. Because the defect involves lipolysis, both saturated and unsaturated fats must be curtailed. The diet should contain at least 5 g of polyunsaturated fat as a source of essential fatty acids, and an ample supply of fat-soluble vitamins must be provided. Careful adherence to this diet will invariably maintain serum triglyceride levels below 1000 mg/dL (11.2 mmol/L) in the absence of pregnancy, lactation, or the administration of exogenous estrogens. Because this is below the level at which pancreatitis usually occurs, compliant patients with these disorders are at low risk.

2. ENDOGENOUS & MIXED LIPEMIAS

Etiology & Pathogenesis

Endogenous lipemia (primary hyperprebetalipoproteinemia) and mixed lipemia probably both result from several genetically determined disorders. The occurrence of multiple cases in a kindred is the basis for considering them primary. Thus, a number of "sporadic cases" may be similar, only lacking evidence of familial occurrence. Because VLDL and chylomicrons are competing substrates in the intravascular lipolytic pathway, saturating levels of VLDL will cause an impedance in the removal of chylomicrons. Therefore, as the severity of endogenous lipemia increases, a pattern of mixed lipemia may supervene. In other cases, the pattern of mixed lipemia appears to be present continuously. Though specific pathophysiologic mechanisms remain obscure, certain familial patterns are known. In all forms, factors that increase the rate of secretion of VLDL from liver aggravate the hypertriglyceridemia—ie, obesity with insulin resistance, or the appearance of fully developed non-insulin-dependent diabetes mellitus (NIDDM); ethanol ingestion; and the use of exogenous estrogens. Studies of VLDL turnover indicate that either increased production or impaired removal of VLDL may be operative in different individuals. It appears that a substantial number of patients with mixed lipemia have partial defects in catabolism of triglyceride-rich lipoproteins. Increases in production rates of VLDL secondary to excess caloric intake, ethanol, or estrogens tend not to be accompanied by increased removal, as in normal individuals, but result in increased levels of circulating triglycerides. Some patients with mixed lipemia have decreased levels of lipoprotein lipase in plasma after a heparin stimulus, which may be of importance in this regard. Most patients with significant endogenous or mixed lipemia have the hypertrophic form of obesity, in which there is a reduced population of insulin receptors on cell membranes associated with impaired effectiveness of insulin. Mobilization of free fatty acids is maintained at a higher than normal rate, providing an increased flux of fatty acids to the liver, in turn increasing the secretion of triglyceride-rich VLDL.

Clinical Findings

Clinical features of these forms of hypertriglyceridemia depend upon severity and include eruptive xanthomas, lipemia retinalis, recurrent epigastric pain, and acute pancreatitis (described above). One constellation of clinical features that may be monogenic is endogenous lipemia with obesity, insulin resistance, elevated baseline levels of insulin, hyperglycemia, and hyperuricemia. There is also a tendency toward the development of hypertension in such patients.

Treatment

The primary mode of treatment is dietary. In the short term, severe restriction of total fat intake will usually result in a rapid decline of serum triglyceride levels to 1000–3000 mg/dL (11.2–33.6 mmol/L), averting pancreatitis. The objective of long-term dietary management is reduction to ideal body weight. Because ethanol causes significant augmentation of VLDL production, abstinence is important.

If weight loss is achieved, the serum triglycerides almost always show a marked response, often approaching normal values. When the fall in triglyceride levels is not satisfactory, gemfibrozil or nicotinic acid, singly or in combination, will usually produce further reductions. (See Treatment of Hyperlipidemia, below.)

3. FAMILIAL COMBINED HYPERLIPIDEMIA

Etiology

Epidemiologic studies of the kindreds of survivors of myocardial infarction revealed this heredofamilial disorder, which is the most common form of hyperlipidemia. The underlying process appears to be overproduction of VLDL. Some of the affected individuals have increased levels of both VLDL and LDL in serum (combined hyperlipidemia); some have increased levels of only VLDL or LDL. Without family studies, the latter two patterns would not be identified as belonging with this syndrome. Patterns in the serum of an individual patient may change with time. It is known that a mating of an individual having any one of the three phenotypic patterns with a normal individual can result in the appearance of one of the other patterns. Children in these kindreds may have hyperlipidemia, but the disorder is usually not fully expressed until adulthood.

Clinical Findings

Neither tendinous nor cutaneous xanthomas other than xanthelasma occur. Available data suggest that this disorder is inherited as a mendelian dominant trait. It appears that the factors that increase the severity of hypertriglyceridemia in other disorders aggravate the lipemia in this syndrome as well.

Treatment

The risk of coronary vascular disease is significantly increased in these patients, and therefore they should be treated aggressively with diet and drugs. Lipemia responds to gemfibrozil, but this may increase LDL levels (beta shift). Hence, niacin may be a better choice. Patients with increased LDL levels respond to bile acid-binding resins but may then have increases in VLDL. Therefore, the combination of a resin and niacin is frequently required. HMG-CoA reductase inhibitors are effective in lowering LDL levels. The addition of niacin to the regimen can then bring VLDL levels under control. (See Treatment of Hyperlipidemia, below.)

4. FAMILIAL DYSBETALIPOPROTEINEMIA (Broad Beta Disease, Type III Hyperlipoproteinemia)

Etiology & Pathogenesis

A permissive genetic constitution for this disease occurs commonly, but expression of hyperlipoproteinemia apparently requires additional genetic or environmental determinants. The molecular basis of this disorder is the presence of isoforms of apo-E that cannot interact normally with high-affinity receptors. In its fully expressed form, the lipoprotein pattern is dominated by the accumulation of remnants of VLDL and chylomicrons. Two populations of VLDL are usually present: normal prebeta-lipoproteins and remnants with beta-electrophoretic mobility. Remnant particles of intermediate density are also present. Characteristically, levels of LDL in serum are decreased, probably reflecting interruption of the normal transformation of VLDL remnants to LDL. The primary defect appears to involve the uptake of remnants of triglyceride-rich lipoproteins from plasma. Chylomicron remnants are frequently present in serum obtained after a 14-hour fast even when total serum triglycerides are only 300–600 mg/dL (3.4–6.7 mmol/L). All the remnant particles are enriched in cholesteryl esters such that the level of cholesterol in serum is often as high as the level of triglycerides. The "broad beta" electrophoretic pattern of VLDL is highly suggestive of familial dysbetalipoproteinemia. However, this pattern is seen also in hypothyroidism, resolving lipemias of other origins, and certain disorders involving immunoglobulin-lipoprotein complexes. Absence of the E-3 and E-4 genes on allele-specific screening of genomic DNA or of the corresponding proteins on isoelectric focusing of VLDL proteins, confirms the diagnosis. Whereas homozygosity for apo-E-2 is present in about 1% of the population, the incidence of clinical hyperlipidemia among these patients is much smaller. Additional mutations of apo-E that cannot be distinguished from E-3 by isoelectric focusing are now known to result in dysbetalipoproteinemia. Some of these cause hyperlipidemia in the heterozygous state, a disorder termed dominant dysbetalipoproteinemia.

Clinical Findings

Hyperlipidemia and clinical stigmas are not usually evident before age 20. In younger patients with hyperlipidemia, hypothyroidism or obesity is likely to be present. Adults frequently have tuberous or tuberoeruptive xanthomas. Both tend to occur on extensor surfaces, especially elbows and knees. Tuberoeruptive xanthomas are pink or yellowish skin nodules 3–8 mm in diameter that often become confluent. Tuberous xanthomas—reddish or orange, often shiny nodules up to 3 cm in diameter—are usually moveable and nontender. Another type, planar xanthomas of the palmar creases, strongly suggests dysbetalipoproteinemia. The skin creases assume an orange color from deposition of carotenoids and other lipids. They occasionally are raised above the level of adjacent skin and are not tender. (Planar xanthomas are also seen in cholestatic disease.) (Figure 20–4.)

Some patients have impaired glucose tolerance, which is usually associated with higher levels of blood lipids. Obesity is commonly present and tends to aggravate the lipemia. Patients with the genetic constitution for dysbetalipoproteinemia often develop severe hyperlipidemia if they are hypothyroid.

Atherosclerotic disease of the coronary and peripheral vessels occurs with increased frequency, and the prevalence of disease of the iliac and femoral vessels is especially high.

Treatment

Management includes a weight reduction diet providing a reduced intake of cholesterol, saturated fat, and alcohol. When the hyperlipidemia does not respond satisfactorily to diet, gemfibrozil or niacin in low doses is usually effective. (See Treatment of Hyperlipidemia, below.)

SECONDARY HYPERTRIGLYCERIDEMIA

1. DIABETES MELLITUS

In patients with insulin-dependent diabetes mellitus (IDDM), levels of VLDL in plasma are frequently elevated despite the regular use of insulin, reflecting the difficulty of control of carbohydrate metabolism in this disorder.

Pathogenesis

The severe lipemia associated with absence or marked insufficiency of insulin is attributable to deficiency of LPL activity, because this enzyme is induced by insulin. The administration of insulin in such cases usually restores triglyceride levels to normal within a few days. However, if massive fatty liver is present, weeks may be required for the VLDL levels to return to normal while the liver secretes its triglyceride into plasma. Conversion of massive amounts of VLDL to LDL, as the impedance of VLDL catabolism is relieved, leads to marked accumulation of LDL that may persist for weeks. This

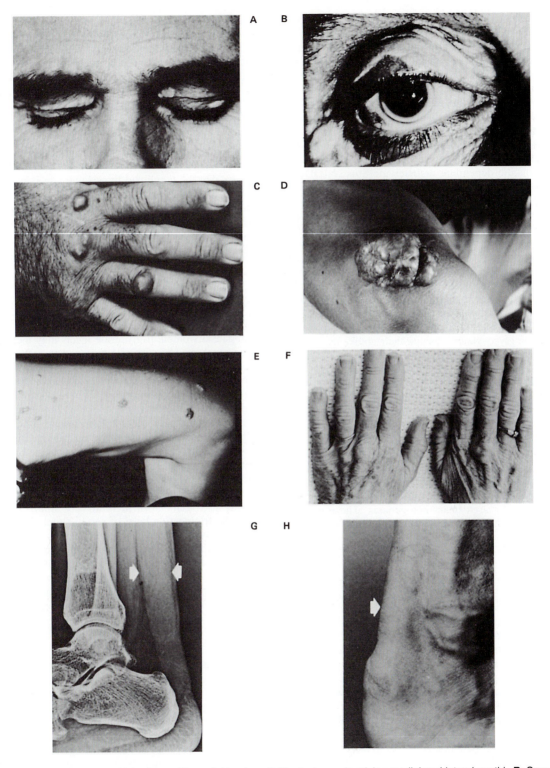

Figure 20–4. Clinical manifestations of hyperlipidemias. ***A:*** Xanthelasma involving medial and lateral canthi. ***B:*** Severe xanthelasma and arcus corneae. ***C:*** Tuberous xanthomas. ***D:*** Large tuberous xanthoma of elbow. ***E:*** Eruptive xanthomas, singly and in rosettes. ***F:*** Xanthomas of extensor tendons of the hands. ***G:*** Xeroradiogram of Achilles tendon xanthoma. ***H:*** Xanthoma of Achilles tendon. (Normal Achilles tendons do not exceed 7 mm in diameter in the region between the calcaneus and the point at which the tendon fibers begin to radiate toward their origins.)

phenomenon may lead to a spurious diagnosis of hypercholesterolemia.

The moderately high levels of VLDL seen in diabetes under average control probably reflect chiefly an increased flux of FFA to liver that stimulates production of triglycerides and their secretion in VLDL. In addition to VLDL, LDL levels are also somewhat increased in insulin-dependent diabetics under poor control, probably accounting in part for their increased risk of coronary heart disease. Mild increases in VLDL and in FFA occur in many individuals with non-insulin-dependent diabetes mellitus (NIDDM). Some have much higher levels of VLDL, suggesting that an additional genetic factor predisposing to lipemia is present. Still another cause of lipemic diabetes is the compromised insulinogenic capacity that can result from acute pancreatitis in individuals with severe primary lipemias. The deficiency may be severe enough to require exogenous insulin, often only in small doses. In diabetics who develop nephrosis as a consequence of their microvascular disease, the secondary lipemia of nephrosis compounds their hypertriglyceridemia. In hyperglycemia, lipoproteins become glycosylated, causing their uptake by macrophages.

Clinical Findings

Lipemia may be very severe, with elevated levels of both VLDL and chylomicrons when control is poor. Lipemic patients usually have ketoacidosis when they are insulin-deficient, but lipemia can occur in its absence. Patients with IDDM who have been chronically undertreated with insulin may have mobilized most of the triglyceride from peripheral adipose tissue, so that they no longer have sufficient substrate for significant ketogenesis. These emaciated individuals may have severe lipemia and striking hepatomegaly.

Treatment

The rigid control of blood glucose levels, which can be attained with continuous subcutaneous insulin infusion, is associated with sustained normalization of levels of both LDL and VLDL.

The lipemia of IDDM responds well to control of the underlying disorder of carbohydrate metabolism. In obese, insulin-resistant individuals, weight loss is the key to treatment. Diets containing a large fraction of calories as carbohydrates are actually well tolerated, allowing a decrease in the burden of chylomicron triglycerides in plasma (see Chapter 18).

2. UREMIA

Uremia is associated with modest isolated increases in VLDL. The most important underlying mechanisms are probably insulin resistance and impairment of catabolism of VLDL. Many uremic patients are also nephrotic. The additional effects of nephrosis upon lipoprotein metabolism may produce a combined hyperlipoproteinemia. Patients who have had renal transplants may be receiving glucocorticoids, which induce elevated concentrations of LDL.

3. CORTICOSTEROID EXCESS

In endogenous Cushing's syndrome, there is insulin resistance, and levels of LDL are increased. It appears that the combined hyperlipidemia is primarily due to increased secretion of VLDL, which is then catabolized to LDL. More severe lipemia ensues when steroidogenic diabetes appears, reducing catabolism of triglyceride-rich lipoproteins via the LPL pathway.

4. EXOGENOUS ESTROGENS

When estrogens are administered to normal premenopausal women, triglyceride levels may increase by as much as 15%. This is believed to reflect increased hepatic production of VLDL. Paradoxically, estrogens increase the efficiency of catabolism of triglyceride-rich lipoproteins. Whereas estrogens tend to induce insulin resistance, it is not clear that this is an important mechanism, because certain nortestosterone derivatives decrease plasma triglyceride levels despite the induction of appreciable insulin resistance.

Certain individuals, usually with preexisting mild lipemia, show marked hypertriglyceridemia when receiving estrogens even in relatively small doses. Thus, the triglyceride level of serum should be measured in any woman receiving exogenous estrogens. Contraceptive combinations with predominant progestational effects produce less hypertriglyceridemia than purely estrogenic compounds. Transdermal delivery of estrogen probably results in lesser increases in VLDL secretion because it avoids the hepatic first-pass effect.

5. ALCOHOL INGESTION

Ingestion of appreciable amounts of alcohol may not necessarily result in significantly elevated levels of triglycerides in serum, but many alcoholics are lipemic. Furthermore, alcohol profoundly increases triglyceride levels in patients with primary and secondary hyperlipemias. In **Zieve's syndrome,** the lipemia is associated with hemolytic anemia and hyperbilirubinemia. Because LCAT originates in liver, severe hepatic parenchymal dysfunction may lead to deficiency in the activity of this enzyme. A resultant accumulation of unesterified cholesterol in erythrocyte membranes may account for the hemolysis seen in Zieve's syndrome.

Ethanol is converted to acetate, exerting a sparing effect on the oxidation of fatty acids. The fatty acids are incorporated into triglyceride in liver, resulting in hepatomegaly due to fatty infiltration and in marked enhancement of secretion of VLDL. In many individuals, there is sufficient adaptive increase in the removal capacity for triglycerides from plasma that triglyceride levels tend to return toward normal if alcohol intake is continued over a period of weeks. In individuals in whom the adaptive response is impaired, marked lipemia may ensue.

6. NEPHROSIS

The hyperlipidemia of nephrosis is biphasic. Before serum albumin levels fall below 2 g/dL, levels of LDL increase selectively. This is probably a result of increased secretion of protein by liver to compensate for that lost in the urine. The synthesis and secretion of VLDL appears to be coupled to that of albumin. The increased flux of VLDL from liver increases production of LDL. As albumin levels fall below 1–2 g/dL, lipemia ensues. Impaired hydrolysis of triglycerides by LPL is due to lack of albumin as an FFA receptor. Free fatty acids, which normally circulate complexed to albumin, bind to lipoproteins when albumin levels are low. The ability of these altered lipoproteins to undergo hydrolysis is thus impaired. In nephrosis, VLDL contain abundant cholesteryl esters.

Because coronary vascular disease is quite prevalent in patients with long-standing nephrotic syndrome, treatment of the hyperlipidemia appears to be indicated, though few studies of the effect of treatment have been reported. The hyperlipidemia is relatively resistant to diet. Gemfibrozil may precipitate myopathy even in relatively small doses. Bile acid-binding resins, niacin, and reductase inhibitors are useful. Nephrotic patients may be deficient in tryptophan, and oral administration of this amino acid has been reported to ameliorate the hypertriglyceridemia.

7. GLYCOGEN STORAGE DISEASE

In type I glycogenosis, insulin secretion is decreased, leading to an increased flux of FFA to liver, where a substantial fraction is converted to triglycerides, causing increased secretion of VLDL. The low levels of insulin in plasma also are the probable cause of reduced activity of LPL, which may cause impaired removal of triglycerides from serum. The fatty liver in these patients tends to progress to cirrhosis.

Frequent small feedings help to maintain blood glucose levels and ameliorate the lipemia. A program of nocturnal nasogastric drip feeding is of considerable benefit in this disease. Other forms of hepatic glycogen storage disease may be associated with elevated levels of VLDL and LDL in serum.

8. HYPOPITUITARISM & ACROMEGALY

Part of the hyperlipidemia of hypopituitarism is attributable to secondary hypothyroidism, but hypertriglyceridemia persists in the face of thyroxine replacement therapy. Dwarfism due to isolated deficiency of growth hormone is associated with higher than normal levels of both LDL and VLDL. Decreased insulin levels may be the major underlying defect; however, deficiency of growth hormone may impair the disposal of FFA by oxidation and ketogenesis in liver, favoring synthesis of triglycerides. Mild hypertriglyceridemia is often associated with acromegaly, probably resulting from insulin resistance. Though growth hormone acutely stimulates lipolysis in adipose tissue, FFA levels are normal in acromegaly.

9. HYPOTHYROIDISM

Whereas significant hypothyroidism tends to produce elevated levels of LDL in serum in nearly all individuals, only a fraction will develop hypertriglyceridemia. The increase in LDL levels results at least in part from decreased numbers of B-100:E receptors on cell membranes, although decreased conversion of cholesterol to bile acids may also contribute. Lipemia, when present, is usually mild, though serum triglyceride levels in excess of 3000 mg/dL (34.5 mmol/L) can occur. The underlying mechanisms are not fully understood, though it is probable that impaired removal of triglycerides from blood is involved, perhaps related to decreased activity of hepatic lipase. Increased content of cholesteryl esters and apo-E in the triglyceride-rich lipoproteins suggests that accumulation of remnant particles occurs. Hypothyroidism, even of very mild degree, causes expression of hyperlipidemia in otherwise latent carriers of familial dysbetalipoproteinemia.

10. IMMUNOGLOBULIN-LIPOPROTEIN COMPLEX DISORDERS

Both polyclonal and monoclonal hypergammaglobulinemias may cause hypertriglyceridemia. IgG, IgM, and IgA have each been involved. Of the underlying monoclonal disorders causing hypertriglyceridemia, myeloma and macroglobulinemia are the most important, but lymphomas and lymphocytic leukemias have also been implicated. Lupus erythematosus and other autoimmune disorders have been associated with the polyclonal type. Binding of heparin by immunoglobulin, with resulting inhibition of LPL, can cause severe mixed lipemia. More commonly, the triglyceride-rich lipoproteins have an abnormally high density, probably as a result of bound immunoglobulin, though some may be remnant-like particles. These complexes, which bind lipophilic stains, usually have gamma mobility on electrophoresis in agarose gel.

Xanthomatosis associated with immunoglobulin complex disease includes tuberous and eruptive xanthomas, xanthelasma, and planar xanthomas of large areas of skin. The latter are otherwise seen only in patients with cholestasis. Deposits of lipid-rich hyaline material can occur in the lamina propria of the intestine, causing malabsorption and protein-losing enteropathy. Circulating immunoglobulin-lipoprotein complexes can fix complement, leading to hypocomplementemia. In such patients, administration of whole blood or plasma can cause anaphylaxis. Hence, washed red cells or albumin are recommended when blood volume replacement is required.

Treatment is directed at the underlying disorder. Because the critical temperature of cryoprecipitation of some of these complexes is close to body temperature, plasmapheresis should be done at a temperature above the critical temperature measured in the serum of individual patients.

THE PRIMARY HYPERCHOLESTEROLEMIAS

FAMILIAL HYPERCHOLESTEROLEMIA

Etiology & Pathogenesis

This disorder, which in its heterozygous form occurs in approximately one in 500 individuals in the USA, is transmitted as a mendelian dominant trait with very high penetrance. Because half of first-degree relatives are affected, including children, all members of a proband's family should be screened for this disorder. Hypercholesterolemia, representing a selective increase in LDL, exists from birth. Levels of LDL tend to increase during childhood and adolescence such that levels of serum cholesterol in adult heterozygotes usually vary from about 260 to 400 mg/dL (6.7–10.4 mmol/L). Aside from an increase in content of cholesteryl esters, the LDL are normal in structure. VLDL levels are usually normal, though some individuals, especially those in kindreds in which hypertriglyceridemia is present, may have higher than normal levels of VLDL and IDL.

The underlying defect is a deficiency of normal high-affinity receptor sites for LDL on cell membranes. A number of genetic defects affecting the structure, translation, modification, or transport of the B-100:E receptor protein have been identified. In some of these defects, the gene product either does not appear on the cell surface or completely lacks receptor function. The gene products associated with other defects appear as kinetically impaired receptors.

Some individuals have combined heterozygosity. In cases in which a kinetic mutant is combined with an ablative mutant, the severity of the hypercholesterolemia is greater than that seen in simple heterozygosity, usually in the range of 500–800 mg/dL (13–20.8 mmol/L). Those patients who are homozygous for genes that produce no effective receptors have extremely severe hypercholesterolemia (approaching 1000 mg/dL [26 mmol/L] or greater) and fulminant arteriosclerosis.

Some patients who are heterozygous for receptor defects may have serum levels of LDL that are only mildly elevated or, even less commonly, in the normal range. Mitigating factors, perhaps involving decreased production rates for VLDL and LDL, may exist in such individuals. Production rates for LDL generally appear to be nearly normal in heterozygotes but are increased in the homozygous state, largely owing to increased conversion of VLDL to LDL. In the heterozygote, a greater fraction of LDL is removed by non-receptor-dependent mechanisms than in normal subjects. In homozygotes, all removal of LDL proceeds through such pathways.

Clinical Findings

One of the most striking clinical features that may be present is tendinous xanthomatosis. The xanthomas, which usually appear in early adulthood, cause a broadening or fusiform mass in the tendon. They can occur in almost any tendon but are most readily detected in the Achilles and patellar tendons and in the extensor tendons of the hands (Figure 20–4). Patients who are physically active may complain of achillodynia. Arcus corneae (Figure 20–4B) may occur as early as the third decade. Xanthelasma (Figure 20–4A) may also be present. Both arcus and xanthelasma are seen in individuals who do not have hyperlipidemia, however. Coronary atherosclerosis tends to occur prematurely in heterozygotes. It is particularly prominent in individuals who are relatively deficient in HDL. It is probable that this represents a coincident inheritance of both traits. The homozygous form of familial hypercholesterolemia is catastrophic. Xanthomatosis progresses rapidly. Patients may have tuberous xanthomas (Figure 20–4C and D) and elevated plaque-like xanthomas of the extremities, buttocks, interdigital webs, and aortic valves.

Homozygotes may have overt coronary disease in the first decade of life.

A serum cholesterol level in excess of 350 mg/dL (9.1 mmol/L) in the absence of significant hypertriglyceridemia makes the diagnosis of heterozygous familial hypercholesterolemia likely. Significantly lower levels can occur in heterozygotes if mitigating genes are present. The presence of affected first-degree relatives is supportive of this diagnosis, especially if no other phenotypes of hyperlipidemia are present in the family that would suggest familial combined disease. The finding of tendon xanthomas is nearly pathognomonic—betasitosterolemia and cerebrotendinous xanthomatosis (cholestanolosis) and ligand-defective apo-B excepted. Although the cholesterol content of serum from umbilical cord blood is usually elevated in patients with this disorder, the diagnosis is most easily established by measuring serum cholesterol levels after the first year of life.

Treatment

Treatment with various single-drug regimens is of moderate benefit in decreasing LDL levels in serum. However, complete normalization of LDL levels can be achieved in most compliant heterozygotes with one of the binary combinations involving reductase inhibitors, niacin, or bile acid sequestrants. Serum cholesterol levels less than 200 mg/dL are often seen with a ternary combination of these drugs. Treatment of homozygotes is extremely difficult. Partial control may be achieved with portacaval shunt or immunopheresis in conjunction with niacin. Reductase inhibitors are only useful if some receptor function is present. Striking reduction of LDL levels is observed after liver transplantation, illustrating the important role of hepatic receptors in LDL clearance. (See Treatment of Hyperlipidemia, below.)

FAMILIAL COMBINED HYPERLIPIDEMIA

In some individuals in kindreds of this disorder (see Primary Hypertriglyceridemia, above), LDL and IDL will be the only lipoproteins that are elevated. This pattern may vary in an individual over time, and elevated VLDL alone or combined elevations of LDL and VLDL may be observed in the patient or the patient's relatives. Some affected children express hyperlipidemia. In contrast to most cases of familial hypercholesterolemia, the serum cholesterol level may often be lower than 350 mg/dL, and neither tendinous nor tuberous xanthomas occur. Studies of kindreds suggest an autosomal dominant mechanism of transmission. Coronary atherosclerosis is accelerated in this disorder, which is sufficiently prevalent to be observed in about 10% of survivors of myocardial infarction. The underlying biochemical mechanism appears to involve increased synthesis of apo-B-100.

Treatment of the hypercholesterolemia should begin with diet and niacin. It may be necessary to add resin or a reductase inhibitor to normalize levels of LDL.

LP(A) HYPERLIPOPROTEINEMIA

A lipoprotein that normally comprises a very minor fraction of circulating lipoproteins, Lp(a), is present in high concentrations in some individuals whose levels of LDL may also be elevated or nearly normal. Upon ultracentrifugation, this lipoprotein ranges on both sides of the density that discriminates LDL from HDL. It contains apo-B-100 and the Lp(a) protein. It is identified in LDL or HDL fractions obtained by ultracentrifugation by its prebeta-electrophoretic mobility. A number of studies implicate it as an independent risk factor for coronary artery disease. Plasma levels of the Lp(a) lipoprotein can be measured by immunoassay. Whereas most individuals have levels below 10 mg/dL, some may have as much as 200 mg/dL. Levels above 30–50 mg/dL clearly present an additional risk of coronary disease. Levels of Lp(a) primarily reflect genetic determinants. Preliminary results indicate that niacin is the most effective drug used in treatment.

FAMILIAL LIGAND-DEFECTIVE APO B

Mutations substituting glutamine for arginine at residue 3500 and cysteine for arginine at residue 3531 in the apo-B protein have been described in patients presenting with elevated levels of LDL. These mutations impair the ability of LDL to bind to the LDL receptor, thus representing a mirror image of familial hypercholesterolemia. These mutations together can be as common as receptor defects and thus may be found in compound states with familial hypercholesterolemia. The hypercholesterolemia with ligand defects alone is generally less severe than in familial hypercholesterolemia because the removal of VLDL remnants is normal, resulting in a lower production of LDL than in familial hypercholesterolemia. The patients may have tendon xanthomas and are at increased risk for coronary disease. Response to reductase inhibitors varies, but many patients show some resistance because up-regulation of receptors cannot correct the defect completely though it can decrease LDL production (because IDL are endocytosed by liver via interaction of the LDL receptor with apo-E).

SECONDARY HYPERCHOLESTEROLEMIA

HYPOTHYROIDISM

The typical disorder of lipoproteins associated with hypothyroidism is high LDL and IDL concentrations. Increased content of apo-E in the VLDL and IDL is consistent with an increase in remnant particles in plasma. In addition to elevated LDL, some patients may have lipemia as described in the section on secondary hyperlipemia. The hyperlipidemia of hypothyroidism may occur in individuals with no overt signs or symptoms of decreased thyroid function. Biliary excretion of cholesterol and bile acids is depressed; however, cholesterol biosynthesis is also decreased. Cholesterol stores in tissues appear to be increased, though the number of B-100:E receptors on cells is decreased. Activity of hepatic lipase is also markedly decreased. Atherogenesis is accelerated by myxedema. The hyperlipidemia responds dramatically to treatment with thyroxine.

NEPHROSIS

As described in the section on secondary hypertriglyceridemias, nephrosis produces a biphasic hyperlipoproteinemia. The earliest alteration of lipoproteins in nephrosis is elevation of LDL. Increased secretion of VLDL by liver is probably involved. Because the lipids of the lipoprotein surfaces are altered by enrichment with sphingomyelin, lysolecithin, and FFA, the catabolism of LDL could be impaired. Perhaps the low metabolic rate in affected patients introduces metabolic changes similar to those associated with hypothyroidism. The hyperlipidemia may be an important element in the markedly increased risk of atherosclerotic heart disease in these patients. The treatment of choice appears to be reductase inhibitors or bile acid-binding resins with niacin.

IMMUNOGLOBULIN DISORDERS

One of the lipoprotein abnormalities that can be associated with monoclonal gammopathy is elevation of LDL. A "gamma lipoprotein" that is a stable complex of immunoglobulin and lipoprotein may be observed in agarose gel electrophoretograms of the sera of some patients. Cryoprecipitation, often in the temperature range encountered in peripheral tissues when the environmental temperature is low, may occur. Patients may have symptoms from the vascular effect of complement fixation resulting from complex formation and may have hyperviscosity syndrome from the elevated immunoglobulins per se. Planar xanthomas may occur.

Treatment is directed at the underlying process. Plasmapheresis is often effective. If cryoprecipitation occurs at critical temperatures near or above room temperature, the procedure must be carried out in a special warm environment. Transfusion of whole blood or serum may be dangerous in these patients because of rapid production of anaphylatoxins from fresh complement in the serum, resulting from interaction with circulating antibody-antigen complexes. This risk can be minimized by the use of packed red blood cells and albumin in place of whole blood.

ANOREXIA NERVOSA

About 40% of patients with anorexia nervosa have elevated LDL in serum, and levels of cholesterol in serum may reach 400–600 mg/dL (10.4–15.6 mmol/L). The hyperlipidemia, which persists despite correction of hypothyroidism, is probably a result of decreased fecal excretion of bile acids and cholesterol.

Serum lipoproteins return to normal when proper nutrition is restored.

CHOLESTASIS

The hyperlipidemia associated with the obstruction of biliary flow is complex. It occurs with either extrahepatic or intrahepatic obstruction, though it tends to be more severe with the former. Levels of cholesterol in serum exceeding 400 mg/dL (10.4 mmol/L) usually are associated with extrahepatic obstruction or with intrahepatic tumor. Several types of abnormal lipoproteins are present in plasma. The most abundant, termed LP-X, is a bilayer vesicle composed of unesterified cholesterol and lecithin, with associated apolipoproteins but not apo-B. LP-X is apparent on electrophoresis of lipoproteins in agarose gel as a band of zero to gamma mobility which shows metachromatic staining with Sudan black. It is these vesicular particles that cause the serum phospholipid and unesterified cholesterol content to be extremely high. There is another abnormal species called LP-Y, which contains appreciable amounts of triglycerides and carries apo-B. It may represent a remnant particle derived from chylomicrons. The LDL in cholestasis also contain an unusually large amount of triglycerides.

Patients with cholestasis may have planar xanthomas of the skin, especially at sites of minor trauma, and xanthomas of the palmar creases. Occasionally, eruptive xanthomas are present. Xanthomatous involvement of nerves may lead to symptoms of peripheral neuropathy, and the abnormal lipoproteins may be atherogenic. Whereas bilirubin levels are nearly normal in some patients with chronic cholestasis, all have elevated serum alkaline phosphatase activity.

Neuropathy is the chief indication for treatment of the hyperlipidemia. Bile acid-binding resins are of some value, whereas fibric acid derivatives may cause an increase in serum cholesterol levels. Plasmapheresis is the most effective treatment. Large doses of vitamin E are indicated to overcome severe impairment of absorption.

THE PRIMARY HYPOLIPIDEMIAS

Although the clinician is confronted infrequently by the problem of a striking deficiency in plasma lipids, it is important to recognize the primary and secondary hypolipidemias. A serum cholesterol level less than 110 mg/dL (2.9 mmol/L) in an adult patient is noteworthy. Since levels of triglycerides in normal fasting serum may be as low as 25 mg/dL (0.29 mmol/L), significance is limited to cases in which they are virtually absent.

PRIMARY HYPOLIPIDEMIA DUE TO DEFICIENCY OF HIGH-DENSITY LIPOPROTEINS

1. TANGIER DISEASE

Etiology & Pathogenesis

Severe deficiency of HDL occurs in the primary disorder known as Tangier disease. Heterozygotes lack clinical signs but have about one-half or less of the normal complement of HDL and apo-A-I in plasma. Homozygotes lack normal plasma HDL, and apo-A-I and apo-A-II are present at extremely low levels. Serum cholesterol levels are usually below 120 mg/dL (3.12 mmol/L) and may be half that value. Mild hypertriglyceridemia is usually present. The genetic defect probably involves alteration of catabolism of HDL. LDL are greatly enriched in triglycerides.

Clinical Findings

The clinical features of this rare autosomal recessive disease include large, orange-colored, lipid-filled tonsils, accumulation of cholesteryl esters in the reticuloendothelial system, and an episodic and recurrent peripheral neuropathy with predominant motor weakness in the later stages. The course of the disease is benign in early childhood, but the neuropa-

thy may appear as early as age 8. Cholesteryl ester accumulates most prominently in peripheral nerve sheaths. Carotenoid coloration may be apparent in pharyngeal and rectal mucous membranes. Splenomegaly and corneal infiltration may also be present. There is some increase in risk of coronary arteriosclerosis.

Treatment

Because much of the lamellar lipoprotein material in plasma is believed to originate in chylomicrons, restriction of dietary fats and cholesterol is suggested.

2. FAMILIAL HYPOALPHALIPOPROTEINEMIA

Etiology & Pathogenesis

This phenotypic pattern is a partial deficiency of HDL in serum that may involve heterogeneous mechanisms. These presumed constitutional disorders must be differentiated from the condition in which moderately low levels of HDL cholesterol are seen in individuals consuming a diet very low in fat, perhaps reflecting decreased generation of HDL from chylomicrons. For example, white and Asian men on such diets usually have HDL cholesterol levels of 38–44 mg/dL (1–1.1 mmol/L) by ultracentrifugal analysis, in contrast to a median value of 49 mg/dL (1.3 mmol/L) when consuming a typical North American diet. Such levels are common in Asiatic populations and among vegetarians, where the risk of coronary disease is small. The physician must further interpret HDL cholesterol levels in the light of the amount of triglyceride-rich lipoproteins in plasma. Because triglyceride is progressively substituted for cholesteryl esters in the core of HDL as the plasma triglyceride level rises, the HDL cholesterol will decrease as an inverse logarithmic function of the triglyceride level. This decrease causes an apparent decrease in HDL levels, since cholesterol is the component of HDL that is commonly measured.

Etiologic Factor in Coronary Disease

Clinical experience suggests that familial hypoalphalipoproteinemia is fairly common and is an important risk factor in coronary vascular disease. This abnormality may be the only apparent risk factor in many cases of premature coronary atherosclerosis. Furthermore, it may accelerate the appearance of coronary disease in patients with familial hypercholesterolemia or other hyperlipidemias. Hypoalphalipoproteinemia shows a strong familial incidence. Although several mechanisms and modes of transmission may be involved, many kindreds show distributions consistent with autosomal dominance.

Treatment

Increases in HDL cholesterol levels in several coronary intervention trials have been independently associated with plaque regression. Only limited means of raising HDL levels are at hand. Recent findings that HDL exist in as many as eight discrete species further complicate this problem. It is not yet known which of these species may be involved in protecting against arteriosclerosis or whether levels of those species can be increased. Thus, though alcohol ingestion can increase total HDL levels in some individuals, it appears that the effect is primarily on the HDL_3 ultracentrifugal fraction, which correlates poorly with decreased risk in epidemiologic studies. Therefore, no recommendation for increased alcohol consumption should be made on this account.

Heavy exercise is associated with increases in HDL in some individuals, but exercise must be approached with caution in patients who may have coronary disease. Niacin increases total HDL levels in many subjects, chiefly in the HDL_2 ultracentrifugal fraction.

Perhaps the most important reason at present for measuring HDL cholesterol levels is to identify patients who are at increased risk. Thus, just as with patients who have premature vascular disease or a family history of early arteriosclerosis, patients with low HDL levels should be treated more aggressively for elevated levels of lipoproteins that appear to be atherogenic (LDL, IDL, and VLDL). Furthermore, vigorous efforts should be directed at the control of other risk factors, such as hypertension. Smoking is known to decrease HDL cholesterol levels significantly. Modest lowering of HDL cholesterol levels by beta-adrenergic blocking agents must be weighed against the need for these drugs in treating cardiovascular disease.

3. DEFICIENCY OF LCAT

Another disorder associated with low serum levels of HDL is lecithin-cholesterol acyltransferase deficiency. This rare autosomal recessive disorder is not expressed in clinical or biochemical form in the heterozygote. In the homozygote, clinical characteristics are variable. The diagnosis is usually made in adult life, though corneal opacities may begin in childhood. Proteinuria may be an early sign. Deposits of unesterified cholesterol and phospholipid in the renal microvasculature lead to progressive loss of nephrons and ultimate renal failure. Many patients have mild to moderate normochromic anemia with target cells. Hyperbilirubinemia or peripheral neuropathy may be present. Red blood cell lipid composition is abnormal, with increased content of unesterified cholesterol and lecithin. Most have elevated plasma triglycerides (200–1000 mg/dL [2.3–11.2

mmol/L]), and levels of serum cholesterol vary from low normal to 500 mg/dL (13 mmol/L), only a small fraction of which is esterified. The large triglyceride-rich lipoproteins, presumably derived from VLDL and chylomicrons, are unusually rich in unesterified cholesterol and appear to have abnormal surface monolayers. The LDL are rich in triglycerides, and abnormal vesicular lipoproteins are present in the LDL density interval. Two abnormal HDL species are present: bilayer disks and small spherical particles. Marked restriction of dietary fat and cholesterol results in a decrease of VLDL-like particles and lamellar LDL in plasma and is the recommended treatment.

PRIMARY HYPOLIPIDEMIA DUE TO DEFICIENCY OF APO-B-CONTAINING LIPOPROTEINS

1. RECESSIVE ABETALIPOPROTEINEMIA

Etiology & Pathogenesis

Recessive abetalipoproteinemia could represent a number of mutations involving the processing of apo-B or the secretion of apo-B-containing lipoproteins. However, the predominant underlying cause appears to be mutations involving the microsomal triglyceride transfer protein (MTTP). Heterozygous patients have no abnormalities of lipoproteins and no clinical signs. In homozygotes, all forms of apo-B are essentially absent. No chylomicrons, VLDL, or LDL are found in plasma, leaving only HDL. Plasma triglyceride levels are usually less than 10 mg/dL (0.12 mmol/L) and fail to rise after a fat load. The plasma cholesterol is usually less than 90 mg/dL (2.3 mmol/L). There is a defect in the incorporation of newly synthesized triglycerides into chylomicron particles. However, at low levels of fat intake, about 80% of the ingested triglycerides are absorbed, probably by direct absorption of fatty acids via the portal vein.

Clinical Findings

Clinical features include a paucity of adipose tissue, associated with malabsorption of long-chain fatty acids due to failure of the intestine to secrete chylomicrons; red blood cells that may be acanthocytic, with a high cholesterol/phospholipid ratio; progressive degeneration of the central nervous system, including cerebellar degeneration and posterior and lateral spinal tract disease; retinal degeneration that may be severe; and, usually, very low levels of fat-soluble vitamins in plasma. The neurologic defects are due to deficiency of vitamin E (normally transported largely in LDL). Patients are apparently normal at birth and develop steatorrhea with impaired growth in infancy. The neuromuscular disorder often appears in late childhood with ataxia, night blindness, decreased visual acuity, and nystagmus. Cardiomyopathy with arrhythmias has been reported and may be a cause of death.

Treatment

Treatment includes administration of fat-soluble vitamins. Very large doses of tocopherol (vitamin E) (1000–5000 IU/d) appear to limit the progressive central nervous system degeneration. Although vitamin A seems to correct the night blindness, it does not alter the course of retinitis pigmentosa. Vitamins D and K may also be indicated. Restriction of dietary fat minimizes steatorrhea.

2. FAMILIAL HYPOBETALIPOPROTEINEMIA

This disorder is usually attributable to defects at the apo-B locus, resulting in decreased production of the protein or in the production of truncated gene products. LDL and apo-B in heterozygotes are often present at about half of normal levels. If a mutant allele resulting in the complete interdiction of apo-B synthesis is present in the homozygous state, the clinical and biochemical features may be indistinguishable from recessive abetalipoproteinemia, and treatment is the same as for that disorder. Very short truncations of apo-B-100 only allow the formation of abnormally dense small LDL. Longer truncations permit the formation of larger lipoproteins, even including VLDL-like particles. The latter may be present in the virtual absence of LDL in some cases.

Clinical features may be absent in patients who secrete at least low levels of LDL-like particles. However, signs and symptoms of tocopherol deficiency may be present. Oral treatment with alpha tocopherol (vitamin E) (800 IU/d) is recommended for all patients with hypobetalipoproteinemia.

3. CHYLOMICRON RETENTION DISEASE

This disorder, which presents in the neonate, appears to be based upon the selective inability of intestinal epithelial cells to secrete chylomicrons. Affected individuals have severe malabsorption of triglycerides with steatorrhea. Levels of LDL and VLDL are about one-half of normal, presumably secondary to malnutrition. Tocopherol levels may be very low and may be associated with neurologic abnormalities. Clinical symptoms diminish somewhat with time if the patient is managed with a low-fat diet and alpha tocopherol (vitamin E) supplementation.

SECONDARY HYPOLIPIDEMIA

Hypolipidemia may be secondary to a number of diseases characterized by chronic cachexia, eg, advanced cancer. Myeloproliferative disorders can lead to extremely low levels of LDL, probably owing to increased uptake related to rapid proliferation and membrane synthesis. A wide variety of conditions leading to intestinal malabsorption produce hypolipidemia. In these situations, levels of chylomicrons, VLDL, and LDL in serum are low but never absent. Because most of the lipoprotein mass of fasting serum is of hepatic origin, massive parenchymal liver failure—eg, in Reye's syndrome—can cause severe hypolipidemia. Secondary hypobetalipoproteinemia occurs in oroticaciduria.

The hypolipidemias associated with immunoglobulin disorders result from diverse mechanisms. Affected patients usually have myeloma or macroglobulinemia but may have lymphomas or lymphocytic leukemia. Any of the major classes of immunoglobulins may be involved. In many cases, the immunoglobulins are cryoprecipitins; thus, the diagnosis may be missed if blood is not drawn and serum prepared at 37 °C and observed for cryoprecipitation. Immunoglobulin-lipoprotein complexes may precipitate in various tissues. When this occurs in the lamina propria of the intestine, a syndrome of malabsorption and protein-losing enteropathy may result. Monoclonal IgA in myeloma may precipitate with lipoproteins, causing xanthomas of the gingiva and cervix. Lesions in the skin are usually planar and xanthomatous and may involve intracutaneous hemorrhage, producing a classic purple xanthoma. Planar xanthomas occurring in cholestasis may be confused with this condition, because the abnormal lipoprotein of cholestasis (LP-X), like the circulating lipoprotein complex of immunoglobulin and lipoprotein, has gamma mobility on electrophoresis.

OTHER DISORDERS OF LIPOPROTEIN METABOLISM

THE LIPODYSTROPHIES

Classification

Current classification of the lipodystrophies is based on their familial or acquired origin and the regional or generalized nature of the fat loss. Among the associated metabolic abnormalities, insulin resistance is the common finding. Two of these disorders are known to be inherited.

Familial generalized lipodystrophy (Seip-Berardinelli syndrome), a rare recessive trait, may be diagnosed at birth and is associated with macrosomia. Genital hypertrophy, hypertrichosis, acanthosis nigricans, hepatomegaly, insulin resistance, hypertriglyceridemia, and glucose intolerance are regularly observed.

Familial lipodystrophy of limbs and trunk (Köbberling-Dunningan syndrome) appears to be transmitted as a dominant gene, affects women predominantly, and is not evident until puberty. The face, neck, and upper trunk are usually spared. Growth is normal, but otherwise this syndrome shares features of the generalized form noted above. It is frequently associated with Stein-Leventhal syndrome.

Acquired forms of lipodystrophy, generalized (Lawrence syndrome) and partial (Barraquer-Simmons syndrome), usually begin in childhood, affect females predominantly, and often follow an acute febrile illness. The generalized type commonly shares the features described above, invariably involving the trunk and extremities but sometimes sparing the face. A sclerosing panniculitis, as seen in Weber-Christian syndrome, may appear at the outset. The partial type usually begins in the face and then involves the neck, upper limbs, and trunk. In this disorder, reduced levels of C3 complement are frequently encountered. Most patients have proteinuria, and some develop overt vascular nephritis.

Associated Disorders

Because a number of patients with disorders resembling both familial and acquired types of lipodystrophy have tumors or other lesions of the hypothalamus, appropriate neurologic evaluation should be obtained. Similarly, the physician should be alert to the association of collagen vascular disorders, including scleroderma and dermatomyositis, with some cases of acquired lipodystrophy.

RARE DISORDERS

Werner's Syndrome, Progeria, Infantile Hypercalcemia, & Sphingolipidoses

These disorders may be associated with hypercholesterolemia, but levels of triglycerides are usually normal. Some patients with Niemann-Pick disease have hypercholesterolemia, but most have hypertriglyceridemia, as do many patients with Gaucher's disease.

Wolman's Disease & Cholesteryl Ester Storage Disease

These recessive lipid storage disorders involve the absence and partial deficiency, respectively, of lysosomal acid lipase, resulting in abnormal cholesteryl ester and triglyceride stores in liver, spleen, adrenal glands, small intestine, and bone marrow. Most patients have elevated levels of both LDL and VLDL in plasma. Wolman's disease is fatal in infancy.

Cerebrotendinous Xanthomatosis

In this recessive disorder, impaired synthesis of bile acids results in increased production of cholesterol and cholestanol, which accumulate in body tissues. Plasma levels of cholesterol and cholestanol are normal or elevated. Cataracts, tendinous xanthomas, progressive neurologic dysfunction, and premature coronary atherosclerosis are hallmarks of this disease. Its central nervous system effects include dementia, spasticity, and ataxia. Death usually ensues before age 50 from neurologic degeneration or coronary disease. Treatment with chenodeoxycholic acid appears useful. Resins must be avoided because they aggravate the underlying defect.

Phytosterolemia

This disorder is distinguished by normal or elevated plasma cholesterol levels; high concentrations of plant sterol in serum, adipose tissue, and skin; and prominent xanthomas of both the tendinous and tuberous types. Individuals with this disorder absorb a substantially larger fraction of phytosterols and cholesterol from the intestine than do normal individuals. A more severe form apparently exists in which serum cholesterol levels may be as high as 700 mg/dL (18.2 mmol/L), reflecting an increase in LDL that contain sitosterol esters in addition to cholesteryl esters. Diagnosis is established by quantitation of phytosterols in plasma by gas-liquid chromatography. Premature coronary arteriosclerosis may be present. Treatment consists of a diet restricted in plant sterols and cholesterol and the use of bile acid-binding resins. HMG-CoA reductase inhibitors may be of some value.

Cholesteryl Ester Transfer Protein Deficiency

Mutations have been identified that impair the function of CETP, resulting in the retention of cholesteryl esters in HDL. Total HDL cholesterol levels are increased by 30–50% in heterozygotes and as high as 200 mg/dL in homozygotes. The risk of atherosclerosis is moderately increased among these patients.

II. TREATMENT OF HYPERLIPIDEMIA

The first therapeutic measure in all forms of hyperlipidemia is institution of an appropriate diet. In most forms of hyperlipidemia, a single "universal" diet (see below) is indicated. In many subjects with lipemia or with hypercholesterolemia of mild to moderate severity, compliance with this diet will be sufficient to control lipoprotein levels. However, many patients with severe hypercholesterolemia or lipemia will require drug therapy. In all of these individuals, the prescribed diet must be continued to achieve the full potential of the medications.

Caution Regarding Drug Therapy

There are insufficient data to evaluate the effects on the fetus of drugs used in treatment of hyperlipoproteinemia. Therefore, women of childbearing age should be advised of the potential risk and should be given these agents only if pregnancy is being actively avoided. If contraceptives are prescribed, estrogens should not be used in patients with hypertriglyceridemia.

In children, hyperlipidemias other than familial hypercholesterolemia rarely require medication. The severity and age at onset of symptomatic coronary disease in the child's family and the presence of other risk factors, especially hypoalphalipoproteinemia and hyper-Lp(a)lipoproteinemia, in the child should be considered in deciding when drug treatment should be started. A resin is the drug of choice. Dietary treatment is indicated for all children with hyperlipidemia and should be started after the second year. The exception is primary chylomicronemia, in which an appropriate diet should be instituted as soon as the disease is detected.

DIETARY FACTORS IN THE MANAGEMENT OF LIPOPROTEIN DISORDERS

Restriction of Caloric Intake

The secretion of VLDL by liver is greatly stimulated by caloric intake in excess of requirements for physical activity and basal metabolism. Therefore, the total caloric content of the diet is of greater importance than its specific composition in treating endogenous hyperlipemia. There is a positive correlation between serum levels of VLDL triglyceride and various measures of obesity, but many obese patients have normal serum lipids. On the other hand, most patients with hypertriglyceridemia—except those with lipoprotein lipase deficiency—are obese. This association is more consistently observed in persons with centripetal obesity whose weight gain occurred in later childhood or adulthood and who have adipocyte hypertrophy with relative insulin resistance. As obese patients lose weight, plasma VLDL stabilize at lower levels. There is a modest correlation of LDL levels with body weight in the general population.

Restriction of Fat Intake

In primary chylomicronemia, saturated and polyunsaturated fats both must be restricted rigidly. Similarly, in the acute management of mixed lipemia with impending pancreatitis, elimination of dietary fat leads to a rapid decrease in chylomicron-borne triglycerides in plasma.

The cholesterol-lowering effect of a significant reduction in total fat content of the diet is well known. It has also been shown that a 10–15% fall in serum cholesterol levels is achieved when many individuals who have been consuming a typical North American diet restrict their intake of saturated fats to 8% of total calories. Most saturated fatty acids cause increased levels of LDL cholesterol by down-regulating hepatic LDL receptors. Whereas polyunsaturated fatty acids do not have this effect, they may reduce levels of HDL and are potentially carcinogenic. Monounsaturated fatty acids do not raise LDL levels and increase HDL levels higher than those observed with markedly restricted fat intake. Thus, moderate use of monounsaturated fats such as olive oil, oleic acid-rich safflower oil, or rapeseed oil from strains of rapeseed that contain little of the cardiotoxic erucic acid, appears to be desirable.

The omega-3 fatty acids found in fish oils have special properties relevant to the treatment of hypertriglyceridemia. Substantial decreases in triglyceride levels can be induced in some patients with severe endogenous or mixed lipemia at doses of 10–15 g/d. In patients with other phenotypes, these fatty acids may increase LDL and decrease HDL levels and therefore are not indicated. Certain members of this class of fatty acids, such as eicosapentaenoic acid, are potent inhibitors of platelet reactivity.

Reduction of Cholesterol Intake

The amount of cholesterol in the diet affects serum cholesterol levels, but individual responses vary. Restriction of dietary cholesterol to less than 200 mg/d (5.2 mmol/d) in normal individuals can result in a decrease of up to 10–15% in serum cholesterol, primarily reflecting a decrease in LDL. This apparently in part reflects the fact that increased cholesterol intake in humans is not completely balanced by reduced cholesterogenesis in the liver. Dietary cholesterol and saturated fat content have independent effects on levels of serum cholesterol.

Role of Carbohydrate in Diet

The role of dietary carbohydrate in lipid metabolism is still being investigated, but certain effects seem to have been uniformly observed. There is great individual variation in these responses. When a high-carbohydrate diet is fed, hypertriglyceridemia develops within 48–72 hours, and levels of triglyceride in serum rise to a maximum in 1–5 weeks. Persons with higher basal triglyceride levels and those consuming hypercaloric diets show the greatest effect. After 1–8 months on a high-carbohydrate diet, triglycerides fall to basal levels in most patients. Similar induction of lipemia by carbohydrate is seen in patients with endogenous and mixed lipemia. There is apparently no type of hyperlipemia that is particularly "carbohydrate-sensitive." It must be emphasized, however, that both of these patterns of lipemia are extremely sensitive to excess total caloric intake. Levels of HDL in serum are lower on a high-carbohydrate intake, but the differences are small.

Alcohol Ingestion

Ingestion of alcohol is a common cause of secondary hypertriglyceridemia, owing to overproduction of VLDL. Some individuals with familial hypertriglyceridemia are particularly sensitive to the effects of alcohol, and abstinence may normalize their triglyceride levels. Chronic alcohol intake may also be associated with hypercholesterolemia. Increased cholesterol synthesis and decreased conversion to bile acids have been observed. Alcohol ingestion may account for alimentary lipemia persisting beyond 12–14 hours. This possibility should be excluded by the history or a repeat lipid analysis. A positive correlation has been found between alcohol intake and HDL cholesterol levels; however, increased HDL levels are not observed in all individuals. Because alcohol-induced changes in HDL appear primarily to involve the HDL_3 subfraction, there does not seem to be an indication for the use of alcohol to increase the "protective effect" of HDL against arteriosclerosis.

Fiber in Diet

Although much attention has been devoted to the possible role of fiber in the development of coronary heart disease, there is little evidence that plasma lipids can be significantly affected by intake of most forms of fiber. A modest reduction in LDL cholesterol is associated with the addition of oat bran to the diet, however.

Other Dietary Substances

Several other nutrients have been studied in relation to atherosclerotic heart disease, including cal-

cium, magnesium, trace elements, vitamins D, E, and C, and pyridoxine. The results of these studies are generally equivocal. Caffeine and sucrose have negligible effects on serum lipids, and their statistical relationship to coronary heart disease is generally unimpressive when data are corrected for cigarette smoking. Ingestion of large amounts of zinc appears to be associated with decreased levels of HDL. Lecithin has no effect on plasma lipoproteins.

The "Universal Diet"

Dietary treatment is an important aspect of the management of all forms of lipoprotein disorders and may in some cases be all that is required. Knowledge of the dietary factors reviewed above allows the physician to select appropriate modifications for an individual patient. However, a basic diet is useful in the treatment of most patients. The elements of this diet are as follows:

(1) Ideal body weight should be achieved and maintained.

(2) Fat should provide less than 30% of total calories. Saturated fat should be less than 7% of total calories.

(3) Cholesterol should be reduced to less than 200 mg/d.

(4) Caloric difference should be made up with complex carbohydrate.

(5) Alcohol should be avoided in any patient with hypertriglyceridemia.

This diet is consistent with the Step-Two Diet recommended by the National Cholesterol Education Program Expert Panel.

Caloric restriction and reduction of adipose tissue mass are particularly important for patients with increased levels of VLDL and IDL. Levels of VLDL and LDL tend to be lower during periods of substantial weight loss than can be maintained under isocaloric conditions, even at ideal body weight.

Sources of Information About Diet

Referral to a local American Heart Association chapter or other source of dietetic consultation is often helpful in ensuring compliance. Several recipe books have been published, and food manufacturers are developing products that add variety and palatability to the restricted diet. Since the prudent diet, as proposed by the American Heart Association and others, is generally recommended, it is helpful to urge the entire family of a hyperlipidemic patient to eat a modified diet, providing greater ease of preparation and an added measure of psychologic support.

DRUGS USED IN TREATMENT OF HYPERLIPOPROTEINEMIA
(Table 20–3)

BILE ACID SEQUESTRANTS

Mechanism of Action

Cholestyramine and colestipol are cationic resins that bind bile acids in the intestinal lumen (Figure 20–5). The resin particles are not absorbed by the bowel and therefore increase the excretion of bile acids in the stool. Excretion of bile acids can be increased up to tenfold when bile acid-binding resins are given. LDL levels decrease as a consequence of increased expression of high-affinity receptors on cell membranes of the liver. These agents are useful only in disorders involving elevated LDL levels. In fact, patients who have increased levels of VLDL may have further increases in serum triglyceride levels during treatment with resins. Thus, in combined hyperlipidemia, where the resins may be given because of high LDL levels, a second agent such as niacin may be required to control the hypertriglyceridemia. Levels of LDL will fall 15–30% in compliant patients with heterozygous familial hypercholesterolemia who are receiving maximal doses of the resins. Larger decrements of LDL cholesterol may be seen in patients with other, less severe forms of hypercholesterolemia, and in some, levels of LDL will be normalized completely.

Drug Dosage

In disorders involving moderately high levels of LDL, 20 g of cholestyramine or colestipol daily may lower cholesterol levels effectively. Treatment should commence at one-half of the above dose to minimize gastrointestinal side effects. Maximum doses of 30 g of colestipol or 32 g of cholestyramine daily are required in more severe cases.

Side Effects

Because the resins are confined to the lumen of the intestine, few systemic side effects are observed. Patients frequently complain of a bloated sensation and constipation, both of which may be relieved by the addition of psyllium to the resin mixture. Malabsorption of fat or fat-soluble vitamins with a daily dose of resin of up to 30 g occurs only in individuals with preexisting bowel disease or with cholestasis. Hypoprothrombinemia has been observed in patients with malabsorption due to these causes. The resins bind thyroxine, digitalis glycosides, and warfarin and impair the absorption of iron, thiazides, beta-blockers, and other drugs. Absorption of all of these substances is ensured if they are administered 1 hour be-

Table 20–3. The primary hyperlipoproteinemias and their drug treatment.

	Single Drug[1]	Drug Combination
Primary chylomicronemia (familial lipoprotein lipase or cofactor deficiency)		
Chylomicrons, VLDL increased	Dietary management	
Familial hypertriglyceridemia		
Severe: Chylomicrons, VLDL increased	Niacin, gemfibrozil	Niacin plus gemfibrozil
Moderate: VLDL and perhaps chylomicrons increased	Gemfibrozil, niacin	
Familial combined hyperlipoproteinemia		
VLDL increased	Niacin	
LDL increased	Resin, niacin, reductase inhibitor	Niacin plus resin or reductase inhibitor
VLDL, LDL increased	Niacin	Niacin plus resin or reductase inhibitor
Familial dysbetalipoproteinemia		
VLDL remnants, chylomicron remnants increased	Niacin, gemfibrozil	
Familial hypercholesterolemia		
Heterozygous: LDL increased	Resin, reductase inhibitor, niacin	Two or three of the single drugs
Homozygous: LDL increased	Niacin	Resin plus niacin plus reductase inhibitor
Lp(a) hyperlipoproteinemia		
Lp(a) increased	Niacin	

[1]Single-drug therapy should be tried before drug combinations are used.

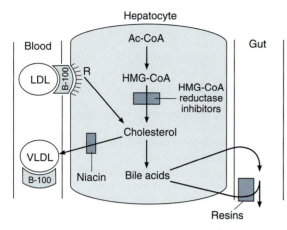

Figure 20–5. Sites of action of HMG-CoA reductase inhibitors, niacin and resins used in treating hyperlipidemias. LDL receptors (R) are increased by treatment with resins and HMG-CoA reductase inhibitors. (Reproduced, with permission, from Katzung BG (editor): *Basic & Clinical Pharmacology,* 5th ed. Appleton & Lange, 1992.)

fore the resin. During long-term treatment with the resins, some patients may complain of dry, flaking skin, which responds to local application of lanolin. Because they change the composition of bile micelles, bile acid sequestrants theoretically may increase the risk of cholelithiasis, particularly in obese subjects. In practice, this risk appears to be very small.

NIACIN
(Nicotinic Acid)

Mechanism of Action

Niacin (but not its amide) is able to effect major reductions in LDL and triglyceride-rich lipoproteins (Figure 20–5). Niacin appears to inhibit the secretion of VLDL by liver and to increase the efficiency of removal of VLDL triglycerides via the LPL pathway. Niacin has several effects on cholesterol metabolism. It increases sterol excretion acutely and mobilizes cholesterol from tissue pools until a new steady state is established. Although it has no effect on the conversion of cholesterol to bile acids, it decreases cholesterol biosynthesis. That it can cause a continued decrease in hepatic cholesterol production even when given with bile acid-binding resins is probably an important feature of the complementary action of these agents. Levels of HDL in plasma, particularly HDL_2, are significantly increased, reflecting a decrease in the fractional catabolic rate of these lipoproteins. Niacin stimulates production of tissue plasminogen activator, an effect that may be of value in preventing thrombotic events.

Drug Dosage

The dose of niacin required for effective treatment varies with the diagnosis. Optimal effect on LDL levels in heterozygous familial hypercholesterolemia is only achieved when a bile acid-binding resin is combined with 4.5–6.5 g of niacin daily (in three doses). For other forms of hypercholesterolemia and for hypertriglyceridemia, a dose of 1.5–3.5 g/d often has a dramatic effect. Because niacin causes cutaneous flushing, it is usually started at a dosage of 100 mg three times daily and increased slowly. Tachyphylaxis to the flushing often occurs within a few days at any dose, allowing stepwise increases. Many patients have no flushing or only occasional minimal flushing when stabilized on a given dose. Because the flushing is prostaglandin-mediated, 0.3 g of aspirin given 20–30 minutes before each dose may mitigate this symptom. It is important to counsel the patient beforehand that the flushing is a harmless cutaneous vasodilation. Patients should be advised to take the drug with meals.

Side Effects

Moderate elevations of aminotransferases are more often observed if the dosage of niacin is increased too rapidly. If a daily dose of 2.5 g is not exceeded by the end of the first month and 6.5 g after the second month, such abnormalities are uncommon. A daily dose of 6.5 g is the maximum under any circumstances. Some patients have reversible elevations of serum glutamic aminotransferase or alkaline phosphatase activities up to three times the upper limit of normal that do not appear to be clinically significant. In a group of patients treated continuously for up to 15 years, no significant liver disease developed despite such enzyme abnormalities. About one-fifth of patients have mild hyperuricemia that tends to be asymptomatic unless the patient has had gout. In such cases, a uricosuric agent can be added to the regimen. A few patients will have moderate elevations of blood glucose during treatment. Again, this is reversible except possibly in some patients who have latent maturity-onset diabetes. A more common side effect is gastric irritation, which responds well to antacids. Rarely, patients develop acanthosis nigricans, which clears if the drug is discontinued. Some patients can have cardiac arrhythmias while taking niacin. Reversible macular degeneration has been described rarely.

Niacin should be avoided in patients with peptic ulcer or hepatic parenchymal disease. It should be discontinued in patients who develop markedly elevated levels of aminotransferases or alkaline phosphatase. Liver function, uric acid, and blood glucose should be evaluated before commencing treatment and periodically thereafter.

Timed-release preparations of niacin should be avoided because of the risk of fulminant hepatic failure. This rare consequence has been associated with several types of sustained-release niacins, suggesting that it could occur with all such preparations.

GEMFIBROZIL

Mechanism of Action

Gemfibrozil, a fibric acid derivative, is excreted chiefly by the kidney. It decreases lipolysis in adipose tissue, reduces levels of circulating triglycerides, and causes modest reductions in LDL cholesterol levels. However, in some patients reductions in VLDL levels are attended by increases in LDL levels. Gemfibrozil causes moderate increases in levels of HDL, including the protein moiety.

Drug Dosage

Gemfibrozil may be useful in the treatment of patients with severe endogenous lipemia and familial dysbetalipoproteinemia. It is not recommended for patients who have overt coronary disease. The usual dose is 600 mg twice daily. Patients with familial dysbetalipoproteinemia may be managed with smaller doses.

Side Effects

Skin eruptions and gastrointestinal and muscular symptoms have been described, as well as blood dyscrasias and elevated plasma levels of aminotransferases and alkaline phosphatase. It enhances the effects of the coumarin and indanedione anticoagulants and increases lithogenicity of bile. Concomitant use of gemfibrozil with reductase inhibitors appears to increase the risk of myopathy.

HMG-CoA REDUCTASE INHIBITORS

Mechanism of Action

Several closely related structural analogs of HMG-CoA act as competitive inhibitors of HMG-CoA reductase, a key enzyme in the cholesterol biosynthetic pathway. Of these, lovastatin, pravastatin, simvastatin, and fluvastatin are approved for use in the USA. Inhibition of cholesterol biosynthesis induces an increase in high-affinity LDL receptors in the liver, increasing removal of LDL from plasma and decreasing production of LDL. The latter results from increased uptake of lipoprotein precursors of LDL by hepatic receptors. Modest increases in HDL cholesterol and limited decreases in VLDL levels occur during treatment (Figure 20–5). Unless LDL levels are increased, these drugs are not indicated for the treatment of hypertriglyceridemias.

Drug Dosage

These drugs are the most effective individual agents for treatment of hypercholesterolemia. Their effects are amplified significantly when combined with niacin or resin. Daily doses of lovastatin vary from 10 mg to 80 mg. A single 20-mg dose, preferably in the evening, may be sufficient to treat moderately elevated LDL levels. Pravastatin dosages vary from 10 mg to 40 mg daily, and simvastatin dosages vary from 10 mg to 40 mg. Fluvastatin, used in doses of 20–40 mg/d, has appreciably less efficacy than the other drugs of this class and is indicated for mild elevations of LDL. Because the rate of cholesterol synthesis is higher at night, reductase inhibitors should be given with the evening meal for greatest effect. At higher doses, a twice-daily regimen is recommended. Patients with heterozygous familial hypercholesterolemia usually require the higher dosage levels. Because information on long-term safety is lacking, use of these agents in children should be restricted to those with homozygous familial hypercholesterolemia who have some receptor function and those heterozygotes over age 10 years who are at particularly high risk. Women who are lactating, pregnant, or likely to become pregnant should not be given these drugs.

Side Effects

These agents are generally well tolerated. Reported side effects, often transient, include changes in bowel function, nausea, headaches, insomnia, fatigue, and rashes. Myopathy with markedly elevated creatine kinase levels occurs in less than 5% of patients. Rarely, myopathy can progress to rhabdomyolysis with myoglobinuria and renal shutdown. There is an increased incidence of myopathy in patients receiving lovastatin with cyclosporine, fibric acid derivatives, erythromycin, and perhaps niacin. Whether the incidence of this side effect will be lower with the other reductase inhibitors is still unclear. The myopathy is rapidly reversible upon cessation of therapy. Minor elevations of creatine kinase activity in plasma are noted more frequently, especially with unusual physical activity. Creatine kinase levels should be measured before starting therapy and monitored at regular intervals.

Moderate, often intermittent elevations of serum aminotransferase (up to three times normal) occur in some patients. Therapy may be continued if aminotransferase levels are measured frequently (at 1- to 2-month intervals). In about 2% of patients, some of whom have underlying liver disease or a history of alcohol abuse, aminotransferase levels may exceed three times the normal limit. This usually occurs after 3–16 months of continuous therapy and may portend more severe hepatic toxicity. Lovastatin should be discontinued in these patients. The drug should be used with caution in patients with a history of liver disease.

COMBINED DRUG THERAPY
(Table 20–3)

Combinations of drugs are indicated (1) when LDL and VLDL levels are both elevated; (2) in cases of hypercholesterolemia in which significant increases of VLDL occur during treatment with bile acid-binding resins; and (3) where a complementary effect is required to normalize LDL levels, as in familial hypercholesterolemia.

Fibric Acid Derivatives
With Other Agents

The combination of gemfibrozil with niacin may be more effective than either drug alone in managing marked hypertriglyceridemia.

Niacin & Resins

Niacin usually normalizes the triglyceride levels in individuals who have increased levels of VLDL while taking resins. The combination of niacin and resins is more effective than either agent alone in decreasing LDL levels in familial hypercholesterolemia. The complementarity of action presumably results from additive effects of increased catabolism of LDL due to the resin and decreased production of VLDL induced by niacin. No additional toxicity or side effects have been described with this regimen beyond those encountered when the agents are used individually. Although the daily dose of niacin required for optimal effect on LDL levels in familial hypercholesterolemia may be 6.5 g in conjunction with 24–30 g of resin, many patients show significant response with niacin doses as low as 1.5 g. On this regimen, levels of HDL cholesterol are significantly elevated, and the diameters of tendon xanthomas are reduced significantly even over a period of only a few months. Patients who have been treated with this combination for 15 years show a sustained effect on lipoprotein levels and have not developed additional side effects or toxicity. The combination is also very useful in the treatment of familial combined hyperlipidemia.

The absorption of niacin from the intestine is unimpeded by the presence of resin; the two medications may therefore be taken together. Because the resins have potent acid-neutralizing properties, there is further reason to give the two medications together when a patient complains of the gastric irritation that sometimes occurs as an adverse effect of niacin.

HMG-CoA Reductase Inhibitors
With Other Agents

The addition of resin or niacin to lovastatin further decreases plasma levels of LDL in patients with primary hypercholesterolemias. Liver function and plasma creatine kinase activity should be monitored frequently when the combination of lovastatin plus niacin is used. These three drugs used together are more effective, frequently at lower doses, than any of their binary combinations in reducing plasma LDL levels. Serum cholesterol levels in patients with severe heterozygous familial hypercholesterolemia usually fall below 200 mg/dL. In some patients, a reduction of as much as 80% has been observed. Effects are sustained, and no compound toxicity is observed. The other reductase inhibitors also behave similarly in binary and ternary combinations with niacin and resins.

POSSIBLE UNTOWARD CONSEQUENCES OF LIPID-LOWERING THERAPY

The risk of coronary heart disease has been found to increase monotonically with LDL cholesterol levels in virtually all epidemiologic surveys, with the lowest incidence at the lowest levels of serum cholesterol. Total mortality tends to be somewhat higher among individuals with serum cholesterol levels below 160 mg/dL, however, raising a question about whether very low levels of serum cholesterol may increase the risk of noncoronary disease. The correlation between deaths from certain digestive and respiratory disorders and low serum cholesterol levels may be a reflection of the effect of wasting illnesses in general upon LDL levels. For instance, the low cholesterol levels seen in hepatic cirrhosis most certainly reflect impaired lipoprotein production by the liver. Furthermore, increased uptake of LDL by malignant cells is known to decrease LDL levels in plasma. However, two studies have shown a modest increase in the risk of hemorrhagic stroke at serum cholesterol levels below 130 mg/dL. In one, the effect was confined to hypertensive patients. In large clinical trials employing niacin or reductase inhibitors, no excess deaths from noncoronary causes occurred in the course of 5 years or more, though impressive reductions in deaths from coronary disease were observed, resulting in significant reduction in all-cause mortality. In a secondary intervention trial (the Four S trial), patients receiving simvastatin had a 37% reduction in new coronary events over a 5- to 6-year period. In the West of Scotland study treatment with pravastatin resulted in a 22% reduction in all cause mortality. In the MRFIT study, a proportionate hazards analysis adjusting for covariance demonstrated that the lowest net death rate occurs at a cholesterol level of 122 mg/dL.

Populations in which many individuals have serum cholesterol levels below 160 mg/dL, such as in Japan, do not have an excess incidence of the noncoronary causes of death under consideration. Of great importance in resolving the question of the relative benefit of lipid-lowering therapy is the fact that about 45% of deaths in the USA and Europe are attributable to cardiovascular disease, predominantly coronary artery disease. Thus, projection of a significant reduction in fatal occlusive coronary events into the age range where coronary disease predominates would be expected to far outweigh the marginal increases that might occur in other causes of death. In the light of the relationship of very low plasma cholesterol levels (< 130 mg/dL) to hemorrhagic stroke, the therapeutic goal for total cholesterol levels in patients with known coronary disease should be 150–160 mg/dL (LDL cholesterol level 90–100 mg/dL) until that relationship is better understood.

REFERENCES

Relationship of Coronary Heart Disease to Disorders of Lipoprotein Metabolism

Castelli WP: Epidemiology of coronary heart disease: The Framingham Study. Am J Med 1984;76(Suppl 2A):4.

Kane JP: High density lipoproteins. In: *Lipoproteins and Coronary Artery Disease.* Kreisberg RA, Segrest J (editors). Blackwell, 1993.

Fuster VL et al: The pathogenesis of coronary artery disease and the acute coronary syndromes. (Two parts.) N Engl J Med 1992;326:242, 310.

Parthasarathy S, Steinberg D, Witztum JL: The role of oxidized low-density lipoproteins in the pathogenesis of atherosclerosis. Annu Rev Med 1992;43:219.

Lipoprotein Metabolism

Brunzell JD: Familial lipoprotein lipase deficiency and other causes of the chylomicronemia syndrome. In: *The Metabolic and Molecular Bases of Inherited Disease,* 7th ed. Scriver CR et al (editors). McGraw-Hill, 1995.

Kane JP, Havel RJ: Introduction: Structure and metabolism of plasma lipoproteins. In: *The Metabolic and Molecular Bases of Inherited Disease,* 7th ed. Scriver CR et al (editors). McGraw-Hill, 1995.

Primary Disorders of Lipoprotein Metabolism

Brown MS, Hobbs HH, Goldstein JL: Familial hypercholesterolemia. In: *The Metabolic and Molecular Bases of Inherited Disease,* 7th ed. Scriver CR et al (editors). McGraw-Hill, 1995.

Grundy SM: Lipids, nutrition, and coronary heart disease. In: *Atherosclerosis and Coronary Artery Disease,* vol 1. Fuster V, Ross R, Topol EJ (editors). Lippincott-Raven, 1996.

Kane JP, Havel RJ: Disorders of the biogenesis and secretion of lipoproteins containing the B apolipoproteins. In: *The Metabolic and Molecular Bases of Inherited Disease,* 7th ed. Scriver CR et al (editors). McGraw-Hill, 1995.

Mahley RW, Rall SC Jr: Type III hyperlipoproteinemia (dysbetalipoproteinemia): The role of apolipoprotein E in normal and abnormal lipoprotein metabolism. In: *The Metabolic and Molecular Bases of Inherited Disease,* 7th ed. Scriver CR et al (editors). McGraw-Hill, 1995.

Treatment of Hyperlipidemia

Brown BG, Fuster V: Impact of management in stabilization and regression of coronary disease. In: *Atherosclerosis and Coronary Artery Disease,* vol 1. Fuster V, Ross R, Topol EJ (editors). Lippincott-Raven, 1996.

Malloy MJ: Disorders of lipoprotein metabolism. In: *Practical Pediatric Therapy,* 3rd ed. Eichenwald HF, Stroder J (editors). Mosby, 1993.

Malloy MJ et al: Complementarity of colestipol, niacin, and lovastatin in treatment of severe familial hypercholesterolemia. Ann Intern Med 1987;107:616.

Malloy MJ, Kane JP: Aggressive medical therapy for the prevention and treatment of coronary artery disease. Adv Intern Med 1997;42:1–38.

Randomized trial of cholesterol lowering in 4444 patients with coronary heart disease: The Scandinavian Simvastatin Survival Study (4S). Lancet 1994;344:1383.

Shepherd J et al: Prevention of coronary heart disease with pravastatin in men with hypercholesterolemia. West of Scotland Coronary Prevention Study Group. N Engl J Med 1995;333:1301.

Summary of the Second Report on the National Cholesterol Education Program (NCEP) Expert Panel on Detection, Evaluation, and Treatment of High Blood Cholesterol in Adults (Adult Treatment Panel II). Arch Intern Med 1992;152:1490.

Regression of Coronary Artery Disease

Brown G et al: Regression of coronary artery disease as a result of intensive lipid-lowering therapy in men with high levels of apolipoprotein B. N Engl J Med 1990;323:1289.

Cashin-Hemphill J et al: Beneficial effects of colestipol-niacin on coronary atherosclerosis. A 4-year follow-up. JAMA 1990;264:3013.

Kane JP et al: Regression of coronary atherosclerosis during treatment of familial hypercholesterolemia with combined drug regimens. JAMA 1990;264:3007.

21

Obesity

George A. Bray, MD

Obesity, like most other chronic human ailments, is a multifactorial disorder; ie, there are a number of factors which influence whether or not obesity—or an abnormal increase in body fat—develops. At the top of the list is genetic susceptibility. Some people and some families appear to be more susceptible to obesity than others. Interacting with this genetic substrate are such factors as gender, age, occupation, and diet. In this chapter a **nutrient balance model** will be used as the framework to describe the normal control of body weight and body fat and as a basis to identify the abnormalities leading to obesity. This nutrient balance model will emphasize the role of the autonomic nervous system and the endocrine glands in nutrient regulation. Obesity can be viewed as an increase of nutrient stores resulting from a failure to balance the intake of nutrients to the daily need for nutrient fuels to stoke the metabolic furnace in a genetically susceptible individual.

GENETIC FACTORS PREDISPOSING TO OBESITY

Genetic susceptibility plays an important role in maintaining nutrient balance and in the development of obesity. Studies using nuclear families, adopted children, and twins suggest that susceptibility genes can account for approximately one-third of the risk of becoming obese. Nongenetic familial transmission from shared environments accounts for up to one-third of the variance, and the remainder is attributed to nontransmissible environmental factors (Figure 21–1). In animals, at least six single genes are known to produce obesity. The gene products for all of these models have been cloned, opening up a new avenue for research into the causes of obesity. The first gene to be cloned was the *agouti* gene, for the dominant yellow obese mouse. The transcription product, a 133-amino-acid protein, is overexpressed in many tissues, and in transgenic mice the *agouti* gene reproduces the syndrome of obesity by modulating the interaction of melanocyte-stimulating hormone (MSH) with its receptor to produce the characteristic yellow

ACRONYMS USED IN THIS CHAPTER	
ARC	Arcuate nucleus
BAT	Brown adipose tissue
cAMP	Cyclic adenosine-3',5'-monophosphate (intracellular second messenger)
CCK	Cholecystokinin
CRH	Corticotropin-releasing hormone
DAG	Diacylglycerol
Dg	Diglyceride
DGP	Diacylglycerol phosphate
DMV	Dorsomotor nucleus of the vagus
End	β-Endorphin
FA	Fatty acid
FABP	Fatty acid-binding protein
FAT	Gene symbol for recessively inherited obesity in FAT mouse
FQ	Food quotient
GR	Glucocorticoid receptor
GABA	Gamma-aminobutyic acid
GLP-1	Glucagon-like peptide-1
GRP	Gastrin-releasing peptide
5-HT	5-Hydroxytryptamine (serotonin)
IP$_3$	Inosine triphosphate
LPL	Lipoprotein lipase
Mg	Monoglyceride
MGP	Monoacylglycerol phosphate
MPG	Motor pattern generator
MSH	Melanocyte-stimulating hormone
NE	Norepinephrine
NPY	Neuropeptide Y
NTS	Nucleus of the tractus solitarius
ob-R	ob (leptin) receptor
ob/ob	Recessive obese mutant (gene symbol ob)
PI	Phosphoinosotide
RMR	Resting metabolic rate
RQ	Respiratory quotient
SNS	Sympathetic nervous system
TEF	Thermic effect of food
TNFα	Tumor necrosis factor-alpha
VMH	Ventromedial hypothalamus

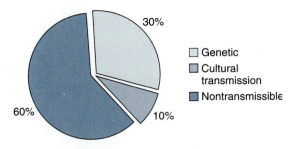

Figure 21–1. Relative importance of transmissible genetic and nongenetic factors and nontransmissible factors in the development of obesity.

coat and the increased food intake. The second gene is from the obese (*ob/ob*) mouse. The *ob* gene protein product (leptin) has 164 amino acids and is produced in adipose cells from which it is secreted to act on many tissues. In the obese mouse, but not the diabetes mouse which lacks the leptin receptor, leptin decreases food intake, increases activity of the sympathetic nervous system and eliminates the infertility. Leptin also reduces the brain peptide, neuropeptide Y (NPY) and may have some of its effects through this neurotransmitter. In animals and human beings, the circulating leptin levels are directly related to the degree of body fat. Clinical trials to treat obesity with leptin are currently underway. The third gene is from the FAT mouse and induces a defect in a carboxypeptidase. Defects in the leptin receptor account for the db/db and fa/fa mutants. There are a variety of chromosomal loci other than these single genes that express genetic information involved in the development of obesity in animals and human beings. As these loci become better understood, they will pro-

vide valuable insights into the defects that produce human obesity.

In addition to single genes associated with obesity, a number of human genes have been shown to contribute to the development of obesity. In spite of these important new genetic insights, the 30% increase in the prevalence of obesity in the USA in the past decade must reflect primarily environmental factors. This is illustrated in the pie chart shown in Figure 21–2. Obesity develops when the susceptible individual interacts with appropriate environmental factors. The nutrient balance model will be presented in this context.

NUTRIENT BALANCE MODEL

The nutrient balance model is a regulated or controlled system consisting of four basic components: a controller located in the brain (Figure 21–3); a controlled system consisting of the intake, digestion, absorption, storage, and metabolism of the nutrients in food; feedback signals that tell the brain (controller) about the state of the controlled system; and efferent control mechanisms that modulate food intake and energy expenditure. This model can be expanded to include key elements in the initiation and termination of a meal.

The Controlled System

The quantities of fat, protein, and carbohydrate in the human body can be expressed in terms of their energy equivalents. Figure 21–4 compares the composition by weight and its equivalent energy value.

Feedback model

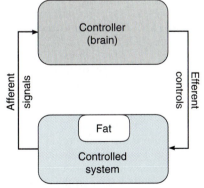

Figure 21–3. Diagram of a controlled system. The controller for food intake is located in the brain, which receives afferent signals from the periphery and integrates them into efferent controls that modulate food intake and the controlled system of nutrient intake storage and oxidation.

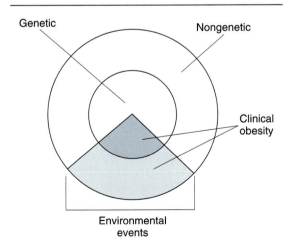

Figure 21–2. Genetic and nongenetic factors in the response to an adverse environmental event.

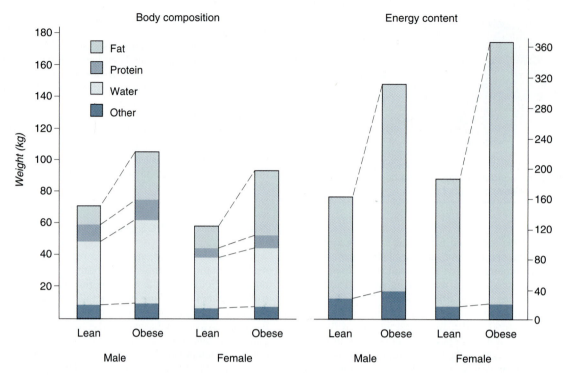

Figure 21–4. Body and energy composition. The four left bars above the lean and obese gender represent the chemical composition of a lean and obese individual expressed as proportion of body weight for a 70-kg and 100-kg man and a 56-kg and 86-kg woman (ie, an extra 30 kg for the obese person of each gender). The corresponding energy contribution from this chemical composition is shown as the right-hand bar of each pair with the ordinate to the right.

On the left side are data on body composition for the standard 70-kg man and 56-kg woman and on the right an overweight man and woman weighing 30 kg more than the lean one. The 150,000 kcal of energy in the body fat of a normal adult human is about six times the quantity of energy stored as protein (24,000 kcal). By comparison, the quantity of carbohydrate is minute (approximately 1000 kcal).

The foods in a normal diet will provide energy equivalent to 1500–3500 kcal/d depending on the age, gender, size, and activity of the individual. An individual eating a 2000-kcal diet of which 40% is carbohydrate will take in an amount of carbohydrate each day that is comparable to the total body stores of carbohydrate. In contrast, the average daily protein intake is only a little over 1% of total stores, and fat intake is considerably less than 1% (Figure 21–5). It should not be surprising, therefore, that in studies of nutrient balance in experimental animals, changes in carbohydrate balance from day to day reciprocally affected carbohydrate intake on the subsequent day. In animals, if carbohydrate balance is positive—ie, if on a given day more carbohydrate is eaten than is oxidized—less carbohydrate will be eaten the next day. Conversely, when carbohydrate balance is negative on a given day, the animal will eat more carbohydrate the next day. For fat balance, on the other hand,

the day-to-day relationship between fat balance and fat intake is very weak. Similar findings have been reported in human beings whose carbohydrate stores are acutely depleted or whose dietary fat is covertly replaced with indigestible fat. The carbohydrate oxidation can be evaluated from measurements of O_2 consumption and CO_2 produced. The ratio of CO_2 produced to O_2 used is the respiratory exchange ratio (RER), or respiratory quotient (RQ). Carbohydrate oxidation has an RQ of 1.0 and fat oxidation an RQ of 0.7. Thus, the higher the RQ, the more carbohydrate is being oxidized. A high RQ is a predictor of future weight gain in human beings.

There are two major pathways for absorption of digested food from the gut. The first pathway for absorption of nutrients across the intestinal tract involves facilitated or active transport of glucose and amino acids as well as short chain fatty acids. On the mucosal side of the intestine, these nutrients enter the portal vein on the way to the liver. The nutrients that enter the body (our controlled system) can be stored, converted to heat through metabolism, or used for work. In addition, small quantities of energy are excreted in the urine as urea and uric acid, the end products of metabolism of amino acids and nucleic acids.

The other pathway of absorption from the intestine

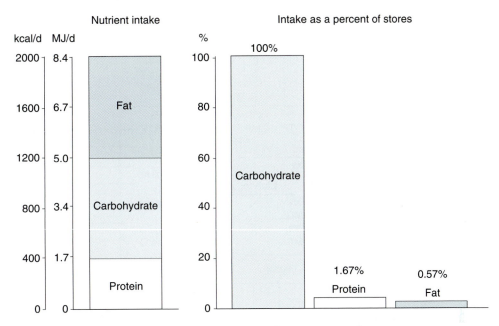

Figure 21–5. Relationship of macronutrient intake to body stores of that macronutrient. A diet containing 40% fat, 40% carbohydrate, and 20% protein is shown on the left. The relationship of each of these components to the body stores of the corresponding nutrient is shown on the left side as a percentage of nutrient stores.

is through the lacteals, which transport triacylglycerols that have been packaged into chylomicrons by the intestinal cells. These chylomicrons enter the venous circulation and are cleared in the periphery by hydrolysis of triacylglycerol catalyzed by the enzyme lipoprotein lipase (LPL). The fatty acids released by LPL enter the fat cell (Figure 21–6), where they are esterified with glycerol 3-phosphate to form triacylglycerols. The activity of LPL and the entry of glucose into the fat cell to form glycerol 3-phosphate are both increased by insulin. Hydrolysis of the stored triacylglycerol is activated through surface receptors by a variety of hormones of which epinephrine is the most important. Epinephrine and norepinephrine interacting with the β-adrenergic receptor (R_β) activates the stimulatory G-proteins, which in turn activate adenylyl cyclase to form cyclic AMP (cAMP). cAMP activates protein kinase A, which activates hormone-sensitive lipase, the rate-limiting step in the hydrolysis of triacylglycerol to release free fatty acids and glycerol from the fat cell (Figure 21–6).

In addition to its role in fat storage and release of fatty acids, adipose tissue also functions as a secretory organ. This role was first suggested when the tissue was shown to synthesize and release lipoprotein lipase. Adipsin, or complement factor D, which is involved in the alternative pathway of coagulation, is synthesized and released from adipose tissue. The adipose tissue can convert steroids into estrogens by aromatizing them. It synthesizes angiotensinogen, which is involved in regulating blood pressure, as well as the cytokine tumor necrosis factor-alpha

(TNFα). Finally, fat cells produce leptin whose absence in the obese (*ob/ob*) mouse leads to obesity.

A reduced response to insulin (insulin resistance) is characteristic of obesity. This insulin resistance involves muscle, liver, and fat cells. One explanation that could account for insulin resistance is the secretion of TNFα by the fat cell. Preventing TNFα action in obese animals by blocking its receptors increases the response to insulin. Increased response to insulin is a predictor of future weight gain. Pima Indians, who are very responsive to insulin, have a greater likelihood of becoming obese than those who are resistant. Insulin resistance may also be related to fatty acid-binding protein (FABP). In transgenic mice with knockout of the *FABP* gene, there is a reduction in insulin resistance (Chapter 18).

For body weight and body fat to remain stable, the body must oxidize the food it eats. Since more oxygen is required to oxidize fat than carbohydrate, the ratio of the carbon dioxide produced to the oxygen consumed (RQ; see above) can be used to estimate the fat and carbohydrates being metabolized. The corresponding ratio of fat to carbohydrate in the diet is called the food quotient (FQ). For stability in fat stores, FQ must equal RQ. When the FQ falls—ie, when more fat than carbohydrate is consumed—there are two mechanisms by which the organism can respond. The first is to reduce carbohydrate oxidation, which will increase fat oxidation at a corresponding rate. The second is to expand fat stores to accommodate the extra fat until the oxidation of fat rises to keep pace with intake.

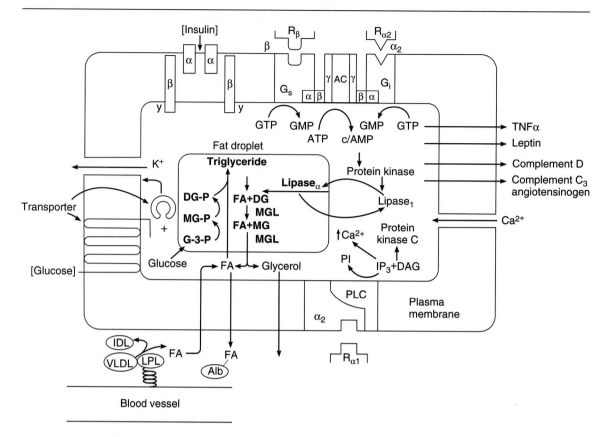

Figure 21–6. Diagram of a fat cell. The biochemical pathways for lipogenesis are shown on the left-hand side, and the pathways for lipolysis are shown on the right. (IDL, intermediate-density lipoprotein; VLDL, very low density lipoprotein; LPL, lipoprotein lipase; FA, fatty acid; MG, monoglyceride; DG, diglyceride; MGL, monoglyceride lipase; DGP, diacyl-glycerol phosphate; MGP, monoglycerol phosphate; G3P, glucose 3-phosphate; Rβ, β-adrenergic receptor; Rα_2, α_2-adrenergic receptor; TNFα, tumor necrosis factor-α.)

Energy expenditure can be divided into three components (Figure 21–7). The first is the resting metabolic rate (RMR), which in human beings is directly related to the amount of fat-free (lean) body mass. RMR has an important familial component and is a predictor for future weight gain.

The second component of energy expenditure is physical work, which accounts for approximately one-third of the energy expended. A number of studies have suggested that body weight and energy stores are well regulated over short intervals in most individuals. For most adults, the change in weight from year to year is less than 1% per year.

The third component of energy expenditure is the thermic effect of food (TEF), which reflects the rise in heat production, ie, increased oxygen consumption following ingestion of food. The TEF has two components: a facultative component, which is blocked by drugs that block β-adrenergic receptors; and an obligatory component, which is not blocked by drugs. TEF is inversely related to fatness—ie, as the percentage of fat rises, the TEF decreases.

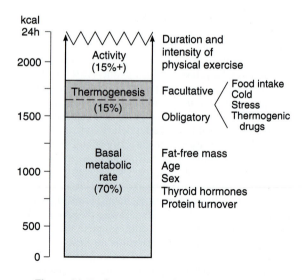

Figure 21–7. Components of energy expenditure.

Some types of obesity in humans and animals are dependent on the composition of the diet and others are not. At one extreme are the types of obesity due simply to hyperphagia or excess food intake regardless of its composition. In these cases, obesity may develop whether the diet consists chiefly of carbohydrates (vegetables, fruits), protein (meat or vegetable protein), or fats. Obesity due to hypothalamic injury or disease of endocrine glands develops regardless of the composition of the diet. At the other extreme are those types of obesity due mainly to the composition of the diet. These include high-fat diets, access to beverages or solutions containing sucrose, or other soluble carbohydrates and diets with an abundance of highly palatable foods.

The key features of the nutrient system can be summarized as follows:

1. Oxidation is continuous; nutrient intake is periodic.
2. Oxidation rate is influenced by age, gender, metabolic size, physical activity, hormonal status, nutritional status and ambient temperature.
3. Diets provide carbohydrate, protein, fat, alcohol and micronutrients.
4. Food intake is influenced by its availability and individual preference.
5. Macronutrient preference may be regulated separately for each macronutrient.
6. Carbohydrate can be oxidized, stored as glycogen, or converted to fat.
7. Lipogenesis from carbohydrate is energy expensive, and can occur in liver or fat.
8. Carbohydrate is the preferred fuel of brain and nerve and is used for bursts of muscular contraction.
9. Fat can be stored or oxidized, but is not converted to carbohydrate.
10. For nutrient balance, i.e. weight stability, fat and carbohydrate oxidized or respiratory quotient (RQ) must equal the carbohydrate to fat ratio or food quotient (FQ) in the diet.
11. When the fat to carbohydrate ratio in the diet rises (FQ falls) the oxidation of carbohydrate falls (RQ falls) and fat oxidation rises.
12. If the fall in carbohydrate oxidation is not sufficient to match the fall in dietary carbohydrate, then food intake will rise to provide carbohydrate.
13. A high RQ (high carbohydrate oxidation) predicts weight gain.
14. A low metabolic rate may predict future weight gain
15. Fat is stored primarily in fat cells.
16. Fat cells synthesize and secrete peptides including complement D (Adipsin), cytokines, angiotensinogen and *ob* protein (leptin).
17. The sympathetic nervous system may modulate adaptation to a low carbohydrate diet.

Afferent Signals to Start & Stop Eating

The brain receives information about nutrient status from several sources. Afferent signals can be transmitted over the somatosensory nervous system, over the autonomic nervous system, or through blood borne signals. These are presented in a cartoon (Figure 21–8) which is an enlargement of the afferent components of the nutrient balance diagram in Figure 21–3.

A. Sensory Signals: The sight and smell of food generate signals transmitted to the brain by sensory nerves. These signals can be positive, stimulating eating of preferred foods; or aversive, as is the case with foods associated with danger or illness. Sounds form a similar distant signaling system that can identify food or danger and permit the organism to make appropriate decisions for eating or for fight or flight.

The texture, palatability, and taste of food in the mouth and the olfactory and other sensory cues about the quality of food serve as more proximate somatosensory input for promoting or inhibiting food intake. The ability of most animals to avoid foods that have previously made them sick—a phenomenon known as bait shyness—is an example of these afferent sensory signals integrated with a central learning system.

B. Metabolic Signals That Stimulate Hunger: In more than 60% of the eating episodes in rodents and in human beings, there is a gradual dip of 7–10% in glucose concentration which is followed by meal-seeking behavior or the request for food after the nadir in glucose has been reached and glucose concentrations have begun to return to normal. If the glucose dip is prevented by infusing glucose before its plasma concentration drops by 5%, the next meal will be substantially delayed. This dip in glucose may be an arousal signal that triggers "metabolic" interest (hunger) in a meal which is then integrated with central somatosensory and other messages in deciding whether to seek food.

Two peptides can increase food intake, though their physiologic significance is unclear. The first is the nonacetylated form of melanocyte-stimulating hormone (desacetyl-MSH). This 13-amino-acid peptide will increase food intake and body weight when injected into experimental animals. Similarly, a 7-amino-acid peptide, β-casomorphin (Try-Pro-Phe-Pro-Gly-Pro-Ileu) formed during the digestion of casein, has opioid-like activity in vitro and will stimulate food intake of animals eating a high-fat diet but will depress food intake of animals eating a low-fat diet.

C. Gastrointestinal Signals That Produce Hunger and Satiety: Hunger is frequently associated with contractions of the stomach. These contractions may be a reflection of the "uneasiness" reported in association with the perception of hunger.

Satiation arising from the gastrointestinal tract

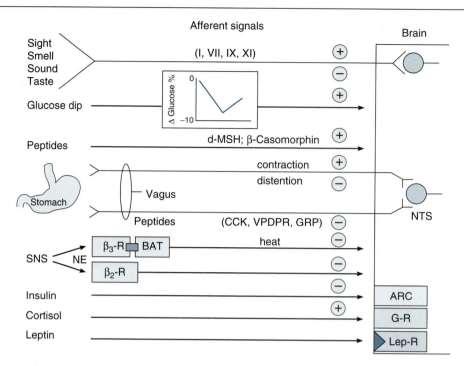

Figure 21–8. Cartoon of afferent signals controlling food intake. (d-MSH, desacetyl-malanocyte-stimulating hormone; CCK, cholecystokinin; VPDPR, enterostatin; GRP, gastrin-releasing peptide; SNS, sympathetic nervous system; NTS, nucleus tractus solitarius; NE, norepinephrine; BAT, brown adipose tissue; ARC, arcuate nucleus; G-R, glucocorticoid receptor; Lep-R, leptin receptor (absent or defective in db mouse).

may be produced by one of three mechanisms: gastrointestinal distention, release of gastrointestinal hormones when nutrients act directly on the gastrointestinal mucosa, and the effects of absorbed nutrients. Both gastric and intestinal distention can terminate meals by negative feedback signals relayed via the autonomic nervous system. The vagus nerve is probably the principal afferent sensory relay for this type of information to the nucleus of the tractus solitarius (NTS) in the hindbrain (medulla). From the NTS these signals are transmitted to many other areas of the brain including the hypothalamus, parabrachial nucleus, amygdala, hippocampus, and cortex.

In addition to the signals generated by distention of the stomach or intestine, there are hormonal messages generated from peptides released during the digestive process. Cholecystokinin, enterostatin, and gastrin-releasing peptide (GRP) are three of these peptides. Cholecystokinin (CCK) injected intraperitoneally decreases food intake in hungry rats, sheep, and human beings as well as inhibiting sham feeding in rats and monkeys. The sequence of events associated with the decrease in food intake after treatment with CCK is similar to the satiety sequence that follows a spontaneous meal. Vagotomy blocks the effect of cholecystokinin, suggesting that its receptors are in the afferent vagal complex in the gastrointesti-

nal tract or liver. One attractive hypothesis is that cholecystokinin may slow gastric emptying by producing pyloric contraction through interacting with CCK-A receptors to contract the pylorus. Drugs that block CCK-A receptors will increase food intake. In clinical studies, CCK inhibits food intake as effectively in patients with obesity due to hypothalamic injury as in obese controls, showing that these hypothalamic nuclei are not involved in the CCK response arc. CCK analogs and drugs that mimic it are attractive possibilities for treatment of obesity.

Enterostatin is a second peptide that will decrease food intake. The pentapeptide Val-Pro-Asp-Pro-Arg (in the rat) and Ala-Pro-Gly-Pro-Arg (in humans) is the signal peptide released from procolipase, which is secreted from the acinar pancreas in response to a fat meal. This peptide will decrease food intake when given into the duodenum, intraperitoneally, intravenously, and into the cerebral ventricles. In the gastrointestinal tract, enterostatin is degraded into two dipeptides (Val-Pro and Asp-Pro), both of which can be absorbed and at least one of which (the latter) can decrease food intake. In studies with animals that could choose their diet, enterostatin specifically decreased the intake of dietary fat.

Gastrin-releasing peptide (GRP) is the third peptide that can decrease food intake. It is related to bombesin, a tetradecapeptide, isolated from the skin of the toad *Bombina bombina*. GRP and bombesin have both been shown to decrease food intake in human beings by a mechanism that does not involve CCK. This satiety effect is only partially blocked by vagotomy but is completely blocked by vagotomy plus cord section, indicating that these afferent signals are relayed over both vagal and nonvagal pathways.

D. Sympathetic Nervous System: The sympathetic nervous system may also be involved in generating satiety signals. β_3-Adrenergic receptors on brown adipose tissue are responsible for mediating heat production when sympathetic nerves to this tissue are stimulated. Part of the thermic effect of a meal may be related to an increase in sympathetic activation of the β_3-adrenergic receptors. The heat produced in this way may in turn be part of a thermogenic stimulus to decrease food intake. There may be a second mechanism involved. Stimulation of peripheral β_2-adrenergic receptors may also decrease food intake but not by producing heat. Doses of clenbuterol, a β_2-adrenergic agonist that significantly decreases food intake, have little or no effect on heat production. The effects of clenbuterol can be blocked by a β_2-adrenergic antagonist, nadolol, which does not cross the blood-brain barrier, suggesting that these β_2-adrenergic satiety receptors may be located outside of the brain. Their precise location has not yet been determined (Figure 21–8).

E. Hormones: Injections of insulin can increase or decrease food intake depending on the dose and route of administration. When sufficient insulin is given to decrease glucose (which is probably the cause of the glucose dip described earlier; see Figure 21–8), hunger is aroused. With continued excess of insulin, food intake increases and weight gain occurs. This is clinically important in patients with diabetes, whose glucose is tightly regulated by injections of insulin. On the other hand, blockade of insulin receptors in the liver with anti-insulin antibodies will increase food intake, and chronic infusions of low doses of insulin peripherally or into the ventricular system of the brain have been reported to reduce food intake. One explanation for the decrease in food intake might be the decrease in neuropeptide Y (NPY) in the arcuate nucleus associated with insulin treatment, since insulin decreases the expression of mRNA for NPY in this region of the brain and NPY is a potent stimulus to eat (see below).

Adrenal steroids also play a role in feeding regulation of body fat stores. Under normal circumstances, the mineralocorticoid or type I receptors in the brain are completely saturated since the brain does not contain enzymes for metabolizing mineralocorticoids. Modulation of the type II receptors by glucocorticoids will increase or decrease food intake and can produce significant obesity with overtreatment in human beings. These effects of steroids are used clinically to increase body weight in cancer patients by treating them with megestrol acetate. Gonadal steroids also modulate body fat. Testosterone decreases total body fat and may reduce visceral fat in men. Estrogens, on the other hand, increase body fat.

The recently identified ob protein (leptin), which is deficient in the genetically obese (*ob/ob*) mouse, produced exclusively by adipose tissue, may form a mechanism for signaling the brain about the state of adipose tissue. This protein might interact with a receptor in brain and other tissues and account for the pleiotropic defects observed in these animals. In obese human beings the mRNA for leptin is increased in adipose tissue, suggesting that it is involved in human obesity.

F. Nutrient Signals: Nutrients absorbed after digestion of food may also act on the liver or brain to induce satiety. Glucose injected into the portal circulation decreases the vagal afferent firing rate, probably by an action on hepatic glucose receptors. Glucose may also act directly on the central nervous system, since this nutrient is the major source of fuel for the brain. It has been demonstrated that glucose modulates the binding of appetite-suppressing drugs, such as amphetamine, to the sodium pump in the hypothalamus. Glucose has also been shown to increase the activity of the peripheral sympathetic nervous system, which might induce satiety by acting on either β_3- or β_2-adrenergic receptors.

Fatty acids and their metabolites may also serve as afferent signals to modulate food intake. Injection of 3-hydroxybutyrate, a metabolite of long-chain free fatty acids, decreases food intake. One possible explanation for this effect is that it changes the electrical potential of the hepatocyte, which may modulate the vagal firing rate. Both mercaptoacetate and palmoxirate, two drugs that interfere with hepatic metabolism of fatty acids, increase food intake. Using diets where animals select between protein, carbohydrate, and fat, it has been shown that these drugs increase the intake of protein. This might have been expected, since the drugs block fat and carbohydrate metabolism, leaving protein as the one that can still be metabolized. In each case, the effect is blocked by vagotomy. Using the appearance of the proto-oncogene, c-*fos*, in brain tissue, it has been possible to trace the afferent neural pathways associated with hepatic vagal activation by mercaptoacetate and enterostatin. Both agents increase c-*fos* activity in the NTS, the lateral parabrachial nucleus, and amygdala as well as a few other sites. Enterostatin activates c-*fos* in several sites not activated by β-mercaptoacetate, suggesting that control of fat and protein intake in the hypothalamus involves different areas.

The Controller

A. Anatomy: Several anatomic regions of the brain appear to play an important role in the control of nutrient balance. Figure 21–9 is a representation of the hypothalamic nuclei with projections to the pitu-

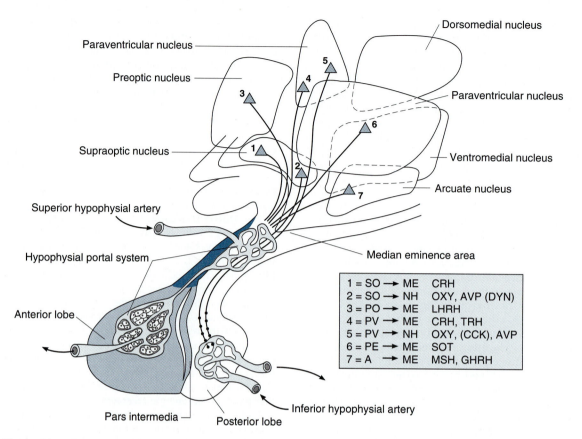

Figure 21–9. Diagram showing the anatomic location of the hypothalamic nuclei. Damage to the ventromedial or paraventricular nucleus will produce obesity. Damage to the more lateral hypothalamus produces weight loss and anorexia. (The numbers 1–7 indicate nerve tracts leading to hormone release, summarized in the box on the right.)

itary gland. Destruction of the ventromedial hypothalamus (VMH) is associated with hyperphagia, decreased activity of the sympathetic nervous system, and obesity in rodents, and it is clear from these studies that the hyperphagia is sufficient to produce obesity. However, it is also clear that hyperphagia is not necessary for the development of obesity after VMH injury or in genetic obesity. Damage to the VMH of weanling rats or small lesions in adult animals can produce obesity without hyperphagia. In genetically obese animals, obesity will also occur when the animals are fed exactly the same amount as lean animals. From a thermodynamic point of view, this nutrient conservation is made possible by reduction of energy expenditure. A similar phenomenon probably occurs in human beings.

Anatomic destruction of the lateral hypothalamus is associated with a decrease in food intake, increased activity of the sympathetic nervous system, and a reduction in body fat. The paraventricular nucleus appears to play a central role in the control of feeding. Food intake, primarily as carbohydrates, increases following topical injection of norepinephrine or NPY into the paraventricular nucleus.

B. Neurotransmitters: A schematic diagram of the monoamines and some of the peptides that modulate food intake is presented in Figure 21–10. The neurotransmitters involved with regulation of feeding can be divided into three groups: (1) the fast-acting amino acids, which modulate ion channels; (2) the monoamines, which act more slowly, primarily through second messengers; and (3) the peptides, which may modulate monoamines and affect intake of specific nutrients. Gamma-aminobutyric acid (GABA) is a fast-acting amino acid neurotransmitter that can increase or decrease food intake depending on where it is injected.

The slower-acting neurotransmitters usually involve a second messenger and include norepinephrine, serotonin, dopamine, and histamine. Serotonin is derived from the dietary amino acid tryptophan. There are seven families of serotonin receptors, and 14 genes in this family have been cloned so far. Only two or three of the seven families appear to be involved in feeding. Serotonin can increase food intake by acting on serotonin-1A receptors (5-HT_{1A}) in the raphe nucleus. When serotonin acts on postganglionic $5\text{-HT}_{1B/D}$ or 5-HT_{2C} receptors, it reduces

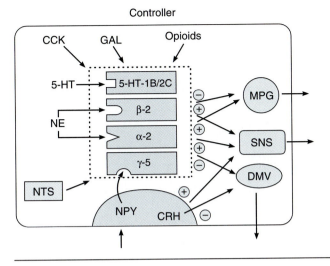

Figure 21–10. Schematic of controller, the peptides and monoamines involved in food intake. See text for details. (NTS, nucleus of the tractus solitarius; CCK, cholecystokinin; 5-HT, serotonin; NE, norepinephrine; CRH, corticotropin-releasing hormone; MPG, motor pattern generator; SNS, sympathetic nervous system; DMV, dorsal motor nucleus of the vagus; NPY, neuropeptide Y; GAL, galanin; 5HT, 5-hydroxytryptamine [serotonin]; Y5, receptor for NPY.)

food intake. Clinically, the effects of drugs that increase serotonin concentrations act at postganglionic sites to decrease food intake.

Norepinephrine can either decrease food intake by activating β_2 adrenoceptors in the perifornical area of the hypothalamus or increase food intake by acting on α_2-adrenergic receptors in the paraventricular or ventromedial nucleus. The tonic level of adrenergic receptor activation in the hypothalamus could account for differences in body fat stores. Increasing the tonic activity of β-adrenergic receptors or decreasing the tonic activity of α_2-adrenergic stimulation (or both) would tend to lower food intake in the hypothalamus.

Dopamine is involved in food reward systems, which may modulate total food intake based on its hedonic value.

Histamine is the fourth monoamine that reduces food intake by activating H_1 histamine receptors in the ventromedial hypothalamus.

Several peptides also modulate food intake (Table 21–1). The concentration of peptides in brain is about 0.1–1% that of the monoamines (picograms per gram versus nanograms per gram). Neuropeptide Y, β-endorphin, dynorphin, growth hormone-releasing hormone, somatostatin, and galanin all stimulate food intake when injected into the lateral cerebral ventricle or the paraventricular nucleus. A variety of other peptides, including bombesin, cholecystokinin, enterostatin, anorectin, calcitonin gene-related peptide, neurotensin, thyrotropin-releasing hormone, and corticotropin-releasing hormone, inhibit feeding when injected into the same regions of the brain.

One hypothesis that can explain the role of neuropeptides on food intake is that they modulate specific types of eating. Thus, neuropeptide Y injected into the paraventricular nucleus preferentially increases carbohydrate intake. Corticotropin-releasing hormone may be an important modulator of stress-re-

lated eating and specifically suppresses fat intake and to some extent carbohydrate intake. The infusion of insulin into the third ventricle will suppress food intake in animals eating a high-carbohydrate diet but not in animals eating a low-carbohydrate (high-fat) diet. Enterostatin specifically reduces fat intake whether the peptide is injected peripherally or into the central nervous system. These examples suggest that one way in which these peptides act may be to modulate specific components of the system regulating individual nutrients and their "appetites." This model or hypothesis can be called the peptide-specific nutrient balance model of eating.

Sensory-specific satiety is a clinical phenomenon whereby subjects offered a choice of preferred foods, including a food that has just been eaten, will choose a new food they have not eaten over one they have just eaten. The nutrient-specific effect of peptides could provide the molecular basis for sensory-specific satiety. Table 21–2 lists the peptides and monoamines that affect specific appetites.

Table 21–1. Peptides that stimulate or suppress feeding.

Increase Food Intake	Decrease Food Intake
Dynorphin	Anorectin
β-Endorphin	Bombesin
Galanin	Calcitonin
Growth hormone-releasing	Cholecystokinin
hormone (low dose)	Corticotropin-releasing
Neuropeptide Y	hormone
Somatostatin (low dose)	Cyclo-His-Pro
	Enterostatin
	Glucagon (GLP-1)
	Insulin
	Neurotensin
	Oxytocin
	Thyrotropin-releasing hormone
	Vasopressin

Table 21–2. Peptides and monoamines affecting specific nutrient appetites.

Nutrient	Increase	Decrease
Fat	Galanin Opiods	Serotonin Enterostatin
Carbohydrate	Norepinephrine Neuropeptide Y	Cholecystokinin
Protein	Growth hormone- releasing hormone	Glucagon
Sodium chloride	Angiotensin	

Table 21–3. Relationship of food intake and sympathetic activity.

	Food Intake	Sympathetic Activity
Lesion		
Ventromedial nucleus	↑	↓
Lateral hypothalamus	↓	↑
Peptides		
Neuropeptide Y	↑	↓
β-Endorphin	↑	↓
Cholecystokinin	↓	↑
Corticotropin-releasing hormone	↓	↑
Glucagon	↓	↑
Fibroblast growth factor	↓	↑
Interleukin 1 β	↓	↑
Neurotensin	↓	↑
Thyrotropin-releasing hormone	↓↓	↑↑
Vasopressin	↓	↑
Drugs and neurotransmitters		
Norepinephrine	↑	↓
Serotonin	↓	↑
Amphetamine	↓	↑
Fenfluramine	↓	↑
2-Deoxyglucose	↑	↓↓
4-Butene-1-olide	↓	↑

Efferent Controls

The efferent controls include the motor activities involved in identifying, obtaining, and ingesting food as well as the efferent effects produced by the autonomic nervous system and several circulating hormones. The complex sequence of motor activities that leads to the initiation of food-seeking behavior, the identification of food, and the killing or gathering and ingesting of food is beyond the scope of this review.

A. Autonomic Nervous System: Both the sympathetic and the parasympathetic nervous system may be involved in the development of obesity. When obesity is produced by hypothalamic lesions, there is increased activity of the efferent parasympathetic nervous system (vagus nerve). This observation may provide part of the explanation of the increase in insulin secretion that characterizes hypothalamic and other forms of obesity.

A reduction in sympathetic activity is also characteristic of obesity and may participate in the enhanced insulin secretion by removing inhibitory controls of insulin release. In experimental animals, there is an inverse relationship between the activity of the sympathetic nervous system and food intake. In spontaneously feeding rats, there is a negative correlation throughout the 24 hours between basal activity of the sympathetic nervous system and spontaneous food intake. In addition, experimental maneuvers that increase food intake, such as genetic obesity or lesions in the ventromedial hypothalamus, decrease the activity of the sympathetic nervous system (Table 21–3). Conversely, experimental maneuvers that decrease food intake, such as lateral hypothalamic lesions, or treatment with the appetite suppressant drug fenfluramine, increases sympathetic activity. This reciprocal relationship between food intake and the efferent sympathetic nervous system can be integrated with the earlier discussion of hypothalamic monoamines as shown in Figure 21–11. Food intake is initiated centrally, perhaps in response to a transient drop in circulating glucose levels, gastric contractions, or both. In anticipation of food intake, vagal activity increases, producing an early phase of insulin release from the pancreas. As food enters the stomach and intestine, the distention leads to satiety. Food in the gastrointestinal tract may also signal satiety by releasing hormones or stimulating the sympathetic nervous system. Stimulation of the sympathetic nervous system releases norepinephrine (NE) which activates β_3-adrenergic or β_2-adrenergic receptors. The β_3-adrenergic receptors may mediate satiety by heat production. β_2-Adrenergic receptors may also be involved in producing satiety. In the postabsorptive period, sympathetic activity slowly declines, but the increased sympathetic activity initiated by food intake may in turn serve to lower the threshold for vagal activation of insulin secretion, resulting in the glucose dip and the increased gastric contractions leading to recurrence of hunger.

B. Efferent Hormonal Mechanisms:

1. Insulin–Increased levels of insulin and resistance to its action on peripheral tissues are characteristic of obesity. Injections of insulin can increase food intake—especially the intake of glucose—probably by lowering glucose concentrations. The increased food intake following insulin injections also produces mild degrees of obesity. Injections of 2-deoxy-D-glucose, an analog of glucose, stimulates food intake by inhibiting intracellular glucose metabolism and producing intracellular glucopenia. Insulin has been proposed as providing information to the brain about the quantity of peripheral fat stores.

2. Adrenal corticosteroids–The development or progression of experimental obesity is either reversed or attenuated by adrenalectomy. In clinical medicine, adrenal insufficiency (Addison's disease)

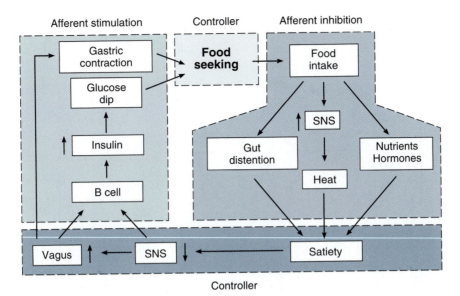

Figure 21–11. A model of food intake and satiety. Food seeking, physiologically, may be initiated by gastric contractions or a dip in glucose. Following ingestion of food, three mechanisms, including nutrient stimulation of hormonal release, gastric distention, and activation of the sympathetic nervous system, serve to signal satiety. In the postabsorptive period, the decline in activity of the sympathetic nervous system may lower the threshold for increasing vagal activity, which in turn stimulates gastric contractions and the rise in insulin leading to the glucose dip. (SNS, sympathetic nervous system.)

is associated with loss of body fat and eventually with death. Cushing's syndrome, the eponym for high levels of adrenal steroid secretion, is associated with obesity. The fact that almost all defects in genetically obese animals are reversed by adrenalectomy and that clinical changes in adrenal status can produce leanness or obesity suggests that glucocorticoids play a key role in the development and maintenance of the obese state.

C. Summary of the Control System for Food Intake: A single model integrating the earlier concepts is shown in Figure 21–12. Neural signal connections are shown as solid lines, hormonal and heat signals as dashed lines, and nutrient flux as parallel solid lines. The afferent signals are shown on the left originating in the sensory system, gut, or liver. The controller is divided into the "receiving" systems, the middle transducers, and the efferent systems. These in turn control food-seeking and ingestion and modulate metabolism. The controlled or metabolic system is sketchily represented by the pituitary adrenal system, brown adipose tissue (BAT), pancreas (B and A cells), muscle, gut, and liver.

TREATMENT OF OBESITY

The model that has been the basis for this chapter suggests three main approaches to treatment. The first is to reduce nutrient intake; the second is to in-

crease energy expenditure; and the third is to modify nutrient metabolism, which secondarily decreases food intake. The first two approaches based on this analysis are diet and exercise, which fit into groups 1 and 2, respectively.

Reduction in food intake is the first approach and the one most widely used. The principal tool is the low-calorie diet, the low-fat diet, and various other diets that have as their goal decreasing available nutrient energy for the body. If energy intake is below physiologic needs, the extra energy will come primarily from fat stores, which are very large. The greatest discrepancy between intake and energy needs is produced by starvation or fasting. With no food intake, 1500–3000 kcal will be withdrawn from fat stores each day. Since body fat contains about 7500 kcal/kg of fat, a negative calorie balance of 1500 kcal/d will produce weight loss of 1 kg every 5 days. Weight losses in the range of 0.5–1 kg/d are appropriate for a weight reduction diet.

Increasing energy expenditure through exercise would serve the purposes of the second approach. As primary treatment for overweight patients, however, exercise does not work well. Heavier people use more energy moving heavier bodies and thus tend to perspire more easily and to injure joints more often. As a strategy for helping people maintain the weight they have lost, however, exercise is an excellent resource. Indeed, if energy expenditure is not increased, maintaining weight loss is very difficult be-

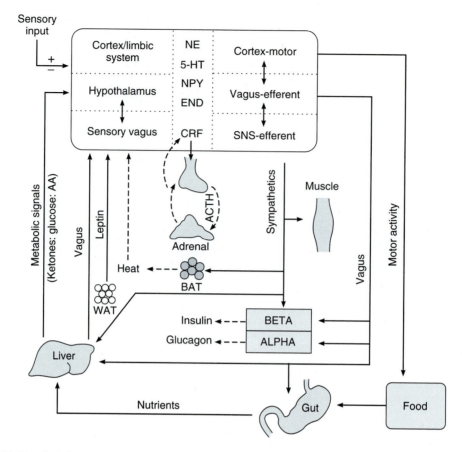

Figure 21–12. Detailed diagram of the controlled system for food intake. Both stimulatory (+) and inhibitory (−) signals are generated and fed to the brain through the sensory system, through circulating nutrients and hormones, or through the vagus and the sympathetic afferent nervous system. All of this information is integrated in the controller, where serotonin (5-HT), the β-adrenergic system, and the α-adrenergic system are important. A number of peptides also modulate feeding. The transduced signals control motor activity for food selection as well as the sympathetic and parasympathetic (vagus) nervous system. These efferent systems in turn modulate the control of food intake and the metabolism within the controlled system. (5-HT, serotonin; NE, norepinephrine; CCK, cholecystokinin; NPY, neuropeptide Y; CRF, corticotropin-releasing factor; NTS, nucleus of the tractus solitarius; F.I., food ingestion; SNS, sympathetic nervous system; DMV, dorsomotor vagal nucleus; BAT, brown adipose tissue; Panc, pancreas; WAT, white adipose tissue.)

cause of the difficulty in maintain a reduced food intake.

One of the key problems with diet and exercise as a means of achieving desired weight loss is that they do not cure the problem. Thus, regain of weight is very common. It is for this reason that growing attention is being paid to the use of medication and surgery for treating people with serious health risks associated with obesity.

Since the controller regulates food intake, drugs aimed at modulating the way the controller functions might be potential targets for drug development. All of the currently approved and available drugs for treatment of obesity are either modulators of noradrenergic receptors (diethylpropion, mazindol, phentermine) or of serotonergic receptors (fenflu-

ramine). Any of these drugs will produce weight loss, but combining them may be more beneficial than using them singly. One such approach has combined fenfluramine (serotonergic) with phentermine (noradrenergic). Because all drugs have potential side effects, appetite suppressants for treatment of obesity should be used only after assessing the risk and benefits of this form of therapy.

The second group of drugs that could be used for treatment of obesity would increase energy expenditure. Some drugs such as thyroid hormone have been used for this purpose, but no agents are currently approved that increase energy expenditure.

The third way of attacking obesity pharmacologically is through the use of drugs that modify nutrient metabolism. This can be done by reducing digestion (lipase inhibition) or by modifying metabolism (androgens, estrogens, growth hormone). None of these approaches have yet been clinically validated. There is thus a need for further research in this field to identify safe, effective, and affordable pharmacologic therapy for obesity.

SUMMARY

Obesity can be most easily conceptualized as a problem of defective control of normal nutrient feedback systems. This homeostatic approach is used as the basis for considering the importance of individual nutrients in this control system. The diet normally consists of about 50% carbohydrate, 35% fat, and 15% protein. Relative to body stores, the amount of carbohydrate eaten each day is very large and nearly equivalent to what is stored as glycogen, whereas the stores of fat and protein are greatly in excess of the daily intake of these macronutrients. Experimental studies suggest that the control of body fat content is more stable on a high-carbohydrate diet than on a high-fat diet. Moreover, maintaining energy balance requires that the average daily intake of carbohydrate and fat must be the same as the mix of carbohydrate and fat, which are used as fuels by the body. Regular physical exercise enhances the oxidation of fat and may in that way play a role in maintaining lower body fat stores. Although body fat usually increases when most animals and probably humans eat a high-fat diet, this is not always the case. There must,

therefore, be mechanisms by which the rate of fat oxidation can be increased in the face of a high-fat diet. Information about the intake of nutrients and about body nutrient stores is relayed to the brain by afferent signals. These signals can be the nutrients themselves, hormones released by interactions of nutrients with the gut, or the effects of food and its nutrients on neural messages to the brain. From this wealth of afferent information, the brain must sort out the relevant signals and make decisions about food intake. These processes are primarily integrated in the hypothalamus and hippocampus. Several neurotransmitters are involved in this intraneural signaling, including gamma-aminobutyric acid, norepinephrine, serotonin, and several peptides. The various peptides used in this process may act to modulate specific types of food intake. Thus, neuropeptide Y stimulates carbohydrate intake, and enterostatin decreases fat intake. Once the brain has made a decision, efferent processes are turned on. The animal or human can search for food or stop eating. When food is ingested, both the autonomic nervous system and the endocrine system are involved in partitioning this intake into body stores. High levels of sympathetic activity are associated with lower levels of body fat. Absence of adrenal glucocorticoid hormones is also associated with lower levels of body fat. On the other hand, high levels of insulin are associated with higher levels of body fat. From this homeostatic model, it is possible to understand the mechanisms involved in the development of obesity and to consider approaches to its treatment.

REFERENCES

Baez M et al: Molecular biology of serotonin receptors. Obes Res 1995;3:441S.

Bouchard C (editor): *The Genetics of Obesity.* CRC Press, 1993.

Bouchard C, Perusse L: Current status of the human obesity gene map. Obes Res 1996;4:81.

Bray GA, York DA, Fisler JS: Experimental obesity: A homeostatic failure due to defective nutrient stimulation of the sympathetic nervous system. Vitam Horm 1989; 45:1.

Campfield LA, Brandon P, Smith FJ: On-line continuous measurement of blood glucose and meal pattern in free-feeding rats: The role of glucose in meal initiation. Brain Res Bull 1985;14:605.

The Diabetes Control and Complications Trial Research Group: The effect of intensive treatment of diabetes on the development and progression of long-term complications in insulin-dependent diabetes mellitus. The Diabetes Control and Complications Trial Research Group. N Engl J Med 1993;329:977.

Flatt JP: Dietary fat, carbohydrate balance, and weight maintenance: Effects of exercise. Am J Clin Nutr 1987; 45:296.

Flier JS: The adipocyte: Storage depot or node on the energy information superhighway. Cell 1995;80:15.

Hotamisligil GS et al: Increased adipose tissue expression of TNF-α in human obesity and insulin resistance. J Clin Invest 1995;95:2409.

Leibowitz SF: Neurochemical-neuroendocrine systems in the brain controlling macronutrient intake and metabolism. (Review.) Trends Neurosci 1992;15:491.

Okada S et al: Enterostatin (Val-Pro-Asp-Pro-Arg), the activation peptide of procolipase selectivity, reduces fat intake. Physiol Behav 1991;49:1185.

Ravussin E et al: Reduced rate of energy expenditure as a risk factor for body-weight gain. N Engl J Med 1988; 318:467.

Reeve JR et al: Cholecystokinin. CCK 1993: International Symposium. Proceedings. Chatham, Massachusetts, May 19–22, 1993. Ann N Y Acad Sci 1994;713:1.

Schwartz MW et al: Insulin in the brain: A hormonal regulator of energy balance. Endocr Rev 1992;13:387.

22

Hormones & Cancer

Debu Tripathy, MD, & Christopher C. Benz, MD

EFFECTS OF HORMONES ON TUMORS

GROWTH PROMOTION & MALIGNANT TRANSFORMATION

It would be logical to suppose that hormones which support normal growth might also promote tumorigenesis. However, although a great deal is known about endocrine factors regulating normal pre- and postnatal growth, very little from that body of information can be applied to our current understanding of tumorigenesis. Growth hormone (GH), thyroid hormone, insulin, and sex and adrenal steroids have permissive roles in prenatal growth (Chapter 6). Of these hormones, only the sex steroids are capable of directly stimulating tissue growth during the postnatal period, and these tropic responses are often augmented by the secondary release of polypeptide growth factors. Genetic rather than endocrine factors play the major role in determining body stature. Gigantism, for example, results from excessive secretion of GH by a pituitary tumor; however, the end-organ tropic responses to GH as well as the responses to thyroxine and insulin are mediated by a family of mitogenic growth factors called somatomedins. Specifically, somatomedins C and A (now known as insulin-like growth factors [IGF]-1 and -2) are polypeptides with structural homology to proinsulin, and their serum concentrations are regulated by hormones. Acting via membrane receptors, these somatomedins and other more recently identified growth factors directly stimulate growth and proliferation of both normal and neoplastic cells. Several of the better characterized growth factors of nonhematopoietic and nonlymphoid tissue origin are shown in Table 22–1; recent reviews on cellular growth factors and their relation to cellular oncogenes are also provided in the reference list that accompanies this chapter.

In brief, many human tumors appear to produce, perhaps constitutively, mitogenic polypeptides that

ACRONYMS USED IN THIS CHAPTER	
ACTH	Adrenocorticotropic hormone
APML	Acute promyelocytic leukemia
APUD	Amine precursor uptake and decarboxylation
CCK	Cholecystokinin
CMF	Cyclophosphamide, methotrexate, fluorouracil
DES	Diethylstilbestrol
DNA	Deoxyribonucleic acid
EGF	Epidermal growth factor
ER	Estrogen receptor
FGF	Fibroblast growth factor
FSH	Follicle-stimulating hormone
GH	Growth hormone
GnRH	Gonadotropin-releasing hormone
hCG	Human chorionic gonadotropin
IGF-1	Insulin-like growth factor-1 (somatomedin C)
IGF-2	Insulin-like growth factor-2 (somatomedin A)
LH	Luteinizing hormone
LTR	Long terminal repeat (segments)
MMTV	Murine mammary tumor virus
NGF	Nerve growth factor
PDGF	Platelet-derived growth factor
PgR	Progesterone receptor
PRL	Prolactin
PSA	Prostate-specific antigen
SIADH	Syndrome of inappropriate secretion of vasopressin (antidiuretic hormone)
TGFα	Transforming growth factor α
TGFβ	Transforming growth factor β
TSH	Thyroid-stimulating hormone (thyrotropin)
VIP	Vasoactive intestinal polypeptide

Table 22–1. Growth factors and receptors potentially involved in the autocrine and paracrine regulation of human tumor growth.

Growth Factor [and Homologous Oncogene]	Tissue Source of Factor	Receptor [and Homologous Oncogene] Expressed by Normal Target
EGF	Submaxillary gland, Brunner's glands	170-kDa tyrosine kinase [c-*erb* B-1] on epithelial and mesenchymal cells
TGFα	Transformed cells, placenta, embryos	Cross-reacts with EGF receptor on same cells
TGFβ	Platelets, kidney, placenta	615-kDa tyrosine kinase on epithelial, epidermal, and mesenchymal cells
PDGF [c-*sis* with beta chain]	Platelets, endothelial cells, placenta	185-kDa tyrosine kinase on smooth muscle, mesenchymal cells, and placenta
IGF-1 (somatomedin C)	Liver, smooth muscle, other cells	450-kDa tyrosine kinase (c-*ros* and c-*src* with beta chain) on epithelial and mesenchymal cells
IGF-2 (somatomedin A)	Fetal liver, placenta	250-kDa glycoprotein on epithelial and mesenchymal cells
FGF [*int*-2 with basic form]	Brain, pituitary, kidney, cartilage	Possible intracellular receptor in endothelial and mesenchymal cells
NGF	Submaxillary gland, keratinocytes	130-kDa protein kinase on sympathetic and sensory neurons, melanocytes
Heregulin	Epithelial and mesenchymal cells, maturing neurons	Heterodimers containing 185-kDa tyrosine kinase (HER2/*neu*) on epithelial cells

are called cellular or transforming growth factors (TGF). In addition, tumor cells synthesize membrane-binding proteins for these same growth factors, and these growth factor receptors commonly possess protein kinase activity that transduces the mitogenic signal from cytoplasm to nucleus. Many of these growth factors and receptors are encoded by DNA sequences that are homologous or identical to normal proto-oncogene sequences (eg, c-*sis* and PDGF beta chain, c-*int*-2 and basic FGF; also, c-*erb* B-1 and EGF receptor, c-*src* and IGF-1 receptor), illustrating the structural relationship that commonly exists between cellular growth-promoting mechanisms and oncogene products (Table 22–1). Proto-oncogenes are cellular genes believed to have been captured and recombined into the transforming genes found in certain oncogenic retroviruses. Strong evidence now exists that the intracellular activation of some of these proto-oncogenes accounts for the development and progression of a variety of human cancers. Carcinogenic mutation, chromosomal rearrangement, sequence deletion, and gene amplification are several of the known genetic mechanisms that can activate normal proto-oncogenes.

Substantial evidence points to the fact that human cancers do not result from a single genetic event. Rather, stepwise genetic changes result in the activation of proto-oncogenes and the inactivation of so-called anti-oncogenes (or tumor suppressor genes), necessary for progression to the fully transformed malignant phenotype. Hormones probably contribute to this process, since many natural and synthetic steroids and steroid-like compounds are known to be carcinogenic. In particular, steroidal estrogens and xenobiotic stilbenes (eg, diethylstilbestrol) can produce DNA damage either directly, by the formation of mutagenic DNA adducts and strand breaks, or indirectly, by the generation of toxic host molecules and intracellular free radicals.

Specific studies have addressed the development of tumors occurring in hormonally regulated tissues. It is known that both chemical carcinogens (including steroidal and nonsteroidal estrogens) and the genomic integration of viral DNA can potentially induce tumorigenesis. Long-term or in utero exposure to exogenous estrogens is epidemiologically associated with an increased incidence of human uterine and breast carcinomas. It is also known that murine mammary cancers are commonly induced by the murine mammary tumor virus (MMTV), which is a weakly oncogenic type B retrovirus. The regional insertion of MMTV DNA activates genomic c-*int*-1, c-*int*-2, and other proto-oncogenes which are then constitutively expressed in mammary epithelium, leading to premalignant hyperplastic lesions and, finally, to infiltrating adenocarcinomas. Since there are closely linked steroid receptor-binding sequences within the integrated MMTV long terminal repeat (LTR) segment, this process of malignant transformation can be promoted by exposure to steroids. In transgenic animal experiments, fusion of the MMTV LTR promoter region to various oncogenes (including c-*myc,* v-Ha-*ras,* c-*int*-1 or c-*int*-2, c-*src,* and activated c-*neu/erb* B-2), and introduction of these fused constructs into viable eggs of female mice leads to breast tumors in otherwise normal mouse offspring. Despite widespread genomic incorporation of the transgene in all mouse tissues, only breast, salivary gland, and epididymal tissues express the incorporated oncogene, and essentially only breast adenocarcinomas occur over a time course and with an increased incidence that depends on the particular oncogene. To date, one of the most effective breast cancer-inducing constructs is the MMTV/c-*neu* transgene, which encodes an activated EGF receptor-like molecule that has potent tyrosine kinase activity. These basic studies have provided important insights into the molecular mechanisms underlying hormone-dependent tumor promotion in humans. One notable finding is an apparent correlation between clinically aggressive disease and the amplification of c-*myc*, *PRAD1* (cyclin D 1), or HER2/*neu* in a significant percentage of human breast tumors.

TUMOR GROWTH MEDIATED BY AUTOCRINE & PARACRINE FACTORS

During human growth and development as well as during normal tissue response to injury, proliferation and invasion of diploid cells is regulated by exogenous and endogenous cellular growth factors. In the absence of these mitogenic factors, normal cells will become reversibly arrested in G_1/G_0 phase, permitting normal expression of the differentiated phenotype. In the process of tumorigenesis, these growth factors become inappropriately or constitutively activated (or both), leading to the invasive and autonomous growth that characterizes malignancy. Ectopic expression of these growth factors may also account for a host of other tumor-related complications. Specific factors such as nerve growth factor (NGF), which are important for the maintenance and differentiation of some normal cells (eg, sensory and sympathetic neurons), may exert mitogenic effects on other related cells (eg, adrenal chromaffin cells). These effects may explain the selective expression of specific factors in certain types of malignant tumors (eg, pheochromocytomas, melanomas, and small-cell carcinomas). The concept that autonomous tumor growth can be driven by unregulated expression of locally produced and locally acting growth factors is exemplified by the mitogenic effect of NGF on cells derived from neural crest. Normal keratinocytes express mitogenic concentrations of NGF, which can stimulate local melanocytes or melanoma cells that possess NGF receptors to overexpress the growth-related oncogenes c-*myc* and c-*fos*. This potential model of tumorigenesis illustrates the functional relationship between growth factors and oncogenes that may exist in addition to the structural relationship described earlier.

There are now abundant in vitro and in vivo models showing growth factor production by a tumor that also possesses receptors for the same autostimulating factor (autocrine loop). Autocrine factors synthesized by some activated oncogenes (eg, c-*sis*) may not even be secreted extracellularly; rather, they may be simply bound to internally sequestered receptors that, when stimulated, result in malignant transformation (intracrine loop). Possibly as important in tumorigenesis as the autocrine loop is a more indirect process of autostimulation in which transformed cells recruit local normal cells of stromal or epithelial origin to secrete growth factors that stimulate the receptor-bearing malignant cells (paracrine loop). This paracrine interdependence between adjacent normal and malignant tissues may also explain a variety of commonly observed neoplastic phenomena, including site-specific metastases, fibroblast and endothelial chemotaxis and proliferation (leading to stromal reactivity and tumor neovascularity), local bone resorption or malignant hypercalcemia, and suppression of normal immune reactions seen with advancing malignancy.

Hormonal influences on tumor-promoting autocrine and paracrine loops have been well described in studies using cultured human breast cancer cell lines. For example, estrogen-induced growth stimulation of receptor-positive tumor cells actually occurs via rapid modulation of autocrine and paracrine growth factor release by estradiol. Estradiol enhances breast cancer cell production of autostimulating mitogens, such as TGFα, EGF, IGF-1, and IGF-2, and of paracrine factors, such as PDGF and FGFs. Additionally, estradiol can depress synthesis of the bifunctional growth factor TGFβ, which normally inhibits proliferation of breast cancer epithelial cells while paradoxically stimulating growth of mesenchymal cells. The net paracrine effect from PDGF, IGF-2, and TGFβ causes a rapid increase in fibroblast expression of several oncogenes (eg, c-*myc*, c-*fos*, c-*jun*) and the release of additional growth factors that can mitogenically stimulate breast cancer cells. Besides inducing a stromal proliferative response, these paracrine influences also stimulate fibroblasts to enzymatically alter the local composition of basement membrane and extracellular matrix, facilitating further invasion and growth by the malignant mammary epithelial cells.

Given the role of growth factors and growth factor receptors in the malignant phenotypes of certain cancers, attempts to modulate their expression and function have been explored as novel therapies. The HER2/*neu* oncogene, which encodes a member of the EGF growth factor receptor family, is amplified and overexpressed in about 20% of human primary breast cancers. Experimental overexpression of this oncogene in breast cells or transgenic mice leads to mammary cancer, and antibodies to this receptor can inhibit the growth of HER2/*neu* overexpressing human cancer cells. Such antibodies to HER2/*neu* are currently in clinical trials for patients with advanced breast cancer whose tumors are known to overexpress this oncogene. Other growth factor receptor systems such as PDGF, somatostatin, and EGF are also being investigated as potential therapeutic targets.

STEROID-DEPENDENT TUMORS

The early studies of Bittner, Huggins, Furth, and others established the concept that sex steroids can cause or at least promote tumor growth. In general, the only cancers frequently promoted by sex steroids include those common tumors arising from breast (male and female), endometrial, and prostatic tissue (Table 22–2).

It may be generally true that endocrine dependency can develop as an associated trait of tumors derived from any tissue whose normal growth is stimulated by a hormone. Studies in fact have demonstrated associations between sex steroids (especially estrogens) as well as vaginal, ovarian, and laryngeal carcinomas as well as hepatomas. It has been suggested that sex steroids alone may play a pathogenic role in almost 30% of all cancer cases in the USA. Thyroid, testicular, and ovarian tumors occur in glands under the tropic influences of TSH, FSH, and LH and may also be putatively included in the list of endocrine-dependent cancers. With increasing epidemiologic data, it is likely that this list will increase. For example, the incidence of osteosarcoma closely parallels the different age-specific growth patterns of men and women, implicating pubertal hormonal changes in the etiology of this tumor. Meningiomas and thyroid and renal cell carcinomas show a marked discrepancy in male-female incidence (and prognosis), also suggesting tropic sex hormone influences on tumor growth.

In contrast to the tropic sex steroids or differentiation-inducing steroids, glucocorticoids are capable of cytolytic responses mediated by steroid-induced enzymatic pathways. Since the realization several decades ago that glucocorticoids could lyse human lymphoblasts, these steroids have been extensively employed in the treatment of leukemia and lymphoma.

TUMORS AFFECTING ENDOCRINE STATUS

Tumors that are not hormone-responsive (or amenable to endocrine therapy) may still affect endocrine status, and these tumor-induced endocrine effects are important for clinical diagnosis and management.

NONSECRETORY TUMORS

Nonsecretory primary or metastatic tumors may invade and replace normal glandular tissue and thereby cause loss of endocrine function. The most common syndrome in this category is hypopituitarism due to pressure necrosis that occurs gradually during tumor growth or that occurs abruptly from tumor infarction and bleeding. Tumors such as breast cancer, leukemia, or lymphoma may be metastatic to the sella; may directly invade, as with a craniopharyngioma or hypothalamic glioma; or may originate from a primary adenoma in the anterior pituitary. Rarely, infarction of the posterior pituitary and the clinical development of diabetes insipidus may be the presenting sign of metastatic cancer (Chapter 5). Adrenal insufficiency can also occur with metastatic infiltration of both glands by a variety of epithelial cancers (eg, lung cancer, breast cancer, melanoma). However, clinical evidence of adrenal insufficiency produced by metastatic infiltration is unusual relative to the high overall incidence of adrenal metastases found at autopsy. Although extensive pancreatic or ovarian replacement can occur with metastatic retroperitoneal tumor spread, diabetes mellitus or ovarian failure virtually never results. Ovarian failure may develop in association with a primary ovarian carcinoma that secretes steroid precursors which in turn inhibit pituitary gonadotropin production.

SECRETORY TUMORS

Several types of benign and malignant tumors secrete hormones or hormone-like substances. When these chemicals are produced ectopically or "inappropriately" (by a tumor arising in a tissue not normally associated with the hormone), the resulting paraneoplastic syndrome may provide a diagnostic clue or

---

Table 22–2. Endocrine-responsive tumors.

Primary treatment involves endocrine therapy
Breast carcinoma
Endometrial carcinoma
Prostatic carcinoma
Leukemia
Lymphoma

Tumor treatment may include endocrine therapy
Renal cell carcinoma
Thyroid carcinoma
Ovarian carcinoma
Pituitary adenoma
Promyelocytic leukemia

Tumor subsets may be endocrine-dependent
Vaginal carcinoma
Meningioma
Melanoma and apudoma
Gastrointestinal carcinoma
Sarcoma

may signify recurrence of an otherwise undetectable lesion (Chapter 23). For example, gynecomastia associated with an elevated titer of human chorionic gonadotropin (hCG) strongly suggests an underlying testicular carcinoma that can be cured with chemotherapy. "Appropriate" hormone production by secretory tumors arising within endocrine tissue may also produce symptoms leading to early tumor detection and cure, as is occasionally observed with insulinomas. On the other hand, endocrine symptoms from secretory tumors may develop in association with advanced disease and result in life-threatening or debilitating clinical complications. Palliation of symptoms of carcinoid or one of the other APUDomas (Chapter 23) can actually become of greater clinical concern than controlling growth of the tumor itself. These secretory tumors are usually well differentiated and may occur in genetic patterns (eg, Klinefelter's syndrome associated with a breast or pituitary tumor) or in familial patterns involving multiple endocrine glands (eg, multiple endocrine neoplasia type I, IIa, or IIb; Chapter 24). Table 22–3 lists the origin of commonly occurring secretory tumors and their associated secretory products.

TREATMENT-INDUCED ENDOCRINOPATHY

With the improved prognosis of patients with leukemia, lymphoma, stage II breast cancer, and

Table 22–3. Secretory tumors of endocrine glands.

Tumor Origin	Secretory Product(s)
Anterior pituitary	GH, PRL, ACTH, TSH, FSH, LH
Adrenal Cortex	Aldosterone, glucocorticoids, androgens, estrogens (rare)
Medulla	Catecholamines
Kidney	Erythropoietin
Gonads Germ cell, trophoblast	hCG
Stroma	Estrogens, androgens, progestins
Pancreas and gut (APUD cells)	Serotonin, kallikrein, prostaglandins, somatostatin, gastrin, glucagon, insulin, VIP, CCK, vasopressin, ACTH, neurotensin
Parathyroids	Parathyroid hormone
Thyroid Parafollicular (medullary) cells	Calcitonin
Follicular cells	Thyroglobulin T_3 and T_4 (rare)

germ cell neoplasms treated with irradiation and chemotherapy, there is a growing awareness of the long-term endocrine complications of treatment. The glands associated with treatment-induced endocrinopathy include the hypothalamus, pituitary, thyroid, parathyroids, and gonads. As shown in Table 22–4, local or regional effects from radiation therapy and the systemic effects of radiomimetic drugs (alkylating agents) produce the greatest clinical problems.

Brain & Pituitary

Children receiving cranial irradiation either to prevent leukemia of the central nervous system or to treat a curable brain tumor have blunted GH responses, impaired growth rates, and some impairment of intellectual function. Less commonly, they may have reduced secretion of TSH, ACTH, FSH, and LH. In adults, apart from the use of hormonal agents, antitumor therapy results in very few abnormalities in the hypothalamic-pituitary-neuroendocrine axis. Adjuvant chemotherapy for breast cancer has been reported to lower serum PRL levels, but the underlying mechanism is unclear. Vincristine and cyclophosphamide have both been associated with a syndrome of inappropriate secretion of vasopressin (antidiuretic hormone), or SIADH. While a direct effect on renal tubules is believed to be the cause of the antidiuresis that occurs with cyclophosphamide, vincristine may increase vasopressin release by disrupting microtubules within the neurohypophysis.

GnRH analogs such as leuprolide and goserelin interfere with the normally pulsatile stimulation of the pituitary by native hypothalamic GnRH. The use of these analogs results in a lack of gonadotropin stimulation of the ovaries or testes and a resultant drop in estrogen or testosterone. This treatment, while successful in a majority of patients with advanced prostate cancer and about half of patients with advanced breast cancer, also results in the expected side effects of sex hormone deprivation, including hot flushes, loss of libido, amenorrhea in women, and some atrophy of sex hormone-dependent tissue.

Thyroid

One-third of patients with cervical lymphomas or carcinomas of the pharynx or larynx treated with curative doses of radiation (which includes the thyroid) develop increased TSH levels, and most of these also develop decreased thyroxine levels. A few become clinically hypothyroid. Both low-dose and (less frequently) high-dose irradiation increase the incidence of thyroid carcinomas occurring 10 or more years after treatment (Chapter 7).

Adrenals

Adrenal gland function appears resistant to the toxic effects of conventional doses of radiation or chemotherapy. However, prolonged busulfan administration for chronic granulocytic leukemia results in

Table 22–4. Treatment-induced endocrinopathy.

	Hormone Abnromality	Clinical Abnormality
Radiation therapy Brain	↓ GH; less commonly, ↓ TSH, ACTH, FSH, LH	Growth retardation.
Head and neck Low-dose (≤ 750 cGy)	↑ Parathyroid hormone	Hyperparathyroidism, thyroid cancer.
High-dose (≥ 1400 cGy)	↓ Thyroxine; ↑ TSH	Hypothyroidism, thyroid cancer.
Abdomen and pelvis (including gonads)	↓ Estrogen; ↑ FSH, LH	Sterility, menopause, azoospermia.
Chemotherapy Alkylating agents, vinblastine, others	↓ Estrogen; ↑ FSH, LH (normal testosterone, adrenal steroids)	Sterility, menopause, azoospermia.
Vincristine	↑ Vasopressin	SIADH[1]
Cyclophosphamide	(Normal vasopressin)	SIADH[1]
Mitotane	↓ Adrenal steroids	Primary adrenal insufficiency.
Aminoglutethimide	↓ Estrogens, adrenal steroids	Primary adrenal insufficiency.
	↓ Thyroxine: ↑ TSH	Hypothyroidism.

[1]Syndrome of inappropriate secretion of vasopressin (antidiuretic hormone).

a clinical syndrome resembling adrenocortical insufficiency. Some investigators believe that pituitary secretion of ACTH—rather than adrenocortical function—is damaged by the drug. This mechanism could be similar to that resulting in impaired PRL secretion, mentioned above. Mitotane (a drug used to treat adrenocortical cancers) and aminoglutethimide (used to treat breast cancers) have as part of their desired therapeutic mechanisms the effect of suppressing steroid production and causing primary adrenocortical insufficiency (Chapter 9).

Gonads

Perhaps the most frequently encountered endocrinopathy resulting from antitumor therapy is gonadal failure. Radiation therapy and chemotherapy can cause infertility in both men and women. In women, amenorrhea (or oligomenorrhea), dyspareunia, decreased libido, and hot flushes may follow either form of therapy. These symptoms are associated with reduced plasma estradiol and increased levels of FSH and LH. In fact, ovarian failure occurs so frequently after adjuvant chemotherapy for breast cancer that some have suggested that the effectiveness of adjuvant therapy results from "chemical oophorectomy." In younger women, there is a greater probability that gonadal function will return to normal. In men, azoospermia (or oligospermia) occurs in association with reduced testicular size, increased FSH, and (occasionally) gynecomastia. Leydig cells are much more resistant to toxic therapy, and serum testosterone levels therefore usually remain normal, although there may be evidence for partial Leydig cell failure compensated for by higher levels of LH. De-

pending on radiation or drug dosage, male gonadal function and fertility may recover. With the aggressive drug combinations used to cure Lymphomas, however, gonadal recovery is unlikely, and men should be offered the opportunity for sperm storage before chemotherapy begins. Recent successes with in vitro fertilization and cryopreservation have provided a similar option for women. GnRH analogs, which decrease serum gonadotropin levels, are currently being investigated for their ability to protect the gonads during cytotoxic therapy. The use of birth control pills to reversibly suppress gonadotropins and suspend ovarian function has reportedly been successful in sparing women from gonadal toxicity during chemotherapy. It should be recognized that gonadal toxicity varies with the type of chemotherapy being used; alkylating agents and procarbazine are the most potent toxins. Certain combinations of drugs used to treat lymphomas may, in fact, cause little permanent gonadal damage.

ENDOCRINE THERAPY FOR CANCER

STEROID RECEPTORS & TREATMENT

At present, endocrine treatment is of major therapeutic value in breast, endometrial, and prostatic cancers. The specific applications of endocrine therapy in these diseases will be discussed later. However, the measurement of steroid receptors has added a further refinement to the technology of determining which tumors are endocrine-sensitive. Estrogen receptors (ER) and progesterone receptors (PgR), useful for predicting the clinical responsiveness of breast cancer, appear to be detectable biochemically in a variety of other human tumors, including ovarian and endometrial carcinomas, hepatomas, sarcomas, meningiomas, renal cell carcinomas, as well as melanomas and colorectal and pancreatic carcinomas. On average, however, most of these tumors have a very low frequency of immunoreactive receptor positivity and a much lower receptor content than that found in breast cancer. Thus, with the exception of endometrial cancer, clinical studies have failed to detect a significant role for endocrine therapy in the management of these other tumors.

The mere presence of a steroid receptor does not ensure either a functioning receptor mechanism or a cytostatic or cytolytic response when endocrine treatment is employed. For example, glucocorticoids are known to alter liver metabolism, but they do not produce the cytolytic effects on hepatocytes that are observed with lymphocytes, although both cell types contain high levels of glucocorticoid receptor. Additionally, ER-positive tumors capable of making PgR are the breast tumors most responsive to endocrine treatment. While most endocrine agents do not exert their antitumor effects by binding to PgR, the mere presence of PgR identifies those tumor subsets with a well-functioning ER mechanism. Even so, 20–30% of ER- and PgR-positive breast tumors may not respond to endocrine treatment, and there is increasing evidence that some of these tumors contain dysfunctional receptors. Both transcriptional and posttranscriptional mechanisms capable of producing defective ER have been detected in human breast tumors. In short, the therapeutic importance of receptors depends on both a functioning receptor mechanism and a growth-regulating receptor response.

Additional comments should be made in reference to the potential clinical significance of the different available means of assaying for tumor ER and PgR content. Biochemical assays have traditionally involved the competitive binding of a radioligand to a cell-free receptor extract prepared by homogenizing fresh tumor specimens. The calculated receptor content (fmol/mg protein cytosol) is very sensitive to procedural conditions, provides no measure of receptor heterogeneity within the tumor specimen, and can be falsely depressed by endogenous or exogenously administered receptor-binding agents. For instance, it has been shown that exogenously administered nonsteroidal antiestrogens can cause a true depression in receptor levels to about 25% of their pretreatment values; thus, it is recommended that at least 2 months elapse after treatment cessation before assaying the tumor if the assay technique utilizes competitive lig-

and binding. Treatment with radiation therapy or chemotherapy may result in a true reduction in receptor levels, independent of the assay procedure, and this may persist for 12–24 months following cessation of therapy. Newer assays utilizing monoclonal antibodies to measure ER and PgR content are easier to perform, and they avoid the problems related to receptor occupation by competing ligands. Monoclonal antibody assays also provide an immunohistochemical means of assessing receptor heterogeneity within tumor tissue and permit the detection of receptor-positive cells in small cytologic samples, eg, fine-needle aspiration biopsies of tumors. Furthermore, immunohistochemical assay enables the unequivocal detection of receptor-positive malignant cells within receptor-positive normal tissue, such as occurs with uterine cancers. Table 22–5 relates the incidence of ER positivity (assayed by monoclonal antibody) of newly diagnosed breast, endometrial, and ovarian cancer samples with the clinical response rates observed when treating unselected advanced cases with endocrine therapy (antiestrogen or progestins). Clinical response rates for selected ER-positive tumor patients are only available for breast cancer, and these will be reviewed in a later section.

PRIMARY MODALITIES OF ENDOCRINE INTERVENTION

The specific applications of endocrine therapy to breast, endometrial, and prostate cancers and the prognostic utility of tumor steroid receptors in predicting therapeutic outcome will be discussed later. For each of the different hormone-responsive tumors, however, different strategies and combinations of endocrine therapies are optimal, even though all endocrine modalities are based on the same hypothalamic-pituitary-gonadal axis of endocrine control. Therapeutic options are commonly categorized as ablative (removing endogenous hormone production), additive (administration of superphysiologic hormone doses), antagonistic (competition for receptor binding by antagonists such as antiestrogens, antiprogestins, or antiandrogens), or inhibitory (block-

Table 22–5. Response to endocrine therapy of tumors known to contain estrogen receptor (ER).

Tumor Type	Percentage Positive for ER	Rate of Response to Endocrine Therapy[1]
Breast carcinoma	50–60%	30%
Endometrial carcinoma	40–50%	30%
Ovarian carcinoma	30–40%	< 20%

[1]Objective clinical response after antiestrogen or progestin therapy in advanced cases unselected with regard to ER status.

ing of steroid metabolizing enzymes). The classic concept has been that hormone antagonists bind to receptors and block the subsequent steps to hormonal response, including the signals to undergo cell division and synthesize proteins. However, clinically effective steroid antagonists such as tamoxifen, clomiphene, cyproterone, and flutamide may or may not share the steroid ring structure of the hormones they antagonize and may bind with high affinity to sites other than steroid receptors within the cytoplasm. Some, in addition to blocking hormonal response, also induce synthesis of bifunctional growth factors and unique proteins with as yet unknown functions. Studies comparing the cellular responses of tumors to either antiestrogen administration or estrogen ablation have shown dissimilar mechanisms of antitumor activity, pointing to the need for further basic studies as well as a revision of present concepts explaining tumor growth control by endocrine therapy. No less confounding to investigators is the therapeutic impact of "spillover" among steroid hormones: the potential cross-reactivity of androgens for ER, progestins for ER and glucocorticoid receptors, and glucocorticoids for androgen receptors.

The concept of endocrine-dependent tumors and ablative endocrine therapy began with Beatson's observation, in the 1890s, of the regression of breast cancer after bilateral oophorectomy. Likewise, Huggins first ushered in the era of hormonal management of advanced prostate cancer by demonstrating the beneficial clinical effect of orchiectomy in 1941. Surgical castration, resulting in over 95% reduction of circulating testosterone in males and a 60% reduction in estrogen levels in females (relative to follicular phase levels in normal premenopausal women), produces the standard response rates for both prostate and premenopausal breast cancers with which all other forms of hormonal therapy must be compared. Sixty to 80 percent of men with metastatic prostate cancer will respond to bilateral orchiectomy. Approximately 30% of unselected premenopausal women—and 60–80% of patients with ER- and PgR-positive breast tumors—will respond to bilateral oophorectomy. As expected, oophorectomy is not beneficial for either postmenopausal patients (< 10% response rates) or perimenopausal patients (< 20% response rates). Ovarian irradiation (450–1000 cGy) as a substitute for surgery can effectively ablate ovarian function but requires several weeks to achieve full effect. These response rates with ablative therapy are consistent with the basic concept that these cancers are induced or stimulated by circulating sex steroids and that tumor regression occurs as a direct result of removing these hormonal stimuli. Ablative therapy is not clinically relevant for endometrial cancer because 80% of these estrogen-sensitive tumors arise in postmenopausal patients.

Residual estrogen levels in castrated or postmenopausal women persist because of adrenally secreted androgenic precursors (DHEA and androstenedione), which are converted to estrogen (estrone) by aromatization in extraglandular tissues. Furthermore, the remaining 5% of androgens circulating in castrated males consists of adrenally synthesized testosterone and androstenedione or its precursor, DHEA; and the influence of these residual androgens on prostate cancer growth may be disproportionate to their circulating levels. Because of this residual androgen production, adrenalectomy and hypophysectomy have been tried with some success in prostate cancer patients who have relapsed after orchiectomy, though these procedures are much more successful in breast cancer patients relapsing after oophorectomy, in whom second responses are commonly seen.

The advent of receptor antagonists and steroid synthesis inhibitors over the past 20 years has reduced the need for all ablative surgical procedures, particularly adrenalectomy and hypophysectomy, which have been replaced by aromatase inhibitors and blockers of gonadotropin-releasing hormones (GnRH), respectively. The additive hormonal agents diethylstilbestrol (DES) and progestins have proved to be effective first-line endocrine therapies for prostate, endometrial, and postmenopausal breast cancers. The number of hormonal agents and endocrine treatment modalities is rapidly increasing as a result of the relatively low toxicity of most endocrine agents and our improved understanding of the cellular and molecular mechanisms mediating hormone-dependent tumor regression. Some of the more promising endocrine agents currently in clinical trials are listed in Table 22–6. Additional discussion will be given to therapeutic decision-making between medical and surgical ablative therapies and the use of receptor antagonists in the following clinical sections.

COMBINATION ENDOCRINE THERAPY

Steroid agonists and antagonists are now being combined with ablative therapies to try to increase endocrine response rates. There can be multiple mechanisms at work when such combinations are employed, and the relative importance of these mechanisms remains uncertain; for instance, besides increasing levels of the estrogen-catabolizing enzyme, 17β-dehydrogenase, medroxyprogesterone acetate is also known to suppress adrenal production of androstenedione and thereby deplete cells of their androgenic substrate for aromatase and reduce conversion to estrogen. Thus, combining medroxyprogesterone acetate with aminoglutethimide brings into play at least two mechanisms of interaction that could result in enhanced inhibition of ER-positive tumors. Furthermore, higher doses of medroxyprogesterone acetate can bind (spill over) to glucocorti-

Table 22–6. Promising new antitumor endocrine agents.

Endocrine Agent(s)	Mechanism	Tumor Targets
ICI-182780, toremifene, dorloxifene, idoxifene, zindoxifene	Estrogen antagonist	Breast
Misopristone (RU-486), onapristone	Progestin antagonists	Breast, endometrium
Anandrone, casodex	Androgen antagonists	Prostate
Goserelin, burerelin; others	GnRH analogs	Prostate, breast, endometrium, ovary
Fadrozole, 4-hydroxy-androstenedione (4-OHA), vorozole, trilostane, examestane	Aromatase inhibitors	Breast, endometrium, ovary
Finasteride, 4-OHA	5α-Reductase inhibitors	Prostate
Octreotide acetate	Somatostatin agonist	Breast, ovary, prostate

coid receptors, obviating the need for administering replacement doses of cortisol to patients receiving aminoglutethimide.

In benign and malignant prostatic tissues, it is believed that ER-positive stromal cells provide the tropic androgens required by the androgen receptor-containing epithelial cells. In the stromal cells, 5α-reductase converts testosterone to the most active androgen, dihydrotestosterone. Strategy for the endocrine treatment of prostatic cancer has recently focused on complete androgen blockade, combining either surgical or medical ablation with an androgen receptor antagonist (antiandrogen). Because of the hormonal interdependence between epithelial and stromal cells and the overall dependence of prostatic tissue on pituitary factors (FSH, LH, and PRL), medical ablation can be accomplished using estrogen agonists and antagonists, GnRH analogs, or inhibitors of 5α-reductase. However, the value of combining these modalities remains controversial.

CHEMO-ENDOCRINE THERAPY

Combining chemotherapy and endocrine therapy is emerging as a popular treatment approach for endocrine-sensitive tumors (especially breast cancer) despite a lack of significant biochemical or cytokinetic rationale. Estramustine and prednimustine are two chemically similar steroid alkylating agents designed to be selectively toxic against receptor-positive cells. At present, it appears that these derivatives are little more effective than their parent compounds, suggesting that impaired receptor binding or systemic drug metabolism is limiting their cytotoxic potential. Simultaneous administration of tamoxifen with drug combinations such as AC (adriamycin cyclophosphamide) or CMF (cyclophosphamide, methotrexate, fluorouracil) may indeed increase response rates in selected groups of breast cancer patients; however, such additive effectiveness has not generally been observed in all patients, in all endocrine-sensitive tumors, or with other drug-hormone combinations. In

fact, the potential for adverse therapeutic effects with chemo-endocrine combinations has also been pointed out. Specifically, by suppressing tumor cell growth, hormonal therapy may protect the tumor from some chemotherapeutic agents that would otherwise be effective against replicating cells.

In summary, endocrine therapy has a long and established history of empiric usefulness; because the mechanism of its antitumor activity is predominantly cytostatic, the duration of endocrine therapy is necessarily longer than that required for cytotoxic chemotherapy. With the recent emergence of some biochemical understanding of the mechanisms underlying endocrine response and hormonal growth promotion, we are now witnessing the advent of more scientifically based applications. The hope is that this new understanding will lead to better tumor control.

CLINICAL PROBLEMS

BREAST CANCER IN WOMEN

Epidemiology

Breast cancer is now the most common life-threatening malignancy in the USA. There are currently about 185,000 new cases of breast cancer annually in the USA, and women have up to a 1:8 lifetime risk of developing the disease. The cause of breast cancer is unknown. Associated risk factors are listed in Table 22–7.

A. Family History: It is well established that the daughters of women with breast cancer are at higher risk of developing the disease than other women in the general population. The highest lifetime risk, 50%, is borne by women whose mothers had bilateral breast cancer with onset before menopause. Inherited mutations on the recently identified genes, *BRCA1* and *BRCA2,* account for an estimated

Table 22–7. Associated risk factors for breast cancer in women.

Family history and genetics
Menstrual history
Parity
Population differences
Endogenous hormones (early menarche, late menopause)
Exogenous hormones (high-dose oral contraceptives or
    estrogen replacement)
Benign breast disease (atypical hyperplasia)
Obesity
Ionizing radiation at a young age.
Prior breast cancer
Prior endometrial or ovarian cancer.

5–10% of all breast cancers, and carriers of these genes have up to an 80% chance of developing breast cancer by age 60. Carriers of *BRCA1* mutations also have a significant risk of ovarian cancer. Whether or not these mutations also confer differential risks due to hormonal factors remains to be determined. Mutations and deletions involving other genes are suspected of conferring increased breast cancer risk, and the identification of these genes is actively being pursued.

B. Menstrual History: Early age at menarche and late age at menopause increase the risk of breast cancer. Conversely, late age at menarche or early menopause (natural or surgical) reduces the risk.

C. Parity: Younger age of the mother at the time of her first pregnancy and history of full-term pregnancy lower the subsequent risk of breast cancer. Possible protective influences of breast feeding are under investigation.

D. Population Differences: There are striking variations across cultures in the incidence of breast cancer. Asian women have a much lower risk than women in Western countries. Women of Japanese descent who grow up in the USA have a higher incidence of breast cancer than those who grow up in Japan. The risk for blacks and whites is approximately 1.5-fold than that for Chinese- or Japanese-American women, 1.7-fold that for Hispanics, and 3.3-fold that for Native American women.

E. Endogenous Hormones: The data on menstrual function and parity in women—and experimental work in animals, where estrogen is clearly permissive or even carcinogenic in the induction of breast cancer—strongly implicate estrogen exposure as an important factor in the development of breast cancer. Many case control studies have examined estrogen profiles as well as PRL levels, but no clear pattern or association has emerged. There is also no linkage with androgens or thyroid hormone levels. An inherent flaw in these studies is that the induction of breast cancer is a long-term process, and if the estrogen profile of a patient or a control were to be related to cancer, it is probable that a short-term analysis of hormones—a snapshot, as it were—when the cancer was detected would not tell enough of the story. One would need instead a longitudinal, integrated profile starting at least at menarche of a large cohort of women in order to reliably detect differences in endocrine physiology and relate them to the development of cancer.

F. Exogenous Hormones: Retrospective analyses of users of birth control pills or of postmenopausal women who take estrogen are contradictory. There is, however, some suggestion that increased duration of estrogen exposure may increase the risk of breast cancer. Prospective studies of birth control pill usage do not indicate an increased risk, and there might even be a slight reduction in risk in some studies; but because of the considerable latent period for induction of breast cancer—presumably decades—further observation will be necessary to resolve the issue. The data certainly do not justify withholding birth control pills, but it would be prudent to limit the overall period of use as much as possible. The administration of estrogen to postmenopausal patients is a hotly debated issue, especially because estrogen use is associated with endometrial cancer. The possibility that prolonged use or high doses can increase the risk of breast cancer warrants further caution. One should keep the dose and duration of exposure to exogenous estrogen to a minimum (Chapter 13).

G. Benign Breast Disease: "Fibrocystic disease" is not a very specific term and usually refers to painful breast nodules that may wax and wane during the menstrual cycle. This commonly diagnosed condition occurs in up to 50% of women and reflects variability in end-organ response to fluctuations in endogenous hormone levels. The condition is less frequent in users of birth control pills and may also respond to the elimination of caffeine from the diet. Histologically, one can see macrocysts, microcysts, adenosis, apocrine change, fibrosis, fibroadenomas, or ductal hyperplasias. These conditions are not found with higher frequency in patients who develop breast cancer, but it has been noted that having had a previous biopsy for benign breast disease increases the relative risk (from 1.86 to 2.13) of developing breast cancer compared with the general population.

Retrospective analysis of a large group of patients was performed to better define who within the benign breast disease category had an increased relative risk for subsequent breast cancer. The presence of a proliferative lesion without atypical hyperplasia (atypia) increased the risk to 1.9 relative to the presence of a nonproliferative lesion without atypia. Atypia increased the risk to 5.3, and patients with atypia plus a family history of breast cancer had a relative risk of 11. It should be noted that the majority of patients (70%) who underwent biopsy for benign breast disease did not have lesions associated with an increased risk of breast cancer.

H. Other Factors: Obese habitus may correlate positively with an increased risk of breast cancer. Ionizing radiation is an established carcinogen.

Atomic bomb survivors, young females who received therapeutic chest radiation (for mastitis or Hodgkin's disease), and those who had repeated diagnostic x-rays for tuberculosis or scoliosis show increased rates of breast cancer. Cancer in one breast is associated with a 10–20% lifetime chance of developing primary cancer in the opposite breast. A history of endometrial or ovarian cancer also increases the chances for developing breast cancer.

It appears from the above data that the hormonal milieu is a critical element in the development of breast cancer. Estrogen seems to be the most important factor. There may be a dose-response effect, as suggested by the correlation with an increased duration of ovulatory cycling or with obesity. In the latter instance, there may be added estrogen contribution by peripheral conversion of sex steroids in adipose tissue. Early pregnancy may cause subtle changes in the set points for estrogen and PRL levels, or it may induce a protective change at a critical time in the breast tissue itself. In women with a strong family history of breast cancer, endogenous estrogen may enhance some inherent genetic susceptibility to breast carcinogenesis. Radiation is clearly a carcinogen for the breast, but other exogenous factors (eg, dietary fat) that might account for population differences in the attack rate of breast cancer are less easy to document. Diet could be influential through specific elements (eg, phytoestrogens), or factors such as fat or fiber content, or it could have a more complex interaction involving specific dietary elements or to-tal caloric intake. The overall calorie content and balance of foodstuffs could produce variations in growth, hormone profiles (anterior pituitary hormones such as GH as well as sex steroids), age at menarche, and the like, and these could influence susceptibility to breast cancer later in life.

Treatment of Metastatic Breast Cancer

A. Steroid Receptors and Other Considerations: While surgery is the mainstay of therapy for primary (localized) breast cancer, chemotherapy and hormonal therapy are the principal modalities for treatment of advanced breast cancer. A fairly straightforward algorithm to guide the selection of treatment utilizes the patient's menopausal status and the ER and PgR profile of the tumor (Figure 22–1). The chance of responding to endocrine therapy increases directly with tumor concentrations of ER and PgR. Table 22–8 shows how breast cancer response rates vary with receptor status when a threshold value for receptor positivity (ER-positive, PgR-positive) is employed. These data also indicate that postmenopausal patients are more apt to have receptor-positive tumors than premenopausal patients and, by implication, to respond more frequently to endocrine therapy.

Important ancillary data include the performance status of the patient, the tempo of tumor growth, the extent of visceral involvement, and the prior treatment history. The better the general condition of the

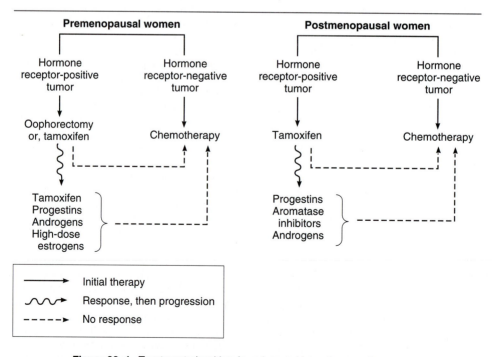

Figure 22–1. Treatment algorithm for advanced breast cancer in women.

Table 22–8. Rates of response to endocrine therapy according to estrogen and progesterone receptors (ER, PgR) in women with breast cancer.[1]

Tumor Receptor Status	Frequency Distribution		Rate of Response to Endocrine Therapy
	Premeno- pausal Women	Postmeno- pausal Women	
ER–, PgR–	30%	19%	11%
ER–, PgR+	9%	3%	46%
ER+, PgR–	12%	23%	27%
ER+, PgR+	49%	55%	77%

[1]Modified and reproduced, with permission, from McGuire WL: Steroid hormone receptors in breast cancer treatment strategy. Recent Prog Horm Res 1980;36:135.

patient and the lower the tumor burden, the more likely that an appropriately chosen hormonal treatment will be effective. Since the response to hormonal treatment is often not evident for several weeks and it can take several months for maximum response to occur, patients who are critically ill from breast cancer and require an immediate antitumor effect should receive chemotherapy. Likewise, patients with explosive tumor growth or with a short interval between tumor resection and the development of metastases are less likely to benefit from hormonal therapy than those with more indolent tumor growth. Skin, soft tissue, lymph nodes, and bone are the metastatic sites most responsive to endocrine maneuvers. Significant lung or liver involvement and brain metastases require chemotherapy and radiation therapy, respectively. Limited lung or liver infiltration may well respond to hormone treatment. The patient who has responded favorably to a prior hormonal maneuver has some likelihood of responding to subsequent endocrine treatment. Conversely, if a patient's tumor is refractory to one form of endocrine therapy, subsequent hormone treatments are usually of little value, and it is better to consider starting chemotherapy.

B. Premenopausal Endocrine Therapy: For premenopausal patients with ER-positive tumors, ablative treatment with oophorectomy is one first-line hormonal maneuver, although the antiestrogen tamoxifen appears to be equally effective in this role. However, because it can lead to increased circulating estrogens and gonadotropins—and because (by mass action effect) it may not adequately block the higher endogenous estrogen level—some clinicians believe that tamoxifen may not be entirely equivalent to oophorectomy as first-line treatment in premenopausal patients. Studies also suggest that women who respond favorably to tamoxifen have some chance of responding to oophorectomy, but the converse is not true. In general, the response rate to either oophorectomy or tamoxifen as initial treatment ranges from 30% to 60%, depending upon the level of ER protein

and the sites of metastatic disease. Responses average 12–15 months in duration. GnRH analogs serve as medical oophorectomy and appear to have equivalent efficacy compared with surgical oophorectomy. Combination endocrine therapy using tamoxifen and a GnRH analog in premenopausal patients is currently undergoing evaluation.

In premenopausal patients who respond to oophorectomy or tamoxifen but whose tumors progress, several options are available. They can next receive a trial of progestational agents or androgens. Progestational agents have few side effects, can increase appetite and sense of well-being, and produce clinical response in 15–30% of patients when used as second-line treatment. Androgens are effective in 10–20% of patients but have masculinizing effects. Attempts to develop less virilizing analogs of testosterone have been only moderately successful, and it is argued that the frequency of virilization may not be all that different between various congeners at equipotent antitumor doses. Another ablative maneuver, adrenalectomy—either surgical or medical (using aminoglutethimide)—can be employed as third-line treatment, with a response rate in the range of 15–30%. Medical adrenalectomy appears equal to surgical ablation in antitumor effect, but its effects are reversible once the drug is stopped. However, like surgical adrenalectomy, it also requires the administration of replacement hydrocortisone. In addition to maintaining vital functions, this replacement therapy also prevents increased pituitary ACTH production and overriding of the adrenal blockade. Since dexamethasone metabolism is augmented by aminoglutethimide, it should not be used as the replacement steroid during treatment. Up to 30% of patients receiving aminoglutethimide will initially experience somnolence or rash, side effects that usually subside with continued treatment and which can be minimized by gradually working up to full doses over several weeks. More potent and selective aromatase inhibitors (Table 22–6) that do not affect adrenal steroid-producing enzymes are currently being tested and becoming available. These agents appear to have fewer side effects and may eventually be used for first-line endocrine therapy.

Finally, the development of transsphenoidal surgery has made hypophysectomy a more feasible ablative maneuver. Before the advent of receptor analyses, hypophysectomy was used as palliative treatment in end-stage patients, especially those with extensive and painful bone metastases. Patients who were responders would often awaken from anesthesia with dramatic pain relief. That it occasionally benefits hormone-refractory cases suggests that its palliative effects are not solely mediated via sex steroid mechanisms. When compared to adrenalectomy in ER-positive tumors as second- or third-line treatment, hypophysectomy is equally effective and may have a slightly longer duration of action. However, the availability of aminoglutethimide, the operative risk, and the requirement for permanent adrenal replacement make hypophysectomy a less desirable and rarely elected option.

Premenopausal patients with ER-negative tumors would bypass endocrine therapy and be placed on a chemotherapy protocol.

C. Postmenopausal Endocrine Therapy: The initial endocrine maneuver in postmenopausal patients with ER-positive tumors is the administration of the antiestrogen tamoxifen. In the recent past, additive therapy with diethylstilbestrol (DES) was used. However, this agent is associated with many more side effects than tamoxifen and has now largely been abandoned. Response rates to tamoxifen or DES range from 30% to 60%, again in proportion to the disease-free interval, metastatic sites, and the ER content of the tumor. Response durations are similar to those for oophorectomy. Once the breast cancer of a patient who has responded to tamoxifen progresses, second-line endocrine therapy is either medical adrenalectomy or administration of an aromatase inhibitor or progestin, with response expected in 15% to 40% of cases. It should be noted that 10–20% of patients initially failing to respond to tamoxifen may have a clinical response to adrenalectomy. Thus, if the tempo of the disease and the clinical status of the patient permit, one can offer a trial of medical adrenalectomy before proceeding to chemotherapy.

When DES was in wider use, induction of therapy in patients with skeletal metastases would occasionally be accompanied by a "flare" with exacerbation of bone pain and hypercalcemia. This phenomenon usually heralded a clinical response and did not necessarily require prolonged interruption of treatment. When the cancer of patients who had responded to DES progressed, drug withdrawal was frequently followed by another clinical remission in up to 30% of patients, and this could last for several months. The flare phenomenon and the response to withdrawal are less frequently seen with tamoxifen; these effects have also been noted to occur with androgen therapy. Postmenopausal patients with ER-negative tumors would bypass hormonal treatment and begin chemotherapy, although with slowly progressive tumors, a trial of tamoxifen may be attempted anticipating only a small chance (10–20%) for clinical response.

Current investigational endocrine agents include congeners of tamoxifen and a variety of GnRH agonists and antagonists.

Treatment of Early Stage Breast Cancer

Following surgery for early stage breast cancer (stage I and stage II), systemic adjuvant hormonal therapy or chemotherapy has been shown to reduce the subsequent likelihood of metastatic recurrence and death from breast cancer. In general, the absolute amount by which the risk can be reduced over time is proportionate to the overall risk of recurrence or death. Therefore, in lower-risk situations, such as with small, node-negative tumors, the absolute benefit may be small—on the order of a 5% reduction in the chances of recurrence over 5 years. In premenopausal women, chemotherapy appears to produce a larger benefit, while in postmenopausal women—especially those with ER-positive tumors—tamoxifen appears to be more effective. Tamoxifen can also be used for premenopausal patients with ER-positive, node-negative tumors. The addition of tamoxifen and/or GnRH analogs to chemotherapy for younger women is currently being studied. Older trials established the effectiveness of oophorectomy in reducing recurrence risk in premenopausal women. With the advent of medical oophorectomy using GnRH analogs, there is a renewed interest in this form of therapy instead of or in addition to chemotherapy for younger women, particularly in the setting of ER-positive tumors. At present, this approach remains investigational. Other forms of hormonal therapy such as progestins or aromatase inhibitors are not currently used for adjuvant therapy.

BREAST CANCER IN MEN

Cancer of the male breast is extremely rare, occurring with a frequency of about 1% of that of cancer of the female breast. There is an association with Klinefelter's syndrome and with exogenous estrogen exposure (eg, in transsexuals), emphasizing the importance of hormonal factors, especially estrogen.

At least 80% of tumors in men are ER-positive. Sixty to 70 percent of patients with metastatic tumors will respond to orchiectomy, and adrenalectomy and hypophysectomy are effective as second-line hormonal treatments. More recently, tamoxifen has shown activity as primary treatment and now offers an alternative to orchiectomy. As in female patients with breast cancer, male patients whose tumors become refractory to hormone therapy go on to receive chemotherapy. Androgens are contraindicated because of their potential for facilitating tumor growth.

ENDOMETRIAL CANCER

Epidemiology

There are approximately 33,000 new cases of endometrial cancer annually in the USA. In contrast to the somewhat equivocal role of estrogen in the induction of breast cancer, its place in the causation of endometrial cancer appears more certain. At the clinical level, as shown in Table 22–9, a variety of conditions have been associated with an increased risk of developing endometrial cancer. Their common denominator is unopposed or increased estrogenic stim-

Table 22–9. Conditions causing prolonged or unopposed estrogen effect on the uterus and associated with an increased risk of developing endometrial cancer.

Exogenous estrogen or partial estrogen agonists
  (eg, tamoxifen)
Late menopause
Obesity (increased peripheral conversion of precursors to
  estrogen)
Polycystic ovary syndrome
Ovarian cortical stromal hyperplasia

---

ulation of the endometrium. This produces endometrial hyperplasia, a condition that can in turn progress to frank cancer. Progesterone antagonizes this effect of estrogen and induces the endometrium to mature or differentiate to a secretory state. Its action may be mediated by augmentation of enzymes in endometrial cells that catabolize estrogen and by decreasing levels of ER in this same tissue. There is a more frequent history of irregular menses in patients who develop endometrial cancer, and while combination birth control pills may have no influence on or may even decrease the risk of uterine cancer, sequential birth control pills may impart an increased risk, possibly because of the days of therapy where only estrogen is being administered.

Epidemiologic studies revealed an upsurge in the incidence of endometrial cancer in the USA in the early 1970s. This followed and paralleled an increase in the number of prescriptions written over the preceding years for replacement estrogen therapy in postmenopausal women. Case control studies of this phenomenon have clearly shown that exogenous estrogen use imparts a three- to eightfold increase in the risk of developing uterine cancer. The higher the dose and the longer the duration of estrogen use, the greater the risk. One follow-up study from the late 1970s reported that a decline in the number of estrogen prescriptions (after the initial recognition of their association with endometrial cancer) was accompanied by a decline in the incidence of endometrial cancer in the same population base. Cyclic or continuous progestin administration has also reduced the incidence of endometrial cancer. Taken together, the above observations strongly support a conservative approach to the use of exogenous estrogens. They should be given in the smallest possible dose, for the shortest duration feasible, and on an intermittent schedule, preferably adding a progestin to the treatment regimen. (See Chapters 8, 13, and 25 for further discussions of estrogen therapy.)

The use of tamoxifen has also been associated with a three- to fivefold increase in the age-adjusted risk of endometrial cancer. This may be a result of the dual antiestrogenic and partial estrogenic activity of tamoxifen. Tamoxifen appears to produce a proliferative effect on the endometrium, and the increased risk of endometrial cancer may be similar in mecha-

nism to that induced by unopposed estrogen. For this reason, the use of tamoxifen needs to be balanced against the risk of endometrial cancer when adjuvant tamoxifen therapy is being considered for low-risk breast cancers (such as node-negative tumors) or in the experimental setting of breast cancer chemoprevention in otherwise healthy individuals who are at increased risk for the development of breast cancer.

Treatment of Metastatic Endometrial Cancer

A. Steroid Receptors: As is true in breast cancer, hormonal therapy is a primary therapeutic modality for advanced endometrial cancer. Unlike the situation in breast cancer, receptor profiles are not used to guide treatment selection in cases of endometrial cancer, although it was from uterine tissue that Jensen first isolated and characterized estrogen receptors in the 1960s. Uterine estrogen receptors increase during the proliferative phase of the menstrual cycle and fall in the presence of exogenous progesterone or with the rise of endogenous progesterone during the luteal phase. Progesterone receptors are induced by estrogen, and their level peaks coincident with the estradiol peak in the menstrual cycle. Many endometrial carcinomas contain ER, and, in contrast to breast cancer, levels are higher and inversely proportionate to the degree of histologic differentiation of the tumor. Progesterone receptors are also present in endometrial cancer, and their presence correlates directly with the degree of differentiation. ER and PgR have little practical application in the management of patients, since immunohistochemical analyses must be performed to distinguish tumor from receptor-positive normal tissue, and these assays are not quantitative. Furthermore, these tumors frequently show an admixture of receptor-positive and -negative tumor cells, the latter accounting for the eventual failure of endocrine treatment.

B. Endocrine Therapy: Approximately one-third of metastatic tumors will respond to progestins. The probability of response is highest in patients with the most differentiated tumors and in those with the longest interval between primary treatment and the appearance of metastases. Responders live an average of 2 years after treatment is started, while nonresponding patients survive only about 6 months. Until recently, parenteral preparations such as hydroxyprogesterone and medroxyprogesterone were used. An orally effective compound, megestrol, has simplified treatment and appears to be as potent as the earlier parenteral formulations. Potential side effects of these compounds include salt retention and an increased predisposition to thrombophlebitis.

In patients who progress on progestational therapy or who do not respond initially, disease may be palliated with chemotherapy. However, in many patients, advanced disease stage, poor general health, and a history of pelvic irradiation limit tolerance to the most effective agents, ie, doxorubicin, cyclophosphamide, fluorouracil, and cisplatin.

PROSTATIC CANCER

Epidemiology

There are approximately 244,000 new cases of prostatic cancer annually in the USA. Prostatic cancer is essentially a disease of men in their 60s and 70s, and autopsy series have shown occult carcinoma in more than one-third of men over age 70 and more than two-thirds of men over age 80.

Several lines of evidence support the idea that testosterone plays a role in the development of prostatic cancer. Testosterone can induce adenocarcinoma of the prostate in rats; castrated men do not develop prostatic cancer; and the disease is less frequent in patients with cirrhosis. Cirrhotic patients tend to be in a stage of relative estrogen excess from decreased hepatic estrogen metabolism, and they frequently exhibit testicular atrophy and gynecomastia. While benign prostatic hypertrophy and prostate cancer are often found concurrently in older men and are associated with the same risk factors, benign hypertrophy is not, in itself, a risk factor for prostate cancer and occurs in an embryologically distinct portion of the gland.

Less clearly understood are racial, familial, and geographic differences. American blacks have a much higher incidence of prostatic cancer than Nigerian blacks, and Japanese-Americans who live in Hawaii have an attack rate intermediate between the low rate seen in Japan and the higher rates seen in whites in the USA. There are inconclusive data suggesting that patients may have higher testosterone production than controls; that viruses with oncogenic potential may play a permissive role; and that the number of sexual partners and a history of sexually transmitted disease also influence the incidence of prostatic cancer. A family history of prostate cancer has been shown to be a risk factor, suggesting that predisposing inherited genetic defects may soon be identified as with breast cancer.

Treatment of Metastatic Prostatic Cancer

A. Steroid Receptors: Cytosol receptors for androgen have been isolated from prostatic cancers, and while they may predict for response, they are not used as a basis for selecting therapy because (1) initial response rates to standard endocrine therapy are high, and alternative choices are far less promising (ie, second-line hormonal maneuvers or chemotherapy); (2) androgen receptor assays are still technically difficult, although these have been simplified by the recent development of monoclonal antibodies; and (3) the volume of tumor specimens from primary sites or metastatic sites (eg, bone) is not usually adequate for quantitative determination of tumor receptor content.

B. Endocrine Therapy: It is difficult to compare the response data and therapies from different treatment centers. Typically, a patient with metastatic disease will complain of bone pain and manifest abnormalities on bone scan or plain x-ray. The acid phosphatase level may be specifically elevated in prostatic cancer, along with increased levels of the relatively nonspecific enzyme, alkaline phosphatase. Response to therapy is hard to quantitate, since subjective complaints are difficult to measure, bone lesions resolve slowly, and the acid phosphatase does not always correlate reliably with variation in tumor volume. Only in less common instances of discrete lung, lymph node, or liver metastases is it possible to objectively and directly measure antitumor response. The advent of an assay for prostate-specific antigen (PSA) has substantially improved the monitoring of therapeutic response, since its serum level and change in titer correlate well with tumor bulk and therapeutic response.

Within these limitations, it appears that one-half to three-fourths of patients will benefit from treatment. Initial therapy is hormonal and is based upon the pioneering work of Huggins, showing that prostatic cancer is a testosterone-dependent tissue. Therapy consists of lowering testosterone levels either by orchiectomy, administration of DES (which suppresses gonadotropins), or use of a GnRH analog such as leuprolide. Since DES has direct suppressive effects on the tumor and inhibits pituitary gonadotropin secretion, some have advocated the use of both DES and orchiectomy. However, the response rates with all hormonal maneuvers are essentially the same. Given the side effects of DES, such as gynecomastia, and the desire to avoid undergoing surgical orchiectomy, GnRH analogs alone or in combination with an androgen receptor antagonist are being utilized more commonly as initial therapy for metastatic prostate cancer. There continues to be rigorous debate over the additional use of an androgen receptor antagonist (like flutamide) with ablative therapy to produce a so-called complete androgen blockade. Antiandrogens are somewhat effective as first-line agents, but it is generally agreed that in combination with GnRH agonists they effectively eliminate painful flare-ups of tumor lesions and may provide added improvements in patients having a minimal burden of metastatic disease. Disease that progresses after initially responding to ablative therapy rarely responds to crossover treatment with other endocrine maneuvers.

The presence of low levels of circulating androgens after orchiectomy has led to trials of adrenalectomy or hypophysectomy in patients with progressive disease. However, subsequent response rates to these ablative therapies are quite low, and responses are short-lived. GnRH analogs alone—or in combination with antiandrogens—with their minimal side effects, have now become front-line agents for treatment of prostatic cancer, with their only limitation being cost. New analogs, including 5α-reductase inhibitors, are being assessed for their comparative efficacy in treating benign prostatic hypertrophy and prostate cancer (Table 22–6).

Chemoprevention of Cancer

Earlier randomized trials assessing the use of adjuvant tamoxifen also showed a decrease in the development of second contralateral breast cancers. This generated interest in the use of tamoxifen as a chemopreventive agent for healthy women felt to be at high risk for developing breast cancer. A large randomized trial is ongoing to assess the efficacy of giving tamoxifen for this purpose for 5 years or longer. The use of steroid hormones, particularly retinoids, has also been studied as these compounds appear to have growth inhibitory and differentiating properties in laboratory models. Animal models of carcinogenesis have also shown promise with the use of tamoxifen and retinoids such as 13-*cis,* all-*trans,* and 9-*cis* retinoic acid as well as combinations of tamoxifen and retinoids. Retinoic acid has been found to be effective in reducing the incidence of occurrence of second cancers in patients treated for a first lung or head and neck cancer. Currently, retinoids are also being evaluated as chemopreventive agents for breast cancer. In addition, the 5α-reductase inhibitor finasteride, currently indicated for the treatment of benign prostatic hypertrophy, is being evaluated as a preventive agent for prostate cancer.

MISCELLANEOUS TUMORS

Steroid hormone receptors have been isolated from tumors arising from organs not usually considered to be under primary endocrine control. Cortico-steroid receptor protein is present in leukemia and lymphoma cells. It shows some correlation with response to steroid therapy, but levels are not used prospectively to guide treatment.

As mentioned earlier, there are reports of low but reproducible levels of ER or ER-like proteins in some human renal, ovarian, hepatic, bone and pancreatic tumors and in melanomas. Progestational agents produce regression in 10% of hypernephromas; there are case reports that tamoxifen and progestins have caused regressions in ovarian cancer; and there are validated studies demonstrating the importance of tamoxifen in chemotherapy regimens effective against melanomas. Hepatomas have responded to progestational agents on occasion, and trials are in progress to determine whether hormonal agents can produce regressions in pancreatic cancer. In summary, it can be said that endocrine treatments for these tumor types either do not appear promising or are believed to be effective for reasons other than the presence of detectable ER.

Several early observations of a transient therapeutic effect in patients with acute promyelocytic leukemia (APML) were reported with the use of retinoic acid. It was later noted that the t(15;17) chromosomal translocation typical of this subtype of leukemia involved a rearrangement of the retinoic acid receptor. The oncogenic fusion protein created by this translocation retains some functional DNA binding but altered localization in the cell cytoplasm rather than the nucleus. Its leukemogenic function is partially overcome by the use of supraphysiologic doses of retinoic acid, producing a temporary but dramatic clinical and hematologic remission. Based on these observations, ongoing clinical trials are assessing the use of retinoids in combination with standard chemotherapy agents to improve the curability of APML.

REFERENCES

Beatson GT: On the treatment of inoperable cases of carcinoma of the mamma: Suggestions for a new method of treatment with illustrative cases. Lancet 1986;2:162.

Benz DD: Hormone responsive tumors. In: *Endocrinology and Metabolism,* 3rd ed. Felig P, Baxter JD, Frohman LA (editors). McGraw-Hill, 1995.

Clarke R et al: Hormonal carcinogenesis in breast cancer: Cellular and molecular studies of malignant progression. Breast Cancer Res Treat 1994;31:237.

Colditz GA et al: The use of estrogens and progestins and the risk of breast cancer in postmenopausal women. N Engl J Med 1995;332:1589.

Dupont WD, Page DL: Risk factors for breast cancer in women with proliferative breast disease. N Engl J Med 1985;312:146.

Early Breast Cancer Trialists' Collaborative Group: Systemic treatment of early breast cancer by hormonal, cy-totoxic, or immune therapy: 133 randomised trials involving 31,000 recurrences and 24,000 deaths among 75,000 women. Lancet 1992;339:71.

Ethier SP: Growth factor synthesis and human breast cancer progression. J Natl Cancer Inst 1995;87:964.

Fisher B et al: A randomized clinical trial evaluating tamoxifen in the treatment of patients with node-negative breast cancer who have estrogen-receptor-positive tumors. N Engl J Med 1989;320:479.

Fisher B et al: Endometrial cancer in tamoxifen-treated breast cancer patients: Findings from the National Surgical Adjuvant Breast and Bowel Program (NSABP) B-14. J Natl Cancer Inst 1994;86:527.

Griffiths K et al: Hormonal treatment of advanced prostate cancer: Some newer aspects. Semin Oncol 1994;21:672.

Henderson BE et al: Endogenous hormones as a major factor in human cancer. Cancer Res 1982;42:3232.

Henderson IC: Risk factors for breast cancer. Cancer 1993; 71(6 Suppl):2127.

Huggins C: Endocrine-induced regression of cancers. Science 1967;156:1050.

Jaiyesimi IA et al: Use of tamoxifen for breast cancer: Twenty years later. J Clin Oncol 1995;13:513.

Jordan VC: Overview from the International Conference on Long-term Tamoxifen Therapy for Breast Cancer. J Natl Cancer Inst 1992;84:231.

Katzenellenbogen BS: Antiestrogen resistance: Mechanisms by which breast cancer cells undermine the effectiveness of endocrine therapy (editorial). J Natl Cancer Inst 1991; 83:1434.

Kimmick G, Muss H: Current status of endocrine therapy for metastatic breast cancer. Oncology 1995;9:877.

Labrie F et al: Combination therapy for prostate cancer. Endocrine and biologic basis of its choice as new standard first-line therapy. Cancer 1993;71(3 Suppl):1059.

Miki Y et al: A strong candidate for the breast and ovarian cancer susceptibility gene *BRCA1*. Science 1994;266:66.

Muller WJ et al: Single-step induction of mammary adenocarcinoma in transgenic mice bearing the activated c-*neu* oncogene. Cell 1988;54:105.

Neijt JP: Systemic treatment in disseminated endometrial cancer. Eur J Cancer 1993;29A:628.

Sporn MB, Roberts AB: Peptide growth factors are multifunctional. Nature 1988;332:217.

Sutherland DJ, Mobbs BG: Hormones and cancer. In: *The Basic Science of Oncology,* 2nd ed. Tannock IF, Hill RP (editors). McGraw-Hill, 1992.

Thompson IM et al: Chemoprevention of prostate cancer. Semin Urol 1995;13:122.

Tripathy D, Benz CC: Activated oncogenes and putative tumor suppressor genes involved in human breast cancers. In: *Oncogenes and Tumor Suppressor Genes in Human Malignancies.* Benz CC, Liu ET (editors). Kluwer, 1993.

Tripathy D, Benz CC: Growth factors and their receptors. Hematol Oncol Clin North Am 1994;8:29.

van Tinteren H, Dalesio O: Systematic overview (meta-analysis) of all randomized trials of treatment of prostate cancer. Cancer 1993;72(12 Suppl):3847.

Wilding G: Endocrine control of prostate cancer. Cancer Surv 1995;23:43.

Wingo PA, Tong T, Bolden S: Cancer statistics 1995. CA Cancer J Clin 1995;45:8.

Humoral Manifestations of Malignancy

23

Gordon J. Strewler, MD

GENERAL CONCEPT OF ECTOPIC HORMONE SECRETION

The idea that tumors can cause endocrine syndromes by secreting hormones inappropriately was first proposed by Fuller Albright, who in 1941 suggested that the cause of hypercalcemia and hypophosphatemia in a patient with renal carcinoma might be production of parathyroid hormone (PTH) by the tumor. The term "ectopic hormonal syndrome" was subsequently coined by Liddle to describe such situations. By now the idea of "ectopic hormone production" is widely held, and some humoral syndromes induced by nonendocrine tumors are recognized as being among the commonest of endocrine disorders. However, the term "ectopic" is probably a poor descriptor of most of these syndromes. Ectopic means "out of place," implying abnormal secretion of a hormone by tissues that do not normally have this function. Yet tumors that produce hormones most often arise from cells that are normally committed to producing the same hormone. For example, adrenocorticotropic hormone (ACTH) is produced by lung carcinomas that develop from ACTH-producing lung cells. Many other examples will be encountered in this chapter. Although truly ectopic secretion of hormones is probably a rarity, the term "ectopic" is firmly ingrained in the vocabulary of our specialty and will not soon be abandoned.

Of all the paraneoplastic syndromes, the ectopic production of hormones is probably the commonest. Virtually all the peptide hormones are produced by nonendocrine tumors (Table 23–1), and a wide variety of neoplasms are associated with syndromes of hormone excess. However, strong associations exist between specific hormones and specific tumors. For example, the PTH-like protein associated with hypercalcemia (see below) is most commonly produced by squamous carcinomas, while ACTH, vasopressin, and calcitonin are most commonly produced by small cell lung carcinoma and other neuroendocrine tumors. It should be noted that nearly all the peptide hormones are represented in Table 23–1, but none of the steroid or thyroid hormones are listed; it is pre-

ACRONYMS USED IN THIS CHAPTER	
ACTH	Adrenocorticotropic hormone
ADH	Antidiuretic hormone (vasopressin)
ANP	Atrial natriuretic peptide
APUD	Amine precursor uptake and decarboxylation
cAMP	Cyclic adenosine monophosphate
CGRP	Calcitonin gene-related peptide
CRH	Corticotropin-releasing hormone
EGF	Epidermal growth factor
FSH	Follicle-stimulating hormone
GH	Growth hormone
GRH	Growth hormone-releasing hormone
GRP	Gastrin-releasing peptide (bombesin)
hCG	Human chorionic gonadotropin
IGF-1	Insulin-like growth factor-1 (somatomedin C)
IGF-2	Insulin-like growth factor-2 (somatomedin A)
LH	Luteinizing hormone
mRNA	Messenger ribonucleic acid
PDGF	Platelet-derived growth factor
PTH	Parathyroid hormone
PTHrP	PTH-related protein
SIADH	Syndrome of inappropriate secretion of vasopressin (antidiuretic hormone)
TRH	Thyrotropin-releasing hormone
TSH	Thyroid-stimulating hormone (thyrotropin)
VIP	Vasoactive intestinal polypeptide

Table 23–1. Hormones produced by tumors.

Hypercalcemia factors
    PTH-related protein (PTHrP)
    Tumor necrosis factor-α
    $1,25(OH)_2D_3$
    Prostaglandins
    PTH
Vasopressin
ACTH
Calcitonin
Human chorionic gonadotrophin (hCG)
Placental lactogen
Growth hormone
Growth hormone-releasing hormone
Corticotropin-releasing hormone
Erythropoietin
Oncogenous osteomalacia factor
Insulin-like growth factor-2 (IGF-2)
Atrial natriuretic peptide
Endothelin
Renin
Other gut hormones (gastrin-releasing peptide, gastrin-
    inhibitory peptide, somatostatin, pancreatic polypeptide,
    vasoactive intestintal polypeptide, substance P, motilin)

Table 23–2. Criteria for determining whether a nonendocrine tumor is a source of hormone.[1]

Association of clinical syndrome or inappropriate hormone
    level with presence of tumor.
Reversal of syndrome with tumor-specific therapy.
Presence of hormone in tumor tissue.
Demonstration of arteriovenous gradient for hormone across
    tumor.
Synthesis or release of hormone by tumor tissue in vitro.
Expression of hormone mRNA by tumor.

[1]Criteria are listed in order of their rigor; the first two are clinical and the rest are primarily investigational.

sumed that steroid hormones are not produced by tumors because their synthesis requires expression of a whole series of enzymes, while synthesis of a peptide requires expression of only a single gene. The exception—secretion of the sterol hormone $1,25(OH)_2D_3$ by certain lymphomas—occurs because its synthesis from the circulating precursor $25(OH)D_3$ requires only a single step.

Secretion of hormones by tumors often differs qualitatively from glandular secretion of hormones. First, secretion by tumors is rarely suppressible. Second, tumors often lack the ability to process peptide hormones normally, and they secrete larger precursor forms whose biologic activity is reduced. Third, tumor-associated syndromes may involve secretion of hormone homologs rather than hormones themselves. For example, in hyperparathyroidism, hypercalcemia is caused by PTH excess, but in malignant disease hypercalcemia may be caused by excess of other physiologically similar peptides, one of which is closely related to PTH.

Criteria for deciding whether a nonendocrine tumor is responsible for producing hormone excess are listed in Table 23–2. Not every criterion has been fulfilled for every hormone listed, but for most of these hormones there is evidence of production by tumor cells in vitro or of mRNA expression.

Cellular Basis of Ectopic Hormone Secretion

It was once held that "derepression" of tumor genes was responsible for ectopic hormone secretion, ie, that tumor cells express a random assortment of genes that are normally repressed, including genes that encode hormones. This hypothesis cannot readily explain the nonrandom association of certain hormonal syndromes (eg, ACTH and vasopressin excess) with specific cancers (eg, small cell lung carcinoma). Moreover, the derepression hypothesis is obviated by the aforementioned finding that tumors typically express the same hormones as their cell of origin. The "dedifferentiation" hypothesis posits a retrograde movement of tumor cells along the pathway of differentiation, leading to the expression of fetal proteins (eg, alpha-fetoprotein, carcinoembryonic antigen) or hormones normally present in immature cells (eg, human chorionic gonadotropin [hCG]). While this hypothesis would account for the nonrandom nature of hormone expression and the presence of low-level expression in mature normal cells, there is no supporting evidence for the occurrence of dedifferentiation. A more sophisticated model is the "dysdifferentiation" hypothesis of Baylin and Mendelsohn, which holds that epithelial malignancy is the result of clonal expansion of a particular cell type along a complex pathway of epithelial differentiation. This is viewed as giving rise to overexpression of hormones, as by clonal expansion of a normally rare population of cells committed to expression of the hormone, or to expression of hormones not present in the mature epithelium, as by clonal expansion of a primitive cell.

Hormone Secretion by APUD Cells

The most celebrated attempt to explain the nonrandom patterns of hormone secretion by tumors is the APUD hypothesis of Pearse. A characteristic shared by many endocrine cells and some tumor cells that secrete hormones is the capacity to synthesize and store biogenic amines (amine precursor uptake and decarboxylation [APUD]). The APUD hypothesis suggests that APUD cells, although widely scattered in many tissues, have a common origin in the neural crest and are specialized for production of peptide hormones. Histologic analysis shows that APUD cells do contain typical neurosecretory granules associated with secretion of peptides and biogenic amines. Besides such endocrine cells as thyroid C cells, pituitary corticotrophs, and adrenal medullary cells, APUD cells are scattered in the bronchial and gastrointestinal mucosa, and hormone-producing neoplasms (carcinoids, small cell lung carcinoma) are frequently composed of APUD cells. Pearse proposed that APUD cells were a "diffuse neuroendocrine system," a third branch of the nervous system.

The APUD theory probably requires modification in two respects. First, it has been clearly shown that not all APUD cells are of neural crest origin—some arise from primitive endoderm. Thus, hormone-producing APUD cells do not necessarily have a common origin. Second, hormones are produced not only by APUD cells but by a variety of non-APUD tumor cells. However, the APUD cell is the type most likely to be associated with the secretion of biologically active hormones that leads to a clinical syndrome of hormone excess. The best example is ACTH in Cushing's syndrome. Although the biologically inactive ACTH precursor proopiomelanocortin is produced by many tumors, Cushing's syndrome is typically associated with APUD tumors containing neurosecretory granules, presumably because these are capable of processing and secreting ACTH. Thus, the rubric APUD identifies cytochemical or ultrastructural features associated not so much with production of hormones as with secretion of active hormones. However, it is preferable to refer to APUD cells as "neuroendocrine cells," a term that denotes the presence of neurosecretory granules that are involved in hormone secretion.

Oncogenes & Growth Factors

The transformation of cells from normal to malignant is thought to involve activation of oncogenes. Oncogenes are aberrant forms of normal genes (proto-oncogenes) that control growth and differentiation, encoding growth factors (*sis* encodes platelet-derived growth factor [PDGF]), growth factor receptors (*erb*-B encodes a portion of the epidermal growth factor [EGF] receptor) or cellular effector systems coupled to growth factor receptors (*src* encodes a tyrosine kinase). The process of transformation thus involves the inappropriate activation of a variety of normal cellular pathways. In many instances, the production of hormones by malignant cells will probably be the consequence of activation of a specific oncogene.

Why should hormone secretion be linked to proto-oncogenes controlling normal growth and differentiation? One possible answer is that production of hormones may have survival value, both for cancer cells and for their normal cells of origin. Among the characteristic tumor products of small cell lung carcinoma is gastrin-releasing peptide (GRP), the mammalian counterpart of the amphibian hormone bombesin. GRP (bombesin) fulfills most criteria as an autocrine growth factor in small cell carcinoma: It is secreted, it can stimulate replication of the cells via specific receptors, and blockade of its action by specific antibodies to GRP inhibits cell replication and tumor formation in vivo. Insulin-like growth factors, transforming growth factor-α, and transforming growth factor-β have also been shown to have autocrine effects on the growth of diverse tumors, including small cell lung carcinoma, breast carcinoma, and bladder carcinoma. Studies may eventually show whether other hormonal products of small cell lung carcinoma (ACTH, vasopressin, calcitonin) also serve as growth factors.

MALIGNANCY-ASSOCIATED HYPERCALCEMIA

Hypercalcemia is the commonest paraneoplastic endocrine syndrome. The incidence is 15 cases per 100,000 person-years, about half the incidence of primary hyperparathyroidism. Hypercalcemia develops as a complication in up to 10% of patients with advanced malignant disease. In hospitalized patients, malignant disease is the commonest cause of hypercalcemia. Table 23–3 shows the frequency with which various tumors cause hypercalcemia. Lung carcinoma, breast carcinoma, and multiple myeloma together account for more than 50%. Among lung carcinomas, hypercalcemia is seen most commonly in squamous carcinoma and is also associated with large cell carcinoma and adenocarcinoma. Small cell lung carcinoma rarely causes hypercalcemia, despite its propensity for other endocrinopathies. Squamous carcinomas of the head, neck, esophagus, and other organs are also strongly associated with hypercalcemia, as is renal cell carcinoma. In contrast, hypercalcemia is rarely seen in gastrointestinal adenocarcinoma or in sarcomas, even lytic sarcomas of bone.

The offending neoplasm is apparent in 98% of cases at the time when hypercalcemia is first detected. Except in patients with multiple myeloma and breast cancer, the course of which can be punctuated by self-limited episodes of hypercalcemia, the prognosis of the cancer patient with hypercalcemia is grim, with a 3-month survival rate of less than 50%.

Table 23–3. Tumors that cause hypercalcemia.[1]

Primary Site	No. (%) of Cases		Known Metastatic Disease (%)
Lung	111	(25.0)	62
Breast	87	(19.6)	92
Multiple myeloma	43	(9.7)	100
Head and neck	36	(8.1)	73
Kidney and urinary tract	35	(7.9)	36
Esophagus	25	(5.6)	53
Female genitalia	24	(5.2)	81
Unknown primary	23	(5.2)	—
Lymphoma	14	(3.2)	91
Colon	8	(1.8)	—
Liver and biliary	7	(1.6)	—
Skin	6	(1.4)	—
Other	25	(5.6)	—
Total	444	(100.0)	

[1]Modified and reproduced, with permission, from Stollerman GH et al (editors): *Advances in Internal Medicine*. Vol. 32. Year Book, 1987.

Differential Diagnosis

The principal entity in the differential diagnosis of hypercalcemia associated with malignancy is primary hyperparathyroidism, which may present as an intercurrent illness in a patient with a malignant tumor. Chronic, long-standing hypercalcemia preceding the diagnosis of cancer or radiographic changes of subperiosteal bone resorption may indicate the presence of primary hyperparathyroidism. The presence of primary hyperparathyroidism may be indicated by an elevated PTH value. In previously used mid region assays, the immunoreactive PTH levels in cancer patients are usually normal. However, PTH levels may be slightly high in some patients with mild hypercalcemia. In two-site assays that measure intact PTH by immunoradiometric techniques, which are now standard, PTH levels are suppressed in malignancy and other forms of nonparathyroid hypercalcemia, greatly facilitating the differential diagnosis of hypercalcemia. Thus, the use of two-site PTH assays is now preferred in hypercalcemic patients. The use of the PTH assay in the differential diagnosis of hypercalcemia is discussed in Chapter 8.

Etiology & Pathogenesis

In patients with cancer, excessive bone resorption is the most important cause of hypercalcemia. The most important stimulus to bone resorption is local or systemic release of tumor-derived mediators, the nature of which is currently under investigation (see below). Direct bone resorption by lytic metastases is less important as a pathogenetic mechanism, as most patients with widespread lytic metastases are not hypercalcemic. Decreased renal calcium excretion may contribute to the pathogenesis of hypercalcemia in many patients. Tumors can secrete hypocalciuric substances, such as the PTH-like protein associated with solid tumors (see below), and the effects of hypercalcemia itself, eg, reduction of the glomerular filtration rate, also contribute to defective renal calcium excretion. The relative roles of excess bone resorption and excess renal reabsorption of calcium are difficult to define, but calcium absorption from the gut probably plays no role in the development of malignancy-associated hypercalcemia, except in patients with lymphoma and elevated levels of $1,25(OH)_2D_3$.

The molecular basis of hypercalcemia associated with cancer involves the production of at least three different hypercalcemic factors (PTHrP, PTH, and $1,25[OH]_2D$), giving rise to several distinct clinical syndromes. In addition, a variety of other mediators have been suggested, eg, prostaglandins. Prostaglandins of the E series are potent bone-resorbing substances. It is clear that prostaglandins are secreted by some tumors, and elevated levels of their metabolites are found in blood and urine in some cancer patients. However, only rare patients with hypercalcemia respond to inhibition of prostaglandin synthesis with nonsteroidal anti-inflammatory agents.

A. Solid Tumors: Solid tumors, especially squamous carcinoma and renal cell carcinoma, produce a characteristic syndrome of hypercalcemia (Table 23–3). This syndrome often occurs in the absence of bone metastases and is characterized by hypophosphatemia and elevated nephrogenous cyclic adenosine monophosphate (cAMP) excretion, both of which occur in hyperparathyroidism. As nephrogenous cAMP is a specific indicator of PTH action, these findings have been thought to implicate a PTH-like substance in the pathogenesis of hypercalcemia. A unique protein has been isolated from both squamous and renal carcinomas (Figure 23–1). The tu-

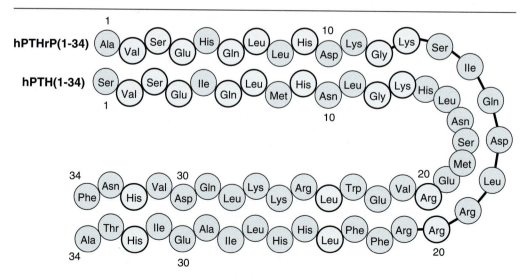

Figure 23–1. Primary structures of the amino terminal part of parathyroid hormone-related protein and of parathyroid hormone. Compared are the human sequences 1–34. Identical amino acids are highlighted.

mor-derived protein, which has been called PTH-related protein (PTHrP) or PTH-like protein (PLP), is expressed in three isoforms, which are identical through amino acid 139 and have 139, 141, or 173 amino acids in toto. PTHrP possesses an amino terminal domain that is strongly homologous with PTH, binds to PTH receptors in both bone and kidney with the same affinity as PTH, and mimics all the classic effects of PTH (eg, excess bone resorption, hypercalcemia, increased renal calcium reabsorption, decreased renal phosphate reabsorption, and increased renal synthesis of 1,25[OH]$_2$D$_3$). PTHrP is the cause of humoral hypercalcemia in most solid tumors. It has recently been shown by immunoassay techniques that the protein is actually present in the circulation in 80% of hypercalcemic patients with tumors. (Figure 23–2). Elevated serum levels of PTHrP are found in over 90% of patients with squamous or renal carcinomas and hypercalcemia. In patients with solid tumors and hypercalcemia, the presence of PTHrP is better correlated with hypercalcemia than the presence of bone metastasis. Thus, even in patients with bone metastases, hypercalcemia may well have a humoral basis. Despite its limited sequence homology with PTH (Figure 23–1), PTHrP does not cross-react with PTH antisera and is not the cause of the PTH-like immunoreactivity often detectable in patients with malignancy-associated hypercalcemia using midregion assays.

Despite the ability of PTHrP to stimulate production of 1,25(OH)$_2$D$_3$, plasma levels of 1,25(OH)$_2$D$_3$ are often normal or even suppressed in patients with cancer, in contrast to the high levels seen in hyperparathyroidism. The reason for this is unclear, but it is known that production of 1,25(OH)$_2$D$_3$ is suppressed by hypercalcemia per se, and it is likely that 1,25(OH)$_2$D$_3$ production is more sensitive to hypercalcemia in cancer patients than in patients with primary hyperparathyroidism.

PTHrP and PTH evolved from a common ancestral gene. PTHrP is expressed in many normal cell types, notably keratinocytes, from which squamous carcinomas arise. Thus, hypercalcemia in squamous carcinoma is another example of hormone production by the cells from which a tumor originates. The PTHrP gene is widely expressed in fetal tissues, and knockout of the gene is lethal in the perinatal period, apparently because of multiple abnormalities of cartilage and bone development. PTHrP is also expressed in the placenta and fetal parathyroid glands and regulates placental calcium transport. In postnatal life, PTHrP appears to have a role in the

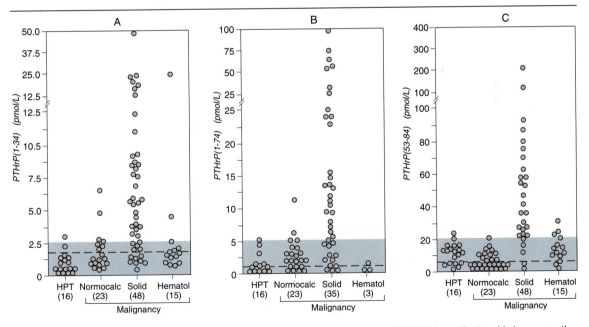

Figure 23–2. Plasma concentrations of parathyroid hormone-related protein (PTHrP) in patients with hyperparathyroidism (HPT), normocalcemic patients with malignancy (Normocalc), and patients with hypercalcemia of malignancy due to a solid tumor (Solid) or a hematologic malignancy (Hematol). Radioimmunoassay (RIA) for amino terminal PTHrP(1–34) (left panel), an IRMA for PTHrP(1–74) (middle panel), and an RIA for midregion PTHrP(53–84) (right panel). The hatched area represents the normal ranges and the dotted line the limits of detection. The numbers attached to each group indicate the number of patients. In the PTHrP(1–74) assay, the group Solid includes five patients classified as local osteolytic type of hypercalcemia (Δ) and two patients with lymphoma. Note the different scales of the y-axes. (Reproduced, with permission, from Blind E, Nissenson RA, Strewler GJ: Parathyroid hormone related protein. In: *Principles and Practice of Endocrinology and Metabolism.* Becker KL [editor]. Lippincott, 1995.)

development of the mammary gland and in the differentiation of skin and the hair follicle. Numerous other physiologic roles have been postulated; some of them may be carried out by unique peptides contained within the PTHrP molecule, but outside the PTH-like amino terminal. Thus, PTHrP may be a polyhormone like proopiomelanocortin, the precursor of multiple biologically active peptides; presumably, multiple receptors are also present to recognize the different peptides. In all cases, PTHrP seems to have local rather than systemic functions, and thus its release into the blood from malignant tumors is inappropriate. More highly conserved during evolution than PTH itself, PTHrP may also be closer in its functions to the primordial hormone from which they evolved, with PTH appearing rather late in evolution to manage systemic calcium homeostasis.

PTHrP is unusual among mediators of paraneoplastic syndromes because it causes a well-defined clinical syndrome by mimicking another hormone that is a distinct gene product. Other tumor products, such as IGF-2, the mediator of tumor-induced hypoglycemia, may well fit the same pattern.

Rarely, hypercalcemia is produced by ectopic secretion of PTH itself. Of the few well-documented cases, most are neuroendocrine tumors, including small cell tumors and thymomas, and one case was an ovarian carcinoma. The diagnosis can be suspected when the PTH level is not suppressed in a patient with a malignant tumor and hypercalcemia, but parathyroid exploration is required to exclude intercurrent primary hyperparathyroidism.

B. Breast Carcinoma: In breast cancer, hypercalcemia occurs almost invariably in patients with extensive bone metastases (Table 23–3). In one study, 35% of patients with advanced breast cancer had hypercalciuria, and 14% developed severe hypercalcemia requiring therapy. Episodes of hypercalcemia are often triggered by estrogen, androgen, or antiestrogen therapy and can be self-limited if hormonal therapy is stopped. These characteristics define a different syndrome from that associated with other solid tumors.

The strong association of hypercalcemia with bone metastases suggests a local osteolytic factor as the etiologic agent. This local factor is probably PTHrP—one of the tumors from which PTHrP was originally isolated was a breast tumor; about one-half of hypercalcemic breast cancer patients have increased levels of PTHrP (Figure 23–2); and PTHrP is demonstrable immunocytochemically in most bone metastases. In some breast cancer metastases, PTHrP is apparently secreted at sufficient levels to produce local osteolysis but not at high enough levels to cause humoral hypercalcemia.

C. Multiple Myeloma: Patients with myeloma are the most likely of all cancer patients to develop hypercalcemia, which occurs at some time in the course of one-third of cases. Hypercalciuria is even more common than hypercalcemia in this group, and hypercalcemia is probably precipitated in many cases by declining renal function with reduced clearance of calcium. As in patients with breast cancer, hypercalcemic episodes in patients with multiple myeloma are sometimes circumscribed, with prolonged subsequent survival. Hypercalcemia in patients with myeloma may respond to glucocorticoids.

The etiologic factor is probably a cytokine produced locally by myeloma cells, and current evidence favors lymphotoxin (tumor necrosis factor-β) or interleukin-1 as the most important of these. It is now clear that leukocytes secrete a variety of cytokines with bone-resorbing activity (eg, interleukin-1, tumor necrosis factor-α, granulocyte-macrophage colony-stimulating factor [GM-CSF], granulocyte colony-stimulating factor [G-CSF]); for example, normal monocytes secrete mostly interleukin-1β. The term "osteoclast-activating factor" was introduced as a rubric for a bone-resorbing factor secreted by normal and malignant leukocytes, but with the discovery of individual bone-resorbing cytokines, it can now be abandoned.

D. Lymphoma: Hypercalcemia occurs in 2–3% of patients with lymphoma, usually those with bone involvement. It is seen in all varieties of lymphoma, but a strong predisposition to hypercalcemia is seen in only one—the adult T cell leukemia-lymphoma syndrome, in which hypercalcemia occurs in two-thirds of cases. The disorder runs an aggressive course, and the associated hypercalcemia responds poorly to steroids and other measures. The causative agent of the syndrome is a retrovirus, the human T cell leukemia-lymphoma virus (HTLV-1). The mediator of hypercalcemia in the adult T cell leukemia syndrome is PTHrP.

The causes of hypercalcemia in other lymphomas are variable. In about one-half of patients, 1,25 $(OH)_2D_3$ appears to be the mediator of hypercalcemia. The latter patients probably have increased intestinal calcium absorption as well as increased bone resorption, and they respond to glucocorticoid therapy. It is recognized that human monocytes in sarcoid granulomas can produce 1,25$(OH)_2D_3$, and it is likely that lymphoma cells are similarly capable of synthesis of this metabolite. The histology of the tumor in patients with high levels of 1,25$(OH)_2D_3$ is diverse; histiocytic, lymphocytic, Hodgkin, and HTLV-positive T cell lymphomas are seen. That a single pathogenetic mechanism would cut across histologic lines of classification in this manner is surprising. In the remaining one-half of lymphoma patients, it is likely that local production of unidentified cytokines is the cause of hypercalcemia.

Treatment

The treatment of hypercalcemia is discussed in Chapter 8.

THE SYNDROME OF INAPPROPRIATE ADH SECRETION

The syndrome of inappropriate secretion of antidiuretic hormone (SIADH) is probably the second most common endocrine complication seen in cancer patients. The syndrome is seen in 10–40% of patients with small cell carcinoma of the lung, the tumor that most commonly produces vasopressin excess. Other causative tumors, many of which are neuroendocrine tumors, include adenocarcinoma and large cell carcinoma of the lung, bronchial carcinoids, carcinoma of the duodenum, small cell carcinoma of the prostate, thymoma, and adrenocortical carcinoma.

Etiology & Pathogenesis

SIADH is now recognized as the most common cause of hyponatremia in hospitalized patients, but most cases result from central (eutopic) secretion of vasopressin, with only 16–50% of cases in different series resulting from ectopic secretion of vasopressin by tumors. The differential diagnosis of hyponatremia is discussed in Chapter 5.

In the presence of vasopressin, excretion of free water is impaired. If the intake of free water exceeds the limited excretion of free water, water intoxication and hyponatremia ensue, with the appearance of symptoms as the serum sodium falls below 125 meq/L. However, if the thirst mechanism is intact and the patient reduces water intake appropriately, a moderate excess of vasopressin may be well tolerated. Thus, the severity of the syndrome depends on water intake as well as on the vasopressin level.

Lung cancer cells have been shown to synthesize a molecule closely resembling propressophysin, the vasopressin precursor, and to secrete immunoreactive vasopressin together with a neurophysin, the other product of its precursor. (Ectopic secretion of the sister octapeptide hormone oxytocin also occurs in small cell lung carcinoma but is not associated with a distinctive clinical syndrome.) In 70–90% of patients with small cell lung carcinoma, the plasma level of at least one of the four neurohypophysial peptides (vasopressin, oxytocin, and their associated neurophysins) is increased, but no more than 10% of these patients have hyponatremia. Many of these patients may in fact have asymptomatic, compensated ectopic secretion of vasopressin, with normal serum osmolality but impaired ability to excrete a water load. However, some cancer patients with hyponatremia and elevated plasma vasopressin levels probably have central or eutopic—rather than ectopic—hypersecretion of vasopressin. For example, in some patients the vasopressin level increases as the plasma osmolality is increased by infusion of hypertonic saline; ie, secretion is under osmotic control. As tumors have not been shown to express an osmoreceptor, these patients probably have a pituitary source of vasopressin. Pituitary secretion of vasopressin could result from stimulation of peripheral baroreceptors by tumor or by hypovolemia.

Many patients with high vasopressin levels also have elevated serum levels of atrial natriuretic peptide (ANP). Small cell carcinomas that produce SIADH often secrete ANP in vitro. An independent role of ANP in causation of SIADH is not proved. However, ANP may well participate in the natriuresis that is characteristic of SIADH.

Clinical Features

Progressive weakness, lethargy, somnolence, and confusion often appear when the serum sodium is less than 125 meq/L; coma, seizures, and death usually occur when the serum sodium is less than 110 meq/L. Patients experience weight gain but no edema, as the retained water is distributed among both intracellular and extracellular spaces. By definition, the urinary osmolality is inappropriately high for the systemic hypo-osmolality. Blood urea nitrogen is often relatively low and the urinary excretion of sodium relatively high, reflecting the expansion of body fluid spaces by retained water. Hypouricemia is often seen. The diagnosis of SIADH is established by excluding other causes of hyponatremia, such as hypovolemia, edematous states, hypothyroidism, and adrenal insufficiency. The presence of inappropriately elevated vasopressin levels can be confirmed by radioimmunoassay, but this test is often unnecessary. The treatment is restriction of water intake. In patients who cannot tolerate a reduction of water intake to correct hypo-osmolality, therapy with hypertonic saline, loop diuretics, or demeclocycline should be started (see Chapter 5). Demeclocycline produces a state of nephrogenic diabetes insipidus that protects the patient from the effects of vasopressin.

CUSHING'S SYNDROME

The ectopic ACTH syndrome (Cushing's syndrome) is strongly associated with neuroendocrine (APUD) tumors. Lung tumors (bronchial carcinoids or small cell lung carcinoma) account for 50% of all cases; 10% are caused by thymic carcinoid tumors (epithelial thymomas), 10% by pancreatic islet cell tumors, 10% by pheochromocytomas, 5% by abdominal carcinoid tumors, and 5% by medullary carcinoma of the thyroid. There is also a strong association of neuroendocrine tumors with secretion of calcitonin and GRP. Neuroendocrine cells are scattered throughout the normal bronchial mucosa, indicating that neuroendocrine cells may represent the cell of origin of small cell carcinomas.

Many (perhaps most) lung tumors contain immunoreactive proopiomelanocortin, the ACTH precursor. However, some tumors that are not associated with Cushing's syndrome use a downstream transcription initiation site in the proopiomelanocortin gene that does not encode a functional protein. In addition, processing of proopiomelanocortin by nonpituitary tumors is frequently abnormal. It is primarily tumors of the neuroendocrine type that process and secrete enough ACTH to cause the clinical manifestations of Cushing's syndrome. It is likely that the ability of neuroendocrine tumors to process and secrete ACTH is related to the dense secretory granules that characterize neuroendocrine cells. However, processing of ACTH is probably abnormal even in a majority of neuroendocrine tumors: It is secreted in a large form that results from incomplete processing of its precursor, and it has reduced biologic activity. At least 25% of patients with small cell lung carcinoma show elevated immunoreactive ACTH levels, but most of these patients have no evidence of cortisol excess. Assays of ACTH in patients with malignancy should employ RIA rather than the newer immunoradiometric assays because the latter may not detect the abnormally processed forms of ACTH that are secreted by malignant neoplasms.

Clinical Features

The classic somatic features of Cushing's syndrome are not present in most patients with Cushing's syndrome associated with nonendocrine tumors. Although cortisol levels are often very high, moon facies, truncal obesity, and cutaneous striae, which reflect the effect of cortisol on protein and fat metabolism, probably do not have time to develop. The syndrome usually develops rapidly and presents with weight loss, wasting, hypokalemia, and muscle weakness. The treatment of Cushing's syndrome is discussed in Chapter 9.

Diagnosis

The differential diagnosis of glucocorticoid excess is presented in Chapter 9. The ectopic ACTH syndrome can usually be distinguished from other forms of Cushing's syndrome by its clinical presentation and by the failure of glucocorticoids to suppress the secretion of ACTH. There is typically no response to administration of corticotropin-releasing hormone (CRH). However, certain slow-growing tumors are associated with chronic secretion of ACTH and produce classic Cushing's syndrome. These tumors are often bronchial or thymic carcinoid tumors, about half of which may be suppressed by administration of dexamethasone in high doses. These tumors are a diagnostic challenge because they are sometimes too small to be detected radiologically and because they may precisely mimic the secretory dynamics of pituitary Cushing's disease. Their suppressibility is rare among ectopic hormone syndromes and is presumably due to their expression of both the glucocorticoid receptor and a glucocorticoid-responsive element in the proopiomelanocortin gene. In cases where the secretory dynamics do not clearly distinguish between pituitary and ectopic sources of ACTH, measurement of ACTH in bilateral samples from the inferior petrosal sinuses, preferably after administration of CRH, may establish whether a pituitary source is present. Ratios of petrosal to peripheral ACTH of > 3.0 after CRH are diagnostic of pituitary Cushing's disease. Inferior petrosal sinus sampling after CRH should be performed in all patients with ACTH-dependent Cushing's syndrome who do not have a pituitary tumor on imaging studies of the gland.

A number of tumors have been reported to secrete both ACTH and CRH; the role of CRH in the pathogenesis of hypercortisolism in patients with such tumors is not clear in all cases. However, in a small number of patients the tumor contained only CRH, and it seems clear that ectopic secretion of CRH stimulated pituitary secretion of ACTH, leading to the development of Cushing's syndrome. CRH-producing tumors do not produce a distinctive clinical syndrome. There is little value in routine determination of CRH levels in ACTH-dependent Cushing's syndrome, but it is appropriate to determine the CRH level in patients who are found to have pituitary corticotroph hyperplasia rather than a pituitary tumor.

NON-ISLET-CELL TUMORS & HYPOGLYCEMIA

Fasting hypoglycemia has been associated with a variety of non-islet-cell tumors. Bulky mesenchymal tumors arising in the retroperitoneum, abdomen, or chest (eg, fibrosarcomas, rhabdomyosarcomas, mesotheliomas, and hemangiopericytomas) account for half of all cases. Hepatocellular carcinomas (hepatomas), gastrointestinal carcinomas, carcinoids, and adrenocortical carcinomas together account for about 25%. A wide variety of carcinomas comprise the remaining 25%.

The clinical presentation and differential diagnosis of fasting hypoglycemia are discussed in Chapter 19. A distinctive feature of hypoglycemia associated with nonpancreatic tumors is that insulin levels are suppressed—there are no authenticated cases of ectopic secretion of insulin. What then is the cause of hypoglycemia? High rates of glucose utilization have been observed in conjunction with impaired hepatic glucose production. It has been suggested that excessive utilization of glucose by extremely large tumors could outstrip hepatic glucose output, but these findings could more readily be accounted for by elaboration of an insulin-like factor that increases peripheral glucose utilization while suppressing glucose output. There is mounting evidence for abnormal secretion and serum binding of IGF-2 in non-islet-cell tumor hypoglycemia. Increased levels of an IGF-2-like substance have been detected in serum, and IGF-2 mRNA has been found in some tumors. In other patients, neither IGF-1 nor IGF-2 levels in serum are increased by radioimmunoassay or by radioreceptor assay. However, the association of IGF-2 with its serum binding proteins is abnormal in patients with non-islet-cell tumors and hypoglycemia. It is possible that the small circulating complexes of IGF-2 in these patients are not sequestered in the blood and are in that way accessible to extravascular receptors, thus accounting for hypoglycemia with minimally increased IGF-2 levels. Factors other than IGF-2 may also contribute to hypoglycemia. Besides increased glucose utilization by the tumor, such factors include deficiency of the glucose counterregulatory hormones (particularly growth hormone) and decreased amino acid flux to the liver as substrate for hepatic gluconeogenesis, resulting from inanition or from the effects of IGF-2.

OTHER HORMONES SECRETED BY TUMORS

Gonadotropins & Other Glycoprotein Hormones

hCG is produced eutopically by trophoblastic and germ cell tumors, including testicular embryonal carcinoma and extragonadal germ cell tumors such as ectopic pinealoma, and in these cases it is highly useful as a tumor marker. hCG is secreted "ectopically" by many tumors. Elevated serum levels are found in 10–30% of patients with lung, breast, gastrointestinal, and ovarian tumors and in some patients with melanoma. hCG has also been detected in low levels in a variety of normal tissues. In one study, elevated levels were found in 9% of patients with various benign diseases, including inflammatory bowel disease, duodenal ulcer disease, and cirrhosis.

Many tumors do not process hCG normally; they secrete free subunits. hCG is a heterodimeric glycoprotein hormone composed of an alpha subunit, which is shared with the other glycoprotein hormones, and a unique beta subunit. One instance in which measurement of subunits is indicated is in patients with pancreatic islet cell tumors. Secretion of intact hCG is rare in islet cell tumors, but about half of malignant functional islet cell tumors secrete alpha subunit while benign islet cell tumors rarely do. Assays of free β-hCG in urine are positive in up to one-half of cases of lung cancer and in advanced and poorly differentiated gynecologic malignancies; the bulk of the immunoreactive material in urine is in the form of a fragment of the beta-subunit known as "beta-core." The sensitivity of these assays for malignancy is too low for any practical use as tumor markers.

The clinical syndromes associated with tumor production of hCG are isosexual precocious pseudopuberty in children and bilateral gynecomastia in adult males. Isosexual precocity occurs in boys with hepatoblastoma. Gynecomastia in adult males is probably due to increased estrogen levels as a consequence of conversion of circulating androgens rather than a di-

rect effect of hCG on the breast. Ectopic secretion of hCG is a relatively uncommon cause of gynecomastia (see Chapter 12).

hCG is the only ectopically secreted hormone composed of multiple subunits, thus requiring the expression of two different genes. The other glycoprotein hormones, follicle-stimulating hormone (FSH), luteinizing hormone (LH), and thyroid-stimulating hormone (TSH), are rarely if ever produced by extrapituitary tumors. Presumably, the propensity of tumors to secrete hCG is related to its expression at low levels in many of their cells of origin in normal tissues.

Growth Hormone-Releasing Hormone, Growth Hormone, & Placental Lactogen

Since 1980, about 50 cases of acromegaly have been associated with extrapituitary production of growth hormone-releasing hormone (GRH). In fact, GRH was first isolated from pancreatic tumors associated with acromegaly. The tumors involved have all been neuroendocrine tumors of the pancreas, lung, or gut (85% involved pancreas or lung; the commonest extrapituitary tumor associated with acromegaly is bronchial carcinoid). The clinical features of acromegaly induced by GRH do not differ from the common form induced by growth hormone (GH) except for the symptoms and signs of the extrapituitary tumor. Although some patients with GRH-induced acromegaly have pituitary somatotroph hyperplasia rather than microadenoma, the radiologic features are often not diagnostic. The response to provocative testing is also unhelpful in detecting GRH-induced acromegaly, but elevated levels of plasma GRH on radioimmunoassay are diagnostic, and this determination should be performed in patients with acromegaly and extrapituitary malignant disease.

Extrapituitary secretion of GH itself is very rare. In one well-documented case, secretion from a pancreatic islet cell carcinoma was confirmed by measurement of an arteriovenous gradient for GH across the tumor and a high tumor content of both GH and GH mRNA.

In contrast to growth hormone, human placental lactogen (chorionic somatomammotropin) is frequently secreted by tumors. In a large series, placental lactogen was detectable in plasma in 9% of patients with malignant disease. Lung carcinoma was the commonest source. Galactorrhea was not present in these patients. The pituitary lactotrophic hormone prolactin is rarely secreted ectopically.

Calcitonin

Like ACTH, vasopressin, and GRP, calcitonin is present in neuroendocrine cells of the normal bronchial epithelium. Calcitonin is frequently secreted by tumors of the neuroendocrine type, including 60% of small cell lung carcinomas. Calcitonin is also secreted by other lung carcinomas (15% of large cell lung carcinomas), breast cancer, leukemia, and a broad spectrum of other cancers. Secretion of calcitonin is not associated with a distinctive clinical syndrome. In part, this may result from incomplete processing of large forms of ectopic calcitonin with reduced biologic activity. However, hypercalcitoninemia is also asymptomatic in medullary thyroid carcinoma, where levels of monomeric calcitonin are sometimes greatly elevated. Secretion of calcitonin by extrathyroidal tumors may respond to secretagogues such as pentagastrin, but the response is smaller than in medullary thyroid carcinoma. By alternative RNA splicing, the calcitonin gene also expresses a distinct calcitonin gene-related peptide (CGRP). CGRP is also produced in lung carcinomas, but less commonly than calcitonin.

Oncogenous Osteomalacia Factor

Osteomalacia (rickets) accompanied by hypophosphatemia occurs in association with tumors of mesenchymal origin, usually small benign tumors of the extremities. Over 50 cases have been reported, making this the commonest cause of late-onset hypophosphatemic rickets. The tumors associated with this syndrome are often highly vascular tumors of mesenchymal origin (hemangiomas, hemangiopericytomas) and frequently include giant cells. The presentation is of osteomalacia with renal phosphate wasting and low levels of $1,25(OH)_2D_3$. The syndrome is rapidly and completely reversed by resection of the tumor, clearly establishing its humoral basis. However, the humor involved has not been identified. The only type of epithelial malignancy associated with a similar syndrome is prostate carcinoma, in which 20% of patients may be hypophosphatemic and a smaller percentage may develop osteomalacia. However, it is possible that in some patients with prostate carcinoma the occurrence of hypophosphatemia and osteomalacia is a direct consequence of rapid new bone formation in metastases rather than a circulating osteomalacia factor.

Hypothalamic-Pituitary Hormones

Ectopic secretion of CRH may cause Cushing's syndrome, and extrapituitary secretion of GRH is a well-documented cause of acromegaly, as discussed above. Beta-endorphin, β-lipotropin, and other products of proopiomelanocortin are associated with the ectopic ACTH syndrome, but they do not produce clinical syndromes other than hyperpigmentation (see Chapter 5). Thyrotropin-releasing hormone (TRH) and somatostatin are detectable in a variety of tumors, mostly of the neuroendocrine type, but clinical disorders associated with their ectopic secretion have not been reported.

Gut Hormones

Vasoactive intestinal polypeptide (VIP) secretion has produced the watery diarrhea-hypokalemia-achlorhydria syndrome in patients with squamous lung carcinoma, ganglioneuroma, and ganglioneuroblastoma, as discussed in Chapter 17. Somatostatin, VIP, GRP (bombesin), motilin, pancreatic polypeptide, and substance P have repeatedly been found in tumors, often of the neuroendocrine type, but have not clearly produced symptoms.

Erythropoietin

One to 3 percent of renal carcinomas, 5% of hepatocellular carcinomas, and 10% of cerebellar hemangioblastomas are associated with erythrocytosis, probably resulting from secretion of erythropoietin. In some cases, production of erythropoietin-like activity or expression of erythropoietin mRNA by tumor cells has been demonstrated. However, serum erythropoietin levels on radioimmunoassay correlate poorly with the presence of erythrocytosis in patients with hepatocellular carcinoma.

Renin

Renin-secreting renal tumors are extremely rare and are associated with severe hypokalemia and hypertension. Removal of the tumor is curative. (See Chapter 10.)

Endothelin

About two-thirds of hepatocellular carcinomas secrete increased levels of a large form of the potent vasoconstrictor peptide endothelin-1. Levels of endothelin-1 are not correlated with blood pressure, but it is possible that the peptide has autocrine mitogenic effects on the tumor, since liver cells have endothelin receptors.

REFERENCES

General

Baylin, SB, Mendelsohn G: Ectopic (inappropriate) hormone production by tumors: Mechanisms involved and the biological and clinical implications. Endocr Rev 1980;1:45.

Daughaday WH, Deuel TF: Tumor secretion of growth factors. Endocrinol Metab Clin North Am 1991;20:539.

LeDouarin NM: On the origin of pancreatic endocrine cells. Cell 1988;53:169.

Russell PJ, O'Mara SM, Raghavan D: Ectopic hormone production by small cell undifferentiated carcinoma. Mol Cell Endocrinol 1990;71:1.

Hypercalcemia of Cancer

Broadus A, Stewart A: Parathyroid hormone-related protein: structure, processing, and physiological actions. In: *The Parathyroids.* Bilezikian J, Levine M, Marcus R (editors). Raven Press, 1994.

Burtis WJ et al: Immunochemical characterization of circulation parathyroid hormone-related protein in patients with humoral hypercalcemia of cancer. N Engl J Med 1990;322:1106.

Halloran BP, Nissenson RA: Parathyroid Hormone-Related Protein: Normal Physiology and Its Role in Cancer. CRC Press, 1992.

Ikeda K et al: Development of a sensitive two-site immunoradiometric assay for parathyroid hormone-related peptide: evidence for elevated levels in plasma from patients with adult T-cell leukemia/lymphoma and B-cell lymphoma. J Clin Endocrinol Metab 1994;79:1322.

Orloff JJ et al: Parathyroid hormone-related protein as a prohormone: Posttranslational processing and receptor interactions. Endocr Rev 1994;15:40.

Seymour JF et al: Calcitriol production in hypercalcemic and normocalcemic patients with non-Hodgkin lymphoma. Ann Intern Med 1994;121:633.

Strewler GJ et al: Production of parathyroid hormone by a malignant nonparathyroid tumor in a hypercalcemic patient. J Clin Endocrinol Metab 1993;76:1373.

Strewler GJ, Nissenson RA: Peptide mediators of hypercalcemia in malignancy. Annu Rev Med 1990;41:35.

Strewler GJ, Nissenson RA: The parathyroid hormone-related protein as a regulator of normal tissue functions. In: Current Opinion in Endocrinology & Diabetes. Kohler PO (editor). Current Science, 1994.

Wysolmerski JJ, Broadus AE: Hypercalcemia of malignancy: The central role of parathyroid hormone-related protein. Annu Rev Med 1994;45:189.

Syndrome of Inappropriate Secretion of ADH

Anderson RJ et al: Hyponatremia: A prospective analysis of its epidemiology and the pathogenetic role of vasopressin. Ann Intern Med 1985;102:164.

Gross AJ et al: Atrial natriuretic factor and arginine vasopressin production in tumor cell lines from patients with lung cancer and their relationship to serum sodium. Cancer Res 1993;53:67.

Kovacs L, Robertson GL: Syndrome of inappropriate antidiuresis. Endocrinol Metab Clin North Am 1992; 21:859.

Moses AM, Scheinman SJ: Ectopic secretion of Neurohypophyseal peptides in patients with malignancy. Endocrinol Metab Clin North Am 1991;20:489.

Shapiro J, Richardson GE: Hyponatremia of malignancy. Crit Rev Oncol Hematol 1995;18:129.

Cushing's Syndrome

Becker M, Aron DC: Ectopic ACTH syndrome and CRH-mediated Cushing's syndrome. Endocrinol Metab Clin North Am 1994;23:585.

Bertagna X: Proopiomelanocortin-derived peptides. Endocrinol Metab Clin North Am 1994;23:467.

Oldfield EH et al: Petrosal sinus sampling with and without corticotropin-releasing hormone for the differential diagnosis of Cushing's syndrome. N Engl J Med 1991;325:897.

Schteingart DE: Ectopic secretion of peptides of the proopiomelanocortin family. Endocrinol Metab Clin North Am 1991;20:453.

Wajchenberg BL et al: Ectopic adrenocorticotropic hormone syndrome. Endocr Rev 1994;15:752.

Hypoglycemia

Baxter RC, Daughaday WH: Impaired formation of the ternary insulin-like growth factor-binding protein complex in patients with hypoglycemia due to non-islet cell tumors. J Clin Endocrinol Metab 1991;73:696.

Daughaday WH, Trivedi B, Baxter RC: Serum "big insulin-like growth factor II" from patients with tumor hypoglycemia lacks normal E-domain O-linked glycosylation, a possible determinant of normal propeptide processing. Proc Natl Acad Sci U S A 1993;90:5823.

Daughaday WH: Hypoglycemia in patients with non-islet cell tumors. Endocrinol Metab Clin North Am 1989;18:91.

Phillips LS, Robertson DG: Insulin-like growth factors and non-islet cell tumor hypoglycemia. Metabolism 1993;42:1093.

Gonadotropins

Kahn CR et al: Ectopic production of chorionic gonadotropin and its subunits by islet-cell tumors: A specific marker for malignancy. N Engl J Med 1977; 297:565.

Neven P et al: Urinary chorionic gonadotropin subunits and beta-core in nonpregnant women: A study of benign and malignant gynecologic disorders. Cancer 1993;71:4124.

Yoshimura M et al: Assessment of urinary beta-core fragment of human chorionic gonadotropin as a new tumor marker of lung cancer. Cancer 1994;73:2745.

GRH, Growth Hormone, & Placental Lactogen

Ezzat S et al: Recurrent acromegaly resulting from ectopic growth hormone gene expression by a metastatic pancreatic tumor. Cancer 1993;71:66.

Melmed S et al: Acromegaly due to secretion of growth hormone by an ectopic pancreatic islet-cell tumor. N Engl J Med 1985;312:9.

Melmed S: Extrapituitary acromegaly. Endocrinol Metab Clin North Am 1991;20:507.

Weintraub BD, Rosen SW: Ectopic production of human chorionic somatomammotropin by nontrophoblastic cancers. J Clin Endocrinol Metab 1971; 32:94.

Calcitonin

Roos BA et al: Plasma immunoreactive calcitonin in lung cancer. J Clin Endocrinol Metab 1980;50:659.

Samaan NA et al: Serum calcitonin after pentagastrin stimulation in patients with bronchogenic and breast cancer compared to that in patients with medullary thyroid carcinoma. J Clin Endocrinol Metab 1980; 51:237.

Oncogenous Osteomalacia Factor

Lyles KW et al: Hypophosphatemic osteomalacia: Association with prostatic carcinoma. Ann Intern Med 1980;93:275.

Ryan EA, Reiss E: Oncogenous osteomalacia: Review of the world literature of 42 cases and report of two new cases. Am J Med 1984;77:501.

Weidner N et al: Neoplastic pathology of oncogenic osteomalacia/rickets. Cancer 1985;55:1691.

Hypothalamic-Pituitary Hormones

Melmed S, Rushakoff RJ: Ectopic pituitary and hypothalamic hormone syndromes. Endocrinol Metab Clin North Am 1987;16:805.

Gut Hormones

Noseda A et al: Increased plasma motilin concentrations in small cell carcinoma of the lung. Thorax 1987; 42:784.

Erythropoietin

Kew MC, Fisher JW: Serum erythropoietin concentrations in patients with hepatocellular carcinoma. Cancer 1986;58:2485.

Endothelin

Ishibashi M et al: Production and secretion of endothelin by hepatocellular carcinoma. J Clin Endocrinol Metab 1993;76:378.

Syndromes Involving Multiple Endocrine Glands

24

Leonard J. Deftos, MD, JD, & John J. Nolan, MB, FRCPI

MULTIPLE ENDOCRINE NEOPLASIA

Astute clinical observation has resulted in the identification of neoplastic syndromes involving multiple endocrine glands. The glands most commonly involved in such syndromes are the parathyroid, pituitary, pancreas, thyroid, and adrenal. The cell types involved in these tumors are postulated to have a common embryologic precursor in the neuroectoderm. This embryologic feature may be accompanied by the presence of the metabolic pathway for *a*mine *p*recursor *u*ptake and *d*ecarboxylation—thus the appellation APUD cells. Oncogenic mutational factors may also influence expression of these tumors. The multiple endocrine neoplasia syndromes are usually transmitted in an autosomal dominant inheritance pattern, but there may be considerable variability in penetrance and in specific tumor incidences among kindreds. Hormonal measurements are used in conjunction with clinical features in the diagnosis of these disorders. Now that some of the genes associated with multiple endocrine disorders have been mapped, genetic testing has begun to revolutionize the diagnosis of inherited endocrine tumors.

There are three well-defined types of multiple endocrine neoplasia (MEN) syndromes (Table 24–1): **MEN type I** (also called Wermer's syndrome), **MEN type IIa** (also called Sipple's syndrome and MEN type II), and **MEN type IIb** (also called MEN type III). The clinical descriptions and terminology for these syndromes have evolved from 1954 to the present. The first MEN syndrome was clearly described by Wermer in 1954 and was characterized by tumors of the parathyroids, pituitary, and pancreas. Shortly thereafter, Zollinger and Ellison described a syndrome that consisted of gastric hypersecretion and severe peptic disease associated with a non-insulin-producing islet cell tumor of the pancreas. This syndrome, the Zollinger-Ellison syndrome, is found in association with MEN type I in some cases but more commonly occurs by itself. In 1961, Sipple re-

ported the association between thyroid cancer and pheochromocytoma. Through the subsequent studies of Williams and Hazard, a distinct thyroid tumor of the calcitonin-producing cells (C cells) of the thyroid—ie, medullary thyroid carcinoma—was defined. Characterization of the second MEN syndrome, consisting of medullary thyroid carcinoma, parathyroid tumors, and pheochromocytoma, evolved from these observations. The additional observation that there were two accompanying somatotypic features—ie, a marfanoid habitus and multiple mucosal neuromas—in some patients with this second type of MEN syndrome led to the classification of the third type of MEN syndrome. In summary, the **major components** of the three syndromes are as follows: **MEN type I**—tumors of the parathyroids, pituitary,

---

ACRONYMS USED IN THIS CHAPTER

ACTH	Adrenocorticotropic hormone
APUD	Amine precursor uptake and decarboxylation
CGRP	Calcitonin gene-related peptide
GH	Growth hormone
HLA	Human leukocyte antigen
LH	Luteinizing hormone
MEN	Multiple endocrine neoplasia
MSH	Melanocyte-stimulating hormone
MTC	Medullary thyroid carcinoma
POEMS	Polyneuropathy, organomegaly, endocrinopathy, M protein, and skin changes
PP	Pancreatic polypeptide
PRL	Prolactin
PTH	Parathyroid hormone
TSH	Thyroid-stimulating hormone (thyrotropin)
VIP	Vasoactive intestinal polypeptide

Table 24–1. Components of the multiple endocrine neoplasias (MEN).

MEN type I
  Parathyroid tumors
  Pituitary tumors
  Pancreatic tumors
MEN type IIa
  Medullary thyroid carcinoma
  Pheochromocytoma
  Hyperparathyroidism
MEN type IIb
  Medullary thyroid carcinoma
  Pheochromocytoma
  Mucosal neuromas

and pancreas, and, in some cases, components of the Zollinger-Ellison syndrome; **MEN type IIa**—medullary thyroid carcinoma, hyperparathyroidism, and pheochromocytoma; and **MEN type IIb**—medullary thyroid carcinoma, pheochromocytoma, marfanoid habitus, and multiple mucosal neuromas.

In general, the clinical and biochemical characteristics of component tumors of MEN syndromes do not differ markedly from characteristics of each tumor when it occurs by itself; therefore, those aspects are only briefly described in this chapter. For example, primary hyperparathyroidism as part of a MEN syndrome has most of the characteristics of multiglandular hyperparathyroidism occurring alone, and the reader should consult Chapter 8 for a more detailed description of the features of primary hyperparathyroidism. However, the presence of multiple endocrinopathies presents a unique clinical picture

(Table 24–2), and the presence of multiple endocrine tumors does have specific implications for therapy.

MULTIPLE ENDOCRINE NEOPLASIA TYPE I

MEN type I—easily remembered as the "PPP" syndrome—is characterized by tumors of the parathyroids, pituitary, and pancreas. The most common pituitary tumor is benign chromophobe adenoma; the most common pancreatic tumor is gastrinoma; and the most common parathyroid lesion is multiglandular primary hyperparathyroidism. Table 24–3 shows the approximate frequency of occurrence of the components of MEN type I. The actual pattern may vary among kindreds. Tumors other than the three principal components of the syndrome (Table 24–3) are rare, and their relationship to the genetic disorder is unclear. The gene for this disorder has been mapped to chromosome 11.

Primary Hyperparathyroidism

Primary hyperparathyroidism is the most common endocrine neoplasia of MEN type I. Thus, upon identifying a patient with primary hyperparathyroidism, it is important to determine whether other components of the syndrome are present. The pathologic characteristics of the parathyroid glands can be best understood by recognizing the multiglandular nature of the disorder. The glands have been described in various terms ranging from adenomatous to hyperplastic. The histologic features necessary to make these classifi-

Table 24–2. Abnormal hormone production by endocrine tumor of MEN syndromes. Measurement of these substances or their metabolites in blood and urine can serve as diagnostic tests.

	Pituitary	Pancreas	Parathyroid	Thyroid	Adrenal
PTH			•		
CT		•		•	
ACTH	•			•	
GH	•				
Somatostatin	•	•			
PRL	•				
VIP		•			
PP		•			
Gastrin		•			
Insulin		•			
Glucagon		•			
Catecholamines					•
Chromagranin A	•	•	•	•	•

Table 24–3. Components of MEN type I and their approximate frequency of occurrence.

Hyperparathyroidism (≈ 80%)
Pancreatic tumors (≈ 75%)
    Gastrinomas
        Benign ≈ 20%
        Malignant ≈ 30%
    Insulinomas
        Benign ≈ 20%
        Malignant ≈ 5%
    Nonfunctioning tumors
        Benign < 5%
        Malignant < 5%
Pituitary tumors (≈ 65%)
    Chromophobe or nonfunctioning adenomas
        Benign ≈ 40%
        Malignant < 5%
    Eosinophilic tumors or acromegaly (benign) ≈ 15%
    Cushing's disease, basophilic ≈ 5%
    Mixed and other types (benign) < 5%
    Prolactin-secreting tumors < 5%
Other tumors (≈ 20%)
    Carcinoid and bronchial adenomas < 5%
    Lipomas and liposarcomas ≈ 5%
    Adrenocortical adenomas ≈ 10%

cations are not always apparent. Although chief cells are usually dominant, clear cells or a mixed picture may also be seen. The most important practical point to be derived from pathologic descriptions is the potential for *all* parathyroid glands to be involved in the neoplastic process, even ectopic glands. This means that aggressive surgical therapy directed toward subtotal parathyroidectomy may be necessary for effective treatment.

Pituitary Tumors

The most common pituitary tumor of MEN type I is chromophobe adenoma. This nonfunctioning tumor is usually benign by histologic criteria but can cause endocrine abnormalities by the effect of its mass on adjacent endocrine cells. Tumors producing growth hormone (GH), adrenocorticotropic hormone (ACTH), prolactin (PRL), and somatostatin have also been described in this syndrome, and their manifestations are classically related to their location and hormonal products. The incidence of pituitary microadenomas is not well defined (see Chapter 5).

Pancreatic Tumors

Gastrin-producing islet cell tumors are the most common pancreatic neoplasias of MEN type I, accounting for at least 50% of all pancreatic tumors. Gastrinomas can also occur at other sites such as the duodenal wall and stomach. Insulinomas are the next most common neoplasias. In addition, there are case reports of tumors producing vasoactive intestinal polypeptide (VIP), glucagon, pancreatic polypeptide (PP), somatostatin, and calcitonin. Measurement by radioimmunoassay of these hormones in serum is an important diagnostic procedure. The "tumors" are

usually composed of hyperplastic islet cells or multiple small tumors. The secretory products of these tumors can explain some of the associated findings. Examples are the peptic ulcer diathesis with gastrin, hypoglycemia with insulin, and secretory diarrhea with VIP and perhaps with PP. Glucagonomas can be associated with bullous dermatitis, but the pathogenesis of this lesion is obscure.

The production of excess gastrin leading to peptic ulceration by a pancreatic islet cell tumor is called **Zollinger-Ellison syndrome.** Zollinger-Ellison syndrome more commonly occurs by itself, but it can also be part of MEN type I. The ulcer diathesis of Zollinger-Ellison syndrome makes gastrointestinal symptoms a dominant clinical feature. Gastrointestinal symptoms may also be dominant in a patient with a VIP-producing islet cell tumor (VIPoma) (see Chapter 17).

Other Tumors

The other tumors indicated in Table 24–3 are also found in patients with MEN type I, but their link to this disorder is not clearly established. Carcinoid tumors associated with MEN type I are more likely to be found in foregut-derived structures such as the thymus and bronchial tree than in midgut-derived structures, where sporadic carcinoid tumors usually occur. Bronchial carcinoid can produce its vasoactive symptoms without metastasizing. Adrenal and thyroid adenomas occurring in MEN type I represent predominantly the results of autopsy findings and are usually nonfunctioning. Lipomas may be present in some kindreds in MEN type I, and when cutaneous they may provide a useful sign of the syndrome.

MULTIPLE ENDOCRINE NEOPLASIA TYPES IIA & IIB

In the early reports of medullary thyroid carcinoma as part of a multiple endocrine disorder, the associated lesions were pheochromocytoma, hyperparathyroidism, and a syndrome consisting of multiple mucosal neuromas and marfanoid habitus (mucosal neuroma syndrome). It is now appreciated that two distinct clinical syndromes can be defined by these associated endocrinopathies: MEN type IIa (Table 24–4) and MEN type IIb (Table 24–5). MEN type IIa consists of medullary thyroid carcinoma, pheochro-

Table 24–4. Components of MEN type IIa and their approximate frequency of occurrence in patients with MEN type IIa.

Component	Frequency
Medullary thyroid carcinoma	97%
Hyperparathyroidism	50%
Phenochromocytoma	30%

Table 24–5. Components of MEN type IIb and their approximate frequency of occurrence in patients with MEN type IIb.

Component	Frequency
Multiple mucosal neuromas	100%
Medullary thyroid carcinoma	90%
Marfanoid habitus	65%
Phenochromocytoma	45%

mocytoma, and hyperparathyroidism; MEN type IIb consists of medullary thyroid carcinoma, pheochromocytoma, multiple mucosal neuromas, and marfanoid habitus. The component tumors of MEN type IIa and MEN type IIb vary in their incidence and prevalence. Since medullary thyroid carcinoma is the central tumor, it will be discussed first. The gene for MEN type IIa has been mapped to chromosome 10.

Medullary Thyroid Carcinoma

Medullary thyroid carcinoma (MTC), a tumor of the calcitonin-producing cells (C cells) of the thyroid gland, is a component of MEN type IIa and IIb. This tumor can also occur sporadically and in familial medullary thyroid carcinoma (FMTC). Sporadic MTC may comprise 0.5% of all thyroid nodular and 15% of all thyroid cancers. The thyroidal C cells are now generally accepted to be of neural crest origin. These cells migrate to the ultimobranchial bodies from the neural crest. In submammals, the cells form a distinct organ, the ultimobranchial organ, which harbors C cells and their secretory product, calcitonin. In mammals, C cells become incorporated into the thyroid gland and perhaps other sites. The neural crest origin of C cells offers an explanation for the association of MTC with other tumors of neural crest origin and also appears to explain the production by these tumors of a wide variety of bioactive substances.

MTC is usually a firm, rounded tumor located in the middle or upper lobes of the thyroid gland. The cells usually are polyhedral or polygonal and are arranged in a variety of patterns. Calcification is commonly found in the tumor, and a characteristic calcification may be visible on x-ray. Although the presence of amyloid has long been considered to be important in the diagnosis of MTC, the diagnosis is best established by the use of specific immunohistochemical procedures for calcitonin that demonstrate the abnormal C cells. The frank malignancy of MTC, at least in familial cases, is preceded by a progressive hyperplasia of C cells referred to as **C cell hyperplasia.** This predecessor of MTC can become manifest in early childhood or as late as the second decade. There may be corresponding changes in the parathyroid and adrenal glands. Several instances of **C cell adenoma** have also been reported. The natural history of MTC can vary greatly, and this may make decisions regarding therapy difficult. The tumor is

generally regarded as intermediate between the aggressive behavior of anaplastic thyroid carcinoma and the more indolent behavior of papillary and follicular thyroid carcinoma. Mixed tumors can also occur, with follicular and papillary elements that display thyroglobulin production. The most common presentation of MTC is a thyroid nodule, and the most common symptom is diarrhea. (See Chapter 7.)

There are two general groups of factors that can contribute to the diarrhea commonly seen in patients with MTC—humoral factors and anatomic ones. Many of the various bioactive substances produced by MTC have been implicated in the pathogenesis of the diarrhea seen with this tumor. These peptide hormones include (1) calcitonin, (2) ACTH and melanocyte-stimulating hormone (MSH), (3) neurotensin, (4) somatostatin, (5) β-endorphin, and (6) nerve growth factor (Table 24–6). The various anatomic abnormalities discussed subsequently that can be found in the gastrointestinal tract of patients with MTC may also account for the diarrhea. These anatomic lesions may reflect and perhaps even produce fundamental abnormalities in gastrointestinal innervation that can produce abnormal motility.

A. Calcitonin and Related Peptides and Proteins: Since MTC is a neoplastic disorder of the C cells of the thyroid gland, the tumor produces abnormally high amounts of calcitonin. As a result, patients with this tumor have elevated concentrations of calcitonin in peripheral blood and urine. In many patients, basal concentrations of the hormone are sufficiently elevated to be diagnostic of the presence of MTC. However, in an increasing percentage of patients with this tumor, basal levels of calcitonin are indistinguishable from normal. Thus, **provocative**

Table 24–6. Products secreted by medullary thyroid carcinoma.

Adrenocorticotropic hormone
Amyloid
Calcitonin
Calcitonin gene-related peptide
Carcinoembryonic antigen
Catecholamines
Chromogranin A
Corticotropin-releasing hormone
Dopa decarboxylase
β-Endorphin
Histaminase
Kallikrein and kinins
Melanin
Melanocyte-stimulating hormone
Nerve growth factor
Neuron-specific enolase
Neurotensin/gastrin release peptide
Prolactin-releasing hormone
Prostaglandins
Serotonin
Somatostain
Substance P
Vasoactive intestinal polypeptide

tests with calcium and pentagastrin have been developed for the diagnosis of MTC and its histologic antecedents. These tests are based on the observation that calcium and pentagastrin are potent calcitonin secretagogues.

Opinion differs regarding the relative clinical value of pentagastrin and calcium infusion in the diagnosis of MTC. One must remember that most tumors respond to either agent and that both infusion procedures sometimes give false-negative results. Therefore, either procedure can be recommended, and if one procedure gives negative results in a patient suspected of having MTC, the alternative procedure should be considered before the diagnosis is excluded. In general, both the sensitivity and the specificity of the calcitonin immunoassay are probably just as important as the choice between calcium and pentagastrin in provocative testing of a patient suspected of having MTC. Selective venous catheterization with measurements of calcitonin can also be useful, but its greatest value is probably not in primary diagnosis but in the location of tumor metastases (or sources of ectopic calcitonin production), since knowledge of the presence of metastatic (or ectopic) disease can greatly influence therapy. The effectiveness of therapy in patients with calcitonin-producing tumors can be monitored by serial measurements of plasma calcitonin. In addition to determining the relatively acute effects of a given treatment regimen, periodic surveillance with appropriate provocative testing can be conducted for recurrence of tumor.

The calcitonin gene encodes other peptides, among them a 37-amino-acid peptide termed CGRP (calcitonin gene-related peptide) (Table 24–6). Although the function of these peptides is unknown, they are secreted by MTC and may thus serve as tumor markers. C cells also secrete chromogranin A, a high-molecular-weight protein originally discovered in the secretory granules of pheochromocytomas and now known to be present in other endocrine tissues, among them the parathyroid, pancreas, and pituitary (Table 24–2). This protein could thus be a marker for each of the endocrine neoplasias encountered in any of the multiple endocrine neoplasias (Table 24–7).

B. Other Secretory Products: In addition to calcitonin, MTC produces other substances, nonpeptides as well as peptides (Table 24–6). Their measurement in blood, eg, chromogranin A or carcinoembryonic antigen (CEA), may also be useful in diagnosis and management. This unusual biosynthetic capacity of MTC may be related to the neural crest origin of C cells.

Pheochromocytoma

Pheochromocytoma is a component of MEN type IIa and IIb. Pheochromocytomas occurring in association with MTC have several distinct features. Bilateral and multifocal pheochromocytomas are very

Table 24–7. Plasma calcitonin and chromogranin A concentrations (mean ± SE) in patients with endocrine tumors.

Group	Chromogranin A (ng/mL)	Calcitonin (pg/mL)
Normal controls (n = 16)	82 ± 16	60 ± 15
Phenochromocytoma (n = 11)	1614 ± 408[1]	. . .
Medullary thyroid carcinoma (n = 6)	789 ± 333[1]	7485 ± 3009[1]
Parathyroid adenoma (n = 7)	218 ± 13[1]	. . .

[1]$P < .01$ compared to control.

common in this clinical setting, with an incidence of over 70%. This contrasts with a bilateral incidence of usually less than 10% for sporadic pheochromocytomas and only 20–50% with familial pheochromocytomas. Pheochromocytomas are much more likely to occur in patients with familial rather than sporadic MTC. The thyroid tumor may antedate the pheochromocytoma by as much as 2 decades. Furthermore, a second pheochromocytoma may become manifest after removal of the first. Thus, there is a greater incidence of pheochromocytomas in older patients with MTC. If hyperparathyroidism also exists, it too is likely to be diagnosed before the pheochromocytoma. **Adrenal medullary hyperplasia** may be a predecessor of the pheochromocytomas seen with MTC, just as C cell hyperplasia may be a predecessor of MTC and chief cell hyperplasia a predecessor of primary hyperparathyroidism in these patients. The increase in adrenal medullary mass results from diffuse or multifocal proliferation of adrenal medullary cells, primarily those found within the head and body of the glands. Diagnostic tests for pheochromocytoma should be pursued vigorously, because the biochemical as well as clinical manifestations of this tumor may be subtle. A high ratio of epinephrine to norepinephrine—rather than absolute levels—is considered an important diagnostic criterion (see Chapter 11).

Hyperparathyroidism

The exact incidence of hyperparathyroidism in patients with MTC is difficult to establish. Hyperparathyroidism is much more common in MEN type IIa than in MEN type IIb. Hyperplasia is more common than adenoma. Despite these uncertainties, the concurrence of hyperparathyroidism and MTC in MEN syndromes is well established, and although it cannot be quantitated, the presence of one tumor should always make one suspect the presence of the other. Hyperparathyroidism does not easily fit into a unitary concept of embryogenesis, since parathyroid cells are not classically considered to be of neural crest origin. However, some authorities have suggested a neural crest origin for the parathyroid gland. An alternative explanation for the hyperparathyroidism is a functional relationship between it and MTC. According to this hypothesis, the abnormal concentrations of calcitonin induce hyperparathyroidism, which is secondary to the hypocalcemic actions of the calcitonin. This type of functional relationship between the neoplasias is unlikely; the most convincing evidence supports a genetic relationship between MTC and hyperparathyroidism (see Chapter 8).

Mucosal Neuromas

The presence of neuromas with a centrofacial distribution is the most consistent component of MEN type IIb. The most common location of neuromas is the oral cavity (tongue, lips, buccal mucosa), but other sites may be involved (Table 24–8). The oral lesions (Figure 24–1) are almost invariably present by the first decade and in some cases even at birth. The most prominent microscopic feature of neuromas is an increase in the size and number of nerves.

Mucosal neuromas can be present in the eyelids,

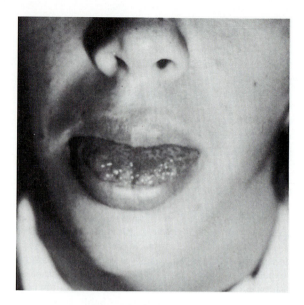

Figure 24–1. Mucosal neuromas on the tongue of a 12-year-old child with MEN type IIb.

Table 24–8. Summary of clinical features in 41 patients with MEN type IIb.

	Number of patients With Findings[1]		
	Positive	Probable	Negative
Family history of MEN type IIb	14	2	15
Neuroma (any type Oral type	41 37		4
Ocular type	24		16
Other type	4		36
"Bumpy" lips	35	2	
Pheochromocytoma	19[2]	4	18
Medullary thyroid carcinoma	38		2
Marfanoid habitus	26	5	
Hypertrophied corneal nerves	23		
Skeletal defects	24		4
Gastrointestinal tract abnormalities	23		10

[1]In some cases, the status of some of the clinical features was not known.
[2]Unilateral in 7 patients; bilateral in 12 patients.
(Reproduced and modified, with permission, from: Khairi MRA, et al: Mucosal neuroma, pheochromocytoma and medullary carcinoma: MEN, type III. Medicine 1975:54:89.)

conjunctiva, and cornea. The thickened medullated corneal nerves traverse the cornea and anastomose in the pupillary area. These hypertrophied nerve fibers are readily seen with a slit lamp but occasionally may be evident even on direct ophthalmoscopic examination.

Gastrointestinal tract abnormalities are part of the multiple mucosal neuroma syndrome. The most common of these is gastrointestinal ganglioneuromatosis. Ganglioneuromatosis is best observed in the small and large intestine but has also been noted in the esophagus and stomach. The anatomic lesions are sometimes associated with functional difficulties in swallowing, megacolon, diarrhea, and constipation. Similar lesions may be present on other mucosal surfaces.

Marfanoid Habitus

The term "marfanoid habitus" denotes a tall, slender body with long arms and legs, an abnormal ratio of upper to lower body segment, and poor muscle development. It is seen commonly in multiple mucosal neuroma syndrome. The extremities are thin, and there may be lax joints and hypotonic muscles. Other features associated with the marfanoid habitus may include dorsal kyphosis, pectus excavatum or pectus carinatum, pes cavus, and high-arched palate. In contrast to patients with true Marfan's syndrome, no patients with multiple mucosal neuromas have been reported to have aortic abnormalities, ectopia lentis, homocystinuria, or, notably, mucopolysaccharide abnormalities.

OTHER MULTIPLE ENDOCRINE NEOPLASIAS

Several additional syndromes exist that are characterized by the autosomal dominant inheritance of multiple endocrine tumors. The **von Hippel-Lindau syndrome** consists of cerebelloretinal hemangioblastomas occurring with pheochromocytomas and pancreatic islet cell tumors along with renal cell carcinoma. It has been linked to a deletion on chromosome 3. In addition to Schwann-cell tumors, patients with neurofibromatosis (**Recklinghausen's disease**) have pheochromocytomas and duodenal carcinoid tumors. This disorder has been mapped to chromosome 17, the location of the nerve growth factor receptor.

As with some other tumors, such as retinoblastoma and small-cell lung carcinoma, the presence of chromosomal deletions in endocrine tumors has led to the hypothesis that the deleted gene encodes an anti-oncogene whose absence allows oncogenesis to occur. Studies with the tools of molecular biology will provide important insights into the pathogenesis of inherited endocrine tumors.

MANAGEMENT OF PATIENTS WITH MULTIPLE ENDOCRINE NEOPLASIA (MEN) SYNDROMES

The individual endocrine components of MEN syndromes have, in general, the same clinical and biochemical manifestations as when they occur as individual entities. The unique clinical aspect of the patient with MEN is the way in which the individual presents to the physician. The patient may be part of a kindred with well-established MEN, and the physician must then evaluate the patient for each potential component of the kindred's syndrome. Or the physician may search for the presence of MEN when a patient presents with one of the endocrine components; in this latter circumstance, the yield will not be great, but when one patient with MEN is discovered, it leads to the identification of other patients.

Surgery is the treatment of choice for the three neoplasias in MEN type IIa. All are potentially lethal—especially MTC and pheochromocytoma—but all can be cured by early diagnosis followed by operation. Aggressive therapy is thus warranted, and special consideration should be given to certain aspects of the treatment, since one is dealing with a patient with three potential endocrine tumors.

Management of the individual components of MEN syndromes generally follows the accepted procedures for each of the neoplasias, and these are discussed in detail elsewhere in this book. Thus, the management of pituitary tumors is guided by the availability of transsphenoidal hypophysectomy and the management of mucosal neuromas by cosmetic factors. However, the clinical setting does influence the sequence and extent of surgical therapy. The sequence of treatment is guided by the presence of multiple endocrine tumors. Pheochromocytomas, which are commonly bilateral, especially in MEN type IIb, should be treated first, medically or surgically, in order to obviate their cardiovascular effects on surgical procedures. Thyroid and parathyroid surgery must be aggressive, because all glandular tissue may be involved.

An essential feature of appropriate clinical management is evaluation of family members, since MEN syndromes are transmitted in an autosomal dominant pattern. Family members must be reevaluated periodically because of the varying penetrance of the component tumors. (See Figure 7–58.)

GENETIC DIAGNOSIS

Mutations in the *RET* proto-oncogene have been established as the genetic basis for MEN type II. Highly specific amino acid substitutions seem to account for most of the abnormalities of the tyrosine kinase product of this gene. Most of the mutations involve substitutions for cysteines. A high percentage of patients with MEN type II can be identified by genetic studies. Abnormalities of this gene also occur in Hirschsprung's disease and familial MTC.

The ethical concerns that surround genetic testing are prominent features of the management of patients with MEN type II and their families. Physicians should also become aware of the range of legal complications that can involve liability in the context of genetic diagnosis, ranging from the failure to diagnose this disease in patients at risk to invasion of the privacy of relatives of patients who do not want to know of any inherited disposition to endocrine cancer. These legal and ethical issues in MEN will be defined further by experience with genetic testing.

FAILURE OF MULTIPLE ENDOCRINE GLANDS

This section deals mainly with the syndromes involving autoimmune destruction of multiple endocrine and specific other tissues. Historically, the first of these associations was Schmidt's syndrome of nontuberculous Addison's disease and lymphocytic thyroiditis. In a 1964 review of Schmidt's syndrome, Carpenter et al found coexisting diabetes mellitus in 10 out of 15 patients with Addison's disease and thyroiditis. They broadened the definition of the syndrome to include diabetes mellitus associated with nontuberculous Addison's disease. However, multiglandular failure may also involve the parathyroids, ovaries, testes, and possibly adenohypophysis. Schmidt's syndrome (the Carpenter definition will be used in this chapter) is thus but one subset of these disorders. In addition, these endocrinopathies are frequently associated with other disorders of tissue-specific autoimmunity, notably pernicious anemia and vitiligo. This discussion will emphasize the evidence for clinical, immunologic, and possibly genetic heterogeneity among groups of patients with these disorders.

Six mechanisms of immunologic tissue injury have been described (Table 24–9). The primary effectors in autoimmune reactions are immunoglobulins, T cells (thymus-dependent lymphocytes that become sensitized to specific antigens and release soluble nonimmunoglobulin mediators), and monocytes (which possess receptors for the Fc region of immunoglobulins and cytotoxic capabilities in the presence of tissue-specific antibody). The role of these mechanisms in autoimmune endocrine disease has been most extensively studied in Hashimoto's thyroiditis and Graves' disease. Although immune complexes are present in the sera of some patients with autoimmune thyroid disease, T cell-mediated immunity and antibody-dependent cell-mediated cytotoxicity have received the greatest attention as mechanisms of target organ destruction in Hashimoto's thyroiditis. Evidence for specifically sensitized T cells has been found in other autoimmune endocrinopathies as well. To explain this apparent break in the immunologically privileged status of autologous tissues, Volpe has proposed a unifying theory of pathogenesis of autoimmune thyroid disease based on a defect in immunoregulation by suppressor T cells (thymus-dependent lymphocytes that suppress immune responses, possibly including recognition of autoantigens). In vitro reconstitution experiments have shown that normal suppressor T cells can depress the production of migration-inhibiting lymphokines by leukocyte cultures from Hashimoto's thyroiditis patients and can also inhibit the differentiation of antithyroid antibody-secreting

cells. Patients with autoimmune thyroid disease, but not other autoimmune diseases, appear to lack suppressor T cells capable of these functions. (See Chapters 4 and 7.)

The events that initiate immune sensitization to antigens of the endocrine system remain unclear. Class II histocompatibility molecules, normally borne only by macrophages and a few other cells, can be expressed on endocrine cells (as manifest by the Ia$^+$ determinant of HLA-DR). This observation has suggested the theory that some environmental event (such as a viral infection) might first cause antigens that are otherwise sequestered to be displayed in conjunction with these essential antigen-presenting molecules. However, Ia antigen expression is also seen in localized areas of lymphocytic reaction in other thyroid diseases such multinodular goiter and thyroid carcinoma. Additional factors must therefore be necessary for progression to established autoimmunity. It remains to be determined for each endocrine cell whether all three factors (display of otherwise sequestered antigens, expression of antigen-presenting molecules, and antigen-specific suppressor cell defect) are necessary and sufficient for the development of autoimmunity.

A number of methods have been used for assessment of tissue-specific immunity in the autoimmune endocrinopathies (Table 24–10). Immunoprecipitation, latex or tanned red cell agglutination, and radioimmunoassay have been used to detect thyroglobulin autoantibodies, the last being the most sensitive method. The indirect immunofluorescence test for autoantibodies to endocrine cells in frozen tissue sections is a versatile technique that has demonstrated autoantibodies to adrenal, thyroid, islet cell, parathyroid, and gonadal "cytoplasmic" antigens. Thyroperoxidase is now recognized as a major component of the thyroid cytoplasmic antigen, which has been localized to microsomal fractions and titered by complement fixation. With the exception of these principal antithyroid antibody tests, the immunofluorescence tests are performed only in specialized laboratories.

Table 24–9. Types of immunologic tissue injury.[1]

IgE-mediated immediate hypersensitivity
Complement-dependent direct humoral cytoxicity
Antigen-antibody complex deposition
T cell-mediated immunity
Receptor autoantibody binding (blocking or stimulating)
Antibody-dependent cell-mediated cytotoxicity

[1]Modified and reproduced, with permission, from Deftos LJ, Catherwood BD, Bone HG: Multiglandular endocrine disorders. In: *Endocrinology and Metabolism,* 3rd ed. Felig P Baxter JD, Frohman LA (editors). McGraw-Hill, 1995.

Table 24–10. Methods for assessment of tissue-specific immunity.

Methods refecting T lymphocyte function
T cell help (for B cell differentiation)
Direct lymphocytotoxicity
Induced lymphocyte proliferation
Induced lymphokine production
Lymphocyte activation (Ia$^+$)

Methods reflecting B lymphocyte function
Precipitin reaction
Complement fixation
Indirect immunofluorescence
Direct serum cytotoxicity
Enablement of cell-mediated cytotoxicity

PROTOTYPICAL AUTOIMMUNE ENDOCRINOPATHY: ADDISON'S DISEASE

Addison's disease plays a central role in several groups of patients with failure of multiple endocrine glands, and there is strong evidence that idiopathic Addison's disease is the end result of autoimmune adrenalitis in most cases. Addison's disease has also provided a good focus for investigation of endocrine autoimmunity (1) because few of these patients should escape medical attention and (2) because tuberculous Addison's disease has provided a natural control group for clinical and immunologic comparison.

Autoimmune Addison's disease is diagnosed when there is no evidence of tuberculosis or any other reasonable explanation for adrenal failure. Pulmonary tuberculosis and adrenal calcification justify a presumptive diagnosis of tuberculous Addison's disease; however, in patients with granulomatous disease on chest film but without adrenal calcification, the cause of adrenal failure is indeterminate. Autoantibodies to adrenal tissue can be detected by indirect immunofluorescence in a high percentage (48–74%) of patients with presumed autoimmune Addison's disease, while the incidence of adrenal autoantibodies is essentially zero in patients with unequivocal tuberculous Addison's disease. Antibodies have been demonstrated against several enzymes of the cytochrome P450 family, including 21-hydroxylase, 17-hydroxylase and side-chain cleavage enzyme. Although comparable data are not available for patients with Addison's disease due to other causes such as histoplasmosis, this information suggests that adrenal autoantibodies are not an epiphenomenon due to tissue destruction. In vitro evidence of T cell activation (increased Ia+ number) and of cell-mediated immunity to adrenal antigen is also present in many patients with autoimmune Addison's disease but not in patients with tuberculous Addison's disease. The autoimmune nature of idiopathic Addison's disease is further substantiated by its specific association with a wide variety of second endocrinopathies with in vitro evidence for tissue-specific autoimmunity. Table 24–11 shows the strikingly higher frequency of second diseases in autoimmune compared with tuberculous Addison's disease. The diseases found with nontuberculous Addison's disease have generally been diabetes mellitus and thyroid disease. These results support the conclusion that idiopathic Addison's disease is part of a larger autoimmune endocrine syndrome.

The presence of adrenal autoantibodies in the blood may be a marker for activity of the autoimmune diathesis. Adrenal autoantibodies tend to have disappeared in patients studied later than 1–5 years after the onset of Addison's disease. Table 24–12 shows the relationship of adrenal autoantibody to the sex of the patient, the age at onset of adrenal insufficiency, and the presence of a second autoimmune disorder. The higher prevalence of autoantibodies in Addison's disease associated with other disorders is particularly striking. Patients with autoimmune Addison's disease with adrenal autoantibodies have a two- to threefold greater incidence of other clinically

Table 24–11. Incidence of other autoimmune disorders in patients with Addison's disease.

	Autoimmune Addison's Disease (n = 419)	Tuberculous Addison's Disease (n = 114)
Diabetes mellitus	10%	. . .
Hyperthyroidism	8%	. . .
Thyroiditis and primary myx-edema	9%	. . .
Pernicious anemia	4%	. . .
Hypogonadism	16%	. . .
Hypoparathy-roidism	5%	. . .
One or more disorders	39%	8%

Table 24–12. Incidence of adrenal autoantibodies in patients with autoimmune Addison's disease accroding to sex, age at onset of adrenal insufficiency, and presence of other disease.[1]

	Sex		Age at Onset		
	Female	Male	< 20	> 20	Total
Addison's disease alone	14/27 (52%)	7/40 (18%)	4/26 (15%)	16/36 (44%)	21/67 (31%)
Addison's disease plus other disease	23/30 (77%)	13/21 (62%)	15/21 (71%)	20/28 (71%)	36/51 (71%)
					57/118 (48%)

[1]Source of data: Blizzard RM, Chee D, Davis W: Clin Exp Immunol 1967;2:19. Modified and reproduced, with permission, from Deftos LJ, Catherwood BD, Bone HG: Multiglandular endocrine disorders. Chapter 28 in: *Endocrinology and Metabolism,* 3rd ed Felig P, Baxter JD, Frohman LA (editors). McGraw-Hill, 1995.

manifest endocrinopathies compared with patients without adrenal autoantibodies. Several investigators have found a higher prevalence of adrenal autoantibodies in women, although this has not been uniformly reported. The frequency of autoantibodies is much less in patients with Addison's disease alone who are male or whose onset of adrenal insufficiency was before age 20 years, which may help in distinguishing between a uniglandular and a polyglandular autoimmune syndrome. Adrenal autoantibodies have been found in 13% of patients with idiopathic hypoparathyroidism alone. They are found rarely in first-degree relatives of patients with autoimmune Addison's disease, in patients with Cushing's disease, and in patients with Hashimoto's thyroiditis or diabetes mellitus alone. The prevalence of adrenal autoantibodies in apparently normal individuals is less than one per 1000 population.

Many investigators have found an increased prevalence of subclinical autoimmunity to other tissues in patients with autoantibody-positive Addison's disease, as evidenced by autoantibodies to parathyroid, islet cell, thyroid, and gastric mucosa. Nerup found a sixfold higher frequency of thyroid autoantibodies and a tenfold increase in parietal cell autoantibodies in patients with adrenal autoantibody-positive Addison's disease, but patients with Addison's disease without adrenal autoantibodies showed no difference from age- and sex-matched controls. When a panel of in vitro immunologic tests was used along with clinical data, 84% of patients with Addison's disease and adrenal autoantibodies were found to have evidence of extra-adrenal autoimmune involvement.

CLINICAL & IMMUNOLOGIC HETEROGENEITY

From what has been said, it can be inferred that autoimmune Addison's disease is not a homogeneous disorder with a random coincidence of other autoimmune endocrine disease and that patients with failure of additional glands might also be heterogeneous. Figure 24–2 supports this thesis, showing the distribution of the age at onset in three clinical subsets of

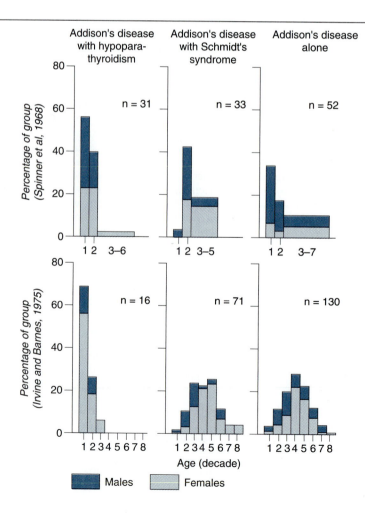

Figure 24–2. Clinical heterogeneity of Addison's disease. Distribution of age at onset *(upper)* or of diagnosis *(lower)* of Addison's disease with hypoparathyroidism, Addison's disease with Schmidt's syndrome, and Addison's disease alone. The lighter color represents females and the darker color represents males. Note that age is measured in decades. (Reproduced, with permission, from Deftos LJ, Catherwood BD, Bone HG: Multiple endocrine disorders. In: *Endocrinology and Metabolism,* 2nd ed. Felig P et al [editors]. McGraw-Hill, 1987.)

patients with Addison's disease studied in the USA and the UK. It is clear that Addison's disease associated with hypoparathyroidism (autoimmune polyglandular syndrome type I) has a much earlier age at onset than Addison's disease associated with Schmidt's syndrome (autoimmune polyglandular syndrome type II) or Addison's disease alone, and the syndromes are readily identified clinically. The former is a rare syndrome, about equally common in males and females, and appears to have an autosomal recessive pattern of inheritance. The latter form of Addison's disease occurring in Schmidt's syndrome is two to three times more common in women and presents later, with age at onset and clinical pattern similar to those of sporadic Addison's disease. The inheritance pattern is autosomal dominant, with incomplete penetrance. Several types of studies have thus led to the concept that polyglandular autoimmune endocrinopathy is not a uniform syndrome nor the random coincidence of a number of individual diseases but that there are at least two distinct patterns of glandular involvement. These ideas are summarized as major types and variations in Figure 24–3. Besides the groups of patients with Addison's disease outlined above, there are groups—sometimes referred to as autoimmune polyglandular syndrome type III—in which a direct association of thyroiditis and diabetes mellitus is found in the absence of Addison's disease. In addition, other endocrine and some nonendocrine disorders occur with increased frequency in these patients.

Addison's Disease With Hypoparathyroidism

In the set of patients with Addison's disease and hypoparathyroidism, male and female patients are usually affected in childhood (Figure 24–2). Chronic mucocutaneous candidiasis frequently precedes both endocrinopathies; conversely, 84% of patients with this infection and an associated endocrinopathy have hypoparathyroidism. The typical sequence of events is shown in Figure 24–4: Hypoparathyroidism develops in the first decade in 88% of patients. Addison's disease follows in about 2 years, and in 75% of patients it occurs within 9 years of the onset of the syndrome. These patients may be affected by a third endocrinopathy, including thyroid disease, diabetes mellitus, pernicious anemia, and ovarian failure in 50% of females. The probability that the sibling of an affected person will have Addison's disease or hypoparathyroidism or any one of the above-mentioned secondary disorders has been estimated to be 0.35. Inheritance follows an autosomal recessive pattern, with no known HLA association.

Patients with idiopathic hypoparathyroidism frequently have circulating autoantibodies to parathyroid tissue; patients with Addison's disease and hypoparathyroidism also have an increased frequency of thyroid and parietal cell autoantibodies. A number

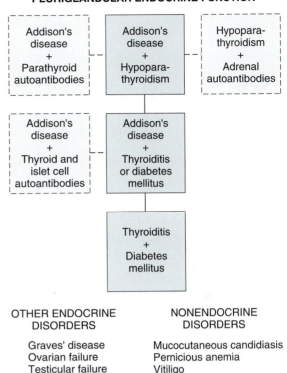

PLURIGLANDULAR ENDOCRINE FUNCTION

Figure 24–3. The three major clinical categories of pluriglandular autoimmune endocrinopathy (center column), with forme fruste variants (dashed boxes) and less frequently associated endocrine disorders and nonendocrine disorders. Graves' disease may substitute for thyroiditis. Gonadal failure is associated with a pan-steroid cell autoantibody in Addison's disease, and candidiasis is strongly associated with hypoparathyroidism. (Modified and reproduced, with permission, from Deftos LJ, Catherwood BD, Bone HG: Multiple endocrine disorders. In: *Endocrinology and Metabolism,* 2nd ed. Felig P et al [editors]. McGraw-Hill, 1987.)

of defective immune responses have been reported in patients with chronic mucocutaneous candidiasis with or without endocrinopathies. These include defective blast transformation, macrophage migration inhibition, and lymphocytotoxicity. The role of these abnormalities in the pathogenesis of immune sensitization to endocrine tissue is unclear.

Isolated Hypoparathyroidism

Patients with isolated hypoparathyroidism are similar to those with Addison's disease plus hypoparathyroidism in having an early onset of disease (73% in the first decade) and associated candidiasis. The frequency of parathyroid autoantibodies in this

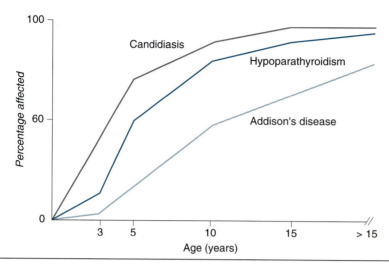

Figure 24–4. Typical sequence for childhood onset of chronic mucocutaneous candidiasis, autoimmune hypoparathyroidism, and Addison's disease. Patients with hypoparathyroidism may not develop Addison's disease, but frequent adrenal autoantibodies suggest that the polyendocrine diathesis is still present. (Source of data: Neufeld et al: Medicine 1981;60:355. Reproduced, with permission, from Deftos LJ, Catherwood BD, Bone HG: Multiple endocrine disorders. In: *Endocrinology and Metabolism*, 2nd ed. Felig P et al [editors]. McGraw-Hill, 1987.)

group is similar to that in the group with Addison's disease. Immunofluorescent adrenal autoantibodies are detected in 7% of patients with hypoparathyroidism, whereas in hypoparathyroidism with candidiasis, most patients have subclinical adrenal autoimmunity. The occurrence of adrenal autoantibodies and candidiasis thus indicates that this subset may represent a forme fruste of pluriglandular endocrine insufficiency.

Isolated Addison's Disease

As noted above, patients with isolated autoimmune Addison's disease still have an increased prevalence of thyroid, parathyroid, and islet cell autoantibodies when compared with control populations. These immunologic findings suggest that despite the absence of clinically evident involvement of other glands, isolated Addison's disease should be considered part of the spectrum of multiple endocrine autoimmunity, since some patients with this disorder may ultimately develop an associated endocrinopathy.

Schmidt's Syndrome

As shown in Figure 24–2, Schmidt's syndrome—or autoimmune polyglandular syndrome type II (defined above)—is more frequent in females, and all of the components including the Addison's disease commonly have their onset in the age range from 20 to 50 years. Table 24–11 shows that the occurrence of diabetes mellitus in autoimmune Addison's disease is 10% and that of Hashimoto's thyroiditis and primary myxedema 9% overall. Although many of these patients may have onset of diabetes in young adulthood, most of them have been treated with insulin. Hashimoto's thyroiditis or diabetes develops an average of 7 years after adrenal insufficiency. Schmidt's syndrome is frequently accompanied by

additional autoimmune diseases, including ovarian failure and pernicious anemia (see below).

Patients with Schmidt's syndrome have the highest rate of thyroid autoantibodies of any group with Addison's disease, which suggests that thyroid autoantibodies in Addison's disease may be predictive of thyroid failure. Activation of cell-mediated immunity is evidenced in Hashimoto's thyroiditis by an increased circulating number of Ia^+ T cells.

Islet cell autoantibodies may also be important in Schmidt's syndrome. These autoantibodies circulate in the majority of patients at the time of diagnosis of type I diabetes mellitus, even in the absence of any other tissue-specific autoimmune disease. The incidence is substantially lower in patients not requiring insulin therapy at the time of diagnosis. In most patients, islet cell autoantibodies disappear with time; their persistence in the blood is associated with the presence of other autoimmune disorders (19%) or autoantibodies to thyroid or gastric tissue (65%). In patients without insulin dependence at the time of diagnosis of their diabetes, the presence of islet cell autoantibodies appears to predict future insulin requirement and failure of oral hypoglycemic agent therapy. (See Chapter 18.)

For about half of index individuals, one or more other family members can be found with autoimmune endocrinopathies. These relatives frequently have only thyroiditis and diabetes without adrenal disease. Such family members may be assigned to this syndrome on the basis of their relative with Addison's disease. Many more family members have been found to have thyroid autoantibodies in the blood. The inheritance of autoimmune polyglandular syndrome type II follows an autosomal dominant pattern with incomplete penetrance. There is a strong HLA association, particularly with HLA types DR3 and DR4.

Other Endocrinopathies Associated With Addison's Disease

Ovarian failure is common in women with autoimmune Addison's disease. In one large series, the prevalence of amenorrhea was 24%, and another 6% had oligomenorrhea. Abnormal reproductive function persists after adrenal replacement therapy and is uncommon in tuberculous Addison's disease, which leads to the conclusion that it is not related to deficiency of adrenal corticosteroids. The presumed autoimmune oophoritis is closely correlated with the onset of the patient's adrenal failure. In girls with Addison's disease and hypoparathyroidism occurring before the age of menarche, the presentation of oophoritis is that of primary amenorrhea, and in some cases streak gonads have been found at laparoscopy.

Ovarian failure in Addison's disease is closely related to a distinctive type of autoantibody against common antigens present in multiple steroid-producing cells, including theca interna, corpus luteum, Leydig cells, placenta, and adrenal cortex. These autoantibodies are cytotoxic for granulosa cells in monolayer cell culture. The presence of such autoantibodies is not only a risk factor for ovarian failure but may also be an independent risk factor for other extra-adrenal endocrinopathies. Steroid cell autoantibodies are uncommon in men with Addison's disease, but several instances of testicular failure associated with Addison's disease have been reported, as has infertility associated with antisperm antibodies.

Although decreased function or failure is the most common consequence of attack on the endocrine glands, Graves' disease is also associated with these disorders; thyrotoxicosis occurs in about 8% of patients with Addison's disease. In patients with autoimmune Addison's disease, clinical atrophic gastritis may occur with or without diabetes, thyroid disease, hypoparathyroidism, or ovarian failure. Pernicious anemia is found in approximately 4% of patients with Addison's disease (Table 24–11).

Direct Association of Thyroid Disease & Diabetes Mellitus

The general frequency of diabetes mellitus and thyroid disease makes the study of a link between these disorders difficult. Nevertheless, an increased frequency of autoimmune thyroid disease in diabetics has been reported by many authors; pernicious anemia is also associated. Comparison of the frequency of tissue-specific autoantibodies in unselected diabetics versus age- and sex-matched controls provides additional support for this association. Table 24–13 provides a representative summary of the interrelationships of autoimmunity against islet, parietal, and thyroid cells.

Table 24–13. Interrelationships of autoimmunity against islet, parietal, and thyroid cells: Representative frequencies of occurrence.[1]

Index Disease	Associated Finding	Frequency
Diabetes mellitus	Thyroid autoantibodies ↑ TSH (males) ↑ TSH (females) Parietal cell autoantibodies	16% 6% 17% 17%
Thyroiditis	Islet cell autoantibodies Intrinsic factor autoantibodies Pernicious anemia	9% 2% 9%
Hyperthyroidism	Islet cell autoantibodies Intrinsic factor autoantibodies Pernicious anemia	3% 3% 3%
Pernicious anemia	Islet cell autoantibodies Thyroid autoantibodies Hypothyroidism Hyperthyroidism	11% 38% 12% 9%

[1]Modified and reproduced, with permission, from Deftos LJ, Catherwood BD, Bone HG: Multiglandular endocrine disorders. Chapter 28 in: *Endocrinology and Metabolism,* 3rd ed. Felig P Baxter JD, Frohman LA (editors). McGraw-Hill, 1995.

Other Disorders

Thirty cases of presumed "autoimmune hypophysitis" have been reported, and several were associated with autoimmune diseases, especially lymphocytic thyroiditis and atrophic gastritis. Twenty-nine of the 30 cases were in women, and all except five cases were diagnosed during or shortly after pregnancy and presented as sellar masses, hypopituitarism, or hypotensive crisis. Panhypopituitarism occurs in up to 50% of these patients. Diabetes insipidus has been associated with a variety of organ-specific autoimmune endocrine diseases, but the pathogenesis of this defect is unclear. (See Chapter 5.)

Vitiligo may occur with any autoimmune endocrinopathy. This disorder probably represents tissue-specific autoimmunity to melanin-producing cells.

MANAGEMENT OF PATIENTS WITH FAILURE OF MULTIPLE ENDOCRINE GLANDS

The history, physical examination, laboratory findings, and treatment of the hormonal disorders discussed in this section are similar to those of the disorders as they occur individually and are discussed in other chapters in this book.

The most serious pitfall in diagnosis of multiple autoimmune endocrinopathy would be to confuse adrenal, thyroid, and ovarian failure with hypopituitarism. In every such case, the integrity of pituitary function should be proved by showing elevated blood levels of TSH, LH, or ACTH. Failure of other glands not dependent on pituitary function (hypoparathyroidism or diabetes mellitus) should be an indicator of autoimmune endocrinopathy.

Patients with Addison's disease should receive particular attention in surveillance for failure of previously uninvolved glands, as these individuals are at greater risk. The physician should be alert for signs of the insidious onset of hypothyroidism and pernicious anemia. Slight elevations of serum TSH may be seen in untreated Addison's disease because of a lack of the normal regulatory effects of the steroid hormone on thyrotroph function and does not necessarily indicate thyroid disease unless it persists on glucocorticoid replacement. In a random population, slight elevation of serum TSH does not necessarily indicate future clinical hypothyroidism, but simultaneous observation of thyroid autoantibodies predicts an incidence of clinical hypothyroidism estimated to be 4% per year, and when autoantibody titers are markedly elevated, the incidence may be as high as 26% per year. These rates may be higher in patients with Addison's disease. First-degree relatives of patients with Addison's disease should also be observed carefully and evaluated with an ACTH stimulation test if they develop any autoimmune disorder. Cases have been reported in which secondary amenorrhea remitted following glucocorticoid replacement therapy of associated Addison's disease. It may thus be important to consider this association in any case of unexplained premature ovarian failure.

The treatment implications of multiglandular endocrine failure are not well characterized. Since cortisol antagonizes the intestinal calcium transport effects of vitamin D, including the vitamin D metabolites used to treat hypoparathyroidism, the development of adrenal failure can result in sudden vitamin D intoxication in hypoparathyroid patients taking vitamin D. Secondary amenorrhea has remitted following treatment of associated Addison's disease. On the other hand, the combination of Addison's disease and loss of ovarian function—even physiologic menopause—may result in more severe postmenopausal osteoporosis if sex steroid replacement therapy is not provided.

GENETIC ASPECTS OF AUTOIMMUNE DISORDERS

Early genetic studies of autoimmune disorders have estimated probabilities of clinical involvement of 0.25–0.35 for siblings of probands with Schmidt's syndrome and Addison's disease with hypoparathyroidism.

Typing of antigens coded by the major histocompatibility (HLA) complex on chromosome 6 has pro-

vided genetic correlations with the clinical and immunopathologic findings in the individual autoimmune endocrinopathies. At least three classes of HLA glycoproteins are displayed by human cells. Class I molecules (antigens of the A and B loci) are expressed on all nucleated cells. They are quantitatively regulated by lymphokines and may play a secondary role in autoimmune disorders. HLA-A and -B typing is useful, primarily because these molecules serve as markers closely linked to the HLA-D locus. Class II HLA molecules (HLA-DR, -DQ, and -DP) are normally displayed only on a few antigen-presenting cells, such as the macrophage, but can be induced on many other cell types. The presence of HLA-DR on cell surfaces can be detected by the reaction of antibodies to common determinants such as Ia. Individuals can be classified into phenotypic groups using panels of antisera to class II antigens. Further polymorphism can be detected functionally by the presence or absence of the mixed lymphocyte culture reaction against homozygous allogeneic lymphocytes, by analysis of restriction endonuclease-digested genomic DNA, and by probing for specific DNA sequences within the HLA-DR and DQ genes. The immunologic defect in immune regulation resulting in autosensitization to endocrine tissue may be a gene in the HLA region genetically linked to certain HLA antigens. The HLA-D antigens are most closely associated with the endocrine disorders (Table 24–14). Common haplotypes such as HLA-A1, -B8, -D3 and HLA-A2, -B15, -D4 occur because of linkage disequilibrium. The presence or absence of specific amino acid residues at positions within the antigen-binding domains of the class II molecule subunits may convey a substantial portion of the genetic risk for autoimmune disease.

Addison's disease occurs three to six times more frequently in individuals who express the HLA-DR3 or HLA-DR4 class II MHC alleles. Subjects who are heterozygous for both HLA-DR3 and HLA-DR4 have a greater than 25-fold increased risk of Addison's disease. However, these HLA associations are not observed if Addison's disease is a feature of type I autoimmune polyglandular syndrome. Thus, there appears to be no significant association between juvenile-onset polyendocrinopathy and the HLA complex. These associations are more common in older patients. (See Figure 24–2 and Chapter 4.)

Table 24–14. HLA antigen association with autoimmune diseases (Caucasians).

Addison's disease	HLA-DR3
Atrophic thyroiditis	HLA-DR3
Graves' disease	HLA-B8 and -DR3
Diabetes mellitus	HL-DR3 and -DR4
Hashimoto's thyroiditis	HLA-DR3 and -DR5
Hypoparathyroidism	?

NONAUTOIMMUNE ENDOCRINE FAILURE

Bardwick et al have reviewed a syndrome, previously reported mostly from Japan, to which they give the acronym POEMS (polyneuropathy, organomegaly, endocrinopathy, M protein, and skin changes) (Table 24–15). Gonadal failure, gynecomastia, and glucose intolerance are frequent endocrine disorders, while adrenal failure is uncommon. Seventy-five percent of affected patients are male, and they have plasma cell dyscrasias with onset in the fourth or fifth decade, usually sclerotic plasmacytomas. In one of the cases reported by Bardwick et al, insulin-dependent diabetes mellitus remitted with irradiation of the patient's plasmacytoma, returned 3 years later with the appearance of a new tumor, and disappeared again with another course of radiation treatment. Neither the polyneuropathy nor the endocrinopathy appears to be due to amyloidosis. In contrast to findings in autoimmune endocrinopathies, Bardwick et al did not find tissue-specific endocrine autoantibodies. The mechanism of this interesting syndrome needs to be elucidated.

Pseudohypoparathyroidism type Ia is due to hereditary deficiency of the guanine nucleotide-binding regulatory protein of the cell membrane-adenylyl cyclase complex and is characterized by resistance to multiple hormones besides parathyroid hormone. This disorder is discussed in Chapter 5. Nonimmunologic forms of familial isolated hypoparathyroidism also exist.

Table 24–15. Incidence of abnormalities in patients with "POEMS" syndrome.[1]

Polyneuropathy	
Peripheral neuropathy	100%
Papilledema	68%
Increased cerebrospinal fluid	94%
Organomegaly	
Hepatomegaly	67%
Splenomegaly	37%
Lymphadenopathy	64%
Endocrinopathy	
Gynecomastia	70%
Impotence	67%
Amenorrhea	100%
Glucose intolerance	48%
Hypothyroidism	10%
M protein	61%
IgG	41%
IgA	20%
Marrow plasma cells	48%
Sclerotic bone lesions	71%
Skin changes	
Hyperpigmentation	98%
Thickening	85%
Hirsutism	78%
Hyperhidrosis	66%
Other	
Peripheral edema	92%
Ascites	68%
Pleural effusions	24%
Fever	48%

[1]Reproduced, with permission, from Bardwick PA et al: Plasma cell dyscrasia with polyneuropathy, organomegaly, endocrinopathy. M protein, and skin changes. Medicine 1980;59:311.

REFERENCES

Multiple Endocrine Neoplasia

Austin LA, Heath H III: Calcitonin: Physiology and pathophysiology. N Engl J Med 1981;304:269.

Carney JA, Sizemore GW, Tyce GM: Bilateral adrenal medullary hyperplasia in MEN, type 2. Mayo Clin Proc 1975;50:3.

Chi DD et al: Predictive testing for multiple endocrine neoplasia type 2A (MEN 2A) based on the detection of mutations in the RET protooncogene. Surgery 1994;116:124.

Chong GC et: Medullary carcinoma of the thyroid gland. Cancer 1975;35:695.

Cole GJ et al: RET protooncogene mutation in MEN type II and MTC. Baillieres Clin Endocrinol Metab 1995;9:609.

Copp DH, Crockroft DW, Kueh Y: Calcitonin from ultimobranchial glands of dogfish and chickens. Science 1967;158:924.

Cushman P Jr: Familial endocrine tumors: Report of two unrelated kindred affected with pheochromocytomas, one also with multiple thyroid carcinomas. Am J Med 1962;32:352.

Deftos LJ, Bone HG, Parthemore JG: Immunohistological studies of medullary thyroid carcinoma and C-cell hyperplasia. J Clin Endocrinol Metab 1980;51:857.

Deftos LJ: *Medullary Thyroid Carcinoma.* Karger, 1983.

Deftos LJ: Radioimmunoassay for calcitonin in medullary thyroid carcinoma. JAMA 1974;227:403.

Fung Y-K T et al: Structural evidence for the authenticity of the human retinoblastoma gene. Science 1987; 236:1657.

Gagel FR et al: Natural history of the familial medullary thyroid carcinoma-pheochromocytoma syndrome and the identification of preneoplastic stages by screening studies: A five-year report. Trans Assoc Am Physicians 1975;88:177.

Gagel RF et al: The clinical outcome of prospective screening for multiple endocrine neoplasia type 2a. N Engl J Med 1988;318:478.

Griffiths DFR, Williams GT, Williams ED: Duodenal carcinoid tumors, phaeochromocytoma and neurofibromatosis: Islet cell tumor, phaeochromocytoma and the Von Hippel-Lindau complex: Two distinctive neuroendocrine syndromes. Q J Med 1987;245:769.

Hazard JB: The C cells (parafollicular cells) of the thyroid gland and medullary thyroid carcinoma: A review. Am J Pathol 1977;88:213.

Hennessey JF et al: A comparison of pentagastrin injection and calcium infusion as provocative agents for the detection of medullary thyroid carcinoma. J Clin Endocrinol Metab 1974;39:487.

Heyningen V: One gene—four syndromes. Nature 1994; 367:319.

Jackson CE et al: The two-mutational-event theory in medullary thyroid carcinoma. Am J Hum Genet 1979;31:704.

Khairi MRA et al: Mucosal neuroma, pheochromocytoma and medullary thyroid carcinoma: MEN, type III. Medicine 1975;54:89.

Ledger GA et al: Genetic testing in the diagnosis and management of multiple endocrine neoplasia type II. Ann Intern Med 1995;122:118.

Melvin KE, Tashjian AH Jr, Miller HH: Studies in familial (medullary) thyroid carcinoma. Recent Prog Horm Res 1972;28:399.

O'Connor DT, Burton D, Deftos LJ: Immunoreactive human chromogranin A in diverse polypeptide hormone-producing human tumors and normal endocrine tissues. Clin Endocrinol Metab 1983;57:1084.

Pacini F et al: Routine measurement of serum calcitonin in nodular thyroid diseases allows the preoperative diagnosis of unsuspected sporadic medullary thyroid carcinoma. J Clin Endocrinol Metab 1994;78: 826.

Parthemore JG et al: A short calcium infusion in the diagnosis of medullary thyroid carcinoma. J Clin Endocrinol Metab 1974;39:108.

Pearse AGE, Ewen SEB, Polak JM: The genesis of APUD amyloid in endocrine polypeptide tumors: Histochemical distinction from immunamyloid. Virchows Arch [Cell Pathol] 1972;10:93.

Ponder BAJ et al: Risk estimation and screening in families of patients with medullary thyroid carcinoma. Lancet 1988;1:397.

Schimke RN, Hartman WH: Familial amyloid-producing medullary thyroid carcinoma and pheochromocytoma: A distinct genetic entity. Ann Intern Med 1965; 63: 1027.

Seizinger BR et al: Genetic linkage of von Recklinghausen neurofibromatosis to nerve growth factor receptor gene. Cell 1987;49:589.

Seizinger BR et al: Von Hippel-Lindau disease maps to the region of chromosome 3 associated with renal cell carcinoma. Nature 1988;332:268.

Sipple JH: The association of pheochromocytoma with carcinoma of the thyroid gland. Am J Med 1961;31: 163.

Steiner AL, Goodman AD, Powers SR: Study of a kindred with pheochromocytoma, medullary thyroid carcinoma, hyperparathyroidism, and Cushing's disease: MEN, type II. Medicine 1968;47:371.

Takai S et al: Loss of genes on chromosomes 22 in medullary thyroid carcinoma and pheochromocytoma. Jpn J Cancer Res 1987;78:894.

Wermer P: Genetic aspects of adenomatosis of endocrine glands. Am J Med 1954;16:363.

Williams ED: A review of 17 cases of carcinoma of the thyroid and phaeochromocytoma. J Clin Pathol 1965; 18:288.

Wolfe HJ et al: C-cell hyperplasia preceding medullary thyroid carcinoma. N Engl J Med 1973;289:437.

Zollinger RM, Ellison EH: Primary peptic ulceration of the jejunum associated with the islet cell tumors of the pancreas. Ann Surg 1955;142:709.

Failure of Multiple Endocrine Glands

Ahmann AJ, Burman KD: The role of T lymphocytes in autoimmune thyroid disease. Endocrinol Metab Clin North Am 1987;16:287.

Ahonen P, Meittinen A, Perheentupa J: Adrenal and steroidal cell antibodies in patients with autoimmune polyglandular disease type I and risk of adrenocortical and ovarian failure. J Clin Endocrinol Metab 1987;64:494.

Bardwick PA et al: Plasma cell dyscrasia with polyneuropathy, organomegaly, endocrinopathy, M protein, and skin changes: The POEMS syndrome. Medicine 1980;59:311.

Betterle C et al: Complement-fixing adrenal autoantibodies as a marker for predicting onset of idiopathic Addison's disease. Lancet 1983;1:1238.

Bottazzo GF et al: Autoimmunity in juvenile diabetics and their families. Br Med J 1978;2:165.

Carpenter CCJ et al: Schmidt's syndrome (thyroid and adrenal insufficiency): A review of the literature and a report of fifteen new cases including ten instances of coexistent diabetes mellitus. Medicine 1964;43: 153.

Chan JY, Walfish PG: Activated (Ia$^+$) T-lymphocytes and their subsets in autoimmune thyroid diseases: Analysis by microfluorocytometry. J Clin Endocrinol Metab 1986;62:403.

Cosman F et al: Lymphocytic hypophysitis: Report of 3 new cases and review of the literature. Medicine 1989;68:240.

Deftos LJ, Catherwood BD, Bone HG: Multiple endocrine disorders. In: *Endocrinology and Metabolism,* 2nd ed. Felig P et al (editors). McGraw-Hill, 1985.

Devogelaer JP, Crabbe J, Nagant de Deuxchaisnes C: Bone mineral density in Addison's disease: Evidence for an effect of adrenal androgens on bone mass. Br Med J 1987 [Clin Res] 294:798.

Dwyer JM: Chronic mucocutaneous candidiasis. Annu Rev Med 1981;32:491.

Eisenbarth GS et al: The polyglandular failure syndrome: Disease inheritance, HLA type, and immune function. Ann Intern Med 1979;91:528.

Foulis AK: Class II major histocompatibility complex and organ specific autoimmunity in man. J Pathol 1986;150:5.

Gordin A, Lamberg BA: Spontaneous hypothyroidism in symptomless autoimmune thyroiditis: A long-term follow-up study. Clin Endocrinol 1981;15:537.

Iitaka M et al: Studies of the effect of suppressor T lymphocytes on the induction of antithyroid microsomal antibody-secreting cells in autoimmune thyroid disease. J Clin Endocrinol Metab 1988;66:708.

Khalil I et al: A combination of HLA-DQ beta Asp57-negative and HLA DQ alpha Arg52 confers susceptibility to insulin-dependent diabetes mellitus. J Clin Invest 1990;85:1315.

Maclaren NK, Riley WJ: Inherited susceptibility to autoimmune Addison's disease is linked to human leukocyte antigens -DR3 and/or -DR4, except when associated with type I autoimmune polyglandular syndrome. J Clin Endocrinol Metab 1986;62:455.

McCarthy-Young S, Lessof MH, Maisey MN: Serum TSH and thyroid antibody studies in Addison's disease. Clin Endocrinol 1972;1:45.

Muir A, McLaren NK: Autoimmune diseases of the adrenal glands, parathyroid glands, gonads and hypothalamic-pituitary axis. Endocrinol Metab Clin North Am 1991;20:619.

Nerup J: Addison's disease. Acta Endocrinol 1974;76:127.

Neufeld M, McLaren N, Blizzard R: Autoimmune polyglandular syndromes. Pediatr Ann 1980;9:154.

Peterson P, Krohn KJE: Mapping of B-cell epitopes on steroid 17-alpha-hydroxylase, an autoantigen in polyglandular syndrome type I. Clin Exp Immunol 1994;98:104.

Pujol-Borrell R et al: Inappropriate major histocompatibility complex class II expression by thyroid follicular cells in thyroid autoimmune disease and by pancreatic beta cells in type I diabetes. Mol Biol Med 1986;3:159.

Rabinowe SL et al: Ia-positive T lymphocytes in recently diagnosed idiopathic Addison's disease. Am J Med 1984;77:597.

Rabinowe SL et al: Lymphocyte dysfunction in autoimmune oophoritis: Resumption of menses with corticosteroids. Am J Med 1986;81:347.

Rapoport B: Recombinant DNA technology in the study of autoimmune thyroid disease. Endocrinol Metab Clin North Am 1987;16:445.

Scherbaum WA, Bottazzo GF: Autoantibodies to vasopressin cells in idiopathic diabetes insipidus: Evidence for an autoimmune variant. Lancet 1983;1:897.

Sridama V, Pacini F, Degroot L: Decreased suppressor T-lymphocytes in autoimmune thyroid diseases detected by monoclonal antibodies. J Clin Endocrinol Metab 1982;54:316.

Todd JA, Bell JI, McDevitt HO: A molecular basis for genetic susceptibility to insulin-dependent diabetes mellitus. Trends Genet 1988;4:129.

Tsatsoulis A, Shalet M: Antisperm antibodies in the polyglandular autoimmune syndrome type I: Response to cyclical steroid therapy. Clin Endocrinol 1991;35:299.

Volpe R: Autoimmune thyroid disease: A perspective. Mol Biol Med 1986;3:25.

Weetman AP: Autoimmunity to steroid producing cells and familial polyendocrine autoimmunity. Baillieres Clin Endocrinol Metab 1995;9:157.

Weetman AP: Regulation and role of thyroid cell class II antigen expression. Immunol Res 1986;5:81.

Winqvist O et al: Identification of the main gonadal autoantigens in patients with adrenal insufficiency and associated ovarian failure. J Clin Endocrinol Metab 1995;80:1717.

Wuepper KD, Wegienka LC, Fudenberg HH: Immunologic aspects of adrenocortical insufficiency. Am J Med 1969;45:206.

25

Geriatric Endocrinology

Susan L. Greenspan, MD, & Neil M. Resnick, MD

Individuals over age 65 comprise the fastest-growing segment of the United States population; each day this group increases by over 1000 people. This increase has led to a remarkable situation—of all the people who have ever lived to the age of 65, more than two-thirds are still alive. Thus, it is becoming increasingly important for the endocrinologist to understand how endocrine physiology and disease may differ in the elderly.

Before considering specific conditions, however, it is worthwhile to review some general principles that account for many of the age-related changes in disease presentation in the elderly. First, aging itself—in the absence of disease—is associated with only a gradual and linear decline in the physiologic reserve of each organ system (Figure 25–1). Since the reserve capacity of each system is substantial, age-related declines have little effect on baseline function and do not significantly interfere with the individual's response to stress until the eighth or ninth decade. Second, because each organ system's function declines at a different physiologic rate and because 75% of the elderly have at least one disease, endocrine dysfunction in the elderly often presents disparately, with initial symptoms derived from the most compromised organ system. For example, hyperthyroidism in an elderly patient with preexisting coronary and conduction system disease may present with atrial fibrillation and a slow ventricular response, while in another equally hyperthyroid patient with a prior stroke, it may present with confusion or depression; neither patient may tolerate hyperthyroidism long enough for the classic thyroid-related manifestations (eg, goiter) to become apparent. Third, elderly patients often have multiple diseases and take many medications that may mimic or mask the usual presentation of endocrine disease.

ACRONYMS USED IN THIS CHAPTER

ACTH	Adrenocorticotropic hormone
AVP	Arginine vasopressin
BMD	Bone mineral density
cAMP	Cyclic adenosine monophosphate
CRH	Corticotropin-releasing hormone
DHEA	Dehydroepiandrosterone
FSH	Follicle-stimulating hormone
hCG	Human chorionic gonadotropin
HPA	Hypothalamic-pituitary-adrenal
LH	Luteinizing hormone
LHRH	Luteinizing hormone-releasing hormone
NPH	Neutral protamine Hagedorn
PSA	Prostate-specific antigen
PTH	Parathyroid hormone
SIADH	Syndrome of inappropriate secretion of antidiuretic hormone
TRH	Thyrotropin-releasing hormone
TSH	Thyroid-stimulating hormone (thyrotropin)

THYROID FUNCTION & DISEASE

The prevalence of thyroid disease in the elderly is approximately twice that in younger individuals, with hypothyroidism ranging from 2% to 7% and hyperthyroidism affecting up to 2% of older individuals. In addition, some studies suggest that up to 9% of hospitalized elderly patients have overt thyroid disease. Furthermore, "subclinical hypothyroidism"—normal serum levels of thyroid hormones (thyroxine, T_4; tri-

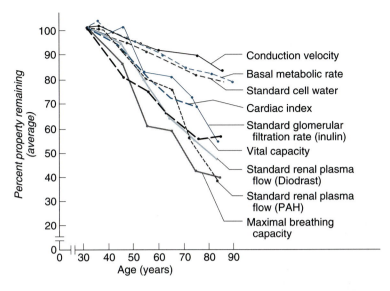

Figure 25–1. Influence of age on physiologic function in humans. (Reproduced, with permission, from Shock NW: Discussion on mortality and measurement. In: *The Biology of Aging: A Symposium.* Strehler BL et al [editors]. American Institute of Biological Sciences, 1960.)

iodothyronine, T_3) but an elevated level of thyrotropin (TSH)—is more prevalent, with estimates of 4–14% in the elderly. "Subclinical hyperthyroidism"—normal serum levels of thyroxine but a suppressed level of serum TSH—may be found in 4% of elderly subjects. Finally, the overall prevalence of thyroid hormone use in older adults is approximately 7% (10% in women and 2% in men).

There are few major age-related changes in the physiology of the hypothalamic-pituitary-thyroid axis (Chapter 7). Serum TSH levels remain constant, and TSH release remains pulsatile (Figure 25–2), though the nocturnal rise in serum TSH appears to be blunted with age. Balanced decreases in T_4 secretion and clearance result in no change in serum T_4; T_3 resin uptake, free T_4, and the free T_4 index are also unchanged. There is a slight age-related decline in serum T_3, but values usually remain within normal limits. The effect of age on the release of TSH by thyrotropin-releasing hormone (TRH) is less clear, but most recent studies show little clinically relevant change in either sex. The 24-hour radioiodine uptake is also not significantly altered with age. Thyroid antibodies are common in older women (prevalence up to 32%), but their presence does not serve as a specific screening test for thyroid disease.

DISORDERS OF THE THYROID GLAND

Although the United States Preventive Services Task Force recommended annual screening thyroid function tests for older women, there is still no consensus among thyroidologists regarding the utility of screening for thyroid dysfunction in the absence of symptoms. However, it is reasonable to measure TSH in older individuals who present with "atypical" symptoms of thyroid disease such as exacerbation of cardiac symptoms, change in mental status, falling, or onset of depression. Despite the sensitivity of the TSH assay, further evaluation with a free T_4 or free T_4 index is often required because up to 98% of elderly subjects with a suppressed TSH levels do not have thyrotoxicosis.

1. HYPERTHYROIDISM

Clinical Features

With age, the prevalence of Graves' disease decreases (though it remains the most common cause of hyperthyroidism), and the prevalence of multinodular goiter and toxic nodules increases. Elderly hyperthyroid patients tend to present with symptoms or complications related to the most vulnerable organ system—usually the cardiovascular system (atrial fibrillation, congestive heart failure, angina, and acute myocardial infarction) or the central nervous system (apathy, depression, confusion, or lassitude). The hypercatabolic state also causes muscle wasting, particularly of the quadriceps, thereby increasing the risk of falls. Occasionally, they present with gastrointestinal symptoms, but these differ from those seen in younger patients because they include constipation, failure to thrive, and anorexia and weight loss. Be-

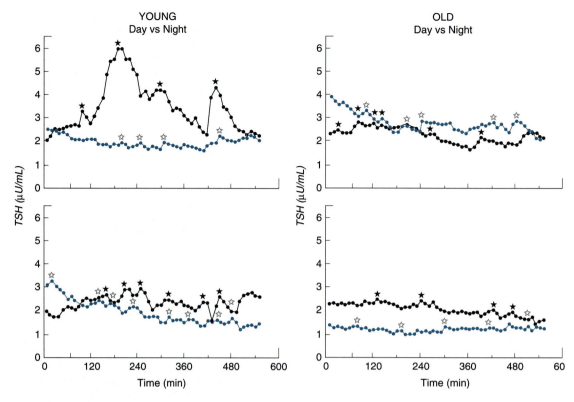

Figure 25–2. Thyrotropin (TSH) pulsation profiles during day and night in two representative young subjects and two representative old subjects. (Open stars, significant daytime pulses; solid stars, significant nighttime pulses as detected by cluster analysis.) (Reproduced, with permission, from Greenspan SL et al: Age-related alterations in pulsatile secretion of TSH: Role of dopaminergic regulation. Am J Physiology 1991;260[3 Part 1]:E486.)

cause of degeneration of the sinus node and fibrotic changes in the cardiac conduction system, older patients are less likely than younger patients to present with palpitations (Table 25–1). However, a low serum TSH concentration is associated with a threefold higher risk of atrial fibrillation in the subsequent decade.

The physical signs of hyperthyroidism also differ in the elderly (Table 25–1). Sinus tachycardia is less frequent; the thyroid feels normal in size or is not palpable in two-thirds of patients; and lid lag is uncommon. Ophthalmopathy is less common, not only because Graves' disease occurs less often, but also because even with Graves' disease ophthalmopathy occurs less frequently in the elderly. However, although they are less common in the elderly, some findings appear to be highly suggestive of hyperthyroidism. These include increased frequency of bowel movements, weight loss despite increased appetite, fine finger tremor, eyelid retraction, and increased perspiration.

Diagnosis

As in younger patients (Chapter 7), the diagnosis is usually confirmed by standard thyroid function tests, beginning with a depressed TSH level as measured by a sensitive immunoradiometric or chemiluminescent assay. A TRH test is rarely required. There are potential pitfalls, however. Hospitalized elderly patients who are acutely ill (but euthyroid) may have a suppressed serum TSH. Further evaluation of other thyroid function tests should help rule out hyperthyroidism. T_3 toxicosis may be more difficult to diagnose because concomitant nonthyroidal illness is common and can depress serum T_3. Euthyroid hyperthyroxinemia (also due to nonthyroidal illness) may also cause confusion. Elderly patients may also be taking medications such as propranolol, which may elevate levels of serum T_4. Furthermore, iodide-induced hyperthyroidism, known also as the jodbasedow effect, is becoming more common in elderly patients with multinodular goiter because of increased exposure to radiocontrast studies; the resultant hyperthyroidism is generally transient. Finally, because of screening tests with sensitive TSH assays, "subclinical hyperthyroidism" (normal T_4, T_3, free T_4 with a suppressed TSH) is being recognized more commonly. This is often found in older subjects with autonomous function of a multinodular goiter or nodule.

Table 25–1. Percentages of patients with symptoms and physical findings attributable to thyrotoxicosis.[1]

	Old[1]	Old[2]	Young
Number	25	85	247
Mean age	81.5	68.6	40[2]
Range	75–95	60–82	5–73
Symptoms (%)			
Weight loss	44	35	85
Palpitations	36	42	89
Weakness	32	28	70
Dizziness, syncope	20	—	—
Nervousness	20	38	99
No symptoms	8	—	—
Memory loss	8	—	—
Tremor	8	—	—
Local symptoms[3]	8	11	—
Pruritus	4	4	—
Heat intolerance	4	63	89
Physical Findings			
Pulse > 100/min	28[4]	58	100
Atrial fibrillation	32	39	10
New-onset atrial fibrillation	20[5]	—	—
Lid lag	12	35	71
Exophthalmos	8	8	—
Fine skin	40	81	97
Tremor	36	89	97
Myopathy	8	39	—
Hyperactive reflexes	24	26	—
Gynecomastia	(1 male)	1	10
None	8	—	—
Thyroid Examination (%)			
Impalpable or normal	68	37	—
Diffusely enlarged	12	22	100
Multinodular goiter	12	20	—
Isolated nodule	8	21	—

[1]Modified and reproduced, with permission, from Tibaldi JM et al: Thyrotoxicosis in the very old. Am J Med 1986;81:619.
[2]Approximated from graph of patients' ages.
[3]Dysphagia, enlarging neck mass, etc.
[4]Includes 5 patients with normal sinus rhythm as well as 2 who had atrial fibrillation.
[5]This was transient in 4 of 5 patients with conversion to normal sinus rhythm.

Old[1] = Tibaldi JM et al: Thyrotoxicosis in the very old. Am J Med 1986;81:619. Old[2] = Davis PJ, Davis FB: Hyperthyroidism in patients over the age of 60 years. Medicine 1974;53:161. Young = Ingbar SH et al: The thyroid gland . In: *Williams' Textbook of Endocrinology.* Williams RH (editor). Saunders, 1981.

Treatment

Beta-blocking agents are useful in alleviating symptoms, but radioactive iodine is the therapy of choice in elderly patients because it is efficient, uncomplicated, and inexpensive. Antithyroid drugs can be used prior to radioactive iodine treatment to render the patient euthyroid and to avoid radiation-induced thyroiditis, but they are not definitive treatment and are more toxic in this age group. Surgery has a more limited role because of its increased morbidity.

Following radioactive iodine treatment, patients become euthyroid over a period of 6–12 weeks. They should receive careful follow-up, because hypothyroidism develops in 80% or more of patients who have been adequately treated. Once hyperthyroidism has abated, the metabolic clearance rate of other medications may decrease, and doses may require readjustment. Older patients with subclinical hyperthyroidism require follow-up, especially if presented with an iodine load.

2. HYPOTHYROIDISM

Hypothyroidism in the elderly is most often due to Hashimoto's thyroiditis or prior radioactive iodine ablative therapy.

Clinical Features

It is easy to overlook hypothyroidism in an older person, because many euthyroid elderly patients have the same symptoms. Moreover, elderly patients with hypothyroidism are more likely than younger patients to present with cardiovascular symptoms (eg, congestive heart failure or angina) or neurologic findings (eg, cognitive impairment, confusion, depression, paresthesias, deafness, psychosis, or coma). Finally, in the older hypothyroid patient, the physical findings are frequently nonspecific, though puffy face, delayed deep tendon reflexes, and myoedema support the diagnosis.

Diagnosis

Serum TSH is the most sensitive indicator of primary hypothyroidism and should be checked first. The diagnosis should then be confirmed with a low serum T_4 or free T_4. Measurement of serum T_3 is unnecessary and potentially misleading, because T_3 is the form of thyroid hormone most likely to decrease in nonthyroidal illness. Serum TSH should not be used alone to diagnose hypothyroidism because it will not always differentiate symptomatic from "subclinical" hypothyroidism. Furthermore, levels of TSH may be higher at night as a result of the nocturnal rise in serum TSH. Moreover, the pulsatile nature of TSH, resulting in serum TSH slightly above the normal ranges, may lead to a diagnosis of subclinical hypothyroidism in a euthyroid subject. Finally, in hypothyroid patients, serum TSH levels can be reduced to within the normal range by treatment with dopaminergic drugs and corticosteroids. In such patients, determination of free T_4 and reverse T_3 may help to differentiate those with true hypothyroidism from those with nonthyroidal illness (Chapter 7).

Treatment

The doses of thyroid hormone required for adequate replacement decrease with age (Tables 25–2 and 7–9). Elderly patients should be started on approximately 25–50 μg of levothyroxine, and the dose should be increased by approximately 25 μg every 3–4 weeks until the serum TSH comes into normal

Table 25–2. Daily doses of thyroxine in hypothyroid patients.[1,2]

	Daily dose of Thyroxine[3] (μg/d)		
	< 40 Years	40–60 Years	>60 Years
All patients	167 ± 62[4] (20)	135 ± 37 (34)	109 ± 42[5] (40)
Men	185 ± 82[6] (5)	149 ± 36 (19)	116 ± 48[4] (16)
Women	148 ± 33[6] (5)	116 ± 15 (15)	105 ± 37[6] (24)

[1]Reproduced, with permission, from Sawin CT et al: Aging and the thyroid. Am J Med 1983;75:206.
[2]Values are mean ± SD; numbers of patients are shown in parentheses.
[3]Current doses of levothyroxine are about 20% lower than the doses reported in this study. [Editor's note.]
[4]$P < .01$ (all P values are compared to ages 40–60).
[5]$P < .05$.
[6]Not significant.

range. In patients with cardiovascular disease, even lower initial doses can be used (12.5 μg) and increased at a slower rate. Desiccated thyroid hormone and preparations containing T_3 should be avoided because T_3 is rapidly absorbed and cleared. The metabolic clearance of other drugs will change as hypothyroidism is corrected, and their dosages may require readjustment. Overtreatment documented by a suppressed serum TSH should be avoided because of the potential adverse effects to the skeleton and cardiovascular system.

It is still not known whether treating "subclinical hypothyroidism" is beneficial in older patients. However, two-thirds of these patients will remain chemically euthyroid for at least 4 years, and low titers of antimicrosomal antibodies may identify patients at lowest risk for progression. Elderly patients previously treated with radioactive iodine are more likely to progress to overt hypothyroidism. At present, careful annual follow-up is recommended.

3. MULTINODULAR GOITER

The prevalence of multinodular goiter increases with age. However, if swallowing and breathing are not compromised and thyroid function tests are normal, the goiter can be observed without treatment. Levothyroxine therapy rarely shrinks the gland, and although it may prevent further enlargement, the risk of inducing hyperthyroidism is significant because multinodular goiters may develop areas of autonomous function.

4. THYROID NODULES & CANCER

Thyroid nodules are more common in the elderly. Ninety percent of these nodules are benign, but the prognosis for elderly patients with malignant nodules

may be worse than that for younger patients with malignant nodules. The approach is similar to the workup in a younger patient. The prognosis correlates with the size of the tumor. The outcome in elderly patients may therefore be substantially improved by early evaluation of nodules in patients who are good surgical candidates.

Papillary carcinoma is more common in young and middle-aged patients. However, it has a poorer prognosis in the elderly, possibly because it is detected at a more advanced stage. Follicular carcinoma accounts for 15% of thyroid cancers and usually occurs in middle-aged and older patients. Anaplastic thyroid carcinoma is found almost exclusively in middle-aged and older patients. It presents as a rapidly growing hard mass which is locally invasive, often associated with metastatic lesions, and has a very poor prognosis (Chapter 7).

CARBOHYDRATE INTOLERANCE & DIABETES MELLITUS

AGING & THE PHYSIOLOGY OF CARBOHYDRATE INTOLERANCE

Even healthy elderly individuals demonstrate an age-related increase in fasting blood glucose (1 mg/dL [0.6 mmol/L] per decade) and a more significant increase in blood glucose (5 mg/dL [0.28 mmol/L] per decade) in response to a standard glucose tolerance test. According to the criteria of the National Diabetes Data Group, nearly 10% of the elderly have some degree of glucose intolerance. The possible causes of this intolerance include changes in body composition, diet, physical activity, insulin secretion, and insulin action.

With aging, lean body mass decreases and body fat increases. The percentage of body fat correlates positively with fasting levels of serum glucose, insulin, and glucagon. When obesity (or the percentage of body fat) is taken into account, the basal levels of glucose, insulin, and glucagon are not influenced by age. However, older individuals have impaired glucose counterregulation to hypoglycemia, associated with higher plasma insulin levels and reduced levels of glucagon.

Decreased physical activity and a low-carbohydrate diet impair glucose tolerance, but the major contribution to glucose intolerance in healthy, active elderly individuals appears to be a decrease in insulin-mediated uptake of glucose in peripheral tissues. This is probably due to a postreceptor defect that has not yet been characterized. Impaired glucose-mediated insulin secretion (decreased B cell sensitivity) and a delayed suppression of hepatic glucose output also contribute to the age-related decline in glucose tolerance. Furthermore, there may be gender-related changes in glucose metabolism with age; healthy older men have an impairment in nonoxidative glucose metabolism but women do not. However, much of the carbohydrate intolerance found in average elderly individuals is caused by diet, drugs, lack of exercise, or environmental factors that may be correctable.

DIABETES MELLITUS

Clinical Features

The prevalence of diabetes mellitus increases with age, affecting 17% of persons over age 65. Most diabetes in the elderly is type II (non-insulin-dependent) diabetes. Diabetes may be difficult to diagnose in the elderly because of its often atypical and asymptomatic presentation. For example, polyuria or polydipsia are not present in many elderly patients, because the glomerular filtration rate and thirst threshold decline with age, while the renal threshold for glycosuria increases. Instead, symptoms in these individuals are usually nonspecific (eg, weakness, fatigue, weight loss, or frequent minor infections). These patients may also present with neurologic findings such as cognitive impairment, acute confusion, or depression.

The diagnosis is established by obtaining a fasting blood glucose above 140 mg/dL (7.8 mmol/L) on two separate occasions (in the absence of acute illness); a 2-hour oral glucose tolerance test is needed rarely, if ever. Because the renal threshold for glycosuria increases in the elderly, the diagnosis should not be based on the presence of glycosuria. Increased blood levels of glycosylated hemoglobin or fructosamine support the diagnosis, but these tests are more useful in monitoring treatment.

Since the complications of diabetes mellitus are related to the duration of disease, elderly patients who live long enough will suffer the same complications of nephropathy, neuropathy, and retinopathy as their younger counterparts. In non-insulin-dependent diabetes mellitus, the risk of subsequent neuropathy is related to the degree of glycemic control and the level of endogenous insulin production rather than age itself. Hypoglycemia in the elderly is associated with important sequelae. Elderly diabetic patients have an impaired counterregulatory response to hypoglycemia. More importantly, the ability to sense hypoglycemia declines, as does the ability to take corrective action. Coupled with the diminished cortical reserve due to higher prevalence of age-associated conditions such as stroke, lacunes, amyloid angiopathy, and Alzheimer's disease, the older brain is apt to be less able to fully recover from hypoglycemic insult. These facts highlight the risks of assuming that the benefits of tight glycemic control will outweigh the risks.

Treatment

A reasonable treatment goal in the elderly patient with diabetes mellitus is to maintain the fasting blood glucose below 150 mg/dL (8.3 mmol/L) and the postprandial blood glucose below 220 mg/dL (12.2 mmol/L). Achieving this goal is often difficult and complicated by other medications commonly prescribed for the elderly, eg, thiazide diuretics, phenytoin, and glucocorticoids, which have hyperglycemic effects. Therapy should decrease hyperglycemic symptoms and prevent infections and the potential progression to nonketotic hyperosmolar coma. Unfortunately, the results of the Diabetes Control and Complications Trial, conducted exclusively in young subjects (mean age 27 years) with insulin-dependent diabetes mellitus, are of limited applicability to older patients who have predominantly non-insulin-dependent diabetes mellitus and other comorbidity.

Similar to the strategy used in younger patients (Chapter 18), initial therapy should include dietary manipulation, weight reduction for the overweight patient, and an exercise program tailored to the individual's capabilities. If mild to moderate hyperglycemia persists (fasting blood glucose < 300 mg/dL [16.7 mmol/L]), an oral hypoglycemic agent should be tried. Chlorpropamide should be avoided because of its long half-life and its propensity to induce both hyponatremia and hypoglycemia. Because of their convenience and potency, second-generation agents such as glipizide and glyburide are often used; these drugs increase insulin secretion and the number of insulin receptors and reduce hepatic glucose production. Both have been shown to be well tolerated in short-term trials. Glipizide, which has a shorter half-life than glyburide, is less likely to cause prolonged hypoglycemia in the elderly, which is poorly tolerated. Few data are available on the efficacy of metformin in this age group; however, it has been associated with gastrointestinal side effects and weight loss.

If the fasting blood sugar remains above 300 mg/dL (16.7 mmol/L), insulin therapy should be started. The usual initial dose is 15–30 units of NPH (neutral protamine Hagedorn, or isophane) or another intermediate-acting insulin. One daily injection is usually sufficient. Since elderly patients often lack symptoms of hypoglycemia, the fasting, postprandial, and bedtime blood glucose levels must be checked initially even if symptoms are absent. Finally, as in younger patients, it is important to control other adverse factors such as hypertension and smoking, which can contribute to vascular complications associated with diabetes.

Diabetic ketoacidosis is rarely seen in the elderly. It should be treated cautiously, following a strategy similar to one used in younger patients (Chapter 18), with particular attention to the correction of electrolytes and water balance.

NONKETOTIC HYPEROSMOLAR COMA

Clinical Features

Nonketotic hyperosmolar coma, also known as nonketotic hypertonicity, occurs almost exclusively in the elderly. Predisposing factors include inadequate insulin secretion in response to hyperglycemia and a reduction in the peripheral effectiveness of insulin. Both factors lead to a progressive increase in serum glucose concentrations. The age-related increased renal threshold prevents osmotic diuresis until significant hyperglycemia is present, while an age-related decline in thirst predisposes to dehydration. Blood glucose concentrations often exceed 1000 mg/dL (55.5 mmol/L) and are coupled with marked elevation of plasma osmolality without ketosis.

This syndrome is frequently seen in elderly patients with type II diabetes who are in nursing homes and have limited access to water. However, one third of such patients have no previous history of diabetes. The most common precipitating event is infection (32–60% of cases); the most common infection is pneumonia. Medications (eg, thiazides, furosemide, phenytoin, glucocorticoids) or other acute medical illnesses can also precipitate this condition. Patients present with an acute confusional state, lethargy, weakness, and occasionally coma. Neurologic findings can be generalized or focal and can mimic an acute cerebrovascular event. Marked volume depletion, orthostatic hypotension, and prerenal azotemia are also usually present.

Treatment

The average extracellular fluid volume deficit is 9 L. It should be replaced initially with normal saline, especially when significant orthostatic hypotension is present. After 1–3 L of isotonic saline have been administered, fluids can be changed to half-normal (0.45%) saline. Half of the fluid and ion deficits should be replaced in the first 24 hours and the remainder over the next 48 hours.

Intravenous insulin in small doses (10–15 units) should be given initially, followed by a drip infusion of 1–3 units/h. Insulin therapy should not be used in lieu of fluids because it will exacerbate intravascular fluid depletion and further compromise renal function as it shifts glucose intracellularly. Potassium deficits should be corrected when the patient is producing urine. Possible precipitating events—such as acute myocardial infarction, pneumonia, or administration of a medication—must be investigated and treated. Although metabolic abnormalities may improve in 1–2 days, mental status deterioration and confusion may persist for 1 week or more. Over one-third of patients can be discharged without insulin treatment, but they are at significant risk for recurrence and should be monitored carefully.

OSTEOPOROSIS & CALCIUM HOMEOSTASIS

OSTEOPOROSIS

Despite the considerable prevalence, morbidity, and expense of osteoporosis, until recently most of our knowledge was derived from studies of perimenopausal women. Yet it is the older woman who typically experiences the ravages of the disease. Twenty-five percent of women have vertebral fractures by age 70; by age 80, the figure is closer to 50%. Over 90% of hip fractures occur in patients over age 70, and by age 90, one woman in three will have sustained such a fracture. Hip fractures are associated with significant morbidity, an increased risk of institutionalization, and up to a 20% increase in mortality rates. Despite the significant differences between perimenopausal and older women, diagnostic and therapeutic approaches for older women are derived largely from studies of perimenopausal women. The relevance of such studies for older women has only recently been questioned.

Definition

The definition of osteoporosis has changed over the years. In 1991, a consensus development conference defined osteoporosis as "a disease characterized by low bone mass and microarchitectural deterioration of bone tissue, leading to enhanced bone fragility and a consequent increase in fracture risk." Recently, the World Health Organization has issued diagnostic criteria for women based on measurements of bone mineral density or bone mineral content. Osteoporosis is defined as a value of bone mineral density more than 2.5 SD below peak bone mass (Table 25–3). This permits numerical standardization of the definition and criteria before a fracture takes place.

Factors Affecting Bone Physiology

There are significant physiologic differences between perimenopausal and older women with respect to maintenance of skeletal integrity. While calcium intake is inadequate in both age groups, calcium absorption declines with age, despite an age-related increase in serum levels of parathyroid hormone (PTH) (Figure 25–3); this increase is not due solely to a decrease in renal clearance, and it is associated with other biochemical evidence of increased PTH activ-

Table 25–3. World Health Organization diagnostic criteria for osteoporosis.[1]

Diagnosis	Criteria
Normal	Bone mineral density or content < 1 SD below the young adult mean value
Osteopenia (low bone mass)	Bone mineral density or content 1–2.5 SD below the young adult mean value (includes individuals in whom prevention of bone loss would be most useful)
Osteoporosis	Bone mineral density or content > 2.5 SD below the young adult mean value
Severe osteoporosis (established osteoporosis)	Bone mineral density or content > 2.5 SD below the young adult mean value in the presence of one or more fragility fractures

[1]Modified and reproduced, with permission, from Kanis JA: The diagnosis of osteoporosis. J Bone Miner Res 1994;9: 1137.

ity, including elevated levels of nephrogenous cyclic adenosine monophosphate (cAMP).

A. Vitamin D: Vitamin D deficiency is common in the elderly, and vitamin D metabolism changes with age. Up to 15% of healthy, elderly residents of communities in the sunny southwestern USA have frank vitamin D deficiency; still more have subclinical vitamin D deficiency; and up to 50% of elderly nursing home residents are deficient in vitamin D. This occurs because elderly individuals experience decreased sun exposure and have an impaired ability to form vitamin D precursors in the skin, a decreased dietary intake of vitamin D, and (possibly) an age-related decline in vitamin D receptors in the duodenum. In addition, the ability to convert vitamin D to its active moiety ($1,25[OH]_2D_3$) is impaired with age. Finally, certain vitamin D receptor alleles have been associated with lower bone density and bone loss in some populations, but further investigations are needed in the elderly in the United States.

B. Bone Loss and Architectural Changes: The rate of bone loss also differs between perimenopausal and older women. Cortical and trabecular bone are lost rapidly at menopause. Older longitudinal studies suggested that bone loss ceased or slowed in older women. Recent longitudinal studies suggest that older women lose an average of 0.7–1% per year at the hip, and femoral bone loss increases with age (Figure 25–4). Vertebral bone density changes assessed by AP measurements can give a misleading assessment of bone mass as a consequence of nonspecific calcifications from osteoarthritis, sclerosis, aortic calcifications, and osteophytes that interfere with and falsely elevate the measurement. Therefore, measurement of femoral bone density is more reliable in the elderly.

In addition, there are changes in bone geometry; cortical bone remodeling in older women is insuffi-

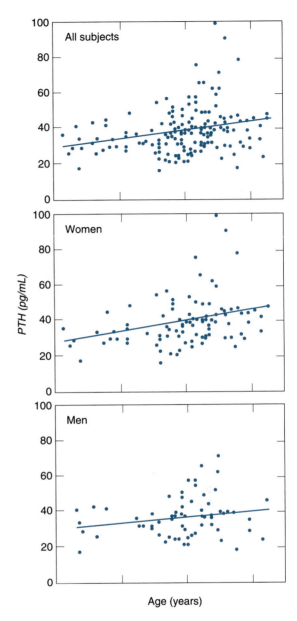

Figure 25–3. The effect of age on serum PTH. **Upper panel:** Entire study group ($P = .27$, $P < .001$). **Middle panel:** Women ($r = 0.31$, $P < .001$). **Lower panel:** Men ($r = 0.21$, $P < .05$). (Reproduced, with permission, from Marcus R et al: Age-related changes in parathyroid hormone and parathyroid action in normal humans. J Clin Endocrinol Metab 1984;58:223.)

cient to compensate for the loss of bone mineral content (Figure 25–5). There are also qualitative changes in trabecular bone, since an age-related reduction in trabecular bone jeopardizes plate integrity or "connectivity"; trabecular plates not only become perforated and disconnected, but with aging they continue to thin, causing further loss of bone

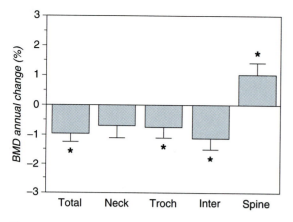

Figure 25–4. Longitudinal annual percentage change in bone mineral density (BMD) (g/cm², mean ± standard error of the mean) of the total hip, femoral neck, trochanter, intertrochanter, and spine in 85 healthy women over age 65 (mean age 77 years) followed for 1 year. (*, $P < 0.05$ difference from zero.) (Modified, with permission, from Greenspan SL et al: Femoral bone loss progresses with age: A longitudinal study in women over age 65. J Bone Min Res 1994;9:1959.)

strength and compromising the bone's ability to regain structural integrity with conventional therapy (Figure 25–6).

C. Risk Factors: Fracture risk factors differ in perimenopausal and older women. While a "fracture threshold" is helpful in determining which perimenopausal women are at risk for fracture, by age 70 most women have bone density measurements below this threshold and there is significant overlap in bone

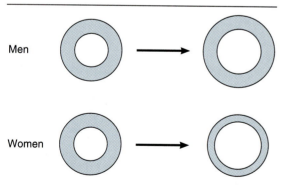

Figure 25–5. Schematic representation of cortical bone remodeling with age in males and females. Note that with age-related bone loss, bone is remodeled in men to increase its diameter and partially offset the loss of strength. In women, bone diameter changes little with age, so that bone strength decreases proportionately more than in men. (Reproduced, with permission, from Ruff CB, Hayes WC: Sex differences in age-related remodeling of the femur and tibia. J Orthop Res 1988;6:886.)

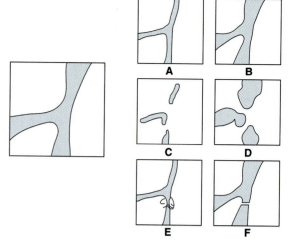

Figure 25–6. Possible effects of osteoporotic treatment regimens on trabecular bone. *Left panel:* Normal trabecular bone mass and architecture. Treatment resulting in anabolic effects on bone volume may restore normal bone volume and architecture in thin trabeculae (A, B). If trabecular integrity is disrupted before treatment, similar effects on bone volume may not reverse architectural abnormalities (C, D), particularly if treatment impairs the repair of microfractures (E, F). (Modified and reproduced, with permission, from Kanis JA: Treatment of osteoporotic fracture. Lancet 1984;1:27.)

density between older patients who fall and fracture and those who fall and do not fracture (Figure 25–7). Falling is often cited as major risk factor for hip fracture in older women. Although more than one-third of elderly women fall annually, however, less than 5% of falls result in a fracture. A fall to the side, a low bone mineral density, low body mass index (an index of obesity), and high fall energy have been shown to be significant independent risk factors for hip fracture in the elderly (Table 25–4). Other fac-

Table 25–4. Multiple logistic regression of factors associated with hip fracture in ambulatory elderly individuals.[1]

Factor	Adjusted Odds Ratio	95% Confidence Interval	P Value
Fall to side	5.7	2.3–14	< 0.001
Femoral neck bone density (g/cm²)*	2.7	1.6–4.6	< 0.001
Fall energy (J)†	2.8	1.5–5.2	≤ 0.001
Body mass index (kg/m²)*	2.2	1.2–3.8	0.003

[1]Modified and reproduced, with permission, from Greenspan SL: Fall severity and bone mineral density as risk factors for hip fracture in ambulatory elderly. JAMA 1994;271:128.
*Calculated for a decrease of 1 SD.
†Calculated for an increase of 1 SD.

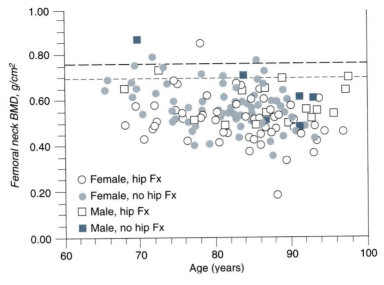

Figure 25–7. Femoral neck bone mineral density (BMD) (g/cm^2) versus age (years) in fallers with and without hip fracture (Fx). The lines represent 2 SD less than peak bone mass (theoretical fracture threshold) for women (dots and lower dashed line) and men (boxes and upper dashed line). Mean (± SD) femoral neck peak bone mass for women, 0.895 (±) and for men, 0.979 (± 0.220) g/cm^2. (Reproduced, with permission, from Greenspan SL et al: Fall severity and bone mineral density as risk factors for hip fractures in ambulatory elderly. JAMA 1994;271:128.)

tors, including a maternal history of hip fracture, previous hyperthyroidism, inability to rise from a chair, poor depth perception, poor contrast vision, and use of anticonvulsants or long-acting benzodiazepines are also associated with hip fractures in elderly women. Furthermore, with multiple risk factors, the risk of hip fracture increases significantly.

Evaluation

Screening older patients by obtaining a bone mineral density measurement is a comfortable, noninvasive, quick technique for determining an individual's bone mass and relative fracture risk. Patients may remain dressed and lie on a comfortable table. Although several methods are available, currently the best technique uses dual energy x-ray absorptiometry (DXA) of the hip or spine. For the patient over 65, the hip is the single most useful measurement because nonspecific calcifications can lead to falsely elevated measurements in the AP spine.

Similar to the evaluation in a younger individual who presents with bone loss or a fracture, the workup in an older patient can be targeted to exclude secondary causes of osteoporosis. Hyperthyroidism and hyperparathyroidism are both more common in older women, can cause bone loss, and can be clinically silent in older individuals. Because 10% of women over age 65 are receiving thyroid hormone replacement therapy and since even long-term "near-physiologic" thyroid hormone replacement results in bone loss in postmenopausal women, true physiologic replacement with a normal serum TSH should be the goal of treatment if possible. Osteomalacia may present as nonspecific muscle or skeletal discomfort and is more common in the elderly. In addition, metastatic carcinoma, multiple myeloma, hepatic and renal disease, and malabsorption (especially secondary to a gastrectomy) should be excluded. Glucocorticoid use and antiseizure medications also can cause significant bone loss in the elderly. Because factors outside the skeleton contribute to fracture risk in the elderly, however, the search for correctable factors must extend beyond those that affect bone density. Particular attention should be devoted to the patient's local environment and medication use.

Older patients presenting with skeletal discomfort should be evaluated by radiography to rule out a fracture. Vertebral osteoporosis usually presents with anterior wedging, involvement of more than one vertebrae, prominent vertebral trabeculae, and vertebral deformities usually occurring below T6. Worrisome signs suggesting that skeletal involvement is not due to osteoporosis alone include nerve root compression, posterior wedging, isolated vertebral involvement (especially above T4), and pedicle destruction. Furthermore, older individuals may complain of persistent groin pain with weight-bearing, while plain radiographs of the hip reveal no fracture. A bone scan may be necessary to confirm the diagnosis of hip fracture.

Treatment

Because the factors that affect bone physiology—the rate of bone loss, the structure of remaining bone, and the risk of fracture—are substantially different in perimenopausal and elderly women, interventions appropriate for perimenopausal women may be inappropriate for older women. Unfortunately, few therapeutic studies include older individuals, and the studies that do generally use bone density (rather than bone fracture) as an end point.

A. Calcium: Considerable controversy surrounds the use of calcium supplementation in perimenopausal women, and few data are available regarding its use in older women. Theoretically, calcium supplementation seems appropriate because calcium intake in the elderly is low and the ability to adapt to a low-calcium diet declines with age. Calcium balance studies suggest that postmenopausal estrogen-deficient women require 1500 mg/d to maintain calcium balance. A reduction in hip fractures and improvement in bone density has been demonstrated in very elderly women (mean age 84) treated with vitamin D, 800 IU, and calcium, 1200 mg daily. Calcium carbonate supplements should be given in divided doses with meals to improve absorption in the elderly, who may suffer from achlorhydria. Calcium citrate can be used as an alternative in such patients. A potential problem with prescribing high doses of calcium in the elderly includes inducing or exacerbating constipation. In addition, since compliance with other drug regimens decreases as the number of drugs increases, calcium tablets may be taken at the therapeutic expense of more important medications. Finally, because supplementary calcium does interfere with absorption of zinc, elderly patients receiving calcium supplementation should be encouraged to take a multivitamin containing zinc. Calcium absorption is not impaired by psyllium.

B. Vitamin D: There are few data to support the use of vitamin D or its metabolites in the treatment of osteoporosis, and results are equivocal. There is a small therapeutic ratio for vitamin D; toxicity from hypercalcemia can occur with doses as low as 50 μg (2000 IU), especially in individuals who are also taking a thiazide diuretic and calcium supplementation. However, because vitamin D deficiency is common in the elderly and vitamin D is needed for calcium absorption and also improves muscle strength, a single daily multivitamin which contains 400 IU is beneficial and will provide a normal vitamin D level even in institutionalized elderly persons. Clinical trials utilizing calcitriol (1,25-dihydroxy vitamin D_3) as a therapeutic option for osteoporosis have shown conflicting results, although one trial found a threefold reduction in vertebral compression fractures. The potential for complications such as hypercalcemia, nephrolithiasis, and

nephrocalcinosis are unknown, and this therapy is currently still under investigation.

C. Estrogen: There is considerable evidence that estrogen therapy, if initiated at menopause, slows bone loss; may temporarily increase bone mass; and may prevent osteoporotic, vertebral, and hip fractures. If therapy is continued, its efficacy is sustained at least until age 70. In addition, some studies have shown that estrogen will increase femoral bone mass. Fewer data are available about elderly persons taking newly prescribed estrogen. Four studies have reported a positive effect of estrogen on bone mass in older women. The observational study of osteoporotic fractures noted a 50% reduction of hip fractures in older women who were currently taking estrogens and had been doing so for a mean period of 14.5 years.

For women with an intact uterus, combined cyclic regimens with estrogen and progesterone may provoke return of menses and are less well tolerated. Despite the need for gynecologic surveillance and possible endometrial sampling to prevent cervical cancer, older women are more tolerant of combined continuous therapy regimens with estrogen and progesterone, which generally provide an atrophic endometrium within 1 year. Similar to younger women, older women receiving estrogen therapy require annual mammograms (Chapter 13).

Estrogen's protective effect against cardiovascular disease is another benefit frequently cited to support its use. Unfortunately, there are few data to support the suggestion that such a benefit will accrue when estrogen is newly prescribed to elderly women, in whom the prevalence of heart disease is already high. Furthermore, because of the possible increased relative risk of breast cancer in older women who have taken estrogen for more than 5 years, physicians must weigh all the individual risks and benefits for each patient.

D. Exercise: Although the rationale for exercise therapy is sound, few data are available on results of exercise in elderly women. One study prescribed exercise for older women and found that forearm bone mineral content increased in those who continued exercising during a 3-year trial. Middle-aged women (mean age 60) participating in high-intensity strength training for 1 year had improvements in femoral bone mass, muscle strength, balance, and activity level compared with controls. Walking—generally 30 minutes three times a week—is often suggested for less frail individuals. However, exercise is potentially dangerous for the reason that sedentary older women who newly engage in exercise may increase their exposure to accidents and subsequent fractures.

E. Other Therapeutic Options: Bisphosphonates—nonhormonal agents that inhibit bone resorption—effectively prevent osteoporosis. The aminobisphosphonate alendronate (an FDA-approved therapy) has been shown to increase bone mass at the spine (10%) and hip (6–8%) over 3 years in prospective clinical trials in postmenopausal women. Moreover, vertebral fractures were reduced by 48% and nonvertebral fractures by 29%. Improvements have also been demonstrated in older women. Furthermore, the medication had few adverse events, an important factor in choosing alternatives for the elderly. Prospective studies with etidronate showed a benefit for the spine, but results were not consistent for the hip. Although calcitonin is an approved therapy for osteoporosis, little data are available about its effect on the incidence of fractures. Given by injection, it is expensive, and it is relatively poorly tolerated by the elderly. Nasal calcitonin may prevent bone loss in early postmenopausal women; more data are needed in the elderly. Fluoride therapy causes significant toxicity in one-third of patients and has been associated with an increase in nonvertebral fractures. Slow-release fluoride is currently under investigation. Although thiazide diuretics have been associated with decreased hip fracture risk in several cross-sectional epidemiologic studies, the results are inconsistent, and the optimal dose and duration are unclear. However, a slight increase in both falls and fractures was noted in the only randomized study of thiazide use, the SHEP trial for hypertension in the elderly. For glucocorticoid-induced bone loss, one study demonstrated that etidronate plus ergocalciferol prevented bone loss.

Summary of Management Recommendations

In summary, there is ample reason to question the validity of extrapolating data from studies of perimenopausal women when formulating a treatment plan for older women. However, given the prevalence of the problem, it is reasonable to recommend an adequate daily intake of vitamin D (10 μg contained in 1 multivitamin tablet), an adequate daily intake of calcium (totaling 800–1500 mg), and judicious participation in an individually tailored exercise program. The use of bisphosphonates, estrogen replacement therapy or other treatment needs to be individually considered.

Perhaps more importantly, the risk of falls should be addressed. The risk can be reduced by reviewing medications (including nonprescription agents) and discontinuing (when possible) those with adverse effects on cognition, balance, or blood pressure. Common offenders include long-acting benzodiazepines, tricyclic antidepressants, antipsychotics, antihypertensives, and agents with anticholinergic side effects. It is also important to correct reversible sensory losses and medical conditions and to educate patients about hazards in their environment, such as throw rugs, extension cords, and poorly illuminated stairways, that could lead to falls and fractures. For patients with gait disorders, physical therapy should be considered.

Patients who have recently sustained a hip fracture should receive the same evaluation and consideration as those without a fracture. Because there is a significant overlap in bone density measurements between those that fracture and those that do not (Figure 25–7), a hip fracture should not be a reason to omit evaluation or treatment (see also Chapter 8).

HYPERPARATHYROIDISM

Clinical Features

The prevalence of hyperparathyroidism increases with age. While its incidence is less than 10 per 100,000 in women under age 40, the incidence increases to 190 per 100,000 in women over age 60. As a result, over half of all cases of hyperparathyroidism occur in individuals over the age of 65. Most cases are mild. Detection is by routine screening of serum calcium, and few or no symptoms are present. However, with relatively minor elevations of serum calcium (up to 11–12 mg/dL [2.8–3 mmol/L]), some elderly subjects may experience weakness, fatigue, depression, and confusion. Failure to thrive and constipation are commonly seen; renal, gastrointestinal, and skeletal complications occur less often. Other causes of hypercalcemia in the elderly—especially multiple myeloma, malignancy, vitamin D intoxication, and thiazide diuretics—must be considered in the differential diagnosis.

Treatment

For symptomatic patients with serum calcium levels above 12 mg/dL (3 mmol/L) and an elevated serum parathyroid hormone level, parathyroidectomy is well tolerated and is the treatment of choice. For those with more modest elevations, treatment decisions are less certain because it is difficult to differentiate symptoms and signs due to the disease from those seen in older individuals without hyperparathyroidism. Moreover, asymptomatic individuals—especially those with levels of serum calcium under 11 mg/dL (2.8 mmol/L)—have been known to remain asymptomatic for over a decade. Until more data become available, the decision to treat asymptomatic individuals surgically should be made on an individual basis.

In patients whose symptoms may be due to hyperparathyroidism, it is worthwhile to observe the response to medical therapy before considering surgery. In women, a course of estrogen may be effective. Ethinyl estradiol (30–50 μg/d) or conjugated estrogens (0.625–1.25 mg/d) reduce serum calcium by an average of 0.8 mg/dL (0.2 mmol/L), diminish urinary calcium excretion, and antagonize the skeletal effect of PTH. In men and in women with higher elevations of serum calcium, oral phosphates can be used, but they are less well tolerated in the elderly because of their gastrointestinal side effects. Furosemide is a less satisfactory alternative in frail elderly patients because it increases the risk of dehydration and resultant hypercalcemia.

CHANGES IN WATER BALANCE

With age, major changes in renal function and homeostatic mechanisms result in significant changes in water balance. Renal blood flow, cortical mass, glomerular number, and tubular function all decline with age, though medullary mass is preserved. Clinically, however, the most relevant change is the age-related decline in creatinine clearance, which is largely due to relative hypertension in the elderly. Because of the decrease in muscle mass associated with aging, however, serum creatinine levels are unchanged and may not accurately reflect the extent of renal functional impairment.

Extrarenal modulators of water balance also change significantly with age. Although there are no changes in the basal level, half-life, volume of distribution, or metabolic clearance of vasopressin, the stimulated responses of vasopressin are significantly altered. Hyperosmolar stimuli increase serum vasopressin levels in older subjects to five times those achieved in younger subjects. On the other hand, the normal vasopressin increase observed in response to overnight dehydration and postural change is impaired in the elderly. Additionally, basal and stimulated levels of serum renin and aldosterone decline with age. In contrast, basal levels of atrial natriuretic factor are three times higher in healthy elderly individuals than in young controls, and elevated levels of atrial natriuretic factor may help identify patients at risk for the development of congestive heart failure. Finally, the thirst sensation appears to be somewhat impaired in healthy elderly individuals and is more impaired in those who are frail.

In addition to physiologic changes, many diseases and drugs further increase the vulnerability of the elderly to changes in water balance. These include kidney disease, hypertension, and congestive heart failure as well as medications that alter water balance (eg, narcotics, diuretics, lithium, chlorpropamide, carbamazepine, amphotericin B, intravenous hypotonic fluids, and hypertonic contrast agents).

HYPERNATREMIA

Clinical Features

The incidence of hypernatremia in elderly patients admitted to the hospital ranges from 1% to 3% and is higher for institutionalized elderly patients. Signs and symptoms are usually nonspecific, eg, lethargy, weakness, confusion, depression, and failure to thrive. The cause is usually multifactorial, including impaired thirst mechanism, renal disease, sedative-induced confusion, use of restraints, reduced access to free water intake, excess water loss due to fever, and decreased response to vasopressin.

Treatment

As in younger patients, initial therapy involves correcting the volume deficit with isotonic saline and then correcting the water deficit with half-normal (0.45%) saline. Roughly 30% of the deficit should be corrected within 24 hours and the remainder within the next 24–48 hours.

HYPONATREMIA

Clinical Features

The prevalence of hyponatremia is approximately 2.5% in the general hospital setting—higher in geriatric units—and rises to 20% in nursing home settings. Presenting symptoms and signs are often nonspecific and include lethargy, weakness, and confusion. The mechanisms predisposing to hyponatremia include the exuberant response of vasopressin to osmolar stimuli, a decreased ability to excrete a water load, and the sodium-wasting tendency of the older kidney. Furthermore, elderly patients often use medications and have diseases that impair free water excretion. Common hyponatremic syndromes in the elderly include the syndrome of inappropriate antidiuretic hormone secretion (SIADH) and thiazide-induced hyponatremia.

Treatment

The treatment of hyponatremia in the elderly does not differ from that in younger patients (Chapter 5).

HYPORENINEMIC HYPOALDOSTERONISM

Hyporeninemic hypoaldosteronism usually occurs in elderly patients with diabetes and mild renal insufficiency. Patients are usually asymptomatic, and hyperkalemia and acidosis are found on routine screening. On the other hand, symptoms of hyperkalemia (eg, heart block) may be provoked by administration of a beta-adrenergic blocking agent, which further compromises extrarenal regulation of potassium homeostasis. After other causes of persistent hyperkalemia are ruled out, patients respond well to administration of small doses of fludrocortisone (0.05 mg/d) or furosemide combined with restriction of potassium.

GLUCOCORTICOIDS & STRESS

Because of equivalent decreases in secretion and clearance, serum cortisol and corticosteroid-binding globulin change little with age. However, the morning peak of cortisol secretion occurs several hours earlier in the elderly (Figure 25–8).

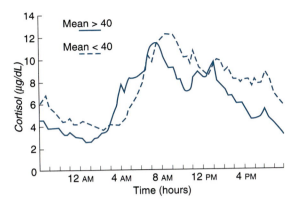

Figure 25–8. Mean 24-hour plasma cortisol concentration derived from 20-minute sampling for 12 subjects more than 40 years of age and for 22 subjects less than 40 years of age. (Reproduced, with permission, from Sherman B et al: Age-related changes in the circadian rhythm of plasma cortisol in man. J Clin Endocrinol Metab 1985;61:439.)

In healthy elderly individuals, dynamic testing of the hypothalamic-pituitary-adrenal axis is normal; expected responses to insulin-induced hypoglycemia, metyrapone, dexamethasone, ACTH, and CRH are preserved (Figure 25–9).

DISORDERS OF THE HYPOTHALAMIC-PITUITARY-ADRENAL AXIS

1. ABNORMAL RESPONSE TO STRESS

In contrast to the normal responses of the hypothalamic-pituitary-adrenal axis in the elderly to dynamic testing, increased stress elicits abnormal responses. For example, although serum cortisol levels increase to the same extent in young and old patients undergoing elective surgery, the increase may be protracted in the elderly. Patients with diabetes mellitus and hypertension have also been found to have an exaggerated and prolonged response to CRH stimulation. Older patients with Alzheimer's disease may also have delayed responses to CRH stimulation. It is not known if these elevated levels may contribute to the increased hypertension, glucose intolerance, muscle atrophy, osteoporosis, and impaired immune function observed in the elderly.

2. ADRENAL HYPERSECRETION

While adrenal hypersecretion (Cushing's syndrome) is uncommon in the elderly, it is easily overlooked because it mimics normal aging processes. Signs such as hypertension, glucose intolerance,

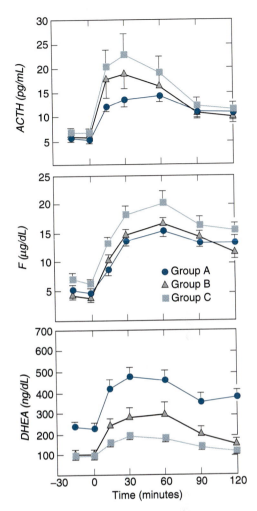

Figure 25–9. Mean values for groups A, B, and C of plasma ACTH *(upper panel),* F or cortisol *(middle panel),* and DHEA *(lower panel)* before and up to 120 minutes after bolus intravenous injection of ovine CRH (1 µg/kg). Group A, 21–49 years, mean age 35.2 years, n = 19. Group B, 50–69 years, mean age 60.7 years, n = 15. Group C, 70–86 years, mean age 77.1 years, n = 15. (Reproduced, with permission, from Pavlov EP et al: Responses of plasma adrenocorticotropin, cortisol, and dehydroepiandrosterone to ovine corticotropin-releasing hormone in healthy aging men. J Clin Endocrinol Metab 1986;62:767.)

weight gain, and osteoporosis are less specific in elderly than in younger patients, but as in younger patients the diagnosis is established or excluded using the usual criteria (Chapter 9).

3. ADRENAL INSUFFICIENCY

Symptoms of adrenal insufficiency in younger patients—eg, failure to thrive, weakness, weight loss, confusion, and arthralgias—are common complaints in adrenally intact elderly patients; the most specific sign of adrenal insufficiency in the elderly is hyperpigmentation. The laboratory findings of adrenal insufficiency are similar to those found in younger patients and include azotemia, hypoglycemia, hyponatremia, hyperkalemia, and eosinophilia. Because the metabolic clearance rate of cortisol decreases with age, older patients generally require lower replacement doses of cortisol.

CHANGES IN REPRODUCTIVE FUNCTION IN MEN

Overall, while sexual activity decreases with age, there are conflicting reports about the physiologic changes in the hypothalamic-pituitary-testicular axis. There is no consensus on the effect of age on the production or metabolism of dihydrotestosterone, estrone, and estradiol. Studies of testosterone economy show that serum testosterone (Figure 25–10), sex hormone-binding globulin, and free testosterone change little, if at all, while testosterone clearance decreases. However, other studies suggest that circulating testosterone and bioavailable testosterone fall with age by 40–65% and are even lower in institutionalized elderly. A decrease in the number or responsiveness of testicular Leydig cells is likely because serum FSH and LH increase with age, and the testosterone response to human chorionic gonadotropin (hCG) decreases. On the other hand, with age there is probably a decrease in the ratio of circulating bioactive to immunoreactive LH. Finally, pituitary changes are suggested by a decreased gonadotropic response to luteinizing hormone-releasing hormone (LHRH) stimulation.

The clinical relevance of these changes is questionable. The correlation between sexual activity and the age-related changes described is weak, and although early studies found decreased concentrations of spermatozoa in the ejaculate of older men, the difference disappeared after corrections were made for frequency of ejaculation. Sperm motility and the volume of ejaculate do decrease with age, and the proportion of abnormal spermatozoa also increases.

Impotence becomes more prevalent with age, but an endocrinologic etiology becomes less likely. The prevalence of impotence in men under age 45 is 5%; the prevalence in men over age 75 is 50%. However, over 90% of men in the latter group have coexistent medical conditions or are taking medications that contribute to the impotence. Furthermore, up to 30% of men over age 76 develop impotence following prostatectomy, compared with 3–11% in younger age

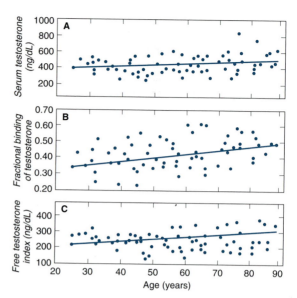

Figure 25–10. Total and free serum testosterone in men in relation to age. **A:** Serum testosterone concentration in men of various ages. The solid line in this and subsequent figures is drawn from least squares linear regression. **B:** Fractional binding of testosterone by column chromatography determined in sera from men of different ages. **C:** Free testosterone index determined from serum testosterone and fractional binders in sera from men of different ages. (Reproduced, with permission, from Harman SM et al: Reproductive hormones in aging men. 1. Measurement of sex steroids, basal luteinizing hormone, and Leydig cell response to human chorionic gonadotropin. J Clin Endocrinol Metab 1980;51:35.)

groups. Often there are multiple overlapping causes of impotence—psychosocial, neurovascular, metabolic (diabetes mellitus), medication-related, and arteriolar—in the same individual.

The evaluation of impotence in the elderly is similar to that in younger individuals (Chapter 12), though more emphasis must be placed on the effects of drugs (both prescribed and nonprescribed) and vascular causes, and a search for multiple causative factors should be undertaken.

BENIGN PROSTATIC HYPERPLASIA

Although the pathogenesis of benign prostatic hyperplasia is incompletely understood, testicular androgens are believed to play a permissive role in the development of prostatic adenomas. This mechanism provides the rationale for the use of antiandrogens in the treatment of benign prostatic hypertrophy. Antiandrogen treatment has been investigated using luteinizing hormone releasing hormone (LHRH) agonists (nafarelin, leuprolide, buserelin), androgen receptor inhibitors (cyproterone acetate, flutamide), and 5α-reductase inhibitors (finasteride). Overall, these agents result in a 25–30% reduction in prostate size, but their effects on the voiding symptoms associated with benign prostatic hypertrophy have been modest, variable, and less immediate and substantial than observed with alpha-adrenergic blockers. For instance, finasteride reduces symptoms by half in only one-third of men, and statistically significant effects in the largest trial occurred only after 11 months. Each of these agents must be continued indefinitely to maintain prostate size reduction, yet many men may find such therapy difficult and undesirable, as well as expensive, and the long-term side effects are largely unknown. The LHRH agonists and cypro-

terone acetate cause impotence; flutamide induces gynecomastia, and one report describes serologic as well as histologic evidence of flutamide-induced hepatotoxicity in a small number of patients. Since finasteride decreases dihydrotestosterone while maintaining the circulating levels of testosterone, undesirable antiandrogenic side effects are lower. Finasteride causes a significant decrease in the level of prostate-specific antigen, a serum marker increasingly used for the clinical detection of prostate adenocarcinoma, the most common cancer in men. Thus, if PSA levels fail to decline in a man compliant with therapy, investigation for prostate cancer should be initiated. Since the effect of finasteride on prostate cancer development and progression is unknown, it is unclear whether any antitumor benefit will mitigate finasteride's effect on the ability to use this important tumor marker in treated men.

REFERENCES

Thyroid Function & Disease

Bagchi N, Brown TR, Parish RF: Thyroid dysfunction in adults over age 55 years: A study in an urban US community. Arch Intern Med 1995;150:785.

Davis PJ, Davis FB: Hyperthyroidism in patients over the age of 60 years. Medicine 1974;53:161.

Faber J, Galloe AM: Changes in bone mass during prolonged subclinical hyperthyroidism due to L-thyroxine treatment: A meta-analysis. Eur J Endocrinol 1994;130:350.

Greenspan SL et al: Age-related alterations in pulsatile secretion of TSH: Role of dopaminergic regulation. Am J Physiol 1991;260(3 Part 1):E486.

Greenspan SL et al: Pulsatile secretion of thyrotropin in man. J Clin Endocrinol Metab 1986;63:661.

Harman SM, Wehman RE, Blackman MR: Pituitary-thyroid hormone economy in healthy aging men: Basal indices of thyroid function and thyrotropin responses to constant infusions of thyrotropin releasing hormone. J Clin Endocrinol Metab 1984;58:320.

Hershman JM et al: Serum thyrotropin and thyroid hormone levels in elderly and middle-aged euthyroid persons. J Am Geriatr Soc 1993;41:823.

Levy EG: Thyroid disease in the elderly. Med Clin North Am 1991;75:151.

Nordyke RA, Gilbert FI, Harada ASM: Graves' disease: Influence of age on clinical findings. Arch Intern Med 1988;148:626.

Rosenthal MJ et al: Thyroid failure in the elderly: Microsomal antibodies as discriminant for therapy. JAMA 1987;258:209.

Sawin CT et al: Low serum thyrotropin (thyroid-stimulating hormone) in older persons without hyperthyroidism. Arch Intern Med 1991;151:165.

Sawin CT et al: Low serum thyrotropin concentrations as a risk factor for atrial fibrillation in older persons. N Engl J Med 1994;331:1249.

Sawin CT et al: The aging thyroid: The use of thyroid hormone in older persons. JAMA 1989;261:2653.

Sawin CT et al: The aging thyroid: Thyroid deficiency in the Framingham study. Arch Intern Med 1985;145:1386.

Sawin CT: Subclinical hypothyroidism in older persons. Clin Geriatr Med 1995;11:231.

Sawin CT: Thyroid dysfunction in older persons. Adv Intern Med 1991;37:223.

Surkse MI et al: American Thyroid Association guidelines for use of laboratory tests in thyroid disorders. JAMA 1990;267:1529.

Tibaldi JM et al: Thyrotoxicosis in the very old. Am J Med 1986;81:619.

Carbohydrate Intolerance & Diabetes Mellitus

Cahill GF: Hyperglycemic hyperosmolar coma: A syndrome almost unique in the elderly. J Am Geriatr Soc 1983;31:103.

Diabetes Control and Complications Trial Research Group: The effect of intensive treatment of diabetes on the development and progression of long-term complications in insulin-dependent diabetes mellitus. N Engl J Med 1993;329:977.

Elahi D et al: Effect of age and obesity on fasting levels of glucose, insulin, growth hormone and glucagon in man. J Gerontol 1982;37:385.

Franssila-Kallunki A, Schalin-Jantti C, Groop L: Effect of gender on insulin resistance associated with aging. Am J Physiol 1992;263:E780.

Harris MI et al: Prevalence of diabetes and impaired glucose tolerance and plasma glucose levels in US population aged 20–74 years. Diabetes 1987;36:523.

Hollenbeck CB et al: Effect of habitual physical activity on regulation of insulin-stimulated glucose disposal in older males. J Am Geriatr Soc 1985;33:273.

Kannel WB: Lipid diabetes in coronary heart disease: Insights from the Framingham Study. Am Heart J 1985;110:1100.

Lorber D: Nonketotic hypertonicity in diabetes mellitus. Med Clin North Am 1995;79:39.

Marker JC, Cryer PE, Clutter WE: Attenuated glucose recovery from hypoglycemia in the elderly. Diabetes 1992;41:671.

Meneilly GS, Cheung E, Tuokko H: Counterregulatory hormone responses to hypoglycemia in the elderly patient with diabetes. Diabetes 1994;43:403.

Morisaki N et al: Diabetic control and progression of retinopathy in elderly patients: Five-year follow-up study. J Am Geriatr Soc 1994;42:142.

Morley JE, Perry HM III: The management of diabetes mellitus in older individuals. Drugs 1991;41:548.

Partanen J et al: Natural history of peripheral neuropathy in patients with non-insulin-dependent diabetes mellitus. N Engl J Med 1995;333:89.

Reaven GM, Reaven EP: Age, glucose tolerance, and non-insulin-dependent diabetes mellitus. J Am Geriatr Soc 1985;33:286.

Zavaroni I et al: Effect of age and environmental factors on glucose tolerance and insulin secretion in a worker population. J Am Geriatr Soc 1986;34:271.

Osteoporosis & Calcium Homeostasis

Cauley JA, Seeley DG, Ensrud K: Estrogen replacement therapy and fractures in older women. Ann Intern Med 1995;122:9.

Chapuy MC et al: Vitamin D_3 and calcium to prevent hip fractures in elderly women. N Engl J Med 1992; 327:1637.

Chesnut CH III et al: Alendronate treatment of the postmenopausal osteoporotic woman: Effect of multiple dosages on bone mass and bone remodeling. Am J Med 1995;99:144.

Chigot J-P, Menegaux F, Achrafi H: Should primary hyperparathyroidism be treated surgically in elderly patients older than 75 years? Surgery 1995;117:397.

Colditz GA et al: The use of estrogens and progestins and the risk of breast cancer in postmenopausal women. N Engl J Med 1995;332:1589.

Consensus development conference: Prophylaxis and treatment of osteoporosis. Am J Med 1991;90:107.

Cummings SR et al: Risk factors for hip fracture in white women. N Engl J Med 1995;332:767.

Dawson-Hughes B et al: A controlled trial of the effect of calcium supplementation in bone density in postmenopausal women. N Engl J Med 1990;323:878.

Diagnostic and therapeutic technology assessment (DATTA). Measurement of bone density with dual-energy x-ray absorptiometry (DEXA). JAMA 1992; 267:286.

Diamond T et al: Cyclical etidronate plus ergocalciferol prevents glucocorticoid-induced bone loss in postmenopausal women. Am J Med 1995;98:459.

Ebeling PR et al: Influence of age on effects of endogenous 1,25-dihydroxyvitamin D on calcium absorption in normal women. Calcif Tissue Int 1994;55:330.

Ebeling PR, Sandgren ME, DiMagno EP: Evidence of an age-related decrease in intestinal responsiveness to vitamin D: Relationship between serum 1,25-dihydroxy vitamin D_3 and intestinal vitamin D receptor concentrations in normal women. J Clin Endocrinol Metab 1992;75:176.

Felson DT et al: The effect of postmenopausal estrogen therapy on bone density in elderly women. N Engl J Med 1993;329:1141.

Greenspan SL et al: Femoral bone loss progresses with age: A longitudinal study in women over age 65. J Bone Miner Res 1994;9:1959.

Greenspan SL et al: Skeletal integrity in pre- and postmenopausal women on long-term L-thyroxine therapy. Am J Med 1991;91:5.

Greenspan SL, Myers ER, Maitland LA: Fall severity and bone mineral density as risk factors for hip fracture in ambulatory elderly. JAMA 1994;271:128.

Grisso JA et al: Risk factors for falls as a cause of hip fracture in women. N Engl J Med 1991;324:1326.

Holick MF: Vitamin D requirements for the elderly. Am J Clin Nutr 1986;5:121.

Hui SL et al: A prospective study of change in bone mass with age in postmenopausal women. J Chron Dis 1982;35:715.

Jones G et al: Thiazide diuretics and fractures: Can meta-analysis help? J Bone Miner Res 1995;10:106.

Kanis JA et al: The diagnosis of osteoporosis. J Bone Miner Res 1994;9:1137.

Kiel DP et al: Hip fracture and the use of estrogens in postmenopausal women: The Framingham study. N Engl J Med 1987;317:1169.

Lindsay R, Tohme JF: Estrogen treatment of patients with osteoporosis. J Obstet Gynecol 1990;76:290.

Lips P et al: The effect of vitamin D supplementation on vitamin D status and parathyroid function in elderly subjects. J Clin Endocrinol Metab 1988;67:644.

Marcus R et al: Conjugated estrogens in the treatment of post-menopausal women with hyperparathyroidism. Ann Intern Med 1984;100:633.

Marcus R, Madvig P, Young G: Age-related changes in parathyroid hormone and parathyroid hormone action in normal humans. J Clin Endocrinol Metab 1984; 58:223.

Morrison NA et al: Prediction of bone density from vitamin D receptor alleles. Nature 1994;367:284.

Quigley MET et al: Estrogen therapy arrests bone loss in elderly women. Am J Obstet Gynecol 1987;156: 1516.

Reginster JY et al: A double-blind, placebo-controlled, dose-finding trial of intermittent nasal salmon calcitonin for prevention of postmenopausal lumbar spine bone loss. Am J Med 1995;98:452.

Resnick NM, Greenspan SL: Senile osteoporosis reconsidered. J Am Med Assoc 1989;261:1025.

Ruff CB, Hayes WC: Sex differences in age-related remodeling of the femur and tibia. J Orthop Res 1988; 6:886.

The SHEP Cooperative Research Group: Prevention of stroke by antihypertensive drug treatment in older persons with systolic hypertension: final results of the Systolic Hypertension in the Elderly Program (SHEP). J Am Med Assoc 1991;265:3255.

Tilyard MW et al: Treatment of postmenopausal osteoporosis with calcitriol or calcium. N Engl J Med 1992;326:357.

Tinetti ME et al: A multifactorial intervention to reduce the risk of falling among elderly people living in the community. N Engl J Med 1994;331:821.

Watts NB et al: Intermittent cyclical etidronate treatment of postmenopausal osteoporosis. N Engl J Med 1990; 323:73.

Changes in Water Balance

Anderson RJ et al: Hyponatremia: A prospective analysis of its epidemiology and the pathogenetic role of vasopressin. Ann Intern Med 1985;102:164.

Borra SI, Beredo R, Kleinfeld M: Hypernatremia in the aging: Causes, manifestations, and outcome. J Natl Med Assoc 1995;87:220.

Cyus JC, Krothapalli RK, Arieff AL: Treatment of symptomatic hyponatremia and its relation to brain damage. N Engl J Med 1987;317:1190.

Davis KM et al: Atrial natriuretic peptide levels in the prediction of congestive heart failure risk in frail elderly JAMA 1992;267:2625.

Ohashi M et al: High plasma concentrations of human atrial natriuretic polypeptide in aged men. J Clin Endocrinol Metab 1987;64:81.

Snyder NA, Feigal DW, Arieff AL: Hypernatremia in elderly patients: A heterogeneous, morbid, and iatrogenic entity. Ann Intern Med 1987;107:309.

Terzian C, Frye EB, Piotrowski ZH: Admission hyponatremia in the elderly: Factors influencing prognosis. J Gen Intern Med 1994;9:89.

Glucocorticoids & Stress

Greenspan SL et al: The pituitary-adrenal glucocorticoid response is altered by gender and disease. J Gerontol 1993;48:M72.

Pavlov EP et al: Response of plasma adrenocorticotropin, cortisol and dehydro-epiandrosterone to ovine corticotropin-releasing hormone in healthy aging men. J Clin Endocrinol Metab 1986;62:767.

Sherman B, Wysham C, Pfohl B: Age-related changes in the circadian rhythm of plasma cortisol in man. J Clin Endocrinol Metab 1985;61:439.

Reproductive Function in Men

Abbasi AA et al: Low circulating levels of insulin-like growth factors and testosterone in chronically institutionalized elderly men. J Am Geriatr Soc 1993;41:975.

DuBeau CE, Resnick NM: Controversies in the diagnosis and management of benign prostatic hyperplasia. Adv Int Med 1992;37:55.

Gormley CJ et al: The effect of finasteride in men with benign prostatic hyperplasia. N Engl J Med 1992;327:1185.

Gormley GJ et al: Effect of finasteride on prostate-specific antigen density. Urology 1994;43:53.

Harman SM et al: Reproductive hormones in aging men. 2. Basal pituitary gonadotropins and gonadotropin responses to luteinizing hormone-releasing hormone. J Clin Endocrinol Metab 1982;54:547.

Korenman SG, Morley JE, Morradian AD: Secondary hypogonadism in older men: its relationship to impotence. J Clin Endocrinol Metab 1990;71:963.

Morley JE, Kaiser FE: Testicular function in the aging male. In: Endocrine Function and Aging. Armbrecht HJ, Coe RM, Wong Surawat N (editors). Springer, 1990.

Rittmaster RS: Finasteride. N Engl J Med 1994;330:120.

Tsitouras PD, Martin CE, Harman SM: Relationship of serum testosterone to sexual activity in healthy elderly men. J Gerontol 1982;37:288

APPENDIX
TABLE OF NORMAL HORMONE REFERENCE RANGES[1,2]

ACTH stimulation test (cosyntropin test): 0.25 mg of synthetic ACTH$_{1-24}$ (cosyntropin) is administered IV or IM, and serum cortisol is measured at 0, 30, and 60 minutes. Normal response: peak cortisol > 20 µg/dL (> 540 nmol/L). A dose of 1 µg of ACTH will give a similar response in the normal individual.

Test	Source	Ages, Conditions, Etc	Conventional Units	Conversion Factor	SI Units	Comments
Adrenocorticotropic hormone (ACTH)	Plasma		10–52 pg/mL	0.222	2–11 pmol/L	Collect in silicone-coated EDTA- containing tubes. Keep iced. Avoid contact with glass during collection and separation. Process immediately. Separate and freeze plasma in plastic tube at –20 °C.
Aldosterone	Plasma (fasting)	Sodium intake 100–200 meq/d: 0700, recumbent 0900, upright Adrenal vein Sodium intake 10 meq/d: 0700, recumbent 0900, upright	3–9 ng/dL 4–30 ng/dL 200–400 ng/dL 12–36 ng/dL 17–137 ng/dL	27.7	83–250 pmol/L 111–832 pmol/L 5548–11,096 pmol/L 333–999 pmol/L 472–3800 pmol/L	Levels in pregnant patients are three to four times higher.
Adlosterone-18-glucuronide	Urine	On normal diet (100–200 meq Na+/d): On low-sodium diet (< 20 meq Na+/d):	5–20 µg/24 h 10–40 µg/24 h	2.77	14–56 nmol/24 h 28–112 nmol/24 h	Refrigerate during collection.
Androstenediol glucuronide	Serum	Male Female	2.6–16 ng/mL 0.6–8.1 ng/mL	2.14	5.7–35.2 nmol/L 1.3–17.8 nmol/L	Freeze serum and store at –20 °C.
Androstenedione	Serum	Male < 6 years 6–8 years 8–10 years 10–12 years 12–14 > 14 years Female < 6 years 6–8 years 8–10 years 10–12 years 12–14 years > 14 years Postmenopausal	0.1–0.2 ng/mL 0.1–0.3 ng/mL 0.1–0.3 ng/mL 0.3–0.7 ng/mL 0.5–1.0 ng/mL 0.8–2.3 ng/mL 0.1–0.2 ng 0.1–0.3 ng/mL 0.2–0.5 ng/mL 0.4–1.0 ng/mL 0.8–1.9 ng/mL 0.8–2.3 ng/mL 0.3–0.8 ng/mL	3.49	0.3–0.7 nmol/L 0.3–1.0 nmol/L 0.3–1.0 nmol/L 1.0–2.4 nmol/L 1.7–3.5 nmol/L 2.0–8.0 nmol/L 0.3–0.7 nmol/L 0.3–1.0 nmol/L 0.7–1.7 nmol/L 1.4–3.5 nmol/L 2.8–6.6 nmol/L 2.8–8.0 nmol/L 1.0–2.8 nmol/L	
Antidiuretic hormone (ADH; vasopressin)	Plasma	If serum osmolality > 290 mosm/kg If serum osmolality < 290 mosm/kg	2–12 pg/mL < 2 pg/mL	0.925	1.85–11.1 pmol/L < 1.85 pmol/L	Collect in EDTA tubes. Keep iced. Contrifuge refrigerated. Store at –70 °C within 2 hours.

Test	Specimen	Detail	Conventional	Factor	SI Units	Collection notes
C peptide of insulin	Serum		0.5–3.0 ng/mL 1.5–9.0 ng/mL	0.331	0.17–1 nmol/L 0.5–3.0 nmol/L	Freeze serum at –20 °C within 8 hours after collection.
Calcitonin	Serum	Male Female	3–26 ng/L 2–17 ng/L	0.293	0.88–7.6 pmol/L 0.58–5 pmol/L	Fasting, nonlipemic specimen. Refrigerate, spin down immediately. Store at –20 °C.

Calcitonin stimulation test:

(1) **Pentagastrin test:** Pentagastrin, 0.5 µg/kg, is administered IV., and serum samples are obtained at 0, 1, 2, and 5 minutes after injection. Normal response at 1 or 2 minutes: male, < 106 pg/mL (31.1 pmol/L); female, < 29 pg/mL (8.5 pmol/L); at 5 minutes: male, < 106 pg/mL (31.1 pmol/L); female, < 23 pg/mL (6.7 nmol/L).

(2) **Pentagastrin and calcium infusion test:** Give 2 mg/kg calcium gluconate IV over 1 minute, followed by 0.5 µg/kg pentagastrin. Collect specimens as above. Normal response at 1 or 2 minutes: male, < 350 pg/mL (< 102.5 nmol/L); female, < 94 pg/mL (< 27.5 nmol/L); at 5 minutes: male, < 244 pg/mL (71.5 nmol/L); female, < 76 pg/mL (< 22.3 nmol/L).

Test	Specimen	Detail	Conventional	Factor	SI Units	Collection notes
Catecholamines (fractionated by HPLC)	Plasma	Norepinephrine Epinephrine Dopamine	110–658 pg/mL < 50 pg/mL < 10 pg/mL	0.00591 0.00546 0.00654	0.65–3.89 nmol/L < 0.27 nmol/L < 0.065 nmol/L	Collect by intravenous catheter after patient has rested 30 minutes. Collect and centrifuge under refrigeration; freeze in plastic tube at –20 °C.
	Urine	Norepinephrine Epinephrine Dopamine	15–80 µg/24 h 1–20 µg/24 h 65–400 µg/24 h	5.91 5.46 6.54	89–473 nmol/d 5.5–109 nmol/d 426–2616 nmol/d	24-hour urine preservative: 25 mL 6N HCl. Aliquot and freeze promptly at –20 °C.
Cholecystokinin	Plasma (fasting)		3.9 ng/mL	0.26	1 pmol/L	
Chorionic gonadotropin, β subunit (β-hCG)	Serum	Males and nonpregnant females Females post conception 7–10 days 30 days 40 days 10 weeks 14 weeks Trophoblastic disease:	Not detectable > 2 mIU/mL > 100 mIU/mL > 2000 mIU/mL 50,000–100,000 mIU/mL 10,000–20,000 mIU/mL > 100,000 mIU/mL	1.00	Not detectable > 2 IU/L > 100 IU/L > 2000 IU/L 50,000–100,000 IU/L 10,000–20,000 IU/L > 100,000 IU/L	See Chapter 16 for further details and interpretation.
Cortisol	Serum	AM PM	3–20 µg/dL 2.5–10 µg/dL	27.59	80–550 nmol/L 70–280 nmol/L	Collect and process under refrigeration. Spin down immediately.
	Urine (free)	24-hour specimen RIA 24-hour specimen HPLC AM 1 hour (0700–0800) PM 1 hour (2200–2300)	20–90 µg/g Cr < 50 µg/24 h 50–200 µg/g Cr 5–45 µg/g Cr	0.312 2.76 0.312 0.312	8–30 µmol/mol Cr < 135 nmol/24 h 16–66 µmol/mol Cr 2–14 µmol/mol Cr	Collect 24-hour specimen with 8 g of boric acid or 10 mL of 6N HCl as preservative.

(continued)

789

Test	Source	Ages, Conditions, Etc	Conventional Units	Conversion Factor	SI Units	Comments
Dehydroepiandrosterone (DHEA)	Serum (fasting preferred)	Male		0.0347		Separate serum immediately and store at –20 °C.
		< 6 years	20–130 ng/dL		0.7–4.5 nmol/L	
		6–8 years	20–275 ng/dL		0.7–9.5 nmol/L	
		8–10 years	31–345 ng/dL		1.1–12.0 nmol/L	
		Pubertal at–				
		Tanner stage 2	110–495 ng/dL		3.8–17.2 nmol/L	
		Tanner stage 3	173–585 ng/dL		5.9–20.3 nmol/L	
		Tanner stage 4	160–640 ng/dL		5.6–22.2 nmol/L	
		Tanner stage 5	250–900 ng/dL		8.7–31.2 nmol/L	
		> 20 years	160–800 ng/dL		5.6–27.8 nmol/L	
		Female				
		< 6 years	20–130 ng/dL		0.7–4.5 nmol/L	
		6–8 years	20–275 ng/dL		0.7–9.5 nmol/L	
		8–10 years	31–345 ng/dL		1.1–12.0 nmol/L	
		Pubertal at–				
		Tanner stage 2	150–570 ng/dL		5.2–19.8 nmol/L	
		Tanner stage 3	200–600 ng/dL		6.9–20.8 nmol/L	
		Tanner stage 4	200–780 ng/dL		6.9–27.1 nmol/L	
		Tanner stage 5	215–850 ng/dL		7.5–29.5 nmol/L	
		> 20 years	160–800 ng/dL		5.6–27.8 nmol/L	
		Postmenopause	30–450 ng/dL		1.0–15.6 nmol/L	
Dehydroepiandrosterone sulfate (DHEAS)	Serum (fasting preferred)	Male		0.0272		Stable 72 hours at 40 °C. Store at –20 °C.
		1–8 years	10–20 µg/dL		0.3–0.5 µmol/L	
		8–10 years	30–50 µg/dL		0.8–1.4 µmol/L	
		10–12 years	30–40 µg/dL		0.8–1.1 µmol/L	
		12–14 years	80–140 µg/dL		2.2–3.8 µmol/L	
		14–50 years	110–690 µg/dL		3.0–18.7 µmol/L	
		> 50 years	40–330 µg/dL		1.1–9.0 µmol/L	
		Female				
		1–8 years	10–20 µg/dL		0.3–0.5 µmol/L	
		8–10 years	30–50 µg/dL		0.8–1.4 µmol/L	
		10–12 years	50–140 µg/dL		1.4–3.8 µmol/L	
		12–14 years	70–170 µg/dL		1.9–4.6 µmol/L	
		14–50 years	80–340 µg/dL		2.2–9.2 µmol/L	
		Postmenopause	17–77 µg/dL		0.5–2.1 µmol/L	
		Pregnancy (term)	23–177 µg/dL		0.6–3.2 µmol/L	
Deoxycorticosterone (DOC)	Serum (fasting preferred)	Cord blood	111–372 ng/dL	30.26	3400–11,300 pmol/L	Process immediately. Store at –20 °C.
		1 week to 12 months	7–49 ng/dL		212–1485 pmol/L	
		Prepubertal child	2–34 ng/dL		61–1030 pmol/L	
		Adults (0800)	2–19 ng/dL		61–576 pmol/L	

Analyte	Specimen	Conventional value	Factor	SI value	Comments
11-Deoxycortisol	Serum	Cord blood 295–554 ng/dL	0.02887	8.56–16.1 nmol/L	Process immediately. Store at –20 °C.
		Premature infants 48–579 ng/dL		1.39–16.8 nmol/L	
		Full-term infants to 3 days 13–147 ng/dL		0.38–4.3 nmol/L	
		1–12 months < 156 ng/dL		< 4.5 nmol/L	
		Prepubertal child 1–10 years 20–155 ng/dL		0.58–4.5 nmol/L	
		Adults (0800) 12–158 ng/dL		0.35–4.6 nmol/L	

Dexamethasone suppression test (low dose) for the diagnosis of Cushing syndrome (see Chapter 9): Obtain a baseline serum cortisol at 0700–0800 hours. Administer 1 mg dexamethasone at 2300 hours that evening and obtain another serum cortisol at 0700–0800 hours the following morning. **Interpretation:** A normal response (normal suppressibility) is a reduction of the postdexamethasone serum cortisol to < 5 µg/dL (< 140 nmol/L).
Dexamethasone suppression test (high dose) for the differential diagnosis of Cushing syndrome (see Chapter 9): Obtain a baseline serum cortisol at 0700–0800 hours. Administer 8.0 mg dexamethasone orally at 2300 hours that evening and obtain another serum cortisol at 0700–0800 hours the following morning. **Interpretation:** A reduction of the postdexamethasone serum cortisol to < 50% of the baseline cortisol indicates suppressibility.

Analyte	Specimen	Conventional value	Factor	SI value	Comments
Dihydrotestoster-one (male)	Serum	Cord blood < 2–8 ng/dL	0.0344	< 0.07–0.28 nmol/L	Separate serum within 1 hour after collection and store at –20 °C.
		Premature infants 10–53 ng/dL		0.34–1.82 nmol/L	
		Full-term newborn 5–60 ng/dL		0.17–2.06 nmol/L	
		30–60 days 12–85 ng/dL		0.42–2.92 nmol/L	
		7 months to puberty at–			
		Tanner stage 1 < 3 ng/dL		< 0.10 nmol/L	
		Tanner stage 2 3–17 ng/dL		0.10–0.58 nmol/L	
		Tanner stage 3 8–33 ng/dL		0.28–1.14 nmol/L	
		Tanner stage 4 22–52 ng/dL		0.76–1.79 nmol/L	
		Tanner stage 5 24–65 ng/dL		0.83–2.24 nmol/L	
		Adult 30–85 ng/dL		1.03–2.92 nmol/L	
Dihydrotestoster-one (female)	Serum	Cord blood < 2–8 ng/dL		< 0.07–0.28 nmol/L	
		Premature infants 2–13 ng/dL		0.07–0.45 nmol/L	
		Full-term newborn < 2–15 ng/dL		< 0.07–0.52 nmol/L	
		30–60 days < 3 ng/dL		< 0.10 nmol/L	
		7 months to puberty at–			
		Tanner stage 1 < 3 ng/dL		< 0.10 nmol/L	
		Tanner stage 2 5–12 ng/dL		0.17–0.41 nmol/L	
		Tanner stage 3 7–19 ng/dL		0.24–0.65 nmol/L	
		Tanner stage 4 4–13 ng/dL		0.14–0.45 nmol/L	
		Tanner stage 5 3–18 ng/dL		0.10–0.62 nmol/L	
		Adult 4–22 ng/dL		0.18–0.76 nmol/L	
Erythropoietin	Serum	4–26 mIU/mL	1.00	4–26 IU/L	
Estradiol	Serum	Male	3.67		
		Prepubertal < 10 pg/mL		< 37 pmol/L	
		12–16 years < 23 pg/mL		< 84 pmol/L	
		> 16 years 20–50 pg/mL		73–184 pmol/L	
		Female			
		< 8 years < 7 pg/mL		< 26 pmol/L	
		8–12 years 8–18 pg/mL		29–66 pmol/L	
		12–14 years 16–34 pg/mL		58–125 pmol/L	
		14–16 years 20–68 pg/mL		73–250 pmol/L	
		Early follicular 20–100 pg/mL		73–367 pmol/L	
		Preovulatory 100–350 pg/mL		367–1285 pmol/L	
		Luteal 100–350 pg/mL		367–1285 pmol/L	
		Postmenopausal 10–30 pg/mL		37–110 pmol/L	

(continued)

Test	Source	Ages, Conditions, Etc	Conventional Units	Conversion Factor	SI Units	Comments
Estriol (pregnancy)	Serum	Pregnant female 30–32 weeks 33–35 weeks 36–38 weeks 39–40 weeks Male and nonpregnant female	 2–12 ng/mL 3–19 ng/mL 5–27 ng/mL 10–30 ng/mL < 2 ng/mL	3.47	 7–42 nmol/L 10–66 nmol/L 17–94 nmol/L 35–104 nmol/L < 7 nmol/L	
Estrone	Serum	Male Female Follicular Ovulatory Luteal Postmenopausal	10–50 pg/mL 30–100 pg/mL > 150 pg/mL 90–160 pg/mL 20–40 pg/mL	3.70	37–185 pmol/L 111–370 pmol/L > 555 pmol/L 333–592 pmol/L 74–148 pmol/L	
Follicle-stimulating hormone	Serum or plasma (heparin)	Male < 8 years 8–12 years 12–14 years 14–18 years Adults Female < 8 years 8–12 years 12–14 years 14–18 years Adult Premenopausal Midcycle peak Pregnancy Postmenopausal	 0.3–1.3 ng/mL 0.8–1.1 ng/mL 1.4–2.0 ng/mL 2.0–3.0 ng/mL 0.5–4.5 ng/mL 0.6–0.8 ng/mL 1.2–2.4 ng/mL 1.7–2.8 ng/mL 2.2–3.0 ng/mL 1.1–5.3 ng/mL 2.6–24 ng/mL Undetectable 11.0–66.0 mg/mL	4.50	 1.4–5.9 IU/L 3.6–5.0 IU/L 6.3–9.0 IU/L 9.0–13.5 IU/L 2.25–20 IU/L 2.7–6.3 IU/L 5.4–10.8 IU/L 7.7–12.6 IU/L 9.9–13.5 IU/L 5–24 IU/L 11.7–108 IU/L Undetectable 50–300 IU/L	
Gastric inhibitory peptide (GIP)	Plasma	Fasting Postprandial	250 pg/mL 1000 pg/mL	0.2	50 pmol/L 200 pmol/L	
Gastrin	Serum	Fasting	21–105 pg/mL	0.475	10–50 pmol/L	Overnight fast required. No heparin. Store at –20 °C.
Glucagon	Plasma		50–200 pg/mL	0.287	14–57 pmol/L	Centrifuge immediately under refrigeration. Store in plastic vial at –20 °C.
Growth hormone	Serum	Fasting Children Adults	 < 10 ng/mL < 5 ng/mL	46.5	 < 460 pmol/L < 230 pmol/L	Store at –20 °C. *Note:* GH values fluctuate widely and functional tests must be utilized for diagnosis of GH deficiency or excess. See Chapter 5 for details of suppression and stimulation tests for GH excess or deficiency.
17-Hydroxy-corticoids	Urine	Adult	3–15 mg/24 h (or 3–7 mg/g Cr)	2.76	8.3–41.4 µmol/24 h (or 0.9–2.2 mmol/mol Cr)	Preservative: 10 mL 6N HCl.

Analyte	Specimen	Reference range	Conversion factor	SI reference range	Comments
5-Hydroxyindole-acetic acid	Urine (24 hours)	< 9 mg/24 h	5.23	< 47.1 μmol/d	Preservative: 10 mL 6N HCl. Refrigerate during collection. For 48 hours prior to and during collection, avoid avocados, alcohol, bananas, passion fruit, pineapple, plaintains, plums, tomatoes, nuts, and berries (falsely high results).
18-Hydroxycorti-costerone	Serum	Recumbent (0800) 25.3 ± 2.4 ng/dL Upright (1200) 48.6 ± 4.9 ng/dL	27.51	657 ± 66 pmol/L 1337 ± 135 pmol/L	Process immediately. Store at −20 °C.
17-Hydroxypreg-nenolone	Serum	Cord blood 50–2121 ng/dL Premature infants 64–2380 ng/dL Full-term infants 3 days 10–829 ng/dL 1–6 months 36–763 ng/dL 6–12 months 42–540 ng/dL Prepubertal child (1–10 years) 15–221 ng/dL Pubertal age groups 44–235 ng/dL Adults 53–357 ng/dL	0.0307	1.5–63.8 nmol/L 1.9–71.6 nmol/L 0.3–25.0 nmol/L 1.1–23.0 nmol/L 1.3–16.3 nmol/L 0.5–6.7 nmol/L 1.3–7.1 nmol/L 1.6–10.7 nmol/L	
17-Hydroxypro-gesterone	Serum (fasting preferred)	Newborn to 1 year < 2.2 μg/L Male Prepubertal < 1.0 μg/L Adult < 2.0 μg/L Female Prepubertal < 1.0 μg/L Adult follicular < 1.0 μg/L Adult luteal < 3.6 μg/L Post menopausal < 0.07 μg/L	3.03	< 6.6 nmol/L < 3.0 nmol/L < 6.0 nmol/L < 3.0 nmol/L < 3.0 nmol/L < 10.8 nmol/L < 2.1 nmol/L	
Hydroxyproline	Urine	Total 25–77 mg/d Free < 2 mg/24 h	7.62	191–588 μmol/24 h < 15 μmol/24 h	Preservative: 25 mL 6N HCl. Freeze at −20 °C.
Insulin	Serum	Fasting Newborn 3–20 μU/mL (0.12–0.8 ng/mL) Adult 5–25 μU/mL (0.2–1 ng/mL)	172.1 (ng/mL→pmol/L)	21–138 pmol/L 34–172 pmol/L	Cold centrifuge. Store at −20 °C.
Insulin (with oral glucose tolerance test)	Serum	0 minutes 7–24 μU/mL (0.28–0.96 ng/mL) 30 minutes 25–231 μU/mL (0.96–9.4 ng/mL) 1 hour 18–276 μU/mL (0.72–11 ng/mL) 2 hours 16–166 μU/mL (0.64–6.6 ng/mL) 3 hours 4–38 μU/mL (0.16–1.5 ng/mL)	172.1 (ng/mL→pmol/L)	48–165 pmol/L 165–1621 pmol/L 124–1893 pmol/L 110–1136 pmol/L 28–258 pmol/L	Cold centrifuge. Freeze at −20 °C.

(continued)

Test	Source	Ages, Conditions, Etc	Conventional Units	Conversion Factor	SI Units	Comments
Insulin-like growth factor (IGF-1)	Serum	Male		1.00		
		2 months–5 years	17–248 µg/L		17–248 µg/L	
		6–8 years	88–474 µg/L		88–474 µg/L	
		9–11 years	110–565 µg/L		110–565 µg/L	
		12–15 years	202–957 µg/L		202–957 µg/L	
		16–24 years	182–780 µg/L		182–780 µg/L	
		25–39 years	114–492 µg/L		114–492 µg/L	
		Female				
		2 months–5 years	17–248 µg/L		17–248 µg/L	
		6–8 years	88–474 µg/L		88–474 µg/L	
		9–11 years	117–771 µg/L		117–771 µg/L	
		12–15 years	261–1096 µg/L		261–1096 µg/L	
		16–24 years	182–780 µg/L		182–780 µg/L	
		25–39 years	114–492 µg/L		114–492 µg/L	
Insulin-like growth factor-2 (IGF-2)	Serum	Prepuberty	334–642 µg/L	1.00	334–642 µg/L	
		Puberty	245–737 µg/L		245–737 µg/L	
		Adult	288–736 µg/L		288–736 µg/L	
Insulin-like growth factor binding protein 3	Serum	Male		1.00		Separate serum with 1 hour. Free serum in plastic vial at –20 °C.
		Newborn	0.4–1.4 µg/L		0.4–1.4 µg/L	
		7–30 days	0.8–2.1 µg/L		0.8–2.1 µg/L	
		1–12 months	1.0–2.8 µg/L		1.0–2.8 µg/L	
		1–9 years	1.1–3.6 µg/L		1.1–3.6 µg/L	
		9–13 years	2.0–4.6 µg/L		2.0–4.6 µg/L	
		13–20 years	2.2–5.2 µg/L		2.2–5.2 µg/L	
		> 20 years	2.0–4.9 µg/L		2.0–4.9 µg/L	
		Female				
		Newborn	0.4–1.4 µg/L		0.4–1.4 µg/L	
		7–30 days	0.8–2.1 µg/L		0.8–2.1 µg/L	
		1–12 months	0.9–2.8 µg/L		0.9–2.8 µg/L	
		1–9 years	1.4–3.9 µg/L		1.4–3.9 µg/L	
		9–13 years	1.8–5.1 µg/L		1.8–5.1 µg/L	
		13–20 years	2.2–5.3 µg/L		2.2–5.3 µg/L	
		> 20 years	2.0–4.9 µg/L		2.0–4.9 µg/L	
17-Ketosteroids	Urine	Birth to 8 years	0–1 mg/24 h	3.47	0–3.5 µmol/d	Preservative: 30 mL 3N HCl.
		8 years to puberty	1–10 mg/24 h		3.5–35 µmol/d	
		Adult male	9–22 mg/24 h		31–76 µmol/d	
		Adult female	5–15 mg/24 h		17–52 µmol/d	

Analyte	Specimen		Reference range	Factor	SI reference range	Note
Luteinizing hormone	Plasma or serum	Male				**Note:** Test measures sum of LH and hCG; high hCG levels in pregnancy or trophoblastic disease will cross-react in the assay, giving falsely high LH levels. Freeze specimen at –20 °C.
		< 8 years	1.0–1.2 µg/L	9.00	9.0–10.8 IU/L	
		8–12 years	1.4–1.7 µg/L		12.6–15.3 IU/L	
		12–14 years	1.5–1.7 µg/L		13.5–15.3 IU/L	
		14–16 years	1.6–1.8 µg/L		14.4–16.2 IU/L	
		16–20 years	1.6–1.8 µg/L		14.4–16.2 IU/L	
		Adult	0.4–1.9 µg/L		3.6–17.1 IU/L	
		Female				
		< 8 years	0.7–0.9 µg/L		6.3–8.1 IU/L	
		8–12 years	0.9–1.4 µg/L		8.1–12.6 IU/L	
		12–14 years	0.9–1.3 µg/L		8.0–11.7 IU/L	
		14–16 years	1.5–1.9 µg/L		13.5–17.1 IU/L	
		16–20 years	1.7–3.0 µg/L		15.3–27.0 IU/L	
		Adult	0.5–2.7 µg/L		4.5–24.3 IU/L	
		Midcycle peak	4.2–15.8 µg/L		38–142 IU/L	
		Postmenopausal	3.2–21.0 µg/L		29–189 IU/L	
Metanephrine (total)	Urine		0.3–0.9 mg/24 h	5.03	1.4–4.5 µmol/24 h	Preservative: 30 mL 3N HCl.
Osmolality	Serum		285–293 mosm/kg	1.00	285–293 mosm/kg	
	Urine	Random specimen	300–900 mosm/kg		300–900 mosm/kg	
Pancreatic polypeptide	Plasma	0–19 years	Not established	0.246	Not established	Process immediately and freeze plama at –60 °C.
		20–29 years	< 228 ng/L		< 56.1 pmol/L	
		30–39 years	< 249 ng/L		< 61.3 pmol/L	
		40–49 years	< 270 ng/L		< 66.4 pmol/L	
		50–59 years	< 291 ng/L		< 71.6 pmol/L	
		60–69 years	< 312 ng/L		< 76.8 pmol/L	
		70–79 years	< 332 ng/L		< 81.7 pmol/L	
Parathyroid hormone	Serum		10–60 pg/mL	0.100	1–6 pmol/L	Intact hormone assay. Freeze serum at –20 °C.
Pregnanetriol	24-hour urine	< 7 years	< 0.2 mg/d	2.97	< 0.6 µmol/d	Preservative: 20 mL 33% acetic acid
		7–16 years	0.3–1.1 mg/d		0.9–3.3 µmol/d	
		> 16 years	< 2.0 mg/d		< 0.6 µmol/d	
Progesterone	Serum	Female:		3.18		Freeze at –20 °C.
		Follicular phase	0.3–0.8 ng/mL		1–3 nmol/L	
		Luteal phase	4–20 ng/mL		13–64 nmol/L	
		Male:	0.12–0.3 ng/mL		0.3–0.9 nmol/L	

(continued)

Test	Source	Ages, Conditions, Etc	Conventional Units	Conversion Factor	SI Units	Comments

Prolactin	Serum	Female
		  Newborn
		  1–5 months
		  Childhood
		  Adult
		    Follicular
		    Luteal
		Male
		  Newborn
		  1–5 months
		  Childhood
		  Adult
			
			<500 ng/mL
			6–14 ng/mL
			4–8 ng/mL
			
			<20 ng/mL
			<40 ng/mL
			
			141–189 ng/mL
			6–14 ng/mL
			4–8 ng/mL
			<15 ng/mL
				0.045	
					<20 nmol/L
					0.27–0.64 nmol/L
					0.18–0.36 nmol/L
					
					<0.9 nmol/L
					<1.8 nmol/L
					
					6.4–8.6 nmol/L
					0.27–0.64 nmol/L
					0.18–0.36 nmol/L
					<0.7 nmol/L
						Freeze serum at –20 °C.

Renin	Plasma	Normal sodium diet (75–150 mmol/d)
		  0800 recumbent
		  1200 upright
		Low-sodium diet (30–75 mmol/d)
		  Upright
			
			0.2–2.3 µg/L/h
			1.3–4.0 g/L/h
			
			4.1–7.7 µg/L/h
				0.278	
					
					0.06–0.64 ng/L/s
					0.36–1.12 ng/L/s
					
					1.14–2.14 ng/L/s
						Draw in cold tube, separate plasma, and freeze in plastic within 15 minutes after collection.

Secretin	Plasma	Fasting Postprandial	3–15 pg/mL 30 pg/mL	0.33	1–5 pmol/L 10 pmol/L	
Somatostatin	Plasma	Fasting Postprandial	<2.35 ng/dL 2.35–7.1 ng/dL	4.26	<10 pmol/L 10–30 pmol/L	

Testosterone, total	Serum	Male
		  Prepubertal
		  Pubertal
		  Adult
		Female
		  Prepubertal
		  Pubertal
		  Adult
			
			8–14 ng/dL
			84–180 ng/dL
			300–1000 ng/dL
			
			5–13 ng/dL
			9–24 ng/dL
			30–70 ng/dL
				0.0347	
					0.28–0.49 nmol/L
					2.91–6.24 nmol/L
					10.4–34.7 nmol/L
					
					0.17–0.45 nmol/L
					0.31–0.83 nmol/L
					1.04–2.43 nmol/L
						Freeze at –20 °C.

Testosterone, free	Serum	Adult male Adult female	50–260 pg/mL 3–13 pg/mL	3.47	174–902 pmol/L 10.4–45.1 pmol/L	Freeze at –20 °C.

Thyroglobulin	Serum	Normal
		After total thyroidectomy
		  On T$_4$
		  Off T$_4$
			<56 ng/mL
			
			<5 ng/mL
			<10 ng/mL
				1.00	<56 µg/L
					
					<5 µg/L
					<10 µg/L
						Freeze at –20 °C. The presence of thyroglobulin autoantibodies in the patient's serum may falsely raise or lower the result.

Test	Specimen	Conventional	Factor	SI Units	Comments
Thyroid autoantibodies	Serum	Microsomal antibodies < 1 unit/mL Thyroid antibodies < 1 unit/mL			
Thyroid-stimulating hormone (TSH)	Serum	0.5–5.0 µU/mL	1.00	0.5–5.0 mU/L	Neonatal and cord blood levels are 2–4 times higher.
Thyroid-stimulating immunoglobulin (TSI) (TSH-R Ab [stim])	Serum	< 130% of basal activity			Based on cAMP generation in thyroid cell tissue culture. Freeze at –20 °C.
Thyroid uptake of radioactive iodine (RAIU)	Activity over thyroid gland	Fractional uptake 2 hours 4–12% 6 hours 6–15% 24 hours 8–30%			Ingestion or administration of iodide will decrease thyroid uptake of RAI.
Thyroxine-binding globulin	Serum	16–34 µg/mL	1.00	16–34 mg/L	
Thyroxine (T₄)	Serum	Cord blood 4.6–13 µg/dL 1–3 days 11.8–23.2 µg/dL 3–10 days 9.9–21.9 µg/dL 10–45 days 8.2–16.2 µg/dL 45–90 days 6.4–14 µg/dL 3–12 months 7.8–16.5 µg/dL 1–5 years 7.3–15.0 µg/dL 5–10 years 6.4–13.3 µg/dL 10–15 years 5.6–11.7 µg/dL 15–20 years 4.2–11.8 µg/dL > 20 years 5.0–12.0 µg/dL	12.87	59.2–167 nmol/L 151.9–298.6 nmol/L 127.4–281.9 nmol/L 105.5–208.5 nmol/L 82.4–180.2 nmol/L 100.4–212.4 nmol/L 94.0–193.1 nmol/L 82.4–171.2 nmol/L 72.1–150.5 nmol/L 54.1–151.9 nmol/L 64.4–154.4 nmol/L	Refrigerate serum. Fasting preferred. Elevated levels in pregnancy due to increased TBG.
Thyroxine, free (FT₄)	Serum	0–4 days 2.2–5.3 ng/dL > 2 weeks 0.9–2.0 ng/dL	12.87	28–68 pmol/L 12–26 pmol/L	By dialysis. FT₄ by two-step immunoassay is comparable.
Resin T₄ uptake (RT₄U)	Serum	25–35%	0.01	0.25–0.35	RT₄U may be expressed as ratio to normal.
Free thyroxine index	Serum	Product of T₄ × RT₄U = 1.3–4.2 arbitrary units. (Expressed as T₄ adjusted for TBG binding = 5–12 arbitrary units.)		Product of T₄ × RT₄U = 16–54 arbitrary units or, adjusted: 64–154.	
Thyroxine:TBG ratio	Serum	T₄ (µg/dL) ÷ TBG (µg/mL) = 0.2–0.5	0.0154	T₄ (nmol/L) ÷ TBG (mg/L) = 2.7–6.4	
Triiodothyronine (T₃)	Serum	Cord blood 15–75 ng/dL 1–3 days 32–216 ng/dL 3–10 days 50–250 ng/dL 1–12 months 105–280 ng/dL 1–5 years 105–269 ng/dL 5–10 years 94–241 ng/dL 10–15 years 83–213 ng/dL 15–20 years 80–210 ng/dL > 20 years 88–160 ng/dL	0.0154	0.23–1.2 nmol/L 0.49–3.3 nmol/L 0.77–3.8 nmol/L 1.6–4.3 nmol/L 1.6–4.1 nmol/L 1.4–3.7 nmol/L 1.3–3.3 nmol/L 1.2–3.2 nmol/L 1.4–2.6 nmol/L	Refrigerate serum. Elevated levels in pregnancy due to increased TBG.

(continued)

Test	Source	Ages, Conditions, Etc	Conventional Units	Conversion Factor	SI Units	Comments
Free T_3 index	Serum	Expressed as product of $T_3 \times TR_4U = 24$–67 (arbitrary units)			0.375–1.02 (arbitrary units)	
Free T_3 (FT$_3$)	Serum		0.2–0.52 ng/dL	15.4	3–8 pmol/L	
Reverse T_3 (RT$_3$)	Serum		25–75 ng/mL	0.0154	0.39–1.5 nmol/L	
Vanillylmandelic acid (VMA)	Urine (24-hour)	Newborn Infant Child Adolescent Adult	< 1 mg/d < 2 mg/d 1–3 mg/d 1–5 mg/d 2–7 mg/d	5.88	< 5.8 nmol/d < 11.7 nmol/d 5.8–17.6 nmol/d 5.8–29.4 nmol/d 11.8–41.2 nmol/d	
	Urine (24-hour or "spot")	1–12 months 1–2 years 2–5 years 5–10 years > 10 years	μg VMA/mg Cr < 36 < 31 < 17 < 15 < 11	0.573	mmol VMA/mol Cr < 20.5 < 17.7 < 9.7 < 8.6 < 6.3	
Vasoactive intestinal polypeptide	Plasma		< 33 pg/mL	0.30	< 10 pmol/L	Freeze at –60 °C.
Vitamin D (25-hydroxy)	Serum		10–50 ng/mL	2.50	25–125 nmol/L	Measures both D_2 and D_3. Freeze serum in plastic tube at –20 °C.
Vitamin D (1,25-dihydroxy)	Serum		20–60 pg/mL	2.50	50–150 pmol/L	Measures both D_2 and D_3. Freeze serum at –60 °C in plastic tube.

[1] Adapted from the *Clinical Laboratories Manual* of the University of California Hospital and Clinics, San Francisco, California, July 28, 1995. The factors used in converting conventional units to SI units were derived, in part, from the *CRC Handbook of Chemistry and Physics*. It is important to emphasize that normal ranges vary among different laboratories; it is essential for the clinician to know the normal range for the test of interest in the laboratory performing the test.
[2] Semen analysis is discussed in Chapter 12.

Index

Abdominal pain, endocrine disease and, 29t
Abetalipoproteinemia, recessive, 700–701
Abortion, threatened, progestins and, 471
Acanthosis nigricans, insulin-resistant diabetes mellitus and, 612
Acarbose, daily dose and duration of action, 624t
Accelerated hypertension, 377
Accessory molecules, 81–83
A cells, 595
    secretory products, 596t
Acetabulum, Paget's disease and, 310f
Acetohexamide
    daily dose and duration of action, 624t
    for diabetes mellitus, 624
Acetylcholine, endocrine system and, 11–12
Achalasia, gut peptides and, 587
Achondroplasia, autosomal dominant, short stature and, 175
Acidosis
    hyperchloremic, 649
    lactic, diabetes mellitus and, 644, 652
Acid secretion, hormones affecting, 589t
Acquired immunodeficiency syndrome. See AIDS
Acromegaly, 136–142, 138f, 139f
    clinical manifestations, 132t
    radiologic signs, 140f
    secondary hypertriglyceridemia and, 695
ACTH. See Adrenocorticotropic hormone
ACTH stimulation test, 332–333
    adrenocortical insufficiency and, 338–339
    hypothalamic-pituitary function and, 119t
    normal reference ranges, 788t
Active suppression, 84
Addison's disease, 334–338, 761–765
    adrenal autoantibodies and, 761t
    autoimmune, 334–335
    autoimmune disorders and, 761t
    causes, 334t
    clinical features, 336–338, 336t
    clinical heterogeneity, 762–765, 762f
    etiology and pathology, 334–336
    hypoparathyroidism and, 763

isolated, 764
    maintenance therapy, 341–342, 341t
    pathophysiology, 336
    sequence for onset, 764f
Addisonian crisis, treatment, 340–341, 341t
Adenoma
    adrenal. See Adrenal adenoma
    aldosterone-producing
        incidental adrenal mass and, 356
        management, 364–366
    C cell, 756
    cortisol-producing, incidental adrenal mass and, 356
    pituitary. See Pituitary adenoma
    toxic, 241–242
Adenylyl cyclase, activation by G proteins, 62
ADH. See Antidiuretic hormone
Adipose tissue
    adrenergic responses, 389t
    glucocorticoids and, 327
    insulin and, 601
Adolescence, constitutional delay, 170–173, 530, 531f
    treatment, 538
Adrenal adenoma, 348
    glucocorticoid-secreting, Cushing's syndrome and, 345
    pathophysiology, 346
    treatment, 353
Adrenal androgens. See Androgens
Adrenal autoantibodies, Addison's disease and, 761t
Adrenal carcinoma, 348
    Cushing's syndrome and, 345
    pathophysiology, 346
    treatment, 353
Adrenal cortex, 319f
    fetal, endocrinology, 559
    pregnancy and, 557
    steroid biosynthesis and, 321f
Adrenal crisis, acute, 337
    clinical features, 337t
    prevention, 342
    treatment, 341t
Adrenalectomy, ACTH-secreting pituitary tumors and, 144–145
Adrenal gland
    ACTH deficiency and, 115
    adenoma. See Adrenal adenoma

AIDS and, 336
anatomy, 318–320
cancer therapy and, 728–729
circulating sex steroids and, 407t
congenital hyperplasia. See Congenital adrenal hyperplasia
cortex. See Adrenal cortex
cortical insufficiency. See Adrenocortical insufficiency
embryology, 317–318
hypersecretion, elderly and, 783
hypertension and, 359–371
insufficiency, 330
    elderly and, 783–784
    hypercalcemia and, 284
location and blood supply, 318f
medulla. See Adrenal medulla
metastatic disease, 335–336
nodular hyperplasia, treatment, 354
steroid biosynthetic pathways, 505f
Adrenal hemorrhage, 337
    adrenal insufficiency and, 335
    clinical features, 337t
Adrenal mass, incidental, 354–356, 355f
Adrenal medulla, 381–401
    anatomy, 381–382
    hormones, 382–392. See also specific type
    hyperfunction, 393
    hypofunction, 392–393
Adrenal medullary hyperplasia, 396
Adrenal rest tissue, incomplete precocious puberty and, 542
Adrenal tumors
    androgen- and estrogen-producing, 367
    Cushing's syndrome and, 343, 345
    etiology and pathogenesis, 345
    prognosis, 354
    treatment, 353–354
Adrenarche, 529
    premature, 543
Adrenergic agonists/antagonists, characteristics interactions, 389t
Adrenergic antagonists, for pheochromocytoma, 399–400
Adrenergic cells, embryonic development, 382f
Adrenergic receptors. See also Alpha-adrenergic receptors; Beta-adrenergic receptors

Adrenergic receptors (*cont.*)
  types and subtypes, 388*t*
Adrenoceptors, types and subtypes, 388*t*
Adrenocortical carcinoma, 355
  aldosterone-producing, 364
Adrenocortical hyperplasia, Cushing's
      syndrome and, 344
Adrenocortical insufficiency, 334–343
  autoimmune, 334–335
  diagnosis, 338–340
  primary, 334–338. *See also* Addison's
      disease
    causes, 334*t*
    clinical features, 336*t*
    evaluation, 339*f*
    maintenance therapy, 341–342,
        341*t*
    prognosis, 343
  secondary, 338
    evaluation, 339*f*
  steroid coverage for surgery and, 342,
      342*t*
  treatment, 340–342
Adrenocortical steroids. *See* Steroid
      hormones
Adrenocorticotropic hormone (ACTH).
      See also Ectopic ACTH
      syndrome
  adrenal cortex and, 322
  biosynthesis, function, measurement,
      secretion, 104–106
  characteristics, 105*t*
  cortisol-secreting cells and, 322*f*
  deficiency, 114–115
    hypopituitarism and, 127
  hypersecretion, 115
    ectopic, 343
  for hypopituitarism, 129
  maternal, changes during pregnancy,
      551*f*
  normal reference ranges, 788*t*
  pituitary adenomas secreting, 142–144
  plasma, 114
    adrenal insufficiency and, 339–340,
        340*f*
    age and, 783*f*
    Cushing's syndrome and, 350
    daily fluctuations, 323*f*
    feedback inhibition, 323–324, 324*f*
    measurement, 330
  secretion, 322
    abnormalities, 345–346
    episodic, pulsatile pattern, 107*f*
  secretory reserve, evaluation, 114–115
  steroidogenesis and, 322–323
Adrenoleukodystrophy, X-linked, adrenal
      insufficiency and, 335
Adrenomedullin, 391
Adult Leydig cell failure, 423
Adults, hypothyroidism and, 227–229,
      227*f*
Adult seminiferous tubule failure,
      421–423
Adult stature, RWT method for
      predicting, 171–172*t*
Age
  physiologic function in humans and,
      771*f*
  serum parathyroid hormone and, 777*f*

Aging. *See also* Elderly
  osteoporosis and, 295–296
  thyroid function and, 216
Agonist, 9
  hormone, 10
AIDS
  adrenal gland and, 336
  pentamidine-induced hypoglycemia
      and, 672
Albright's hereditary osteodystrophy, G
      protein-coupled receptors and,
      65
Albumin
  binding site for thyroid hormones,
      203
  cortisol binding and, 325
Alcohol ingestion
  lipoprotein disorders and, 704
  secondary hypertriglyceridemia and,
      694–695
Aldosterone
  basal levels, Cushing's syndrome and,
      368*f*
  maternal, changes during pregnancy,
      550*f*
  mineralocorticoid activity, 359–360
  normal reference ranges, 788*t*
  secretion, ACTH stimulation test and,
      333
  synthesis of, pathway of, 50*f*
  trivial and chemical names, 51*t*
Aldosterone-18-glucuronide, normal ref-
      erence ranges, 788*t*
Aldosterone-producing adenoma
  incidental adrenal mass and, 356
  management, 364–366
Aldosterone-producing adrenocortical
      carcinoma, 364
Aldosteronism
  glucocorticoid-remedial, 364
  primary, 362–366
    clinical features, 362–363
    diagnosis, 363–364
    management, 364–366
    postural stimulation and, 364*f*
    rare forms, 364
Alendronate disodium, for osteoporosis,
      303
Alimentary hypoglycemia
  functional, 677–678
  postgastrectomy, 677
Allergy, insulin, 640
Allopregnanolone, trivial and chemical
      names, 51*t*
Alpha-adrenergic receptor blockers,
      pheochromocytoma and,
      397–398
Alpha-adrenergic receptors, 389
Alpha-glucosidase inhibitors, for diabetes
      mellitus, 626–627
Aluminum deposition,
      hypoparathyroidism and, 288
Amenorrhea
  in absence of sexual maturation,
      454–455
  with androgen excess, 461–463
  athletes and, 459
  causes, 454*t*
  diagnostic evaluation, 456*f*

endocrine disease and, 29*t*
  galactorrhea and, 460
  hypothalamic, 459
  post-pill, 460
  in presence of sexual maturation,
      455–460
  primary, normal secondary sexual
      development and, 537
  prolactinoma and, 132
AMH. *See* Anti-mullerian hormone
Amines. *See also* Catecholamines
  rate of secretion
    asphyxia and, 385*f*
    insulin injection and, 385*f*
Amino acids, glucagon release and,
      603
Aminoglutethimide, for Cushing's
      disease, 144
Amiodarone, for toxic multinodular
      goiter, 242
Amitriptyline, for sensory neuropathy,
      657
Amplifiers, 600
Amylin, 602
Amyotrophy, diabetic, 657
Anabolic agents, for osteoporosis,
      303–304
Anabolism, insulin and, 601
Anandrone, mechanism and tumor target,
      732*t*
Anaplastic carcinoma, thyroid. *See*
      Thyroid cancer
Androblastoma, amenorrhea and,
      458–459
Androgen(s)
  adrenal tumors producing, 367
  for androgen deficiency, 414
  autonomous secretion, incomplete pre-
      cocious puberty and, 541
  biologic effects, 329–330
  biosynthesis, 320–324
  circulation, 324–325
    women and, 461*t*
  conversion and excretion, 325–
      326
  end-organ resistance, 512–514
  excess
    amenorrhea and, 461–463
    Cushing's disease and, 346
  for hypopituitarism, 129
  laboratory evaluation, 330–334
  maternal, female
      pseudohermaphroditism and,
      508
  measurement, 334
  mechanism of action, 407*f*
  metabolism, 325–326
    disorders in women, 460–463
  ovarian
    menstrual cycle and, 443–444
    physiologic effects, 441
  pregnancy and, 557
  prenatal exposure, female
      pseudohermaphroditism and,
      504*f*
  production, adrenocorticotropic
      hormone and, 324
  release, 40
  synthesis/secretion by preovulatory

follicle, pathways involved, 445*f*

testicular, biosynthetic pathways, 406*f*

use in therapy, 22*t*

Androgen receptor, defects, 512–514

Androgen receptor gene, 513*f*

Andropause, 423

Androstenediol glucuronide, normal reference ranges, 788*t*

Androstenedione

circulating, women and, 461*t*

maternal, changes during pregnancy, 551*f*

normal ranges in men, 411*t*

normal reference ranges, 788*t*

ovarian

concentrations, production and secretion rates, 438*t*

percentage distribution, 438*t*

serum concentrations, menopause and, 473*t*

Anemia

endocrine disease and, 29*t*

hypothyroidism and, 228–229

Anergy, 84

Aneuploidy, prenatal screening and, 552

Angiotensin converting enzyme, 373

Angiotensin II, 373

effects in brain, 373–374

sequence of formation, 372*f*

Angiotensinogen, 372–373

Anorchia, 535–536

bilateral, 417–418

congenital, 516

Anorexia nervosa

amenorrhea and, 460

endocrine disease and, 29*t*

hypogonadotropic hypogonadism and, 534

hypothalamic-pituitary axis and, 118

secondary hypercholesterolemia and, 698

Anosmia, 455

Anovulation, pathophysiology in polycystic ovary syndrome, 462*f*

Anovulatory bleeding, 468–469

ANP. *See* Atrial natriuretic peptide

Antagonists, hormone, 10

Antiandrogens

for hirsutism, 466–468

ovarian function inhibition and, 472–473

Antibodies, 76, 83

Antidiuretic hormone (ADH), 102

actions, 146–147

normal reference ranges, 788*t*

radioimmunoassay, 151–152

secretion, control, 148–149

syndrome of inappropriate secretion, 152–153

cancer and, 747

conditions associated, 153*t*

Antiestrogens, ovarian function inhibition and, 471

Anti-mullerian hormone (AMH), 491–492

defects in synthesis and secretion, 516

Antiprogestins, ovarian function inhibition and, 472

Antithyroid drug therapy, for Graves' disease, 238–239

Antral follicle, 444

Antral G cell hyperplasia, gut peptides and, 587

Antrum, 444

Anxiety, menopause and, 474

"Apathetic hyperthyroidism", 238

Apolipoprotein(s), 681–682

Apolipoprotein A-1, 682

Apolipoprotein A-II, 682

Apolipoprotein A-IV, 682

Apomorphine, growth hormone secretion and, 108

APUD cells, 579

hormone secretion and, 742–743

Arachidonic acid, 6

eicosanoid derivation and, 53–54

Arborization, 450

Arginine, growth hormone levels and, 116

Arginine infusion test, hypothalamic-pituitary function and, 119*t*

Arginine vasopressin. *See also* Vasopressin

structure, 101*t*

Arnold-Healy-Gordon syndrome, 371

Arrhenoblastoma, amenorrhea and, 458–459

Arteriosclerosis, 680–681

Asherman's syndrome, amenorrhea and, 457

Aspartame, diabetes mellitus and, 621–622

Atherogenicity, triglyceride-rich lipoproteins and, 689

Atherosclerosis, reversal, 681

Athletes, amenorrhea and, 459

Athyreotic cretins, 247

Atrial natriuretic peptide (ANP), hypertension and, 378

Atrophic thyroiditis, 247

Autacoids, hypertension and, 379

Autoantibodies, thyroid, measurement, 223–224

Autoantigens, thyroid, 217*t*

Autocrine, 3

Autocrine delivery, 576

Autocrine factors, tumor growth and, 726–727

Autocrine hormone, 87

Autoimmune adrenocortical insufficiency, 334–335

Autoimmune disease, 88–93

Addison's disease and, 761*t*

animal models, 93

environment and, 90–91

genetic aspects, 88–89, 766

HLA antigen association, 766*t*

HLA genotype and, 89*t*

induction models, 91–93

major histocompatibility complex and, 89–90

pregnancy and, 23

T and B cells and, 91

thyroid, 247*f*

Autoimmune endocrinopathy, 761–762

clinical categories, 763*f*

Autoimmune hypoglycemia, 672

Autoimmune hypoparathyroidism, sequence for onset, 764*f*

Autoimmune hypophysitis, 765

Autoimmune response, development by molecular mimicry, 92, 92*f*

Autoimmunity

interrelationships against islet, parietal, and thyroid cells, 765*t*

thyroid, 217–218

Autonomic hyperactivity, hypoglycemia and, 641

Autonomic insufficiency, disorders associated, 393*t*

Autonomic nervous system (ANS)

obesity and, 720

response to hypoglycemia, 667*t*

Autonomic neuropathy, diabetes mellitus and, 657–658

Autosomal karyotypic disorders, short stature and, 175

Autosomal recessive hypophosphatemic rickets, 307

B7, 82

B apolipoprotein, 681–682

deficiency, primary hypolipidemia and, 700–701

familial ligand-defective, 697

Bardet-Biedl syndrome, hypogonadotropic hypogonadism and, 533

Barraquer-Simmons synrome, 702

Barr body, 489*f*

Basal layer, 448

Basal metabolic rate (BMR), thyroid hormones and, 223

Basal-parabasal cells, 451

B cells

autoimmunity and, 91

immune response and, 88

thyroid regulation and, 212

B cells (pancreatic), 595–596

insulin release, sulfonylurea stimulation and, 623*f*

preproinsulin biosynthesis and, 596–597, 597*f*

secretory products, 596*t*

tumors, hypoglycemia and, 672–676

type I diabetes mellitus and, 606–607

Beckwith-Wiedemann syndrome, tall stature and, 188–189

Benign prostatic hyperplasia, 784–785

Beta-adrenergic antagonists, use in therapy, 22*t*

Beta-adrenergic receptors, 389

signaling in cytoplasmic and nuclear compartments, 63*f*

thyroid hormones and, 214

Betamethasone, chemical name, 51*t*

Biedl-Bardet syndrome, short stature and, 175

Biguanides, for diabetes mellitus, 625–626

Bilateral anorchia, 417–418

Bilateral nodular hyperplasia, Cushing's syndrome and, 344
Bile acid sequestrants, for hyper-lipoproteinemia, 705–706
Bioamines, endocrine system and, 11–12
Biopsy
  fine-needle aspiration, 223
  testicular, male hypogonadism and, 412
  thyroid, 223
  thyroid nodule, 251
Birth weight, diabetic mothers and, 189
Bisphosphonates
  for osteoporosis, 303
  for Paget's disease of bone, 311
  rickets/osteomalacia and, 307
Blood cells, glucocorticoids and, 328
Blood glucose monitoring
  diabetes mellitus and, 615–616
  insulin dosage during pregnancy and, 569*t*
Blood pressure, pheochromocytoma and, 398*f*
Blood vessels, adrenergic responses, 389*t*
Blood volume
  osmolality and, 148–149
  plasma vasopressin and, 149*f*
BMD. *See* Bone mineral density
BMR. *See* Basal metabolic rate
Body composition, 712*f*
Body fluids, calcium concentrations, 264*t*
Bombesin, properties, 582–583
Bone. *See also* Fractures
  age, 170
  cells, 292–294
  demineralization, diabetes mellitus and, 659
  densitometry, osteoporosis and, 300
  density, of lumbar spine and femoral neck, 300*f*
  diabetes mellitus and, 659
  disease
    chronic renal failure and, 311–313
    hyperparathyroid, 279, 280*f*
  functions, 290–291
  glucocorticoids and, 328
  mass, delayed puberty and, 539
  mineral, 292
  Paget's disease, 308–311, 309*f*, 310*f*
    complications, 311*t*
  physiology, factors affecting, 776–779
  remodeling, 294–295
  resorption
    osteoclast-mediated, 293*f*
    thyroid hormones and, 215
  structure, 291–295, 291*f*
  vitamin D and, 274
Bone mineral density (BMD), 296*f*
  annual percentage change in, 778*f*
  femoral neck, versus age, 779*f*
Brain
  cancer therapy and, 728
  effects of angiotensin II, 373–374
Brain-gut axis, 578–579, 579*t*
Breast cancer, 732–736
  hypercalcemia and, 746
  in men, 736
  pregnancy and, 563–564
  in women, 732–736

  associated risk factors, 733*t*
  treatment, 734–736, 734*f*
Breast development, 521
  stages, 522*f*
Breast disease, benign, breast cancer and, 733
Bromocriptine
  growth hormone secretion and, 108
  ovulation induction and, 470
  for prolactinoma, 134–135
Bronchioles, adrenergic responses, 389*t*
Buserelin, ovarian function inhibition and, 471

Cabergoline, for prolactinoma, 135
Calcitonin, 269–271. *See also* Salmon calcitonin
  amino acid sequence, 270*f*
  medullary thyroid carcinoma and, 756–757
  normal reference ranges, 789*t*
  for osteoporosis, 303
  plasma, endocrine tumors and, 757*t*
  tumors secreting, 749–750
Calcitonin gene, alternative processing, 270*f*
Calcitonin gene-related peptide (CGRP), 269–270
  distribution, 579*t*
  hypertension and, 379
  mode of delivery, 576*t*
  properties, 583
Calcitonin stimulation test, normal reference ranges, 789*t*
Calcitriol, for renal osteodystrophy, 313
Calcium
  absorption, vitamin D and, 273–274
  concentrations in body fluids, 264*t*
  fluxes in state of zero external mineral balance, 264*f*
  insulin release and, 599
  metabolism
    cellular and extracellular, 263–264
    glucocorticoids and, 328
  nutrition, osteoporosis and, 297*t*
  for osteoporosis, 780
  for renal osteodystrophy, 313
  serum, parathyroid hormone and, 265*f*
Calcium carbonate supplements, menopause and, 477
Calnexin, 43
Caloric intake, restriction, lipoprotein disorders and, 703
Campomelic dysplasia, 491
Cancer
  breast. *See* Breast cancer
  chemoprevention, 739
  Cushing's syndrome and, 747–748
  endocrine therapy, 729–732
  endometrial. *See* Endometrial cancer
  hormones and, 21–22, 724–739
  hypercalcemia and, 743–746
  prostatic, 738–739
  syndrome of inappropriate ADH secretion and, 747
  thyroid. *See* Thyroid cancer

Candidiasis, mucocutaneous, sequence for onset, 764*f*
Capillary morphometry, diabetes mellitus and, 617
C apolipoprotein, 682
Carbimazole, structure, 201*f*
Carbohydrate
  lipid metabolism and, 704
  metabolism
    oral contraceptives and, 479
    thyroid hormones and, 215
Carbohydrate intolerance, aging and, 774–775
Carcinoid syndrome, 589–590
Carcinoid tumors, 589–590
Carcinoma. *See specific type*; Cancer
Cardiac muscle contractility, thyroid hormones and, 214, 223
Cardiac output
  glucocorticoids and, 329
  oral contraceptives and, 479
Cardiomyopathy, hypothyroid, 228*f*
Cardiovascular disease, menopause and, 475–476
Cardiovascular system, functions, hormones and, 22
Casodex
  mechanism and tumor target, 732*t*
  ovarian function inhibition and, 472–473
Catabolism, insulin and, 601
Cataracts, diabetes mellitus and, 655
Catecholamines, 382–391
  biosynthesis, 382–384, 383*f*
  conjugation, 387–388
  counterregulatory response to hypoglycemia and, 665
  hormone secretion and, 391
  mechanism of action, 388–389
  metabolism, 56, 386, 386*f*
  metabolism and elimination, 20
  normal reference ranges, 789*t*
  parturition and, 560
  physiologic effects, 390–391
  plasma levels
    pheochromocytoma and, 398*f*
    range in healthy subjects, 396*t*
  present as norepinephrine in various species, 384*t*
  regulation of activity, 390
  secretion, 49, 384–386
  storage, 384
  transport, 386
  uptake, 386–387
  urinary, maximal normal concentrations, 397*t*
Catechol-*O*-methyltransferase (COMT), catecholamine metabolism and, 386*f*
Caveolae, 48
CBG. *See* Corticosteroid-binding globulin
C cell adenoma, 756
C cell hyperplasia, 756
CCK. *See* Cholecystokinin
CD3, 82
CD4, 82
CD8, 82

CD28, 82
CD40 ligand, 88
Celiac disease, short stature and, 175–176
Cell growth, hormones and, 21–22
Cell-mediated immunity, 76
Cell surface receptors, for hormones, 6
Cellular dehydration, thirst/ADH secretion and, 148
Central lymphoid organ, 84
Central nervous system (CNS)
  disorders
    hypogonadotropic hypogonadism and, 530–532
    precocious puberty and, 540–541
  glucocorticoids and, 329
  hormones and, 22
  oral contraceptives and, 478
Cerebral gigantism, 188
Cerebrotendinous xanthomatosis, 702
Cerebrovascular disease, oral contraceptives and, 481
Cervical mucus
  menstrual cycle and, 450, 451f
  patterns, 452f
CF. See Cystic fibrosis
CGRP. See Calcitonin gene-related peptide
CHAOS, 609
Chemical mediators, intercellular communication and, 96f
Chemo-endocrine therapy, 732
Chemotherapy, gonadal failure and, 535
Children, hypothyroidism and, 227
Chlorpropamide
  daily dose and duration of action, 624t
  for diabetes mellitus, 623–624
  hypoglycemia and, 671
Chlorthalidone, hypercalcemia and, 284
Cholangitis, oral contraceptives and, 481
Cholecystitis, oral contraceptives and, 481
Cholecystokinin (CCK)
  carboxyl terminal polypeptides, 580f
  distribution, 579t
  mode of delivery, 576t
  normal reference ranges, 789t
  properties, 580–581
Cholera, G protein-coupled receptors and, 65
Cholera toxin, G protein transduction system and, 62
Cholestasis, secondary hypercholesterolemia and, 698–699
Cholestatic jaundice, oral contraceptives and, 481
Cholesterol
  elevated serum levels, 688–689
  homeostasis in cell, 685f
  intracellular storage and transport, 52
  metabolism, 320–321
  synthesis and uptake, 51–52, 320
Cholesterol economy, 686
Cholesterol intake, reduction, lipoprotein disorders and, 703–704
Cholesteryl ester storage disease, 702

Cholesteryl ester transfer protein deficiency, 702
Cholestyramine, for hyperlipoproteinemia, 705
Cholinergic neurotransmitters, counterregulatory response to hypoglycemia and, 667
Chorionic gonadotropin, for cryptorchidism, 420
Chorionic gonadotropin stimulation test, male hypogonadism and, 411–412
Chorionic peptides, pregnancy and, 553
Chromaffin cells, 382
Chromaffin tissue, extra-adrenal in newborn, 395f
Chromogranin(s), 384
Chromogranin A, plasma, endocrine tumors and, 757t
Chromosome(s)
  abnormalities, fetal growth and, 158
  metaphase, 488f
  sex. See Sex chromosomes
Chromosome 11, type I diabetes mellitus and, 607
Chronic disease, short stature and, 175–176
Chylomicron(s)
  metabolism, 682f
  secretion, 682–683
Chylomicron retention disease, 701
CI-164,384, ovarian function inhibition and, 471
Circadian rhythm, CRH/ACTH secretion and, 323
Circumventricular organs, 103, 103f
Cisapride, for diabetic gastroparesis, 658
Clomiphene citrate, ovulation induction and, 469
Clomiphene citrate stimulation test
  hypothalamic-pituitary function and, 117, 120t
  male hypogonadism and, 412
Clonal deletion, 84
Clone, 78
Clonidine suppression test, pheochromo-cytoma and, 397
Cognate antigen, 84
Colestipol, for hyperlipoproteinemia, 705
Colles' fracture, indices in relation to age, 475f
Colloid, 49
Coma
  diabetic, 644–645
    laboratory abnormalities and, 644t
  hyperglycemic, 644
  hypoglycemic, 644, 651–652
  myxedema
    hypothyroidism and, 230–231
    treatment, 232
  nonketotic hyperosmolar, elderly and, 776
Compact layer, 448
COMT. See Catechol-O-methyl-transferase
Congenital adrenal hyperplasia (CAH), 330

adult-onset, amenorrhea/hirsutism and, 463
clinical manifestations, 506t
enzyme deficiencies and, 505f
female pseudohermaphroditism and, 504
11beta-hydroxylase deficiency and, 366
Congenital anorchia, 516
Congenital lipoid adrenal hyperplasia, male sexual differentiation and, 509–510
Congenital malformations, maternal diabetes mellitus and, 569–570, 570t
Connective tissue
  disorders, osteoporosis and, 298
  glucocorticoids and, 328
Constipation, endocrine disease and, 29t
Constitutional delay, 530, 531f
  treatment, 538
Constitutional short stature, 170–173
Constitutional tall stature, 188
Constitutive secretory pathway, 46
Contraception
  hormonal, 477–482
    noncontraceptive advantages, 481–482
  progestins and, 482
Contraceptives
  oral. See Oral contraceptives
  postcoital, 482
    schedules for use, 482f
Controlled system, food intake and, 711–715, 711f, 722f
COP I, 46
COP II, 46
Copper deposition, hypoparathyroidism and, 288
Co-receptors, 81–83
  T cell, 82t
Coronary disease, familial hypoalphalipoproteinemia and, 699
Corpus albicans, 445
Corpus luteum, 444–445
  function markers, 549
Cortical bone
  formation, stages involved, 294f
  remodeling with age, 778f
Corticosteroid(s)
  excess, secondary hypertriglyceridemia and, 694
  obesity and, 720–721
  urinary, measurement, 331
Corticosteroid-binding globulin (CBG)
  aldosterone binding, 359
  cortisol and, 324–325
  progesterone binding, 437
  steroid hormones and, 17
Corticosterone, trivial and chemical names, 51t
Corticotroph, 99
Corticotropin, counterregulatory response to hypoglycemia and, 666
Corticotropin-releasing hormone (CRH), 101–102
  secretion, 322

Corticotropin-releasing hormone (CRH)
(*cont.*)
structure, 101*t*
Corticotropin-releasing hormone (CRH)
test
ACTH responses and, 333
hypothalamic-pituitary function and,
120*t*
Cortisol
for adrenocortical insufficiency, 341
basal levels, Cushing's syndrome and,
368*f*
biosynthesis, 320–324
circulation, 324–325
classification of action, 9*f*
conversion and excretion, 325
excess, effects, 346
free and bound, 324–325
laboratory evaluation, 330–334
maternal, changes during pregnancy,
550*f*
metabolism, 325–326
pathways, 370*f*
mineralocorticoid activity, 359
normal reference ranges, 789*t*
ovarian, percentage distribution, 438*t*
plasma
adrenal insufficiency and, 340*f*
age and, 783*f*
measurement, 330–331
responses to surgery, 323*f*
syndrome of primary resistance,
367
synthesis, pathway, 50*f*
thyrotropin and, 111
trivial and chemical names, 51*t*
urinary
Cushing's syndrome and, 349–350
measurement, 331
urinary metabolites, syndrome of
apparent mineralcorticoid
excess and, 370*f*
Cortisol-producing adenoma, incidental
adrenal mass and, 356
Cortisol resistance, adrenal gland and,
336
Cortisone, trivial and chemical names, 51*t*
Co-stimulatory signals, 84
Cosyntropin test, hypothalamic-pituitary
function and, 119*t*
C peptide, 597–598
normal reference ranges, 789*t*
structure, 598*f*
Cranial nerve palsy, diabetes mellitus
and, 657
Craniopharyngioma, 124
delayed puberty and, 531
Craniotomy, transfrontal, for
prolactinoma, 134
Cretinism, 226–227, 227*f*
CRH. *See* Corticotropin-releasing
hormone
Cryptorchidism, 419–420, 535–536
CTLA-4, 82
Cushing's disease, 142–144, 343, 348
etiology and pathogenesis, 345
pathophysiology, 345–346
prognosis, 354
treatment, 353

Cushing's syndrome, 343–354
adrenal CT scans, 352*f*
basal mineralocorticoid levels and,
368*f*
cancer and, 747–748
childhood, 343
classification and incidence, 343
clinical features, 346–348, 347*t*
dexamethasone suppression test and,
331–332
diagnosis, 348–350, 349*f*
differential, 343*t*, 350–353
problems, 350
elderly and, 783
etiology and pathogenesis, 345
hypertension and, 367–368
pathology, 344–345
pathophysiology, 345–346
plasma ACTH and, 330
prognosis, 354
short stature and, 185–186
treatment, 353–354
Cutaneous xanthoma, eruptive, 690
Cyclic AMP, insulin release and,
599–600
Cyclic AMP response element binding
protein (CREB), bound to
consensus CRE, 63*f*
Cyclosporine, interleukin-2 production
and, 87
Cyproterone, ovarian function inhibition
and, 472
Cyproterone acetate
for hirsutism, 466–468
ovarian function inhibition and,
472
Cystic fibrosis (CF)
membrane protein mutations and,
49
short stature and, 175
Cytochrome P450, 52
Cytokine(s), 83–84
properties, 85–86*t*
Cytokine receptors, 67–68

DAG. *See* Diacylglycerol
Danazol, ovarian function inhibition and,
472
D apolipoprotein, 682
Dawn phenomenon, 638
DCCT. *See* Diabetes Control &
Complications Trial
D cells, 595–596
secretory products, 596*t*
Decidua, 549
Definitive zone, 317
Dehydration
plasma vasopressin and, 152*f*
thirst/ADH secretion and, 148
Dehydroepiandrosterone (DHEA)
circulating, women and, 461*t*
maternal, changes during pregnancy,
551*f*
normal reference ranges, 790*t*
ovarian, concentrations, production
and secretion rates, 438*t*
serum concentrations, menopause and,
473*t*

structure, 320*f*
trivial and chemical names, 51*t*
Dehydroepiandrosterone (DHEA) sulfate
circulating, women and, 461*t*
normal reference ranges, 790*t*
serum concentrations
childhood and, 529*t*
menopause and, 473*t*
Delayed puberty, 530–539
classification, 530*t*
differential diagnosis, 537–538, 537*t*
treatment, 538–539
Delivery, insulin management and,
571–572, 571*t*
Dent's disease, 307
Deoxycorticosterone (DOC)
basal levels, Cushing's syndrome and,
368*f*
excess production, syndromes due to,
366–367
maternal, changes during pregnancy,
550*f*
mineralocorticoid activity, 359–360
normal reference ranges, 790*t*
11-Deoxycorticosterone, trivial and
chemical names, 51*t*
11-Deoxycortisol, normal reference
ranges, 791*t*
11-Deoxy-17-hydroxycorticosterone,
trivial and chemical names,
51*t*
Depression
hypothalamic-pituitary axis and,
118
menopause and, 474
oral contraceptives and, 481
Dermopathy, Graves' disease and, 235*f*
Desipramine, for sensory neuropathy,
657
Desmopressin acetate, for central
diabetes insipidus, 152
Development
defects, hypogonadotropic
hypogonadism and, 532
glucocorticoids and, 328
hormones and, 21
Dexamethasone, chemical name, 51*t*
Dexamethasone-remedial aldosteronism,
364
Dexamethasone suppression test,
331–332
Cushing's syndrome and, 348–349,
351
Diabetes Control & Complications Trial
(DCCT), 619–620
Diabetes insipidus, 149–152
central, 149–150, 152
nephrogenic, 150, 152
causes, 149*t*
neurogenic
causes, 147*t*
pituitary-hypothalamic disorders and,
123
short stature and, 187
Diabetes mellitus, 595, 605–661
classification, 605–612, 606*t*
complications
acute, 641–652
chronic, 653–659, 653*t*

diagnosis, 617–619
elderly and, 775–776
familial inheritance, 89*t*
gestational, 567–568
  diagnosis, 568*t*
  diet management and, 568*t*
glucocorticoid therapy and, 24
hypothalamic-pituitary axis and,
  117
insulin-resistant, acanthosis nigricans
  and, 612
laboratory findings, 614–617
management, 632–641
maturity-onset of young, 609–610,
  610*t*
nonpregnant women and, diagnostic
  criteria, 569*t*
occult, 678
osteoporosis and, 298
pregnancy and, 566–572
  classification, 567*t*
  fetal development/growth and,
    569–570, 570*t*
prognosis, 660–661
secondary, 611–612
secondary hypertriglyceridemia and,
  692–694
short stature and, 186–187
thyroid disease and, 765
treatment, 619–641
  diet and, 620–622
  insulin and, 627–632
  oral hypoglycemic drugs and,
    622–627, 624*t*
type I, 605–608
  clinical features, 612–613, 612*t*
  diet and, 621
  early morning hyperglycemia and,
    638–639
  genetics, 606–607
  immunosuppression and, 607–608
  overnight blood glucose levels,
    638*t*
  therapy, 634–639
type II, 608–611
  clinical features, 612*t*, 613–614
  diet and, 621
  nonobese, 609–611
  obese, 609
  subgroups, 609
  therapy, 639–640
Diabetic amyotrophy, 657
Diabetic coma, 644–645
  laboratory abnormalities and, 644*t*
Diabetic diarrhea, 658
Diabetic gastroparesis, 657–658, 671
Diabetic ketoacidosis, 645–649
  treatment flow sheet, 647*f*
Diabetic mother, birth weight and size
  and, 189
Diabetic nephropathy, 655–656
Diabetic neuropathy, 656–658
Diabetic patient, surgery and, 659–660
Diabetic retinopathy, 654–655
Diabetic vascular disease, classification,
  653
Diabinese. *See* Chlorpropamide
Diacylglycerol (DAG), protein kinase C
  activation and, 63

Diarrhea
  diabetic, 658
  endocrine disease and, 29*t*
Diazoxide, for insulinoma, 675–676
Diet
  diabetes mellitus and, 620–622
  nonobese diabetic patient and, 639
Dietary fat
  absorption, 682–683
  restriction, effects, 684–685
Dietary fiber
  diabetes mellitus and, 621
  lipoprotein disorders and, 704
Diffuse toxic goiter. *See* Graves'
  disease
DiGeorge syndrome, neonatal
  hypoparathyroidism and, 287
Dihydrotestosterone
  circulating, women and, 461*t*
  male reproductive function and, 405
  normal ranges in men, 411*t*
  normal reference ranges, 791*t*
  ovarian
    concentrations, production and
      secretion rates, 438*t*
    percentage distribution, 438*t*
  synthesis, pathway, 50*f*
Dihydroxyphenylalanine. *See* Dopa
Diiodothyronine, chemical structures and
  biologic activity, 205*t*
Diiodotyrosine (DIT), structure, 196*f*
Direct stimulants, 600
DIT. *See* Diiodotyrosine
Diuretics
  hypercalcemia and, 284
  syndrome of inappropriate secretion of
    antidiuretic hormone and, 153
Diurnal rhythm, Cushing's syndrome
  and, 350
DNA analysis. *See also* Recombinant
  DNA technology
  genetic disease diagnosis and, 31–33
DOC. *See* Deoxycorticosterone
Dolichols, 43
Dopa
  conversion to dopamine, 383–384
  tyrosine conversion to, 382–383
Dopamine, 101
  in adrenal medulla, 382
  conversion of dopa to, 383–384
  conversion to norepinephrine, 384
  endocrine system and, 11–12
  food intake and, 719
  structure, 101*t*
Dopamine agonists, for prolactinoma,
  135
Dopamine agonists/antagonists, prolactin
  secretion and, 110
Dopamine receptors, 389
Dorloxifene, mechanism and tumor
  target, 732*t*
Down-regulation, 600
Down's syndrome, prenatal screening
  and, 552
Drospirenome, ovarian function
  inhibition and, 473
Drugs
  insulin-treated diabetics and, 671
  short stature and, 176

toxicity, secondary diabetes mellitus
  and, 612
Duodenal pH, hormones affecting, 589*t*
Duodenal ulcer, gut peptides and,
  586–587
Dupuytren's contracture, diabetes
  mellitus and, 659
Dwarfism
  hypopituitary, 532–533, 534*f*
  psychosocial, 184, 185*f*
Dymelor. *See* Acetohexamide
Dynorphin, food intake and, 719
Dysbetalipoproteinemia, familial, 692
Dysgerminoma, amenorrhea and, 458
Dyshormonogenesis, 200
Dyslipidemia, insulin resistance
  syndrome and, 608
Dysmenorrhea, 453

E apolipoprotein, 682
Early phase, 599
Eating, afferent signals to start and stop,
  715–717
Eclampsia, 564–565
Ectopic ACTH syndrome, 348
  Cushing's syndrome and, 344
  etiology and pathogenesis, 345
  neuroendocrine tumors and, 747–748
  pathophysiology, 346
  prognosis, 354
  treatment, 353
EDRF. *See* Endothelium-derived relaxing
  factor
Effectors, G protein-coupled receptors
  and, 62–64
EGF. *See* Epidermal growth factor
EI. *See* Eosinophilic index
Eicosanoids, 5–6
  export, 53–54
  metabolism, 20, 56
  release, 40
  synthesis, pathways, 54*f*
Elderly
  benign prostatic hyperplasia and,
    784–785
  carbohydrate intolerance and,
    774–775
  diabetes mellitus and, 775–776
  glucocorticoids and stress and,
    782–784
  hyperparathyroidism and, 781
  nonketotic hyperosmolar coma and,
    776
  osteoporosis and, 776–781
  reproductive function in men and,
    784
  thyroid function and disease and,
    770–774
  water balance and, 782
Electrolyte replacement, for
  hyperglycemic, hyperosmolar,
  nonketotic state, 651
Embryonal carcinoma, amenorrhea and,
  458
Empty sella syndrome, 123–124
  amenorrhea and, 459
Endocrine cell, 578*f*
Endocrine delivery, 576, 577*f*

Endocrine disease
approach to patient and, 27–35
central diabetes insipidus and, 152
genetic, 13–14
manifestations, 29t
screening and, 33–34
treatment, 34–35
Endocrine effects, 601, 601t
Endocrine failure, nonautoimmune, 767
Endocrine function tests, pregnancy and,
556t
Endocrine glands
control of function, 12f
destruction, autoimmune disease and,
24
disorders not associated with disease,
27
evolution, 16
failure of multiple, 759–766
hyperplasia, 25
Endocrine pancreas, 595–605
anatomy and histology, 595–596
hormones, 596–605
Endocrine status, tumors and, 727–729
Endocrine system, 1–3
disorders, 24–27
evolution, 14–16, 14f
genes involved, 15–16
hyperfunction, 25
causes, 24f
hypofunction, 24–25
causes, 24f
immune system and, 5f
molecules involved, relationships of
species, 4f
nervous system and, 10–14
regulation, 20–21, 56–57
Endocrine testing
hypopituitarism and, 128–129
hypothalamic-pituitary axis and, 118,
119–120t
Endocrine therapy
antitumor agents, 732t
for cancer, 729–732
combination, 731–732
for endometrial cancer, 737–738
for metastatic breast cancer in women,
735–736
for prostatic cancer, 738–739
Endocrine tissue, steroidogenic
pathways, 53f
Endocrine tumors
hypercalcemia and, 284
nonsecretory, 727
secretory, 727–728, 728t
Endocrinology, recombinant DNA
technology and, 13–14, 14t
Endocrinopathy
autoimmune, 761–762
clinical categories, 763f
hypercalcemia and, 284
treatment-induced, 728–729, 729t
Endocytosis, 39, 48
Endometrial cancer, 736–738
estrogen effects and, 737t
metastatic, treatment, 737–738
Endometrium, menstrual cycle and,
448–450, 449f

Endoplasmic reticulum (ER)
hormone export and, 40–42
polypeptide hormone translocation
across, 41f
beta-Endorphin
characteristics, 105t
food intake and, 719
measurement, 330
Endothelin
hypertension and, 378–379
tumors secreting, 750
Endothelium-derived relaxing factor
(EDRF), hypertension and, 378
Energy content, 712f
Energy expenditure, components,
713–714, 714f
Enkephalins
distribution, 579t
mode of delivery, 576t
properties, 585
Enteroglucagon
distribution, 579t
mode of delivery, 576t
properties, 586
Environment, autoimmune disease and,
90–91
Eosinophilic index (EI), 451
Epidermal growth factor (EGF), tumor
growth and, 725t
Epinephrine, 381
in adrenal medulla, 382
conversion of norepinephrine to, 384
endocrine system and, 11–12
plasma
cardiovascular/metabolic effects
and, 391t
insulin administration and, 392f
in vena cava blood samples, 400f
Epinine, 384
Epitopes, 81
Epostane, ovarian function inhibition
and, 472
ER. See Endoplasmic reticulum
Erectile dysfunction, 423–425
organic causes, 424t
Eruptive cutaneous xanthoma, 690
Erythrocytes, glucocorticoids and, 328
Erythropoiesis, thyroid hormones and,
215
Erythropoietin
normal reference ranges, 791t
tumors secreting, 750
Essential hypertension, 374–375
Estradiol. See also Ethinyl estradiol
binding to sex hormone-binding globulin, 437
chemical name, 51t
levels, evaluation, 117
male reproductive function and, 405
maternal, changes during pregnancy,
551f
menstrual cycle and, 442f
normal ranges in men, 411t
normal reference ranges, 791t
ovarian
concentrations, production and
secretion rates, 438t
percentage distribution, 438t

plasma, stage of puberty and, 527f
secretory pattern during menstrual
cycle, 113f
serum concentrations, menopause and,
473t
synthesis, pathway, 50f
synthesis/secretion by preovulatory
follicle, pathways involved,
445f
Estriol
maternal, changes during pregnancy,
551f
normal reference ranges, 792t
Estrogen(s)
adrenal tumors producing, 367
biosynthesis and metabolism, 437f
endocrinologic management and, 35t
endometrial cancer and, 737t
exogenous, secondary
hypertriglyceridemia and, 694
exogenous administration, incomplete
precocious puberty and, 542
for hypopituitarism, 129
levels, evaluation, 117
menstrual cycle and, 443
metabolism, 438
for osteoporosis, 780
pharmacologic effects, 477–479
physiologic effects, 440
pregnancy and, 553–554
release, 40
secretion, progesterone and, 471
testicular, biosynthetic pathways,
406f
thyrotropin and, 111
use in therapy, 22t
Estrogen receptors, 72–73
breast cancer and, 563–564
endocrine therapy in breast cancer and,
735t
endocrine therapy of tumors
containing, responses, 730t
Estrogen replacement therapy
aldosterone levels and, 377
for menopause, 476–477
for osteoporosis, 302–303
decision-making algorithm, 303f
Estrone
maternal, changes during pregnancy,
551f
normal ranges in men, 411t
normal reference ranges, 792t
ovarian
concentrations, production and
secretion rates, 438t
percentage distribution, 438t
serum concentrations, menopause and,
473t
Ethanol hypoglycemia, 676–677
Ethinyl estradiol. See also Estradiol
for permanent hypogonadism, 539
Etidronate disodium
for Paget's disease of bone, 311
rickets/osteomalacia and, 307
Euglycemia, maintenance, postabsorptive
state and, 667–668, 668t
Euglycemic clamp, insulinoma and, 674
Euthyroid sick syndrome, 216–217

Examestane, mechanism and tumor target, 732*t*
Exercise
  diabetic patient and, 633, 670
  osteoporosis and, 780
Exocrine pancreas, 595
Exocytosis, hormone release after, regulation of, 47–48
Exons, 80
Exophthalmometer, 236*f*
Extracellular calcium, 263
Extracellular fluid dehydration, thirst/ADH secretion and, 148
Extrasellar tumors, sexual infantilism and, 532

Fadrozole, mechanism and tumor target, 732*t*
Familial benign hypocalciuric hypercalcemia (FBHH), 282–283
Familial combined hyperlipidemia, 691–692, 697
Familial dysalbuminemic hyperthyroxinemia, 238
Familial dysbetalipoproteinemia, 692
Familial generalized lipodystrophy, 702
Familial hypercholesterolemia, 696–697
Familial hypoalphalipoproteinemia, 699–700
Familial hypobetalipoproteinemia, 701
Familial ligand-defective apo B, 697
Familial lipodystrophy of limbs and trunk, 702
Fanconi's syndrome, 307
Fat, dietary
  absorption, 682–683
  effects of restriction, 684–685
Fat cell, diagram, 714*f*
Fatigue, endocrine disease and, 29*t*
Fat intake, restriction, lipoprotein disorders and, 703
FBHH. *See* Familial benign hypocalciuric hypercalcemia
F cells, 595–596
  secretory products, 596*t*
Fed state, 566
Feedback inhibition, CRH/ACTH secretion and, 323–324, 324*f*
Female reproductive system
  cyclic changes, 448–452
  internal organs, 435*f*
  oxytocin and, 147
  postpartum changes, 561
Femoral neck, bone density, 300*f*
  versus age, 779*f*
Femur, Paget's disease and, 310*f*
Ferning, 450
Fertilization, 548–549
Fetal development
  maternal diabetes mellitus and, 569–570, 570*t*
  thyroid hormones and, 214
Fetal endocrinology, 558–559
Fetal-placental-decidual unit, 549–552
Fetal zone, 317

Fetus
  intrauterine growth, 157–158
  sexual differentiation, 493*f*
  testicular and ovarian differentiation, 491–493
  thyroid function and, 215
Fever, endocrine disease and, 29*t*
FGF. *See* Fibroblast growth factor
Fibric acid derivatives, for hyperlipoproteinemia, 708
Fibroblast growth factor (FGF), tumor growth and, 725*t*
Finasteride, mechanism and tumor target, 732*t*
Fine-needle aspiration biopsy, 223
Fludrocortisone acetate, for diabetic gastroparesis, 658
Fluid replacement
  for diabetic ketoacidosis, 648
  for hyperglycemic, hyperosmolar, non-ketotic state, 650–651
Fluid restriction, syndrome of inappropriate secretion of antidiuretic hormone and, 153
Fluorescent scanning, thyroid and, 222
Fluoride, rickets/osteomalacia and, 307
Flutamide, ovarian function inhibition and, 472–473
Follicle-stimulating hormone (FSH)
  biosynthesis, function, measurement, secretion, 112–114
  characteristics, 105*t*
  maternal, changes during pregnancy, 551*f*
  menstrual cycle and, 441–442, 442*f*
  normal ranges in men, 411*t*
  normal reference ranges, 792*t*
  plasma, stage of puberty and, 527*f*
  secretory pattern during menstrual cycle, 113*f*
  secretory reserve, evaluation, 117
Follicular carcinoma, thyroid. *See* Thyroid cancer
Follicular cysts, incomplete precocious puberty and, 542
Food intake
  afferent signals controlling, 716*f*
  controlled system, 711–715, 711*f*, 722*f*
  inadequate, insulin-treated diabetics and, 670
  model, 721*f*
  neurotransmitters and, 718–719
  sympathetic activity and, 720*t*
Formestane, ovarian function inhibition and, 472
Fractures
  Colles', indices in relation to age, 475*f*
  hip, in elderly, 778*t*
  osteoporotic, incidence rates, 295*f*
  risks in 50-year-old white women and men, 295*t*
Free radical formation, thyroid hormones and, 214
Free thyroxine index (FTI), 218–219
  levothyroxine therapy and, 231*f*
  normal reference ranges, 797*t*
Fructose, diabetes mellitus and, 622
FSH. *See* Follicle-stimulating hormone

Functional layer, 448
Functional ovarian hyperandrogenism, 461–463

GABA. *See* Gamma-aminobutyric acid
GAD. *See* Glutamic acid decarboxylase
Galactopoiesis, 562
Galactorrhea
  amenorrhea and, 460
  prolactinoma and, 132
Galanin
  food intake and, 719
  properties, 584
Gallbladder disease, oral contraceptives and, 481
Gamete intra-follicular transfer (GIFT), 484
Gamma-aminobutyric acid (GABA)
  endocrine system and, 11–12
  food intake and, 718
  secretion, 49
Gamma-knife radiosurgery
  for Cushing's disease, 144
  for pituitary adenoma, 131
Gangrene, diabetes mellitus and, 658
Gastric inhibitory peptide (GIP)
  distribution, 579*t*
  mode of delivery, 576*t*
  normal reference ranges, 792*t*
  properties, 583
Gastric outlet obstruction, gut peptides and, 587
Gastrin
  carboxyl terminal polypeptides, 580*f*
  distribution, 579*t*
  mode of delivery, 576*t*
  normal reference ranges, 792*t*
  properties, 579–580
Gastrinoma, gut peptides and, 587
Gastrin-releasing peptide (GRP)
  distribution, 579*t*
  mode of delivery, 576*t*
  properties, 582–583
Gastrointestinal disease, gut peptide abnormalities and, 586–591
Gastrointestinal hormones. *See* Gut peptides
Gastroparesis, diabetes mellitus and, 657–658, 671
GDM. *See* Gestational diabetes
Gemfibrozil, for hyperlipoproteinemia, 707
Gender identity, 493–497
Gender orientation, 493
Gender role, 493
Gene expression, endocrinology and metabolism and, 13–14
Genes, involved in endocrine system, evolution, 15–16
Genetic disease
  diagnosis, 32*f*
  membrane trafficking defects and, 49
Genetic short stature, 173–174
Genetic tall stature, 188
Genetic variability, 77
Genital(s), external, differentiation, 492–493, 495*f*

Genital ducts, differentiation, 491–492, 494f
Genital system, male, 404f
Genital tract infection, male infertility and, 427
Genitourinary system, menopause and, 474
Geriatric endocrinology, 770–785. *See also* Elderly
Germ cell tumors, 431–432
  ovarian, 458
Germinal cell(s), maturation, familial gonadotropin-independent premature, 541
Germinal cell aplasia, 535
Germinal epithelium, 435
Germinoma, amenorrhea and, 458
Gestational diabetes (GDM), 567–568
  diagnosis, 568t
  diet management and, 568t
GH. *See* Growth hormone
GI. *See* Glycemic index
GIFT. *See* Gamete intra-follicular transfer
Gigantism, 136–142
  cerebral, 188
  pituitary, 189
GIP. *See* Gastric inhibitory peptide
Glaucoma, diabetes mellitus and, 655
Glibenclamide. *See* Glyburide
Glimeperide
  daily dose and duration of action, 624t
  for diabetes mellitus, 625
Glipizide
  daily dose and duration of action, 624t
  for diabetes mellitus, 625
Glomerulus, diagram, 372f
Glucagon, 602–604
  action, 603–604
  biochemistry, 602–603
  counterregulatory response to hypoglycemia and, 665
  normal reference ranges, 792t
  secretion, 603
Glucagonoma, 589
Glucagon stimulation test
  insulinoma and, 673–674
  pheochromocytoma and, 397
Glucocorticoid(s)
  agonists/antagonists, 327
  biologic effects, 326–329
  elderly and, 782–784
  endocrinologic management and, 35t
  excess, poor growth and, 185–186
  familial deficiency, adrenal gland and, 336
  for hirsutism, 466
  intermediary metabolism and, 327–328
  osteoporosis and, 298, 304
  plasma, daily fluctuations, 323f
  postnatal growth and, 163
  pregnancy and, 557
  release, 40
Glucocorticoid hypertension, mechanisms involved, 369f
Glucocorticoid receptor, 73, 326–327
Glucocorticoid-remedial aldosteronism, 364

Glucocorticoid therapy, 22t
  diabetes mellitus and, 24
Gluconeogenesis, hepatic, reduced, disorders associated, 676
Glucose
  blood testing
    diabetes mellitus and, 615–616
    insulin dosage during pregnancy and, 569t
  glucagon secretion and, 603
  impaired counterregulation in diabetics, 670–671
  metabolism, glucocorticoids and, 327
  nondiabetic glycosuria and, 614
  pancreas stimulation and, 599f
  plasma
    documentation of low levels, 669–670
    fasting, diabetes mellitus and, 617
    insulin administration and, 392f, 667f
    response to food intake, 599f
    response to stepwise reduction, 665f
  suppression, acromegaly and, 140
Glucose-growth hormone suppression test, hypothalamic-pituitary function and, 120t
Glucose tolerance test
  intravenous, diabetes mellitus and, 618–619
  oral
    diabetes mellitus and, 618
    insulinoma and, 674
Glucose transporter, 601–602, 602t
  glycemic regulation, 666f
Glutamic acid decarboxylase (GAD), islet cell antibodies and, 607
Glyburide
  daily dose and duration of action, 624t
  for diabetes mellitus, 625
Glycemic index (GI), 621
Glycogen storage disease, secondary hypertriglyceridemia and, 695
Glycohemoglobin assay
  diabetes mellitus and, 616–617
  factors interfering, 616–617, 616t
  insulinoma and, 674
Glycoprotein hormones, tumors secreting, 749
Glycosuria, 614
Glydiazinamide. *See* Glipizide
GnRH. *See* Gonadotropin-releasing hormone
Goiter
  diffuse toxic. *See* Graves' disease
  multinodular
    elderly and, 774
    toxic, 242, 242f
  nontoxic, 244–246
    etiology, 244t
  toxic nodular, serum thyrotropin responses, 210f
Golgi apparatus, 40
Gonad(s)
  cancer therapy and, 729
  fetal, endocrinology, 559
  steroid biosynthetic pathways, 505f
Gonadal agenesis, amenorrhea and, 455

Gonadal dysfunction, Cushing's syndrome and, 347
Gonadal dysgenesis
  ambiguous genitals and, 515–516
  amenorrhea and, 455
  45,X, 489–491, 499–500
  46,XX, 498–499, 501–502
    familial and sporadic forms, 537
  46,XY, 502–503
    familial and sporadic forms, 537
Gonadal dysgenesis syndrome, 499–501, 536
  treatment, 539
  X and Y chromosome structural abnormalities and, 500t
  X chromatin-negative variants, 501
  X chromatin-positive variants, 500–501
Gonadal neoplasms, dysgenetic gonads and, 503
Gonadal steroids, 405–407. *See also* Sex steroids
  biosynthetic pathways, 406f
  measurements, 410–411
  normal ranges in men, 411t
Gonadoblastomas, amenorrhea and, 458
Gonadorelin, LH and FSH secretory reserves and, 117
Gonadotrophs, 99
Gonadotropin(s)
  biosynthesis, function, measurement, secretion, 112–114
  deficiency, hypopituitarism and, 127
  glucocorticoids and, 329
  human menopausal, ovulation induction and, 469–470, 470t
  for hypopituitarism, 129
  for male gonadal disorders, 414–415
  measurements, male hypogonadism and, 411
  normal responses, 114t
  pituitary, menstrual cycle and, 441–442
  pituitary adenomas secreting, 145–146
  secretion
    mid-childhood nadir, 526
    ovarian steroids and, 447
    pattern during menstrual cycle, 113f
    peripubertal increase, 526–527
  tumors secreting, 749
Gonadotropin-releasing hormone (GnRH), 102
  for cryptorchidism, 420
  for male gonadal disorders, 415
  menstrual cycle and, 446–447
  ovulation induction and, 470
  pubertal development and, 528–529, 528f
  structure, 101t
  use in therapy, 22t
Gonadotropin-releasing hormone (GnRH) analogs
  for hirsutism, 466
  ovarian function inhibition and, 471
  for precocious puberty, 543–545

Gonadotropin-releasing hormone (GnRH) test
  hypothalamic-pituitary function and, 117, 120*t*
  male hypogonadism and, 412
Gonadotropin-secreting tumors, incomplete precocious puberty and, 541
Gonocytoma, amenorrhea and, 458
G protein(s)
  interactions with receptor/effector mechanisms, 61*t*
  signal transduction mediated by, 62*f*
G protein-coupled receptors
  effectors linked to, 62–64
  human disease and, 65–66
G protein transducers, 61–62
Graafian follicle, 444
Granulomatous disorders, hypercalcemia and, 284
Granulosa cell tumors, incomplete precocious puberty and, 542
Granulosa-theca cell tumors, amenorrhea and, 458
Graves' disease, 233–241
  classification of eye changes, 235*t*
  clinical features, 234–237
  complications, 238
  dermopathy and, 235*f*
  differential diagnosis, 237–238
  etiology, 233
  HLA genotype and, 89
  neonatal, 241
  onycholysis and, 237*f*
  ophthalmopathy and, 234*f*, 236*f*, 240–241
  pathogenesis, 233–234, 233*f*
  pregnancy and, 565–566
  treatment, 238–241
GRH. *See* Growth hormone-releasing hormone
Growth, 157–189
  abnormal
    causes, 173*t*
    plotted on height velocity chart, 182*f*
  constitutional delay, 170–173, 530, 531*f*
    treatment, 538
  disorders, 170–189
  extremes, 183*f*
  glucocorticoids and, 328
  intrauterine, 157–158
  measurement, 168–170
  midparental stature and, 164*f*, 165*f*
  parent-specific adjustments for stature, 166*f*, 167*f*
  postnatal, 158–168
Growth chart
  abnormal, 181*f*
  for boys in USA, 159*f*
  for girls in USA, 160*f*
  incremental for boys and girls, 162*f*
Growth factor(s)
  malignant transformation and, 743
  pregnancy and, 553
  tumor growth and, 725*t*
Growth factor-dependent pathway, 67*f*
Growth factor receptors, 66–67
  signaling by, 66*f*

Growth hormone (GH)
  biosynthesis, function, measurement, secretion, 106–108
  characteristics, 105*t*
  counterregulatory response to hypoglycemia and, 666–667
  deficiency, 127, 176–184
    acquired, 178
    congenital, 177–178
    constitutional delayed puberty and, 539
    diagnosis, 179–180
    treatment, 180–184
  endocrinologic management and, 35*t*
  hypersecretion, 116, 136–142
  for hypopituitarism, 129
  intrauterine growth and, 157
  maternal, changes during pregnancy, 551*f*
  normal reference ranges, 792*t*
  postnatal growth and, 161–163
  secretion
    ectopic, acromegaly and, 141
    factors affecting, 108*t*
    sleep-associated changes, 109*f*
  secretory reserve, evaluation, 115–116
  tumors secreting, 749
Growth hormone receptors, signaling by, 68*f*
Growth hormone-releasing hormone (GRH), 100
  food intake and, 719
  growth hormone secretion and, 107
  secretion, ectopic, acromegaly and, 141
  structure, 101*t*
  tumors secreting, 749
Growth hormone-releasing hormone (GRH) test, hypothalamic-pituitary function and, 120*t*
Growth spurt, 524–525
GRP. *See* Gastrin-releasing peptide
Guanylyl cyclase-linked receptors, 68–69
Gut
  adrenergic responses, 389*t*
  endocrine cell, 578*f*
  neuroendocrine tumors, 588
Gut motility, thyroid hormones and, 215
Gut peptides, 575–591
  abnormalities, gastrointestinal disease and, 586–591
  clinical uses, 591
  distribution, 578, 579*t*
  families, 578*t*
  mechanisms of action, 576–577
  modes of delivery, 576, 576*t*
  structure, 577
  tumors secreting, 750
Gynecomastia, 427–429
  adolescent, 543
  causes, 428*t*
    diagnostic evaluation, 428*f*
  Klinefelter's syndrome and, 498

Hair
  endocrine disease and, 29*t*
  menopause and, 474

"Hamburger thyrotoxicosis", 243
Hashimoto's thyroiditis, 247–249
HDL. *See* High-density lipoprotein
Headache, endocrine disease and, 29*t*
Head trauma, hypopituitarism and, 126
Heart, adrenergic responses, 389*t*
Heart disease
  diabetes mellitus and, 658
  myxedema and, 231, 232
Heat production, thyroid hormones and, 214
Heavy chain constant region, 83
Heavy particle irradiation
  for growth hormone hypersecretion, 141
  for pituitary adenoma, 131
Height, 168–169
  adjustment based on midparental stature, 164*f*, 165*f*
Helicobacter pylori, 586
Hemochromatosis, hypopituitarism and, 126
Hemodialysis, diabetic nephropathy and, 656
Hemoglobin, glycosylated, assays, 616–617, 616*t*
Hepatic gluconeogenesis, reduced, disorders associated, 676
Heredity, osteoporosis and, 296–297
Heregulin, tumor growth and, 725*t*
Hermaphroditism, true, 503
Hernia, cryptorchidism and, 420
Hertel exophthalmometer, 236*f*
High-density lipoprotein (HDL)
  deficiency, primary hyperlipidemia and, 699–700
  metabolism, 685–686
Hilar cell tumors, amenorrhea and, 459
Hip fracture, in elderly, factors associated, 778*t*
Hirschsprung's disease, gut peptides and, 587
Hirsutism, 354, 463–468
  androgen-dependent, development factors, 461*f*
  causes, 461*t*
  Cushing's syndrome and, 347
  evaluation, 465–466
    hormone measurements and, 464*f*
  pathophysiology, 463–465
  treatment, 466–468
Histamine
  endocrine system and, 11–12
  food intake and, 719
Histiocytosis X, hypopituitarism and, 126
Histrelin, for precocious puberty, 544
HLA. *See* Human leukocyte antigen
HLA-A, 77
HLA-B, 77
HLA-C, 77
HLA-DP, 77
HLA-DQ, 77
HLA-DR, 77
HMG-CoA reductase inhibitors
  for hyperlipoproteinemia, 707, 708
  sites of action, 706*f*
Homeostasis, mineral, control, 274

Homocystinuria, tall stature and, 188
Hormonal contraception, 477–482
　noncontraceptive advantages, 481–482
Hormone(s)
　actions, 6–8, 21–23, 58–74
　actions and interrelationships, 2f
　adrenal medullary, 382–392. *See also*
　　　specific type
　assays
　　nonimmunologic, 31
　　pheochromocytoma and, 397
　autocrine, 87
　basal levels, measurements, 28–29
　biosynthesis, 39–40
　　defects, endocrine hypofunction
　　　and, 25
　cancer and, 724–739
　chemical composition, 3–4
　classification of action, 8–10, 9f
　　ligands and, 9–10
　　receptors and, 8–9
　defects in sensitivity, 25–27
　deficiency, hypogonadotropic hypogo-
　　nadism and, 532
　effects on tumors, 724–727
　elimination, 19–20
　endogenous, breast cancer and, 733
　exogenous, breast cancer and, 733
　export
　　membrane vesicle-mediated, 40–49
　　non-membrane-vesicle-mediated,
　　　49–54
　food intake and, 717
　free levels, 30
　gastrointestinal. *See* Gut peptides
　hypophyseotropic, 100–102
　　structure, 101t
　hypothalamic, 100–103
　immune system and, 5
　immunoassays, 30–31, 31f
　malignant transformation and,
　　724–726
　metabolism, 18f, 19–20
　metabolism, transport, elimination,
　　regulation, 54–57
　mineralocorticoid. *See*
　　Mineralocorticoids
　neurotransmitters and, 10–11
　nonendocrine disease therapy and,
　　35–36, 35t
　normal reference ranges, 788–798t
　oncogenes and, 5
　origins, 15
　ovarian, 435–441
　　pregnancy and, 549
　　therapeutic uses, 470–471
　pancreatic, endocrine, 596–605
　paracrine/autocrine actions, 3
　peptide. *See* Peptide hormones
　pituitary. *See* Pituitary hormones
　plasma and urine assays, 29–30
　polypeptide. *See* Polypeptide
　　hormones
　precursors, 3f
　receptors, 6–7, 58–73
　　ligand saturation/Scatchard analysis
　　　of interactions, 59f
　　structural schematics, 60f

　regulation of responsiveness, 7, 7f
　release after exocytosis, regulation,
　　47–48
　secretion
　　catecholamines and, 391
　　ectopic, 741–743
　　modes, 40f
　　regulated, 47
　steroid. *See* Steroid hormones
　syndromes of excess, 27
　synthesis and release, 17
　thyroid. *See* Thyroid hormones
　transmission of signals. pathways, 8f
　transport, 17–19
　tumor-produced, 742t
　vitamins and, 4–5
Hormone-binding proteins, regulation in
　plasma, 56
Hormone-recognition element (HRE), 7,
　71
　for nuclear hormone receptors, 72t
Hormone response, synergistic, 8f
Hormone-response system, interactions,
　7–8
Hormone-secreting cells, membrane traf-
　fic, 44f
Hot flushes, menopause and, 474
hPL. *See* Human placental lactogen
HRE. *See* Hormone-recognition
　element
Human chorionic gonadotropin (hCG)
　maternal, changes during pregnancy,
　　551f
　normal reference ranges, 789t
　pregnancy and, 552
　testicular unresponsiveness, male
　　sexual differentiation and,
　　508–509
　tumors secreting, 749
Human leukocyte antigen (HLA), 77
　antigen specificities, 78t
　autoimmune disease and, 89t, 766t
　type I diabetes mellitus and, 606–607
Human leukocyte antigen (HLA)
　　molecule, class I, diagrammatic
　　structure, 79f
Human menopausal gonadotropins,
　ovulation induction and,
　469–470, 470t
Human placental lactogen (hPL)
　maternal, changes during pregnancy,
　　551f
　pregnancy and, 552–553
　tumors secreting, 749
Humoral immunity, 76
Hunger
　gastrointestinal signals producing,
　　715–717
　metabolic signals stimulating, 715
Hydatidiform mole, 243
Hydralazine, for preeclampsia, 565
Hydrocortisone
　for adrenocortical insufficiency, 341
　counterregulatory response to
　　hypoglycemia and, 666
4-Hydroxyandrostenedione
　mechanism and tumor target, 732t
　ovarian function inhibition and, 472

17-Hydroxycorticosteroids
　measurement, 331
　normal reference ranges, 792t
18-Hydroxycorticosterone, normal refer-
　ence ranges, 793t
5-Hydroxyindoleacetic acid, normal
　reference ranges, 793t
1alpha-Hydroxylase
　regulators, 272t
17alpha-Hydroxylase deficiency
　amenorrhea and, 455
　hypertension and, 366
　male pseudohermaphroditism and,
　　510–511
　treatment, 367
11beta-Hydroxylase deficiency
　treatment, 367
　congenital adrenal hyperplasia and,
　　366
17-Hydroxypregnenolone, normal
　reference ranges, 793t
17-Hydroxyprogesterone
　corpus luteum function and, 549
　maternal, changes during pregnancy,
　　550f
　menstrual cycle and, 442f
　normal reference ranges, 793t
Hydroxyproline, normal reference
　ranges, 793t
3beta-Hydroxysteroid dehydrogenase de-
　ficiency, male pseudohermaph-
　roditism and, 510
11beta-Hydroxysteroid dehydrogenase
　deficiency, 369
17beta-Hydroxysteroid oxidoreductase
　deficiency, male pseudo-
　hermaphroditism and, 511
Hygiene, diabetic patient and, 633
Hyperalphalipoproteinemia, 688
Hyperandrogenism, ovarian, functional,
　461–463
Hypercalcemia, 276–286
　aggravation, 277t
　causes, 277–285, 277t
　gut peptides and, 587
　hypocalciuric, benign, familial,
　　282–283
　infantile, 702
　malignancy-associated, 283, 743–746,
　　743t
　treatment, 285–286
Hyperchloremic acidosis, 649
Hypercholesterolemia
　familial, 696–697
　primary, 696–697
　secondary, 698–699
Hypercortisolism, hypertension and,
　367
Hypergastinemia, evaluation, 586
Hyperglycemia, insulin resistance
　syndrome and, 608
Hyperglycemic coma, 644
Hyperglycemic, hyperosmolar,
　nonketotic state, 650–651
Hypergonadotropic hypogonadism,
　535–537
Hyperinsulinemia, insulin resistance syn-
　drome and, 608

Hyperinsulinism, symptomatic fasting hypoglycemia and, 670–677

Hyperlipidemia
clinical manifestations, 693f
familial combined, 691–692, 697
treatment, 703

Hyperlipoproteinemia
Lp(a), 697
treatment, drugs used, 705–709, 705t

Hypermenorrhea, causes, 454t

Hypermetabolism, disorders presenting with features, 394t

Hypernatremia, elderly and, 782

Hyperparathyroidism
elderly and, 781
multiple endocrine neoplasia and, 757–758
primary, 277–283
clinical features, 279–281
etiology and pathogenesis, 278–279
multiple endocrine neoplasia and, 754–755
treatment, 281–282
variants, 282–283
secondary, renal osteodystrophy and, 311–312

Hyperphosphatemia, hypocalcemia and, 289

Hyperprolactinemia, 133–135

Hypersensitivity response, 88

Hypertension, 359–379
accelerated, 377
adrenal origin, 359–371
atrial natriuretic peptide and, 378
autacoids and, 379
Cushing's syndrome and, 347, 367–368
endothelin and, 378–379
endothelium-derived relaxing factor and, 378
essential, 374–375
excess deoxycorticosterone production and, 366
glucocorticoid, mechanisms involved, 369f
insulin and, 377
insulin resistance syndrome and, 608
kallikrein-kinin system and, 379
mineralocorticoid
mechanisms involved, 361f
pathogenesis, 361–362
pheochromocytoma causing, common symptoms, 393t
pregnancy and, 564–565
primary aldosteronism and, 362–366
renal origin, 371–377
renin-angiotensin system and, 374–377
renovascular, 275–277
clinical index of suspicion and, 376t
suggested workup, 377f
sympathetic nervous system and, 379

Hyperthyroidism, 233–243
apathetic, 238
differential diagnosis, 237f
elderly and, 771–773
osteoporosis and, 298
pregnancy and, 565–566

serum thyrotropin responses, 210f
spontaneously resolving, 248–249

Hyperthyroxinemia, dysalbuminemic, familial, 238

Hypertriglyceridemia, 689–696
primary, 690–692
secondary, 692–696

Hypoalbuminemia, hypocalcemia and, 289

Hypoaldosteronism, hyporeninemic, elderly and, 782

Hypoalphalipoproteinemia, familial, 699–700

Hypobetalipoproteinemia, familial, 701

Hypocalcemia, 286–290
causes, 286t, 287–289
treatment, 290

Hypocalcemic tetany, 286f

Hypocortisolism, insulin-treated diabetics and, 671

Hypoglycemia, 664–678. *See also* Insulin-induced hypoglycemia
alimentary
functional, 677–678
postgastrectomy, 677
asymptomatic, 668–669
autoimmune, 672
autonomic nervous system and, 667t
classification, 668–669
clinical presentation, 669–670
counterregulatory responses, 641–642, 642t, 664–667
diabetes mellitus and, 641–644
ethanol, 676–677
factitious, 672
insulin reaction and, 670–671
late, 678
non-islet-cell tumors and, 748–749
pancreatic B cell tumors and, 672–676
pentamidine-induced, 672
reactive, 677
sulfonylurea overdose and, 671
symptomatic, 668
causes, 668t
symptomatic fasting
with hyperinsulinism, 670–676
without hyperinsulinism, 676–677
treatment, 643–644

Hypoglycemic awareness, human insulin and, 642

Hypoglycemic coma, 644, 651–652

Hypoglycemic drugs
obese diabetic patient and, 639
oral, 622–627, 624t
diabetic patient and, 633
nonobese diabetic patient and, 639–640

Hypoglycemic unawareness, management, 642–643, 643t

Hypogonadism
female, causes, 455
hypergonadotropic, 535–537
hypogonadotropic, 530–535
male
classification, 415t
clinical presentation, 409, 410f
evaluation, 412–414, 413f
genital examination and, 409–410

measurement of gonadal steroids and, 117
permanent, treatment, 538–539
primary, treatment in women, 470
prolactinoma and, 132–133

Hypogonadotropic hypogonadism, 530–535
hypopituitarism and, 126

Hypogonadotropism, 455

Hypokalemia, primary aldosteronism and, 363

Hypolipidemia
primary, 699–701
secondary, 701

Hypomenorrhea, causes, 454t

Hyponatremia, elderly and, 782

Hypoparathyroidism
Addison's disease and, 763
autoimmune, sequence for onset, 764f
hypocalcemia and, 287–288
isolated, 763–764

Hypophosphatasia, rickets/osteomalacia and, 307

Hypophosphatemic rickets, 307

Hypophyseotropic hormones, 100–102
structure, 101t

Hypophysitis
autoimmune, 765
lymphocytic, hypopituitarism and, 126–127

Hypopituitarism, 125–129
congenital, 174f
secondary hypertriglyceridemia and, 695

Hypopituitary dwarfism, 532–533, 534f

Hyporeninemic hypoaldosteronism, elderly and, 782

Hypospadias, 516–517
pseudovaginal perineoscrotal, 514–515

Hypotension, orthostatic, diabetes mellitus and, 658

Hypothalamic amenorrhea, 459

Hypothalamic hormones, 100–103
structure, 101t
tumors secreting, 750

Hypothalamic-hypophysial-thyroid axis, 207f

Hypothalamic nuclei, anatomic location, 718f

Hypothalamic-pituitary-adrenal axis, 106f
disorders, elderly and, 783–784

Hypothalamic-pituitary axis
endocrine tests and, 118, 119–120t
endocrinologic evaluation, 114–122
neuroradiologic evaluation, 118–122, 121f
pharmacologic agents and, 118
problems in evaluation, 117–118

Hypothalamic-pituitary-gonadal interactions, menstrual cycle and, 448f

Hypothalamic-pituitary-Leydig cell axis, 408, 408f

Hypothalamic-pituitary-seminiferous tubular axis, 408–409, 408f

Hypothalamic-pituitary-thyroid axis, 111f
evaluation, 219–220

Hypothalamus, 95–153
  anatomy and embryology, 96*t*
  blood supply, 97–98
  disorders, 122–146. *See also specific disorder*
  neuroendocrinology, 102–103
  neurotransmitters, 11–12
  pituitary relationships, 11–13
  portal hypophysial vessels, 97*f*
Hypothermia, endocrine disease and, 29*t*
Hypothyroid cardiomyopathy, 228*f*
Hypothyroidism, 225–233
  complications, 230–231
  daily doses of thyroxine, 774*t*
  diagnosis, 229–230, 229*t*
  elderly and, 773–774
  etiology, 225–226, 226*t*
  hypogonadotropic hypogonadism and, 534–535
  incomplete precocious puberty and, 542
  pathogenesis, 226–229
  pregnancy and, 566
  secondary hypercholesterolemia and, 698
  secondary hypertriglyceridemia and, 695
  serum thyrotropin responses, 210*f*
  short stature and, 184
  treatment, 231–233

IAPP. *See* Islet amyloid polypeptide
ICI-182780
  mechanism and tumor target, 732*t*
  ovarian function inhibition and, 472
IDDM. *See* Diabetes mellitus, type I
Identification bracelet, diabetic patient and, 633
Idoxifene, mechanism and tumor target, 732*t*
IgA, 84
IgD, 84
IgE, 84
IGF. *See* Insulin-like growth factor
IgG, 84
IgM, 84
Immobilization
  hypercalcemia and, 285
  osteoporosis and, 298
Immune cells, 76
  co-receptors and accessory molecules, 81–83
Immune insulin resistance, 640–641
Immune recognition, molecules, 76–81
Immune response, 84–88
  activation, 84–87
  soluble components, 83–84
Immune response cascade, 87*f*
Immune system
  components, 76–88
  endocrine system and, 5*f*
  glucocorticoids and, 328–329
  hormones and, 5, 23
Immunity
  cell-mediated, 76
  humoral, 76

tissue-specific, assessment methods, 760*t*
Immunoassay, hormone, 30–31, 31*f*
Immunoglobulin(s), 76, 77, 83–84
  disorders, secondary hypercholesterolemia and, 698
  isotypes, 84
  surface-bound, transformation, 83*f*
Immunoglobulin-lipoprotein complex disorders, 695–696
Immunoglobulin superfamily, 83
Immunologic tissue injury, types, 760*t*
Immunosuppression, treatment of recent-onset type I diabetes mellitus and, 607–608
Implantation, 549
Impotence, 423–425
  aging and, 784
  diabetes mellitus and, 657–658
  organic causes, 424*t*
Incidental adrenal mass, 354–356, 355*f*
Incidental findings, 396
Indapamide, hypercalcemia and, 284
Infantile hypercalcemia, 702
Infantile hypertrophic pyloric stenosis, gut peptides and, 587
Infection
  diabetes mellitus and, 633, 659
  hypopituitarism and, 127
Inferior petrosal sinus sampling (IPSS), Cushing's syndrome and, 351–353
Infertility, 482–484
  causes, 483*t*
  cryptorchidism and, 420
  male, 425–427
    causes, 426*t*
  prolactinoma and, 132
Inflammatory bowel disease, gut peptides and, 587–588
Inhibitors, 600
Insoluble fibers, 621
Insulin, 596–602
  action, 600
  administration
    methods, 631–632
    plasma glucose and, 667*f*
  allergy, 640
  analogs, 630–631
  assay, insulinomas and, 673
  bioavailability characteristics, 627*t*, 628–631
  biosynthesis, 596–597
  concentrations, 628, 629*t*
  counterregulatory response to hypoglycemia and, 664–665
  for diabetes mellitus, 627–632
  diabetes mellitus during pregnancy and, 568–569
  for diabetic ketoacidosis, 648
  diabetic patient and, 633
  endocrine effects, 601, 601*t*
  hypertension and, 377
  intermediate-acting, 630
  intrapartum infusion, 571*t*
  intrauterine growth and, 158
  levels, glucose tolerance test and, 618
  long-acting, 630

  metabolic effects, 600–601
  mixtures, 630
  molecule, abnormalities, 611
  mutant, 610–611, 610*t*
  normal reference ranges, 793*t*
  obesity and, 720
  paracrine effects, 600–601
  plasma, response to food intake, 599*f*
  plasma glucose, epinephrine, norepinephrine and, 392*f*
  purity, 628
  regulation of release, 600*t*
  responses, factors reducing, 608*t*
  secretion, 598–600
    basal, 598
    stimulated, 598–599
  short-acting, 629–630
  species, 627–628
  type II diabetic patient and, 640
Insulin-dependent diabetes mellitus (IDDM). *See* Diabetes mellitus, type I
Insulin hypoglycemia test, hypothalamic-pituitary function and, 119*t*
Insulin-induced hypoglycemia
  growth hormone secretion and, 116
  pituitary ACTH reserve and, 115
  pituitary-adrenal reserve and, 333
Insulin-like growth factor (IGF)
  intrauterine growth and, 158
  normal reference ranges, 794*t*
  postnatal growth and, 161–163
  tumor growth and, 725*t*
Insulin-like growth factor-1 (IGF-1)
  acromegaly and, 140
  endocrinologic management and, 35*t*
Insulin-like growth factor binding protein 3, normal reference ranges, 794*t*
Insulinoma, 672–676
  clinical findings, 673
  diagnosis, 673–674
  treatment, 675–676, 675*f*
Insulin pump
  insulin therapy and, 635
  perioperative diabetes management and, 660*t*
Insulin reaction, symptomatic fasting hypoglycemia and, 670–671
Insulin receptors, 600
Insulin resistance, immune, 640–641
Insulin resistance syndrome, 608–609
Insulin sensitizers, for diabetes mellitus, 627
Insulin therapy
  for hyperglycemic, hyperosmolar, non-ketotic state, 651
  immunopathology, 640–641
  for type I diabetes mellitus, 634–638
    advantages/disadvantages, 634*t*
    guidelines, 636*f*
Integrative networks, 16
Integrins, 83
Interleukin(s), properties, 85–86*t*
Interleukin-2 (IL-2), 87
Interleukin-4 (IL-4), 88
Interleukin-5 (IL-5), 88
Interleukin-6 (IL-6), 88
Intermediate cells, 451

Intersexuality
  diagnostic steps, 518f
  management, 517–519
Interstitial cells, 403
Intestinal pseudo-obstruction, chronic,
    gut peptides and, 587
Intracellular calcium, 263
Intracellular communication, 15
Intracellular vesicular traffic, SNARE
    hypothesis and, 45f
Intrathyroidal deiodinase, 200
Intrauterine growth, 157–158
Intrauterine growth retardation (IUGR)
  maternal diabetes mellitus and, 570
  prematurity and, 174
Introns, 80
In vitro fertilization, 484
Iodide
  deficiency, hormone biosynthesis and,
    200
  thyroidal organification, thiocarbamide
    inhibitors, 201f
Iodide transporter, 198–199, 198f
Iodide trap, 198–199
Iodine
  excess, hormone biosynthesis and,
    201
  metabolism, 194–196, 197f, 220
    thyrotropin and, 211
  radioactive
    for Graves' disease, 239
    uptake in subacute thyroiditis,
      246f
  thyroidal inorganic, perchlorate
    discharge, 199f
Iodothyronine, representative values in
    euthyroid human, 207t
Iodothyronine deiodinases, 206t
Ionizing radiation, thyroid and, 249–250,
    249t
IPSS. See Inferior petrosal sinus
    sampling
Iron deficiency, short stature and,
    176
Iron deposition, hypoparathyroidism and,
    288
Iron storage disease, hypopituitarism and,
    126
Irradiation
  for Cushing's disease, 144
  for growth hormone hypersecretion,
    141
  for pituitary adenoma, 130–131
  thyroid lesions after, 249t
Irritable bowel syndrome, gut peptides
    and, 587
Islet amyloid polypeptide (IAPP), 602
Islet cell autoantibodies, type I diabetes
    mellitus and, 607
Islets of Langerhans, 595–596, 596f
  autoimmunity against, 765t
  cell types, 596t
  transplantation, diabetes mellitus and,
    632
  vascularization, 596
Isotype(s), 84
Isotype switching, 84
IUGR. See Intrauterine growth
    retardation

Jaundice, cholestatic, oral contraceptives
    and, 481
Joints, diabetes mellitus and, 659
Jugular vein, plasma osmolality, water
    intake and, 148f
Juvenile diabetic "cheirarthropathy", dia-
    betes mellitus and, 659

Kallikrein-kinin system, hypertension
    and, 379
Kallmann's syndrome, 455, 532, 533f
Karyopyknotic index (KPI), 451
Karyotype, normal 46,XY, G bands, 488f
Karyotypic disorders, autosomal, short
    stature and, 175
Ketoacidosis, diabetic, 645–649
  treatment flow sheet, 647f
Ketoconazole
  for Cushing's disease, 144
  ovarian function inhibition and, 473
  for precocious puberty, 545
Ketone(s), serum determinations,
    diabetes mellitus and, 616
Ketone bodies, 615
Ketonuria, diabetes mellitus and, 615
17-Ketosteroids, normal reference
    ranges, 794t
Kidney
  adrenergic responses, 389t
  antidiuretic hormone and, 146–147
  cortisol inactivation and, 325
  functions, hormones and, 22
  glucocorticoids and, 329
  parathyroid hormone and, 268
  vitamin D and, 274
Kidney disease, hyperparathyroid, 280
Kidney failure
  gut peptides and, 587
  hypercalcemia and, 285
Klinefelter's syndrome, 415–417, 416f,
    497–499, 535
  tall stature and, 189
  variants, 498
Kobberling-Dunningan syndrome,
    702
KPI. See Karyopyknotic index

Labor, insulin management and,
    571–572, 571t
Lactation, 561–562
  oxytocin and, 147
Lactic acidosis, diabetes mellitus and,
    644, 652
Lactotrophs, 99
Late phase, 599
Laurence-Moon syndrome
  hypogonadotropic hypogonadism and,
    533
  short stature and, 175
Lawrence syndrome, 702
LCAT. See Lecithin-cholesterol
    acyltransferase
LDL. See Low-density lipoprotein
Lecithin-cholesterol acyltransferase
    (LCAT), deficiency, primary
    hypolipidemia and, 700

Letrozole, ovarian function inhibition
    and, 472
Leukocytes, glucocorticoids and, 328
Leukotrienes, 5–6
  synthesis of, pathways for, 54f
Leuprolide
  ovarian function inhibition and, 471
  for precocious puberty, 544
Levodopa, growth hormone secretion
    and, 108, 116
Levodopa test, hypothalamic-pituitary
    function and, 119t
Levothyroxine
  dosage, 231–232, 232t
  serum free thyroxine index and, 231f
  toxic effects, 232
Leydig cell(s), 403
  adult failure, 423
  maturation, familial gonadotropin-
    independent premature, 541
Leydig cell aplasia, 418–419
Leydig cell tumors, 431–432
LH. See Luteinizing hormone
Libido, endocrine disease and, 29t
Licorice, chronic ingestion, pseudohyper-
    aldosteronism and, 369
Liddle's syndrome, 370–371
Lifestyle, osteoporosis and, 297
Ligand, hormone classification and, 9–10
Ligand-receptor complex, kinase-
    dependent desensitization,
    65f
Lipemia, endogenous, 691
Lipemia retinalis, 690
Lipid(s)
  laboratory analyses, 687
  metabolism
    oral contraceptives and, 478–479
    thyroid hormones and, 215
  oral estrogen therapy and, 476f
  transport, 681–686
Lipid-lowering therapy, untoward conse-
    quences, 708–709
Lipodystrophy
  classification, 701–702
  insulin injection sites and, 641
Lipoid cell tumors, amenorrhea and,
    459
Lipoprotein(s)
  diabetes mellitus and, 617
  disorders, dietary factors in
    management, 703–704
  half-lives, 684
  high-density
    metabolism, 685–686
    primary hyperlipidemia and,
      699–700
  laboratory analyses, 687
  low-density, catabolism, 685, 685f
  metabolism, disorders, 680–709
  oral estrogen therapy and, 476f
  plasma, 681, 681t
    abnormal patterns, 687–689
  triglyceride-rich
    atherogenicity, 689
    metabolism in plasma, 684–685
  very low density
    formation, 683–684
    metabolism, 683f

Lipoprotein lipase
    deficiency, 690–691
    metabolism of triglyceride-rich
        lipoproteins and, 684
beta-Lipotropin
    characteristics, 105t
    measurement, 330
Lithium therapy, primary hyper-
    parathyroidism and, 283
Liver
    adrenergic responses, 389t
    cortisol metabolism and, 325
    glucose metabolism and,
        glucocorticoids and, 327
    glucose output, disorders associated
        with low, 676
    oral contraceptives and, 478
Low-density lipoprotein (LDL),
        catabolism, 685, 685f
Lp(a) hyperlipoproteinemia, 697
Lp(a) protein, 682
Lumbar spine, bone density, 300f
Luteal phase, inadequate, ovarian
        hormones and, 471
Luteinizing hormone (LH)
    biosynthesis, function, measurement,
        secretion, 112–114
    characteristics, 105t
    maternal, changes during pregnancy,
        551f
    menstrual cycle and, 441–442, 442f
    normal ranges in men, 411t
    normal reference ranges, 795t
    plasma, pubertal stage 2 and, 527f
    secretory pattern during menstrual
        cycle, 113f
    secretory reserve, evaluation, 117
    testicular unresponsiveness, male
        sexual differentiation and,
        508–509
17,20-Lyase deficiency, male pseudoher-
        maphroditism and, 511
Lymphocyte antigen receptors, 77–81,
        80f
Lymphocyte self-reactivity, controls
        against, 84, 86f
Lymphocytic hypophysitis,
        hypopituitarism and, 126–127
Lymphoma
    hypercalcemia and, 746
    thyroid, 254
Lypressin, for central diabetes insipidus,
        152
Lysosomal enzyme sorting, 46–47
Lysosomes, 45

Macroadenoma, 122, 130
Macronutrients, relationship of intake to
        body stores, 713f
Macrovascular disease, diabetic, 653
Magnesium depletion,
        hypoparathyroidism and, 288
Magnetic resonance imaging (MRI)
    Cushing's syndrome and, 351
    hypothalamic-pituitary axis and,
        118–121
    thyroid and, 222

Major histocompatibility complex
        (MHC), 76
    autoimmune disease and, 89–90
    gene organization, 77f
Major histocompatibility complex
        (MHC) molecules, 77
    class I and II, schematic
        representation, 78f
    inappropriate expression, 93
Male infertility, 425–427
    causes, 426t
Male reproductive function, aging and,
        784
Male reproductive system, 404f
    accessory structures, 405
    anatomy, 403–405, 404f
    disorders
        clinical, 415–432
        pharmacology of drugs used to treat,
            414–415
    evaluation of function, 409–414
    physiology, 405–409
Male Turner's syndrome, 420–421,
        537
Malformation syndromes, intrauterine
        growth retardation and, 158
Malignancy
    adrenocortical, 355
    humoral manifestations, 741–750
Malignancy-associated hypercalcemia,
        283, 743–746, 743t
Malignant transformation, hormones and,
        724–726
Malnutrition
    hypogonadotropic hypogonadism and,
        533–534
    short stature and, 176
MAO. See Monoamine oxidase
Marfanoid habitus, multiple endocrine
        neoplasia and, 758
Marfan's syndrome, tall stature and,
        188
Maturation index (MI), 451
Mayer-Rokitansky-Kuster-Hauser
        syndrome, 457
McCune-Albright syndrome
    G protein-coupled receptors and, 65
    incomplete precocious puberty and,
        542
Medroxyprogesterone
    for inadequate luteal phase, 471
    for menopause, 476–477
Medroxyprogesterone acetate
    ovarian suppression and, 470
    for precocious puberty, 545
Medullary thyroid carcinoma (MTC). See
        Thyroid cancer, medullary
        carcinoma
Melatonin, formation and metabolism,
        104f
Membrane trafficking
    disease and, 49
    hormone-secreting cells and, 44f
    prior to sorting of cargo, 45–46
    SNARE hypothesis and, 45f
Membrane vesicles
    hormone export and, 40–49
    hormone storage and, 39
MEN. See Multiple endocrine neoplasia

Menarche, 529
    premature, 542–543
Meninges, relationship to pituitary,
        123f
Menopause, 473–477
    clinical manifestations, 474–476
    hormonal changes, 473–474, 473t
    management, 476–477
Menorrhagia, causes, 454t
Menotropins, ovulation induction and,
        469–470, 470t
Menstrual cycle, 441–447
    cervical mucus and, 450, 451f
    endometrium and, 448–450, 449f
    hormone interaction and regulation
        during, 446–447
    hormone profiles during, 441–444
    median lengths during reproductive
        life, 442f
    menopause and, 474
    menstrual phase, 450
    neural regulation, 447, 448f
    ovarian cycle, 444–446
    proliferative phase, 448
    secretory phase, 448–450
    vaginal epithelium and, 450–452
Menstrual function
    disorders, 453–469
    extragenital symptoms associated,
        452–453
Menstrual phase, 450
Metabolism
    catecholamines and, 391
    hormones and, 22
    recombinant DNA technology and,
        13–14, 14t
Metanephrine, normal reference ranges,
        795t
Metaphase chromosomes, 488f
Metformin
    daily dose and duration of action, 624t
    for diabetes mellitus, 625–626
Methimazole
    for Graves' disease, 238–239
    structure, 201f
    for thyrotoxic crisis, 240
Methyldopa, for hypertension in
        pregnancy, 565
Metoclopramide, for diabetic gastropare-
        sis, 658
Metolazone, hypercalcemia and, 284
Metrorrhagia, causes, 454t
Metyrapone, ACTH secretory reserve
        and, 115
Metyrapone test
    adrenal insufficiency and, 333
    hypothalamic-pituitary function and,
        119t
MHC. See Major histocompatibility com-
        plex
MI. See Maturation index
Microadenoma, 122, 130
Microalbuminuria, diabetes mellitus and,
        615, 655–656
Microphallus, 517
    response to testosterone therapy, 517f
Microsurgery, transsphenoidal. See
        Transphenoidal microsurgery
Microvascular disease, diabetic, 653

Mifepristone, ovarian function inhibition and, 472
Milk-alkali syndrome, hypercalcemia and, 285
Mineral homeostasis, control, 274
Mineral metabolism, hormones and, 23
Mineralocorticoid(s)
  biosynthetic pathways, 360f
  pregnancy and, 557
  release, 40
  syndrome of apparent excess, 369
    ratio of urinary cortisol metabolites and, 370f
  synthesis, metabolism, action, 359–360, 361f
  use in therapy, 22t
Mineralocorticoid hypertension
  mechanisms involved, 361f
  pathogenesis, 361–362
Misopristone, mechanism and tumor target, 732t
MIT. See Monoiodotyrosine
Mitochondria, steroid hormone synthesis and, 52
Mitotane
  for adrenal tumors, 353
  for Cushing's disease, 144
Molecular chaperones, 43
Molecular mimicry
  autoimmune pancreatic B cell destruction and, 607
  autoimmune response and, 92, 92f
Monoamine(s)
  food intake and, 718–719, 719f
  nutrient appetites and, 720t
Monoamine oxidase (MAO), catecholamine metabolism and, 386f
Monoiodotyrosine (MIT), structure, 196f
Mononeuritis multiplex, 657
Motilin
  distribution, 579t
  mode of delivery, 576t
  properties, 585–586
Motility disorders, gut peptides and, 587
Motor neuropathy, diabetes mellitus and, 657
MRI. See Magnetic resonance imaging
Mucin-like molecules, 83
Mucocutaneous candidiasis, sequence for onset, 764f
Mucosal neuroma, multiple endocrine neoplasia and, 758, 758f
Mullerian defects, amenorrhea and, 457
Multinodular goiter
  elderly and, 774
  toxic, 242, 242f
Multiple endocrine neoplasia (MEN), 274–276, 283, 394–395, 588, 753–759
  abnormal hormone production, 754t
  components, 754t
  genetic diagnosis, 759
  management, 759
  type I, 753, 754–755
    components, 755t
  type IIa, 753, 754, 755–758
    components, 755t

type IIb, 753, 754, 755–758
  clinical features, 758t
  components, 756t
Multiple myeloma, hypercalcemia and, 746
Muscle, insulin and, 601
Muscle weakness, Cushing's syndrome and, 347
Myocardial infarction, oral contraceptives and, 481
Myocardium
  adrenergic responses, 389t
  catecholamines and, 390
Myopathy, thyroid hormones and, 215
Myotonic dystrophy, 421
Myxedema, 225
  heart disease and, 231, 232
Myxedema coma
  hypothyroidism and, 230–231
  treatment, 232

NAC. See Nascent chain-associated complex
Nafarelin, ovarian function inhibition and, 471
Nascent chain-associated complex (NAC), 42
National Cholesterol Education Program, 688
  adult treatment guidelines, 688t
Necrotizing papillitis, diabetes mellitus and, 656
Needle biopsy, thyroid nodules and, 251
Negative selection, 84
Nelson's syndrome, 144–145
Neoplasms, cryptorchidism and, 420
Nephrolithiasis, hypercalciuric, 307
Nephropathy, diabetic, 655–656
Nephrosis
  secondary hypercholesterolemia and, 698
  secondary hypertriglyceridemia and, 695
Nerve growth factor (NGF), tumor growth and, 725t
Nervousness, endocrine disease and, 29t
Nervous system, endocrine system and, 10–14
Neural hormones, substances functioning as, 96t
Neurocrine delivery, 576, 577f
Neuroeffector junction, 387f
Neuroendocrine messengers, 96t
Neuroendocrine tumors, gut, 588
Neuroendocrinology, 10–14
Neuroglycopenia
  counterregulatory response, 664–668
  hypoglycemia and, 641
Neuroma, mucosal, multiple endocrine neoplasia and, 758, 758f
Neurons, amine uptake and, 386
Neuropathy, diabetic, 656–658
Neuropeptide(s), endocrine system and, 12
Neuropeptide Y (NPY)
  distribution, 579t

food intake and, 719
mode of delivery, 576t
Neuropsychiatric disease, hypothyroidism and, 231
Neurosteroidogenesis, 52
Neurotensin
  distribution, 579t
  mode of delivery, 576t
  properties, 585
Neurotransmitters
  actions and interrelationships, 2f
  counterregulatory response to hypoglycemia and, 667
  food intake and, 718–719
  hormones and, 10–11
  hypothalamic, 11–12
  receptors, 60–61
    subdivisions of, 60t
  substances functioning as, 96t
Newborn, hypothyroidism and, 226–227, 227f
NGF. See Nerve growth factor
Niacin
  for hyperlipoproteinemia, 706–707, 708
  sites of action, 706f
Nicotinic acid, for hyperlipoproteinemia, 706–707
NIDDM. See Diabetes mellitus, type II
Nitric oxide (NO), parturition and, 560
Nitric oxide synthase (NOS)
  neural, inducible, endothelial forms, structural schematics, 68f
  signaling through, 69f
NO. See Nitric oxide
Nonfasting hypoglycemia, 677
Non-insulin-dependent diabetes mellitus (NIDDM). See Diabetes mellitus, type II
Nonketotic hyperosmolar coma, elderly and, 776
Nonproliferative retinopathy, diabetes mellitus and, 654
Noonan's syndrome, 420–421, 537
  short stature and, 175
Norepinephrine, 381
  in adrenal medulla, 382
  catecholamines present as, 384t
  conversion of dopamine to, 384
  conversion to epinephrine, 384
  endocrine system and, 11–12
  food intake and, 719
  plasma
    cardiovascular/metabolic effects, 391t
    insulin administration and, 392f
    in vena cava blood samples, 400f
  release, substances altering, 385t
NOS. See Nitric oxide synthase
NPY. See Neuropeptide Y
Nuclear receptors, 70
  hormone-recognition elements for, 72t
  for hormones, 6–7
Nutrient(s)
  balance, controller, 717–719, 718f
  satiety signaling and, 717
  storage of ingested, insulin and, 600
Nutrient balance model, 710, 711–721

Nutrition
  osteoporosis and, 297–298
  postnatal growth and, 164–165
  vitamin D, 272–273

Obesity, 710–723
  Cushing's syndrome and, 346
  genetic factors and, 710–711, 711*f*
  hypothalamic-pituitary axis and, 117
  nutrient balance model and, 710,
    711–721
  treatment, 721–723
  type II diabetes mellitus and, 609
Obstructive sleep apnea, short stature
    and, 176
Occult diabetes, 678
Occupation, diabetic patient and, 633
Octreotide, 582
  therapeutic uses, 591
Octreotide acetate
  for acromegaly, 141–142
  endocrinologic management and, 35*t*
  mechanism and tumor target, 732*t*
  thyrotropin secretion and, 111
4-OHA, mechanism and tumor target,
    732*t*
Oligomenorrhea
  causes, 454*t*
  endocrine disease and, 29*t*
  prolactinoma and, 132
Onapristone, mechanism and tumor
    target, 732*t*
Oncogenes, 743
  hormones and, 5
Oncogenous osteomalacia, 307
Oncogenous osteomalacia factor, 750
Onycholysis, Graves' disease and, 237*f*
Ophthalmopathy, Graves' disease and,
    234*f*, 236*f*, 240–241
Oral contraceptives, 477–482
  adverse effects, 479–481
  clinical uses, 479
  contraindications, 482
  hirsutism and, 466, 467–468*t*
  pharmacologic effects, 477–479
Orinase. *See* Tolbutamide
Orthostatic hypotension, diabetes
    mellitus and, 658
Osmolality
  blood volume and, 148–149
  normal reference ranges, 795*t*
  plasma/urine, diabetes
    insipidus/primary polydipsia
    and, 151
Osmoregulatory defects, 153
Osteitis deformans, 308–311
Osteoarthritis, Paget's disease and, 310
Osteoblast, 292
Osteoclast, 292–294
  cells in lineage, 293*f*
Osteocyte, 292
Osteodystrophy, renal, 311–313
  adynamic, 312
  pathogenesis, 312*f*
Osteomalacia, 304–308, 306*f*
  causes, 305*t*
  clinical features, 305–306
  diagnosis, 307

drug-induced, 307
oncogenous, 307
pathology, 304
pathophysiology, 304–305
treatment, 307
vitamin D deficiency and, 274
Osteomalacia factor, oncogenous, 750
Osteopathy, thyroid, 235*f*
Osteoporosis, 295–304, 299*f*
  calcium nutrition and, 297*t*
  calcium preparations and, 302*t*
  causes, 297*t*
  clinical features, 298–300
  Cushing's syndrome and, 347
  diagnosis, 301
  diagnostic criteria, World Health Orga-
    nization, 777*t*
  elderly and, 776–781
  epidemiology, 295
  etiology, 295–298
  menopause and, 475, 475*f*
  pathogenesis, 300–301
  secondary, 298
  treatment, 301–304
Ovarian cycle, 444–446
Ovaries, 434–484
  anatomy, 434–435
  differentiation, 491–493
  disorders of function, 453–469
  failure
    autoimmune Addison's disease and,
      765
    primary, 536–537
  follicles
    changes during growth and develop-
      ment, 444*f*
    control of growth and steroidogene-
      sis and, 445–446
  functional hyperandrogenism,
    461–463
  hormones, 435–441
    pregnancy and, 549
    therapeutic uses, 470–471
  inhibitors, 471–473
  mammalian, 436*f*
  nonsteroidal regulatory factors, 446
  number of germ cells at different ages,
    435*f*
  ovulation induction, 469–470
  premature failure, amenorrhea and,
    457
  structure, 444–445
  suppression, estrogen-progestin combi-
    nations and, 470–471
  tumors
    amenorrhea and, 457–459
    classification and clinical features,
      458*t*
Ovulation
  disorders, infertility and, 483
  induction, 469–470
    hypothalamic-pituitary dysfunction
      and, 129
Oxandrolone, for permanent
    hypogonadism, 538–539
Oxygen consumption, thyroid hormones
    and, 214
Oxytocin, 102
  actions, 147

parturition and, 560
structure, 101*t*

P450 aromatase deficiency, female
    pseudohermaphroditism and,
    508
P450c17 deficiency, male
    pseudohermaphroditism and,
    510–511
P450c21 hydroxylase deficiency, female
    pseudohermaphroditism and,
    504–507
Paget's disease of bone, 308–311, 309*f*,
    310*f*
  complications, 311*t*
Pain, abdominal, endocrine disease and,
    29*t*
Palsy, cranial nerve, diabetes mellitus
    and, 657
Pancreas. *See also* Islets of Langerhans
  adrenergic responses, 389*t*
  disease, secondary diabetes mellitus
    and, 611–612
  endocrine. *See* Endocrine pancreas
  exocrine, 595
  pregnancy and, 556–557
  response during glucose stimulation,
    599*f*
  transplantation, diabetes mellitus and,
    632
  tumors, multiple endocrine neoplasia
    and, 755
Pancreatic cholera, 589
Pancreatic polypeptide (PP), 605'
  distribution, 579*t*
  mode of delivery, 576*t*
  normal reference ranges, 795*t*
  properties, 586
Pancreatitis, plasma triglycerides and,
    689
Papillary carcinoma, thyroid. *See*
    Thyroid cancer
Paracrine, 3
Paracrine delivery, 576, 577*f*
Paracrine effects, 600–601
Paracrine factors, tumor growth and,
    726–727
Parathyroidectomy, for primary
    hyperparathyroidism, 281–282
Parathyroid gland
  anatomy and physiology, 264
  cells, parathyroid hormone production
    and, 267*f*
  congenital aplasia, 287–288
  fetal, endocrinology, 559
  pregnancy and, 556
Parathyroid hormone (PTH), 264–269
  amino terminal part, 844*f*
  assay, 267–268
    two-site, 268*t*
  biologic effects, 268–269
  clearance and metabolism, 267
  endocrinologic management and, 35*t*
  intact, immunoradiometric assay, 278*f*
  mechanism of action, 269
  normal reference ranges, 795*t*
  production within parathyroid cell,
    267*f*

secretion, 264–266
serum
  calcium and, 265f
  effect of age, 777f
synthesis and processing, 266
Parathyroid hormone-related protein
  (PTHrP), 269
  amino terminal part, 744f
  concentrations in malignancy, 745f
  hypercalcemia and, 745–746
Parietal cells, autoimmunity against, 765t
Parity, breast cancer and, 733
Partial agonist-partial antagonist, 10
Parturition
  endocrine control, 559–560
  oxytocin and, 147
Pathogens, processing and presentation,
  80t
Pathologic short stature, criteria, 169
PCR. See Polymerase chain reaction
PDGF. See Platelet-derived growth factor
Pelvis, Paget's disease and, 310f
Penis, anatomic defects, male infertility
  and, 427
Pentamidine-induced hypoglycemia,
  672
Peptic ulcer, glucocorticoids and, 329
Peptide(s)
  food intake and, 718–719, 719f, 719t
  nutrient appetites and, 720t
Peptide hormones
  metabolism and elimination, 19
  nuclear action, 70
  receptors, 60–61
    subdivisions, 60t
Peptide YY (PYY)
  distribution, 579t
  mode of delivery, 576t
Pergolide, for prolactinoma, 135
Peripheral sensory neuropathy, diabetes
  mellitus and, 656–657
Peripheral vascular disease, diabetes mellitus and, 658–659
Persistent Mullerian duct syndrome, 516
Pertussis toxin, G protein transduction
  system and, 62
Phenformin, for diabetes mellitus, 625
Phenoxybenzamine, pheochromocytoma
  and, 397–398, 400
Phentolamine, growth hormone secretion
  and, 108
Pheochromocytes, 382
Pheochromocytoma, 393–401
  clinical features, 393–394, 393t
  complications, 396
  diagnostic tests and procedures,
    397–398
  differential diagnosis, 396–397
  hypercalcemia and, 284
  incidental adrenal mass and, 356
  localization of tumors, 398–399, 399f
  malignant, distribution of metastases
    and, 401t
  management, 399–401
  multiple endocrine neoplasia and,
    757
  pathology, 395–396, 395f
  screening and, 398, 398t
  unsuspected, causes of death and, 396t

Phosphate, for diabetic ketoacidosis, 649
Phospholipase C beta
  activation, 62
  receptor signaling and, 64f
Photocoagulation, for diabetic
  retinopathy, 655
Photomotogram, 223
Physical activity, hypogonadotropic
  hypogonadism and, 534
Phytosterolemia, 702
PIH. See Prolactin-inhibiting hormone
Pineal gland, 13, 103
Pituitary, 95–153
  ACTH hormone reserve, 115
  amenorrhea and, 459
  anatomic relationships, 98f
  anatomy and embryology, 96t
  anterior, Cushing's syndrome and,
    344
  blood supply, 97–98, 98f
  cancer therapy and, 728
  disorders, 122–146. See also specific
    disorder
  histology, 98–100
  hormones. See Pituitary hormones
  hypersecretion, 122
  hypothalamic relationships, 11–13
  insufficiency, 122–123
  pregnancy and, 554
  relationship to meninges, 123f
  tumors
    amenorrhea and, 459
    multiple endocrine neoplasia and,
      755
  venous drainage, 99f
Pituitary adenoma, 130–146. See also
  Prolactinoma
  ACTH-secreting, 142–145
  alpha subunit-secreting, 146
  Cushing's syndrome and, 344
  gonadotropin-secreting, 145–146
  nonfunctional, 146
  pregnancy and, 562–563
  thyrotropin-secreting, 145, 243
Pituitary-adrenal reserve, measurement,
  332–334
Pituitary gigantism, 189
Pituitary hormones
  anterior, 104–114
    characteristics, 105t
    fetal, 558
  posterior, 102, 146–153
    fetal, 559
    structure, 101t
  postpartum levels, 561
  tumors secreting, 750
PKC. See Protein kinase C
Placenta, function, 549
Placental lactogen. See Human placental
  lactogen
Plasma, regulation of hormone-binding
  proteins and, 56
Plasma binding, delivery of hormones
  and, 18–19, 19f
Plasma-binding proteins
  cortisol/androgens and, 324
  regulation, 18–19
Plasma volume, catecholamine infusion
  and, 390f

Platelet-derived growth factor (PDGF),
  tumor growth and, 725t
Plicamycin, for Paget's disease of bone,
  311
Plummer's disease, 241–242
PMS. See Premenstrual syndrome
POEMS syndrome, 767
  incidence of abnormalities, 767t
Polycystic ovary syndrome, 461–463
  clinical findings, 462t
  pathophysiology of chronic
    anovulation, 462f
Polydipsia, primary, 150
Polymenorrhea, causes, 454t
Polymerase chain reaction (PCR), 31–32
Polymorphism, 77
Polypeptide hormones
  metabolism, 55
  pregnancy and, 552–553
  secretion, 39
  translocation across ER membrane,
41f
  transport, 18
Polyuria
  Cushing's syndrome and, 347
  differential diagnosis, 151t
  endocrine disease and, 29t
  results of diagnostic studies, 150t
POMC. See Proopiomelanocortin
Positive selection, 84
Postabsorptive state, 566
  maintenance of euglycemia and,
    667–668, 668t
Postcoital contraceptives, 482
  schedules for use, 482f
Postnatal growth, 158–168
Potassium, for diabetic ketoacidosis,
  648–649
PP. See Pancreatic polypeptide
Prader orchidometer, 411f
Prader-Willi syndrome
  hypogonadotropic hypogonadism and,
    533
  short stature and, 175
Prazosin, for pheochromocytoma, 400
Preantral follicle, 444
Precocious puberty, 539–545
  classification, 539t
  complete, 540–541, 540f
  incomplete, 540, 541–542
  tall stature and, 189
Prednisolone, chemical name, 51t
Prednisone, chemical name, 51t
Preeclampsia, 564–565
  treatment, 565
Pregnancy
  autoimmune disease and, 23
  breast cancer and, 563–564
  diabetes mellitus and, 566–572
    classification, 567t
  endocrine disorders and, 562–572
  endocrine function tests and, 556t
  endocrinology, 548–572
  hypertensive disorders and, 564–565
  hyperthyroidism and, 565–566
  hypothyroidism and, 566
  insulin-treated diabetics and, 671
  maternal adaptations, 554–557,
    555–556f

Pregnancy (*cont.*)
  maternal serum hormone changes during, 550–551*f*
  ovarian hormones and, 549
  pituitary adenomas and, 562–563
  polypeptide hormones and, 552–553
  steroid hormones and, 553–554
  symptoms and signs, 549
  thyroid function and, 215–216
  thyrotoxicosis and, 241
Pregnanetriol, normal reference ranges, 795*t*
Pregnenolone
  chemical name, 51*t*
  steroids derived, 49
Prematurity, intrauterine growth retardation and, 174
Premenstrual syndrome (PMS), 452–453
Preocious puberty
  differential diagnosis, 543, 544*t*
  treatment, 543–545
Preovulatory follicle, 444
  androgen/estradiol synthesis and secretion, pathways involved, 445*f*
Preparathyroid hormone, primary structure, 266*f*
Preproinsulin, 596
  biosynthesis and release, pancreatic B cells and, 596–597, 597*f*
Primary follicle, 444
PRL. *See* Prolactin
Progeria, 702
Progesterone
  binding to corticosteroid-binding globulin, 437
  chemical name, 51*t*
  classification of action, 9*f*
  endocrinologic management and, 35*t*
  estrogen secretion and, 471
  for hypopituitarism, 129
  for inadequate luteal phase, 471
  maternal, changes during pregnancy, 550*f*
  menstrual cycle and, 442*f*, 443
  normal reference ranges, 795*t*
  ovarian
    concentrations, production and secretion rates, 438*t*
    metabolism, 438
    percentage distribution, 438*t*
  parturition and, 560
  physiologic effects, 440
  pregnancy and, 553
  secretory pattern during menstrual cycle, 113*f*
  serum concentrations, menopause and, 473*t*
  structure, 320*f*
  synthesis, pathway, 50*f*
  use in therapy, 22*t*
Progesterone receptors, endocrine therapy in breast cancer and, 735*t*
Progestins
  contraception and, 482
  for hirsutism, 466

synthetic, pharmacologic effects, 477–479
  threatened abortion and, 471
Progestogens, maternal, female pseudohermaphroditism and, 508
Proglucagon, tissue-specific secretory products, 603*f*
Proinsulin, 597
  assay, insulinoma and, 674
  molecule, abnormalities, 611
  mutant, 610–611, 610*t*
  structure, 598*f*
Prolactin (PRL)
  biosynthesis, function, measurement, secretion, 108–110
  characteristics, 105*t*
  deficiency, hypopituitarism and, 128
  hypersecretion, 116
  indications for measurement, 125*t*
  lactation and, 561–562
  maternal, changes during pregnancy, 551*f*
  measurements, male hypogonadism and, 411
  menstrual cycle and, 443
  normal ranges in men, 411*t*
  normal reference ranges, 796*t*
  normal responses, 116*t*
  postpartum levels, 561
  reserve, 116
  secretion
    factors affecting, 110*t*
    sleep-associated changes, 109*f*
Prolactin-inhibiting hormone (PIH), 101
  structure, 101*t*
Prolactinoma, 131–136
  pathology, 131–132
Prolactin-releasing factors, 101, 110
Proliferative phase, 448
Proliferative retinopathy, diabetes mellitus and, 654–655
Proopiomelanocortin (POMC)
  processing, 105*f*
  processing and secretion, 48
Propranolol, for pheochromocytoma, 400
Propylthiouracil
  for Graves' disease, 238–239
  for hyperthyroidism in pregnancy, 565–566
  structure, 201*f*
  for thyrotoxic crisis, 240
Prostacyclins, synthesis, pathways, 54*f*
Prostaglandins, 5–6
  endocrinologic management and, 35*t*
  parturition and, 560
  release, 40
  synthesis, pathways, 54*f*
  use in therapy, 22*t*
Prostate gland, benign hyperplasia, 784–785
Prostatic cancer, 738–739
  androgen therapy and, 414
Protein kinase C (PKC), activator, 63
Proteins, co- and posttranslational modification, 42–43
Proteinuria, diabetes mellitus and, 615
Protirelin, thyrotropin and, 116

Provocative tests, 756–757
Pseudofracture, 306*f*
Pseudohermaphroditism
  female, 503–508, 504*f*
  male, 491, 508–516
    dysgenetic, 515–516
Pseudohyperaldosteronism, 368–371
  type II, 371
Pseudohypoparathyroidism (PHP), 288*f*
  features, 289*t*
  hypocalcemia and, 288–289
  short stature and, 186
  type I, G protein-coupled receptors and, 65
  type Ia, 767
Pseudopseudohypoparathyroidism, 288
Pseudo-Turner's syndrome, 537
  short stature and, 175
Pseudovaginal perineoscrotal hypospadias, 514–515
Psychosexual differentiation, 493–497
Psychosocial dwarfism, 184, 185*f*
PTH. *See* Parathyroid hormone
PTHrP. *See* Parathyroid hormone-related protein
Puberty, 521–545
  delayed, 530–539
    classification, 530*t*
    differential diagnosis, 537–538, 537*t*
    treatment, 538–539
  physiology, 521–530
  precocious, 539–545
    classification, 539*t*
    complete, 540–541, 540*f*
    incomplete, 540, 541–542
    tall stature and, 189
  variations in development and, 542–543
Pubic hair development
  female, 522, 523*f*
  male, 522, 524*f*
Puerperium, endocrinology, 560–562
Pyloric stenosis, infantile hypertrophic, gut peptides and, 587
PYY. *See* Peptide YY

Quingolide, for prolactinoma, 135

Radiation, ionizing, thyroid and, 249–250, 249*t*
Radiation therapy. *See also* Radiotherapy
  hypogonadotropic hypogonadism and, 532
  hypopituitarism and, 127
Radioactive iodine therapy, for Graves' disease, 239
Radioactive iodine uptake (RAIU), 220
  normal reference ranges, 797*t*
  subacute thyroiditis and, 246*f*
Radioimmunoassay
  diabetes insipidus/primary polydipsia and, 151–152
  gonadal steroids and, 410–411
Radioiodine, 24-hour uptake, 197*f*, 220
Radionuclide imaging, thyroid and, 220–222, 222*f*

Radiosurgery
  for Cushing's disease, 144
  for pituitary adenoma, 131
Radiotherapy. *See also* Radiation therapy
  for Cushing's disease, 144
  for growth hormone hypersecretion, 141
  for prolactinoma, 135
Radius, osteomalacia and, 306*f*
RAIU. *See* Radioactive iodine uptake
Rapid ACTH stimulation test, hypothalamic-pituitary function and, 119*t*
Reactive hypoglycemia, 677
Receptors. *See specific receptor*
Recessive abetalipoproteinemia, 700–701
Recklinghausen's disease, 759
Recombinant DNA technology. *See also* DNA analysis
  endocrinology and metabolism and, 13–14, 14*t*
5alpha-Reductase deficiency, male pseudohermaphroditism and, 514–515
Regulated secretory pathway, 46
Regulatory chemicals, origins, 15
Reifenstein's syndrome, 514
Relaxin, 441, 549
Renal calculi, Cushing's syndrome and, 347
Renal cell carcinoma, hypercalcemia and, 744
Renal failure, gut peptides and, 587
Renal insufficiency, insulin-treated diabetics and, 671
Renal osteodystrophy, 311–313
  adynamic, 312
  pathogenesis, 312*f*
Renal transplantation, diabetic nephropathy and, 656
Renal tubular acidosis, short stature and, 176
Renin, 371–372
  normal reference ranges, 796*t*
  tumors secreting, 750
Renin-angiotensin-aldosterone system, assessment, 363–364
Renin-angiotensin system, 371–374
  hypertension and, 374–377
  pregnancy and, 557
Renin-secreting tumors, 377
Renovascular hypertension, 375–377
  clinical index of suspicion and, 376*t*
  suggested workup, 377*f*
Reproduction, hormones and, 23
Reproductive system
  female. *See* Female reproductive system
  male. *See* Male reproductive system
Resistant ovary syndrome, amenorrhea and, 457
Restriction fragment length polymorphism (RFLP), 32–33
Retained antrum syndrome, gut peptides and, 587
Retinoic acid, receptors, 72–73
Retinopathy, diabetic, 654–655
Retrograde ejaculation, male infertility and, 427

RFLP. *See* Restriction fragment length polymorphism
Rickets, 304–308, 750
  causes, 305*t*
  clinical features, 305–306
  hypophosphatemic, 307
  pathology, 304
  pathophysiology, 304–305
  short stature and, 186
  treatment, 308
Riedel's struma, 247
RU-486, mechanism and tumor target, 732*t*
Rudimentary testes syndrome, 516
Ruffled border, 292

Saccharin, diabetes mellitus and, 621
Saline infusion test, primary aldosteronism and, 364
Salmon calcitonin, for Paget's disease of bone, 311
Salt intake, primary aldosteronism and, 363
Sarcoidosis
  hypercalcemia and, 284
  hypopituitarism and, 126
Satiety
  gastrointestinal signals producing, 715–717
  model, 721*f*
Schmidt's syndrome, 247–248, 764
Secondary follicle, 444
Secondary sexual characteristics, development, 521–525
  sequence, 525*f*
Secretin
  distribution, 579*t*
  mode of delivery, 576*t*
  normal reference ranges, 796*t*
  properties, 581
Secretory granules, 40
Secretory pathway
  constitutive, 46
  post-ER vesicular traffic and, 43–45
  regulated, 46
Secretory phase, 448–450
Seip-Berardinelli syndrome, 702
Selectins, 83
Self-monitoring, diabetic patient and, 633
Self-tolerance, 76
Sella turcica, enlarged, 123
Semen analysis
  gonadal dysfunction and, 410
  infertility and, 482–483
Seminiferous tubule(s), 403–405
  adult failure, 421–423
Seminiferous tubule dysgenesis, 497–499, 535
Seminoma, amenorrhea and, 458
Senile cataract, diabetes mellitus and, 655
Sensory neuropathy, peripheral, diabetes mellitus and, 656–657
Serotonin
  endocrine system and, 11–12
  food intake and, 718
Sertoli cell(s), 403–405

Sertoli cell only syndrome, 535
Sertoli-Leydig cell tumors, amenorrhea and, 458–459
Seven-transmembrane receptors, 61
Sex chromosomes, 487–489
  abnormalities, nomenclature, 489*t*
  structural abnormalities, syndrome of gonadal dysgenesis and, 500*t*
  X, G-banded, 490*f*
  X chromatin and Y bodies and, 491*t*
  Y, G-banded, 490*f*
Sex cord-mesenchymal tumors, amenorrhea and, 458–459
Sex determination, 489–491
Sex differentiation
  anomalous, 497, 497*t*
  diagrammatic summation, 496*f*
  female, abnormal, 517
  male
    abnormal, 516–517
    hormones involved, 492*f*
  normal, 487–491
Sex hormone-binding globulin (SHBG)
  binding capacity, measurement, 334
  estradiol binding, 437
  serum concentration, factors affecting, 465*t*
  steroid hormones and, 17
  testosterone binding, 405–406
Sex hormone deficiency, osteoporosis and, 296
Sex steroids. *See also* Gonadal steroids; Steroid hormones
  circulating, contributions of testes, adrenals, peripheral tissues, 407*t*
  for constitutional delay in growth, 538
  parturition and, 560
  postnatal growth and, 163
  secretion
    pattern during menstrual cycle, 113*f*
    puberty and, 527–528
Sexual characteristics, secondary, development, 521–525, 525*f*
Sexual infantilism, 530–539
Sexual precocity. *See* Precocious puberty
SF-1. *See* Steroidogenic factor-1
SHBG. *See* Sex hormone-binding globulin
Short stature
  causes, 173*t*
    endocrine, 176–187
    nonendocrine, 170–176
  constitutional, 170–173
  diagnosis, 187–188
  genetic, 173–174
  pathologic, criteria, 169
  syndromes, 174–175
SIADH. *See* Syndrome of inappropriate secretion of antidiuretic hormone
Sickle cell anemia, short stature and, 176
Signal patch, 46
Signal recognition particle (SRP), protein translocation across ER membrane and, 41–42
Signal sequence, 41

Signal transduction, G protein-mediated, 62*f*

Sipple's syndrome, 394, 588, 753

Skeletal age, 170

Skeletal dysplasia, short stature and, 175

Skeleton
  bone remodeling rates, 294*t*
  functions, hormones and, 23

Skin
  adrenergic responses, 389*t*
  Cushing's syndrome and, 346–347
  diabetes mellitus and, 659
  endocrine disease and, 29*t*
  menopause and, 474
  oral contraceptives and, 479

Skull, Paget's disease and, 310*f*

Sleep apnea, short stature and, 176

Small bowel resection, gut peptides and, 587

Small intestine, wall, 577*f*

Smooth muscle, catecholamines and, 390–391

SNARE hypothesis, for intracellular vesicular traffic, 45*f*

Sodium bicarbonate, for diabetic ketoacidosis, 648

Soluble fibers, 621

Soluble mediators, 83–84

Somatic recombination, 78

Somatomammotropin, characteristics, 105*t*

Somatostatin, 100–101, 604–605
  amino acid sequence, 604*f*
  distribution, 579*t*
  food intake and, 719
  growth hormone secretion and, 107
  mode of delivery, 576*t*
  normal reference ranges, 796*t*
  properties, 582
  structure, 101*t*
  thyrotropin and, 111

Somatostatinoma, 590–591

Somatotrophs, 99

Somatotropin. *See* Growth hormone

Somogyi effect, 638

Spermatogenesis
  defects, 427
  gonadotropins and, 415
  hypopituitarism and, 129

Spermaturia, 523

Sphingolipidoses, 702

Spine, Paget's disease and, 310*f*

Spinnbarkeit, 450

Spiral arteries, 448

Spironolactone
  classification of action, 9*f*
  for hirsutism, 468
  trivial and chemical name, 51*t*

Spongiosa layer, 448

Squamous carcinoma, hypercalcemia and, 744

SRP. *See* Signal recognition particle

SRP receptor, 41–42

Starch blockers, diabetes mellitus and, 622

StAR deficiency, male sexual differentiation and, 509–510

Starvation, hypothalamic-pituitary axis and, 118

Stature. *See also* Short stature; Tall stature
  adult, RWT method for predicting, 171–172*t*
  midparental height and, 169
  parent-specific adjustments, 166*f*, 167*f*

Steroid-dependent tumors, 727, 727*t*

Steroid hormones. *See also* Sex steroids
  biosynthesis, 320–324, 321*f*, 322*f*
    pathways in adrenal and gonads, 505*f*
  chemistry, 49–51
  export, 49–52
  gonadal, 405–407
    biosynthetic pathways, 406*f*
    measurements, 410–411
    normal ranges in men, 411*t*
  metabolism, 55
  metabolism and elimination, 19–20
  nongenomic effects, 73–74
  ovarian, 435–441
    biosynthesis, 435–436, 437*f*
    concentrations, production and secretion rates, 438*t*
    gonadotropin secretion and, 447
    menstrual cycle and, 443–444
    metabolism, 438, 439*f*
    percentage distribution, 438*t*
    physiologic effects, 438–441
    secretion, 436–437
    transport, 437
  postpartum levels, 561
  pregnancy and, 553–554
  receptor resistance syndrome, 74
  release, 40
  serum concentrations, menopause and, 473*t*
  steps in action, 326*f*
  structure, 320*f*
  synthesis, 52
    pathways, 50*f*
  transport, 17
  trivial and chemical names, 51*t*

Steroidogenesis, 320–322
  ovarian, control, 445–446

Steroidogenic factor-1 (SF-1), 489–491

Steroid receptor complex, 70–72
  signaling through, 71*f*

Steroid receptors
  endocrine therapy and, 729–732
  endometrial cancer and, 737
  metastatic breast cancer in women and, 734–735, 735*t*
  prostatic cancer and, 738

Stimulation tests, insulinomas and, 673–674

Straight artery, 448

Stress
  CRH/ACTH secretion and, 323
  diabetic patient and, 633, 671
  elderly and, 782–784

Struma ovarii, 243

Subcapsular cataract, diabetes mellitus and, 655

Substance P
  distribution, 579*t*

mode of delivery, 576*t*
  properties, 584

Sulfonylureas
  for diabetes mellitus, 622–625
  hypoglycemia and, 671–672
  insulin release and, 623*f*
  type II diabetic patient and, 640

Superficial cells, 451

Suppression tests, insulinomas and, 673

Suppressor cells, 84

Sweeteners, diabetes mellitus and, 621–622

Sympathetic nervous system
  hypertension and, 379
  neuroeffector junction, 387*f*
  satiety signals and, 717

Syndrome of gonadal dysgenesis, 499–501, 536
  treatment, 539
  X and Y chromosome structural abnormalities and, 500*t*
  X chromatin-negative variants, 501
  X chromatin-positive variants, 500–501

Syndrome of inappropriate secretion of antidiuretic hormone (SIADH), 152–153
  cancer and, 747
  conditions associated, 153*t*

Syndrome of inappropriate secretion of thyrotropin, 243

Syndrome X, 608–609

Tacrolimus, interleukin-2 production and, 87

Tall stature
  causes, 173*t*
    endocrine, 189
    nonendocrine, 188
  constitutional, 188
  genetic, 188
  syndromes, 188–189

Tamoxifen
  classification of action, 9*f*
  ovarian function inhibition and, 471

Tangier disease, 699

TBG. *See* Thyroxine-binding globulin

TBPA. *See* Thyroxine-binding prealbumin

T cell(s)
  autoimmunity and, 91
  co-receptors, 82*t*
  cytotoxic, immune response and, 88
  model for antigen recognition, 82*f*

T cell receptor (TCR), 76, 77
  alpha and beta genes, rearrangement, 81*f*

TCR. *See* T cell receptor

TDF. *See* Testis-determining factor

Teratomas, amenorrhea and, 458

Tertiary follicle, 444

Testes, 403–432
  biopsy, male hypogonadism and, 412
  circulating sex steroids and, 407*t*
  control of function, 408–409
  differentiation, 491–493
  failure, primary, 535

laboratory tests of function, 410–414
tumors, 429–432
Testicular feminization, 457, 512–514
Testicular regression syndrome, 516
Testis-determining cascade, 489, 492*f*
Testis-determining factor (TDF), 488,
    489
Testosterone
    biosynthesis, inborn errors, 509–511
    biosynthetic pathway, enzymatic
        defects, 509*f*
    chemical name, 51*t*
    circulating, women and, 461*t*
    endocrinologic management and, 35*t*
    free, measurement, 334
    for Klinefelter's syndrome, 417,
        498
    levels, evaluation, 117
    male reproductive function and, 405
    maternal, changes during pregnancy,
        551*f*
    mechanism of action, 512*f*
    metabolism, 515*f*
        defects, 514–515
    normal ranges in men, 411*t*
    normal reference ranges, 796*t*
    ovarian
        concentrations, production and
            secretion rates, 438*t*
        percentage distribution, 438*t*
    for permanent hypogonadism, 538
    plasma, pubertal stage 2 and, 527*f*
    serum
        menopause and, 473*t*
        relation to age, 784*f*
Tetany, hypocalcemic, 286*f*
Tetraiodothyroacetic acid, chemical
        structures and biologic activity,
        205*t*
Tetraiodothyronine
    chemical structures and biologic activ-
        ity, 205*t*
    decreased conversion to triio-
        dothyronine, associated
        factors/conditions, 207*t*
    free, at pituitary and peripheral tissue
        level, 201*f*
    intramolecular formation, 200*f*
    radioactive, distribution, 202*f*
    structure, 196*f*
    uptake in subacute thyroiditis, 246*f*
TGF. *See* Transforming growth factor
TGN. *See* Trans-Golgi network
Thalassemia, short stature and, 176
THBR. *See* Thyroid hormone-binding ra-
    tio
Theca cell tumors, incomplete precocious
        puberty and, 542
Thelarche, premature, 542
Thiazide diuretics, hypercalcemia and,
        284
Thiazolidinediones, for diabetes mellitus,
        627
Thiocarbamide inhibitors, thyroidal
        iodide organification and, 201*f*
Thiouracil, structure, 201*f*
Thirst
    control, 148–149
    Cushing's syndrome and, 347

Thromboembolism, oral contraceptives
        and, 478, 480–481
Thromboxane, 5–6
    synthesis, pathways, 54*f*
Thyrocardiac disease, 238
Thyroglobulin, 49
    coupling of iodotyrosyl residues, 199
    iodination, 198*f*
    measurement, 219
    normal reference ranges, 796*t*
    proteolysis, 199–200
    reabsorption and digestion, 195*f*
    structure and function, 217*t*
    synthesis and iodination, 195*f*
    synthesis and secretion, 197–198
    tyrosyl iodination, 199
Thyroglossal duct, 192
Thyroid, 192–259
    anatomy and histology, 192–194, 193*f*
    autoantibodies
        measurement, 223–224
        normal reference ranges, 797*t*
    autoantigens, 217*t*
    autoimmune disease spectrum, 247*f*
    autoimmunity, 217–218
    autoregulation, 212
    biopsy, 223
    blood supply, 194*f*
    cancer. *See* Thyroid cancer
    cancer therapy and, 728
    cells
        autoimmunity against, 765*t*
        effects of thyrotropin, 211–212
        iodide transporter, 198*f*
    disorders, 224–258. *See also specific
        disorder*
        diabetes mellitus and, 765
        elderly and, 770–774
    examination, 225*f*
    fetal, endocrinology, 559
    function
        acute and chronic illness and,
            216–217, 216*f*
        control, 207–213
        function tests, 218–224
        clinical use, 224
    glucocorticoids and, 329
    imaging, 220–222
    ionizing radiation and, 249–250,
        249*t*
    magnetic resonance imaging and, 222
    nodules. *See* Thyroid nodules
    physiology, 194–218
    pregnancy and, 554
    rat, normal, 195*f*
    relationships, 193*f*
    ultrasonography and, 222
Thyroidal iodide, organification, thiocar-
        bamide inhibitors, 201*f*
Thyroidal peroxidase, synthesis and
        secretion, 198
Thyroid cancer, 243, 252–258
    anaplastic carcinoma, 254
        management, 257
    classification and staging, 257*t*
    course and prognosis, 257–258
    elderly and, 774
    follicular carcinoma, 253–254
        management, 255–256

frequency, 253*t*
    management, 253*t*, 255–257
    management decision matrix, 255*f*,
        256*f*
    medullary carcinoma, 254, 274–276
        management, 257
        multiple endocrine neoplasia and,
            756–757
        products secreted, 756*t*
    molecular defects associated, 255*f*
    papillary carcinoma, 252–253
        management, 255–256
    pathology, 252–255
    survival post-radioiodine therapy,
        259*f*
    survival post-thyroidectomy, 258*f*
Thyroidectomy, subtotal, for Graves' dis-
    ease, 239
Thyroid hormone
    actions, 213–215
    chemical structures and biologic activ-
        ity, 205*t*
    deficiency. *See* Hypothyroidism
    effects on peripheral tissues, 223
    intrauterine growth and, 158
    maternal, changes during pregnancy,
        550*f*
    metabolism, 55–56, 204–206
    metabolism and elimination, 20
    physiologic effects, 214–215
    postnatal growth and, 163
    protein-bound, factors influencing con-
        centration, 202*t*
    receptor resistance syndrome, 74
    receptors, 72–73, 213
        protein structure, 213*f*
        triiodothyronine actions and, 214*f*
    resistance syndromes, 243–244
    secretion, 49
        factors controlling, 208*t*
    structure, 194, 196*f*
    synthesis and secretion, 196–200
        abnormalities, 200–201
    synthesis in thyroid follicle, 197*f*
    tests in blood, 218–219
    transport, 17–18, 201–203
Thyroid hormone-binding proteins,
        203
    free and protein-bound hormone
        concentrations and, 203*f*
Thyroid hormone-binding ratio (THBR),
        218–219
Thyroiditis, 246–249
    atrophic, 247
    chronic, 247–249
    subacute, 246–247
        tetraiodothyronine/radioactive
            iodine uptake and, 246*f*
    subacute or chronic, 242–243
Thyroid nodules
    benign, 250–252
        differentiation, 251*t*
        etiology, 250*t*
    elderly and, 774
    workup decision matrix, 252*f*
Thyroid osteopathy, 235*f*
Thyroid peroxidase, structure and
        function, 217*t*
Thyroid receptor family, 72–73

Thyroid-stimulating hormone (TSH). *See* Thyrotropin

Thyroid-stimulating immunoglobulin (TSI), normal reference ranges, 797*t*

Thyroid storm, 238

Thyrotoxic crisis, 238
treatment, 240

Thyrotoxicosis, 233–243
aging and, 773*t*
conditions associated, 233*t*
hamburger, 243
hypercalcemia and, 284
pregnancy and, 241
tall stature and, 189

Thyrotoxicosis factitia, 243

Thyrotoxic periodic paralysis, 238

Thyrotrophs, 99

Thyrotropin
actions, 209–211
biosynthesis, function, measurement, secretion, 110–111
characteristics, 105*t*
deficiency, hypopituitarism and, 127–128
effects on thyroid cell, 211–212
for hypopituitarism, 129
maternal, changes during pregnancy, 551*f*
normal reference ranges, 797*t*
normal responses, 116*t*
pituitary adenomas secreting, 145, 243
pulsation profiles, aging and, 772*f*
secretion
circadian rhythms, 209*f*
control, 212
secretory reserve, evaluation, 116–117
serum, 212
serum responses to disease, 210*f*
subunit genes, 210*f*
syndrome of inappropriate secretion, 243

Thyrotropin receptor
model, 211*f*
structure and function, 217*t*

Thyrotropin receptor gene, mutations, 244

Thyrotropin-releasing hormone (TRH), 101, 111
actions, 207–209
chemical structure, 208*f*
structure, 101*t*

Thyrotropin-releasing hormone (TRH) test, 116–117
hypothalamic-pituitary function and, 120*t*

Thyroxine
daily doses for hypothyroidism, 774*t*
metabolism
deiodinative pathway, 206*f*
pathways, 204*f*
normal reference ranges, 797*t*
structure, 196*f*

Thyroxine:TBG ratio, normal reference ranges, 797*t*

Thyroxine-binding globulin (TBG)
normal reference ranges, 797*t*
synthesis and secretion, 202

Thyroxine-binding prealbumin (TBPA), synthesis and secretion, 202–203

Tibia, lytic Paget's disease and, 309*f*

Tissue injury, immunologic, types, 760*t*

Tissue-specific immunity, assessment methods, 760*t*

Tolazamide
daily dose and duration of action, 624*t*
for diabetes mellitus, 624

Tolbutamide
daily dose and duration of action, 624*t*
for diabetes mellitus, 622–623

Tolbutamide stimulation test, insulinoma and, 673

Tolinase. *See* Tolazamide

Toremifene, mechanism and tumor target, 732*t*

Torsion, cryptorchidism and, 420

Total triiodothyronine, measurement, 219

Toxic adenoma, 241–242

Toxic multinodular goiter, 242, 242*f*

Toxic nodular goiter, serum thyrotropin responses, 210*f*

Trabecular bone
osteoporotic treatment regimens and, 778*f*
remodeling, 292*f*

Transcortin. *See* Corticosteroid-binding globulin

Transcytosis, 49

Transforming growth factor (TGF), tumor growth and, 725*t*

Transfrontal craniotomy, for prolactinoma, 134

Trans-Golgi network (TGN)
formation of vesicles and, 45
sorting of vesicle cargo and, 46

Transhepatic portal vein sampling, insulinoma and, 674

Transsphenoidal microsurgery
for Cushing's disease, 143–144
for prolactinoma, 134

Transthyretin, synthesis and secretion, 202–203

Trauma, cryptorchidism and, 420

TRH. *See* Thyrotropin-releasing hormone

Triamcinolone, chemical name, 51*t*

Triglycerides, elevated serum levels, 689

Triiodothyroacetic acid, chemical structures and biologic activity, 205*t*

Triiodothyronine
chemical structures and biologic activity, 205*t*
normal reference ranges, 797*t*
structure, 196*f*
total, measurement, 219

Trilostane, mechanism and tumor target, 732*t*

Trisomy 21. *See* Down's syndrome

True hermaphroditism, 503

TSH. *See* Thyrotropin

TSI. *See* Thyroid-stimulating immunoglobulin

t-SNARES, 45, 47

Tubal patency, tests, 483–484

Tuberculosis, primary adrenal insufficiency and, 335

Tumors. *See also specific type*
antitumor endocrine agents, 732*t*
effects of hormones, 724–727
endocrine
nonsecretory, 727
secretory, 727–728, 728*t*
endocrine status and, 727–729
growth, autocrine/paracrine regulation, 725*t*
hormones produced, 742*t*
hypercalcemia and, 743–746, 743*t*
multiple endocrine neoplasia and, 755
non-islet-cell, hypoglycemia and, 748–749
steroid-dependent, 727, 727*t*

Turner's syndrome, 499–500, 536
amenorrhea and, 455
male, 420–421, 537
short stature and, 174–175

Tyramine, 385

Tyrosine, conversion to dopa, 382–383

Tyrosine hydroxylase, 383

Ulcer
duodenal, gut peptides and, 586–587
peptic, glucocorticoids and, 329

Ullrich's syndrome, 537

Ulna, osteomalacia and, 306*f*

Ultrasonography, thyroid and, 222

Uremia
hypothalamic-pituitary axis and, 117–118
secondary hypertriglyceridemia and, 694

Urinalysis, diabetes mellitus and, 614–615

Urinary bladder, atonic, diabetes mellitus and, 658

Urine, concentration, 147

Uterine synechia, amenorrhea and, 457

Uterus, adrenergic responses, 389*t*

Vagina, absent, 457

Vaginal bleeding, abnormal, types, 454*t*

Vaginal epithelium, menstrual cycle and, 450–452

Vanillylmandelic acid (VMA), normal reference ranges, 798*t*

Vanishing testes syndrome, 417–418, 516

Variable region, 80, 83

Variocele, male infertility and, 427

Vascular disease, diabetic, classification, 653

Vas deferens, obstruction, 427

Vasoactive intestinal polypeptide (VIP)
distribution, 579*t*
mode of delivery, 576*t*
normal reference ranges, 798*t*
properties, 583–584

Vasopressin. *See also* Arginine vasopressin
actions, 137*t*, 146–147
plasma
blood volume and, 149*f*
dehydration and, 152*f*

osmolality during dehydration and, 148f
Vasopressin test, diabetes insipidus/primary polydipsia and, 151
Verner-Morrison syndrome, 589
Very low density lipoprotein (VLDL)
  formation, 683–684
  metabolism, 683f
VIP. See Vasoactive intestinal polypeptide
VIPoma, 589
Virilism, 354
Virilization, 541, 542
  P450c21 hydroxylase deficiency and, 504–507
Visual field defects, pituitary-hypothalamic disorders and, 123
Vitamin(s), hormones and, 4–5, 23
Vitamin A intoxication, hypercalcemia and, 285
Vitamin D, 271–274
  abnormalities, 306–307
  actions, 273–274
  deficiency
    elderly and, 776–777
    nutritional, 306
  export, 52–53
  hypercalcemia and, 284
  malabsorption, 306
  for menopause, 477
  metabolism, 55
    abnormal, 306
    elimination and, 19–20
    short stature and, 186
  metabolites, 272
    assay, 273
  normal reference ranges, 798t
  nutrition, 272–273
  for osteoporosis, 780
  peripheral resistance, 306–307

pharmacology, 290t
receptors, 72–73
synthesis and activation, 271–272, 271f
transport, 17
Vitiligo, 765
VLDL. See Very low density lipoprotein
VMA. See Vanillylmandelic acid
von Hippel-Lindau syndrome, 759
Vorozole, mechanism and tumor target, 732t
v-SNARES, 45, 47

Water
  balance
    aging and, 782
    control, 147–149
  deprivation, diabetes insipidus/primary polydipsia and, 151
  intake, jugular vein plasma osmolality and, 148f
  requirements, 147
  routes of loss, 146t
Weakness, endocrine disease and, 29t
Weber-Christian syndrome, 702
Weight, 170
Weight gain, endocrine disease and, 29t
Weight loss, endocrine disease and, 29t
Weight reduction, obese diabetic patient and, 639
Wermer's syndrome, 588, 753
Werner's syndrome, 702
Wolff-Chaikoff effect, 201, 201f
Wolman's disease, 702
World Health Organization (WHO), diagnostic criteria for osteoporosis, 777t

Xanthoma, cutaneous, eruptive, 690
Xanthomatosis, cerebrotendinous, 702

X chromatin body, 489f
  sex chromosomes and, 491t
X chromosome
  G-banded, 490f
  structural abnormalities, syndrome of gonadal dysgenesis and, 500t
X-linked adrenoleukodystrophy, adrenal insufficiency and, 335
X-linked recessive hypophosphatemic rickets, 307
X-ray therapy, for thyroid cancer, 257
XX gonadal dysgenesis, 501–502
XXY seminiferous tubule dysgenesis, 415–417
XY agonadism, 516
XY gonadal dysgenesis, 489–491, 502–503
XYY syndrome, tall stature and, 189

Y chromosome
  G-banded, 490f
  structural abnormalities, syndrome of gonadal dysgenesis and, 500t

Zieve's syndrome, 694–695
Zinc deficiency, short stature and, 176
Zinc fingers, schema, 72f
Zindoxifene, mechanism and tumor target, 732t
ZK 98,734, ovarian function inhibition and, 472
Zollinger-Ellison syndrome, 755
  gut peptides and, 588–589
Zona fasciculata, 318, 321f
Zona glomerulosa, 318, 322f
Zona reticularis, 318–320, 321